Pediatric ENT Infections

Cemal Cingi • Emin Sami Arısoy
Nuray Bayar Muluk

Editors

Pediatric ENT Infections

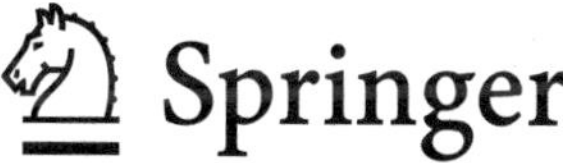 Springer

Editors
Cemal Cingi
Department of Otorhinolaryngology
Faculty of Medicine
Eskişehir Osmangazi University
Eskişehir, Turkey

Nuray Bayar Muluk
Department of Otorhinolaryngology
Faculty of Medicine
Kırıkkale University
Kırıkkale, Turkey

Emin Sami Arısoy
Division of Pediatric Infectious Diseases
Department of Pediatrics
Faculty of Medicine
Kocaeli University
Kocaeli, Turkey

ISBN 978-3-030-80693-4   ISBN 978-3-030-80691-0   (eBook)
https://doi.org/10.1007/978-3-030-80691-0

This Springer imprint is published by the registered company Springer Nature Switzerland AG
The registered company address is: Gewerbestrasse 11, 6330 Cham, Switzerland

Preface

We, the editors, are deeply honored and humbled for the opportunity to provide the *Pediatric Ear, Nose, and Throat Infections* textbook to physicians and healthcare providers working in this field as a comprehensive and up-to-date reference book, which will be available both online and in printed format.

Humankind, world history, and, more recently, globalization have sarcastically failed at equally scattering health opportunities and solutions for all children on behalf of a fair life in all corners of the world. In this context, during the last century, morbidity and mortality rates in children due to infectious diseases have been dramatically reduced in high-income countries. On the other side, pediatric infectious diseases in low- and middle-income countries remain among the leading causes of morbidity and mortality. Children in these countries also experience disproportionate rates of ear, nose, and throat (ENT) infections, often with more frequency and severity than those in the high-income world.

The knowledge and experience in the field of pediatric ENT infections are widening, deepening, and ever-changing. And so are the responsibilities and roles of physicians and other healthcare providers. The goal of preparing the *Pediatric Ear, Nose, and Throat Infections* is to provide a comprehensive, evidence-based, up-to-date reference book presenting current medical information required in the daily practice for those who care for children with infections in the ENT area and related issues. With the release of *Pediatric Ear, Nose, and Throat Infections*, we have aimed to guide the family physician, pediatrician, pediatric infectious diseases expert, and ENT specialists in the diagnosis and treatment of these conditions and to manage the neonate, infant, children, and adolescents with optimal care and outcomes, no matter what part of the world they live in.

Total 222 author colleagues from 34 countries collaborated with their willingness, enthusiasm, cooperation, effort, and time dedicated to preparing this book. The *Pediatric Ear, Nose, and Throat Infections* could not have been created without the mentorship, professional expertise, co-authorship, and enthusiastic support of our authors, including worldwide-known experts in the fields of pediatric infectious diseases and otorhinolaryngology. We have been exceptionally fortunate to have been able to work with them and count on their collaboration. Not enough words could be written to sufficiently express our heartfelt gratitude towards them.

Finally, we would like to wholeheartedly thank our teachers, mentors, parents, and families for providing us education, guidance, encouragement, help, patience, time, and a convenient environment in support of our intellectual aims and work.

<table>
<tr><td>Eskişehir, Turkey</td><td>Cemal Cingi</td></tr>
<tr><td>Kocaeli, Turkey</td><td>Emin Sami Arısoy</td></tr>
<tr><td>Kırıkkale, Turkey</td><td>Nuray Bayar Muluk</td></tr>
<tr><td>October 29, 2021</td><td></td></tr>
</table>

Contents

Part II   Symptoms and Signs

Contributors

Mustafa Acar, MD The Acar Ear, Nose, and Throat Diseases and Surgery Clinic, Eskişehir, Turkey

Murat Acat, MD Department of Pulmonology, Faculty of Medicine, Karabük University, Karabük, Turkey

İbrahim Aladağ, MD Department of Otorhinolaryngology, Faculty of Medicine, Katip Çelebi University, İzmir, Turkey

Fatih Alaşan, MD Department of Pulmonology, Faculty of Medicine, Muğla Sıtkı Koçman University, Muğla, Turkey

Naif Yaseen Albar, MD Department of Otorhinolaryngology, Head and Neck Surgery, College of Medicine, King Abdulaziz University, Rabigh, Saudi Arabia

Lyalikov Sergey Aleksandrovich, MD Department of Pediatrics, Grodno State Medical University, Grodno, Belarus

Marwan Alqunaee, MBBCH Division of Otolaryngology, Head and Neck Surgery, Saint Paul's Sinus Center, Vancouver General Hospital, University of British Columbia, Vancouver, BC, Canada

Fazilet Altın, MD Section of Otorhinolaryngology, Haseki Training and Research Hospital, University of Health Sciences, İstanbul, Turkey

Mustafa Altıntaş, MD Section of Otorhinolaryngology, Antalya Training and Research Hospital, University of Health Sciences, Antalya, Turkey

Nitin R. Ankle, MD Department of Otorhinolaryngology, Head and Neck Surgery, Jawaharlal Nehru Medical College, KLE Academy of Higher Education and Research (KAHER), Belagavi, Karnataka, India

Mehmet Surhan Arda, MD Department of Pediatric Surgery, Faculty of Medicine, Eskişehir Osmangazi University, Eskişehir, Turkey

Mehmet Arıcı, MD Section of Otorhinolaryngology, Adıyaman Training and Research Hospital, University of Health Sciences, Adıyaman, Turkey

Kamile Arıkan, MD Section of Pediatric Infectious Diseases, İzmir Dr. Behçet Uz Children's Hospital, University of Health Sciences, İzmir, Turkey

Ayşe Engin Arısoy, MD Division of Neonatology, Department of Pediatrics, Faculty of Medicine, Kocaeli University, Kocaeli, Turkey

Emin Sami Arısoy, MD Division of Pediatric Infectious Diseases, Department of Pediatrics, Faculty of Medicine, Kocaeli University, Kocaeli, Turkey

Ali Arslantaş, MD Department of Neurosurgery, Faculty of Medicine, Eskişehir Osmangazi University, Eskişehir, Turkey

Nihal Yaman Artunç, MD Section of Pediatrics, Dr. Sami Ulus Children's Hospital, University of Health Sciences, Ankara, Turkey

Hale Aslan, MD Department of Otorhinolaryngology, Faculty of Medicine, Katip Çelebi University, İzmir, Turkey

Emine Atağ, MD Division of Pediatric Pulmonology, Department of Pediatrics, Faculty of Medicine, Medipol University, İstanbul, Turkey

Metin Aydoğan, MD Division of Pediatric Allergy and Immunology, Department of Pediatrics, Faculty of Medicine, Kocaeli University, Kocaeli, Turkey

Fatma Deniz Aygün, MD Division of Pediatric Infectious Diseases, Department of Pediatrics, Cerrahpaşa Faculty of Medicine, İstanbul University-Cerrahpaşa, İstanbul, Turkey

İsmail Aytaç, MD Department of Otorhinolaryngology, Faculty of Medicine, Gaziantep University, Gaziantep, Turkey

Zeynep Arıkan Ayyıldız, MD Section of Pediatric Allergy and Immunology, Medical Park Hospital, İzmir Economy University, İzmir, Turkey

Sema Başak, MD Department of Otorhinolaryngology, Faculty of Medicine, Aydın Adnan Menderes University, Aydın, Turkey

Yeşim Başal, MD Department of Otorhinolaryngology, Faculty of Medicine, Aydın Adnan Menderes University, Aydın, Turkey

Gülsüm İclal Bayhan, MD Section of Pediatric Infectious Diseases, Ankara City Hospital, Ankara Yıldırım Beyazıt University, Ankara, Turkey

Ali Bayram, MD Section of Otorhinolaryngology, Kayseri City Training and Research Hospital, Kayseri, Turkey

Nuri Bayram, MD Section of Pediatric Infectious Diseases, İzmir Dr. Behçet Uz Children's Hospital, University of Health Sciences, İzmir, Turkey

Jeffrey C. Bedrosian, MD St. Luke's Medical Center, Rhinology and Skull Base Surgery, Bethlehem Otolaryngology Office of Specialty Physician Associates, Bethlehem, PA, USA

Nurşen Belet, MD Division of Pediatric Infectious Diseases, Department of Pediatrics, Faculty of Medicine, Dokuz Eylül University, İzmir, Turkey

Gülbin Bingöl, MD Division of Pediatric Allergy and Immunology, Department of Pediatrics, Faculty of Medicine, Acıbadem University, İstanbul, Turkey

Fuat Bulut, MD Section of Otorhinolaryngology, Reyap Çorlu Hospital, İstanbul Rumeli University, Çorlu, Tekirdağ, Turkey

Nicolas Busaba, MD Department of Otolaryngology, Head and Neck Surgery, Harvard Medical School, Harvard University, Boston, MA, USA

Ayşe Büyükçam, MD Section of Pediatric Infectious Diseases, Gaziantep Cengiz Gökçek Maternity and Children's Hospital, Gaziantep, Turkey

Kerimcan Çakıcı, MD Department of Otorhinolaryngology, Faculty of Medicine, Muğla Sıtkı Koçman University, Muğla, Turkey

Judith R. Campbell, MD Section of Infectious Diseases, Department of Pediatrics, Baylor College of Medicine, and Infectious Disease Service, Texas Children's Hospital, Houston, TX, USA

Demet Can, MD Division of Allergy and Immunology, Department of Pediatrics, Faculty of Medicine, Balıkesir University, Balıkesir, Turkey

Mustafa Çanakçı, MD Department of Emergency Medicine, Faculty of Medicine, Eskişehir Osmangazi University, Eskişehir, Turkey

Peter Catalano, MD, FACS, FARS Department of Otolaryngology, School of Medicine, St. Elizabeth's Medical Center, Tufts University, Boston, MA, USA

Erdinç Çekiç, MD Section of Otorhinolaryngology, İstanbul Haseki Training and Research Hospital, İstanbul, Turkey

Melda Çelik, MD Division of Social Pediatrics, Department of Pediatrics, Faculty of Medicine, Hacettepe University, Ankara, Turkey

Ümit Çelik, MD Section of Pediatric Infectious Diseases, Adana City Training and Research Hospital, University of Health Sciences, Adana, Turkey

Hakan Çelikhisar, MD Section of Pulmonology, İzmir Metropolitan Multicipality Eşrefpaşa Hospital, İzmir, Turkey

Can Celiloğlu, MD Department of Pediatrics, Faculty of Medicine, Çukurova University, Adana, Turkey

Benhur Şirvan Çetin, MD Division of Pediatric Infectious Diseases, Department of Pediatrics, Faculty of Medicine, Erciyes University, Kayseri, Turkey

Erdem Atalay Cetinkaya, MD Section of Otorhinolaryngology, Antalya Training and Research Hospital, University of Health Sciences, Antalya, Turkey

Pelin Duru Çetinkaya, MD Section of Pulmonology, Adana City Training and Research Hospital, University of Health Sciences, Adana, Turkey

Mehmet Emrah Ceylan, MD Section of Otorhinolaryngology, Davraz Yaşam Hospital, Davraz, Isparta, Turkey

Dennis Chua, MD Section of Otorhinolaryngology, and Ear, Nose, and Throat Surgeons Medical Centre, Mount Elizabeth Hospital, Singapore, Singapore

Tuğçe Küçükoğlu Çiçek, MD Section of Otorhinolaryngology, Adana City Training and Research Hospital, University of Health Sciences, Adana, Turkey

Ergin Çiftçi, MD Division of Pediatric Infectious Diseases, Department of Pediatrics, Faculty of Medicine, Ankara University, Ankara, Turkey

Can Cemal Cingi, MD Department of Communication Design and Management, Faculty of Communication Sciences, Anadolu University, Eskişehir, Turkey

Cemal Cingi, MD Department of Otorhinolaryngology, Faculty of Medicine, Eskişehir Osmangazi University, Eskişehir, Turkey

Funda Çipe, MD Section of Pediatric Allergy and Immunology, Bahçelievler Medical Park Hospital, İstinye University, İstanbul, Turkey

Haluk Çokuğraş, MD Division of Pediatric Infectious Diseases, Department of Pediatrics, Cerrahpaşa Faculty of Medicine, İstanbul University-Cerrahpaşa, İstanbul, Turkey

Armando G. Correa, MD Section of Academic General Pediatrics, Department of Pediatrics, Baylor College of Medicine, and Section of International and Destination Medicine, Texas Children's Hospital, Houston, TX, USA

Özlem Yüksel Coşar, MD Section of Otorhinolaryngology, Dr. Ersin Arslan Training and Research Hospital, Şahinbey, Gaziantep, Turkey

İbrahim Güven Coşğun, MD Section of Pulmonology, Afyonkarahisar University of Health Sciences Hospital, Afyonkarahisar, Turkey

İbrahim Çukurova, MD Section of Otorhinolaryngology, Tepecik Training and Research Hospital, İzmir University of Health Sciences, İzmir, Turkey

Nazan Dalgıç, MD Section of Pediatric Infectious Diseases, İstanbul Şişli Etfal Training and Research Hospital, İstanbul, Turkey

Valerio Damiani, MD Drugs Minerals and Generics (DMG) Italia Medical Department, Pomezia, Rome, Italy

Eugenio De Corso, MD Department Head and Neck Surgery, Institute of Otorhinolaryngology, Catholic University of Sacred Heart, Rome, Italy

Deniz Demir, MD Department of Otorhinolaryngology, Faculty of Medicine, Sakarya University, Sakarya, Turkey

Emine Demir, MD Department of Otorhinolaryngology, Faculty of Medicine, Recep Tayyip Erdoğan University, Rize, Turkey

Necdet Demir, MD Section of Otorhinolaryngology, VM Medical Park Pendik Hospital, Pendik, İstanbul, Turkey

Gail J. Demmler-Harrison, MD Section of Infectious Diseases, Department of Pediatrics, Baylor College of Medicine, and Infectious Disease Service, Texas Children's Hospital, Houston, TX, USA

İlker Devrim, MD Section of Pediatric Infectious Diseases, İzmir Dr. Behçet Uz Children's Hospital, University of Health Sciences, İzmir, Turkey

Khassan M. Diab, MD, PhD Federal State Budgetary Institution, Scientific and Clinical Center of Otorhinolaryngology of the Medico-Biological Agency, and Ministry of Health, Pirogov Russian National Research Medical University, Moscow, Russia

Muhammet Dilber, MD The Dilber Ear, Nose, and Throat Diseases and Surgery Clinic, İstanbul, Turkey

Fatih Dilek, MD Division of Pediatric Allergy and Immunology, Department of Pediatrics, School of Medicine, Atlas University, İstanbul, Turkey

Ener Çağrı Dinleyici, MD Department of Pediatrics, Faculty of Medicine, Eskişehir Osmangazi University, Eskişehir, Turkey

Sertaç Düzer, MD Section of Otorhinolaryngology, Elazığ Fethi Sekin City Hospital, Elazığ, Turkey

İsmail Zafer Ecevit, MD Division of Pediatric Infectious Diseases, Department of Pediatrics, Faculty of Medicine, Başkent University, Ankara, Turkey

Morven S. Edwards, MD Section of Infectious Diseases, Department of Pediatrics, Baylor College of Medicine, and Infectious Disease Service, Texas Children's Hospital, Houston, TX, USA

Nur Yücel Ekici, MD Section of Otorhinolaryngology, Adana City Training and Research Hospital, University of Health Sciences, Adana, Turkey

Sena Genç Elden, MD Section of Otorhinolaryngology, Hendek State Hospital, Hendek, Sakarya, Turkey

Ahmed El-Saggan, MD Department of Otolaryngology, Stavanger University Hospital, Stavanger, Norway

Erhan Eroğlu, PhD Department of Communication Design and Management, Faculty of Communication Sciences, Anadolu University, Eskişehir, Turkey

Refika Ersu, MD Section of Pediatric Sleep Medicine, Children's Hospital of Eastern Ontario, University of Ottawa, Ottawa, ON, Canada

Aylin Eryılmaz, MD Department of Otorhinolaryngology, Faculty of Medicine, Aydın Adnan Menderes University, Aydın, Turkey

Emine Ünal Evren, MD Department of Infectious Diseases and Microbiology, University of Kyrenia, School of Medicine, Kyrenia, Turkish Republic on Northern Cyprus (TRNC), Cyprus

Hakan Evren, MD Department of Infectious Diseases and Microbiology, University of Kyrenia, School of Medicine, Kyrenia, Turkish Republic on Northern Cyprus (TRNC), Cyprus

Pietro Ferrara, MD Department of Pediatrics, Faculty of Medicine and Surgery, University of Rome, Campus Bio-Medico, Rome, Italy

Oren Friedman, MD Department of Otorhinolaryngology, Head and Neck Surgery, Perelman School of Medicine, University of Pennsylvania, Philadelphia, PA, USA

Hülya Maraş Genç, MD Section of Pediatric Neurology, Ümraniye Training and Research Hospital, University of Health Sciences, İstanbul, Turkey

Koray Gençay, Dt, PhD Department of Pedodontics, Faculty of Dentistry, İstanbul University, İstanbul, Turkey

Laura Gochicoa-Rangel, MD National Institute of Respiratory Diseases, Mexico City, Mexico

Ozan Gökdoğan, MD Department of Otorhinolaryngology, Faculty of Medicine, Muğla Sıtkı Koçman University, Muğla, Turkey

Aylin Gül, MD Section of Otorhinolayngology, Medical Park Gaziantep Hospital, Gaziantep, Turkey

Belgin Gülhan, MD Section of Pediatric Infectious Diseases, Ankara City Training and Research Hospital, University of Health Sciences, Ankara, Turkey

Ceren Günel, MD Department of Otorhinolaryngology, Faculty of Medicine, Aydın Adnan Menderes University, Aydın, Turkey

Melek Kezban Gürbüz, MD Department of Otorhinolaryngology, Faculty of Medicine, Eskişehir Osmangazi University, Eskişehir, Turkey

Sibel Laçinel Gürlevik, MD Division of Pediatric Infectious Diseases, Department of Pediatrics, Faculty of Medicine, Hacettepe University, Ankara, Turkey

Sheng-Po Hao, MD Department of Otorhinolaryngology, Shin Kong Wu Ho-Su Memorial Hospital, Fu Jen Catholic University, Taipei, Taiwan

Biray Harbiyeli, MD Section of Pulmonology, Adana Seyhan State Hospital, Adana, Turkey

Nevin Hatipoğlu, MD Section of Pediatric Infectious Diseases, Bakırköy Dr. Sadi Konuk Training and Research Hospital, University of Health Sciences, İstanbul, Turkey

Eda Çabuk Horoz, MD Department of Otorhinolaryngology, Faculty of Medicine, Katip Çelebi University, İzmir, Turkey

Abdulkadir İmre, MD Department of Otorhinolaryngology, Faculty of Medicine, Katip Çelebi University, İzmir, Turkey

Ş. Armağan İncesulu, MD Department of Otorhinolaryngology, Faculty of Medicine, Eskişehir Osmangazi University, Eskişehir, Turkey

Kamil Janeczek, MD Department of Lung Diseases and Rheumatology, Medical University of Lublin, Lublin, Poland

Olcay Y. Jones, MD, PhD School of Medicine and Health Sciences, George Washington University, Washington, DC, USA

Ljiljana Jovancevic, MD, PhD Department of Otorhinolaryngology, Head and Neck Surgery, Faculty of Medicine, Clinical Centre of Vojvodina, University of Novi Sad, Novi Sad, Serbia

Z. Begüm Kalyoncu, PhD Department of Nutrition and Dietetics, Faculty of Health Sciences, Atılım University, Ankara, Turkey

Yunus Kantekin, MD Section of Otorhinolaryngology, Kayseri City Training and Research Hospital, Kayseri, Turkey

Sheldon L. Kaplan, MD Section of Infectious Diseases, Department of Pediatrics, Baylor College of Medicine, and Infectious Disease Service, Texas Children's Hospital, Houston, TX, USA

Murat Kar, MD Alanya Education and Research Hospital, Alanya Alaaddin Keykubat University, Alanya, Antalya, Turkey

Ateş Kara, MD Division of Pediatric Infectious Diseases, Department of Pediatrics, Faculty of Medicine, Hacettepe University, Ankara, Turkey

Bülent Kara, MD Division of Pediatric Neurology, Department of Pediatrics, Faculty of Medicine, Kocaeli University, Kocaeli, Turkey

Emine Manolya Kara, MD Division of Pediatric Infectious Diseases, Department of Pediatrics, Faculty of Medicine, İstanbul University, İstanbul, Turkey

Tuğçe Tural Kara, MD Division of Pediatric Infectious Diseases, Department of Pediatrics, Faculty of Medicine, Akdeniz University, Antalya, Turkey

Bülent Karadağ, MD Division of Pediatric Pulmonology, Department of Pediatrics, Faculty of Medicine, Marmara University, İstanbul, Turkey

Muhammed Evvah Karakılıç, MD, PhD Department of Emergency Medicine, Faculty of Medicine, Eskişehir Osmangazi University, Eskişehir, Turkey

Recep Karamert, MD Department of Otorhinolaryngology, Faculty of Medicine, Gazi University, Ankara, Turkey

Adem Karbuz, MD Section of Pediatric Infectious Diseases, Prof. Dr. Cemil Taşçıoğlu City Hospital, İstanbul, Turkey

Sergei Karpischenko, MD Department of Otorhinolaryngology, The First Pavlov State Medical University of Saint Petersburg, Saint Petersburg, Russia

Ercan Kaya, MD Department of Otorhinolaryngology, Faculty of Medicine, Eskişehir Osmangazi University, Eskişehir, Turkey

Alev Ketenci, MD Section of Pulmonology, Başakşehir Pine and Sakura City Hospital, İstanbul, Turkey

Ulugbek S. Khasanov, MD Department of Otorhinolaryngology and Stomatology, Tashkent Medical Academy, Tashkent, Uzbekistan

Oleg Khorov, MD Department of Otorhinolaryngology, Grodno State Medical University, Grodno, Belarus

Ahmet Erdem Kilavuz, MD Department of Otorhinolaryngology, Faculty of Medicine, Acıbadem Mehmet Ali Aydınlar University, İstanbul, Turkey

Abdullah Kınar, MD Section of Otorhinolaryngology, Afyonkarahisar State Hospital, Afyonkarahisar, Turkey

Furkan Kırık, MD Department of Ophthalmology, Faculty of Medicine, Bezmialem Vakıf University, İstanbul, Turkey

Bilge Aldemir Kocabaş, MD Section of Pediatric Infectious Diseases, Antalya Training and Research Hospital, University of Health Sciences, Antalya, Turkey

Murat Koçyiğit, MD Section of Otorhinolaryngology, Kanuni Sultan Süleyman Training and Research Hospital, University of Health Sciences, İstanbul, Turkey

Iordanis Konstantinidis, MD, PhD Second Academic Department of Otorhinolaryngology, Academic Faculty of Medicine, Aristotle University of Thessaloniki, Thessaloníki, Greece

Gabriela Kopacheva-Barsova, MD, PhD Department of Otorhinolaryngology, Faculty of Medicine, Cyril and Methodius University of Skopje, Skopje, Republic of North Macedonia

Gary L. Kreps, PhD Department of Communication, Center for Health and Risk Communication, George Mason University, Fairfax, VA, USA

Nagehan Küçükcan, MD Section of Otorhinolaryngology, Adana Çukurova State Hospital, Çukurova, Adana, Turkey

Senem Çengel Kurnaz, MD Department of Otorhinolaryngology, Faculty of Medicine, Ondokuz Mayıs University, Samsun, Turkey

Yücel Kurt, MD Section of Otorhinolaryngology, Finike State Hospital, Finike, Antalya, Turkey

Zafer Kurugöl, MD Division of Pediatric Infectious Diseases, Department of Pediatrics, Faculty of Medicine, Ege University, İzmir, Turkey

Sinem Gökçe Kütük, MD Section of Otorhinolaryngology, Aydın State Hospital, Aydın, Turkey

Stephan Lang, MD Department of Otorhinolaryngology, Head and Neck Surgery, University Hospital Essen, Essen, Germany

Anu Laulajainen-Hongisto, MD, PhD Department of Otorhinolaryngology, Head and Neck Surgery, University of Helsinki, and Helsinki University Hospital, Helsinki, Finland

Fatma Levent, MD Division of Pediatric Infectious Diseases, Department of Pediatrics, School of Medicine, Texas Tech University, Lubbock, TX, USA

Enrico Lombardi, MD Pediatric Pulmonary Departmental Unit, Department of Pediatrics, Florence Meyer Pediatric Hospital, University of Florence, Florence, Italy

Andrey Lopatin, MD Policlinic №1, Medical Department, Business Administration of the President of Russian Federation, Moscow, Russia

Torello M. Lotti, MD Department of Dermatology and Venereology, University of Studies Guglielmo Marconi, Rome, Italy

Jacques Magnan, MD Department of Otolaryngology, Head and Neck Surgery, Aix-Marseille University and NORD Hospital, Marseille, France

Felicia Manole, MD Department of Otorhinolaryngology, Faculty of Medicine and Pharmacy, University of Oradea, Oradea, Bihor, Romania

Feride Marim, MD Section of Pulmonology, Evliya Çelebi Training and Research Hospital, Kütahya Dumlupınar University, Kütahya, Turkey

Utku Mete, MD Section of Otorhinolaryngology, Bursa City Hospital, Bursa, Turkey

Mario Milkov, MD Department of Otorhinolaryngology, Faculty of Medicine, Varna University, Varna, Bulgaria

Nuray Bayar Muluk, MD Department of Otorhinolaryngology, Faculty of Medicine, Kırıkkale University, Kırıkkale, Turkey

Charles M. Myer III, MD Department of Otolaryngology, Head and Neck Surgery, College of Medicine, and Cincinnati Children's Hospital and Medical Center, University of Cincinnati, Cincinnati, OH, USA

Hesham Negm, MD Department of Otorhinolaryngology, Faculty of Medicine, Cairo University, Cairo, Egypt

Pamela Nguyen, MD Department of Radiology, Irving Medical Center, Columbia University, New York, USA

Marina Maintinguer Norde, PhD Department of Nutrition, Faculty of Public Health, University of São Paulo, São Paulo, Brazil

Fatma Ceyda Akın Öçal, MD Section of Otorhinolaryngology, Gülhane Training and Research Hospital, University of Health Sciences, Ankara, Turkey

Fatih Öner, MD Section of Otorhinolaryngology, Erzurum Regional Training and Research Hospital, University of Health Sciences, Erzurum, Turkey

Ümran Öner, MD Section of Dermatology, Erzurum Regional Training and Research Hospital, University of Health Sciences, Erzurum, Turkey

Mehmet Hakan Özdemir, MD Department of Ophthalmology, Faculty of Medicine, Bezmialem Vakıf University, İstanbul, Turkey

Hülya Gökmen Özel, PhD Department of Nutrition and Dietetics, Faculty of Health Sciences, Hacettepe University, Ankara, Turkey

Çiğdem Öztunalı, MD Department of Radiology, Faculty of Medicine, Eskişehir Osmangazi University, Eskişehir, Turkey

Erkan Özüdoğru, MD Department of Otorhinolaryngology, Faculty of Medicine, Eskişehir Osmangazi University, Eskişehir, Turkey

Desiderio Passali, MD, PhD Department of Medical, Surgical and Neuroscience Sciences, and Department of Otorhinolaryngology, University of Siena, Siena, Italy

Francesco Maria Passali, MD, PhD Department of Clinical Sciences, Translational Medicine University, Tor Vergata, Rome, Italy

Giulio Cesare Passali, MD, PhD Department of Otorhinolaryngology, Catholic University of Sacred Heart, Roma, Italy

Kevin A. Peng, MD Section of Otolaryngology and Neurotology, Burbank, Providence Saint Joseph Medical Center, Los Angeles, CA, USA

Mehmet Özgür Pınarbaşlı, MD Department of Otorhinolaryngology, Faculty of Medicine, Eskişehir Osmangazi University, Eskişehir, Turkey

Gülru Polat, MD Dr. Suat Seren Chest Diseases and Chest Surgery Training and Research Hospital, University of Health Sciences, İzmir, Turkey

Kostas Priftis, MD Third Pediatric Department of Athens, Respiratory and Allergy Unit, National and the Kapodistrian University of Athens, University General Hospital "Attikon", Athens, Greece

Emmanuel P. Prokopakis, MD, PhD Department of Otorhinolaryngology, School of Medicine, University of Crete, Heraklion, Crete, Greece

William Reisacher, MD Department of Otolaryngology, Head and Neck Surgery, Weill Cornell Medical College, New York, NY, USA

Ali Seyed Resuli, MD Department of Otorhinolaryngology, Faculty of Medicine, İstanbul Yeni Yüzyıl University, İstanbul, Turkey

Chae-Seo Rhee, MD, PhD Department of Otorhinolaryngology, Head and Neck Surgery, College of Medicine, Seoul National University, Seoul, Korea

Philippe Rombaux, MD Department of Otorhinolaryngology, and Institute of Neurosciences, Saint Luc University Clinics, Catholic University of Louvain, Brussels, Belgium

Michael Rudenko, MD, PhD, FAAAAI Section of Pediatric Allergy and Immunology, The London Allergy and Immunology Centre, London, UK

Bülent Saat, MD Section of Otorhinolaryngology, Ankara Occupational and Environmental Diseases Hospital, Ankara, Turkey

Mustafa Şahin, MD Department of Otorhinolaryngology, Faculty of Medicine, Aydın Adnan Menderes University, Aydın, Turkey

Özlem Naciye Atan Şahin, MD, PhD Department of Pediatrics, Faculty of Medicine, Acıbadem Mehmet Ali Aydınlar University, İstanbul, Turkey

Mustafa Salış, MD Department of General Surgery, Faculty of Medicine, Eskişehir Osmangazi University, Eskişehir, Turkey

Suela Sallavaci, MD, MSc, PhD Department of Otorhinolaryngology, University Hospital Centre "Mother Teresa", Tirana, Albania

Codrut Sarafoleanu, MD Department of Otorhinolaryngology, Head and Neck Surgery, Sfanta Maria Hospital, Carol Davila University of Medicine and Pharmacy, Bucharest, Romania

Nazan Sarper, MD Division of Pediatric Hematology, Department of Pediatrics, Faculty of Medicine, Kocaeli University, Kocaeli, Turkey

Suzan Şaylısoy, MD Department of Radiology, Faculty of Medicine, Eskişehir Osmangazi University, Eskişehir, Turkey

Glenis Scadding, MD, FRCP University College London, Royal National Throat, Nose, and Ear Hospital (Honorary Consultant Physician in Allergy and Rhinology), London, UK

Bert Schmelzer, MD Section of Otorhinolaryngology, Head and Neck Surgery, Ziekenhuis Netwerk Antwerpen (ZNA), Antwerpen, Belgium

Semra Şen, MD Division of Pediatric Infectious Diseases, Department of Pediatrics, Faculty of Medicine, Manisa Celal Bayar University, Manisa, Turkey

Tania Sih, MD, PhD, (Hon) FACS Department of Pediatric Otolaryngology, School of Medicine, University of São Paulo, São Paulo, Brazil

Işıl Eser Şimşek, MD Division of Pediatric Allergy and Immunology, Department of Pediatrics, Faculty of Medicine, Kocaeli University, Kocaeli, Turkey

Bilal Sizer, MD Section of Otorhinolaryngology, Memorial Diyarbakır Hospital, Diyarbakır, Turkey

Ayper Somer, MD Division of Pediatric Infectious Diseases, Department of Pediatrics, Faculty of Medicine, İstanbul University, İstanbul, Turkey

Murat Songu, MD Section of Otorhinolaryngology, Medicana International İzmir Hospital, İzmir, Turkey

Gordon Soo, MD Department of Otorhinolaryngology, Head and Neck Surgery, Hong Kong Special Administrative Region, The Chinese University of Hong Kong, Hong Kong, People's Republic of China

Michael B. Soyka, MD Department of Otorhinolaryngology, Head and Neck Surgery, University and University Hospital Zurich, Zurich, Switzerland

Slobodan Spremo, MD Department for Otorhinolaryngology, Faculty of Medicine, University of Banja Luka, University Clinic Center Banja Luka, Banja Luka, Bosnia and Herzegovina

Georg Mathias Sprinzl, MD Department of Otorhinolaryngology, Head and Neck Surgery, University Clinic Saint Poelten, Saint Poelten, Austria

Jeffrey R. Starke, MD Section of Infectious Diseases, Department of Pediatrics, Baylor College of Medicine, and Infectious Disease Service, Texas Children's Hospital, Houston, TX, USA

Nihat Susaman, MD Section of Otorhinolaryngology, Elazığ Fethi Sekin City Hospital, Elazığ, Turkey

Emel Tahir, MD Department of Otorhinolaryngology, Faculty of Medicine, Ondokuz Mayıs University, Samsun, Turkey

Zeynep Tamay, MD Division of Pediatric Allergy and Immunology, Department of Pediatrics, Faculty of Medicine, İstanbul University, İstanbul, Turkey

Anıl Aktaş Tapısız, MD Division of Pediatric Infectious Diseases, Department of Pediatrics, Faculty of Medicine, Gazi University, Ankara, Turkey

Tobias Tenenbaum, MD Division of Pediatric Infectious Diseases, University Children's Hospital Mannheim, Heidelberg University, Mannheim, Germany

Hasan Tezer, MD Division of Pediatric Infectious Diseases, Department of Pediatrics, Faculty of Medicine, Gazi University, Ankara, Turkey

Baran Tokar, MD Department of Pediatric Surgery, Faculty of Medicine, Eskişehir Osmangazi University, Eskişehir, Turkey

Taşkın Tokat, MD Department of Otorhinolaryngology, Faculty of Medicine, Sakarya University, Sakarya, Turkey

Sanna Toppila-Salmi, MD, PhD Skin and Allergy Hospital, University of Helsinki and Helsinki University Hospital, Helsinki, Finland

Vedat Topsakal, MD, PhD Department of Otorhinolaryngology, Head and Neck Surgery, Vrije Universiteit Brussel (VUB), University Hospital UZ Brussel, Brussels Health Campus, Brussels, Belgium

Sema Zer Toros, MD Section of Otorhinolaryngology, Head and Neck Surgery, İstanbul Haydarpaşa Numune Training and Research Hospital, İstanbul, Turkey

Mümtaz Taner Torun, MD Section of Otorhinolaryngology, Bandırma State Hospital, Bandırma, Balıkesir, Turkey

Selda Hançerli Törün, MD Division of Pediatric Infectious Diseases, Department of Pediatrics, Faculty of Medicine, İstanbul University, İstanbul, Turkey

Edhem Ünver, MD Department of Pulmonology, Faculty of Medicine, Erzincan Binali Yıldırım University, Erzincan, Turkey

Zeynep Seda Uyan, MD Division of Pediatric Pulmonology, Department of Pediatrics, Faculty of Medicine, Koç University, İstanbul, Turkey

Yvan Vandenplas, MD Department of Pediatrics, University Hospital Brussels, Vrije University Brussels, KidZ Health Castle, Brussels, Belgium

Klara Van Gool, MD Department of Otorhinolaryngology, Head and Neck Surgery, University Hospital Antwerpen, Antwerpen, Belgium

Evda Vevecka, MD Division of Pediatric Pneumology, Department of Pediatrics, Faculty of Medicine, University of Medicine, Tirana, Albania

Claudio Vicini, MD Unit of Otolaryngology, Ferrara, and Hospital Morgagni Pierantoni, Unit of Otolaryngology, University of Ferrara, Forli, Italy

Andrew A. Winkler, MD Department of Otolaryngology, University of Colorado School of Medicine, Aurora, CO, USA

Çiçek Wöber-Bingöl, MD Department of Child and Adolescent Psychiatry, Medical University of Vienna (former affiliation), Vienna, Austria

Adem Yaşar, MD Division of Pediatric Allergy and Pulmonology, Department of Pediatrics, Faculty of Medicine, Manisa Celal Bayar University, Manisa, Turkey

Hüsamettin Yaşar, MD Section of Otorhinolaryngology, İstanbul Haseki Training and Research Hospital, İstanbul, Turkey

Selçuk Yıldız, MD Section of Otorhinolaryngology, Head and Neck Surgery, İstanbul Haydarpaşa Numune Training and Research Hospital, İstanbul, Turkey

Orhan Yılmaz, MD Department of Otorhinolaryngology, Faculty of Medicine, Karabük University, Karabük, Turkey

Özge Yılmaz, MD Division of Pediatric Allergy and Pulmonology, Department of Pediatrics, Faculty of Medicine, Manisa Celal Bayar University, Manisa, Turkey

Ümit Yılmaz, MD Section of Otorhinolaryngology, Selahaddin Eyyubi State Hospital, Diyarbakır, Turkey

Yavuz Fuat Yılmaz, MD Section of Otorhinolaryngology, Gülhane Training and Research Hospital, University of Health Sciences, Ankara, Turkey

Cüneyt Yılmazer, MD Section of Otorhinolaryngology, Adıyaman Training and Research Hospital, Adıyaman, Turkey

Fatih Yücedağ, MD Section of Otorhinolaryngology, Karaman State Hospital, Karaman, Turkey

Gül Yücel, MD Section of Pediatric Neurology, Konya Training and Research Hospital, University of Health Sciences, Konya, Turkey

Hasan Yüksel, MD Division of Pediatric Allergy and Pulmonology, Department of Pediatrics, Faculty of Medicine, Manisa Celal Bayar University, Manisa, Turkey

Dmytro Illich Zabolotny, MD, PhD Institute of Otorhinolaryngology, National Academy of Medical Sciences of Ukraine, Kyiv, Ukraine

Part I

General Overview

Immunological Responses to Infection

Funda Çipe, Emin Sami Arısoy, and Armando G. Correa

1.1 Introduction

The immune system exists to protect against the invasion of pathogens into the body. This function can only be achieved if the immune system can distinguish self from non-self, whether a microorganism, toxin, or allergenic substance. The immune system is vital in the response against severe, potentially fatal, infective episodes. In most cases, the immune system incapacitates the pathogen, and the individual recovers, but any defective immunological defense may give rise to primary immunodeficiency [1, 2]. Individuals with primary immunodeficiency are at risk of chronic or recurrent infection. Different categories of pathogens provoke different immune responses; therefore, an infection's clinical features may provide clues about which aspect of the immunological response is deficient [1, 2].

On occasion, there may be an abnormal response by the immune system, such as occurs in hypersensitivity, where inflammation results in injury to the tissues. Pathogens may also bear antigens resembling components of the self, which may lead to autoimmunity via cross-reactivity [2–5].

There are two main branches of the immune system: innate immunity and adaptive immunity. Both of these branches are employed to identify and destroy

F. Çipe (✉)
Section of Pediatric Allergy and Immunology, Bahçelievler Medical Park Hospital, İstinye University, İstanbul, Turkey

E. S. Arısoy
Division of Pediatric Infectious Diseases, Department of Pediatrics, Faculty of Medicine, Kocaeli University, Kocaeli, Turkey

A. G. Correa
Section of Academic General Pediatrics, Department of Pediatrics, Baylor College of Medicine, and Section of International and Destination Medicine, Texas Children's Hospital, Houston, TX, USA

© The Author(s), under exclusive license to Springer Nature Switzerland AG 2022
C. Cingi et al. (eds.), *Pediatric ENT Infections*,
https://doi.org/10.1007/978-3-030-80691-0_1

invading pathogens, and are geared to differentiate between foreign matter and components of the self. Innate immunity comprises physical barriers, humoral proteins, secreted components, and particular cellular populations. A mechanical barrier, such as the skin or the bony skull, first acts to exclude microorganisms from entry into the body. Secreted enzymes and other molecules suppress bacterial multiplication. Gastric or vaginal acidity prevents the overgrowth of bacteria. Tears contain the natural antibiotic lysozyme. Secretions need to drain away if they are not to form pools where pathogens may multiply. The drainage of lacrimal fluid, saliva, intestinal bile, mucus, and pancreatic juice keeps mucosae free from injury. Impaired drainage often results in the risk of infection [1, 2, 6].

If normal, healthy bacterial flora is present on an epithelial surface, it may prevent pathogenic bacterial invasion. Immune function needs to achieve a difficult equilibrium between being alert to the presence of invasive microorganisms while not over-reacting to cause autoimmunity or allergy [7]. Antibiotic pharmacotherapy may upset the healthy bacterial flora, leading to opportunistic infections by pathogenic microbes. Humoral elements and cells capable of engulfing pathogens (i.e., phagocytosis) are also part of natural immunity. Complement plays a significant role in preserving homeostatic balance and inhibiting autoimmune dysfunction [8].

The immune destruction of intracellular and extracellular bacteria is accomplished by different types of effector cells belonging to the adaptive immunity division. It was first recognized in the 1950s that antibodies assisted in destroying extracellular bacteria. While antibodies alone cannot lyse bacteria, they do inhibit the bacteria from attaching to the host. Furthermore, antibodies interact with complement proteins to opsonize bacteria, allowing them to be phagocytosed. Natural immunity occurs before adaptive immunity and is fast, although lacking specificity. Many microbes activate the toll-like receptors (TLRs) found embedded in plasma membranes [9, 10]. Lysozyme either destroys or damages bacteria, which leads to leakage of bacterial contents, such as peptidoglycans, which can be recognized as alien by receptors borne on cells of the innate system [11]. Neutrophils target bacteria, while macrophages are effective against intracellular microbes, including both bacteria and protozoa. Eosinophils accomplish defense against helminthic invasion.

Polymorphonucleocytes (PMNs) form the first wave of immune defensive response and are intimately connected with developing inflammation. PMNs work by engulfing bacteria and destroying them within the PMN's cytoplasm. They also release granules and produce neutrophil extracellular traps (NETs) if they sense harmful conditions [12]. Knowledge of the mechanisms controlling the release of these NETs is revolutionizing the understanding of how immunity functions, the triggering of the inflammatory process, and the development of autoimmunity and malignant neoplasia [13, 14].

Adaptive immune mechanisms target intracellular microbes (virus, bacterium, protozoa, or fungus). In particular, CD8+ T-lymphocytes release cytokines that signal macrophages to destroy infected cells. Langerhans cells phagocytose molecular debris from the lysis of viruses, bacteria, or other pathogens. They move to the lymph nodes, where they present the antigens to lymphocytes; this is the first stage in the body, becoming specifically immune, tolerant, or hypersensitive [15].

The T helper cells (CD4+) were defined as two types initially, Th1 and Th2. The former are proinflammatory T lymphocytes that release interferon-gamma (IFN-γ) and interleukin (IL) -12. IL-12 stimulates differentiation into Th1 lymphocytes [16]. Recent researches have uncovered other subpopulations of the CD4+ cell line, particularly Th9, Th17, Th22, T follicular-helper (Tfh), and Treg (T-regulatory) lymphocytes. These findings have led to a more complete understanding of immune pathology [17]. Th9 lymphocytes are capable of synthesizing IL-9 and IL-21. Their precursors are naive CD4+ T-lymphocytes. Transformation occurs following exposure to *transforming growth factor*-beta (TGF-β) and IL-4 [18, 19]. Th22 lymphocytes differ from Th17 and all other recognized offspring of CD4+ precursors by virtue of their distinctive gene expression and specific function [20]. Although a necessary reappraisal of the numbers of T-helper progeny (CD4+) and the range of variability that these recent discoveries have necessitated, the fundamental division into Th1 and Th2 type immune reactions retains explanatory value [21].

There is marked heterogeneity among CD4+ T-lymphocyte subpopulations. T helper type 1 (Th1), type 2 (Th2), type 17 (Th17), type 9 (Th9), and type 22 (Th22), follicular T helper cells (Tfh), induced regulatory T cells (iTreg), and type 1 regulatory T cells (Tr1) are posited to exist on the basis of the number of cytokines that have been identified. Cells that secrete a range of cytokines include Langerhans cells and macrophages, among others [21].

Th1-associated immune responses are most effective against protozoans, intracellular bacteria, and viral infections, while the Th2-associated defense targets helminthic organisms and extracellular bacteria. These two patterns of immune response interact with each other, so that, for example, Th1 lymphocytes secrete IFN-γ, which exerts opposite effects to IL-4 and 10, which Th2 lymphocytes release. Tregs that have positivity for CD4 and CD25 act in concert to release IL-10 with or without TGF-β (from Tr1 and Th3 subpopulations). The secretion of these mediators assists in suppressing hypersensitive or autoimmune reactions [17, 21]. Table 1.1 lists the cytokines and their primary functions.

Innate lymphoid cells (ILCs) have been recently identified; they are lymphocytes, but they do not express antigen receptors that normally are expressed on T or B cells. They are tissue-resident cells and play a role in tissue integrity and protection against tissue-infiltrating pathogens. ILCs are divided into three subsets, ILC1, ILC2, and ILC3. Different signals can activate each subset. ILCs are present in lymphoid and nonlymphoid organs, especially at the mucosal barriers. ILC1s produce IFN-γ after secretion of IL-12, IL-15, and IL-18 in a similar way that Th1 cells do. ILC2s resemble Th2 cells and secrete type-2 cytokines such as IL-5, IL-9, and IL-13. Of these cytokines, IL-13, in particular, appears to have a significant role in immunity against helminth infections. ILC3s secrete IL-22 and IL-17 in response to IL-23 and IL-1β as Th17 cells. IL-22 stimulates the differentiation of epithelial cells from intestinal stem cells [22–24].

Table 1.1 Cytokines and their primary functions

Cytokines	Main Cell Source	Functions
IL-1ß	Macrophages, monocytes	Pro-inflammatory, proliferation, apoptosis, differentiation
IL-2	Activated T cells	Proliferation and activation of T cells
IL-3	T cells	Growth of blood precursors
IL-4	Th cells, mast cells	Anti-inflammatory, B cell proliferation, apoptosis, differentiation
IL-5	Th cells, mast cells	Growth of eosinophils
IL-6	Macrophages, T cells, adipocytes	Pro-inflammatory, cytokine production, differentiation
IL-7	Thymus, bone marrow, stromal cells	Development of T-B cell precursors
IL-8	Macrophages, epithelial cells, endothelial cells	Pro-inflammatory, chemotaxis, angiogenesis
Il-9	Activated T cells	Growth of T and mast cells
IL-10	Monocytes, T-B cells	Anti-inflammation, inhibition of pro-inflammation
IL-12	Dendritic cells, macrophages, neutrophils	Pro-inflammatory, differentiation, activates NK cells
IL-11	Fibroblasts, neurons, epithelial cells	Anti-inflammatory, differentiation, induces acute phase reaction
IL-13	Th2 cells	Anti-inflammatory, B cell proliferation, apoptosis, differentiation
IL-15	Epithelial cells, monocytes	Proliferation and activation of T cells
IL-16	CD8+ cells	Chemotaxis of CD4+ cells
IL-17	Activated memory T cells	T cell proliferation
IL-18	Macrophages	Production of IFN-γ
TNF-α	Macrophages, CD4+ T cells, adipocytes, NK cells	Pro-inflammatory, cytokine production, differentiation apoptosis, anti-infectious
IFN-γ	T cells, NK cells, NKT cells	Pro-inflammatory, anti-viral innate-adaptive immunity
GM-CSF	Macrophages, T cells, fibroblasts	Pro-inflammatory, monocyte, macrophage, neutrophil activation
TGF-ß	Macrophages, T cells,	Anti-inflammation, inhibition of pro-inflammation

GM-CSF indicates granulocyte-macrophage colony-stimulating factor; IFN-γ, interferon-gamma; IL, interleukin; NK, natural killer; NKT, natural killer T; TGF-ß, *transforming growth factor*-beta; Th, T helper; TNF-α, tumor necrosis factor-alpha

1.2 Bacterial Infections and Immunity

The immune response to bacterial invasion consists of contributions from the natural barriers and both innate and acquired immune systems. If extracellular bacterium gets into the body through a breach in the barrier, such as an injury, the complement system is first activated. Cleaved complement proteins (e.g., C3a and C5a) attract neutrophils and stimulate mast cells. This results in vasodilatation and secretion of messengers that encourage the inflammatory response [25].

Intracellular bacterial pathogens include most mycobacteria (e.g., *Mycobacterium tuberculosis, Mycobacterium leprae*) and *Listeria monocytogenes, Salmonella enterica,* and *Brucella* species, among others. These organisms enter macrophages and thus evade the usual immune defense mechanisms. Neutrophils are unable to lyse intracellular bacteria. Only active cytotoxic activity by macrophages can produce an effective immune response. The organism triggers a robust inflammatory reaction by entering the host cells, which causes widespread tissue injury in the host. Intracellular pathogenic bacteria cause activation of either CD4+ T-lymphocytes expressing MHC class II or CD8+ T-lymphocytes expressing MHC class I. The latter are directly cytotoxic, whereas CD4+ T-lymphocytes release IFN-γ after antigen is presented to them. CD4+ T-lymphocytes activate macrophages, synthesize nitrous oxide, and destroy the bacterial invaders. It is apparent from this explanation why individuals with human immunodeficiency virus (HIV) infection, which weaken cellular immune defenses, are at risk of mycobacterial diseases [26, 27].

T cell involvement results in the tissues secreting cytokines involved in Th1 responses (IFN-γ, IL-2) and cytokines that promote inflammation, such as *tumor necrosis factor-alpha* (TNF-α) [28]. Under prompting by these messengers, Langerhans cells undergo differentiation into dendritic cells and move towards the regional lymph nodes, where they perform antigen presentation to T-lymphocytes. T-lymphocytes circulating between the blood and the lymphatics are presented with the antigen by the dendritic cells.

"Priming" refers to the activation of T-lymphocytes through antigen presentation, co-stimulatory molecule release, and signaling by cytokines. There is infiltration by CD4+ T cells in the infected area, while HLA-DR is expressed at elevated levels alongside the receptor for IL-2 [25, 27]. After priming, T-lymphocytes can assist other cell types of the immune system. Failure of secretion of IFN-γ by Th1 cells positive for CD4+ and CD8+ is the essential step by which infection by intracellular bacteria becomes a chronic situation that does not resolve. Administering IFN-γ to patients is thus one potential treatment option [29].

Extracellular bacterial infections are more common than those caused by intracellular species. The critical defensive components against extracellular bacteria are physical barriers and immunoglobulins. The skin and mucosae secrete substances intended to inhibit bacteria from clinging to the surface and passing through the barrier. In the respiratory tree, the mucociliary circulation clears away bacteria. Gastric acid kills bacteria entering the gut from the mouth. Saliva is one of several secreted substances that are toxic to bacteria [1, 2, 6].

The complement proteins C5a, C3a, and C4a lead to the activation of all cell types capable of phagocytosis. These include basophils and mast cells. The complement proteins also recruit white cells to infected tissues and assist with crossing out of the capillaries into the tissues. Eosinophils possess certain substances, such as major basic protein (MBP) and eosinophil cationic protein (ECP), capable of killing microorganisms. Activated PMNs and macrophages engulf bacteria opsonized by complement. PMNs lyse phagocytosed bacteria utilizing superoxide radicals, notably N_2O or H_2O_2. Despite sharing the feature of phagocytotic ability, macrophages and PMNs are otherwise quite different. PMNs in the circulation or tissues have a considerably shorter life span than macrophages. The presence of neutrophils indicates infection, whereas macrophages are located in both diseased and normal tissues. Neutrophils are responsible for pus formation, but macrophages produce granulomas. The neutrophilic response is key to defense against extracellular bacteria. Macrophages, in contrast, target intracellular infections [12, 13, 16].

The membrane attack complex is produced by the association of complement proteins C5 to C9 and disrupts bacteria membranes. Complement protein C3b is responsible for opsonization. C3b attaches to bacterial membranes and forms the ligand for phagocytic cell receptors. The complement cascade's innate disorders may result in grave infective episodes, mainly through the *Neisseria* genus [25].

Natural immunity relies on phagocytes and the alternative pathway to complement activation. Macrophages secrete IL-1 and IL-6, which activate a hepatic acute phase response. This response leads to the more outstanding production of complement precursors, alongside other serum proteins. Many chemical messengers orchestrate the immune response to bacterial invasion, including chemokines, cytokines, and other proteins, notably C-reactive protein (CRP). CRP can attach to the membrane of bacteria similarly to opsonin, marking it a target for a phagocytic attack. CRP is an activator of complement as well as stimulating TNF-α production. The latter leads to raised levels of N_2O. These processes should result in the elimination of bacterial pathogenic organisms [28, 29].

Inflammation may simultaneously produce tissue injury. Tissue damage frequently is not particularly significant. Gram-negative bacteria contain lipopolysaccharides in their cell walls, powerful stimulants to release proinflammatory cytokines by PMNs, macrophages, and vascular endothelium. The balance between chemical messengers promoting inflammation and those dampening the response dictates how sepsis presents clinically [29]. The release of TNF-α, IL-1, IL-6, IL-8, and N_2O produce hypotension, which prevents adequate perfusion of the tissues. Necrosis may then ensue [28, 29].

Effector cells respond to cytokines and chemokines in enacting their immune roles [17]. The initial stages of infection are marked by synthesizing the proinflammatory cytokines IL-1 and IL-6, plus TNF-α. These messengers stimulate the hypothalamus, which resets the thermoregulation network and results in an increase in body temperature in an attempt to kill the pathogen; this is clinically manifested as pyrexia. The adhesion molecules, P-selectin and intercellular adhesion molecules (ICAMs) are increasingly expressed by the endothelium, facilitating the extravascular migration of inflammatory cells. Bacteria are engulfed by PMNs and macrophages and lysed by the action of superoxides. Macrophages also release cytokine messengers that call on the acquired immune response. IL-12 assists the maturation of precursor Th0 cells into Th1 lymphocytes [17]. IL-4, synthesized in basophils, mast cells, and macrophages, encourages Th0 cells to become Th2 lymphocytes. The arrival of Th1 and Th2 lymphocytes stimulates B lymphocytes to synthesize immunoglobulins [21]. Plasma cells then release messengers that encourage the maturation of CD4+ cells into Th2 lymphocytes. T-lymphocyte participation enables B-lymphocytes to expand as clones and refines their affinity for the target. This whole process leads to raised levels of immunoglobulins of high target-affinity capable of opsonizing bacteria, activating complement particles, destroying bacteria, or the toxins they produce [11, 30].

Within mucosae, immunoglobulin A (IgA) is the primary antibody synthesized; IgA neutralizes bacteria more effectively than inflammation alone. However, IgA cannot prevent sepsis development; only immunoglobulin G (IgG) can do so. In pulmonary tissues, immunoglobulin production is mainly in IgG, allowing neutrophils to destroy bacterial invaders. If IgG is deficient or absent, respiratory infections may develop [31, 32].

During opsonization, immunoglobulins bind to particular fragments of the bacteria. The antibody molecule has a region, Fc, which can attach to a specific membrane-bound receptor found on neutrophils and macrophages. The Fc region of the molecule additionally activates complement pathways, particularly in the case of IgA. The complement then forms the membrane attack complex to destroy the pathogen. Immunoglobulins can hinder bacterial attachment to mucosal surfaces of the gut or respiratory tree. Immunoglobulins also help eliminate toxins synthesized by bacteria, such as *Clostridium tetani* or *Corynebacterium diphtheriae* [31, 32].

1.2.1 Bloodstream Infections

PMNs may be unable to neutralize blood-borne bacteria. The spleen may destroy bacteria that have evaded antibody attachment within the circulation. Thus, individuals without a functioning spleen may be at risk of developing sepsis and septic shock from bacterial infection. Hepatic stellate macrophages can phagocytose bacteria to which the antibody has bound. Hepatic failure leads to ineffective phagocytic activity and a reduction in acute-phase protein secretion, which may cause secondary immunodeficiency [33].

1.2.2 Encapsulated Bacteria

Certain bacteria (*Neisseria meningitidis*, *Streptococcus pneumoniae*, and *Haemophilus influenzae*) possess a polysaccharide coat that protects them from phagocytosis. This coat leads to the activation of B-lymphocytes without any T cell involvement. Activated B cells then move to T-lymphocytic regions in the secondary lymphoid tissue. Healthy individuals produce immunoglobulins that attach to encapsulated bacteria, opsonizing them. However, children below the age of 2 years mount inadequate responses to encapsulated bacteria. Conjugated vaccines have been created wherein carbohydrate antigenic sites are placed alongside specific protein epitopes. Infants can then mount adequate immune responses to *H. influenzae*, *S. pneumoniae*, and *N. meningitidis*, reflected in the lower death rate and morbidity in vaccinated infants [34].

1.3 Viral Infections and Immunity

Infections due to viruses are frequent and range in severity from mildly symptomatic to potentially fatal. The immune response to viral infection is sophisticated, and several elements are involved, especially CD8+ cytotoxic T-lymphocytes, natural killer (NK) cells, and virus-specific immunoglobulins. Immunoglobulins are crucial to protecting against viable viruses. Antigenic processing occurs in the same fashion as for the antibacterial response. Following viral entry, the first line of defense is via macrophages and NK cells, orchestrated by IFNs of type 1 (alpha and beta) [35]. The majority of cell types release IFNs alpha and beta, which suppress the production of viral copies within the cell. Double-stranded RNA acts as the principal trigger for IFN expression [36]. CD8+ cytotoxic T-lymphocytes provide the second line of defense. Partial proteins of both self and viral types are taken up from the cytosol by the endoplasmic reticulum, binding to class I molecules. The class I molecules migrate to the external plasma membrane, becoming visible to the CD8+ cytotoxic T-lymphocytes [16].

Cells that are virally infected release type 1 IFNs. In addition, IFN-γ, which is synthesized by T-lymphocytes, mobilizes macrophages and NK cells against viruses. At first, IL-12 is released by macrophages and other cells capable of antigen presentation. This cytokine induces a cell-killing response by NK cells, which also release IFN-γ. NK cell cytotoxicity is accomplished through their production of granzyme and perforin [16, 35, 36].

Although CD8+ T-lymphocytes are the leading group of effectors in the adaptive immune system tasked with viral defense, they do not usually act alone. Cells undergoing apoptosis due to viral infection may be engulfed by Langerhans cells. There are special features to how Langerhans cells process antigen captured in this way. Recognition of antigen derived from virus particles occurs via MHC class I receptors in affected cells. Following such recognition, granzyme and perforin are released, destroying cells containing the virus or the virus itself. B cells switch to IgG synthesis when CD4+ T-lymphocytes have activated them. Although viral reproduction occurs within cells, they need to exit one cell to infect another. When viruses leave the cell, they become susceptible to immunoglobulin binding, and this is one way for the immune system to halt the viral spread. Immunoglobulins can also attach to virally infected cells and assist with killing by NK cells. Immunoglobulins play a particularly significant role in individuals with previous exposure to viral antigen, either through infection or vaccination. Viruses of poliomyelitis, measles, hepatitis B, or varicella-zoster virus cannot attach to the host cells once they have been bound by antibody [16].

These responses are typically adequate to combat viral infections, ensuring that most viruses either produce no symptoms or give only mild symptoms, such as pyrexia or exanthems. However, a few infective episodes do progress, resulting in tissue injury and systemic involvement. Viral infections may ultimately cause cytopathy, hypersensitivity, and autoimmunity [37]. In various viral infection cases, several mechanisms operate at once to bring the disease under control of the immune system. In HIV and hepatitis B virus (HBV) infections, the viruses cause a cyto-pathic effect. NK cells and CD8+ T-lymphocytes are vital to killing virally infected cells. If an individual is immunodeficient due to T-lymphocyte dysfunction, viruses, such as Herpesviridae, cytomegalovirus, or the Epstein-Barr virus (EBV), may be able to multiply in an uncontrolled manner. The non-clearance of viral infections by these agents is found when T-lymphocytic immune responses are functionally exhausted and thus incapable of being effectively mounted [36].

HIV has a tropism for CD4+ T-lymphocytes. Destruction of these cells results from viral cytopathy and accelerated apoptosis. CD4+ T-lymphocytes present virus-derived antigens on their surface and thus become a target for cytotoxic CD8+ T-lymphocytes. Therefore, the CD4+ cell count falls. Because CD4+ T-lymphocyte numbers are low, the acquired immune functions become deficient, resulting in a drop of IL-2, IFN-γ, and TNF-α [38]. This situation paves the way for invasion by opportunistic and intracellular microbes, notably *M. tuberculosis*, cytomegalovirus, *Candida albicans, Pneumocystis jirovecii,* and *Cryptosporidium* spp., leading to AIDS. Because this situation also interferes with CD4+ T-lymphocytic regulation of B cell immunoglobulin function, extracellular bacteria may also become invasive, as immunoglobulin production is not triggered despite the presence of B memory cells [38].

The human T-cell lymphocytotrophic virus-1 (HTLV-1) infects Th1 cells, which are thereby triggered to proliferate and become active significantly. This prolifera-tion appears as adult T-cell leukemia [39]. The predominance of Th1 cells in HTLV-1 infection switches off the production of Th2-associated messengers, e.g., IL-4 and IL-5, plus prevents the synthesis of immunoglobulin molecules of class E. Helminths may take advantage of this situation. Infection with *Schistosoma* or *Strongyloides* spp. is correspondingly higher in individuals infected with the virus [40].

Human papillomavirus (HPV) is the causative agent for verruca vulgaris, condy-loma accuminatum, and epidermodysplasia verruciformis, which may undergo malignant transformation into cervical or skin cancer [40]. Cellular effectors of the immune system target HPV. Studies of condylomata and cervical neoplasia indicate the involvement of macrophages, T-lymphocytes (both CD4+ and CD8+), alongside antibodies of classes A and G [41, 42].

The severe acute respiratory syndrome coronavirus 2 (SARS CoV-2), respon-sible for the pandemic of coronavirus disease 2019 (COVID-19) in 2020 and 2021, causes infection in the respiratory tract with mild to severe clinical mani-festations and can potentially be fatal. SARS-CoV-2 can infect alveolar epithelial and immune cells in the lung but cannot replicate in immune cells. Viral spikes and proteins trigger an immune response in the host to eliminate the virus [43]. These viral antigens can be either recognized by the B cells, macrophages, and dendritic cells, then MHC-Class I-II complexes recognize and present these viral antigens to the CD4+ helper and CD8+ cytotoxic T cells. This presentation results in cytolytic activity, antibody production, and cytokine secretion. After improvement, protective memory T-cell responses develop but are not persistent in the long term [44, 45].

1.4 Fungal Infections and Immunity

Phagocytic cells are the mainstay of immune defense against fungal pathogens. Fungal killing is accomplished by nitrous oxide and other mechanisms. T-lymphocytes secrete IFN-γ, which activates PMNs and macrophages [46]. One of the consequences of severe neutropenia (<500 PMNs/mm^3) is susceptibility to recurrent fungal infections, ranging from mild to severe, typically by opportunistic organisms. This also occurs where cellular immunity is compromised by *Candida* spp. [47].

The fungal membrane contains β (1 → 6) glucans on its surface, which can be recognized by macrophage-1 antigen (formed by a combination of CD11b and CD18) [41]. Human cells also produce pattern recognition receptors (PRRs), e.g., toll-like receptors, C-type lectin receptors, and the galectin family's proteins. These molecules can act to detect pathogen-associated molecular patterns (PAMPs) associated with fungal organisms [47, 48].

Despite the numerous fungal species that can potentially cause infections in humans, most fail to result in any disease. *C. albicans* is part of the normal commensal flora and causes only mild infective episodes unless the patient is already infected with HIV or has a primary immunodeficiency disease. C. albicans may infect the pulmonary tissues, skin, esophagus, stomach, and elsewhere in the gut in such cases. *C. albicans* is recognized by toll-like receptors present on fully differentiated immune cell types, e.g., phagocytes, setting off intracellular signals that result in the synthesis of proinflammatory cytokines. These cytokines need to be present for the efficient functioning of the natural immune response and coordination of acquired immune defensive measures [47, 48]. Chronic mucocutaneous candidiasis refers to disseminated candida infection occurring alone due to defective cell-based immune defenses or widespread endocrine dysfunction (APECED: autoimmunity, polyendocrinopathy, enteropathy, candidiasis, ectodermal dysplasia) [49].

Primary immune deficiency syndromes may cause any of the following: chronic mucocutaneous candidiasis, invasive candidiasis, invasive aspergillosis, deep dermatophytosis, pneumocystis, and endemic mycoses. Specific immunodeficiency syndromes are strongly associated with particular infections. Thus, if no other risk factors are present, a child or younger adult presenting with a fungal infection of this type should be suspected of an innate immunodeficiency syndrome caused by a single gene mutation and investigated accordingly [50].

Recurrent candidiasis affecting the vagina is observed in up to 5% of pregnant women, associated with reduced levels of IFN-γ. Although no evidence exists to show Th2 cell involvement in combatting *C. albicans*, it is worth noting that allergy is common in this group of patients [51].

Cryptococcus neoformans invades the lungs and the brain in patients with immunosuppression. If a Th2 response does not occur, the organism can spread into the lungs. IL-4 prevents fungal organisms from causing severe lung infections [47, 52].

1.5   Protozoal Infections and Immunity

Protozoal parasitic organisms typically possess a high degree of complexity and invade the body via the mucosae or skin. The most effective defense against them is primary prevention [53, 54].

The immunoglobulin E (IgE) response that features in anaphylaxis appears to have evolved originally as a defense against parasites. Mast cells release vasoactive granules, mainly histamine. IL-4, produced by Th2 lymphocytes, activate IgE synthesis. Th2 cells also release IL-5, which draws eosinophils to the infection site, where they release ECP, killing the protozoa. IL-4 enhances the effectiveness of the Th2 response by preventing Th1 lymphocytes from maturing [53, 54].

The principal protozoa causing infection in humans are *Leishmania* spp., *Plasmodium* spp., *Toxoplasma* spp., and amoebae. Protozoa live intracellularly for extensive periods, but signs of disease only appear in a portion of those so infected. This is because protozoa are confined in place by the immune system. A protozoal organism may remain within the host without causing any symptoms, but if the host becomes immunosuppressed, disseminated infection and inflammatory response may occur [55, 56].

Defense against protozoal infection calls on various effectors within the immune system [54]. The disease-causing *Leishmania* spp. and *Trypanosoma cruzi* can withstand attack by complement. *Leishmania* may enter into macrophages and provoke a neutrophilic response. Neutrophils can destroy *Leishmania* with superoxide radicals, namely nitrous oxide and hydrogen peroxide. CD4+ and CD8+ T-lymphocytes of the acquired immune system undergo activation after being presented with the protozoal antigen by macrophages and dendritic cells. When the primary infection has been defeated, effector T cells persist transiently, but memory T-cells (including in the skin) persist long term, ready to respond if a subsequent infection occurs [53, 57].

The response against protozoa also crucially depends upon humoral mechanisms. If immunoglobulin-based deficiencies occur, patients are at risk of infection by *Giardia lamblia* [53].

Since the Th1-orchestrated response is effective against intracellular pathogens, if the response is Th2-orchestrated, tissue damage may occur, and the protozoon may spread around the body. Overactivity of the immune system in protozoal diseases is responsible for tissue injury. For disease not to happen, even given a parasite within the body, the immune system needs to be working very efficiently [53].

As a particularly illustrative example, the Th1-orchestrated response is key to controlling granuloma formation in leishmaniasis. Individuals unable to synthesize IFN-γ and whose macrophages remain inactive suffer the disseminated spread of *Leishmania* when they enter the skin. If mononuclear cells taken from the circulation are cultured and exposed to IL-10 and IL-12, the individual recovers its immunocompetence [55, 57].

Immune defenses cannot entirely eradicate *Leishmania,* and a prolonged and violent Th1-orchestrated reaction leads to ulceration of the skin and mucosal surfaces. Even early treatment fails to prevent ulcer appearance [56]. These ulcers are characterized by a potent immune response with the increased secretion of IFN-γ and TNF-α, and few *Leishmania* organisms present [58].

1.6 Helminths and Immunity

Helminths are large, and the structure of their antigens is complex. These features determine how the immune system responds to infection by them. Helminths can live for several years within the host. How this can occur is illustrated by the case of *Schistosoma mansoni*, which becomes coated with the antigens of the infected host and thereby eludes immune defenses [59].

Helminthic infestation is associated with the phenomenon of "concomitant immunity." The immune response to the initial infection creates immunity to subsequent parasitic infection, while the initial invading organisms evade the host defenses. The parasite's adult stage has ways to avoid the immune response, although the larvae cannot escape attack in this fashion. The initial parasitic infection alters the patient's anatomical and physiological aspects to deprive parasites coming later of the chance to establish themselves within the host [60, 61].

Defense against helminthic infection includes effector cells of the innate immune system, the complement cascade, immunoglobulins, and particular cytokines. Th2-associated cytokines, notably IL-4, IL-5, and IL-13, stimulate IgE synthesis while mobilizing eosinophils, mast cells, and basophils. Histamine release is a crucial action, as are other activities also associated with hypersensitivity reactions [62]. Successful defense against *S. mansoni*, *Strongyloides stercoralis,* and *Ascaris lumbricoides* depends on Th2 function. IL-4 and IL-13 promote IgE synthesis, which triggers the release of other proinflammatory mediators, increased mucus production, and more significant contraction of gut-associated smooth muscle, helping to expel the adult parasite from the gut [59]. However, IL-4, IL-5, and IL-13 also stimulate granulomatous lesion formation and fibrotic repair, which feature in response to chronic helminthic infections [63].

References

1. David D, Chaplin MD, Overview of the immune response. J Allergy Clin Immunol. 2010;125(2):S3–S23.
2. Tosi MB. Normal and impaired immunologic responses to infection. In: Cherry J, Harrison GJ, Kaplan SL, Steinbach WJ, Hotez PJ, editors. Feigin and Cherry's textbook of pediatric infectious diseases. 8th ed. Philadelphia: Elsevier; 2019. p. 15–40.
3. Smatti MK, Cyprian FS, Nasrallah GK, et al. Viruses and autoimmunity: a review on the potential interaction and molecular mechanisms. Viruses. 2019;11(8):762.
4. Steed AL, Stappenbeck TS. Role of viruses and bacteria-virus interactions in autoimmunity. Curr Opin Immunol. 2014;31:102–7.
5. Park HJ, Kim DH, Lim SH, et al. Insights into the role of follicular helper T cells in autoimmunity. Immune Netw. 2014;14:21–9.
6. Turvey SE, Broide DH. Innate immunity. J Allergy Clin Immunol. 2010;125(2):S24–32.

7. Felix KM, Tahsin S, Wu HJ. Host-microbiota interplay in mediating immune disorders. Ann N Y Acad Sci. 2018;1417:57–70.
8. Bajic G, Degn SE, Thiel S, et al. Complement activation, regulation, and molecular basis for complement-related diseases. EMBO J. 2015;34:2735–57.
9. Vijay K. Toll-like receptors in immunity and inflammatory diseases: past, present, and future. Int Immunopharmacol. 2018;59:391–412.
10. Silva MT. When two is better than one: macrophages and neutrophils work in concert in innate immunity as complementary and cooperative partners of a myeloid phagocyte system. J Leukoc Biol. 2010;87:93–106.
11. Ragland SA, Criss AK. From bacterial killing to immune modulation: recent insights into the functions of lysozyme. PLoS Pathog. 2017;13(9):e1006512.
12. Yang F, Feng C, Zhang X, et al. The diverse biological functions of neutrophils, beyond the defense against infections. Inflammation. 2017;40:311–23.
13. Kubelkova K, Macela A. Innate immune recognition: an issue more complex than expected. Front Cell Infect Microbiol. 2019;9:241.
14. Papayannopoulos V. Neutrophil extracellular traps in immunity and disease. Nat Rev Immunol. 2018;18:134–47.
15. Merad M, Ginhoux F, Collin M. Origin, homeostasis and function of Langerhans cells and other langerin-expressing dendritic cells. Nat Rev Immunol. 2008;8:935–47.
16. Bedoui S, Heath WR, Mueller SN. CD4(+) T-cell help amplifies innate signals for primary CD8(+) T-cell immunity. Immunol Rev. 2016;272:52–64.
17. Hirahara K, Nakayama T. CD4+ T-cell subsets in inflammatory diseases: beyond the Th1/Th2 paradigm. Int Immunol. 2016;28:163–71.
18. Ma CS, Tangye SG, Deenick EK. Human Th9 cells: inflammatory cytokines modulate IL-9 production through the induction of IL-21. Immunol Cell Biol. 2010;88:621–3.
19. Jabeen R, Kaplan MH. The symphony of the ninth: the development and function of Th9 cells. Curr Opin Immunol. 2012;24:303–7.
20. Mirshafiey A, Simhag A, El Rouby NM, et al. T-helper 22 cells as a new player in chronic inflammatory skin disorders. Int J Dermatol. 2015;54:880–8.
21. Carbo A, Hontecillas R, Andrew T, et al. Computational modeling of heterogeneity and function of CD4+ T cells. Front Cell Dev Biol. 2014;2:31.
22. Trabanelli S, Gomez-Cadena A, Salomé B, et al. Human innate lymphoid cells (ILCs): toward a uniform immune-phenotyping. Cytometry B Clin Cytom. 2018;94:392–9.
23. Fan X, Rudensky AY. Hallmarks of tissue-resident lymphocytes. Cell. 2016;164:1198–211.
24. Panda SK, Colonna M. Innate lymphoid cells in mucosal immunity. Front Immunol. 2019;10:861.
25. Killick J, Morisse G, Sieger D, Astier AL. Complement as a regulator of adaptive immunity. Semin Immunopathol. 2018;40:37–48.
26. Chen L, Deng H, Cui H, et al. Inflammatory responses and inflammation-associated diseases in organs. Oncotarget. 2018;9:7204–18.
27. Montoya D, Modlin RL. Learning from leprosy: insight into the human innate immune response. Adv Immunol. 2010;105:1–24.
28. Chen K, Bao Z, Tang P, et al. Chemokines in homeostasis and diseases. Cell Mol Immunol. 2018;15:324–34.
29. Abbas AK, Lichtman AH, Pillai S. Properties and overview of immune responses. In: Cellular and molecular immunology. 9th ed. Philadelphia: Elsevier; 2018. p. 1–11.
30. Giamarellos-Bourboulis EJ, Raftogiannis M. The immune response to severe bacterial infections: consequences for therapy. Expert Rev Anti-Infect Ther. 2012;10:369–80.
31. Liew PX, Kim JH, Lee WY, Kubes P. Antibody-dependent fragmentation is a newly identified mechanism of cell killing in vivo. Sci Rep. 2017;7(1):10515.
32. Katzenmeyer KN, Szott LM, Bryers JD. Artificial opsonin enhances bacterial phagocytosis, oxidative burst and chemokine production by human neutrophils. Pathog Dis. 2017;75(6):75.
33. Chong J, Jones P, Spelman D, et al. Overwhelming post-splenectomy sepsis in patients with asplenia and hyposplenia: a retrospective cohort study. Epidemiol Infect. 2017;145:397–400.

34. González-Fernández A, Faro J, Fernández C. Immune responses to polysaccharides: lessons from humans and mice. Vaccine. 2008;26:292–300.
35. Yang Q, Shu HB. Deciphering the pathways to antiviral innate immunity and inflammation. Adv Immunol. 2020;145:1–36.
36. Beltra JC, Decaluwe H. Cytokines and persistent viral infections. Cytokine. 2016;82:4–15.
37. Lin GL, McGinley JP, Drysdale SB, et al. Epidemiology and immune pathogenesis of viral sepsis. Front Immunol. 2018;9:2147.
38. Bergantz L, Subra F, Deprez E, et al. Interplay between intrinsic and innate immunity during HIV infection. Cell. 2019;8(8):922.
39. Nozuma S, Jacobson S. Neuroimmunology of human T-lymphotropic virus type 1-associated myelopathy/tropical spastic paraparesis. Front Microbiol. 2019;10:885.
40. Porto AF, Neva FA, Bittencourt H, et al. HTLV-1 decreases Th2 type of immune response in patients with strongyloidiasis. Parasite Imunol. 2001;23:503–7.
41. Hufbauer M, Akgül B. Molecular mechanisms of human papillomavirus induced skin carcinogenesis. Viruses. 2017;9(7):187.
42. Hernández-Montes J, Rocha-Zavaleta L, Monroy-García A, et al. Peripheral blood lymphocytes from low-grade squamous intraepithelial lesions patients recognize vaccine antigens in the presence of activated dendritic cells and produced high levels of CD8 + IFNγ + T cells and low levels of IL-2 when induced to proliferate. Infect Agent Cancer. 2012;7(1):12.
43. Azkur AK, Akdis M, Azkur D, et al. Immune response to SARS-CoV-2 and mechanisms of immunopathological changes in COVID-19. Allergy. 2020;75:1564–81.
44. Shah VK, Firmal P, Alam A, et al. Overview of immune response during SARS-CoV-2 infection: lessons from the past. Front Immunol. 2020;11:1949.
45. Liang Y, Wang ML, Chien CS, et al. Highlight of immune pathogenic response and hematopathologic effect in SARS-CoV, MERS-CoV, and SARS-Cov-2 infection. Front Immunol. 2020;11:1022.
46. Brakhage AA, Bruns S, Thywissen A, et al. Interaction of phagocytes with filamentous fungi. Curr Opin Microbiol. 2010;13:409–15.
47. Romani L. Immunity to fungal infections. Nat Rev Immunol. 2011;11:275–88.
48. Luisa Gil M, Murciano C, Yáñez A, et al. Role of foll-like receptors in systemic Candida albicans infections. Front Biosci. 2016;21:278–302.
49. Constantine GM, Lionakis MS. Lessons from primary immunodeficiencies: autoimmune regulator and autoimmune polyendocrinopathy-candidiasis-ectodermal dystrophy. Immunol Rev. 2019;287:103–20.
50. Abers MS, Lionakis MS. Chronic mucocutaneous candidiasis and invasive fungal infection susceptibility. In: Sullivan KE, Stiehm ER, Cunningham Rundles C, et al., editors. Stiehm's immune deficiencies, inborn errors of immunity. 2nd ed. London: Elsevier Academic Press; 2020. p. 961–89.
51. Khosravi AR, Shokri H, Darvishi S. Altered immune responses in patients with chronic mucocutaneous candidiasis. J Mycol Med. 2014;24:135–40.
52. Smith N, Sehring M, Chambers J, et al. Perspectives on non-neoformans cryptococcal opportunistic infections. J Community Hosp Intern Med Perspect. 2017;7:214–7.
53. Mukai K, Tsai M, Starkl P, et al. IgE and mast cells in host defense against parasites and venoms. Semin Immunopathol. 2016;38:581–603.
54. Zambrano-Villa S, Rosales-Borjas D, Carrero JC, et al. How protozoan parasites evade the immune response. Trends Parasitol. 2002;18:272–8.
55. Sarkar SR, Ray NC, Nahar S, et al. Role of immune cells and cytokines for immune response in kala-azar. Mymensingh Med J. 2018;27:904–11.
56. Kumar R, Bhatia M, Pai K. Role of cytokines in the pathogenesis of visceral leishmaniasis. Clin Lab. 2017;63:1549–59.
57. Glennie ND, Scott P. Memory T cells in cutaneous leishmaniasis. Cell Immunol. 2016;309:50–4.
58. Boelaert M, Sundar S. Leishmaniasis. In: Farrar J, Hotez PJ, Junghanss T, Kang G, Lalloo D, White NJ, editors. Manson's tropical diseases. 23rd ed. Philadelphia: Elsevier Saunders; 2014. p. 631–51.

59. Motran CC, Silvane L, Chiapello LS, et al. Helminth infections: recognition and modulation of the immune response by innate immune cells. Front Immunol. 2018;9:664.
60. Maizels RM, Smits HH, McSorley HJ. Modulation of host immunity by helminths: the expanding repertoire of parasite effector molecules. Immunity. 2018;49:801–18.
61. Mabbott NA. The influence of parasite infections on host immunity to co-infection with other pathogens. Front Immunol. 2018;9:2579.
62. Caldas IR, Campi-Azevedo AC, Oliveira LF, et al. Human schistosomiasis mansoni: immune responses during acute and chronic phases of the infection. Acta Trop. 2008;108:109–17.
63. Gazzinelli-Guimaraes PH, Nutman TB. Helminth parasites and immune regulation. F1000Res. 2018;7:F1000.

Pathophysiology of Pediatric Ear, Nose, and Throat Infections

2

Recep Karamert, Anıl Aktaş Tapısız,
and Iordanis Konstantinidis

2.1 Introduction

Infections of the upper respiratory tract are the most common infectious diseases in the general population. Including acute pharyngitis, they account for about 5% of ambulatory care visits, which make them the most common acute diagnosis in office settings [1]. They range from self-limiting viral infections like common cold to severe infections related to serious complications like acute bacterial pharyngitis, rhinosinusitis, and otitis media. In this chapter, we present the pathophysiology of acute pharyngitis, acute rhinosinusitis, and acute otitis media.

2.2 Acute Pharyngitis

Pharyngitis is the inflammation of the pharynx most commonly originated from infectious agents. Infectious pharyngitis generally occurs as a part of the common cold, presenting a low risk for complications. Bacterial pharyngitis is less common, but it is related to serious complications and sequelae. The pathophysiology of pharyngitis varies according to the etiology. Pathogens may directly invade the

R. Karamert (✉)
Department of Otorhinolaryngology, Faculty of Medicine, Gazi University, Ankara, Turkey
e-mail: recepkaramert@gazi.edu.tr

A. A. Tapısız
Division of Pediatric Infectious Diseases, Department of Pediatrics, Faculty of Medicine, Gazi University, Ankara, Turkey

I. Konstantinidis
Second Academic Department of Otorhinolaryngology, Academic Faculty of Medicine, Aristotle University of Thessaloniki, Thessaloníki, Greece

pharyngeal mucosa as seen in streptococcal pharyngitis or can cause irritation on the pharyngeal mucosa along with increased nasal secretions only [2].

Both pathogenic and nonpathogenic bacteria form a commensal flora in the oropharyngeal cavity. Protection from these microorganisms is achieved by the potent local immune defense system of the oropharyngeal cavity. Saliva takes the most important role in the innate immunity of the oropharynx. Primary antibacterial functions of saliva are neutralization and transportation of the pathogens to the stomach. Saliva constantly baths the oral cavity and neutralizes the bacteria with numerous antibacterial properties it contains. Lysozyme, lactoferrin, and immunoglobulins are secreted into the saliva and contribute to the inhibition of the metabolism, adherence, and viability of the microorganisms. The sputum continuously moves and carries pathogens towards the stomach where they are killed by the effective enzymes in combination with low pH [3].

Lysozyme and lactoferrin seem to be the most important components of the innate immunity of the oropharynx. They are found at significant levels in saliva. Lysozyme aggregates bacteria through muramidase activity which is causing hydrolysis of the pathogens. Lysozyme by itself has a high impact against gram-positive bacteria but requires a co-factor like lactoferrin or an antibody-complement complex to be effective against gram-negative pathogens. Unlike lysozyme, the major effect of lactoferrin in human saliva is thought to be bacteriostatic but not bactericidal. Streptococci, staphylococci, candida, and enteric microorganisms are affected by lactoferrin. Lysozyme and lactoferrin can also potentiate the antibacterial effect of the humoral immunity of the mucosal membranes [4].

The major immunoglobulin on mucosal membranes is secretory (S)-immunoglobulin (Ig) A. IgA can prevent the binding of viruses to cells as well as their endocytosis and replication. Palatine tonsils produce a substantial amount of IgG that has an important role in the humoral immune defense of the oropharynx. IgG antibodies participate in opsonization and enhance phagocytosis. Similarly, nasal secretions contain lactoferrin and components of innate immunity. There are significant levels of IgA and IgG present in nasal secretions, originating from the submucosal plasma cells which contribute to adaptive immunity [5, 6]. Considering that nasal secretions follow a pathway towards the nasopharynx and oropharynx before swallowing they are an additional antimicrobial film for the pharyngeal mucosa.

2.2.1 Viral Pharyngitis

Viral pharyngitis usually presents with mild symptoms. Tonsillar exudates, cervical lymphadenitis, and leukocytosis are infrequent. The presence of cough, coryza, hoarseness, conjunctivitis, and/or stomatitis is usually related to viral infection.

The most common causes of viral pharyngitis are rhinoviruses which are responsible for approximately 20% of all infectious pharyngitis cases. Rhinovirus transmits by large particle aerosols, does not invade the mucosa, causing only a local inflammatory reaction. As in rhinovirus infections, pharyngitis caused by coronavirus usually is a part of the common cold and the virus does not invade the mucosa. Recently there are some studies about the evidence that severe acute respiratory syndrome coronavirus 2 (SARS-CoV-2), the etiologic agent of coronavirus disease 19 (COVID-19), invades the nasal and olfactory mucosa where ACE2 receptors exist. Adenoviral infections are also common in children. Unlike rhinovirus and coronavirus, adenovirus invades the pharyngeal mucosa and has a cytopathic effect on epithelial cells. Hyperemia and exudates are seen frequently and can mimic streptococcal infection. Adenovirus is also associated with pharyngoconjunctival fever in children [6–9].

Among viral pharyngitis causes Epstein-Barr virus (EBV) to have the most dangerous clinical course particularly in adolescents. EBV spreads with oropharyngeal secretions by person-to-person contact. It is the cause of infectious mononucleosis syndrome, which is characterized by hyperplasia in lymphoid tissues including Waldeyer's ring, lymph nodes, liver, and spleen. Tonsillopharyngitis is present in 70–90% of the cases [10, 11].

Both herpes simplex virus (HSV) type 1 and 2 can cause pharyngitis as a primary infection in immunocompetent patients. HSV enters the mucosal surface and affects nerve endings. The viral capsid is transported to the ganglia and the virus can spread to other mucosal surfaces from the nerve cell bodies through peripheral nerves. Latent virus reactivation can occur in immunocompromised hosts [6, 12].

Influenza virus, especially Influenza A, is another cause of pharyngitis. The virus invades the mucosa and causes necrosis, which predisposes to secondary bacterial infections. Parainfluenza virus is also a frequent cause of common cold and accompanying pharyngitis. It is a self-limiting infection and can occur either epidemically or sporadically.

Enteroviruses, especially coxsackievirus and echovirus, can also cause pharyngitis. Enteroviruses are transmitted predominantly by the fecal-oral route. Vesicular enanthems that progress to ulcers on an erythematous base on oral mucosa are the distinctive manifestations of coxsackievirus infections which are also self-limited [13].

Respiratory syncytial virus (RSV) can cause severe infections in infants. Transmission occurs by aerosols and contact with secretions. Cytomegalovirus (CMV) is transmitted usually by direct and prolonged contact with saliva, urine, and breast milk of an infected person or via respiratory droplets. The clinically apparent disease is rarely presented in immunocompetent hosts. A mononucleosis-like syndrome with mild pharyngitis can be seen infrequently [4].

Finally, pharyngitis is one of the symptoms of acute retroviral syndrome which is the most common initial manifestation of the human immunodeficiency virus (HIV) infection. Fever, lymphadenopathy, maculopapular rash, myalgia, arthralgia, and mucocutaneous ulcerations can be accompanying symptoms. Nonexudative pharyngitis occurs in 50–70% of patients [4, 6].

2.2.2 Bacterial Pharyngitis

Bacterial pharyngitis is less common but can result in severe complications and sequelae, requiring usually a specific antimicrobial therapy. *Streptococcus pyogenes* (Group A beta-hemolytic streptococcus; GABHS) is the most common cause of bacterial pharyngitis and contributes to about 15–30% of all cases [6]. Fever, exudative tonsillopharyngitis, odynophagia, anterior cervical adenitis, and leukocytosis are the main symptoms and signs of GABHS pharyngitis. None of these symptoms are specific for this infection with variable symptomatology between patients. Half of the children do not present with tonsillar or pharyngeal exudates despite the positive throat culture [4, 14].

S. pyogenes spread from person to person by large droplet nuclei. The incidence of streptococcal pharyngitis peaks during winter and early spring, probably due to increased indoor activities. Children are the major reservoir of *S. pyogenes* and spread among family members is common [4, 6].

M protein located on the cell membrane gives GABHS its invasive character. It also takes an important role in the development of rheumatic heart disease, which is a consequence of the cross-reaction with human cardiac myosin that mimics M-protein [15].

There are more than 100 serotypes of M-protein. Immunity to one serotype is not protective for the rest and infection can reoccur with a different serotype. The virulence of *S. pyogenes* correlates with its hyaluronic acid capsule in addition to M-protein. Capsule plays an important role in adherence and epithelial internalization [16]. Adhesin is another surface component that allows attachment to the pharyngeal mucosa and enables colonization and competition with normal host flora.

S. pyogenes produces highly potent exotoxins which act as superantigens. Production of such toxins enhances inflammatory reactions that can lead to severe hypotension and multi-organ failure. During tonsillopharyngitis, the immune response against GABHS is thought to be impaired by superantigens, while other less well-equipped mucosal commensals are still eliminated with the evoked hostile innate immune response [17].

2.3 Acute Rhinosinusitis

Acute rhinosinusitis (ARS) is one of the most common infectious diseases in childhood. ARS has three forms recognized as acute viral, acute post-viral, and acute bacterial rhinosinusitis. Viral rhinitis or the common cold is known to trigger the process by post-viral inflammation that causes damage to nasal and sinus epithelium. This damage affects mechanical, humoral, and cellular defense mechanisms of the upper airway, resulting in increased bacterial superinfection risk. All ARS types present this common pathogenic background, clinical presentation, and inflammatory pathways making differential diagnosis challenging particularly in the early stages of the disease [18].

The most common causes of viral upper airway infections are rhinoviruses which constitute about 50% of the cases. Coronaviruses take second place followed by influenza viruses and the other respiratory viruses [8, 18].

Streptococcus pneumoniae, Haemophilus influenzae, and *Moraxella catarrhalis* which are also called as *"infernal trio"* and *Staphylococcus aureus* are the most common causes of acute bacterial rhinosinusitis (ABRS). These are also the most common bacteria isolated from the maxillary sinus and middle meatus. Widespread use of the pneumococcal conjugate vaccine caused a reduction in the incidence of *S. pneumoniae* and a relative increase in the incidence of non-typeable *H. influenzae, S. pyogenes,* and *S. aureus* was reported [18].

The mucociliary clearance function of the upper airway mucosa is the first barrier and elimination mechanism against the infectious agents. Microorganisms are trapped in the mucus secreted by the goblet cells and removed mechanically by the ciliated epithelial cells. If a viral agent passes this barrier, it binds to the cell membrane and penetrates the cell. Viruses bind only to specific receptors on the cell membrane and these cells and receptors differ from one to another. This is also the reason for the specificity of a certain type of viruses regarding the involvement of specific organ systems [19].

The type of tissue damage also varies in viral infections. Specifically, rhinoviruses impair ciliary activity. However, influenza and parainfluenza viruses can destroy the respiratory epithelium [20].

As mentioned before, viral infections of the upper airway increase the risk of bacterial superinfection. Increased risk of ABRS is also related to the impaired mucociliary activity (due to primary ciliary dyskinesia or cystic fibrosis), allergy, and laryngopharyngeal reflux [18].

These factors cause multiple changes in the mucosal layer of the upper airway and contribute to the sinus ostial obstruction. The pressure into the sinus first increases depending on mucus accumulation but due to decreased sinus aeration and absorption of the residual oxygen in the sinus, a negative pressure develops afterward. Negative pressure aggravates further local congestion, increases mucus accumulation, and finally the mucociliary clearance of the sinus is impaired [18, 21]. All these changes in the mucosal environment increase the risk of a second bacterial infection by facilitating bacterial colonization and growth.

Viral infections also predispose secondary bacterial infections by triggering excessive adhesion molecule expression on the host cell. Adhesion of the common bacterial pathogens on rhinovirus-infected cells is significantly higher than on healthy cells. This can also partially explain the pathophysiology of ABRS following rhinovirus infections [22].

Characteristics of bacteria are also involved in superinfections. Encapsulated bacteria like *S. pneumoniae* and *H. influenza*e have invasive activity depending on their capsules, while other common bacterial pathogens like *S. pyogenes, S. aureus,* and gram-negative strains produce exotoxins against the defense system.

The two main defensive strategies against the microorganisms that succeed to enter the body are innate and adaptive immune systems. The innate or nonspecific immunity highly depends on the mucus barrier and antimicrobial proteins like lysozyme and lactoferrin. Adaptive immunity consists of immune response and inflammatory reaction. Most of the viral infections are eliminated by innate immunity alone, while bacterial infections often require adaptive immunity [23].

The innate immune system depends on phagocytic cells: neutrophils, monocytes, and macrophages. Cell-mediated immune responses are activated both in viral and in bacterial infections. Cell-mediated immunity is essential in the eradication of viral infections, because of its intracellular nature. Bacterial infections also activate the innate immune system and release chemotactic factors stimulating macrophages and neutrophils [23].

Antigen-presenting cells present specific antigens to T lymphocytes and activate the adaptive immune system. The antiviral response is thought to be Th1 cell mediated. Cytotoxic T lymphocytes kill the infected cells by recognizing the proteins expressed on the cell surface. Natural killer (NK) cells can also induce the death of the cells infected with viruses. T lymphocytes (especially Th1) and antibodies take an important place also in bacterial infections. T lymphocytes can increase phagocytic activity by releasing cytokines. They also stimulate B lymphocytes to produce specific antibodies [18, 23].

As mentioned before, allergy is an important predisposing factor in ARS. Allergic rhinitis is related to more abnormal nasal airflow and reduced mucociliary clearance during viral upper airway infections. These facts impair the functions of the sinus and increase the risk of ABRS [18].

2.4 Acute Otitis Media

Acute otitis media (AOM) is one of the most common infectious diseases in children. It affects nearly 80% of children by the age of 3 years and often requires antibiotic treatment [24]. There are various interacting factors in the pathophysiology of otitis media, including anatomy, infectious agents, and the environment.

2.4.1 Anatomy

The eustachian tube is shorter, more horizontal, and less rigid in infants. These anatomic characteristics are related to impaired function and the high rate of otitis media in children. The configuration of the tube changes and functions improve with age and the prevalence of otitis media reduces. The primary functions of the eustachian tube are the ventilation of the tympanic cavity, protection of the middle ear from the reflux of the nasopharyngeal content, and drainage of the middle ear secretions. Impairment of any of these functions may cause otitis media.

Tensor veli palatini (TVP) muscle controls ventilation and pressure regulation of the tympanic cavity by opening up the pharyngeal end of the eustachian tube during swallowing, jaw movements, and yawning. There is a correlation between active tubal function impairment and predisposition to AOM in children. The eustachian tube is collapsed passively at rest. This closure protects the middle ear from the nasopharyngeal reflux. The closure starts at the proximal part of the tube and continues through the nasopharyngeal end like a pump. Together with the mucociliary activity, this pumping action provides the discharge of the secretions from the tympanic cavity to the nasopharynx. Anatomic abnormalities of the musculature which are common in patients with a cleft palate may also cause eustachian tube dysfunction [24].

2.4.2 Infectious Causes

AOM is caused by bacteria and less commonly by viruses. Bacterial superinfections after viral upper airway infections take an important place in the etiology of AOM with viral-bacterial coinfections being common [25].

2.4.2.1 Viruses

Viral etiology without co-infecting bacteria corresponds to only about 10% of all AOM cases. However, common respiratory viruses are isolated in 20–70% of cases. AOM is usually a coinfection of viruses and bacteria. Viral upper airway infections facilitate bacterial colonization in the nasopharynx and may yield to reflux of pathogen bacteria to the middle ear cavity by impairing the mucociliary activity and the eustachian tube functions. The most common viruses related to AOM are RSV, coronavirus, adenovirus, human bocavirus, and rhinovirus [25].

2.4.2.2 Bacteria

Bacteria colonize the nasopharynx usually without causing an obvious infection. It is the viral upper airway infection that initiates the bacterial involvement and infection of the middle ear. Viral infections trigger an inflammatory response in the nasopharynx and eustachian tube. Bacterial colonization and adherence are increased in the infected nasopharyngeal mucosa. Silent bacteria are activated and their virulence is increased during this viral infection. The inflammation causes impaired mucociliary clearance of the nasopharyngeal and tympano-mastoid mucosa. Impairment of the clearance causes eustachian tube dysfunction and obstruction, yielding to negative pressure in the tympanic cavity. Negative pressure makes a vacuum effect and causes the reflux of colonized bacteria and viruses into the tympanic cavity from the nasopharynx. Infection of the middle ear initiates immune responses, resulting in inflammatory changes in the mucosa and middle ear effusion. Finally, the symptoms and signs of AOM occur [25].

The most common bacterial causes of AOM are the *"infernal trio"* S. pneumoniae, H. influenzae, and *M. catarrhalis* as in ABRS. After the introduction of the pneumococcal conjugate vaccines, an overall decrease in AOM prevalence was documented. However, *S. pneumoniae* remains the most common pathogen among children hospitalized with AOM due to increased non-vaccinated strains of *S. pneumoniae* infections, especially serotype 19A which is an invasive and multidrug-resistant strain [26, 27].

2.4.2.3 Environment

The most common environmental risk factor for the development of AOM is tobacco smoke exposure. Tobacco smoke has toxic effects on the respiratory epithelium and causes inflammation and congestion in the upper airway mucosa. Mucociliary activity in the mucosal surfaces of the nasopharynx and eustachian tube is also impaired due to tobacco smoke. Exposure also may facilitate the adherence of the pathogens to the respiratory tract epithelium. The combination of the abovementioned effects predisposes to middle ear infections like viral infections. It is also possible that tobacco smoke exposure may impair local immune defense like IgA production [24].

Daycare and allergy are also well-known risk factors for AOM. Breastfeeding is related to increased serum IgG and lower incidence of AOM [28].

References

1. Hing E, Hall MJ, Xu J. National hospital ambulatory medical care survey: 2006 outpatient department summary. Natl Health Stat Report. 2008;6:1–31.
2. Weber R. Pharyngitis. Prim Care. 2014;41:91–8.
3. Dawes C, Pedersen AM, Villa A, et al. The functions of human saliva: a review sponsored by the world workshop on Oral medicine VI. Arch Oral Biol. 2015;60:863–74.
4. Flores AR, Caserta MT. Pharyngitis. In: Bennett JE, Dolin R, Blaser MJ, editors. Mandell, Douglas, and Bennett's principles and practice of infectious diseases. 9th ed. Philadelphia: Elsevier; 2020. p. 824–31.
5. Pedan H, Janosova V, Hajtman A, Calkovsky V. Non-reflex defense mechanisms of upper airway mucosa: possible clinical application. Physiol Res. 2020;69:55–67.
6. Alcaide ML, Bisno AL. Pharyngitis and epiglottitis. Infect Dis Clin N Am. 2007;21:449–69.
7. Hildreth AF, Takhar S, Clark MA, Hatten B. Evidence-based evaluation and management of patients with pharyngitis in the emergency department. Emerg Med Pract. 2015;17:1–16.
8. Allan GM, Arroll B. Prevention and treatment of the common cold: making sense of the evidence. CMAJ. 2014;186:190–9.
9. Li Z, Liu T, Yang N, et al. Neurological manifestations of patients with COVID-19: potential routes of SARS-CoV-2 neuroinvasion from the periphery to the brain. Front Med. 2020;14:533–41.
10. Ebell MH, Call M, Shinholser J, Gardner J. Does this patient have infectious mononucleosis?: the rational clinical examination systematic review. JAMA. 2016;315:1502–9.
11. Rezk SA, Zhao X, Weiss LM. Epstein-Barr virus (EBV)-associated lymphoid proliferations, a 2018 update. Hum Pathol. 2018;79:18–41.
12. Clarke RW. Forces and structures of the herpes simplex virus (HSV) entry mechanism. ACS Infect Dis. 2015;1:403–15.
13. Saguil A, Kane SF, Lauters R, Mercado MG. Hand-foot-and-mouth disease: rapid evidence review. Am Fam Physician. 2019;100:408–14.
14. Lamagni TL, Darenberg J, Luca-Harari B, et al. Epidemiology of severe Streptococcus pyogenes disease in Europe. J Clin Microbiol. 2008;46:2359–67.
15. Guilherme L, Kalil J, Cunningham M. Molecular mimicry in the autoimmune pathogenesis of rheumatic heart disease. Autoimmunity. 2006;39:31–9.
16. Stollerman GH, Dale JB. The importance of the group a streptococcus capsule in the pathogenesis of human infections: a historical perspective. Clin Infect Dis. 2008;46:1038–45.
17. Sriskandan S, Faulkner L, Hopkins P. Streptococcus pyogenes: insight into the function of the streptococcal superantigens. Int J Biochem Cell Biol. 2007;39:12–9.
18. Fokkens WJ, Lund VJ, Hopkins C, et al. European position paper on rhinosinusitis and nasal polyps 2020. Rhinology. 2020;58(Suppl S29):1–464.

19. Cauwenberge PV, Ingels K. Effects of viral and bacterial infection on nasal and sinus mucosa. Acta Otolaryngol. 1996;116:316–21.
20. Barclay W, Al-Nakib W, Higgins P, Tyrrell D. The time course of the humoral immune response to rhinovirus infection. Epidemiol Infect. 1989;103:659–69.
21. Lund VJ. Therapeutic targets in rhinosinusitis: infection or inflammation? Medscape J Med. 2008;10:105.
22. Wang JH, Kwon HJ, Jang YJ. Rhinovirus enhances various bacterial adhesions to nasal epithelial cells simultaneously. Laryngoscope. 2009;119:1406–11.
23. Stambas J, Lu C, Tripp RA. Innate and adaptive immune responses in respiratory virus infection: implications for the clinic. Expert Rev Respir Med. 2020;14:1141–7.
24. Minovi A, Dazert S. Diseases of the middle ear in childhood. GMS Curr Top Otorhinolaryngol Head Neck Surg. 2014;13:1–29.
25. Nokso-Koivisto J, Marom T, Chonmaitree T. Importance of viruses in acute otitis media. Curr Opin Pediatr. 2015;27:110–5.
26. Coticchia JM, Chen M, Sachdeva L, Mutchnick S. New paradigms in the pathogenesis of otitis media in children. Front Pediatr. 2013;1:1–7.
27. Isturiz R, Sings HL, Hilton B, Arguedas A, Reinert RR, Jodar L. Streptococcus pneumoniae serotype 19A: worldwide epidemiology. Expert Rev Vaccines. 2017;16:1007–27.
28. Tignor E, Bailey LeConte DY, Makishima T. Update on the management of otitis media. In: Ulualp S, editor. Recent advances in pediatric medicine: synopsis of current general pediatrics practice, vol. 1. 1st ed. Sharjah: Bentham Science Publishers; 2017. p. 1–18.
29. Hiemstra PS, McCray PB Jr, Bals R. The innate immune function of airway epithelial cells in inflammatory lung disease. Eur Respir J. 2015;45:1150–62.

Laboratory Diagnosis for Paediatric Ear, Nose and Throat Infections

3

Hakan Evren, Emine Ünal Evren, and Codrut Sarafoleanu

3.1 Introduction

In children, the most frequent type of infection is one affecting the upper respiratory tract (URTI). Whilst a great deal of such infections do not require medical assistance, finding out which pathogen is involved at the start can prove essential to treating with an appropriate antibiotic and organising infection control measures. There have been considerable advances in how pathogens are identified. The latest assays are swift, possess a high sensitivity and specificity and are progressively substituting the previous gold standard methods [1].

3.2 Specimen Collection

Gathering a suitable sample is tied to a number of different considerations. Specimens need to be gathered no later than 5 days after the patient shows signs of illness and should precede giving antibiotics. It is only worthwhile obtaining samples after this point if the clinical situation fails to resolve or deteriorates or if the child is an infant or has immunocompromise [2, 3]. A usable sample needs to contain viable pathogens and should not have been contaminated. For URTIs, the

H. Evren (✉) · E. Ü. Evren
Department of Infectious Diseases and Microbiology, University of Kyrenia,
School of Medicine, Kyrenia, Turkish Republic on Northern Cyprus
(TRNC), Cyprus

C. Sarafoleanu
Department of Otorhinolaryngology, Head and Neck Surgery, Sfanta Maria Hospital,
Carol Davila University of Medicine and Pharmacy, Bucharest, Romania

C. Cingi et al. (eds.), *Pediatric ENT Infections*,
https://doi.org/10.1007/978-3-030-80691-0_3

most frequent specimens obtained are swabs from the throat or nasopharynx, nasopharyngeal washing, oral swabs or scrapings. If the laboratory is planning to use a rapid antigen detection test (RADT), the swab taken needs to match the kit used [4]. Identification of the pathogen in sinusitis cannot be reliably performed using a nasopharyngeal swab or wash, and a paranasal aspirate is needed. In fact, however, aspirates from the paranasal sinuses or middle ear cavity do not often reach laboratories, except where clinical issues arise, since empirical trials without pathogenic identification is usually sufficient. Aspirates from the nasopharynx have usually been considered gold standard for viral URTIs [5]. The ideal specimen collection technique involves gathering material from both left and right tonsil and the rear throat, and avoiding contamination from the mouth or elsewhere in the pharynx [6]. In cases of bacterial pharyngitis, throat swabs are examined solely for Group A Streptococci (*Streptococcus pyogenes*) unless other organisms are suspected [7]. Whilst a range of different microbes are typically cultured from a specimen, depending on how well it was taken, if the colony numbers are small, this has potential diagnostic significance. If a clinician suspects infection is not due to Group A Streptococci, but another pathogen, e.g. *S. dysgalactiae, Arcanobacterium haemolyticum, Neisseria gonorrheae, Clostridium diphtheriae, Francisella tularensis* or *Mycoplasma pneumoniae*, then this should be stated on the laboratory request form [6].

3.3 Direct Microscopic Examination

Direct microscopic examination of specimens is quick, but lacks specificity. Where only a small volume of specimen is available, microscopy requires supplementation with further diagnostic methods. A stained smear from within the mouth usually yields more information on microscopy than swabs from the surface of the throat. The smear may be stained with fluorescent immunoglobulins to directly identify particular bacterial pathogens and can identify isolated microbes. Current practice is to use direct fluorescent antibody (DFA) staining mainly to identify viral, rather than bacterial, pathogens. There are DFA stains available for certain bacterial species, i.e. *S. pyogenes*, Legionella spp. and *Bordetella pertussis*, and these are used in a few settings. For the most part, DFA testing of *S. pyogenes* is now done via RDA testing [8].

3.4 Culture Methods

The gold standard in diagnosing viral URTI is the finding of haemadsorption and cytopathic changes in cell culture. The viral pathogens most frequently identified via this technique are adenovirus, influenza A/B, RSV, and human parainfluenza viruses [9, 10]. Many of the frequently encountered viral pathogens (such as rhinovirus and coronavirus) are not readily tissue-cultured, however [11]. Cell culture of viruses has several drawbacks when compared with molecular techniques, and therefore cell culture has been discontinued in many settings [12, 13]. It has been found that where viral cell cultures only gradually show positivity, the result did not influence the management of otherwise healthy children [14].

Bacterial culture and RAD testing have value solely where Group A Streptococci, *B. pertussis* or *C. diphtheriae* of the nose is the diagnosis. Culture suffers from a delay of 24–48 h before reporting is reliable. Furthermore, up to 20% of culture positives during the winter represent carriage rather than an active infective episode [15]. Usually positive cultures for Group A Streptococci are not tested against different antibiotics as they are invariably penicillin sensitive.

For other pathogens which result in pharyngitis, special media and methods are required. A clinical suspicion of diphtheria should be communicated to the laboratory, which will then culture on selective growth media. Culture of other bacterial pathogens cannot explain rhinitis or sinusitis. If there is loculated pus, it may be aspirated via an extraoral surgical approach and any aspirate sent in an anaerobic packaging to microbiology without delay [6].

3.5 Antigen Detection Assays

RAD testing produces an answer within half an hour [16]. The procedure needs little time and the cost is low. However, RAD tests are less sensitive and specific than other techniques in the case of certain pathogens. Off-the-shelf RAD kits are generally confined to identifying influenza A and B and respiratory syncytial virus, but they suffer from a low detection rate of between 44% and 95% in these circumstances. Their median specificity of between 90% and 95% does, however, compare favourably with tissue culture [17, 18].

3.6 Direct Fluorescent Antibody Tests

Direct fluorescent antibody (DFA) may be applied to washings from the nasopharynx and is a swift and reliable method to diagnose viral URTIs. DFA testing is effective even if the virus is non-viable, and is performed very rapidly, two aspects in which it is superior to viral tissue culture [19]. Shafik et al. [20], examining paediatric cases of suspected RSV, demonstrated DFA testing is highly specific (99–100%), and can be relied on to detect viral pathogens, especially in the initial stages of an URTI. Fluorescent antibody assay testing, performed in conjunction with RT-PCR, renders highly probable the correct detection of acute viral infections. This combined technique has been employed to accurately identify pathogens other than influenza in a group of children [1, 21, 22].

3.7 Serology

Prior to viral antigen tests and nucleic acid amplification tests (NAATs) becoming available, the majority of pathology departments relied on serology. Even now, it enjoys widespread employment in viral detection. How the assay is performed, the viral antigens targeted, the state of the patient's immune system and when the sample is gathered, all have an effect on how sensitive and specific serology can be. Immunoglobulins targeting pathogenic viruses are produced within few weeks of the start of an URTI and their presence is detectable by serology. Serology can identify immunoglobulins produced in response to the majority of pathogens affecting the respiratory system, e.g. RSV, adenovirus, influenza A and B, and parainfluenza virus. In paediatric cases within hospital, serology can pick up mixed type acute respiratory infective episodes, unless the patient is an immunocompromised infant [23, 24].

For parainfluenza virus and adenovirus detection, however, serology has a markedly lower sensitivity than molecular techniques, e.g. RT-PCR [25]. Serology has no benefit in detecting viral episodes that recur often, where vaccine exposure and circulating viruses complicate the picture [26]. Serology is difficult to use effectively to identify bacterial infections, particularly where an unusual pathogen, e.g. *M. pneumoniae*, is involved. In these types of cases, serology is between 14% and 77% sensitive and 49–97% specific and cannot compete with PCR in terms of clinical usefulness [27].

3.8   Molecular Tests

With the advent of molecular detection methods, URTI pathogenic identification has advanced greatly and they have become the new gold standard. Despite their considerable popularity, it is still important to bear in mind various factors before implementing novel testing. These factors include which group of patients are to be screened (children, adults, immunocompromised individuals), how big the laboratory is, the aim of testing (routine or emergency) and the probable costs compared to potential advantages. A broad variety of novel nucleic acid amplification tests (NAATs) now exists to detect pathogens affecting the respiratory tract. The results obtained from molecular testing are determined not simply by the reaction itself, but also on how well the sample is taken, how much material is available and of what quality, as Dunn noted [26]. Taking a nasopharyngeal swab, particularly from a severely affected paediatric patient, is more straightforward than nasal aspiration or nasal washing [28]. The window of opportunity for obtaining a specimen with the optimal concentration of viral particles is 3–5 days following the beginning of the infective episode. Specimens must be conveyed to the laboratory in an appropriate transport medium and kept at a low temperature of 2 8 °C [29].

Molecular testing is capable of high sensitivity and specificity, and an improved rate of identifying pathogens; thus, doctors should consider test results prior to commencing a particular antimicrobial therapy. Molecular tests are appropriate routinely for diagnosis. In contrast, the older techniques, e.g. cell culture or electron microscopy, may be needed to identify new strains of pathogens [30].

The older techniques, e.g. rapid antigen detection techniques, DFA tests, and viral culture, have for the most part been superseded by NAATs, which are swifter and possess higher sensitivity. NAATs have revolutionised the laboratory management of URTIs.

References

1. Zhang Y, Sakthivel SK, Bramley A, Jain S, Haynes A, Chappell JD, Hymas W, Lenny N, Patel A, Qi C. Serology enhances molecular diagnosis of respiratory virus infections other than influenza in children and adults hospitalized with community-acquired pneumonia. J Clin Microbiol. 2017;55(1):79–89.
2. Ginocchio CC, McAdam AJ. Current best practices for respiratory virus testing. J Clin Microbiol. 2011;49(9 Suppl):S44–8.
3. Harper SA, Bradley JS, Englund JA, File TM, Gravenstein S, Hayden FG, McGeer AJ, Neuzil KM, Pavia AT, Tapper ML. Seasonal influenza in adults and children—diagnosis, treatment, chemoprophylaxis, and institutional outbreak management: clinical practice guidelines of the Infectious Diseases Society of America. Clin Infect Dis. 2009;48(8):1003–32.
4. Scansen KA, Bonsu BK, Stoner E, Mack K, Salamon D, Leber A, Marcon MJ. Comparison of polyurethane foam to nylon flocked swabs for collection of secretions from the anterior nares in performance of a rapid influenza virus antigen test in a pediatric emergency department. J Clin Microbiol. 2010;48(3):852–6.
5. Meerhoff T, Houben M, Coenjaerts F, Kimpen J, Hofland R, Schellevis F, Bont L. Detection of multiple respiratory pathogens during primary respiratory infection: nasal swab versus nasopharyngeal aspirate using real-time polymerase chain reaction. Eur J Clin Microbiol Infect Dis. 2010;29(4):365–71.
6. Bennett JE, Dolin R, Blaser MJ. Mandell, Douglas, and Bennett's principles and practice of infectious diseases. 8th ed. Philadelphia, PA: Elsevier/Saunders; 2015.
7. Bisno AL, Gerber MA, Gwaltney JM Jr, Kaplan EL, Schwartz RH. Practice guidelines for the diagnosis and management of group a streptococcal pharyngitis. Clin Infect Dis. 2002;35(2):113–25.
8. She RC, Billetdeaux E, Phansalkar AR, Petti CA. Limited applicability of direct fluorescent-antibody testing for Bordetella sp. and Legionella sp. specimens for the clinical microbiology laboratory. J Clin Microbiol. 2007;45(7):2212–4.
9. Olsen MA, Shuck K, Sambol AR, Flor S, O'Brien J, Cabrera B. Isolation of seven respiratory viruses in shell vials: a practical and highly sensitive method. J Clin Microbiol. 1993;31(2):422–5.
10. Winn WC. Koneman's color atlas and textbook of diagnostic microbiology. Philadelphia, PA: Lippincott Williams & Wilkins; 2006.
11. Ieven M, Goossens H. Relevance of nucleic acid amplification techniques for diagnosis of respiratory tract infections in the clinical laboratory. Clin Microbiol Rev. 1997;10(2):242–56.
12. Freymuth F, Vabret A, Galateau-Salle F, Ferey J, Eugene G, Petitjean J, Gennetay E, Brouard J, Jokik M, Duhamel J-F. Detection of respiratory syncytial virus, parainfluenzavirus 3, adenovirus and rhinovirus sequences in respiratory tract of infants by polymerase chain reaction and hybridization. Clin Diagn Virol. 1997;8(1):31–40.
13. Lin C, Ye R, Xia Y. A meta-analysis to evaluate the effectiveness of real-time PCR for diagnosing novel coronavirus infections. Genet Mol Res. 2015;14:15634–41.
14. Shetty AK, Treynor E, Hill DW, Gutierrez KM, Warford A, Baron EJ. Comparison of conventional viral cultures with direct fluorescent antibody stains for diagnosis of community-acquired respiratory virus infections in hospitalized children. Pediatr Infect Dis J. 2003;22(9):789–94.
15. Kliegman R, Marcdante KJ. Nelson essentials of pediatrics. Amsterdam: Elsevier; 2019.
16. Weinberg A, Walker ML. Evaluation of three immunoassay kits for rapid detection of influenza virus a and B. Clin Diagn Lab Immunol. 2005;12(3):367–70.
17. Leland DS, Ginocchio CC. Role of cell culture for virus detection in the age of technology. Clin Microbiol Rev. 2007;20(1):49–78.
18. World Health Organization. Recommendations on the use of rapid testing for influenza diagnosis. Geneva: WHO; 2018.
19. Charlton CL, Babady E, Ginocchio CC, Hatchette TF, Jerris RC, Li Y, Loeffelholz M, McCarter YS, Miller MB, Novak-Weekley S. Practical guidance for clinical microbiology laboratories: viruses causing acute respiratory tract infections. Clin Microbiol Rev. 2018;32(1):e00042.

20. Shafik CF, Mohareb EW, Youssef FG. Comparison of direct fluorescence assay and real-time RT-PCR as diagnostics for respiratory syncytial virus in young children. J Trop Med. 2011;2011:781919.
21. Feikin DR, Njenga MK, Bigogo G, Aura B, Gikunju S, Balish A, Katz MA, Erdman D, Breiman RF. Additional diagnostic yield of adding serology to PCR in diagnosing viral acute respiratory infections in Kenyan patients 5 years of age and older. Clin Vaccine Immunol. 2013;20(1):113–4.
22. Sawatwong P, Chittaganpitch M, Hall H, Peruski LF, Xu X, Baggett HC, Fry AM, Erdman DD, Olsen SJ. Serology as an adjunct to polymerase chain reaction assays for surveillance of acute respiratory virus infections. Clin Infect Dis. 2012;54(3):445–6.
23. Chkhaidze I, Manjavidze N, Nemsadze K. Serodiagnosis of acute respiratory infections in children in Georgia. Indian J Pediatr. 2006;73(7):569–72.
24. Hall CB, Walsh EE, Long CE, Schnabel KC. Immunity to and frequency of reinfection with respiratory syncytial virus. J Infect Dis. 1991;163(4):693–8.
25. Kuypers J, Wright N, Ferrenberg J, Huang M-L, Cent A, Corey L, Morrow R. Comparison of real-time PCR assays with fluorescent-antibody assays for diagnosis of respiratory virus infections in children. J Clin Microbiol. 2006;44(7):2382–8.
26. Dunn JJ. Specimen collection, transport, and processing: virology. In: Manual of clinical microbiology. 11th ed. Washington, DC: American Society of Microbiology; 2015. p. 1405–21.
27. Beersma MF, Dirven K, van Dam AP, Templeton KE, Claas EC, Goossens H. Evaluation of 12 commercial tests and the complement fixation test for mycoplasma pneumoniae-specific immunoglobulin G (IgG) and IgM antibodies, with PCR used as the "gold standard". J Clin Microbiol. 2005;43(5):2277–85.
28. Hammitt LL, Murdoch DR, JAG S, Driscoll A, Karron RA, Levine OS, O'Brien KL, Group PMW. Specimen collection for the diagnosis of pediatric pneumonia. Clin Infect Dis. 2012;54(Suppl_2):S132–9.
29. Grys TE, Smith TF. Specimen requirements: selection, collection, transport, and processing. In: Clinical virology manual. 4th ed. Washington, DC: American Society of Microbiology; 2009. p. 18–35.
30. Tang Y-W, Das S, Dunbar S. Laboratory diagnosis of respiratory tract infections in children-the state of the art. Front Microbiol. 2018;9:2478.

Imaging of Pediatric Ear, Nose, and Throat Infections

4

Çiğdem Öztunalı, Suzan Şaylısoy, and Pamela Nguyen

4.1 Sinonasal Infections

Infections of the sinonasal mucosa (rhinosinusitis) are mostly caused by upper respiratory infections (URIs) in children. Most infections are due to viral pathogens and follow an uncomplicated, self-limited course. In 6–13% of pediatric patients, however, viral disease can be complicated by acute bacterial disease that can spread to the orbits or the cranium. The other causes of sinonasal infections include immune-deficiency syndromes, cystic fibrosis, and anatomical abnormalities that obstruct the drainage of the sinuses [1, 2].

4.2 Imaging Considerations

Imaging in uncomplicated infectious sinonasal disease is not indicated in children. The mucosal swelling and thickening of the paranasal sinuses seen on radiographic, computed tomography (CT) or MR (magnetic resonance) images of children is a frequent finding and does not necessarily equate to sinonasal infection. Also, imaging is not helpful in differentiating viral from bacterial disease, and the mucosal changes observed in imaging studies can persist after an acute infection [2, 3].

For persistent, recurrent, or chronic sinusitis, or for defining the paranasal sinus anatomy before functional sinus surgery, initial imaging with non-enhanced CT is usually appropriate. CT and MRI of the head and the paranasal sinuses with

Ç. Öztunalı (✉) · S. Şaylısoy
Department of Radiology, Faculty of Medicine, Eskişehir Osmangazi University, Eskişehir, Turkey

P. Nguyen
Department of Radiology, Irving Medical Center, Columbia University, New York, USA

© The Author(s), under exclusive license to Springer Nature Switzerland AG 2022
C. Cingi et al. (eds.), *Pediatric ENT Infections*,
https://doi.org/10.1007/978-3-030-80691-0_4

intravenous contrast are usually appropriate for clinically suspected orbital or intracranial complications [3–6].

4.2.1 Acute Sinusitis

Both CT and MRI show inflamed mucosa as peripheral soft tissue thickenings. This appearance is, however, a nonspecific finding and can also be seen in chronic sinusitis or in the course of normal nasal cycle. Air-fluid levels in the sinuses and the presence of gas air bubbles within the sinusal fluid are more commonly seen in the acute disease. On MR images, both mucosal thickening and fluid within the sinuses appear hyperintense on T2-weighted images. Post-contrast images will show enhancement of the inflamed peripheral mucosa on T1-weighted images; fluid within the sinuses will not enhance [2, 5, 7].

4.2.2 Chronic Sinusitis

Mucosal thickening resulting from multiple episodes of sinusitis is commonly seen as peripheral linear soft tissue in paranasal sinuses. The degree and the location of the mucosal thickening may give information on the pattern of the sinonasal disease or may point out to the presence of an obstructive anatomical variation, and can help the surgeon select the most effective surgery [5]. Chronic, inspissated fluid collections of the sinuses may look denser than the acute fluid collections of sinusitis on CT. On MRI, higher protein content of the inspissated fluid causes an increase in

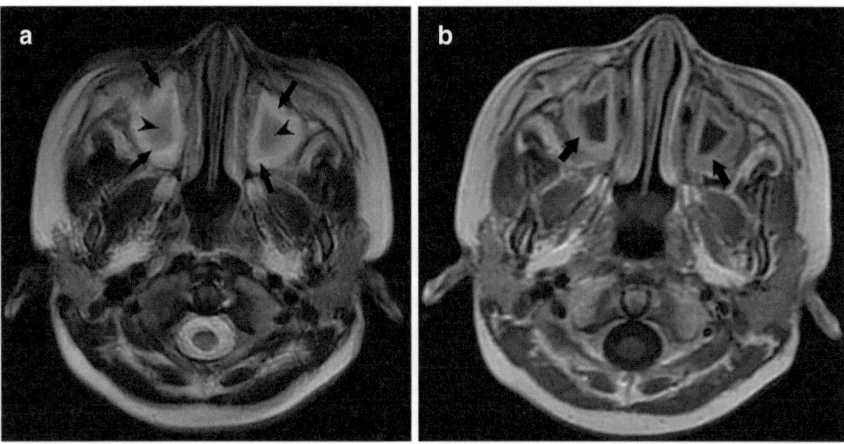

Fig. 4.1 (**a**) Axial T2-weighted image of a child with chronic sinusitis demonstrates increased thickness and hyperintensity of the mucosal surfaces at the periphery of the maxillary sinuses (arrows). Chronic inspissated fluid at the center exhibits decreased signal intensity (arrowheads). (**b**) Post-contrast T1-weighted image of the same patient as shown in (**a**) demonstrates enhancement of the peripheral mucosal surfaces (arrows)

signal intensity on T1-weighted images; the signal intensity of the protein-rich fluid will be decreased on T2-weighted images [2] (Fig. 4.1). Although less commonly observed in pediatric population, long-standing infection may cause wall thickening, wall sclerosis, osteitis, or new bone formation, with hypoaeration and/or contraction of the affected sinus(es). Sclerotic wall changes are best seen on CT images as increased density of the sinus walls. Osteitis is seen as laminated density increase of the sinus walls, and may be associated with periosteal reaction and/or osteoneogenesis. Nasal turbinates may show similar bony changes [5, 7].

4.2.3 Allergic Sinusitis

Systemic allergic diseases often cause hypertrophy and thickening of the sinonasal mucosa. On imaging, mucosal changes may be indistinguishable from that of infectious sinusitis, and infection may coexist. Although not specific, polyps, which are formed by hypertrophy and infolding of the mucosa with some fluid retention, are commonly seen on CT and MR images of allergic sinusitis patients, and present as polypoid, non-enhancing soft tissue masses with convex borders. The signal intensity of a polyp on MRI can vary according to its water and protein composition. Polyps in allergic sinusitis tend to be large and multiple. An aggressive polyposis pattern may be present with expansion of the sinonasal cavities and/or bony distortion, bone erosion or thinning. In such cases, the presence of a thin hypodense zone of secretion material between the polypoid masses on CT may be helpful in distinguishing polyposis from a neoplasm [2, 5, 7].

4.2.4 Fungal Sinusitis

Fungal infections can present as invasive and noninvasive forms, depending on the patient's immune system. Invasive form of the disease is mostly seen in immunosuppressed children, and can be further categorized into acute, subacute, granulomatous, and chronic forms [2, 7]. When acute, invasive fungal sinusitis may exhibit a rapidly progressive and aggressive imaging pattern. On CT, the involved sinuses show mucosal thickening and soft tissue opacification. Sinus contents will often be hyperdense with a peripheral rim of hypodense mucous. Hyperdensity of the contests on CT is usually a sign of benign disease and helps to differentiate from tumor. Tumor is not hyperdense. Bone erosion/destruction is best depicted on CT, if present. However, bony changes may be subtle or inapparent, and the fungal infection may extend through an intact bone via vascular invasion. In such cases, T1- and fat-suppressed T2-weighted images may show the spread of the infection as stranding of the fat planes outside the sinuses. A contrast-enhanced MRI of the head should be added to imaging protocol in all cases with suspected intracranial complications. Spread through the neuronal and vascular routes can cause cavernous sinus thrombosis, mycotic aneurysms, or cerebral infarctions. Intracranial spread of the infection can cause leptomeningeal involvement, epidural abscess formation, and subdural empyemas [1, 4].

Noninvasive fungal infections may present with mycotic colonization (fungus ball, or mycetoma) or allergic fungal rhinosinusitis. Fungus balls result from benign fungal colonization of a sinus. Most patients have an underlying impaired mucociliary clearance and/or chronic inflammatory changes of the mucosa. On CT images, involvement of a single or a few sinus(es) is seen as soft tissue opacification of the sinus(es), which can be of increased density [1, 2]. Punctate calcifications can be observed within the soft tissue density. Associated chronic inflammatory changes include sclerosis and thickening of the sinus walls. On MR images, presence of calcium and ferromagnetic elements in cases of fungal colonization may cause decreased signal intensity within the sinus on T2-weighted images (Fig. 4.2). Contrast enhancement of the peripheral mucosa can also be seen and reflects chronic mucosal changes. Allergic fungal rhinosinusitis commonly affects multiple sinuses in the form of sinonasal polyposis. A non-enhanced CT demonstrates expansion of the involved sinuses with a high-density soft tissue mass. Thinning of the sinus walls, bone remodelling, and erosions can be present. On MRI, T2-weighted images demonstrate low-signal areas within the soft tissue masses, due to the presence of fungal ferromagnetic elements. T1-weighted signal intensity may vary, depending on the protein and free water content of the masses. Post-contrast T1-weighted images frequently show the enhancement of the peripheral mucosa. No enhancement is expected in the center of the fungal soft tissue component and this feature may aid in differentiating allergic fungal from neoplastic sinonasal disease [4, 7].

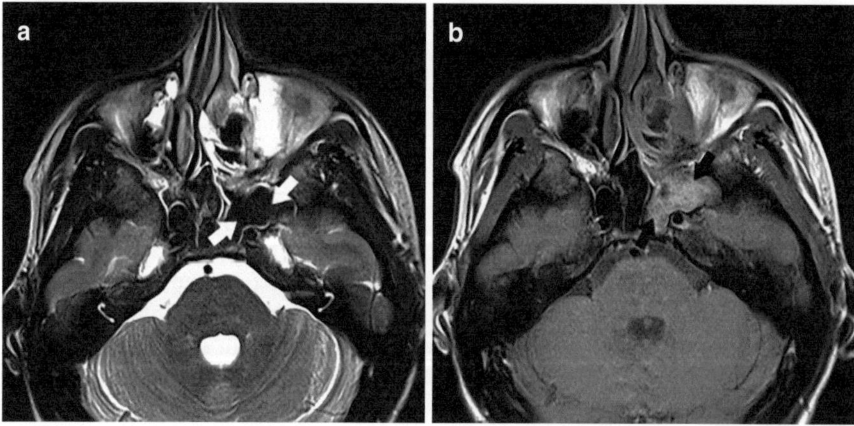

Fig. 4.2 (a) Axial T2-weighted MR image of an adolescent with fungal colonization of the sphenoid sinus demonstrates markedly decreased signal intensity of the left sphenoid (white arrows). (b) Axial T1-weighted MR image obtained at the same level as shown in A demonstrates increased signal intensity of left half of the sphenoid sinus (black arrows)

4.2.5 Complications of Rhinosinusitis

Rhinosinusitis may be complicated by orbital and/or intracranial spread of the sinonasal infection. This may result from delayed diagnosis and treatment, incomplete treatment, or from infection with antibiotic resistant or aggressive pathogens [1, 2].

4.2.5.1 Imaging

Imaging protocols for the orbit and/or the cranium should be included in evaluation of the paranasal sinuses if orbital and/or intracranial extension of the sinonasal infection is suspected clinically.

For suspected orbital and/or intracranial complications, CT is often the modality of first choice, since it is widely available, usually does not require sedation, and depicts the bony anatomy best. However, use of ionizing radiation is a major disadvantage of CT [1, 2, 4].

Contrast-enhanced MRI is more sensitive than CT in depicting the spread of infection to the orbital fat planes, leptomeninges, cerebral parenchyma, or to the bone marrow, and should be preferred over CT, especially in children who do not require sedation. MR angiography with or without intravenous (IV) contrast may be added to the imaging protocol if any vascular complications are suspected.

An MRI protocol for the imaging of orbital complication should include at least fat-suppressed T2- and T1-weighted images with a slice thickness of 3 mm or less. If not contraindicated, IV contrast medium should be administered, and axial and coronal fat-suppressed T1-weighted images should be obtained. Diffusion-weighted (DW) imaging may be particularly useful in detecting an abscess formation. In addition to contrast-enhanced T1-weighted and DW images, an MRI protocol for the imaging of the head should also include fluid-attenuated inversion recovery (FLAIR) images [1, 4, 5].

4.2.5.2 Orbital Complications

Orbital spread of the sinonasal infection can cause preseptal (periorbital) cellulitis, postseptal (orbital) cellulitis, subperiosteal/orbital abscess, or cavernous sinus thrombosis.

4.2.5.3 Preseptal (Periorbital) Cellulitis

Preseptal cellulitis occur anterior to the orbital septum and involve superficial tissues such as the conjunctiva and the eyelid. On CT, preseptal spread of the infection presents with soft tissue thickening and stranding anterior to the orbital septum [1, 2] (Fig. 4.3). Orbital septum is a fibrous membrane that extends between the periorbital periosteum and the tarsal plates of the eyelids. It is not clearly visible in cross-sectional imaging; however, its location can be imagined as a line that is connecting the anterior border of the globe with the orbital rim on both sides on axial sections. MRI shows T2 hyperintense and T1 hypointense soft tissue thickening that is limited anterior to the orbital septum [4, 8] (Fig. 4.4).

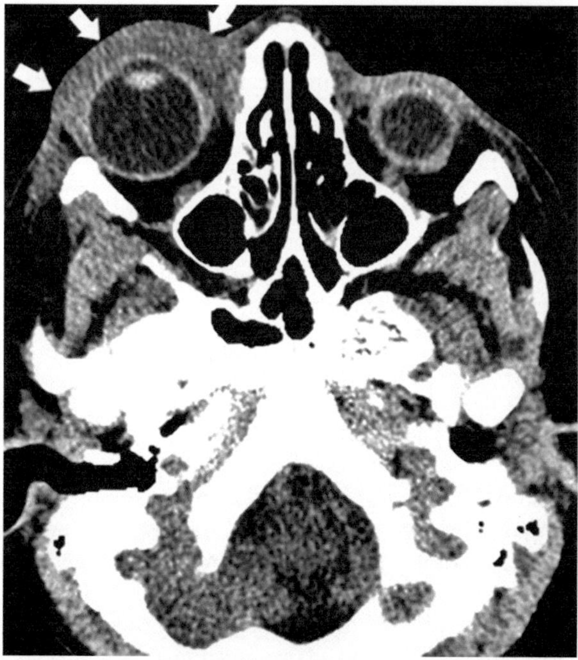

Fig. 4.3 Axial CT image shows right orbital preseptal cellulitis as soft tissue thickening that is limited anterior to the orbital septum (arrows)

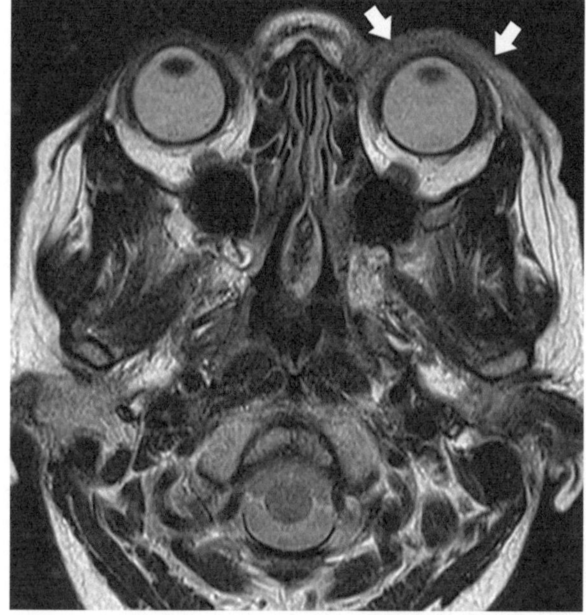

Fig. 4.4 Axial T2-weighted image of another patient with left preseptal cellulitis shows increased thickness and signal intensity of the soft tissue planes anterior to the orbital septum (arrows)

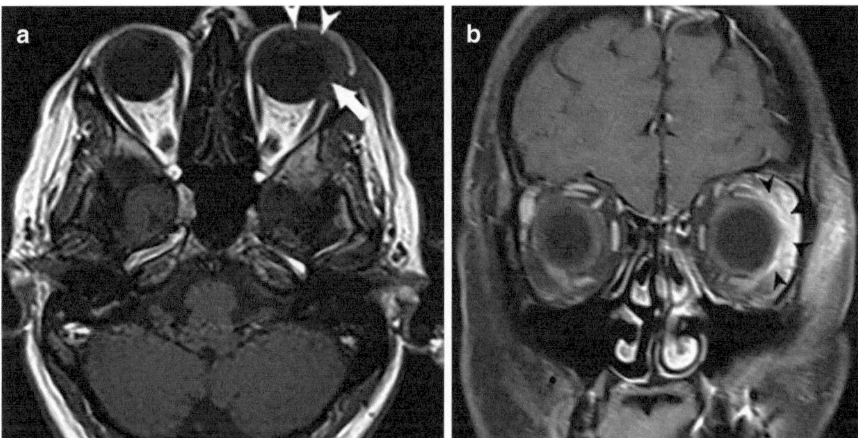

Fig. 4.5 (**a**) Axial T1-weighted MR image shows preseptal hypointense soft tissue thickening anterior to left orbital septum (arrowheads). Orbital cellulitis is seen as extension of the soft tissue thickening posterolaterally into the extraconal orbital fat (arrow). (**b**) Coronal fat-suppressed contrast-enhanced T1-weighted image of the same patient as shown in (**a**) demonstrates enhancement of the lateral orbital fat planes

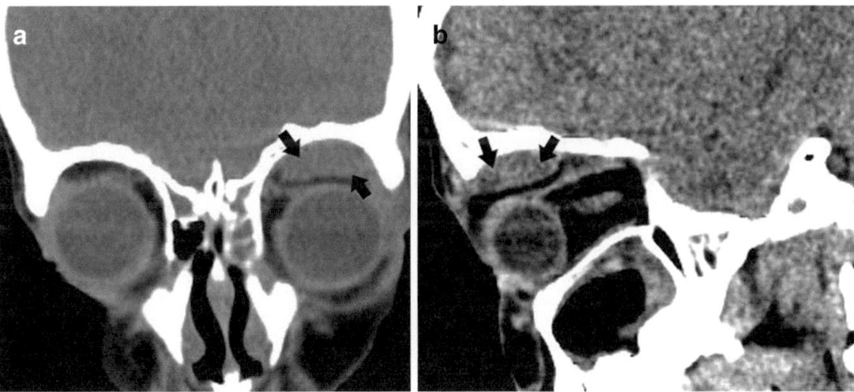

Fig. 4.6 Coronal (**a**) and sagittal (**b**) CT images of a child with subperiosteal abscess show an oval fluid collection along the left superior orbital wall (arrows)

4.2.5.4 Postseptal (Orbital) Cellulitis

Postseptal cellulitis occur posterior to the orbital septum. On CT, orbital spread of the infection is seen as soft tissue stranding in extraconal and/or intraconal orbital fat planes, posterior to the orbital septum. Infectious changes are most conspicuous on fat-suppressed images on MRI; spread of the infection shows T2 hyperintense signal changes and contrast enhancement of orbital fat planes on post-contrast T1-weighted images [1, 3, 4, 8] (Fig. 4.5a and b).

4.2.5.5 Subperiosteal Abscess

Intraorbital abscesses due to sinonasal infections most frequently occur subperiosteally. They originate between the bone and the periorbita. On cross-sectional images, a subperiosteal abscess presents as a lenticular- or oval-shaped fluid collection along the involved bone (Fig. 4.6). On MRI, subperiosteal abscess shows peripheral contrast enhancement and diffusion restriction on post-contrast and DW images, respectively. The extraocular muscles may be displaced [1, 7].

4.2.5.6 Cavernous Sinus Thrombosis

Orbital spread of the sinonasal infection can affect the valveless veins of the orbit and cause superior ophthalmic vein thrombosis. This, in turn, can lead to thrombosis of the cavernous sinus. Non-contrast CT may show a thrombosed superior ophthalmic vein as an enlarged and hyperdense vascular structure. Thrombosed cavernous sinus will look distended and hyperdense. Contrast-enhanced CT may demonstrate a nonfat density filling defect. Contrast-enhanced MRI is the modality of choice in cases of suspected cavernous sinus. In addition to cavernous sinus distention, MRI can show heterogeneous signal intensity changes in the expected location of the cavernous sinus fat signal intensity. The signal intensity of the thrombus may change, depending on its stage (acute, subacute, and chronic). Subacute thrombi often show high signal on T1- and T2-weighted images. On contrast-enhanced images, thrombi may be seen as filling defects. However, this finding may not always be present, as an organizing or subacute thrombus can also enhance heterogeneously. In such cases, MR venography can be helpful and shows the intra-cavernosal thrombus as a filling defect [1, 2, 4].

4.2.5.7 Extra- and Intracranial Complications

Intracranial spread of the sinonasal infection can result in meningitis, subdural/epidural empyema, cerebritis, and cerebral abscess. With the exception of the cavernous sinus thrombosis, intracranial complications often occur secondary to frontal sinusitis [1].

4.2.5.8 Pott's Puffy Tumor

While most frontal sinus infections spread to the anterior cranial fossa, in rare cases, the infection spreads outward and causes osteomyelitis and/or subperiosteal abscess formation (Pott's puffy tumor). In such cases, in addition to the signs of frontal sinusitis and erosive/destructive frontal bone changes, CT and MR images show a subperiosteal fluid collection that is located anterior to the frontal bone and enhances peripherally (Fig. 4.7a and b). DW images demonstrate diffusion restriction in the anterior fluid collection [1, 3].

4.2.5.9 Intracranial Complications

Infectious spread to the leptomeninges results in meningitis. A contrast-enhanced CT will show enhancement of the leptomeninges as curvilinear hyperdensities overlying the sulci and gyri. On MRI, non-contrast FLAIR, contrast-enhanced T1-weighted, and contrast-enhanced FLAIR images all may demonstrate thickened and edematous

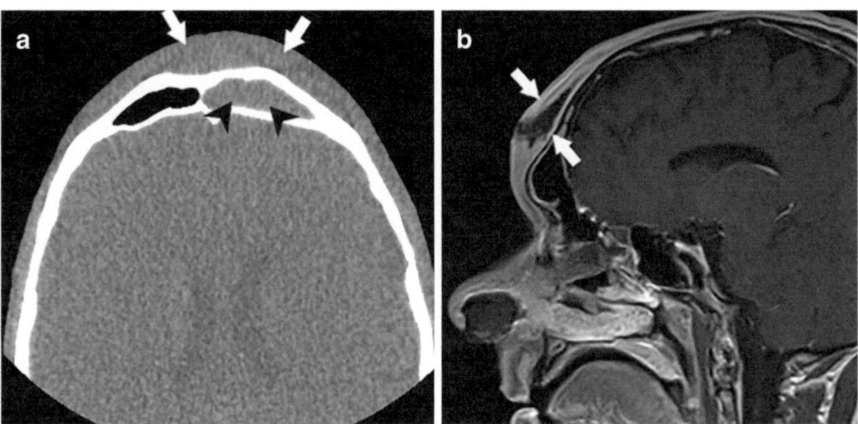

Fig. 4.7 Pott's puffy tumor. (**a**) Axial CT image shows soft tissue opacification of the left compartment of the frontal sinus (arrowheads). Note the increased thickness of the frontal soft tissue planes (arrows). (**b**) Post-contrast sagittal T1-weighted image of the same patient demonstrates a subperiosteal abscess as a fluid collection located anterior to the anterior wall of the frontal sinus (arrows). Note the peripheral enhancement of the subperiosteal fluid collection

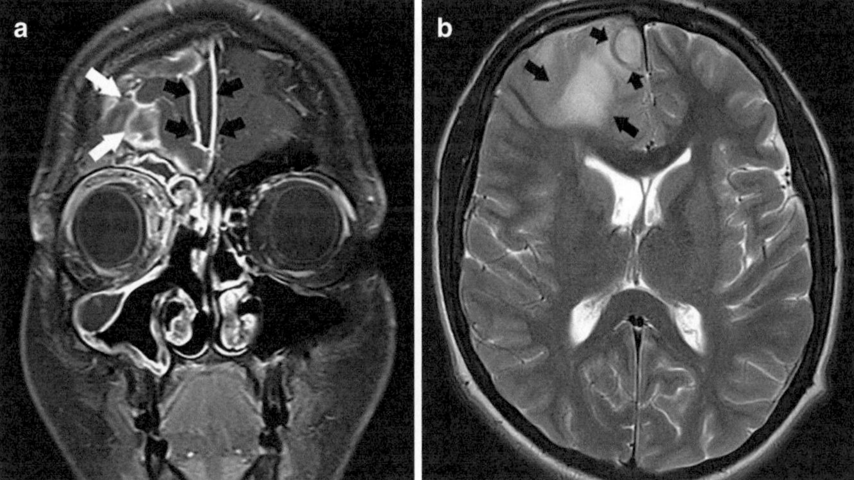

Fig. 4.8 (**a**) Post-contrast coronal T1W image of a child with invasive fungal sinusitis shows intracranial spread of right frontal infection as leptomeningeal contrast enhancement (white arrows). Note the right frontal parafalcine subdural fluid collection with peripheral contrast enhancement (black arrows). (**b**) Axial T2W image of the same patient as shown in A demonstrates right frontal cerebritis as increased signal intensity and edema of the frontal lobe (long arrows). The right parafalcine empyema demonstrates high signal (short arrows)

meninges as curvilinear hyperintensities that are extending into the sulci. Of these, contrast-enhanced FLAIR images have shown to be more sensitive in demonstrating leptomeningeal involvement. Epidural and subdural empyemas represent infected extra-axial fluid collections that are located between the cranium and the brain parenchyma. On MRI, both collections exhibit mass effect on the brain parenchyma, show peripheral rim enhancement and restrict diffusion (Fig. 4.8a). Epidural collections do not cross the suture lines, but they can cross falx cerebri.

Spread of the infection to the brain parenchyma first results in focal cerebritis, that is best seen as focal edema of the brain parenchyma on T2-weighted and FLAIR MR images (Fig. 4.8b). A cerebral abscess will demonstrate a parenchymal fluid collection that is surrounded by a well-defined peripheral rim. Pronounced vasogenic edema of the adjacent parenchyma is often seen. On contrast-enhanced images, the rim of the cerebral abscess will show enhancement, and the central pus within the abscess cavity will show diffusion restriction on DW images [1, 2, 7].

4.2.6 Ear Infections

Infections of the ear can be grouped into external, middle, and inner infections, according to dominantly involved temporal bone compartment. Spread of infection often develops between these compartments, and also between these and the skull base, neck spaces, and intra- and extra-cranial spaces [9, 10].

4.2.6.1 Imaging

In evaluation of persistent/recurrent otitis media, acute mastoiditis, chronic otomastoiditis, acquired cholesteatoma, and late labyrinthitis, a high-resolution temporal bone CT is often the initial imaging method of choice. CT nicely demonstrates acute and chronic bony changes, shows the extent of the middle ear and/or mastoid involvement. Contrast-enhanced temporal bone MRI is better than CT in evaluation of complications. Contrast-enhanced images of the head should be acquired to evaluate intracranial spread of the infection. MRI shows early changes of osteomyelitis and skull base and/or cranial nerve involvement better than CT. MR angiography may also be needed if venous or arterial vascular complications are suspected [9–11].

4.2.6.2 External Otitis and Necrotizing Otitis Externa

Uncomplicated external otitis is a clinical diagnosis and usually does not warrant imaging. When imaged, CT may show soft tissue thickening that is limited to external ear canal [11].

In addition to more extensive soft tissue changes in and around the external canal, rapidly progressive necrotizing otitis externa (malignant otitis externa) can show bony destruction of the walls of the external canal. The infection can contiguously spread to temporomandibular joint fossa posteriorly, infratemporal fossa inferiorly, parotid region laterally, and the petrous apex and the middle cranial fossa medially [9, 12]. MRI shows signs of osteomyelitis as bone marrow edema on

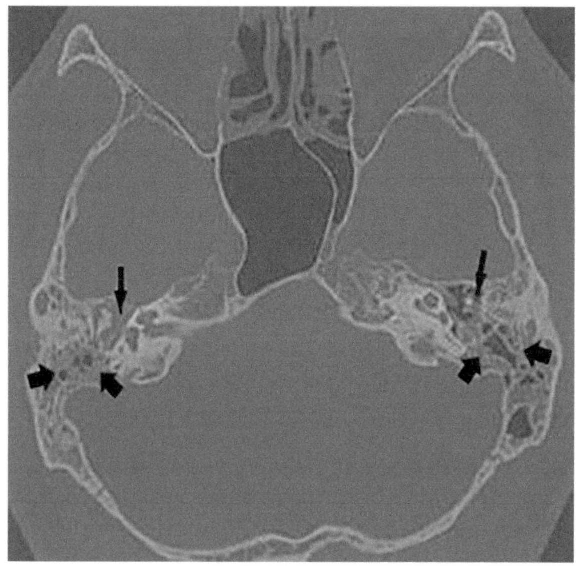

Fig. 4.9 Axial CT image of a child with bilateral acute otitis media shows soft tissue opacification of the mastoid air cells (short arrows) and the right middle ear cavity (long arrows)

fat-suppressed T2-weighted images. Post-contrast images demonstrate abnormal enhancement of the affected bones, soft tissues, and cranial nerves [3, 9].

4.2.6.3 Acute Otitis Media

Imaging in non-complicated acute otitis media is not indicated. On CT, involvement of mucoperiosteum of the middle ear presents with nonspecific soft tissue opacification of the middle ear cavity, with or without associated fluid collections (Fig. 4.9). The middle ear ossicles remain unaffected and do not show any signs of erosion or sclerosis [3, 11].

4.2.6.4 Mastoiditis

Uncomplicated mastoiditis often accompany otitis media, and is seen as soft tissue opacification of the mastoid air cells on CT, with or without air-fluid levels. The mastoid trabeculae remain intact and this imaging pattern of mastoid opacification with no osseous resorption or periostitis is defined as incipient mastoiditis [3, 10].

4.2.7   Complications of Acute Otomastoiditis

4.2.7.1 Coalescent Mastoiditis

Coalescent mastoiditis occurs when suppurative infection of the mastoid cells results in absorption of mastoid osseous trabeculae and empyema formation. On CT, early bony changes of the mastoiditis can be seen as soft tissue opacification of the mastoid cells and decreased conspicuity of the mastoid septa.

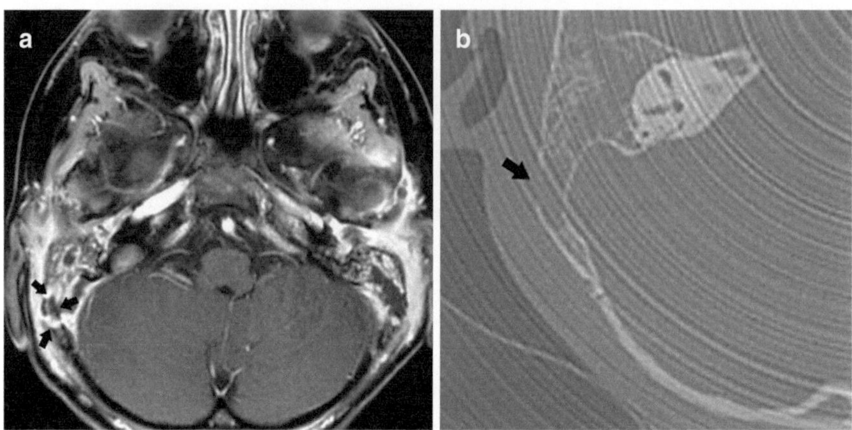

Fig. 4.10 (**a**) Contrast-enhanced axial T1-weighted MR image of a patient with bilateral coalescent mastoiditis shows a right-sided subperiosteal abscess as a peripherally enhancing hypointense fluid collection that is located immediately lateral to the right lateral cortical plate of the mastoid (arrows). (**b**) Axial CT image of the same patient as shown in (**a**) demonstrates eroded right lateral mastoid wall as focal cortical discontinuity (arrow)

Progressive infection results in erosion of the mastoid septa and/or mastoid wall. Coalescing purulent fluid collections can be seen as soft tissue areas within the residual mastoid septa [9].

4.2.7.2 Subperiosteal Abscess

Lateral spread of the infection often occurs towards the posterior auricular region, where the mastoid wall is thin. This results in subperiosteal abscess formation that can be seen as an oval- or lenticular-shaped fluid collection overlying an intact or focally eroded lateral mastoid wall. On MRI, both intramastoid fluid collections and subperiosteal abscesses can show peripheral rim enhancement and diffusion restriction (Fig. 4.10a and b). Inferior spread of the mastoid infection in adults often causes abscess formation at the mastoid tip (Bezold abscess). This condition occurs less frequently in children, due to poor pneumatization of the mastoid tip [3, 10].

4.2.7.3 Petrous Apicitis and Skull Base Involvement

Contiguous spread of the infection can involve pneumatized or non-pneumatized petrous apex, as well as the skull base. In its early stage, petrous apex infection, or petrous apicitis, can present with fluid collection within the petrous apex. At this stage, MRI best demonstrates signs of bone marrow edema/osteomyelitis as increased signal intensity of the petrous apex on fat-suppressed fluid-sensitive sequences. A central apical fluid collection can be seen as an expansile, T2-hyperintense fluid collection (Fig. 4.11). Peripheral enhancement and diffusion restriction may accompany the findings. Involvement of the adjacent dura and the nerves of the skull base results in abnormal contrast enhancement [9, 12].

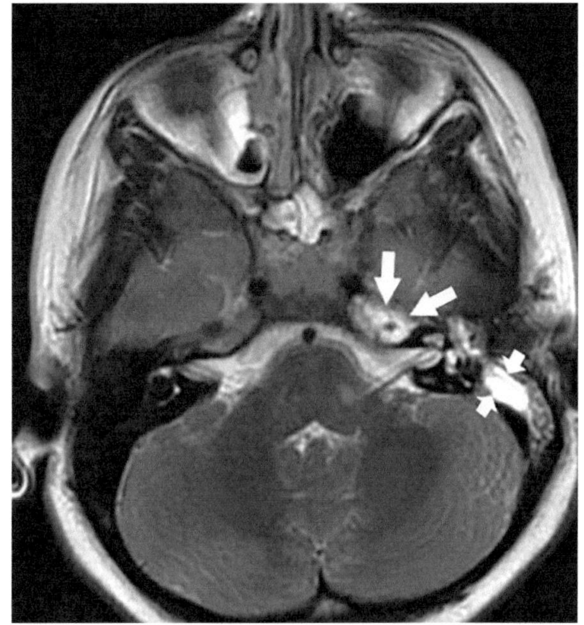

Fig. 4.11 Left petrous apicitis in a child with left mastoiditis. Axial T2-weighted MR image shows increased signal intensity and mild expansion of the left petrous apex (long arrows). Note the hyperintense fluid collection at the level of the left mastoid air cells (short arrows)

4.2.7.4 Labyrinthitis

Labyrinthitis can occur from spread of infection via preformed pathways such as the oval and round windows (tympanogenic spread), internal acoustic canal, or vestibular and cochlear aqueducts (meningogenic spread). Alternatively, it can result from contiguous spread of infection to the bony labyrinth. On MRI, contrast-enhanced images can show abnormal enhancement of the internal acoustic canal and/or of the membranous labyrinth. At the acute stage, high-resolution T2-weighted MR images may not demonstrate any signal abnormalities of the cochlea and vestibule. The subacute (fibrous) stage is characterized by the loss of normally high T2-weighted signal intensity of the membranous labyrinth. At the chronic stage (labyrinthitis ossificans), ossification within the membranous labyrinth causes marked signal intensity loss on T2-weighted images. CT will show the chronic changes as increased density and ossification of the membranous labyrinth [9–11].

4.2.7.5 Intracranial Complications

Intracranial spread of the infection commonly occurs via the relatively thin plates of the temporal bone. Erosion of the tegmen tympani may result in middle cranial fossa involvement. Posteriorly, erosion of the thin sigmoid plate of the temporal bone usually results in posterior cranial fossa involvement. Intracranial spread of the infection into these fossae can be seen in the form of meningitis, epidural or subdural empyema, cerebritis, cerebellitis, or cerebral and/or cerebellar abscesses. Transvenous spread may occur via emissary veins and may cause thrombophlebitis or dural venous sinus thrombosis [10, 12]. Sinus thrombosis most commonly involves the sigmoid sinus, and the petrous apex infection may cause cavernous sinus and/or

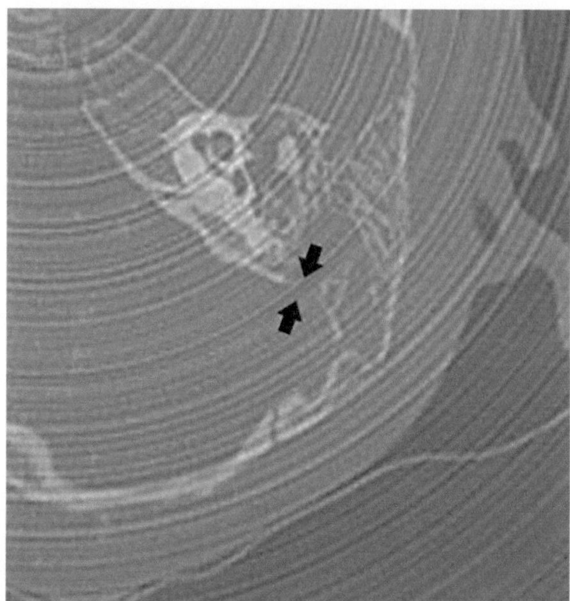

Fig. 4.12 Axial CT image of a child with coalescent mastoiditis shows discontinuity of the cortical bone at the level of the medial sigmoid plate (arrows)

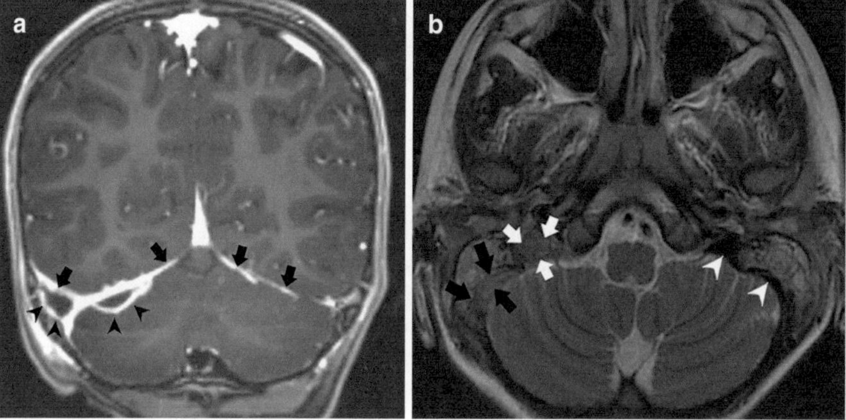

Fig. 4.13 (**a**) Contrast- enhanced T1-weighted coronal image of a child with bilateral coalescent mastoiditis shows abnormal enhancement and thickening of the dura at the level of the tentorium cerebelli and the right transvers dural sinus (arrows). Subdural empyemas are seen as peripherally enhancing hypointense fluid collections (arrowheads). (**b**) Axial T2-weighted image of the patient as shown in A demonstrates thrombosis of the right jugular vein (white arrows) and the right sigmoid sinus (black arrows) as absence of the normal venous flow-void signal. Note the signal void at the level of the normal left jugular vein and sigmoid sinus (arrowheads)

petrosal sinus thrombosis. Venous thrombosis in turn may lead to hemorrhagic venous infarctions. CT in these cases may show erosion/destruction of the tegmen tympani or the sigmoid plate of the temporal bone (Fig. 4.12). Contrast-enhanced MR images may demonstrate pachymeningitis as abnormal enhancement and thickening of the meninges and the dura along the sigmoid sinus and the floor of the middle cranial fossa in cases of sigmoid and tegmen tympani region involvement, respectively. An epidural or subdural empyema can be seen as an extra-axial fluid collection that enhances peripherally and restricts diffusion. Dural vein thrombosis can be seen as a filling defect on contrast-enhanced CT images (Fig. 4.13a and b). On non-contrast MRI, absence of the normal venous flow void on spin-echo images can be suspicious for thrombosis. However, this can also occur due to slow venous flow or significant compression of the involved sinus. Definitive diagnosis frequently necessitates the use of contrast-enhanced MR venography, which will demonstrate the thrombosis as a filling defect within the sinus lumen [10, 12].

4.2.8 Neck Infections

Superficial and deep infections comprise the most common disease group in the pediatric neck. A detailed evaluation of the airways, neck compartments, and vascular structures can be necessary, since direct spread of the infection can rapidly occur to involve multiple neck compartments and vessels [13].

4.2.8.1 Imaging

Imaging in pediatric neck infections should be tailored according to clinical findings and the information needed. Ultrasonography with color Doppler is usually the first imaging modality employed in detection and characterization of superficial infections. US can also be helpful in guiding interventions such as aspiration or drainage. Contrast-enhanced CT is the imaging modality of deep neck space infections in an acute setting, since most modern CT scanners now allow fast imaging with multiplanar reconstructions. A contrast-enhanced CT can be useful in localizing a suspected deep neck infection, as well as in detection of infection spread through multiple deep neck compartments and in evaluation of any vascular complications. Despite the employment of low-dose protocols, the use of ionizing radiation remains as the main disadvantage of CT. Contrast-enhanced MRI provides better soft tissue contrast and may help further assessment of a complicated infection. Its drawbacks include longer scan times and the need for sedation for many young children [13–15].

4.2.8.2 Cervical Adenitis

Acute cervical adenitis does not necessitate imaging evaluation. Imaging can be required in subacute or chronic cases that are unresponsive to therapy, to determine if there is an underlying cause. Although some imaging characteristics such as vascularity, size, and contrast enhancement can aid in differentiating infectious from malignant lymphadenopathy, biopsy or surgery may be required [13].

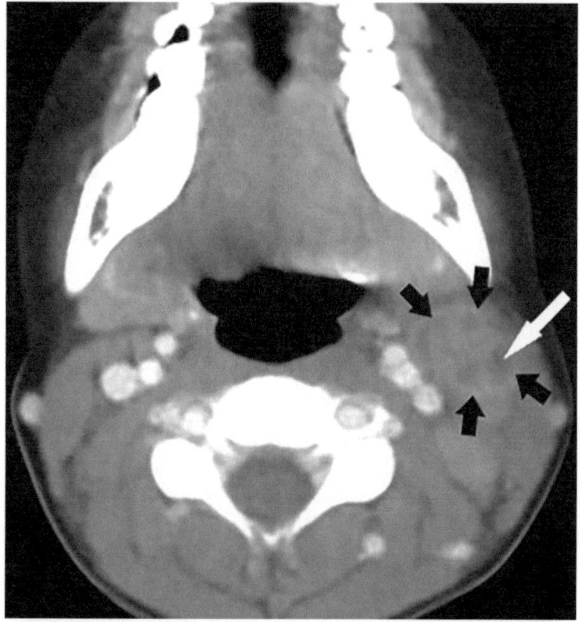

Fig. 4.14 Axial contrast-enhanced CT of a child with tuberculous adenitis shows a left-sided enlarged lymph node (black arrows) with small hypodense necrotic areas (white arrow)

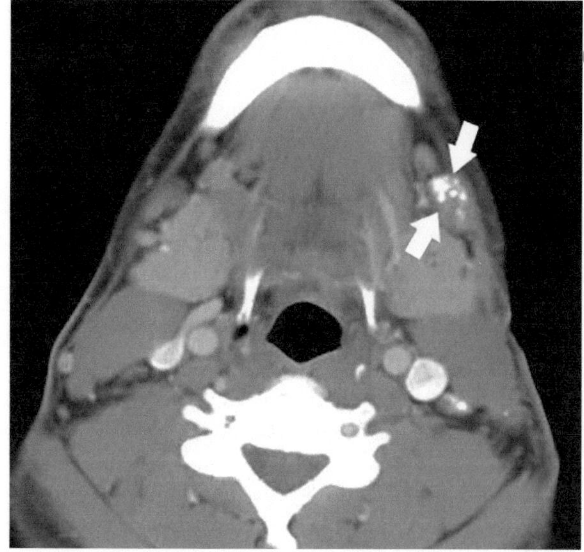

Fig. 4.15 Axial contrast-enhanced CT image of an adolescent with chronic tuberculous lymphadenitis demonstrates a normal-sized left submandibular lymph node with internal hyperdense calcifications (arrows)

At US, reactive lymph nodes are seen as enlarged, ovoid-shaped, hypoechoic nodes with a central hyperechogenic fatty hilum. They may exhibit increased vascularity on color Doppler imaging. Involvement of the surrounding tissues can cause stranding of the adjacent fat planes. Suppurative and necrotic lymph nodes mostly contain centrally located fluid-filled areas on US. The central fluid collection

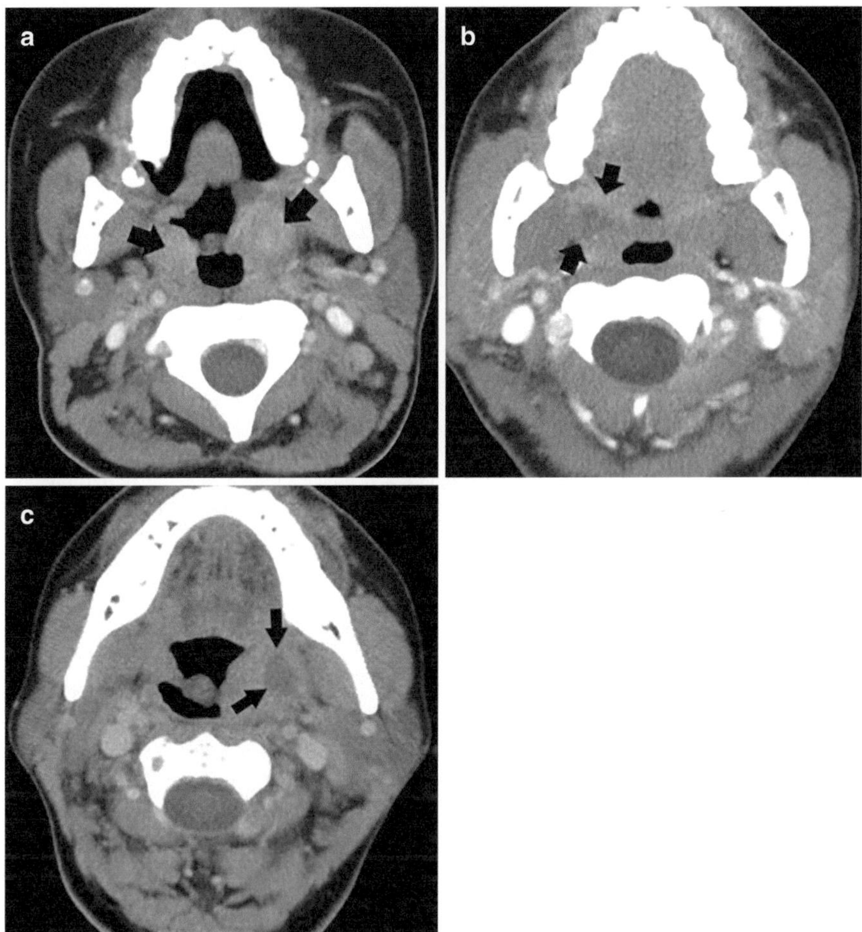

Fig. 4.16 (**a**) Axial contrast-enhanced CT at the level of the oropharynx demonstrates enlargement and increased contrast enhancement of the palatine tonsils (arrows). (**b**) A right-sided tonsillar abscess is seen as a hypodense area of fluid collection with peripheral contrast enhancement on post-contrast CT (arrows). (**c**) A left-sided paratonsillar abscess is seen as an area of fluid collection with peripheral rim enhancement, located immediately adjacent to the left tonsil (arrows)

demonstrates low-attenuation on CT and appears hypointense and markedly hyperintense on T1- and T2- weighted images, respectively. The periphery of the lymph node shows contrast enhancement [3, 13] (Fig. 4.14). In the chronic stage of fungal and tuberculous infections, calcifications can be seen as US hyperechogenic and CT hyperdense foci within the infected nodes [14] (Fig. 4.15).

4.2.8.3 Tonsillitis and Tonsillar/Peritonsillar Abscess

Uncomplicated tonsillitis does not require imaging. If imaged, CT may demonstrate diffuse enlargement and intense enhancement of the tonsils, with stranding

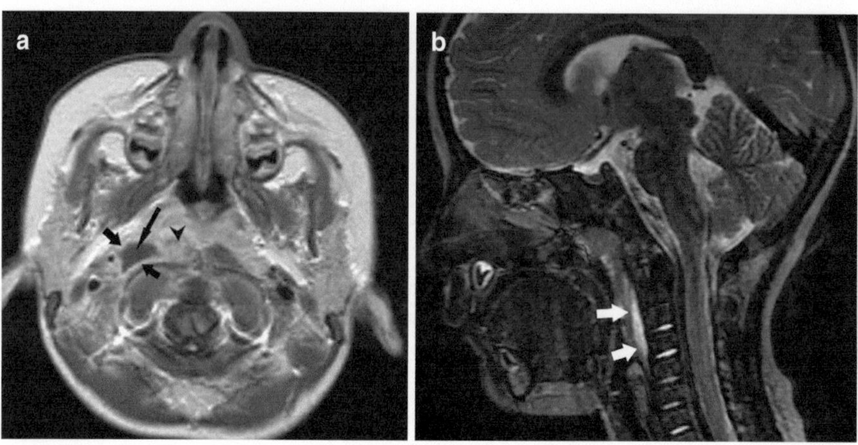

Fig. 4.17 (**a**) Axial contrast-enhanced T1-weighted MR image shows a suppurative retropharyngeal lymph node with a hypointense necrotic center and peripheral contrast enhancement. Note the enhancement of the prevertebral muscles and the perinodal soft tissues. (**b**) Sagittal T2-weighted image shows edema of the retropharyngeal soft tissues as increased signal intensity at the level of the C2 and C3 vertebrae

of the peritonsillary fat planes (Fig. 4.16a). Therapy-unresponsive cases may require evaluation with contrast-enhanced CT for a diagnosis of intratonsillar or peritonsillar abscess. When present, CT shows a hypodense fluid collection with peripheral contrast enhancement within the tonsil in cases of tonsillar abscess (Fig. 4.16b). Alternatively, a peritonsillar abscess can form outside the tonsil, and shows the same imaging findings, only immediately adjacent to tonsils (Fig. 4.16c). A peritonsillar abscess can spread to parapharyngeal and retropharyngeal spaces. Direct involvement of the internal jugular vein may result in septic thrombus formation and suppurative thrombophlebitis of the internal jugular vein, which can be seen as luminal filling defects on contrast-enhanced CT images [13, 15].

4.2.8.4 Retropharyngeal Phlegmon and Retropharyngeal Abscess

Retropharyngeal spread of infection can occur from middle ear, nasopharyngeal, or oropharyngeal infections. Retropharyngeal infection can present with retropharyngeal lymphadenopathy, phlegmon, or abscess formation [3, 13]. Infected lymph nodes are usually increased in size and may demonstrate suppurative/necrotic centers. Perinodal soft tissues usually show thickening and edema (Fig. 4.17a and b). Retropharyngeal soft tissue involvement can initially be seen as retropharyngeal phlegmon formation, that is characterized by thickening/edema of the retropharyngeal soft tissues on CT or MRI. A phlegmon then can proceed to an abscess formation, which is seen as a hypodense fluid collection with peripheral contrast enhancement on post-contrast CT. In cases of prevertebral extension of the infection, MRI can better demonstrate bone involvement/osteomyelitis as increased signal intensity and contrast enhancement of the vertebrae on T2-weighted and contrast-enhanced T1-weighted images, respectively [12, 13].

References

1. Dankbaar JW, van Bemmel AJ, Pameijer FA. Imaging findings of the orbital and intracranial complications of acute bacterial rhinosinusitis. Insights Imaging. 2015;6(5):509–18.
2. Rodriguez DP. Imaging of specific sinonasal disease entities, nose and sinonasal cavities. In: Coley BD, editor. Caffey's pediatric diagnostic imaging. 12th ed. Philadelphia: Saunders; 2013. p. 79.
3. Ludwig BJ, Foster BR, Saito N, Nadgir RN, Castro-Aragon I, Sakai O. Diagnostic imaging in nontraumatic pediatric head and neck emergencies. Radiographics. 2010 May;30(3):781–99.
4. Ho ML, Courtier J, Glastonbury CM. The ABCs (airway, blood vessels, and compartments) of pediatric neck infections and masses. AJR Am J Roentgenol. 2016;206(5):963–72.
5. Eggesbo HB. Radiological imaging of inflammatory lesions in the nasal cavity and paranasal sinuses. Eur Radiol. 2006;16(4):872–88.
6. Tekes A, Palasis S, Durand DJ, Pruthi S, Booth TN, Desai NK, Jones JY, Kadom N, Lam HFS, Milla SS, Mirsky DM, Partap S, Robertson RL, Ryan ME, Saigal G, Setzen G, Soares BP, Trout AT, Whitehead MT, Karmazyn B. ACR appropriat fgeness criteria® sinusitis-child. Expert panel on pediatric imaging. J Am Coll Radiol. 2018;15(11S):403–12.
7. Ahmed A. Imaging of the paediatric paranasal sinuses. S Afr J Rad. 2013;17(3):91–7.
8. Burns NS, Iyer RS, Robinson AJ, Chapman T. Diagnostic imaging of fetal and pediatric orbital abnormalities. AJR Am J Roentgenol. 2013 Dec;201(6):797–808.
9. Juliano AF, Ginat DT, Moonis G. Imaging review of the temporal bone: Part I. anatomy and inflammatory and neoplastic processes. Radiology. 2013;269(1):17–33.
10. Vazquez E, Castellote A, Piqueras J, Mauleon S, Creixell S, Pumarola F, Figueras C, Carreño JC, Lucaya J. Imaging of complications of acute mastoiditis in children. Radiographics. 2003;23(2):359–7.
11. Booth TN. Infection and inflammation, ear and temporal bone. In: Coley BD, editor. Caffey's pediatric diagnostic imaging. 12th ed. Philadelphia: Saunders; 2013. p. 102.
12. Gopal N, Vilanilam GK, Gupta V, Vibhute P, Bhatt AA. A comprehensive review of imaging of skull base infections – part II. Radiol Infect Dis. 2019;6(3):87–94. https://doi.org/10.1016/j.jrid.2019.09.001.
13. Meuwly JY, Lepori D, Theumann N, Schnyder P, Etechami G, Hohlfeld J, Gudinchet F. Multimodality imaging evaluation of the pediatric neck: techniques and spectrum of findings. Radiographics. 2005;25(4):931–48.
14. Lowe LH, Smith CJ. Infection and inflammation, neck. In: Coley BD, editor. Caffey's pediatric diagnostic imaging. 12th ed. Philadelphia: Saunders; 2013. p. 136.
15. von Kalle T, Koitschev A. Pediatric radiology in oto-rhino-laryngology. GMS Curr Top Otorhinolaryngol Head Neck Surg. 2014;13:Doc03.

Recurrent Respiratory Infections in Childhood: The Importance of Local Microbiota Modulation

Desiderio Passali, Francesco Maria Passali, and Valerio Damiani

5.1 Introduction

Respiratory infections ever represented a major problem for humankind since ancient times, strongly impacting on the development of humankind itself. Still today, millions of people die, every year, because of infections or because of their complications.

The COVID-19 pandemic is just an actual example of how infections can affect health and socioeconomic issues worldwide.

Respiratory infections in children significantly affect the healthcare system and represent a relevant problem for the family and society, in both developing and industrialized countries [1–3]. Respiratory infections represent a common reason for frequent physician office and emergency room visits, improper use of antibiotics and antipyretic drugs, and scholastic and/or working absenteeism. As a result, pediatricians and otolaryngologists face very frequently this issue in daily practice [4].

It has been estimated that approximately 6% of children suffer from RRI worldwide. Several risk factors can promote RRI, including prematurity, preschool age (for a relative immaturity of the immune system), early attending at nursery school, air pollution, home dampness, passive exposure to tobacco, or vape fumes, low socioeconomic level, overcrowding, and allergy [5].

D. Passali (✉)
Department of Medical, Surgical and Neuroscience Sciences, and Department of Otorhinolaryngology, University of Siena, Siena, Italy

F. M. Passali
Department of Clinical Sciences, Translational Medicine University, Tor Vergata, Rome, Italy

V. Damiani
Drugs Minerals and Generics (DMG) Italia Medical Department, Pomezia, Rome, Italy

© The Author(s), under exclusive license to Springer Nature Switzerland AG 2022   55
C. Cingi et al. (eds.), *Pediatric ENT Infections*,
https://doi.org/10.1007/978-3-030-80691-0_5

Moreover, allergy is characterized by an unbalanced type 2 immune response, which predisposes to infections [6, 7]. Allergic subjects have a functional defect of type 1 immune response involved in fighting infections, and are, consequently, prone to have more numerous and severe infections than nonallergic subjects [8]. Consistently, allergen immunotherapy restores a physiological immune response and reverts susceptibility to RRI [9].

Furthermore, viral infections may per se represent a cause of RRI as they lower host immune defense [10]. Bacterial super-infections may be frequently associated with viral infections and entail overuse/misuse of antibiotics by primary care doctors [11]. As a consequence, antibiotic resistance is an overwhelming problem in every country [12].

Moreover, bacteria create a biofilm, such as thinly layered colonies, which causes antibiotic failure and need to surgery, especially in case of chronic rhinosinusitis [13]. Biofilm has been considered an "influencer of infections" as it is able to increase and optimize pathogens survival and to promote unfavorable host-bacteria interactions [14].

Despite the frequency and prevalence of these pathologies, the definition of recurrent respiratory infections (RRI) is still controversial and, during decades, various sub-definition of the single nosological entities had been developed.

Namely, the recurrent pharyngotonsillitis can be defined as >7 episodes of pharyngotonsillitis in 1 year, or >5 episodes/year for two consecutive years, or >3 episodes/year for three consecutive years [15]. Recurrent otitis media includes >3 episodes of otitis media in 6 months or >4 episodes/year [16]. Recurrent lower RI occurs when there are >3 episodes/year of bronchitis, bronchiolitis, or pneumonia [17].

In clinical practice, to differentiate lower and upper respiratory tract infections may be difficult because symptoms and signs overlap, and both may be present at the same time [18].

Therefore, the possibility of preventing the recurrence of RI could significantly reduce complications and medical costs and improve the social and family burden. At present, there is no consolidated evidence of effective treatment able to prevent RRI. However, several options are used in clinical practice.

In recent years, much attention has been paid to the concept of the microbioma. The word "microbioma" means an ecological community of commensal, symbiotic, and pathogenic microorganisms found in and on all multicellular organisms studied to date, from plants to animals [19].

The importance of the normal microbiota in the protection against RRI has been widely demonstrated [20, 21]. However, an imbalance in the physiological flora composition may lead to the colonization and infection of the mucosae by opportunistic pathogens [22]. For instance, it has been noted that otitis-prone children were characterized by a significantly lower number of α-hemolytic streptococci in their nasopharyngeal flora than non-otitis-prone ones, opening the possibility to administer living microorganisms as probiotics to confer health benefits to the host. As a proof of concept, the recolonization with "interfering" bacteria could restore the physiological microbioma and prevent RRI [23].

A possible mechanism is the capacity of some strains of α Streptococci of producing bacteriocin-like inhibitory substances (BLIS) able to contrast pathogens [24]. Therefore, modulation of upper airways microbioma could represent an intriguing option [25].

The term "bacteriotherapy" has been used for the first time over 70 years ago [26], and first clinical experiences were performed in the early '50s [27, 28].

After some decades of forgetfulness, in which scientists were more focused in developing new antibacterial drugs that in treating the local environment, bacteriotherapy has been re-evaluated, and the idea of using bacteria as probiotics throughout the maintenance or restoration of a physiological microbiome get ever more and more consensus. The mechanism involves the interference and/or inhibition of pathogens from the production of antimicrobial proteins and immunomodulating mediators [24].

Local bacteriotherapy approach is aimed at recolonizing upper airways, in particular nasopharyngeal and oropharyngeal districts, with healthy bacteria, in order to displace potential pathogens by bacterial interference [22]. The first clinical use of streptococcal probiotics in the treatment of halitosis and/or S. pyogenes infections was reported by Tagg and colleagues, who attributed the inhibition of the S. pyogenes species to S. salivarius K12 [29].

Our last 10 years' experience on this field focused, on the contrary, on other two very interesting strains: the Streptococcus salivarius 24SMB and the Streptococcus oralis 89a.

In particular, the strain 24SMB was isolated in 2012 and selected as a promising probiotic due to the absence of virulence traits and antibiotic resistance genes and its ability to inhibit S. pneumoniae growth [30]. Santagati et al. demonstrated its safety and tolerability, and its capability to colonize the nasopharynx when administrated as a nasal spray [31].

Conversely, S. oralis 89a was isolated from a recalcitrant healthy child during a tonsillitis outbreak and it was found to be able to inhibit the growth of group A streptococci in vitro [32]. Table 5.1 summarizes most significant collaborative studies on these two bacteria.

From a chronological viewpoint, the first evidence of efficacy derived from a prospective, randomized, double-blind, placebo-controlled study that enrolled 100 children (aged 1–5 years) with recurrent acute otitis media [33]. Streptococcus salivarius 24SMB, administered as a nasal spray, reduced the recurrence of otitis media and the usage of antibiotics during the treatment period (3 months) and during the post-treatment follow-up period (other 3 months).

A confirmative real-life study on 267 children included 108 otitis-prone as control and 159 actively treated with a nasal spray containing Streptococcus salivarius 24SMB and Streptococcus oralis 89a [32]. Local bacteriotherapy reduced both the recurrence rate of otitis media and the severity of the single episodes.

Meanwhile, an in vitro study explored the potential mechanisms of action of these two strains; in particular, the anti-biofilm activity was tested against *S. pneumoniae*, *S. pyogenes* and *M. catarrhalis* being the most common bacterial

Table 5.1 Clinical studies on local bacteriotherapy with Streptococcus salivarius 24SMB and Streptococcus oralis 89a, administered as a nasal spray or oral spray

Authors (ref)	Disease	Patients	Schedule	Duration	Outcomes for treatment
Nasal bacteriotherapy					
Marchisio et al. [33]	RAOM	50 treated 50 controls (1–5 years)	Twice/daily For 5 days/ month	3 courses	Less AOM Fewer antibiotics
La Mantia et al. [32]	RAOM	159 treated 108 controls (3–10 years)	Twice/daily for 7 days/ month	3 courses	Less AOM Reduced severity
Bellussi et al. [34]	RRI SDB	42 (<18 years)	Twice/daily for 7 days/ month	3 courses	Sleep and nasal symptoms improvement
Tarantino et al. [35]	RRI	80 (3–14 years)	Twice/daily for 7 days/ month	3 courses	Less RI, school absence, and working days
La Mantia et al. [36]	AH OME	44 (3–6 years)	Twice/daily for 7 days/ month	3 courses	Reduction surgery need, adenoid size, improved tympanometry
Passali et al. [37]	RRI	202 (m7.5 years)	Twice/daily for 7 days/ month	3 courses	Less RI
Cantarutti et al. [38]	RAOM	79 treated 70 controls (1–6 years)	Twice/daily for 7 days/ month	5 courses	Less AOM
Manti et al. [39]	RRI	91 (1–12 years)	Twice/daily for 7 days/ month	3 courses	Less RI Reduction symptoms severity
Oral bacteriotherapy					
Andaloro et al. [40]	RPT	41 treated 41 placebo (6–11 years)	Once/daily for 30 days/ month	3 courses	Less PT Shorter duration Fewer antibiotics Fewer school absences
Tarantino et al. [41]	RRI	51 (3–10 years)	Once/daily for 30 days/ month	3 courses	Less RI Fewer school absences

(*RAOM* recurrent acute otitis media, *RRI* recurrent respiratory infections, *SDB* sleep-disordered breathing, *AH* adenoid hypertrophy; *OME* otitis media with effusion, *m* median, *RPT* recurrent pharyngotonsillitis).

pathogens causing acute otitis media and bacterial pharyngotonsillitis. Moreover, the anti-biofilm effect was assessed on S. aureus, involved in 50% of recalcitrant chronic rhinosinusitis. Both strains interfered with biofilm formation and dispersed the preformed biofilms [42].

Later, Bellussi and coworkers performed a prospective study on 42 children with sleep-disordered breathing and RRI [34]. In this pilot study, sleep clinical records significantly diminished after the 3-month treatment. Moreover, treated children experience a significant improvement of nasal patency and oral breathing.

Tarantino and colleagues provided real-world experience in 80 children with RRI [35]. Local bacteriotherapy halved the number of RI, reduced the number of school days and parental working days missed per month.

La Mantia and coworkers investigated an intriguing issue, such as avoiding adenoidectomy, in children with adenoid hypertrophy, caused by RRI [36]. This open study included 44 children candidates for adenoidectomy and tympanocentesis as a treatment for adenoid hypertrophy and otitis media with effusion. Twenty-two children were treated with both strains administered by nasal spray. Control children were treated with hypertonic saline. Bacteriotherapy significantly reduced the need for surgery (70% of spared surgical procedures in the treated group) and improved tympanometry outcomes.

A more recent study confirmed previous results: Passali and colleagues enrolled 202 children with RRI [37]. All children were treated with local bacteriotherapy, including both strains. Bacteriotherapy significantly reduced the number of RI in comparison with the previous year.

Another observational study included 79 otitis-prone children (1–6 years old) treated with local bacteriotherapy and 70 controls [38]. Streptococcus salivarius 24SMB and Streptococcus oralis 89a, intranasally administered, reduced the number of acute otitis media episodes.

Manti and coworkers performed a similar study in 91 children with RRI [39]. Both strains administered by nasal spray reduced fever, cough, bronchial obstruction, rhinorrhea, and otalgia. The efficacy of local bacteriotherapy was quicker in older children than in younger.

More recently, a new product was available, such as the oral formulation containing the same strains. At present, two studies were performed using oral bacteriotherapy with Streptococcus salivarius 24SMB and Streptococcus oralis 89a.

The first study evaluated a group of 82 children with recurrent streptococcal pharyngotonsillitis due to group A β-hemolytic Streptococcus (GHABS) and was conducted as randomized and placebo-controlled [40].

Oral bacteriotherapy reduced the number and duration of GABHS infections, the use of antibiotics, and school absences.

A second real-life study enrolled 51 children (mean age 4.8 years) with RRI [41]. Consistently, oral bacteriotherapy reduced the number of RI and school absences due to infections.

5.2 Conclusion

In conclusion, microbiota modulation through local bacteriotherapy is a feasible, safe, and reliable approach. Local administration of safe living bacteria represents an opportunity of directly modulating the immune response, which may be impaired by several environmental or individual factors. Overuse/abuse of large-spectrum antibiotics indiscriminately alters microbioma equilibrium with an ecological vacuum promoting the overgrowth of pathogens.

Therefore, restoring therapy, i.e., the local recolonization of nasopharyngeal and oropharyngeal micro-environment with "good" bacteria, results in a competition against pathogens and provides a favorable, cheap, and long-lasting prevention of infections.

References

1. Mansback AI, Brihave P, Casimir G, et al. Clinical aspects of chronic ENT inflammation in children. B ENT. 2012;8(Suppl 19):83–101.
2. Orlandi RR, Kingdom TT, Hwang PH, et al. International consensus statement on allergy and rhinology: rhinosinusitis. Int Forum Allergy Rhinol. 2016;6(Suppl 1):S22–S209.
3. Fokkens WJ, Lund VJ, Mullol J, et al. EPOS 2012: European position paper on rhinosinusitis and nasal polyps 2012. A summary for otorhinolaryngologists. Rhinology. 2012;50(1):1–12.
4. de Martino M, Vierucci A, Appendino C. Children with recurrent respiratory infections. Immunol Ped. 1981;4:76–81.
5. Patria MF, Esposito S. Recurrent lower respiratory tract infections in children: a practical approach to diagnosis. Paediatric Respir Rev. 2013;14:53–60.
6. Fahy JV. Type 2 inflammation in asthma– present in most, absent in many. Nat Rev Immunol. 2015;15:57–65.
7. Ciprandi G, Tosca MA, Silvestri M, Ricciardolo FLM. Inflammatory biomarkers for asthma endotyping and personalized therapy. Exp Rev Clin Immunol. 2017;13:715–21.
8. Cirillo I, Marseglia G, Klersy C, Ciprandi G. Allergic patients have more numerous and prolonged respiratory infections than non-allergic subjects. Allergy. 2007;62:1087–90.
9. Ciprandi G, Sormani MP, Cirillo I, et al. Upper respiratory infections and SLIT: preliminary evidence. Ann Allergy. 2009;102:262–3.
10. Griffin MR, Walker FJ, Iwane MK, et al. New vaccine surveillance network study group: epidemiology of respiratory infections in young children: insights from the new vaccine surveillance network. Pediatr Infect Dis J. 2004;23:188–92.
11. Li J, Song X, Yang T, et al. A systematic review of antibiotic prescription associated with upper respiratory tract infections in China. Medicine. 2016;95:e3587.
12. Alexandrino AS, Santos R, Melo C, et al. Caregivers' education vs. rhinopharyngeal clearance in children with upper respiratory infections: impact on children's health outcomes. Eur J Pediatr. 2017;176:1375–83.
13. Nazzari E, Torretta S, Pignataro L, et al. Role of biofilm in children with recurrent upper respiratory tract infections. Eur J Clin Microbiol Infect Dis. 2015;34:421–9.
14. Drago L, Pignataro L, Torretta S. Microbiological aspects of acute and chronic pediatric rhinosinusitis. J Clin Med. 2019;8:149.
15. Paradise JL, Bluestone CD, Colborn DK, Bernard BS, Rockette HE, Kurs-Lasky M. Tonsillectomy and adenotonsillectomy for recurrent throat infection in moderately affected children. Pediatrics. 2002;110:7–15.
16. Greenberg D, Bilenko N, Liss Z. The burden of acute otitis media on the patient and family. Eur J Pediatr. 2003;162:576–81.
17. de Benedictis FM, Bush A. Recurrent lower respiratory tract infections in children. BMJ. 2018;362:k2698.
18. Karevold G, Kvestad E, Nafstad P, Kvaerner KJ. Respiratory infections in schoolchildren: co-morbidity and risk factors. Arch Dis Child. 2006;91:391–5.
19. Yamanishi S, Pawankar R. Current advances o the microbiome and role of probiotics in upper airways. Curr Opin Allergy Clin Immunol. 2020;20:30–5.
20. Faden H, Waz MJ, Bernstein JM, Brodsky L, Stanievich J, Ogra PL. Nasopharyngeal flora in the first three years of life in normal and otitis-prone children. Ann Otol Rhinol Laryngol. 1991;100:612–5.

21. Bernstein JM, Faden HF, Dryia DM, Wactawski-Wende J. Micro-ecology of the naso-pharyngeal bacterial flora in otitis-prone and non-otitis prone children. Acta Otolaryngol. 1993;113:88–92.
22. Gao Z, Kang Y, Yu J, Ren L. Human pharyngeal microbiome may play a protective role in respiratory tract infections. Genom Proteom Bioinform. 2014;12:144–50.
23. Roos K, GrahnHakansson E, Holm S. Effect of recolonization with "interfering" α strepto-cocci on recurrences of acute and secretory otitis media in children: randomised placebo-controlled trial. BMJ. 2001;322:1–4.
24. Walls T, Power D, Tagg J. Bacteriocin-like inhibitory substances (BLIS) production by the normal flora of the nasopharynx: potential to protect against otitis media? J Med Microbiol. 2003;52:829–33.
25. Marsh RL, Aho C, Beissbarth J, Bialasiewicz S, Binks M, Cervin A, et al. Recent advances in understanding the natural history of the otitis media microbiome and its response to environ-mental pressures. Int J Ped Otorhinolaryngol. 2020;130(Suppl 1):109836.
26. Torrent H. La bacteriothérapie lactique; ses applications actuelles. Vie Med. 1949;30:39.
27. Lanza Castelli RA, Elkeles G. Bacteriology and Bacteriotherapy in otorhinolaryngology. Ann Otolaryngol. 1950;67:152–60.
28. Lopez LaCarrere E, Viale del Carril A. Remote results of bacteriotherapy in otorhinolaryngol-ogy. Rev Fac Cienc Med. 1953;11:453–61.
29. Wescombe PA, Heng NC, Burton JP, Chilcott CN, Tagg JR. Streptococcal bacteriocins and the case for Streptococcus salivarius as model oral probiotics. Future Microbiol. 2009;4:819–35.
30. Santagati M, Scillato M, PatanèF AC, Stefani S. Bacteriocin-producing oral streptococci and inhibition of respiratory pathogens. FEMS Immunol Med Microbiol. 2012;2012:1–9.
31. Santagati M, Scillato M, Muscaridola N, Metoldo V, La Mantia I, Stefani S. Colonization, safety, and tolerability study of the Streptococcus salivarius 24SMBc nasal spray for its appli-cation in upper respiratory tract infections. Eur J Clin Microbiol Infect Dis. 2015;34:2075–80.
32. La Mantia I, Varricchio A, Ciprandi G. Bacteriotherapy with Streptococcus salivarius 24SMB and Streptococcus oralis 89a nasal spray for preventing recurrent acute otitis media in chil-dren: a real-life clinical experience. Int J Gen Med. 2017;10:171–5.
33. Marchisio P, Santagati M, Scillato M, Baggi E, Fattizzo M, Rosazza C, et al. Streptococcus salivarius 24SMB administered by nasal spray for the prevention of acute otitis media in otitis-prone children. Eur J Clin Microbiol Infect Dis. 2015;34:2377–83.
34. Bellussi LM, Villa MP, Degiorgi G, Passali FM, Evangelisti M, Innocenti Paganelli I, et al. Preventive nasal bacteriotherapy for the treatment of upper respiratory tract infections and sleep-disordered breathing in children. Int J Ped Otorhinolaryngol. 2018;110:43–7.
35. Tarantino V, Savaia V, D'Agostino R, Silvestri M, Ciprandi G. Bacteriotherapy for preventing recurrent upper respiratory infections in children: a real-world experience. Otolaryngol Pol. 2018;72:33–8.
36. La Mantia I, Varricchio A, Di Girolamo S, Minni A, Passali GC, Ciprandi G. The role of bac-teriotherapy in the prevention of adenoidectomy. Eur Rev Med Pharmacol Sci. 2019;23(Suppl 1):44–7.
37. Passali D, Passali GC, Vesperini E, Cocca S, Visconti IC, Ralli M, et al. The efficacy and toler-ability of Streptococcus salivarius 24SMB and Streptococcus oralis 89° administered as nasal spray in the treatment of recurrent upper respiratory tract infections in children. Eur Rev Med Pharmacol Sci. 2019;23(Suppl 1):67–72.
38. Cantarutti A, Rea F, Donà D, Cantarutti L, Passarella A, Scamarcia A, et al. Preventing recurrent acute otitis media with Streptococcus salivarius 24SMB and Streptococcus oralis 89a five months intermittent treatment: an observational prospective cohort study. Int J Ped Otorhinolaryngol. 2020;132:109921.
39. Manti S, Parisi GF, Papale M, Licari A, Salpietro C. Miraglia del Giudice M, et al. Bacteriotherapy with Streptococcus salivarius 24SMB and Streptococcus oralis 89a nasal spray for treatment of upper respiratory tract infections in children: a pilot study on short-term efficacy. Ital J Pediatr. 2020;46:42.

40. Andaloro C, Santagati M, Stefani S, La Mantia I. Bacteriotherapy with Streptococcus salivarius 24SMB and Streptococcus oralis 89a oral spray for children with recurrent streptococcal pharyngotonsillitis: a randomized placebo-controlled clinical study. Eur Arch Ohtorhinolaryngol. 2019;276:879–87.
41. Tarantino V, Savaia V, D'Agostino R, Damiani V, Ciprandi G. Oral bacteriotherapy in children with recurrent respiratory infections: a real-life study. Acta Biomed. 2020;91(Suppl 1):73–6.
42. Bidossi A, De Grandi R, Toscano M, Bottagisio M, De Vecchi E, Gelardi M, et al. Probiotics Streptococcus salivarius 24SMB and Streptococcus oralis 89a interfere with biofilm formation of pathogens of the upper respiratory tract. BMC Infect Dis. 2018;18:653.

Role of Allergy in ENT Infections

6

Fatih Dilek, Zeynep Tamay, Anu Laulajainen-Hongisto, and Sanna Toppila-Salmi

6.1 Introduction to Atopic Diseases

Allergy is an unusual reaction to a generally harmless substance called an allergen. An allergen is an antigen that is recognized by the immune system and able to initiate an allergic inflammation. Most of the major clinically important allergens are commonly encountered in nature such as tree, weed, and grass pollen, dust mite, mold, as well as food allergens milk, egg, wheat, soy, nut, or fish proteins. Atopy is defined as the tendency to produce specific immunoglobulin E (IgE) against allergens; it is clinically proven by the presence of at least one allergen-specific IgE [1]. Allergic diseases include allergic rhinitis (AR), allergic conjunctivitis (AC), atopic dermatitis (AD), food allergy (FA), and allergic asthma. AR, AC, and allergic asthma are typically caused by aeroallergens, whereas FA by orally ingested allergens [2]. The prevalence of allergic diseases has increased in the Western world during the past decades, and is estimated at 8.5–14.6% for AR [3], 20.7% for AC [4], 13% for AD [5], 5% for FA [6], and 9.5% for asthma [7] in children. The corresponding percentages in adults are about 13% for AR [8], 20–40% for AC [9],

F. Dilek (✉)
Division of Pediatric Allergy and Immunology, Department of Pediatrics, School of Medicine, Atlas University, İstanbul, Turkey

Z. Tamay
Division of Pediatric Allergy and Immunology, Department of Pediatrics, Faculty of Medicine, İstanbul University, İstanbul, Turkey

A. Laulajainen-Hongisto
Department of Otorhinolaryngology, Head and Neck Surgery, University of Helsinki, and Helsinki University Hospital, Helsinki, Finland

S. Toppila-Salmi
Skin and Allergy Hospital, University of Helsinki and Helsinki University Hospital, Helsinki, Finland

© The Author(s), under exclusive license to Springer Nature Switzerland AG 2022 63
C. Cingi et al. (eds.), *Pediatric ENT Infections*,
https://doi.org/10.1007/978-3-030-80691-0_6

11% for AD [10], 3–4% for FA [6], and 7.7% for asthma [7]. The increased occurrence of asthma, AR, or both after AD onset in children has been called the atopic march. However, recent studies show that the atopic march is not always detected [11, 12]. Mechanisms for developing atopic comorbidities after AD onset are poorly understood; they are thought to involve impairment of the cutaneous barrier, facilitating cutaneous sensitization [13].

The risk factors of allergic airway diseases include genetic predisposition and environmental/clinical factors, such as exposure to tobacco smoke pre- and postnatally, breastfeeding, obesity, sedentary lifestyle, dietary exposure, pollution, and altered microbiome [14]. Both multiple allergen sensitization and allergic multimorbidity (e.g., the presence of at least two allergic diseases) have been shown to associate with higher risk of disease severity in children [15], or risk of disease onset both in chidren and adults [16].

Up to date, genome-wide association studies (GWASs) have identified over 1500 allergy-related associations in over 100 studies (https://www.ebi.ac.uk/gwas/). In connection with asthma or AR, 267 single nucleotide polymorphisms (SNPs) and 170 protein coding genes, functioning in airway epithelial cells or immunity, were determined in 31 GWASs [17]. Well-replicated allergy/asthma-related loci are at 17q12-21(GSDMB, ORMDL), 6p21.32 near HLA-, 5q22.1 near TSLP, 2q12 near IL1RL1/IL18R, and 9p24.1 near IL33 [18] . There is a genetic overlap between (childhood-onset) asthma and allergic diseases (in barrier biology and HLA region) [19].

The estimated heritability of asthma and AR ranged from 25% to 75% reflecting the roles of environmental exposure [20]. Polygenetic character of allergic diseases and the contribution of modifying environmental factors have led to epigenome-wide association studies (EWASs) [21]. EWASs in asthma revealed thousands of differentially methylated sites in adults and over 400 CpG sites (CpGs) in children. SMAD3, SERPINC1, PROK1, IL13, RUNX3, and TIGIT were found as differentially methylated genes associated with asthma [22]. A genome-wide consortium meta-analysis including 13 cohorts with 6700 newborns demonstrated differential methylation on more than 6000 CpGs in relation to maternal smoking [23]. In a recent epigenome-wide meta-analysis, postnatally acquired 14 methylated CpGs were identified in association with childhood asthma [24]. In the near future, genetic and epigenetic analyses conducted together may yield new diagnostic markers for allergic diseases, and therapeutic and protective interventions [21].

6.1.1 Allergic Rhinitis

Allergic rhinitis (AR) is an IgE-mediated chronic disease of the nasal mucosa characterized by nasal blockage, rhinorrhea, sneezing, and nasal itching [25, 26]. AR is the most common chronic disease of childhood in the United States with increasing prevalence, currently about 20% [27, 28]. There are large variations in the prevalence of AR in other parts of the world, ranging from 4.5% (Georgia and Latvia) to 45.1% (Paraguay) in children aged 13–14 years [29].

The clinical diagnosis of the AR is made combining typical history with typical symptoms caused by allergen exposure, as well as physical examination findings, including nasal mucosal edema accompanied by pallor or a pale bluish color, a clear nasal secretion which may be seen anteriorly or posteriorly, cobblestone appearance of the nasopharyngeal mucosa, a transverse nasal crease (allergic salute) and infraorbital edema and discoloration (allergic shiners) [30]. The diagnosis is confirmed by elevated levels of serum allergen-specific IgE, and/or by positive skin prick test result to allergen(s) [30, 31]. AR is classified as intermittent or persistent according to the duration of the symptoms, and mild or moderate/severe according to the severity level of the symptoms [31, 32]. In the past decade, researchers have described a group of patients who have similar clinical picture to AR but have negative skin tests and/or in vitro specific-IgE assays for aeroallergens [33]. They responded positively to nasal provocation tests with common aeroallergens. It was found that IgE was locally produced in the nasal mucosa of these patients; this entity was named as local allergic rhinitis (LAR) [33].

Currently, the AR treatment approach combines environmental control measures, pharmacotherapy, and allergen-specific immunotherapy (ASIT) [33, 34].

6.1.2 Unified Airway Concept

The association between diseases affecting the upper and lower airways was first noticed almost 100 years ago, but not much attention were paid to this fact until the last two decades [35]. Data from several epidemiological, pathophysiological, and treatment studies have shown that all segments of the respiratory tract (including mucosa of the middle ears, nose, nasopharynx, sinuses, and lungs) act as an integrated, organized, functional unit [35]. The pathophysiological events or disease processes affecting one part of the airways also affect other segments, causing disease progression. Likewise, treatment of a pathological process in one segment of the unified airways also provides therapeutic benefit in other parts of the respiratory tract [35].

Asthma and AR frequently coexist; 80% of asthmatics have rhinitis and 40% of AR patients have concomitant asthma [31, 33]. It has been shown that 30% of patients with AR, who do not have coexisting asthma, have bronchial hyperreactivity [35]. AR is an important risk factor for asthma development; several prospective studies demonstrate that the risk of developing asthma in children increases threefold to fourfold in the presence of AR [36–38].

Several mechanisms have been proposed to explain the unified airway concept (UAC), but the "common inflammation" hypothesis prevails. Both upper and lower respiratory tracts consist of the same structural elements including pseudostratified columnar epithelium, basement membrane, lamina propria, goblet cells, and glands [35, 37]. A study demonstrated that when segmental bronchial provocation was applied to nonasthmatic AR patients, the procedure resulted in peripheral blood eosinophilia and allergic inflammation of the nose [38]. However, no significant changes could be observed in healthy controls [38]. Nasal antigen provocation can induce bronchial inflammation also in nonasthmatic AR patients [39]. These findings suggest an inflammatory crosstalk of the respiratory tract [35].

Treatment of AR may alleviate asthma symptoms and airway hyperresponsiveness [40]. ASIT is not only a treatment option for AR but can also modify the natural course of allergic diseases. ASIT can reduce new sensitizations in monosensitized patients with AR and risk of developing asthma [41, 42]. Studies show that successful treatment of chronic rhinosinusitis (CRS) reduces asthma symptoms and improves lung functions [43, 44].

The aim of this chapter is to provide a literature review of the UAC within pediatric otorhinolaryngology. Allergy and AR can have significant impact on the pathogenesis of diseases including otitis media with effusion (OME), CRS, and chronic laryngitis [45, 46].

6.2 Role of Allergy in Pediatric Otitis Media

Otitis media (OM) is a disease spectrum that includes acute otitis media (AOM), otitis media with effusion (OME), and chronic suppurative otitis media (CSOM) [47]. Patients with OME have an increased prevalence of atopic disease such as AD, AR, and asthma compared to healthy controls [48]. Alles et al. studied 209 children with a history of chronic and recurrent OME, and found AR in 89%, asthma in 36%, and eczema in 24% [48]. Kwon et al. evaluated 370 children diagnosed with OME and 100 healthy controls and found the incidence of AR twofold higher in children with OME (34%) than their healthy counterparts (16%) [49]. A meta-analysis also concluded that AR and allergy are important risk factors for the development of OME [50]. Many studies show that the prevalence of AR in patients with OME is significantly increased compared to the general population [51, 52].

Middle ear mucosa is a part of unified airways and responds to allergen stimulations in similar ways as the nasal mucosa or bronchi [51]. Allergic inflammation has been demonstrated in both the middle ear and nasopharynx of atopic patients with OME [53]. Wright et al. demonstrated the expression of IL-5 mRNA, CD3+ cells, and eosinophils in the middle ears of patients with OME; this supports the presence of Th-2 type allergic inflammation in patients with OME [54]. Hurst et al. also showed that atopic patients with OME have elevated levels of eosinophil cationic protein (ECP), myeloperoxidase, and tryptase in their middle ear effusions compared to non-atopic patients with OME [55].

Eustachian tube dysfunction (ETD) plays a prominent role in the pathophysiology of OME [51, 56]. Ciliary dysmotility, cleft palate, gastroesophageal reflux, and adenoid hypertrophy are some of the reasons of ETD [51]. Additionally, several studies have showed that patients with AR have a higher risk of ETD, particularly during childhood [57, 58]

Friedman et al. demonstrated that intranasal pollen challenge applied to AR patients leads to ETD [59]. Presumably, exposure to allergens leads to inflammation, disturbing middle ear pressure via the induction of mucosal edema and obstruction of the eustachian tube [50, 51].

Several studies have investigated the impact of AR on OME. The authors of a Cochrane meta-analysis, including 945 patients in 12 clinical trials, concluded that oral steroids have some impact on improvement of OME in the short term, but no long-term effects in terms of hearing loss and resolution of OME. They also found no evidence of beneficial short- or long-term effects of topical intranasal steroids on symptoms of OME [60]. On the contrary, one prospective, randomized, double-blinded, placebo-controlled study showed some beneficial effect of intranasal mometasone furoate for the OME resolution, improvement of hearing and quality of life in children with adenoid hypertrophy and OME [61]. Another Cochrane meta-analysis, including 16 studies and 1880 participants, concluded that antihistamines or decongestants combined or alone are of no benefit in the management of OME [62]. Leukotriene receptor antagonist studies have failed to reach a conclusion of their effect in the treatment of OME [46].

A prospective study by Hurst included 89 atopic patients (52 children <15 years old and 37 adults with chronic OME) of whom 68 underwent ASIT for an average of 4 years, whereas the 21 refusing the therapy formed the control group. At the end of the study, 85% of the affected ears were completely resolved in the ASIT group, 5.5% significantly improved, whereas none of the ears in the control group were resolved [63]. Hurst suggested that patients with refractory OME deserve evaluation for allergy, since most of them respond to ASIT [63].

In conclusion, OME is a multifactorial disease for which AR may be an important predisposing risk factor [51]. There is a need for further well-designed prospective interventional studies focusing on evaluating comorbid allergies like AR in children with OME.

6.3 Role of Allergy in Pediatric Rhinosinusitis

Rhinosinusitis is an inflammation of the mucosa of the nose and paranasal sinuses which may be triggered by viral, bacterial, or fungal infections [64]. It is a major health problem which causes a significant financial burden, healthcare consumption, and productivity loss [65]. European Position Paper on Rhinosinusitis and Nasal Polyps 2020 (EPOS) classifies acute rhinosinusitis (ARS) as acute viral rhinosinusitis (common colds), acute post-viral rhinosinusitis, and acute bacterial rhinosinusitis according to duration and severity of symptoms [66]. Most of ARSs are viral upper respiratory infections (URTIs), those persist for more than 10 days (acute post-viral sinusitis) usually requires no antibiotic treatment; less than 2–4% of patients (bacterial ARS) may require antibiotic treatment for bacterial infection [64, 66].

Rhinosinusitis in children is defined as presence of two or more symptoms one of which should be either nasal blockage/obstruction/congestion or nasal discharge (anterior/posterior nasal drip) ± facial pain/pressure ± cough and either endoscopic signs of nasal polyps, and/or mucopurulent discharge primarily from middle meatus and/or oedema/mucosal obstruction primarily in middle meatus and/or CT changes including mucosal changes within the ostiomeatal complex and/or sinuses [66, 67]. Rhinosinusitis is classified as ARS and chronic rhinosinusitis (CRS) depending on whether the duration of symptoms is shorter or longer than 3 months [66].

6.3.1 Allergy and Pediatric Acute Rhinosinusitis, Upper Respiratory Tract Infections

URTIs are very common in children but precise incidence of which is difficult to estimate [66]. It has been estimated that school children may suffer seven to ten URTIs per year [65, 66]. Rhinoviruses, which include more than 100 serotypes, cause nearly half of URTIs in children and adults [68]. Influenza viruses, coronaviruses, respiratory syncytial virus (RSV), parainfluenza viruses, adenoviruses, coxsackievirus, and human metapneumovirus are the other viruses that are leading causes of URTIs in children [68]. The course of most uncomplicated viral URTIs is 7–10 days [68]. Worsening symptoms after 5 days or prolonged illness beyond 10 days with less than 12 weeks duration is classified as acute post-viral rhinosinusitis by EPOS [66]. Only a very small proportion of ARSs (0.5–2%) are of bacterial origin [66]. Signs of acute bacterial rhinosinusitis are: discolored mucus, severe local pain (often unilateral), fever >38 °C, raised CRP/ESR, and "double" sickening [66]. Acute otitis media, asthma exacerbation, and bacterial pneumonia are some other complications of viral URTIs [68].

The prevalence of ARS in general pediatric practice is 9% in children between 1 and 5 years of age [69]. It is estimated that approximately 6–9% of viral URTIs in children are complicated by the development of ARS [70]. In a population-based study conducted in the Netherlands, reflecting national general practice database of 7 years interval (2002–2008), the incidence rates of ARS (for 1000 children per year) ranged from 2 to 18 in children (2 in 0–4 years, 7 in 5–14 years, and 18 in 12–17 years), with a decreasing trend (7/1000 in 2002 reducing to 4/1000 in 2008) in 5–14 years [71].

Most studies report some role of allergy in pediatric ARS [72, 73]; however not all authors agree with this opinion [74, 75]. Mbarek et al. reported significant association between allergy and rhinosinusitis in children with recurrent URTIs compared to healthy controls [73]. AR patients are 4.4 times more likely to have an episode of ARS compared to healthy controls [76]. In another study, Vlastos et al. showed that the sinusitis-prone AR patients had a significantly longer mucociliary clearance time than did those who were not sinusitis-prone [77]. Impaired mucociliary clearance may be a factor that predisposes these patients to ARS [77]. However, another study conducted on young adults concluded that no relationship between allergic status and ARS exists [78]. The conflicting results may be attributable as the most common predisposing risk factor is acute viral infections. Besides seasonal variations, severity, type of AR, and disease control may affect the likelihood of ARS. The current knowledge about the role of allergy in pediatric ARS is not sufficient to make a clear decision; further well-designed studies are needed.

6.3.2   Allergy and Pediatric Chronic Rhinosinusitis

CRS is a heterogeneous and multifactorial disorder; its pathogenesis has not yet been fully understood. In adults two phenotype of CRS are defined: with nasal polyps (CRSwNP) or without nasal polyps (CRSsNP) [79]. Especially the CRSwNP phenotype is closely related with a Th2-skewed eosinophilic inflammation [79]. Studies evaluating CRSwNP in pediatric populations are scarce; CRSwNP is a rare finding in young children and if present, other comorbidities like allergic fungal rhinosinusitis (AFRS) or cystic fibrosis should be investigated [80]. There are also significant differences in the histopathology of CRS in adults compared with children. Pediatric CRS tissue tends to have more monocytes/macrophages, lymphocytes, neutrophils, and natural killer cells, fewer submucosal glands, thinner epithelium, and less eosinophils infiltration in mucosa and submucosa when compared with adult CRS [80]. Thus, information on CRS pathogenesis obtained from adult studies may not be always valid for pediatric CRS.

Elevated levels of TNF-α, TGF-β, epidermal growth factor, eotaxin, fibroblast growth factor-2, sIL-2R, MMP-2, MMP-9, and TIMP-1 have been shown in tissue samples obtained from sinus mucosa or adenoids of children with CRS [81, 82]. The released mediators can induce vasodilatation, increased mucus secretion, plasma extravasation leading to defective mucociliary clearance, obstruction of sinus drainage as well as decrease in oxygenation leading to an environment prone to infection being formed [83].

According to a new published study, chronic rhinosinusitis (CRS) is diagnosed in 2.1% of patients younger than 20 years in ambulatory healthcare visits per year and the visit burden from CRS exceeds that of ARS in US [84].

EPOS 2020 guideline describes four symptoms (nasal blockage, nasal discharge, fascial pain/pressure, and cough) and presence of at least two of these symptoms are essential for CRS diagnosis in children [66]. Most common complaints are cough (45%) and rhinorrhea (37%) [85, 86]. The most common presenting symptoms are rhinorrhea (95%), cough (91%), postnasal drip (86%), nasal congestion (83%), and snoring (65%), respectively [86]. Cough is usually productive (75%) and increases at night [85].

Diagnosis of CRS in children is based on clinical manifestations. Symptoms should be continued for at least 12 weeks in association with endoscopic or imaging signs [85]. But often nasal endoscopy is not tolerated by children and computed tomography is only necessary in patients scheduled for surgical treatment [85]. Medical therapy is the mainstay of management of pediatric CRS. The most commonly used therapies include saline nasal irrigation, intranasal steroids, and antibiotics [66]. Saline irrigation washes the nasal cavities, reduces postnasal drainage, removes secretions, and rinses away allergens and irritants [87]. A Cochrane meta-analysis on this issue also concluded that the saline irrigation is beneficial in the treatment of CRS when used as the sole modality of treatment or adjunctive treatment [66, 88].

Nowadays, intranasal steroids have become the cornerstone of CRS treatment because of their powerful anti-inflammatory properties [66]. But, a Cochrane review rated the overall quality of evidence in CRS as very low, specifically in adults, as well as to date, there is no evidence from randomized controlled trials to support the efficacy of intranasal steroids in pediatric CRS [66, 87, 89]. Antibiotic treatment for CRS is controversial because of a lack of evidence from well-conducted clinical trials [66, 90]. Nevertheless, it is frequently used in both adults and children, especially in the treatment of acute exacerbations [66, 87].

Currently, surgical treatment options in children only come into question in case of unresponsiveness to appropriate medical treatment [66]. Adenoidectomy is the first-choice procedure and complete or near-complete symptom resolution was reported in 58% of children with CRS [66, 91]. Functional endoscopic sinus surgery is an effective surgical technique with reported success rates of up to 80% in children with CRS [92]. Major complication rate is reported as 0.6% and minor complication rate as 2% [93].

The relationship between allergy and CRS is a much more studied than that between allergy and ARS. Over half of the patients with AR have clinical or radiographic evidence of CRS, and 50-84% of the patients with CRS have aeroallergen sensitization [94, 95]. The overall prevalence of inhalant allergy is reported between 39–80% in CRS patients who underwent sinus surgery [96, 97].

In a large survey conducted in 12 European countries, a strong association of asthma with CRS (OR: 3.47) at all ages was seen [98]. Over 80% of children with CRS have a family history of allergy [83]. Emanuel and Shah demonstrated that 84% of CRS patients had aeroallergen sensitivity, 58% of patients were polysensitized, and the vast majority of patients, who required sinus surgery, had concomitant allergy [99]. Newman et al. showed that CRS severity determined by computerized tomography is correlated well with the presence of asthma, specific IgE antibodies, and eosinophilia [100].

Ramadan et al. reported that treatment of AR with oral antihistamines, intranasal steroids, and ASIT (25% of patients) before sinus surgery significantly improved outcomes in pediatric patients with AR who suffered from CRS [101]. In another study conducted on pediatric age group, allergic patients with CRS who were treated with ASIT additionally showed better subjective symptom scores and radiographic improvement compared to patients who were treated medically [102]. DeYoung et al. also reviewed the efficacy of ASIT in atopic patients with CRS and concluded that there is not enough high-quality work to say the last word in this matter [103].

Elevated local IgE levels are detected in CRSwNP patients without systemic allergy but with local allergic inflammation [104, 105]. Studies focusing on local allergic inflammation in CRS may provide new insights into relationship between allergy and CRS. Wise et al. also showed increased local IgE production in patients with AFRS [106]. Although the number of patients in studies are low, there is encouraging evidence that both subcutaneous and sublingual ASIT are effective in AFRS [97, 107]. AFRS typically affects atopic young individuals and has close relation with AR and asthma. It is a unique subtype of CRS and characterized by type 1 hypersensitivity to fungal allergens. AFRS has many clinicopathologic analogies to allergic bronchopulmonary aspergillosis, so some authors believe that these two entities are similar examples of the disease of unified airways [108].

In adults, several well-designed placebo-controlled studies show that mepolizumab (anti-IL 5 monoclonal antibody) reduces blood and sputum eosinophil counts as well as asthma exacerbations and improves quality of life of patients with severe eosinophilic asthma [95, 109]. Mepolizumab treatment can also reduce nasal polyp size in patients with severe nasal polyposis [110]. Reslizumab (anti-IL 5 monoclonal antibody) is also a useful treatment option for both eosinophilic asthma and nasal polyposis [111, 112]. Omalizumab (anti IgE monoclonal antibody) is approved for use in moderate-to-severe asthma and its clinical efficiency has been shown in patients with CRSwNP [113]. These monoclonal antibody treatments have not been studied as much in pediatric populations; currently the use of biologics is confined to patients with recalcitrant severe cases where other therapies have failed [114].

CRS is a complex inflammatory disease for which the exact pathophysiologic etiology remains elusive, even more so in the pediatric population [115]. Thus, also the role of allergy in CRS warrants further studies.

6.4   Role of Allergy in Pediatric and Adult Laryngitis

Croup, viral laryngitis, is typically a self-limited, common disease affecting children aged from 6 months to 3 years [116]. Of children under the age of 4 years, 6% are reported to have two or more croup attacks [117]. Recurrent laryngitis is a separate clinical entity characterized by repeated, relapsing episodes of croup-like cough [118].

Aslan et al. reported that atopy, AD, and previous history of wheezing increase the risk of recurrent croup episodes in children [119]. Children who have croup at an older age of 7–9 years have elevated risk of asthma development and should be monitored [120]. A study involving young adults with AR reported allergic patients having more vocal complaints compared to healthy controls; this study also suggested that ASIT decreased these vocal symptoms [121]. Also Krouse et al. reported that currently asymptomatic mite-sensitive adult patients had increased vocal complaints compared to non-allergic counterparts [122].

Laryngitis is the inflammation of the mucosa and other tissues of the larynx [123]. Whether inhalant allergens are the cause of laryngitis has been a matter of debate for decades [123]. The reason of this: both symptoms including hoarseness, throat clearing, and coughing and signs including vocal fold edema, hyperemia, and dense endolaryngeal mucus of allergic laryngitis (AL) are not specific for this disease [123, 124]. There is no study focusing specifically on this clinical entity in childhood, yet.

Brook et al. reported in their study that 52% of patients with chronic laryngeal symptoms (cough, throat clearing, hoarseness, increased secretions) had positive in vitro allergen-specific IgE tests; mites were the most common allergen [125]. Dworkin et al. had to prematurely terminate their graded laryngeal allergen challenge protocol on mite-sensitive patients due to two patients having serious adverse effects, including cough, chest tightness, and voice difficulties; both also showed viscous endolaryngeal secretions and vocal fold edema [126].

There is an overlap in clinical presentation and physical examination findings of patients with laryngopharyngeal reflux (LPR) disease and AL [127]. It has been suggested that patients may often be overdiagnosed with LPR and underdiagnosed with AL [46]. Characteristic examination signs in AL are sticky, viscid mucus within endolarynx and mucosal hyperemia [127]. Especially, thick endolaryngeal mucus has been accepted a significant predictor of allergy [128].

The treatment of AL has not been studied enough, but one study showed ASIT may reduce vocal symptoms in patients with AR [121]. Epidemiological evidence, however, suggests that allergy may have an important role on the pathogenesis of recurrent croup and a part of chronic laryngitis, but a clear need for more high-quality clinical studies exists.

6.5 Conclusions and Future Needs

AR is the most common chronic disease of the upper airways in children. Coexistence of AR with asthma shared pathophysiological mechanisms of the two diseases, and improvement in asthma control with proper AR treatment supports UAC that the respiratory tract is considered an integrated system acting as a functional unit with upper and lower airways, middle ear, and larynx. Allergy and AR can have significant impact on the pathogenesis of chronic or recurrent upper airway tract diseases including OME, CRS, and chronic laryngitis. There are convincing studies showing correlation between AR and OME, as well as conflicting studies showing no therapeutic benefit of AR treatment in the course of OME. Pediatric CRS has a considerable clinical correlation with asthma, whereas a weak association with AR. Knowledge about chronic laryngitis in children and also in adults is very scarce to make a conclusion.

One of the pitfalls of this conflicting results is that symptoms of AR overlap with acute and chronic rhinosinusitis; it is not easy to distinguish these entities from each other. Secondly, because AR is the most prevalent form of chronic rhinitis in children with a prevalence of up to 40%, it can coincide with CRS and also with OME. Plenty of risk factors exist in the ethiopathogenesis of OME, ARS, and CRS, in which allergy and AR is one of them.

To establish a clear, definite casual relationship between AR and OME, CRS, there is a need for further randomized, placebo-controlled well-designed prospective interventional studies focusing on evaluating comorbid allergies like AR in children with OME, the role of allergy in ARS and CRS, and prevalence, diagnostics, and treatment of AL in children and adults.

References

1. Holloway JW. 022 Genetics and epigenetics of allergic diseases and asthma. In: Middleton's allergy, vol. 2. Amsterdam: Elsevier; 2000. p. 343–63.
2. Burks W SS. Clinical manifestations of food allergy: an overview—Uptodate. 2020. https://www.uptodate.com/contents/clinical-manifestations-of-food-allergy-an-overview?search=clinicalmanifestationsoffoodallergy&source=search_result&selectedTitle=1~150&usage_type=default&display_rank=1.

3. Mallol J, Crane J, von Mutius E, Odhiambo J, Keil U, Stewart A. The international study of asthma and allergies in childhood (ISAAC) phase three: a global synthesis. Allergol Immunopathol. 2013;41(2):73–85.

4. Geraldini M, Neto HJC, Riedi CA, Rosário NA. Epidemiology of ocular allergy and comorbidities in adolescents. J Pediatr. 2013;89(4):354–60.

5. Silverberg JI, Simpson EL. Associations of childhood eczema severity: a US population-based study. Dermatitis. 2014;25(3):107–14.

6. Sicherer SH, Sampson HA. Food allergy. J Allergy Clin Immunol. 2010;125:S116–25.

7. Akinbami LJ, Moorman JE, Bailey C, Zahran HS, King M, Johnson CA, et al. NCHS Data Brief, Number 94, 2001. http://www.cdc.gov/nchs/data/databriefs/db94_tables.pdf#2.

8. Bauchau V, Durham SR. Prevalence and rate of diagnosis of allergic rhinitis in Europe. Eur Respir J. 2004;24(5):758–64.

9. Rosario N, Bielory L. Epidemiology of allergic conjunctivitis. Curr Opin Allergy Clin Immunol. 2011;11:471–6.

10. Rönmark EP, Ekerljung L, Lötvall J, Wennergren G, Rönmark E, Torén K, et al. Eczema among adults: prevalence, risk factors and relation to airway diseases. Results from a large-scale population survey in Sweden. Br J Dermatol. 2012;166:1301–8.

11. van der Hulst AE, Klip H, Brand PLP. Risk of developing asthma in young children with atopic eczema: a systematic review. J Allergy Clin Immunol. 2007;120(3):565–9.

12. Belgrave DCM, Granell R, Simpson A, Guiver J, Bishop C, Buchan I, et al. Developmental profiles of eczema, wheeze, and rhinitis: two population-based birth cohort studies. PLoS Med. 2014;11(10):e1001748.

13. Paller AS, Spergel JM, Mina-Osorio P, Irvine AD. The atopic march and atopic multimorbidity: many trajectories, many pathways. J Allergy Clin Immunol. 2019;143:46–55.

14. Doll RJ, Joseph NI, McGarry D, Jhaveri D, Sher T, Hostoffer R. Epidemiology of allergic diseases. In: Mahmoudi M, editor. Allergy and asthma. Cham: Springer; 2019. p. 31–51.

15. Ha EK, Baek JH, Lee S-Y, Park YM, Kim WK, Sheen YH, et al. Association of polysensitization, allergic multimorbidity, and allergy severity: a cross-sectional study of school children. Int Arch Allergy Immunol. 2016;171(3–4):251–60.

16. Siroux V, Boudier A, Nadif R, Lupinek C, Valenta R, Bousquet J. Association between asthma, rhinitis, and conjunctivitis multimorbidities with molecular IgE sensitization in adults. Allergy. 2019;74(4):824–7.

17. Laulajainen-Hongisto A, Lyly A, Hanif T, Dhaygude K, Kankainen M, Renkonen R, et al. Genomics of asthma, allergy and chronic rhinosinusitis: novel concepts and relevance in airway mucosa. Clin Transl Allergy. 2020;10:45.

18. Demenais F, Margaritte-Jeannin P, Barnes KC, Cookson WOC, Altmüller J, Ang W, et al. Multiancestry association study identifies new asthma risk loci that colocalize with immune-cell enhancer marks. Nat Genet. 2018;50(1):42–50.

19. Schoettler N, Rodríguez E, Weidinger S, Ober C. Advances in asthma and allergic disease genetics: is bigger always better? J Allergy Clin Immunol. 2019;144(6):1495–506.

20. Duffy DL, Martin NG, Battistutta D, Hopper JL, Mathews JD. Genetics of asthma and hay fever in Australian twins. Am Rev Respir Dis. 1990;142(6):1351–8.

21. Potaczek DP, Harb H, Michel S, Alhamwe BA, Renz H, Tost J. Epigenetics and allergy: from basic mechanisms to clinical applications. Epigenomics. 2017;9:539–71.

22. Edris A, den Dekker HT, Melén E, Lahousse L. Epigenome-wide association studies in asthma: a systematic review. Clin Exp Allergy. 2019;49:953–68.

23. Joubert BR, Felix JF, Yousefi P, Bakulski KM, Just AC, Breton C, et al. DNA methylation in newborns and maternal smoking in pregnancy: genome-wide consortium meta-analysis. Am J Hum Genet. 2016;98(4):680–96.

24. Xu CJ, Söderhäll C, Bustamante M, Baïz N, Gruzieva O, Gehring U, et al. DNA methylation in childhood asthma: an epigenome-wide meta-analysis. Lancet Respir Med. 2018;6(5):379–88.

25. Seidman MD, Gurgel RK, Lin SY, Schwartz SR, Baroody FM, Bonner JR, et al. Reviewers list. Otolaryngol Neck Surg. 2015;152(1):1–2.

26. Okubo K, Kurono Y, Ichimura K, Enomoto T, Okamoto Y, Kawauchi H, et al. Japanese guidelines for allergic rhinitis 2017. Allergol Int. 2017;66(2):205–19.
27. Seidman MD, Gurgel RK, Lin SY, Schwartz SR, Baroody FM, Bonner JR, et al. Clinical practice guideline. Otolaryngol Neck Surg. 2015;152(2):197–206.
28. Settipane RA. Demographics and epidemiology of allergic and nonallergic rhinitis. Allergy and asthma proceedings : the official journal of regional and state allergy societies. Allergy Asthma Proc. 2001;22:185–9.
29. Asher MI, Montefort S, Björkstén B, Lai CK, Strachan DP, Weiland SK, et al. Worldwide time trends in the prevalence of symptoms of asthma, allergic rhinoconjunctivitis, and eczema in childhood: ISAAC phases one and three repeat multicountry cross-sectional surveys. Lancet. 2006;368(9537):733–43.
30. Tharpe CA, Kemp SF. Pediatric allergic rhinitis. Immunol Allergy Clin N Am. 2015;35(1):185–98.
31. Bousquet J, Khaltaev N, Cruz AA, Denburg J, Fokkens WJ, Togias A, et al. Allergic rhinitis and its impact on asthma (ARIA) 2008 update (in collaboration with the World Health Organization, GA2LEN and AllerGen). Allergy. 2008;63:8–160.
32. Bousquet J, Van Cauwenberge P, Khaltaev N, Aria Workshop Group; World Health Organization. Allergic rhinitis and its impact on asthma. J Allergy Clin Immunol. 2001;108(5 Suppl):S147–334.
33. Corren J, Baroody FM, Togias A. 40 - Allergic and nonallergic rhinitis. In: Wesley BA, Holgate Stephen T, O'Hehir Robyn E, Broide David H, Bacharier Leonard B, Hershey Gurjit K, PRSJ K, editors. Middleton's allergy, vol. 2. 9th ed. Amsterdam: Elsevier; 2020. p. 636–58.
34. Bousquet J, Pfaar O, Togias A, Schünemann HJ, Ansotegui I, Papadopoulos NG, et al. 2019 ARIA care pathways for allergen immunotherapy. Allergy. 2019;74(11):2087–102.
35. Krouse JH. The unified airway-conceptual framework. Otolaryngol Clin N Am. 2008;41(2):257–66.
36. Corren J. The connection between allergic rhinitis and bronchial asthma. Curr Opin Pulm Med. 2007;13(1):13–8.
37. Giavina-Bianchi P, Aun MV, Takejima P, Kalil J, Agondi RC. United airway disease: current perspectives. J Asthma Allergy. 2016;9:93–100.
38. Braunstahl GJ, Kleinjan A, Overbeek SE, Prins JB, Hoogsteden HC, Fokkens WJ. Segmental bronchial provocation induces nasal inflammation in allergic rhinitis patients. Am J Respir Crit Care Med. 2000;161(6):2051–7.
39. Braunstahl GJ, Overbeek SE, KleinJan A, Prins JB, Hoogsteden HC, Fokkens WJ. Nasal allergen provocation induces adhesion molecule expression and tissue eosinophilia in upper and lower airways. J Allergy Clin Immunol. 2001;107(3):469–76.
40. Agondi RC, MacHado ML, Kalil J, Giavina-Bianchi P. Intranasal corticosteroid administration reduces nonspecific bronchial hyperresponsiveness and improves asthma symptoms. J Asthma. 2008;45(9):754–7.
41. Niggemann B, Jacobsen L, Dreborg S, Ferdousi HA, Halken S, Høst A, et al. Five-year follow-up on the PAT study: specific immunotherapy and long-term prevention of asthma in children. Allergy Eur J Allergy Clin Immunol. 2006;61(7):855–9.
42. Des Roches A, Paradis L, Menardo JL, Bouges S, Daurès JP, Bousquet J. Immunotherapy with a standardized Dermatophagoides pteronyssinus extract. VI. Specific immunotherapy prevents the onset of new sensitizations in children. J Allergy Clin Immunol. 1997;99(4):450–3.
43. Ikeda K, Tamura G, Shimomura A, Suzuki H, Nakabayashi S, Tanno N, et al. Endoscopic sinus surgery improves pulmonary function in patients with asthma associated with chronic sinusitis. Ann Otol Rhinol Laryngol. 1999;108(4):355–9.
44. Batra PS, Kern RC, Tripathi A, Conley DB, Ditto AM, Haines GK, et al. Outcome analysis of endoscopic sinus surgery in patients with nasal polyps and asthma. Laryngoscope. 2003;113(10):1703–6.
45. Feng CH, Miller MD, Simon RA. The united allergic airway: connections between allergic rhinitis, asthma, and chronic sinusitis. Am J Rhinol Allergy. 2012;26(3):187–90.

46. Platt MP, Brook CD, Kuperstock J, Krouse JH. What role does allergy play in chronic ear disease and laryngitis? Curr Allergy Asthma Rep. 2016;16(10):76.
47. Schilder AGM, Chonmaitree T, Cripps AW, Rosenfeld RM, Casselbrant ML, Haggard MP, et al. Otitis media. Nat Rev Dis Prim. 2016;2:16063.
48. Alles R, Parikh A, Hawk L, Darby Y, Romero JN, Scadding G. The prevalence of atopic disorders in children with chronic otitis media with effusion. Pediatr Allergy Immunol. 2001;12(2):102–6.
49. Kwon C, Lee HY, Kim MG, Boo SH, Yeo SG. Allergic diseases in children with otitis media with effusion. Int J Pediatr Otorhinolaryngol. 2013;77(2):158–61.
50. Cheng X, Sheng H, Ma R, Gao Z, Han Z, Chi F, et al. Allergic rhinitis and allergy are risk factors for otitis media with effusion: a meta-analysis. Allergol Immunopathol (Madr). 2017;45(1):25–32.
51. Hurst DS. The role of allergy in otitis media with effusion. Otolaryngol Clin N Am. 2011;44(3):637–54.
52. Luong A, Roland PS. The link between allergic rhinitis and chronic otitis media with effusion in atopic patients. Otolaryngol Clin N Am. 2008;41(2):311–23.
53. Nguyen LHP, Manoukian JJ, Sobol SE, Tewfik TL, Mazer BD, Schloss MD, et al. Similar allergic inflammation in the middle ear and the upper airway: evidence linking otitis media with effusion to the united airways concept. J Allergy Clin Immunol. 2004;114(5):1110–5.
54. Wright ED, Hurst D, Miotto D, Giguere C, Hamid Q. Increased expression of major basic protein (MBP) and interleukin-5(IL-5) in middle ear biopsy specimens from atopic patients with persistent otitis media with effusion. Otolaryngol Head Neck Surg. 2000;123(5):533–8.
55. Hurst DS, Venge P. Evidence of eosinophil, neutrophil, and mast-cell mediators in the effusion of OME patients with and without atopy. Allergy. 2000;55(5):435–41.
56. Fireman P. Otitis media and eustachian tube dysfunction: connection to allergic rhinitis. J Allergy Clin Immunol. 1997;99(2):S787–97.
57. Lazo-Sáenz JG, Galván-Aguilera AA, Martínez-Ordaz VA, Velasco-Rodríguez VM, Nieves-Rentería A, Rincón-Castañeda C. Eustachian tube dysfunction in allergic rhinitis. Otolaryngol - Head Neck Surg. 2005;132(4):626–9.
58. Ma Y, Liang M, Tian P, Liu X, Dang H, Chen Q, et al. Eustachian tube dysfunction in patients with house dust mite-allergic rhinitis. Clin Transl Allergy. 2020;10(1):30.
59. Friedman RA, Doyle WJ, Casselbrant ML, Bluestone C, Fireman P. Immunologic-mediated eustachian tube obstruction: a double-blind crossover study. J Allergy Clin Immunol. 1983;71(5):442–7.
60. Simpson SA, Lewis R, van der Voort J, Butler CC. Oral or topical nasal steroids for hearing loss associated with otitis media with effusion in children. Cochrane Database Syst Rev. 2011;5:CD001935.
61. Bhargava R, Chakravarti A. A double-blind randomized placebo-controlled trial of topical intranasal mometasone furoate nasal spray in children of adenoidal hypertrophy with otitis media with effusion. Am J Otolaryngol. 2014;35(6):766–70.
62. Griffin G, Flynn CA. Antihistamines and/or decongestants for otitis media with effusion (OME) in children. Cochrane database Syst Rev. 2011;9:CD003423.
63. Hurst DS. Efficacy of allergy immunotherapy as a treatment for patients with chronic otitis media with effusion. Int J Pediatr Otorhinolaryngol. 2008;72(8):1215–23.
64. Bachert C, Zhang N, Gevaert P. 41 - Rhinosinusitis and nasal polyps. In: Wesley BA, Holgate Stephen T, O'Hehir Robyn E, Broide David H, Bacharier Leonard B, Hershey Gurjit K, Khurana PRSJ, editors. Middleton's allergy, vol. 2. 9th ed. Elsevier; 2020. p. 659–72.
65. Bachert C, Hörmann K, Mösges R, Rasp G, Riechelmann H, Müller R, et al. An update on the diagnosis and treatment of sinusitis and nasal polyposis. Allergy. 2003;58:176–91.
66. Fokkens WJ, Lund VJ, Hopkins C, Hellings PW, Kern R, Reitsma S, et al. European position paper on rhinosinusitis and nasal polyps 2020. Rhinology. 2020;58(Suppl S29):1–464.
67. Fokkens WJ, Lund VJ, Hopkins C, Hellings PW, Kern R, Reitsma S, et al. Executive summary of EPOS 2020 including integrated care pathways. Rhinology. 2020;58(2):82–111.

68. Pappas DE, Taveras EM, Torchia M. The common cold in children: Clinical features and diagnosis—uptodate. 2020. https://www.uptodate.com/contents/the-common-cold-in-children-clinical-features-and-diagnosis?search=Upperrespiratorytractinfections&topicRef=16629&source=see_link.

69. Aitken M, Taylor JA. Prevalence of clinical sinusitis in young children followed up by primary care pediatricians. Arch Pediatr Adolesc Med. 1998;152(3):244–8.

70. Wald ER, Kaplan SL, Wood RA, Isaacson GC, Torchia MM. Acute bacterial rhinosinusitis in children: clinical features and diagnosis—uptodate. 2020. https://www.uptodate.com/contents/acute-bacterial-rhinosinusitis-in-children-clinical-features-anddiagnosis?sectionName=CLINICALFEATURES&search=Upperrespiratorytractinfections&topicRef=5978&anchor=H7&source=see_link#H4.

71. Uijen JH, Bindels PJ, Schellevis FG, Van Der Wouden JC. ENT problems in Dutch children: trends in incidence rates, antibiotic prescribing and referrals 2002-2008. Scand J Prim Health Care. 2011;29(2):75–9.

72. Lin SW, Wang YH, Lee MY, Ku MS, Sun HL, Lu KH, et al. Clinical spectrum of acute rhinosinusitis among atopic and nonatopic children in Taiwan. Int J Pediatr Otorhinolaryngol. 2012;76(1):70–5.

73. Mbarek C, Akrout A, Khamassi K, Ben Gamra O, Hariga I, Ben Amor M, et al. Recurrent upper respiratory tract infections in children and allergy. A cross-sectional study of 100 cases. Tunis Med. 2008;86(4):358–61.

74. Leo G, Incorvaia C, Cazzavillan A, Consonni D, Zuccotti GV. Could seasonal allergy be a risk factor for acute rhinosinusitis in children? J Laryngol Otol. 2018;132(2):150–3.

75. Pant H, Ferguson BJ, Macardle PJ. The role of allergy in rhinosinusitis. Curr Opin Otolaryngol Head Neck Surg. 2009;17:232–8.

76. Schatz M, Zeiger RS, Chen W, Yang S-J, Corrao MA, Quinn VP. The burden of rhinitis in a managed care organization. Ann Allergy Asthma Immunol. 2008;101(3):240–7.

77. Vlastos I, Athanasopoulos I, Mastronikolis NS, Panogeorgou T, Margaritis V, Naxakis S, et al. Impaired mucociliary clearance in allergic rhinitis patients is related to a predisposition to rhinosinusitis. Ear Nose Throat J. 2009;88(4):E17–9.

78. Savolainen S. Allergy in patients with acute maxillary sinusitis. Allergy. 1989;44(2):116–22.

79. Van Crombruggen K, Zhang N, Gevaert P, Tomassen P, Bachert C. Pathogenesis of chronic rhinosinusitis: inflammation. J Allergy Clin Immunol. 2011;128(4):728–32.

80. Mahdavinia M, Grammer LC. Chronic rhinosinusitis and age: is the pathogenesis different? Expert Rev Anti-Infect Ther. 2013;11(10):1029–40.

81. Shin S-Y, Choi G-S, Park H-S, Lee K-H, Kim S-W, Cho J-S. Immunological investigation in the adenoid tissues from children with chronic rhinosinusitis. Otolaryngol Head Neck Surg. 2009;141(1):91–6.

82. Anfuso A, Ramadan H, Terrell A, Demirdag Y, Walton C, Skoner DP, et al. Sinus and adenoid inflammation in children with chronic rhinosinusitis and asthma. Ann Allergy Asthma Immunol. 2015;114(2):103–10.

83. Veling MC. The role of allergy in pediatric rhinosinusitis. Curr Opin Otolaryngol Head Neck Surg. 2013;21(3):271–6.

84. Gilani S, Shin JJ. The burden and visit prevalence of pediatric chronic rhinosinusitis. Otolaryngol Neck Surg. 2017;157:1048–52.

85. Snidvongs K, Sangubol M, Poachanukoon O. Pediatric versus adult chronic rhinosinusitis. Curr Allergy Asthma Rep. 2020;20:29.

86. Poachanukoon O, Nanthapisal S, Chaumrattanakul U. Pediatric acute and chronic rhinosinusitis: comparison of clinical characteristics and outcome of treatment. Asian Pac J Allergy Immunol. 2012;30:146–51.

87. Hamilos DL, Holbrook EH, Corren J, Descheler DG, Feldweg AM. Chronic rhinosinusitis: management—uptodate. 2020. https://www.uptodate.com/contents/chronic-rhinosinusitis-management?source=history_widget#H4.

88. Harvey R, Hannan SA, Badia L, Scadding G. Nasal saline irrigations for the symptoms of chronic rhinosinusitis. Cochrane Database Syst Rev. 2007;18:CD006394.

89. Chong LY, Head K, Hopkins C, Philpott C, Schilder AGM, Burton MJ. Intranasal steroids versus placebo or no intervention for chronic rhinosinusitis. Cochrane Database Syst Rev. 2016;4:CD011996.

90. Peters AT, Spector S, Hsu J, Hamilos DL, Baroody FM, Chandra RK, et al. Diagnosis and management of rhinosinusitis: a practice parameter update. Ann Allergy Asthma Immunol. 2014;113(4):347–85.

91. Vandenberg SJ, Heatley DG. Efficacy of adenoidectomy in relieving symptoms of chronic sinusitis in children. Arch Otolaryngol Head Neck Surg. 1997;123(7):675–8.

92. Lusk RP, Muntz HR. Endoscopic sinus surgery in children with chronic sinusitis. Laryngoscope. 1990;100(6):654–8.

93. Vlastarakos PV, Fetta M, Segas JV, Maragoudakis P, Nikolopoulos TP. Functional endoscopic sinus surgery improves sinus-related symptoms and quality of life in children with chronic rhinosinusitis: a systematic analysis and meta-analysis of published interventional studies. Clin Pediatr. 2013;52:1091–7.

94. Kennedy JL, Borish L. Chronic sinusitis pathophysiology: the role of allergy. Am J Rhinol Allergy. 2013;27(5):367–71.

95. Rosati MG, Peters AT. Relationships among allergic rhinitis, asthma, and chronic rhinosinusitis. Am J Rhinol Allergy. 2016;30(1):44–7.

96. Batra PS, Tong L, Citardi MJ. Analysis of comorbidities and objective parameters in refractory chronic rhinosinusitis. Laryngoscope. 2013;123:S1–11.

97. Melzer JM, Driskill BR, Clenney TL, Gessler EM. Sublingual immunotherapy for allergic fungal sinusitis. Ann Otol Rhinol Laryngol. 2015;124(10):782–7.

98. Jarvis D, Newson R, Lotvall J, Hastan D, Tomassen P, Keil T, et al. Asthma in adults and its association with chronic rhinosinusitis: the GA2LEN survey in Europe. Allergy. 2012;67(1):91–8.

99. Emanuel IA, Shah SB. Chronic rhinosinusitis: allergy and sinus computed tomography relationships. Otolaryngol Head Neck Surg. 2000;123(6):687–91.

100. Newman LJ, Platts-Mills TA, Phillips CD, Hazen KC, Gross CW. Chronic sinusitis. Relationship of computed tomographic findings to allergy, asthma, and eosinophilia. JAMA. 1994;271(5):363–7.

101. Ramadan HH, Hinerman RA. Outcome of endoscopic sinus surgery in children with allergic rhinitis. Am J Rhinol. 2006;20(4):438–40.

102. Asakura K, Kojima T, Shirasaki H, Kataura A. Evaluation of the effects of antigen specific immunotherapy on chronic sinusitis in children with allergy. Auris Nasus Larynx. 1990;17(1):33–8.

103. DeYoung K, Wentzel JL, Schlosser RJ, Nguyen SA, Soler ZM. Systematic review of immunotherapy for chronic rhinosinusitis. Am J Rhinol Allergy. 2014;28(2):145–50.

104. Zhang Y-N, Song J, Wang H, Wang H, Zeng M, Zhai G-T, et al. Nasal IL-4(+)CXCR5(+) CD4(+) T follicular helper cell counts correlate with local IgE production in eosinophilic nasal polyps. J Allergy Clin Immunol. 2016;137(2):462–73.

105. Cheng K-J, Zhou M-L, Xu Y-Y, Zhou S-H. The role of local allergy in the nasal inflammation. Eur Arch Otorhinolaryngol. 2017;274(9):3275–81.

106. Wise SK, Ahn CN, Lathers DMR, Mulligan RM, Schlosser RJ. Antigen-specific IgE in sinus mucosa of allergic fungal rhinosinusitis patients. Am J Rhinol. 2008;22(5):451–6.

107. Mabry RL, Marple BF, Folker RJ, Mabry CS. Immunotherapy for allergic fungal sinusitis: three years' experience. Otolaryngol Neck Surg. 1998;119(6):648–51.

108. Ryan MW, Clark CM. Allergic fungal rhinosinusitis and the unified airway: the role of antifungal therapy in AFRS. Curr Allergy Asthma Rep. 2015;15(12):75.

109. Haldar P, Brightling CE, Hargadon B, Gupta S, Monteiro W, Sousa A, et al. Mepolizumab and exacerbations of refractory eosinophilic asthma. N Engl J Med. 2009;360(10):973–84.

110. Gevaert P, Van Bruaene N, Cattaert T, Van Steen K, Van Zele T, Acke F, et al. Mepolizumab, a humanized anti–IL-5 mAb, as a treatment option for severe nasal polyposis. J Allergy Clin Immunol. 2011;128(5):989–95.

111. Castro M, Mathur S, Hargreave F, Boulet L-P, Xie F, Young J, et al. Reslizumab for poorly controlled, eosinophilic asthma. Am J Respir Crit Care Med. 2011;184(10):1125–32.
112. Gevaert P, Langloidolt D, Lackner A, Stammberger H, Staudinger H, Vanzele T, et al. Nasal IL-5 levels determine the response to anti–IL-5 treatment in patients with nasal polyps. J Allergy Clin Immunol. 2006;118(5):1133–41.
113. Gevaert P, Calus L, Van Zele T, Blomme K, De Ruyck N, Bauters W, et al. Omalizumab is effective in allergic and nonallergic patients with nasal polyps and asthma. J Allergy Clin Immunol. 2013;131(1):110–6.
114. Shinee T, Sutikno B, Abdullah B. The use of biologics in children with allergic rhinitis and chronic rhinosinusitis: current updates. Pediatr Investig. 2019;3(3):165–72.
115. Schwartz JS, Tajudeen BA, Cohen NA. Medical management of chronic rhinosinusitis – an update. Expert Rev Clin Pharmacol. 2016;9(5):695–704.
116. Hiebert JC, Zhao YD, Willis EB. Bronchoscopy findings in recurrent croup: a systematic review and meta-analysis. Int J Pediatr Otorhinolaryngol. 2016;90:86–90.
117. Hide DW, Guyer BM. Recurrent croup. Arch Dis Child. 1985;60(6):585–6.
118. Kwong K, Hoa M, Coticchia JM. Recurrent croup presentation, diagnosis, and management. Am J Otolaryngol Head Neck Med Surg. 2007;28(6):401–7.
119. Arslan Z, Çipe FE, Özmen S, Kondolot M, Piskin IE, Yöney A. Evaluation of allergic sensitization and gastroesophageal reflux disease in children with recurrent croup. Pediatr Int. 2009;51(5):661–5.
120. Lin S-C, Lin H-W, Chiang B-L. Association of croup with asthma in children. Medicine. 2017;96(35):e7667.
121. Simberg S, Sala E, Tuomainen J, Rönnemaa A-M. Vocal symptoms and allergy--a pilot study. J Voice. 2009;23(1):136–9.
122. Krouse JH, Dworkin JP, Carron MA, Stachler RJ. Baseline laryngeal effects among individuals with dust mite allergy. Otolaryngol Head Neck Surg. 2008;139(1):149–51.
123. Spantideas N, Bougea A, Drosou E, Assimakopoulos D. The role of allergy in phonation. J Voice. 2019;33(5):811.
124. Campagnolo A, Benninger MS. Allergic laryngitis: chronic laryngitis and allergic sensitization. Braz J Otorhinolaryngol. 2019;85:263–6.
125. Brook CD, Platt MP, Reese S, Noordzij JP. Utility of allergy testing in patients with chronic laryngopharyngeal symptoms. Otolaryngol Neck Surg. 2016;154(1):41–5.
126. Dworkin JP, Reidy PM, Stachler RJ, Krouse JH. Effects of sequential Dermatophagoides pteronyssinus antigen stimulation on anatomy and physiology of the larynx. Ear Nose Throat J. 2009;88(2):793–9.
127. Krouse JH. Allergy and laryngeal disorders. Curr Opin Otolaryngol Head Neck Surg. 2016;24(3):221–5.
128. Eren E, Arslanoğlu S, Aktaş A, Kopar A, Ciğer E, Önal K, et al. Factors confusing the diagnosis of laryngopharyngeal reflux: the role of allergic rhinitis and inter-rater variability of laryngeal findings. Eur Arch Oto-Rhino-Laryngology. 2014;271(4):743–7.

Ear, Nose, and Throat Infections in Immunocompromised Children

Kerimcan Çakıcı, Ozan Gökdoğan, and Gülbin Bingöl

7.1 Introduction

Immunocompromised children constitute a heterogeneous patient population. Patients with primary immunodeficiency have undergone solid organ transplantation or hematopoietic stem cell transplantation. Patients who receive biological immunomodulators and immunosuppressive therapy due to various diseases (gastrointestinal diseases such as rheumatological, neurological, inflammatory bowel disease) are included in this group.

With the increasingly widespread application of solid organ transplantation (SOT), hematopoietic stem cell transplantation (HSCT), and immunomodulatory therapies, conditions that put the immune system at risk are common among children [1].

Immunodeficiencies in the pediatric age can be overlooked due to the high frequency of upper respiratory tract (URI) infections in daily practice. For early detection of these diseases, consultations with pediatric immunologists and pediatric disorders are very important in cases where all physicians are suspected of immunodeficiency. Thus, treatments can be managed correctly, and treatment costs can be reduced.

K. Çakıcı (✉) · O. Gökdoğan
Department of Otorhinolaryngology, Faculty of Medicine, Muğla Sıtkı Koçman University, Muğla, Turkey

G. Bingöl
Division of Pediatric Allergy and Immunology, Department of Pediatrics, Faculty of Medicine, Acıbadem University, İstanbul, Turkey

7.2   Primary Immunodeficiencies

Primary immunodeficiency disorders (PID) refer to a heterogeneous group of more than 130 disorders that result from defects in immune system development and/or function. Primary immune deficiencies are extremely rare. Immunoglobulin A (IgA) deficiency, a humoral immunodeficiency, is quite familiar with a prevalence of 1 /300–1/600.

Early diagnosis of PIDs is essential to prevent morbidity and mortality associated with the disease. Delays in diagnosis and treatment may cause medical treatment failure and inappropriate antibiotic use, and increased complications in surgical interventions [2, 3].

Among the criteria used for the diagnosis of PID are [4]:

1. ≥8 new ear infection within 1 year.
2. severe sinus infection within 1 year.
3. Minimal antibiotics effect despite 2 months of use.
4. ≥2 episodes of pneumonia within 1 year.
5. A baby not gaining weight or growing normally.
6. Recurrent deep skin or organ abscesses.
7. Persistent thrush in the mouth or skin after the age of 1.
8. Need for IV antibiotics.
9. ≥2 Deep infections.
10. PID's family history is included.

Although more than 40% of patients with these disorders reported severe or chronic health conditions (such as sinusitis, bronchitis, and pneumonia), it was observed that their diagnosis was not diagnosed until adulthood. The importance of immediate recognition and management of PIDs affects the hospitalization rate before and after the diagnosis. At the same time, 70% of the patients had a history of hospitalization before diagnosis, and it was observed that this rate decreased to 50% after diagnosis. In some forms of PID, URTI (upper respiratory tract infection) does not show symptoms initially, but URTI findings can be observed in the later stages of the disease [2, 5].

This disease has different subtypes.

7.3   Humoral Immunodeficiencies

The most common forms of primary immunodeficiencies are humoral immunodeficiencies. Although there are various diseases and syndromes under this heading, conditions related to USR diseases will be mentioned. These are:

1. Transient hypogammaglobulinemia (THI) of the infant.
2. Common variable immune deficiency (CVID).
3. X-linked agammaglobulinemia (XLA).

4. Selective IgA deficiency (IgAD).
5. Ig G subclass deficiency.
6. Hyper IgM syndrome (HIgMS).

7.3.1   Transient Hypogammaglobulinemia (THI) of the Infant

It is accepted as a prolongation of physiological hypogammaglobulinemia that occurs from 3 to 6 months due to the loss of maternal transplacental IgG and the baby's IgG's slow increase levels [6].

Prolonged hypogammaglobulinemia can be seen in many children, so there are criteria for diagnosis.

According to the ESID (European Society for Immunodeficiencies) diagnostic criteria: With the detection of IgG below the standard value due to age in at least two measurements in the first 3 years of life, there should be no other defined hypogammaglobulinemia and spontaneous resolution after 4 years of age [7].

These infants have inadequate antibody responses to one or more vaccine antigens. Several different reasons have been suggested for the occurrence of this disorder. The first of these is that maternal immunoglobulins suppress fetal immunoglobulin production [8]. Another theory is the familial genetic heterozygous inheritance hypothesis [9]. In another study, the cause was observed as T helper dysfunction [10]. Cytokine imbalance is one of the hypotheses put forward in pathophysiology [11]. Some of other hypothesis, which is generally seen in premature babies who have been in the neonatal intensive care unit for a long time due to various diseases are; low IgG levels due to stress, plasma loss to the gastrointestinal or respiratory system, steroid use and frequent blood intake [12].

Acute otitis media (AOM), sinusitis, bronchitis, and pneumonia are frequently observed among the infections. Rarely, there may be sepsis, meningitis, or soft tissue cellulitis. Atopic findings and oral candidiasis are also uncommon findings.

Development is normal on physical examination. Tonsil and lymph nodes are small. Thymic shadow is not seen in radiological examination with direct radiography. Generally, there is a decrease in all three major immunoglobulins. There is no molecular test for a definitive diagnosis.

In symptomatic patients, a conservative approach to avoiding crowded environments, especially during winter months, rapid treatment of respiratory tract infections, and prophylactic antibiotic treatment are required. In rare THI patients with severe infections or inadequate antibody responses to vaccine antigens, IVIG (intravenous immune globulin) therapy can be used, usually for 6–12 months, at 400–500 mg/kg/month. After IVIG therapy, immunoglobulin levels and antibody responses are retested 3 months later [12].

The disease has a good prognosis, and consequently most patients recover by the age of 2. Low IgG levels can persist in some patients up to 5 years (rarely even longer) [12].

7.3.2   Common Variable Immune Deficiency (CVID)

In North America and Europe, it is the most common primary immunodeficiency symptomatically, with an incidence of 1: 25,000 to 1: 66,000 [13, 14]. CVID is a disease characterized by low serum immunoglobulin concentration, defective specific antibody production, and increased susceptibility to bacterial infections. In affected patients, common respiratory tract infections are usually observed with autoimmune cytopenia, lymphoproliferative syndrome, and granuloma.

Diagnostic criteria for CVID diagnosis [7] (It should be at least one of the following):

- Increased susceptibility to infection.
- Autoimmune symptoms.
- Granulomatous disease.
- Unexplained polyclonal lymphoproliferation.
- An affected family member with antibody deficiency.

Furthermore, there should be a significant decrease in IgG and a significant reduction in IgA with or without low IgM levels (measurement at least twice; <2SD of normal levels for their age), and must be at least one of the following:

- Inadequate antibody response (and/or absence of isohemagglutinins) to vaccines, i.e., lack of protective levels despite vaccination.
- Low differentiated memory B cells (<70% of standard age-related value).
- Furthermore, they should not have secondary causes of hypogammaglobulinemia (e.g., infection, protein loss, drug therapy, malignancy).

Bacterial infections can be seen as well as viral, fungal, and parasitic infections. Serum IgM concentration is expected in about half of the patients. Abnormalities in T cell numbers or function are common. Most patients have standard numbers of B cells; however, some have low or no B cells. About 50% of patients have autoimmune symptoms. There is an increased risk of malignancy [13, 14].

Mucus accumulating in the airways can lead to airway obstruction, bacterial colonization, and recurrent infections. Especially in children, due to specific developmental differences such as Eustachian tube anatomy, the most common infection site in childhood is the upper respiratory tract [9, 15].

The most common infections observed in patients diagnosed with CVID are acute bronchitis, pneumonia, acute otitis, chronic bronchitis, and chronic sinusitis. The rate of recurrent or chronic airway infection was 88%, sinusitis 78%, and recurrent otitis 78% in children before CVID diagnosis in childhood [16]. However, urinary infections, cutaneous abscesses, and bacterial meningitis can be seen. The prevalence of chronic rhinosinusitis in patients with CVID was found to be 36–78% [16, 17]. Acute recurrent rhinosinusitis was reported in 41% of cases and chronic rhinosinusitis in 40% [18, 19].

According to different sources, CVID patients are diagnosed after an average of 5.8–8.9 years after the onset of symptoms. The high incidence of recurrent minor infections in children with intact immune systems and significant clinical overlap with atopic diseases make it difficult to recognize this disease [14, 17].

In the presence of atopy or autoimmune disease, it is necessary to evaluate immunoglobulin levels to provide specific treatment as early as possible in case of recurrent infection. Thus, diagnosis can be made as early as possible and specific treatment can be started. This will ultimately reduce the risks associated with a severe infection and the decline in quality of life caused by chronic infection [16, 17]. Children with recurrent rhinosinusitis that do not improve after three should be evaluated in terms of PID. Rhinosinusitis secondary to an IgA or IgG subclass deficiency is usually treated medically. Sinus surgery may be required in cases resistant to medical treatment [20].

IVIG treatment can be very useful in these patients. With IVIG treatment, we can replace the only IgG. In contrast, IgA, which are principal secretory antibodies on mucosal surfaces, and IgM, which is significantly responsible for primary immunity, cannot be replaced. However, the percentage of CVID patients affected by acute respiratory infections, pneumonia, and otitis is significantly reduced with IVIG therapy.

A constant level of antibodies is mandatory to protect against infections. Serum immunoglobulins include low- and high-affinity antibodies with different isotypes; they are produced either without prior immunization (natural antibodies) or after antigenic stimulation (adaptive antibodies). In CVID patients with fewer symptoms, innate immunity is preserved: while it can produce low but detectable IgM levels, defective adaptive immunity can be compensated by IgG substitution therapy. IgM levels cannot be detected in more symptomatic CVID patients, and chronic lung disease and intestinal diseases are more common [21, 22].

Both IVIG therapy and better diagnosis and treatment strategies have a major impact on CVID mortality. B cell abnormalities are the most important factor in the developing and prognosis of chronic diseases in CVID patients [23–25].

7.3.3 X-Linked Agammaglobulinemia (XLA)

X-linked (Bruton's) agammaglobulinemia is a disease characterized by the complete absence of B lymphocytes and plasma cells. Children do not show any disease symptoms in the first 6 months due to antibodies from the mother. After the first 6 months, recurrent pyogenic upper respiratory tract infections (*Pseudomonas aeruginosae*, *H. influenzae*, Pneumococci, and other streptococci) begin to be observed [26].

A critical clinical clue during examination in these patients is the absence of tonsils. In some cases, the tonsils are observed very small, and usually the cervical lymph nodes cannot be detected. Approximately 50% of patients with clinical and laboratory findings of XLA have a positive family history [27] because the disease is observed in the population with new mutations in the XLA gene, Bruton tyrosine kinase (Btk) [16, 28]. Btk is a hematopoietic specific tyrosine kinase expressed during B cell differentiation [28, 29].

Almost all patients with XLA have recurrent otitis or sinusitis during the first year of life. It was observed that some of these patients were diagnosed with immunodeficiency with a few episodes of otitis. Some of them were treated by hospitalization many times without being diagnosed with immunodeficiency despite the widespread otitis episode [17, 30].

The absence of cervical lymph nodes and tonsillar tissue in XLA patients is pathognomic and should alert the physician to immunodeficiency states. If the tonsils and cervical lymph nodes are tiny in a patient with frequent otitis and sinusitis attacks, serum Ig (Immunoglobulin) concentrations should be examined. Suppose at least two of the three primary serum Ig classes (IgM, IgG, and IgA) are below the normal range. In that case, the patient should be referred for further evaluation, including determining the percentage of B cells in the peripheral circulation [30].

In the treatment of XLA patients, vaccination with live vaccines should be avoided, and IVIG treatment should be planned when necessary [26]. Loss of treatment for XLA patients is associated with significant morbidity and mortality. Delayed or inadequate treatment can also cause chronic problems such as chronic pulmonary diseases and hearing loss.

Gammaglobulin replacement and, when necessary, the use of aggressive antibiotics form the basis of treatment. Acute life-threatening infections are rarely observed in XLA patients receiving IVIG [31].

7.3.4 Selective IgA Deficiency (IgAD)

IgA is the primary mediator that provides mucosal immunity in the gastrointestinal and respiratory systems [32]. The exact pathology in selective IgA deficiency is not understood. The probable reason is that B lymphocytes do not differentiate into IgA-secreting plasma cells, and the immunoglobulin class cannot be changed [33].

IgA deficiency is defined as a serum IgA level of <0.07 g/L in individuals aged 4 years or older [18, 34]. This immunodeficiency is the most common antibody-dependent defect. It can be seen in a broad spectrum from partial to complete [32]. The complete absence of IgA disrupts the mucosa's immune barrier property, and susceptibility to infections occurs. However, susceptibility to autoimmune diseases and allergies also occurs.

Frequent rhinosinusitis, otitis media, mastoiditis, adenotonsillitis, and recurrent parotitis are common in this group of patients [35]. Patients with IgA deficiency associated with decreased serum antibodies to pneumococcal polysaccharides, decreased serum IgG subclasses (IgG2 and IgG4), or some polymorphisms of Manos binding lectin 2 (MBL2) are more likely to have recurrent infections [36–40].

Although most patients are asymptomatic, one-third of patients with IgA deficiency may have recurrent infections, such as frequent sinopulmonary and gastrointestinal tract infections.

Attempts to treat these patients with heterologous IgA are dangerous because many anti-IgA antibody expression can easily have fatal anaphylaxis [41, 42].

7.3.5   IgG Subclass Deficiency

IgG1, IgG2, IgG3, and IgG4 account for approximately 70%, 20%, 7%, and 3% of total IgG levels, respectively. Each subclass has its own structural, antigenic, and biological differences. The most critical biological difference is observed in IgG2, and it is the primary antibody against polysaccharide antigens [12]. Laboratory diagnosis of IgG subclass deficiency is made in humans with normal or near-normal total IgG levels when one or more of the IgG subclasses is <2 SD below the relevant average age subclass [12].

Recurrent respiratory infections such as otitis, sinusitis, and bronchitis caused by common respiratory bacterial pathogens are observed in adults and children. Although severe systemic infections such as sepsis, pneumonia, meningitis, and cellulitis are less common, most of these patients are either atopic or have lower respiratory tract comorbid conditions such as asthma bronchitis [42]. Selective IgG2 deficiency is the most common subclass associated with recurrent infection and may accompany IgA and IgG4 deficiencies. The failure of long-term antibiotics, the presence of severe symptoms, and the development of permanent radiographic abnormalities may sometimes require IVIG treatment at therapeutic doses.

Conservative treatment is successful in most patients, but treatment can be extended and lifelong. However, symptomatic adults can progress to CVID. Subclass checks are required at annual intervals [12].

7.3.6   Hyper-IgM Syndrome (HIgM)

Normal or elevated IgM levels are present in patients with the hyper-IgM syndrome. Recurrent bacterial sinopulmonary infections usually begin after the 6th month of life with maternal immunoglobulins' protective effect. Peritonsillar and other soft tissue infections may be evident in the neck. Periodic antigenic stimulation can lead to significant adenotonsillar hypertrophy and, consequently, upper airway obstruction [21, 43].

Besides the humoral defect, neutropenia may be observed in patients. However, chronic stomatitis and oral ulcers can be seen. Patients tend to develop autoimmune and malignant diseases [26].

The surface molecules on T cells are required for interaction with B cells in the CD40 ligand. Without this ligand, T cells cannot dock properly with B cells to stimulate further antibody isotype production. As a result, these patients' B cells primarily produce IgM, and patients with this deficiency have hyper-IgM syndrome [44].

Typically, recurrent otitis media, respiratory tract infections, and Pneumocystis carinii pneumonia can be observed in children younger than 2 years of age.

7.4   Lack of Components

Among all PIDs, complement deficiencies account for less than 1% of detected cases. There are many complement deficiency subtypes. Looking at their general characteristics, patients with these disorders tend to show a systemic autoimmune disease similar to lupus erythematosus or severe or recurrent infections with encapsulated organisms.

Complement deficiencies that can lead to clinically significant immunodeficiency are rare. Defects of opsonizing complement components (C2, C3; H, I, P) can predispose the patient to encapsulated bacterial infections.

The deficiency of components that make up the membrane attack complex (C5, C6, C7, C8) is associated with an immune defect against Neisseria species leading to meningococcal meningitis or sepsis [45].

There is no specific treatment for complement deficiencies. The treatment of these disorders focuses on antibiotic prophylaxis to prevent recurrent infections. Due to the high risk of Neisseria meningitis and meningococcal infections, multivalent meningococcal vaccines should also be recommended for some patients with complement disorders [43].

7.5   Phagocytosis Disorders

7.5.1   Myeloperoxidase Deficiency (MPO)

It is the most common hereditary neutrophil defect. Most MPO patients are asymptomatic, as the oxidative killing pathways remain functional. However, recurrent candidiasis can be observed in diabetic patients with MPO deficiency [46]. Severe fungal osteomyelitis of the skull base has been described as an unusual complication of MPO deficiency [47].

In general, prophylactic antibiotics are not recommended as patients with MPO deficiency are asymptomatic. However, patients with comorbid diabetes mellitus with a high incidence of localized and systemic infections may require rapid and aggressive treatment with antimicrobials to control infections. These patients should be followed up in terms of complications that may develop in treatments that may increase the tendency of fungal infections such as long-term use of antibiotics or steroids [48].

7.5.2   Chronic Granulomatous Disease (CGD)

Multiple genetic defects cause chronic granulomatous disease in phlox genes that produce adenine dinucleotide phosphate (NAPDH) oxidase; the reduced nicotinamide enzyme catalyzes the formation of oxygen radicals that mediate the killing of bacteria and fungi by phagocytes. The deficiency can be quantitative and/or qualitative. The severity of the disease depends on the amount of functional NADPH oxidase expressed [49].

Recurrent infections are usually mediated by catalase-positive microorganisms such as S. aureus, Aspergillus, Nocardia, and Serratia. Recurrent pneumonia, skin infections, and cervical lymphadenopathy can be observed in these patients [49].

Outer ear and mastoid infections can progress rapidly and require aggressive surgery. Oral symptoms are gingivitis and aphthous ulcers. Facial infections can result in severe acne, cellulitis, ulcers, and chronic inflammation of nostrils. Although inflammation may cause large granulomas, if these granulomas occur in the head and neck, they may obstruct the larynx or esophagus [50–54]. Although the mycobacterial disease is not common, vaccination with the bacillus Calmette-Guerin (BCG) vaccine may cause permanent lymphadenopathy or fistula.

In addition to aggressive management of infections with antibiotics, treatment may sometimes require surgical incision and drainage. Trimethoprim/sulfamethoxazole prophylactic administration has been shown to reduce the incidence of severe bacterial infections, and interferon-gamma (IFN-g) therapy has been shown to reduce both bacterial and fungal infections [53].

7.5.3 Chediak-Higashi Disease (CHD)

It is a rare disease that causes neutrophil dysfunction. As a result of mutation in the LYST gene, defects occur in the chemotaxis and degranulation functions of neutrophils, resulting in susceptibility to bacterial infections. Serious periodontal infections can be seen [55]. Especially there is a predisposition to S. aureus and beta-hemolytic streptococcal infections.

Peripheral neuropathy, platelet defects, and mental retardation are other findings that can be observed in this disease [43].

The disease can progress to an accelerated phase in which macrophages and T-lymphocytes infiltrate into the liver, spleen, and bone marrow leading to pancytopenia and thus death. When the disease reaches its final stage, bone marrow transplantation may be required [56].

7.5.4 Hyper-IgE Syndrome (HIgES)

Although the name seems to be a humoral immune disorder, the disease consists of a phagocytosis defect.

It has autosomal dominant and recessive forms. The autosomal dominant form, the most common disease in this group, is caused by STAT3 mutations. Various connective tissue and skeletal abnormalities can be observed in these patients. The genetic etiology of the more rare autosomal recessive forms has not been clearly revealed yet [57].

There is a problem with neutrophil and monocyte chemotaxis. S. aureus is the most common pathogen seen in this syndrome and patients have high levels of anti S. aureus serum IgE antibody [58, 59].

Nasal septal perforation due to severe cervicofacial infections and abscess can be observed [60]. They have typical facial morphologies related to craniosynostosis [61]. Common eczema can be observed. As in humoral immune deficiencies, otitis media is frequently observed in HGES. In addition, other URTIs, such as recurrent and chronic sinusitis, severe pharyngitis, laryngitis, and/or tonsillitis, have been reported in HGES patients [62].

In treatment, early antimicrobial initiation and skin protection are important.

7.6 Cellular Disorders

7.6.1 Di George Syndrome

DiGeorge syndrome is a disease caused by a 22q11.2 (del22) genetic mutation. With this mutation, a defect occurs in the development of the third and fourth pharyngeal clefts. Under normal conditions, parathyroid and thymus glands form from these pharyngeal arches [63–65].

With a defect in the thymus, T lymphocyte maturation deteriorates. With this deterioration, recurrent diarrhea, mucocutaneous candidiasis, pneumonia (especially Pneumocystis carinii pneumonia), chronic rhinosinusitis, and otitis media can be observed [66, 67].

These infections start early in life and may be accompanied by developmental disorders. Patients with the complete DiGeorge form are similar to patients with severe combined immunodeficiency disease (SCID) in terms of susceptibility to infection.

However, in many cases a partial form is observed in which the immunodeficiency is less severe and the clinical symptoms are less severe [65–67].

Most patients do not require treatment in DiGeorge syndrome. Treatment methods ranging from thymus tissue transplantation or bone marrow transplantation can be used in patients with more severe symptoms and SCID-like symptoms [66, 67].

Non-immunological morphological findings of DiGeorge syndrome may progress with facial morphological anomalies. Among these findings are abnormal helix development, low localized ears micrognathia, hypertelorism, antimongoloid sloping eyes, high arched palate, and bifid uvula [68]. Various congenital heart defects and large vessel anomalies such as truncus arteriosus can also be observed in patients [69].

7.6.2 Chronic Mucocutaneous Candidiasis (CMC)

Chronic mucocutaneous candidiasis usually occurs in early childhood [70–72]. Chronic mucocutaneous candidiasis; Sporadic form, familial variant, and the type associated with endocrinopathy (the most common being autoimmune polyendocrinopathy candidiasis ectodermal dystrophy), and a heterogeneous group of diseases with late onset types [71].

Mutations in interleukin-17 (IL-17) pathways are mainly blamed in the pathophysiology. Cellular response to IL-17 is very important for C. Albicans. Autosomal recessive mutation in the cytokine receptor of interleukin-17 receptor A (IL-17RA) completely abolishes the cellular response to IL-17A and IL-17F. Another mutation is the IL17F mutation and it is inherited autosomal dominantly. There is a partial response in this defect and it does not eliminate cellular activity [73].

Recurrent or severe infections may be observed, including viral, bacterial, and other fungal pathogens. Low iron blood levels and decreased storage iron are observed in some patients associated with reduced absorption. Iron replacement should be initiated in these patients [26]. URI evaluation may be requested for oral candidiasis or dysphagia secondary to esophageal or hypopharyngeal involvement.

There are secondary causes of chronic candidiasis. Among them are infancy, long-term use of antibiotics or inhaled steroids, immunosuppressive therapy, diabetes mellitus, some neoplasms (lymphoreticular malignancy), HIV infection, AIDS, SCID, and other combined immune deficiencies.

The clinical picture, including the presence of other infections for diagnosis, helps to distinguish the primary cause of CMC.

Recommended treatment includes systemic antifungals such as fluconazole, ketoconazole, itraconazole, voriconazole or posaconazole or amphotericin B. In severe cases antifungal therapy containing azole is recommended for a long time [74].

7.6.3 T-Helper-1 Cytokine Signal Impairment

Several genetic defects are blamed in the pathogenesis. There is a problem with Interleukin 12 (IL-12) and Interferon gamma (IF-g) receptors. These cytokines are responsible for cell-mediated immunity against intracellular pathogens.

Recurrent Mycobacterial infections and Salmonella infections are observed in these patients. Since the immune response to mycobacterial infections is weak, granuloma formation is weak [75]. The first application of children can be with cervical suppurative abscess formation. Development of mycobacterial infection can be observed after BCG vaccination [76].

Exogenous IF can be given as cytokine therapy in treatment [76].

7.7 Primary Combined Immunodeficiencies

7.7.1 Severe Combined Immunodeficiency (SCID)

The genetics of severe combined immunodeficiency (SCID) are variable, with 42% X-linked recessive inheritance (X-SCID) and 20% autosomal recessive inheritance [25, 77, 78]. Generally, X-SCID occurs earlier and with severe symptoms. While patients with SCID experience problems with both humoral and cellular immunity, severe defects can be observed, including lymphopenia, reduced delayed-type hypersensitivity, low serum immunoglobulins, and weak specific antibody formation against immunogens. However, patients usually have a normal number of B cells [79].

The clinical presentation is generally characterized by frequent and recurrent lung and digestive system infections in the first few months of life. Recurrent diarrhea, sepsis, pneumonia, and skin infections can lead to growth retardation. Recurrent upper respiratory tract infections such as pharyngitis, acute otitis media and mastoiditis, adenotonsillitis, sinusitis, rhinitis, oral ulcers, and thrush are common. URF infections are observed in more than 70% of patients before diagnosis as a result of immunodeficiency in SCID patients [80].

Patients with SCID are susceptible to a variety of organisms, including Candida, Pneumocystis carinii pneumonia, Varicella, measles, parainfluenza virus, Cytomegalovirus, and EBV.

In these patients, the thymus is small and does not descend into the mediastinum. Lymph nodes and adenotonsillar tissue are often hypoplastic [81]. Like other patients with severe T-cell deficiencies, SCID patients are highly susceptible to graft-versus host disease caused by transfusion with non-irradiated blood products. There is a 95% chance of survival if bone marrow transplantation is performed in the first 3 months of life. If diagnosis is delayed, high mortality rates are observed between the ages of 1 and 2 years.

7.7.2 Wiscott-Aldrich Syndrome

Wiscott-Aldrich syndrome: Although it involves both cell-mediated and humoral immune problems, it can also cause additional systemic problems such as thrombocytopenia, eczema, and susceptibility to malignant and autoimmune diseases [82, 83]. Mutations in the Wiscott-Aldrich syndrome protein (WASP), an intracellular protein expressed in lymphocytes and megakaryocytes, are inherited in an X-linked recessive fashion. There are impaired cellular immunity and decreased antibody response (IgM and sometimes IgG) against polysaccharide and protein antigens [83].

Infections (pneumonia, sepsis, meningitis, otitis media) usually occur in the first year of life and are often caused by pneumococci and other encapsulated bacteria. Besides P. carinii and Herpesvirus, other common pathogens can also be observed. In these patients, otitis media, atopic asthma, and eczema are common. Patients who survive infancy are susceptible to autoimmune vasculitis and malignancy [82, 84].

Intravenous immunoglobulin intake can reduce the frequency of serious infections. Thrombocytopenia is treated with thrombocyte transfusions or splenectomy [26, 85]. Bone marrow transplantation can be performed if there is a matching sibling donor; otherwise, death rates are high in the second decade [86].

7.8 Secondary Immunodeficiencies

7.8.1 Human immunodeficiency virus (HIV) and Acquired Immunodeficiency Syndrome (AIDS)

Symptoms related to HIV in URI are very common and are seen in approximately 10% of infected patients. Oral candidiasis is the most common mucocutaneous manifestation of HIV in the pediatric population. It has been reported in approximately 60–75% of symptomatic pediatric patients [87, 88]. In the treatment of oral candidiasis, Clotrimazole lozenge, nystatin oral suspension, and lozenges are used. Fluconazole, intraconazole, and voriconazole can be used systemically in mild and moderate infections [89].

Recurrent otitis media associated with HIV infection is common in children. Generally responsible organisms are Staphylococcus epidermidis, Pneumococcus, Enterococcus, Escherichia coli, and Pseudomonas aeruginosa. Broad spectrum antibiotherapy is used in treatment. Mastoidectomy may be required in cases resistant to medical treatment. Unilateral and bilateral facial paralysis are more likely to occur in HIV patients [89].

55% of children present with the first URI symptom before the age of 3. 98% of the patients show URI symptoms at the age of 9. Common URI findings include cervical, lymph adenopathy (70%), otitis media (46%), oral candidiasis (35%), and adenotonsillar disease (31%) [90].

Masses in the head and neck in pediatric patients may be HIV related. Cervical lymph adenopathies may be observed. In case of rapid growth or pain in the mass under close observation, further investigation and treatment may be required in terms of lymphoma or secondary infection.

An enlarged unilateral or bilateral parotid gland can be an early sign of HIV disease. Most are multilocular, but can also be monolocular [31]. Understanding that the mass is a lymphoepithelial cyst should be warning for HIV infection [91].

7.8.2 Secondary Immune Deficiencies Non-HIV Infection

Among the conditions that cause immunodeficiency other than HIV infection are chemotherapy treatment, autoimmune disorders, malignancies, nephrotic syndrome, splenectomy, long-term corticosteroid use, diabetes mellitus.

Patients undergoing bone marrow transplantation (BMT) have their immune systems almost completely ablated before the donor marrow is vaccinated, leaving the body defenseless.

Solid organ transplant recipients often undergo subtotal immunosuppression. However, although immunosuppressive regimens are reduced, the immunodeficiency state may persist for years after transplantation.

In transplant patients, factors are mostly caused by opportunistic infections in the organs of the donor or recipient waiting to be reactivated. In investigating the etiology of the infections that develop in these patients, it is very important at what stage of transplantation the infection occurs [78]. Accordingly, the pathogen can possibly be predicted and guided in the treatment to be initiated against the infection. Prophylactic antiviral and antibacterial therapy is generally recommended (Table 7.1).

Bone marrow transplant patients are extremely susceptible to acute bacterial and fungal rhinosinusitis, with a reported incidence of up to 30% [92]. The most common cause of fungal sinusitis is Aspergillus. Although the incidence of invasive fungal sinusitis is reported as 0.5–4%, mortality reaches 50–90% [93]. Treatment of invasive

Table 7.1 Ear, Nose, and Throat Infections in Immunocompromised Children

The disease	Sub-Class	Pathophysiology	Diagnosis age	ENT findings and infections	Potential Pathogens	Treatment of the disease
1.Transient hypogammaglobulinemia of the infant (THI)	Humoral immune deficiency	It is not clear. There are different theories.	After 3.-6. Months	Sinusitis, bronchitis, Oral candidiasis, rarely pneumonia	Non-specific bacterial infections	Observation, during the infection or prophylactic antibiotherapy, rarely IVIG
2.Common variable immune deficiency (CVID)	Humoral immune deficiency	Low serum immunoglobulin concentration, defective specific antibody production. Probably polygenic.	Variable related to symptom severity	Chronic respiratory tract infections, sinusitis, otitis media, intestinal tract infections	Encapsulated bacteria, herpesvirus family	IVIG treatment and antibiotic prophylaxis
3. X-linked (Bruton's) agammaglobulinemia (XLA)	Humoral immune deficiency	Defect in B cell differentiation by mutation in Bruton tyrosine kinase (BTK)	After 6 months	No tonsillar or coexisting cervical lymph nodes, recurrent pyogenic upper respiratory tract infections	*Pseudomonas aeruginosa, H. influenzae, pneumococcus and other streptococci*	IVIG treatment, Antibiotherapy
4.Selective IgA deficiency (IgAD)	Humoral immune deficiency	It is not clear. Probably flaw in IG grade change.	After 4 years	Rhinosinusitis, otitis media, mastoiditis, adenotonsillitis and recurrent parotitis	*Streptococcus pneumoniae, Haemophilus influenzae.* (encapsulated bacteria)	During the infection period or prophylactic antibiotherapy should be given. IgA replacement should not be done due to the risk of anaphylaxis

5. IgG subclass deficiencies	Humoral immune deficiency	It is not clear. There may be a B cell differentiation disorder.	Usually in childhood	Recurrent ear infections, sinusitis, bronchitis and pneumonia	Especially encapsulated bacteria	IVIG treatment, Antibiotherapy
6. Hyper IgM syndrome (HIgMS)	Humoral immune deficiency	CD40 ligand defect. IgM production as a result of differentiation in B cells	6 months-2 years	Peritonsillar and other soft tissue infections of the neck, adenotonsillar hypertrophy, pneumonia	*Pneumocystis carinii pneumonia*	IVIG therapy, Antibiotherapy, G-CSF if required
7. Myeloperoxidase deficiency (MPO)	Phagocytosis disorders	Neutrophil phagocytosis disorder with MPO deficiency enzyme deficiency	Variable (even at adulthood)	Recurrent candidiasis, invasive fungal sinusitis	*Candida albicans and Aspergillus hyphae*	Antibiotherapy, antifungal
8. Chronic granulomatous disease (CGD)	Phagocytosis disorders	Phox gene mutation that produces NAPDH oxidase.	2 years	Pneumonia, skin infections, and cervical lymphadenopathy	*S. aureus, Aspergillus, Nocardia &Serratia*	Trimethoprim / sulfamethoxazole prophylaxis, interferon-gamma therapy
9. Chediak-Higashi disease (CHD)	Phagocytosis disorders	Chemotaxis degranulation defect of neutrophils with mutations in the LYST gene	Usually under the age of 5 (can also be diagnosed in adulthood)	Pyogenic upper respiratory tract infections, periodontitis, Oculocutaneous albinism	*S. aureus and beta-hemolytic streptococcus*	Bone marrow transplantation
10. Hyper-IgE syndrome (HIgES)	Phagocytosis disorders	There is a problem with neutrophil and monocyte chemotaxis STAT 3 mutation	Variable (can also be diagnosed in adulthood)	Otitis media, chronic sinusitis, tonsillitis, typical facial morphology	*S. aureus*	Antibiotherapy, IVIG, skin protection

(continued)

Table 7.1 (continued)

The disease	Sub-Class	Pathophysiology	Diagnosis age	ENT findings and infections	Potential Pathogens	Treatment of the disease
11. DiGeorge syndrome	Cellular disorders	22q11.2 deletion. Deterioration in T lymphocyte maturation	After 3 months	Mucocutaneous candidiasis, pneumonias, chronic rhinosinusitis and otitis media, typical facial appearance	*Candida, Pneumocystis carinii*	Thymus or bone marrow transplantation
12. Chronic mucocutaneous candidiasis	Cellular disorders	IL-17RA and IL-17F mutations. Disruption in IL-17 pathway	In early childhood	Oral candidiasis, candida esophagitis	*Candida albicans, Staphylococcus aureus*	Local or systemic antifungals
13. T-helper-1 cytokine signaling defects	Cellular disorders	Problem with interleukin 12 (IL-12) and interferon gamma (IF-g) receptors	In early childhood	Suppurative abscess formations	Mycobacterial infections and Salmonella infections	Antibiotherapy, exogenous IF-g
14. Severe combined immunodeficiency (SCID)	Combined immunodeficiency	Genes responsible for the function of T and B cells are affected.	1st week of life	Pharyngitis, acute otitis media, mastoiditis, adenotonsillitis, sinusitis, rhinitis, oral ulcers, thrush, pneumonia, Sepsis	Candida, Pneumocystis carinii, varicella, measles, parainfluenza virus, CMV, EBV	Bone marrow transplant in the first 3 months of life
15. Wiscott-Aldrich syndrome	Combined immunodeficiency	WASP mutations	1st year of life	Pneumonia, sepsis, meningitis, otitis media	Encapsulated bacteria, P. carinii and herpesvirus	IVIG, splenectomy, bone marrow transplant

fungal sinusitis almost always involves aggressive medical and surgical therapy; however, the extent of surgical debridement is controversial. Although radical excision of all involved tissue is not necessary, surgical intervention is always indicated to reduce infectious burden and eliminate anatomical barriers to sinus drainage. Medical treatment includes the potent antifungal agent amphotericin B and granulocyte colony stimulating factor (GCSF) or granulocyte transfusions of the neutrophil count. Like BMT patients, solid organ transplant (SOT) recipients are susceptible to bacterial and fungal sinusitis, but the incidence of invasive fungal sinusitis is much lower. In these patients, the incidence of invasive fungal sinusitis was observed to be 0.25% [94]. Most cases of bacterial sinusitis in this population can be managed on an outpatient basis with oral antibiotics, but patients should be evaluated for fungal co-infection when severe symptoms or resistance to treatment are observed. Antibiotics used in the treatment of these patients should be in a broad spectrum, including Staphylococcus and Pseudomonas. It is recommended that paranasal sinus CT should be performed before transplantation and close follow-up of patients during the transplantation phase for sinusitis in pediatric and adult patients who underwent allogeneic bone marrow transplant. It may cause complications in a short time [95]. An increase in infections caused by encapsulated bacteria can be seen in patients with splenectomy. Steroid use causes susceptibility to infection, especially in treatments taken at 20–40 mg doses lasting 4–6 weeks or longer. This regimen is generally used in transplant patients and rheumatologic diseases. Steroids disrupt phagocyte migration and affect T-lymphocyte functions [56]. Vaccination in immunocompromised children: The severity of the primary disease may limit efforts to vaccinate pediatric patients early in the disease process, prior to immunosuppression. According to our classical knowledge, inactivated vaccines are safe and immunogenic after administration of immunosuppression, but live vaccines are contraindicated. Recent data support the safety and efficacy of live vaccines in certain immunosuppressed individuals [1].

References

1. Miller K, Leake K, Sharma T. Advances in vaccinating immunocompromised children. Curr Opin Pediatr. 2020;32:145–50. https://doi.org/10.1097/MOP.0000000000000846.
2. Immune Deficiency Foundation. Diagnostic and clinical care guidelines for primary immunodeficiency diseases. Available at: http://www.primaryimmune.org/publications/book_diag/IDF_Diagnostic_and_Clinical_Care_Guidelines-Final.pdf2006. Accessed 6 Oct 2008.
3. Manning SC, Wasserman RL, Leach J, Truelson J. Chronic sinusitis as a manifestation of primary immunodeficiency in Adults. Am J Rhinol. 1994;8:29–36. https://doi.org/10.2500/105065894781882657.
4. Jeffrey Modell Foundation: Primary Immunodeficiency Resource Centre., Available at: http://www.info4pi.org/aboutPI/index.cfm?section=aboutPI&content=warningsigns&TrkId=24&CFID=40303331&CFTOKEN=79353748. Accessed 4 July 2020.
5. Bonilla FA, Bernstein IL, Khan DA, et al. Practice parameter for the diagnosis and management of primary immunodeficiency. Ann Allergy Asthma Immunol. 2005;94 https://doi.org/10.1016/S1081-1206(10)61142-8.
6. Dalal, I., and Roifman, C. H. 2006. Transient hypogammaglobulinemia of infancy. UpToDate www.uptodate.com, pp. 1–10.

7. Seidel MG, Kindle G, Gathmann B, et al. The European Society for Immunodeficiencies (ESID) registry working definitions for the clinical diagnosis of inborn errors of immunity. J Allergy Clin Immunol Pract. 2019;7:1763–70. https://doi.org/10.1016/j.jaip.2019.02.004.
8. Fudenberg HH, Fudenberg BR. Antibody to hereditary human gamma-globulin (Gm) factor resulting from maternal-fetal incompatibility. Science. 1964;145(80):170–1. https://doi.org/10.1126/science.145.3628.170.
9. Nathenson G, Schorr J, Litwin SD. Gm Factor Fetomaternal Gamma Globulin I ncompatibility. Pediatr Res. 1971;5:2–9.
10. Siegel RL, Issekutz T, Schwaber J, et al. Deficiency of T Helper cells in transient Hypogammaglobulinemia of infancy. N Engl J Med. 1981;305:1307–13. https://doi.org/10.1056/nejm198111263052202.
11. Kowalczyk D, Mytar B, Zembala M. Cytokine production in transient hypogammaglobulinemia and isolated IgA deficiency. J Allergy Clin Immunol. 1997;100:556–62. https://doi.org/10.1016/S0091-6749(97)70150-7.
12. Stiehm ER. The four most common pediatric immunodeficiencies. J Immunotoxicol. 2008;5:227–34. https://doi.org/10.1080/15476910802129646.
13. Schroeder HW, Schroeder HW, Sheikh SM. The complex genetics of common variable immunodeficiency. J. Investig. Med. 2004;52:90–103.
14. Cunningham-Rundles C. Common variable immunodeficiency. Curr Allergy Asthma Rep. 2001;1:421–9.
15. Magliulo G, Iannella G, Granata G, et al. Otologic evaluation of patients with primary antibody deficiency. Eur Arch Oto-Rhino-Laryngol. 2016;273:3537–46. https://doi.org/10.1007/s00405-016-3956-y.
16. Urschel S, Kayikci L, Wintergerst U, et al. Common variable immunodeficiency disorders in children: delayed diagnosis despite typical clinical presentation. J Pediatr. 2009;154:888–94. https://doi.org/10.1016/j.jpeds.2008.12.020.
17. Quinti I, Soresina A, Spadaro G, et al. Long-term follow-up and outcome of a large cohort of patients with common variable immunodeficiency. J Clin Immunol. 2007;27:308–16. https://doi.org/10.1007/s10875-007-9075-1.
18. Aghamohammadi A, Moazzami K, Rezaei N, et al. ENT manifestations in Iranian patients with primary antibody deficiencies. J Laryngol Otol. 2008;122:409–13. https://doi.org/10.1017/S0022215107008626.
19. Yew KC, Decker PA, O'Byrne MM, Weiler CR. Clinical and laboratory characteristics of 75 patients with specific polysaccharide antibody deficiency syndrome. Ann Allergy Asthma Immunol. 2006;97:306–11. https://doi.org/10.1016/s1081-1206(10)60794-6.
20. Manning SC. Surgical management of sinus disease in children. Ann Otol Rhinol Laryngol Suppl. 1991;155:42–5.
21. Roifman CM, Levison H, Gelfand EW. High-dose versus low-dose intravenous immunoglobulin in Hypogammaglobulinaemia and chronic lung disease. Lancet. 1987;329:1075–7. https://doi.org/10.1016/S0140-6736(87)90494-6.
22. Busse PJ, Razvi S, Cunningham-Rundles C. Efficacy of intravenous immunoglobulin in the prevention of pneumonia in patients with common variable immunodeficiency. J Allergy Clin Immunol. 2002;109:1001–4. https://doi.org/10.1067/mai.2002.124999.
23. Carsetti R, Rosado MM, Donnanno S, et al. The loss of IgM memory B cells correlates with clinical disease in common variable immunodeficiency. J Allergy Clin Immunol. 2005;115:412–7. https://doi.org/10.1016/j.jaci.2004.10.048.
24. Warnatz K, Denz A, Dräger R, et al. Severe deficiency of switched memory B cells (CD27+IgM-IgD-) in subgroups of patients with common variable immunodeficiency: A new approach to classify a heterogeneous disease. Blood. 2002;99:1544–51. https://doi.org/10.1182/blood.V99.5.1544.
25. Ko J, Radigan L, Cunningham-Rundles C. Immune competence and switched memory B cells in common variable immunodeficiency. Clin Immunol. 2005;116:37–41. https://doi.org/10.1016/j.clim.2005.03.019.

26. De Vincentiis GC, Sitzia E, Bottero S, et al. Otolaryngologic manifestations of pediatric immunodeficiency. Int J Pediatr Otorhinolaryngol. 2009;73:S42–8. https://doi.org/10.1016/S0165-5876(09)70009-6.
27. Conley ME, Mathias D, Treadaway J, et al. Mutations in Btk in patients with presumed X-linked agammaglobulinemia. Am J Hum Genet. 1998;62:1034–43. https://doi.org/10.1086/301828.
28. Genevier HC, Hinshelwood S, Gaspar HB, et al. Expression of Bruton's tyrosine kinase protein within the B cell lineage. Eur J Immunol. 1994;24:3100–5. https://doi.org/10.1002/eji.1830241228.
29. Smith CI, Baskin B, Humire-Greiff P, et al. Expression of Bruton's agammaglobulinemia tyrosine kinase gene, BTK, is selectively down-regulated in T lymphocytes and plasma cells. J Immunol. 1994;152:557–65.
30. Conley ME, Howard V. Clinical findings leading to the diagnosis of X-linked agammaglobulinemia. J Pediatr. 2002;141:566–71. https://doi.org/10.1067/mpd.2002.127711.
31. Quartier P, Debré M, De Blic J, et al. Early and prolonged intravenous immunoglobulin replacement therapy in childhood agammaglobulinemia: A retrospective survey of 31 patients. J Pediatr. 1999;134:589–96. https://doi.org/10.1016/S0022-3476(99)70246-5.
32. Latiff AHA, Kerr MA. The clinical significance of immunoglobulin A deficiency. Ann. Clin. Biochem. 2007;44:131–9.
33. Abolhassani H, Aghamohammadi A, Hammarström L. Monogenic mutations associated with IgA deficiency. Expert Rev. Clin. Immunol. 2016;12:1321–35.
34. Singh K, Chang C, Gershwin ME. IgA deficiency and autoimmunity. Autoimmun Rev. 2014;13:163–77.
35. Ballow M. Primary immunodeficiency disorders: Antibody deficiency. J Allergy Clin Immunol. 2002;109:581–91. https://doi.org/10.1067/mai.2002.122466.
36. Bossuyt X, Moens L, Van Hoeyveld E, et al. Coexistence of (partial) immune defect and risk of recurrent respiratory infections. Clin Chem. 2007;53:124–30. https://doi.org/10.1373/clinchem.2007.075861.
37. Edwards E, Razvi S, Cunningham-Rundles C. IgA deficiency: clinical correlates and responses to pneumococcal vaccine. Clin Immunol. 2004;111:93–7. https://doi.org/10.1016/j.clim.2003.12.005.
38. French MAH, Denis KA, Dawkins R, Peter JB. Severity of infections in IgA deficiency: correlation with decreased serum antibodies to pneumococcal polysaccharides and decreased serum IgG2 and/or IgG4. Clin Exp Immunol. 1995;100:47–53. https://doi.org/10.1111/j.1365-2249.1995.tb03602.x.
39. Cunningham-Rundles C. Physiology of Iga and Iga deficiency. J Clin Immunol. 2001;21:303–9.
40. Kimmelman CP, Potsic WP. Immunodeficiency in pediatric otolaryngology. Am J Otolaryngol Neck Med Surg. 1979;1:33–8. https://doi.org/10.1016/S0196-0709(79)80006-X.
41. Burks AW, Sampson HA, Buckley RH. Anaphylactic reactions after Gamma globulin administration in patients with hypogammaglobulinemia. N Engl J Med. 1986;314:560–4. https://doi.org/10.1056/nejm198602273140907.
42. Shackelford PG, Polmar SH, Mayus JL, et al. Spectrum of IgG2 subclass deficiency in children with recurrent infections: Prospective study. J Pediatr. 1986;108:647–53. https://doi.org/10.1016/S0022-3476(86)81035-6.
43. McCusker C, Warrington R. Primary immunodeficiency. Allergy Asthma Clin Immunol. 2011;7:S11. https://doi.org/10.1186/1710-1492-7-s1-s11.
44. Notarangelo LD, Duse M, Ugazio AG. Immunodeficiency with hyper-IgM (HIM). Immunodefic: Rev. 1992;3:101–21.
45. Haddad J, Brager R, Bluestone CD. Infections of the ears, nose, and throat in children with primary immunodeficiencies. Arch Otolaryngol Neck Surg. 1992;118:138–41. https://doi.org/10.1001/archotol.1992.01880020030011.
46. Winkelstein JA, Marino MC, Johnston RB, et al. Chronic granulomatous disease: Report on a national registry of 368 patients. Medicine. 2000;79:155–69. https://doi.org/10.1097/00005792-200005000-00003.

47. Weber ML, Abela A, de Repentigny L, et al. Myeloperoxidase deficiency with extensive candidal osteomyelitis of the base of the skull. Pediatrics. 1987;80:876–9.
48. Pahwa R, Modi P, Jialal I. Myeloperoxidase deficiency. Treasure Island, FL: Stat Pearls Publishing; 2020.
49. Lekstrom-Himes JA, Gallin JI. Immunodeficiency diseases caused by defects in phagocytes. N Engl J Med. 2000;343:1703–14. https://doi.org/10.1056/nejm200012073432307.
50. Gray S. Otolaryngologic manifestations of chronic granulomatous disease. Am J Otolaryngol-Head Neck Med Surg. 1988;9:79–82. https://doi.org/10.1016/S0196-0709(88)80011-5.
51. Blayney AW, Bunch C. Mastoid surgery in chronic granulomatous disease. J Laryngol Otol. 1984;98:187–8. https://doi.org/10.1017/S0022215100146390.
52. Daley AJ, McIntyre P, Kakakios A, et al. Ulcerative lesion of the nasal bridge in a five-month-old infant. Pediatr Infect Dis J. 1999;18(10):936–7. https://doi.org/10.1097/00006454-199910000-00019.
53. Gallin JI. Interferon-γ in the treatment of the chronic granulomatous diseases of childhood. Clin Immunol Immunopathol. 1991;61:S100–5. https://doi.org/10.1016/S0090-1229(05)80044-3.
54. Gallin JI, Farber JM, Holland SM, Nutman TB. Interferon-γ in the management of infectious diseases. Ann Intern Med. 1995;123(3):216–24.
55. Delcourt-Debruyne EMC, Boutigny HRA, Hildebrand HF. Features of Severe Periodontal Disease in a Teenager With Chédiak-Higashi Syndrome. J Periodontol. 2000;71:816–24. https://doi.org/10.1902/jop.2000.71.5.816.
56. Sikora AG, Lee KC. Otolaryngologic manifestations of immunodeficiency. Otolaryngol Clin North Am. 2003;36:647–72. https://doi.org/10.1016/S0030-6665(03)00034-3.
57. Freeman AF, Holland SM. The Hyper-IgE Syndromes. Immunol Allergy Clin North Am. 2008;28:277–91.
58. Grimbacher B, Holland SM, Gallin JI, et al. Hyper-IgE syndrome with recurrent infections — an autosomal dominant multisystem disorder. N Engl J Med. 1999;340:692–702. https://doi.org/10.1056/nejm199903043400904.
59. Hatori M, Yoshiya M, Kurachi Y, Nagumo M. Prolonged infection of the floor of the mouth in hyperimmunoglobulinemia E (Buckley's syndrome). Report of a case. Oral Surg Oral Med Oral Pathol. 1993;76:289–93. https://doi.org/10.1016/0030-4220(93)90255-3.
60. Fernandez M, Roman J, Latasa M, et al. Perforation of the nasal wall and hyper-IgE syndrome. J Investig Allergol Clin Immunol. 1993;3:217–20.
61. Barges WG, Hensley T, Carey JC, et al. The face of Job. J Pediatr. 1998;133:303–5. https://doi.org/10.1016/s0022-3476(98)70243-4.
62. Wu J, Hong L, Chen TX. Clinical manifestation of hyper IgE syndrome including otitis media. Curr Allergy Asthma Rep. 2018;18.
63. Schubert M, Moss R. Selective polysaccharide antibody deficiency in familial DiGeorge syndrome. Ann Allergy. 1992;69:231–8.
64. Müller W, Peter HH, Wilken M, et al. The DiGeorge syndrome - I. Clinical evaluation and course of partial and complete forms of the syndrome. Eur J Pediatr. 1988;147:496–502. https://doi.org/10.1007/BF00441974.
65. Junker AK, Driscoll DA. Humoral immunity in DiGeorge syndrome. J Pediatr. 1995;127:231–7. https://doi.org/10.1016/S0022-3476(95)70300-4.
66. Müller W, Peter HH, Kallfelz HC, et al. The DiGeorge sequence II. Immunologic findings in partial and complete forms of the disorder. Eur J Pediatr. 1989;149:96–103. https://doi.org/10.1007/BF01995856.
67. Matsumoto T, Amamoto N, Kondoh T, et al. Complete-type DiGeorge syndrome treated by bone marrow transplantation. Bone Marrow Transplant. 1998;22:927–30. https://doi.org/10.1038/sj.bmt.1701475.
68. Hong R. The DiGeorge anomaly. Immunodeficiency Rev. 1991;3(1):1–14.
69. Goldmuntz E, Emanuel BS. Genetic disorders of cardiac morphogenesis: The DiGeorge and velocardiofacial syndromes. Circ. Res. 1997;80:437–43.
70. Kirkpatrick CH, Hill HR. Chronic mucocutaneous candidiasis. Pediatr Infect Dis J. 2001;20:197–206. https://doi.org/10.1097/00006454-200102000-00017.

71. Lilic D, Gravenor I. Immunology of chronic mucocutaneous candidiasis. J Clin Pathol. 2001;54:81–3. https://doi.org/10.1136/jcp.54.2.81.
72. Jagtap S, Saple J, Dhaliat S. Congenital cutaneous candidiasis: A rare and unpredictable disease. Indian J Dermatol. 2011;56:92. https://doi.org/10.4103/0019-5154.77564.
73. Puel A, Cypowyj S, Bustamante J, et al. Chronic mucocutaneous candidiasis in humans with inborn errors of interleukin-17 immunity. Science. 2011;332(80):65–8. https://doi.org/10.1126/science.1200439.
74. Firinu D, Massidda O, Lorrai MM, et al. Successful treatment of chronic mucocutaneous candidiasis caused by azole-resistant Candida albicans with posaconazole. Clin Dev Immunol. 2011;2011:283239. https://doi.org/10.1155/2011/283239.
75. Gollob JA, Veenstra KG, Jyonouchi H, et al. Impairment of STAT Activation by IL-12 in a Patient with Atypical Mycobacterial and Staphylococcal Infections. J Immunol. 2000;165:4120–6. https://doi.org/10.4049/jimmunol.165.7.4120.
76. Nylén O, Berg-Kelly K, Andersson B. Cervical lymph node infections with non-tuberculous mycobacteria in preschool children: interferon gamma deficiency as a possible cause of clinical infection. Acta Paediatr. 2000;89:1322–5. https://doi.org/10.1080/080352500300002507.
77. Buckley RH. Primary immunodeficiency diseases: Dissectors of the immune system. Immunol Rev. 2002;185:206–19.
78. Steele RW. Managing infection in cancer patients and other immunocompromised children. Ochsner J. 2012;12:202–10.
79. Buckley RH, Schiff RI, Schiff SE, et al. Human severe combined immunodeficiency: Genetic, phenotypic, and functional diversity in one hundred eight infants. J Pediatr. 1997;130:378–87. https://doi.org/10.1016/S0022-3476(97)70199-9.
80. Stocks RMS, Thompson JW, Kun S, et al. Severe combined immunodeficiency: Otolaryngological presentation and management. Ann Otol Rhinol Laryngol. 1999;108:403–7. https://doi.org/10.1177/000348949910800415.
81. Stephan JL, Vlekova V, Le Deist F, et al. Severe combined immunodeficiency: A retrospective single-center study of clinical presentation and outcome in 117 patients. J Pediatr. 1993;123:564–72. https://doi.org/10.1016/S0022-3476(05)80951-5.
82. Sullivan KE, Mullen CA, Blaese RM, Winkelstein JA. A multiinstitutional survey of the Wiskott-Aldrich syndrome. J Pediatr. 1994;125:876–85. https://doi.org/10.1016/S0022-3476(05)82002-5.
83. Ochs HD. The Wiskott-Aldrich syndrome. Seminars in hematology. 1998;35(4):332–45.
84. Akman IO, Ostrov BE, Neudorf S. Autoimmune manifestations of the Wiskott-Aldrich syndrome. Semin Arthritis Rheum. 1998;27:218–25. https://doi.org/10.1016/S0049-0172(98)80002-4.
85. Litzman J, Jones A, Hann I, et al. Intravenous immunoglobulin, splenectomy, and antibiotic prophylaxis in Wiskott-Aldrich syndrome. Arch Dis Child. 1996;75:436–9. https://doi.org/10.1136/adc.75.5.436.
86. Ozsahin H, Le Deist F, Benkerrou M, et al. Bone marrow transplantation in 26 patients with Wiskott-Aldrich syndrome from a single center. J Pediatr. 1996;129:238–44. https://doi.org/10.1016/S0022-3476(96)70248-2.
87. Prose NS. Mucocutaneous disease in pediatric human immunodeficiency virus infection. Pediatr Clin North Am. 1991;38:977–90. https://doi.org/10.1016/S0031-3955(16)38163-9.
88. Cooper ER, Pelton SI, LeMay M. Acquired immunodeficiency syndrome: A new population of children at risk. Pediatr Clin North Am. 1988;35(6):1365–87. https://doi.org/10.1016/S0031-3955(16)36589-0.
89. Iacovou E, Vlastarakos PV, Papacharalampous G, et al. Diagnosis and treatment of HIV-associated manifestations in otolaryngology. Infect Dis Rep. 2012;4:9. https://doi.org/10.4081/idr.2012.e9.
90. Singh A, Georgalas C, Patel N, Papesch M. ENT presentations in children with HIV infection. Clin Otolaryngol Allied Sci. 2003;28:240–3. https://doi.org/10.1046/j.1365-2273.2003.00698.x.

91. Som PM, Brandwein MS, Silvers A. Nodal inclusion cysts of the parotid gland and parapharyngeal space: A discussion of lymphoepithelial, aids-related parotid, and branchial cysts, cystic Warthin's tumors, and cysts in Sjögren's syndrome. Laryngoscope. 1995;105:1122–8. https://doi.org/10.1288/00005537-199510000-00020.
92. Shibuya TY, Momin F, Abella E, et al. Sinus disease in the bone marrow transplant population: Incidence, risk factors, and complications. Otolaryngol-Head Neck Surg. 1995;113:705–11. https://doi.org/10.1016/S0194-5998(95)70009-9.
93. Kennedy CA, Adams GL, Neglia JR, Giebink GS. Impact of Surgical Treatment on Paranasal Fungal Infections in Bone Marrow Transplant Patients. Otolaryngol Head Neck Surg. 1997;116:610–6. https://doi.org/10.1016/S0194-5998(97)70236-5.
94. Patel R, Portela D, Badley AD, et al. Risk factors of invasive Candida and non-Candida fungal infections after liver transplantation. Transplantation. 1996;62:926–34. https://doi.org/10.1097/00007890-199610150-00010.
95. Drozd-Sokolowska JE, Sokolowski J, Wiktor-Jedrzejczak W, Niemczyk K. Sinusite em pacientes submetidos a transplante alogênico de medula óssea – uma revisão. Braz J Otorhinolaryngol. 2017;83:105–11. https://doi.org/10.1016/j.bjorl.2016.02.012.

Immunization for Prevention of Ear, Nose, and Throat Infections in Children

8

Sibel Laçinel Gürlevik, Ateş Kara, and Emin Sami Arısoy

8.1 Introduction

Disease prevention methods such as vaccine programs play an essential role in ensuring individual and community health. Vaccination is the most critical and effective primary measure promoted and encouraged by all healthcare professionals.

According to the World Health Organization (WHO) data, 60% of hearing loss occurs due to preventable causes [1]. About 466 million people, including 34 million children, are estimated to have a hearing impairment [2]. Vaccination can prevent infections such as rubella, measles, mumps, and diseases like meningitis, and good healthcare is estimated to prevent 30% of childhood hearing losses [2]. Hearing impairment associated with otitis media is also a significant health problem. It affects the quality of life in approximately one-third of the population in low- and middle-income countries [2]. By strengthening immunization programs and improving healthcare services, hearing impairment due to infections can be precluded [3–5].

In this chapter, vaccines effective for preventing ear, nose, and throat (ENT) infections and hearing loss in pediatric patients will be highlighted.

S. L. Gürlevik (✉) · A. Kara
Division of Pediatric Infectious Diseases, Department of Pediatrics, Faculty of Medicine, Hacettepe University, Ankara, Turkey

E. S. Arısoy
Division of Pediatric Infectious Diseases, Department of Pediatrics, Faculty of Medicine, Kocaeli University, Kocaeli, Turkey

8.2 Measles, Mumps, Rubella, and Varicella Infections and Vaccines

8.2.1 Measles, Mumps, Rubella, and Varicella Infections

Rubella causes mild fever and rashes that last about 2 or 3 days. Rashes initially occur on the face and neck. Although it is a mild disease, it may cause serious complications, such as fetal death or congenital rubella syndrome, if it develops mostly during early pregnancy.

Congenital rubella syndrome can cause malformations in the heart, brain, eyes, and ears. During the first trimester, rubella infection, especially in the first 8–10 weeks, may lead to severe cardiac and ocular problems. Rubella may cause isolated hearing loss if women have rubella infection towards the end of the first half of the pregnancy [6, 7]. Due to congenital rubella infection, generally sensorineural and bilateral hearing loss occurs. Hearing impairment can exist at birth and may be progressive. Despite a worldwide plan to reduce the incidence of congenital rubella syndrome, still many babies are born annually with congenital rubella syndrome [8, 9].

Measles and mumps infections may cause acquired deafness by damaging the eighth cranial nerve and cochlear system [10]. Measles has many complications, and otitis media is among the most common ones. The measles infection can result in permanent bilateral hearing loss.

Mumps mainly causes parotitis, but also meningoencephalitis and deafness. It may cause harm to the cochlear ducts and inner ear. Mumps-related deafness, usually unilateral, occurs with or without meningoencephalitis and may also develop after asymptomatic infection [11]. Vertigo is also noted occasionally in patients with mumps, and it occurs most commonly in those who develop deafness [12–14].

Varicella-zoster virus (VZV) can cause hearing loss by causing neuro-labyrinthitis during the acute infection period [15, 16]. After vaccination and improvement of healthcare opportunities, the incidence of hearing loss due to varicella infection has declined [17].

8.2.2 Measles, Mumps, Rubella, and Varicella Vaccines

Two different vaccine combinations containing live attenuated measles, mumps, and rubella (MMR) vaccines are the trivalent MMR vaccine and the quadrivalent MMRV (MMR plus varicella) vaccine [18].

It is thought that measles and rubella vaccines have lifelong protection [19]. However, mumps vaccination should be repeated during mumps outbreaks. The trivalent MMR vaccine is administered to children over 12 months of age. Still, it can be applied to children over 6 months in international travel and an epidemic. The quadrivalent MMRV vaccine is given to children over 12 months and up to 12 years of age [18]. Both lyophilized vaccines should be prepared and applied as described by the manufacturer and administered subcutaneously.

Most of the committees, such as the United States (US) Centers for Disease Control and Prevention (CDC) Advisory Committee on Immunization Practices (ACIP), American Academy of Pediatrics (AAP), American College of Obstetricians and Gynecologists (ACOG), and American College of Physicians (ACP), state that if there is no evidence that adults are immune, 1 or 2 doses of MMR vaccine should be administered [20, 21].

The MMR vaccine is routinely administered to children in two doses. The first dose should be applied between the ages of 12 and 15 months and the second dose between the ages of 4 and 6 before attending school. If the second dose is administered before the age of 4, at least 28 days should be between the first and the second doses [21]. Two doses of MMR vaccine are also recommended for high-risk groups, such as students attending colleges or other post-high school educational institutions, healthcare workers, and international travelers.

Two doses of MMR vaccine should be administered to those serologically not found immune. Most people may have adequate immune responses for mumps after vaccination; however, some people may not respond adequately [22–25]. Because of this, some people may need a third dose of MMR vaccine during an outbreak [26].

Varicella vaccine, recommended in two doses, contains live, attenuated VZV. The first varicella vaccine dose is administered at 12–15 months of age for the routine vaccination, and the second, as a booster dose at age 4–6 years. However, the second dose can be given as early as 4 weeks after the first dose.

Vaccination with MMR or MMRV vaccines is contraindicated if a severe allergic reaction (e.g., anaphylaxis) occurs towards any of the vaccine's substances, including neomycin and if vaccine-related serious events occurred due to previous vaccination [27]. Vaccination with MMR or MMRV vaccines is also contraindicated for severely immunocompromised patients (e.g., congenital immune deficiencies, those with malignancies receiving chemotherapy, patients with AIDS) and pregnant women [27].

8.3 Vaccination to Prevent Acute Otitis Media

Acute otitis media (AOM) is one of the common infectious diseases of childhood. Viral and bacterial infections are the most common causes of AOM. Bacterial and viral causative microorganisms can co-occur. Maternal antibodies acquired transplacentally may be protective against AOM in the first 6 months of age. Otitis media incidence increases mostly in 6–24 months. *Streptococcus pneumoniae*, non-typeable *Haemophilus influenzae*, *Moraxella catarrhalis*, *Staphylococcus aureus*, and *Streptococcus pyogenes* are the most common pathogens causing otitis media [28].

During viral upper respiratory tract infections (URTIs), mucus production increases, motility of cilia decreases, resulting in the cause of an inflammatory environment in the nasopharynx. Viral URTIs also cause edema of the eustachian tube and its closure, which causes otitis media development easier. Respiratory syncytial virus (RSV), coronavirus, influenza virus, adenovirus, human metapneumovirus, and picornaviruses are the most common AOM agents.

Severe morbidity such as hearing loss can occur due to AOM, so disease prevention is an important issue. Since otitis media is a polymicrobial disease, vaccines against the most common bacteria and viruses can be applied. Routine administration of vaccines and their effect in preventing AOM will also be discussed below.

8.4 Pneumococcal Vaccines

S. pneumoniae has more than 90 serotypes. However, among a large number of *S. pneumoniae* serotypes, very few cause mucosal and invasive diseases in children. Pneumococcal conjugate vaccines (PCVs) have proven to be effective in preventing AOM caused by pneumococcal vaccine serotypes. Studies show that AOM incidence in children under 2 years of age who received the PCV7 vaccine was decreased [29–31].

PCVs also licensed containing the capsule polysaccharides of some other serotypes are now available. The seven-valent PCV (PCV7, Prev[e]nar®) was the first licensed vaccine in 2000. Later on, the 10-valent (PCV10, Synflorix®) and the 13-valent (PCV13, Prevenar 13®) vaccines were licensed. PCV7 was replaced by PCV13 in the USA in 2010 and then in other countries [32]. A series of three or four doses of PCV is given to infants at ages of 2, 4, (±6), and 12 through 15 months.

The 23-valent pneumococcal polysaccharide vaccine (PPSV23, Pneumovax 23®) can produce antibody responses in children 2 years of age or older. Hence, PPSV23 is administered to children over 2 years of age at risk of invasive pneumococcal disease. Children with an immunocompromising condition, cochlear implant, cerebrospinal fluid (CSF) leak, and functional or anatomic asplenia are indicated to have both a PCV (PCV10, PCV13) and PPSV23. There should be at least 8 weeks between the PCV and the PPSV. It is recommended that PPSV23 be applied to the high-risk children aged 2 years and older after $\geq$8 weeks of PCV13 to prevent AOM [33].

Hypersensitivity to diphtheria toxin, when the carrier protein is a nontoxic diphtheria toxin, or anaphylaxis against the previous dose of pcv13 or any vaccine containing diphtheria toxoid is a contraindication for the pcv13. Pneumococcal vaccination is contraindicated if a severe allergic reaction (e.g., anaphylaxis) occurs towards any substances in the vaccine

8.5 *Haemophilus influenzae* Type B Conjugate Vaccines

H. influenzae type b (Hib) was among the most common microorganisms causing pneumonia, meningitis, and epiglottitis, and also causes AOM and sinusitis. In 1990, after the Hib conjugate vaccine was included in the childhood vaccination programs, the epidemiology and clinical presentation of the invasive Hib disease has shifted to adults. In 2011, invasive Hib disease incidence in Europe had been reported as 0.58 cases per 100,000 population [34]. *H. influenzae* type b related epiglottitis rate was around 17% between 2009 and 2012 [35]. In the USA, after the

Hib conjugate vaccine was introduced, a significant decrease in invasive Hib disease has occurred [36, 37].

In the prevaccine era, children under the age of 5 years were the main reservoirs of Hib, with nasopharyngeal colonization rates of 3–9%. By reducing carriage, the Hib conjugate vaccine also reduces transmission to susceptible individuals of all ages, thus providing herd protection [38, 39]. *H. influenzae* type b vaccine is now recommended for all children under the age of 5 years. Currently, there are three monovalent conjugate Hib vaccines and combination vaccines containing those. ActHIB® (PRP-T), Hiberix® (PRP-T), and PedvaxHIB® (PRP-OMB) are three monovalent conjugated vaccines. They can be used in infants as young as 6 weeks of age. Combination vaccines decrease the number of injections needed, are used from 6 weeks of age, and should not be used after 5 years of age.

H. influenzae type b containing vaccines are administered in 4 doses at 2, 4, 6, and 12–18 months. The interval between doses should be at least 28 days. The booster dose should be applied after 1 year of age and at least 6 months after completing the primary series of the first 3 doses.

8.6   Pertussis Vaccines

Pertussis, also known as whooping cough, is caused by *Bordetella pertussis* or *Bordetella parapertussis*. They are found in the mouth, nose, and throat of an infected person. Initially, symptoms resemble those of a common cold, including sneezing, runny nose, low-grade fever, and a mild cough. Later on, pertussis causes severe coughing attacks that can lead to difficulty breathing, vomiting, and sleep disturbance. Acute otitis media can be seen as a complication, a secondary bacterial infection. Whooping cough can spread from person to person through secretions while coughing and sneezing.

There are two types of pertussis vaccines, acellular and whole-cell vaccines [40]. While the number of whooping cough cases was high before introducing pertussis vaccines, it decreased considerably after vaccination programs. As a result of vaccination, complications due to pertussis also reduced. Childhood pertussis vaccines are in combination with tetanus, diphtheria, polio, and/or Hib vaccines. The primary series of pertussis vaccines are administered at 2, 4, and 6 months of age. The fourth dose is applied at 15 to 18 months of age. The fifth one, a booster dose, is applied at 4–6 years of age. The first pertussis vaccine dose may be applied as early as 6 weeks of age [41, 42].

8.7   Diphtheria Vaccines

Diphtheria, caused by *Corynebacterium diphtheria* settled in the throat, nose, eyes, and skin, can lead to severe consequences and death [43]. Diphtheria is characterized by a membranous inflammation of the upper respiratory tract structures, including the pharynx, posterior nasal passages, larynx, and trachea. Within 2 or 3 days, a grayish, thick, and firmly adherent membrane may cover the whole pharynx, and surrounding tissue becomes edematous. It may also give harm to peripheral nerves and the myocardium through diphtheria toxin.

Diphtheria has a more significant mortality and morbidity rate [44]. It may cause upper airway obstruction, and an urgent need for tracheostomy may develop. Secondary AOM may occur due to edematous pharyngeal structures [45]. Because diphtheria has life-threatening complications, it is crucial to prevent the disease.

Even if people had the disease, there is a risk of getting sick again because a complete protective response is not produced. Therefore, not only healthy people but also patients should be vaccinated after the disease. The clinical efficacy of the vaccines is estimated to be 97%. Diphtheria toxoid-containing vaccines are among the oldest vaccines in current use. Diphtheria vaccine is usually in a combination vaccine that includes tetanus and pertussis vaccines [46, 47]. Twelve combination vaccines, 9 of which contain the pertussis vaccine, have been approved by the US Food and Drug Administration (FDA). Some combination vaccines may contain poliovirus, Hib, and hepatitis B vaccines. The diphtheria vaccine is administered at ages 2, 4, and 6 months with the fourth dose at 15–18 months of age. The fifth dose is applied at 4–6 years of age [48].

8.8 Influenza Vaccines

Although AOM is usually due to bacteria, it also occurs as a complication of viral URTI. In most children, AOM is self-limiting, but it does carry a risk of complications. Antibiotic therapy for AOM significantly increases the risk of antibiotic resistance. Influenza vaccines may decrease the risk of AOM by preventing development due to seasonal influenza [49].

Annually applied influenza vaccines should be part of the strategy to reduce the frequency of AOM for children with recurrent and severe disease as recommended by the guidelines [50]. Routine annual influenza vaccination with age-appropriate vaccines should be administered to all children aged ≥ 6 months who do not have contraindications.

8.9 Immunization to Prevent RSV Infection

RSV, a significant infectious agent mostly in infancy, may have substantial morbidity and mortality rates. It is a respiratory infection virus with one serotype and two major antigenic subgroups, A and B. It is believed that most children will experience at least one RSV infection by the age of 2 years [51].

Passive immunization with high titers of the anti-RSV immunoglobulin (palivizumab) has proved beneficial for prophylaxis in high-risk infants, such as premature babies or babies with cyanotic heart disease or chronic lung disease (bronchopulmonary dysplasia).

An effective vaccine against RSV is likely to have a higher impact on the occurrence of AOM following URTI. However, no vaccine effective against RSV infection is currently available as a preventive measure other than palivizumab applied to the risk groups [52]. Studies for a vaccine against RSV have been unsuccessful.

8.10 Immunization Recommendations for Cochlear Implant Patients

Especially in children under 3 years of age, Cochlear implants' application is increasing. Postoperative wound infection, device-related infections, meningitis, and AOM may develop in patients with cochlear implants [53, 54]. All age-appropriate vaccines such as PCV, PPSV23, Hib, and influenza vaccines are recommended for patients with Cochlear implants [55].

Children with cochlear implants are not included in the risk group for invasive meningococcal diseases. Meningococcal vaccination is administered according to routine immunization recommendations.

8.10.1 Pneumococcal Vaccines

Two vaccines are currently available that generate antibodies to the polysaccharide capsule of *S. pneumoniae,* as mentioned above. These vaccines are the 23-valent pneumococcal polysaccharide vaccine (PPSV23) composed of pure capsular antigens and a 13-valent pneumococcal conjugate vaccine (PCV) that contains the capsules of 13 pneumococcal serotypes conjugated to a nontoxic variant of diphtheria toxin (PCV-13, Prevenar 13®). However, PPSV-23 is not recommended for children under 2 years of age because the immune system is not mature enough to respond to pure capsular antigen [56].

Cochlear implant candidate children such as those with the middle ear malformation with a central nervous system connection should be vaccinated with PSV13 and PPSV23 [57, 58]. It is better if the vaccine doses are completed 14 days before implant surgery. PPSV23 should be administered at least 8 weeks after the last dose of PCV13 as a single dose to children older than 24 months old [59].

If the fourth dose of the PCV was administered as PCV13 in children older than 12 months, there is no need for additional PCV13. Regardless of previous pneumococcal vaccination status, an additional single booster dose of PCV13 is recommended for children over 6 years of age planned to be implanted or have an implant.

8.10.2 *Haemophilus influenzae* Type B Conjugate Vaccines

H. influenzae type b disease causes serious public health problems in countries where the Hib vaccine is not administered. During the first year of life, Hib is one of the leading causes of bacterial meningitis and pneumonia. *H. influenzae* type b conjugate vaccine is also very effective in preventing AOM caused by Hib. After immunization, anti-capsular antibody concentrations are likely to be protective [60]. However, the Hib vaccine does not prevent non-serotype b strains, which may cause colonization or infection.

H. influenzae type b containing vaccines are administered in 4 doses at 2, 4, 6, and 18 months. The first dose may be applied as early as 6 weeks of age. The interval between the first 3 doses should be at least 4 weeks. A booster dose should be applied at least 6 months after completing the primary series and the first year of age.

8.10.3 Influenza Vaccines

Influenza seasonal vaccine administration to healthy children may decrease the incidence of AOM during the influenza season. Annual administration of the influenza vaccine may reduce the number of episodes of AOM. Therefore, influenza vaccination is recommended every year for those with cochlear implantation. Influenza vaccination for household contacts also should be applied [61].

References

1. World Health Organization. WHO global estimates on prevalence of hearing loss. Geneva: World Health Organization. 2012. https://www.who.int/pbd/deafness/WHO_GE_HL.pdf. Accessed 1 Nov 2020.
2. World Health Organization. Deafness and hearing loss. Geneva: World Health Organization. 2020. https://www.who.int/news-room/fact-sheets/detail/deafness-and-hearing-loss. Accessed 30 Dec 2020.
3. Lambert N, Strebel P, Orenstein W, Icenogle J, Poland GA. Rubella. Lancet. 2015;385(9984):2297–307.
4. Mongua-Rodriguez N, Diaz-Ortega JL, Garcia-Garcia L, et al. A systematic review of rubella vaccination strategies implemented in the Americas: impact on the incidence and seroprevalence rates of rubella and congenital rubella syndrome. Vaccine. 2013;31:2145–51.
5. Cohen BE, Durstenfeld A, Roehm PC. Viral causes of hearing loss: a review for hearing health professionals. Trends Hearing. 2014;18:1–17.
6. Simons EA, Reef SE, Cooper LZ, et al. Systematic review of the manifestations of congenital rubella syndrome in infants and characterization of disability-adjusted life years (DALYs). Risk Anal. 2016;36:1332–56.
7. Mansi N, de Maio V, Della Volpe A, et al. Ear, nose and throat manifestation of viral systemic infections in pediatric patients. Int J Pediatr Otorhinolaryngol. 2009;73:S26–32.
8. World Health Organization. Rubella: key facts. 2019. https://www.who.int/news-room/fact sheets/detail/rubella. Accessed 30 Dec 2020
9. Grant GB, Reef S, Dabbagh A, et al. Global progress toward rubella and congenital rubella syndrome control and elimination 2000-2014. MMWR. 2014;64:1052–5.
10. McKenna MJ. Measles, mumps, and sensorineural hearing loss. Ann N Y Acad Sci. 1997;830:291–8.
11. Chuden HG, Michtl W, Stehr K. Hearing loss due to mumps. Laryngol Rhinol Otol. 1978;57:745–50.
12. Hviid A, Rubin S, Muhlemann K. Mumps. Lancet. 2008;371(9616):932–44.
13. Hyden D, Odkvist LM, Kylen P. Vestibular symptoms in mumps deafness. Acta Otolaryngol Suppl. 1979;360:182–3.

14. Casey JR, Bluestone CD. Mumps. In: Cherry JD, Harrison GJ, Kaplan SL, Steinbach WJ, Hotez PJ, editors. Feigin and Cherry's textbook of pediatric infectious diseases. Philadelphia: Elsevier; 2019. p. 1771–9.
15. Pitaro J, Bechor-Fellner A, Gavriel H, Marom T, Eviatar E. Sudden sensorineural hearing loss in children: etiology, management, and outcome. Int J Pediatr Otorhinolaryngol. 2016;82:34–7.
16. Tarshish Y, Leschinski A, Kenna M. Pediatric sudden sensorineural hearing loss: diagnosed causes and response to intervention. Int J Pediatr Otorhinolaryngol. 2013;77:553–9.
17. Zhang BY, Young YH. Declining prevalence of pediatric sudden deafness during the past two decades. Int J Pediatr Otorhinolaryngol. 2019;119:118–22.
18. American Academy of Pediatrics. Measles. In: Kimberlin DW, Brady MT, Jackson MA, Long SS, editors. Red book: 2018 Report of the committee on infectious diseases. 31st ed. Itasca, IL: American Academy of Pediatrics; 2018. p. 537–50.
19. Wellington K, Goa KL. Measles, mumps, rubella vaccine (Priorix; GSK-MMR): a review. Drugs. 2003;63:2107–26.
20. Centers for Disease Control and Prevention Immunization Practices Advisory Committee (ACIP). Rubella prevention: recommendations of the Immunization Practices Advisory Committee. MMWR. 2013;62(RR04):1–34.
21. Centers for Disease Control and Prevention. Documentation and verification of measles, rubella, and congenital rubella syndrome elimination in the region of the Americas, United States National Report, March 28, 2012. Atlanta, GA: CDC; 2012. p. 1–62.
22. Takla A, Bohmer MM, Klinc C, et al. Outbreak-related mumps vaccine effectiveness among a cohort of children and young adults in Germany 2011. Hum Vaccin Immunother. 2014;10:140–5.
23. Cordeiro E, Ferreira M, Rodrigues F, et al. Mumps outbreak among highly vaccinated teenagers and children in the central region of Portugal, 2012-2013. Acta Medica Port. 2015;28:435–41.
24. Greenland K, Whelan J, Fanoy E, et al. Mumps outbreak among vaccinated university students associated with a large party, the Netherlands, 2010. Vaccine. 2012;30:4676–80.
25. Rubin S, Plotkin S. Mumps vaccine. In: Plotkin S, Orenstein W, Offit P, Edwards MK, editors. Plotkin's vaccines. Philadelphia, PA: Elsevier; 2017. p. 663–88.
26. Gouma S, Schurink-Van't Klooster TM, de Melker HE, et al. Mumps serum antibody levels before and after an outbreak to assess infection and immunity in vaccinated students. Open Forum Infect Dis. 2014;1:ofu101.
27. Centers for Disease Control and Prevention. Varicella. In: Hamborsky J, Kroger A, Wolfe S, editors. Epidemiology and prevention of vaccine-preventable diseases. 13th ed. Washington, DC, Public Health Foundation; 2015. p. 353–76.
28. Coker TR, Chan LS, Newberry SJ, et al. Diagnosis, microbial epidemiology, and antibiotic treatment of acute otitis media in children: a systematic review. JAMA. 2010;304:2161–9.
29. Fortanier AC, Venekamp RP, Hoes AW, Schilder AGM. Does pneumococcal conjugate vaccination affect the onset and risk of first acute otitis media and recurrences? A primary care-based cohort study. Vaccine. 2019;37:1528–32.
30. Pavia M, Bianco A, Nobile CG, Marinelli P, Angelillo IF. Efficacy of pneumococcal vaccination in children younger than 24 months: a meta-analysis. Pediatrics. 2009;123:e1103–10.
31. Hammitt LL, Campbell JC, Borys D, et al. Efficacy, safety and immunogenicity of a pneumococcal protein-based vaccine co-administered with 13-valent pneumococcal conjugate vaccine against acute otitis media in young children: A phase IIb randomized study. Vaccine. 2019;37:7482–92.
32. Johnson HL, Deloria-Knoll M, Levine OS, et al. Systematic evaluation of serotypes causing invasive pneumococcal disease among children under five: The Pneumococcal Global Serotype Project. PLoS Med. 2010;7(10):e1000348.
33. Centers for Disease Control and Prevention. Use of 13- valent pneumococcal vaccine and 23-valent pneumococcal polysaccharide vaccine among children aged 6–18 years with immunocompromising conditions: recommendations of Advisory Committee on Immunization Practices (ACIP). MMWR. 2013;62(25):521–4.

34. Rubin LG. Prevention and treatment of meningitis and acute otitis media in children with cochlear implants. Otol Neurotol. 2010;31:1331–3.
35. European Centre for Disease Prevention and Control. Surveillance of invasive bacterial diseases in Europe. 2011. https://ecdc.europa.eu/sites/portal/files/media/en/publications/Publications/invasive-bacterial-diseases-surveillance-2011.pdf. Accessed 30 Dec 2020.
36. Collins S, Ramsay M, Campbell H, Slack MP, Ladhani SN. Invasive Haemophilus influenzae type b disease in England and Wales: who is at risk after 2 decades of routine childhood vaccination? Clin Infect Dis. 2013;57:1715–21.
37. Morris SK, Moss WJ, Halsey N. Haemophilus influenzae type b conjugate vaccine use and effectiveness. Lancet Infect Dis. 2008;8:435–43.
38. Ladhani S, Slack MP, Heath PT, von Gottberg A, Chandra M, Ramsay ME. Invasive Haemophilus influenzae disease, Europe, 1996–2006. Emerg Infect Dis. 2010;16:455–63.
39. McVernon J, Howard AJ, Slack MP, Ramsay ME. The long-term impact of vaccination on Haemophilus influenzae type b (Hib) carriage in the United Kingdom. Epidemiol Infect. 2004;132:765–7.
40. Ladhani S, Ramsay M, Flood J, et al. Haemophilus influenzae serotype B (Hib) seroprevalence in England and Wales in 2009. Euro Surveill. 2012;15(17):20313.
41. World Health Organization. WHO immunological basis for immunization series: pertussis vaccines. Geneva: World Health Organization; 2017. p. 1–60.
42. Centers for Disease Control. Pertussis: United States, January–June 1995. MMWR. 1995;44(28):528–9.
43. Kline JM, Lewis WD, Smith EA, Tracy LR, Moerschel SK. Pertussis: a reemerging infection. Am Fam Physician. 2013;8:507–14.
44. Murakami H, Phuong NM, Thang HV, et al. Endemic diphtheria in Ho Chi Minh City; Viet Nam: a matched case-control study to identify risk factors of incidence. Vaccine. 2010;28:8141–6.
45. Centers for Disease Control and Prevention. Summary of notifiable diseases: the United States, 2009. MMWR. 2011;58:64.
46. Leichtle A, Hoffmann TK, Wigand MC. Otitis media: definition, pathogenesis, clinical presentation, diagnosis and therapy. Laryngorhinootologie. 2018;97:497–508.
47. Liang JL, Tiwari T, Moro P, et al. Prevention of pertussis, tetanus, and diphtheria with vaccines in the United States: Recommendations of the Advisory Committee on Immunization Practices (ACIP). MMWR. 2018;67(RR-2):1–44.
48. Desai S, Scobie HM, Cherian T, Goodman T. Expert group on the use of td vaccine in childhood. Use of tetanus-diphtheria (td) vaccine in children 4-7 years of age: World Health Organization consultation of experts. Vaccine. 2020;38:3800–7.
49. Aris E, Montourcy M, Esterberg E, Kurosky SK, Poston S, Hogea C. The adult vaccination landscape in the United States during the affordable care act era: results from a large retrospective database analysis. Vaccine. 2020;38:2984–94.
50. Norhayati MN, Ho JJ, Azman MY. Influenza vaccines for preventing acute otitis media in infants and children. Cochrane Database Syst Rev. 2017;2017(10):CD010089.
51. Leiberthal AS, Carroll AE, Chonmaitree T, et al. Clinical practice guideline: the diagnosis and management of acute otitis media. Pediatrics. 2013;13:e964–99.
52. Heikkinen T, Ojala E, Waris M. Clinical and socioeconomic burden of respiratory syncytial virus infection in children. J Infect Dis. 2017;215:17 23.
53. Schuster JE, O'Leary S, Kimberlin DW. Update from the advisory committee on immunization practices. J Pediatric Infect Dis Soc. 2016;5:349–55.
54. Farinetti A, Ben Gharbia D, Mancini J, Nicollas R, Triglia JM, Farinetti A. Cochlear implant complications in 403 patients: a comparative study of adults and children and review of the literature. Eur Ann Otorhinolaryngol Head Neck Dis. 2014;131:177–82.
55. Piotrowska A, Paradowska-Stankiewicz I, Skarżyński H. Rates of vaccination against Streptococcus pneumoniae in cochlear implant patients. Med Sci Monit. 2017;23:4567–73.
56. Rubin LG, Papsin B, Bocchini JA, et al. Cochlear implants in children: surgical site infections and prevention and treatment of acute otitis media and meningitis. Pediatrics. 2010;126:381–91.

57. Daniels CC, Rogers PD, Shelton CM. A review of pneumococcal vaccines: current polysaccharide vaccine recommendations and future protein antigens. J Pediatr Pharmacol Ther. 2016;21:27–35.
58. Kahue CN, Sweeney AD, Carlson ML, Haynes DS. Vaccination recommendations and risk of meningitis following cochlear implantation. Curr Opin Otolaryngol Head Neck Surg. 2014;22:359–66.
59. Centers for Disease Control and Prevention, Advisory Committee on Immunization Practices. Pneumococcal vaccination for cochlear implant candidates and recipients: updated recommendations of the Advisory Committee on Infectious Practices. MMWR. 2003;52:739–40.
60. Centers for Disease Control and Prevention, Advisory Committee on Immunization Practices. Update recommendation of the Advisory Committee on Immunization Practices (ACIP) for use of 7-valent pneumococcal conjugate vaccine (PCV7) in children aged 24–59 months who are not completely vaccinated. MMWR. 2008;57:343–5.
61. Jin L, Téllez P, Chia R, et al. Improving vaccination uptake in pediatric cochlear implant recipients. J Otolaryngol Head Neck Surg. 2018;47(1):56.

The Role of Surgery in Protection and Treatment of Ear, Nose and Throat Infections

Fuat Bulut, Orhan Yılmaz, and Ljiljana Jovancevic

9.1   Introduction

There is an ongoing debate around what role surgical interventions should play in protecting and/or treating children suffering from infections of the ear, nose and throat. ENT specialists tend to favour operating in such circumstances, whilst paediatricians generally favour a more conservative approach, relying on pharmacotherapy.

The operations that are carried out with the highest frequency in paediatric patients are tonsillectomy, adenoidectomy or adenotonsillectomy. By their ability to remove a focus of infection, these operations play a major part in prevention of further ENT infections and in treating existing infections. Procedures that have a mainly protective role in children rather than as therapy for infections include septoplasty for septal deviation, turbinoplasty for remodelling of the airway within the nose and myringotomy +/− grommet insertion.

F. Bulut (✉)
Section of Otorhinolaryngology, Reyap Çorlu Hospital, İstanbul Rumeli University, Çorlu, Tekirdağ, Turkey

O. Yılmaz
Department of Otorhinolaryngology, Faculty of Medicine, Karabük University, Karabük, Turkey
e-mail: orhanyilmaz@karabuk.edu.tr

L. Jovancevic
Department of Otorhinolaryngology, Head and Neck Surgery, Faculty of Medicine, Clinical Centre of Vojvodina, University of Novi Sad, Novi Sad, Serbia
e-mail: ljiljana.jovancevic@mf.uns.ac.rs

9.2   Tonsillectomy

Once tonsils become infected, they act as a reservoir for further infections in paediatric patients. Repeated episodes of infective pharyngitis and sleep-disordered breathing are indications for tonsillectomy [1].

In tonsillectomy, the tonsil is excised in its entirety (i.e. plus the capsule) through a dissection of the peritonsillar space, the boundaries of which are the tonsillar capsule and the surrounding muscle. It may be accompanied by adenoidectomy. Whether adenoidectomy is performed at the same time or not depends on the indication for tonsillectomy. Sleep-disordered breathing usually calls for adenotonsillectomy [1–3].

Pharyngitis may occur due to infection of viral or bacterial origin of the pharynx and/or the faucial tonsils. Swabs obtained from cases of pharyngitis often produce a positive culture for Group A beta-haemolytic streptococci. The phrase "sore throat" thus encompasses a variety of other diagnoses, namely "strep throat", acute tonsillitis, pharyngitis, adenotonsillitis or tonsillopharyngitis.

The principal rationale for carrying out a tonsillectomy is because it improves the child's quality of life. Repeated episodes of infective pharyngitis in children have an association with more somatic pain and deterioration in overall health as well as impairment of physical functioning than healthy peers [3]. There are several ways in which tonsillectomy improves children's quality of life, in particular through decreasing the frequency of infective pharyngitis, clinician consultations and requirements for antimicrobial pharmacotherapy [4, 5]. There are considerable differences in the frequency with which tonsillectomy is performed in different countries as reported in the literature for Japan [6], Canada [7], the United Kingdom [8] and the USA [9]. These various rates are typically considered to reflect differences in surgeons' professional practice and familiarity rather than patient-level differences [10]. Even within the USA, there is little agreement on when tonsillitis is indicated and how cases should be managed perioperatively, which highlights the pressing requirement for guidelines to be developed, drawing on the evidence base available.

9.2.1   Structure and Function of the Tonsils

The faucial tonsils are found at the point where the oral cavity gives way to the oropharynx. They are composed of both lymphoid and epithelial cells. They occupy a key defensive position and are part of the immune defences guarding the entrance into the body via the oral and nasal cavities. The tonsils are most active in immune defence in patients aged over three and under 10 years [11]. The tonsils have their greatest prominence at these ages, after which they begin to involute as the child matures into adulthood [12].

The tonsillar epithelium is shaped like a net, with many crypts. There are multiple channels within the tonsils, where the microfold (M) cells are located [13]. M cells phagocytose antigenic material, which they then carry to the extrafollicular areas or the lymphoid follicles. Within the extrafollicular zones there are dendritic cells with interdigitations, as well as macrophages. These cells are specialised for antigen presentation to T cells of the helper subset (T_h cells). The T_h cells cause appropriate B lymphocytes within the follicle to undergo a clonal expansion, producing both plasmacytes and memory cells. The plasmacytes then travel to the site where the antigen was first encountered and begin secreting immunoglobulins into the cryptic lumens [13].

The faucial tonsil are capable of synthesising all five classes of antibody, but the key class produced at this location is immunoglobulin A (IgA). IgA dimerises prior to binding to a transmembrane secretory component, thereby creating secretory IgA (SIgA), which plays an essential role in the immunological defensive functions undertaken by the mucosae which line the upper airway. The secretory component is not made within the tonsil itself, but immune cells within the tonsil do possess the J chain composed of carbohydrates which is needed for the dimerisation of IgA molecules and the formation of SIgA. Expressing the J chain is one of the key functions undertaken by the follicular B lymphocytes within the tonsil.

9.2.2   Effects of Tonsillitis and Tonsillectomy on Immunity

Repeated episodes of tonsillitis prevent the orderly mechanism by which M cells carry antigen to the dendritic cells and macrophages, as M cells are lost from the epithelial surface of the tonsil [13, 14]. Antigens now directly stimulate the mature plasmacytes to an exaggerated degree and there is a reduction in B lymphocytes devoted to expressing J-chain carbohydrates. The constant stimulus provided by antigen to the lymphocytic cells of the tonsil may leave few available to respond to different types of antigen. The tonsil ceases therefore to respond appropriately to defend the pharyngeal entrance and no longer plays a role in ensuring the secretion of immunoglobulin by cells within the upper part of the airway [13, 14]. This is the logic behind surgical excision of tonsils which keep becoming inflamed. It has been shown in some studies, nonetheless, that there are small changes in serum and pharyngeal tissue levels of immunoglobulin after removal of the tonsils [15–18]. At present, though, no research indicates that tonsillectomy has a lasting and important effect on immunological functioning [19].

9.3   Adenoidectomy

ENT specialists have been carrying out adenoidectomy frequently for many years [20, 21]. The American Academy of Otolaryngology/Head and Neck Surgery in 2017 published online a number of circumstances where adenoidectomy was appropriate, as listed in Table 9.1 [22].

Table 9.1 American Academy of Otolaryngology/Head and Neck Surgery guideline criteria for when adenoidectomy may be suitable in children with ENT-related infections [22]

- At least four episodes in which a child has had a pus-filled nasal discharge in the year prior to surgery and is still under 12 years old.
- Inflammation of the adenoids which fails to resolve completely despite two separate courses of antimicrobial pharmacotherapy, one of which should involve an agent resistant to degradation by beta-lactamase and have been prescribed for a minimum of 14 days.
- Effusive middle ear infection lasting more than 3 months or needing a second set of grommets to be inserted.
- Any effusive middle ear infection in a child who is at least 4 years old.

9.3.1 Epidemiology and Incidence

The frequency with which adenoidectomy is performed varies considerably between countries, as reported in the literature [23–25]. A number of researchers have observed that it is more common to operate on male than female children [26–28]. The most frequently cited reasons for carrying out adenoidectomy are reported as acute middle ear infection (with or without an effusion), otitis and adenoidal enlargement [26].

In 2010, one study from the United States examined the popularity of adenoidectomy over the decade 1996 to 2006. When adenoidectomy was carried out without tonsillar removal, there was no significant alteration in the frequency of operation between 1996 (when it was 183 per 100,000 paediatric population) and 2006 (when it was 176 per 100,000). When performed alongside removal of the tonsils, however, the rate had risen significantly, from 370 per 100,000 to 687 per 100,000 over the period in question [29].

Research conducted in Sweden in 2016 established a frequency of adenoidectomy of 740 per 100,000 children up to the age of 10 years. The most common age at which primary adenoidectomy was performed was 3 years. If a child was under the age of 2 years, it was most common for adenoidectomy only to be carried out, whereas over this age, it was more common to perform an adenotonsillectomy. The countries which perform adenoid removal most often are, according to the literature, Finland, with a rate of 1290 per 100,000 children, and Belgium, with a rate of 1270 per 100,000 children [30].

Data obtained by researchers in Taiwan [28] indicate that adenoidectomy was carried out on 20,599 paediatric patients between 1997 and 2012. The average age was 7.4 years, with twice as many males as females and a frequency of 24.5 per 100,000 children. The peak age range for adenoidectomy was between the age of 3 and 5 years when both sexes were considered together ($p < 0.001$), and was even higher for the male children ($p < 0.001$). The researchers identified that the frequency of adenoidectomy had increased between 1997 and 2012, from an annual rate of 14.8 per 100,000 to 26.9 per 100,000 children. Along with this increased rate, there was an alteration in the frequency of the stated surgical indication. It became more common to perform adenoidectomy to relieve sleep-disordered breathing (up from 10.1% to 35.6% of cases), whereas infection as the indication became less frequent (down from 32.3% to 8.0% of cases), with an associated *p* value of less than 0.001 [28].

9.3.2   Assessment for Adenoid Hypertrophy

Ideally, to assess for potential hypertrophy of the adenoids, the clinician should first obtain a targeted history, examine the patient physically and evaluate the size of the adenoids either by directly visualising them or through imaging studies. The standard of care for this procedure is nasopharyngoscopy, according to the literature [31–33]. There remains a limited role for lateral views obtained using cervical X-ray, although some scholars dispute this. The utility of this imaging modality was assessed by Feres et al. [34], in a systematic review of 11 previous studies. This review highlighted the limitations in the current published evidence base, such as the considerable variety in imaging methods and in how nasopharyngoscopy was performed, and the limited information available detailing exactly how the investigation was performed, or information which revealed an absence of objective standards in assessment. Feres et al. did, however, acknowledge that lateral X-ray may still play a role in assessment, despite the unclear nature of the evidence [34].

9.3.3   Assessment for Adenoid Hypertrophy

There are a number of other reasons why adenoidectomy may need to be carried out, all related to ear disease, namely effusive middle ear disease, repeated episodes of acute otitis media (3 episodes within 6 months, or 4 within a year) or malfunctioning eustachian tubes. Adenoidectomy is beneficial in shortening the duration of effusive disease of the middle ear, decreasing recurrence of otitis media following extrusion of grommets, and reducing the frequency of grommet reinsertion. In the past, it was thought that there was an association between the volume of the adenoids and the benefit obtainable. However, it is now known that this relates instead to a reduction in the numbers of pathogenic bacteria located within the nasopharynx.

The existing trial evidence on the benefits of adenoidectomy were reviewed by Wallace et al. in 2014 [35]. These researchers noted that adenoidectomy led to a 27% improvement in the rate of resolution at 6 months, as assessed by otoscopy, whereas, when assessed by tympanometry, the improvement was 22% and 29% at 1 year. In the same year, Mikals and Brigger published a systematic review and meta-analysis [36] of 15 studies, either randomised trials or observational in methodology, in which adenoidectomy was performed for the indication of acute otitis media or otitis media with effusion. Performing adenoidectomy resulted in a reduction in the frequency of grommet reinsertion in children aged at least 4 years, from 36% to 17%. They concluded, however, that there was no significant benefit below the age of 4 years.

Boonacker et al. [37] undertook a meta-analysis of nine randomised trials involving 1761 paediatric cases. The treatment allocations were adenoidectomy

+/− myringotomy and grommet insertion versus no operation or only myringotomy with grommet insertion. Below the age of 4 years, adenoidectomy was not associated with any clinical benefit. Above this age, the duration of effusive otitis media decreased by 50 days, the failure rate over the following year fell from 70% to 51%, and the need for further surgical intervention also went down (from 19% to 2% of cases).

The findings from this research are incorporated in the decision by the joint committee of the American Academy of Otolaryngology—Head and Neck Surgery Foundation (AAO-HNSF), the American Academy of Pediatrics, and the American Academy of Family Physicians [38, 39] not to recommend adenoidectomy in cases where otitis media is the main rationale for surgery and the patient is below the age of 4 years. The recommendation not to operate also applies to children with preexisting grommets, as long as there is no other reason to perform surgery (such as to relieve an obstructed nose, or for chronic adenoiditis).

9.3.4 Adenoidectomy for Chronic Rhinosinusitis in Children

The definition of chronic rhinosinusitis (CRS) in children is an episode lasting a minimum of 90 days without interruption where there are symptoms of pus-filled nasal discharge, a blocked nose, pain or pressure over the face and coughing. Furthermore, to diagnose CRS, there should be swollen mucosae, drainage of pus and polyps within the nose visible on endoscopy, or CT should indicate altered mucosa in the area of the ostiomeatus and the sinuses [20]. Although the condition occurs frequently in children, it causes considerable problems. Fortunately, the majority of cases are responsive to the initial treatment of choice, namely irrigation of the nose with saline, intranasal corticosteroid sprays and antimicrobial pharmacotherapy targeting the most frequently occurring bacteria within the sinuses and nasal cavity. Taking a child away from nursery is an intervention of high efficacy in preventing a child being exposed to infections of the upper airways and reducing the incidence of sinusitis. There is considerable published evidence showing that adenoidectomy is efficacious in treating paediatric CRS resistant to medical therapy.

The adenoids are believed to play a role in sinus infections by harbouring pathogenic bacteria that can form biofilms. Coticchia et al. [40] looked at the extent to which biofilms covered the adenoids excised at operation, comparing cases where the indication was paediatric CRS with those for sleep-disordered breathing. In the first group, fully developed biofilms were found to envelop 94.9% of the adenoidal surface, compared to only 1.9% in cases of sleep-disordered breathing. These researchers came to the conclusion that the presence of a biofilm on the adenoidal surface accounted for the persistence of CRS after pharmacotherapy. They therefore suggested that unless the adenoids were physically removed, there was little possibility of disrupting the reservoir of infection represented by the biofilm.

Shin et al. [41] retrospectively reviewed the medical record in cases of paediatric CRS, looking at the adenoidal volume and the results of pathogen isolation. There was a correlation between positive bacterial culture from swabs of the adenoids and more severe disease within the sinuses, assessed radiologically from an occipito-mental view ($p < 0.001$). Overall, some 79.3% of adenoid samples had a positive bacterial culture. Cases were consistently rated as more severe on radiological assessment where *Haemophilus influenzae* or *Streptococcus pneumoniae* were isolated, a result that was statistically significant. However, the volume of the adenoids was not correlated with how severe CRS was. This last result may be interpreted to indicate that the significance of the adenoids to the pathogenesis relates to them harbouring biofilms rather than physically hindering sinus drainage [41, 42].

A meta-analysis also exists [42] looking at the situation in which children underwent adenoid removal due to treatment-resistant CRS and where the principal outcome evaluated was the caregiver's account of the child's symptoms. It was calculated that the statistical probability of symptoms being better after adenoid removal was 83.4% (95% CI 574.5–92.2%, $p < 0.001$). Brietzke and Brigger therefore strongly recommend that treatment-resistant CRS in children be managed by adenoid removal as the first surgical option [42].

A statement regarding the consensus views held by clinicians was published in 2014 by the AAO-HNSF [39], which concluded about adenoidectomy specifically that:

- Adenoidectomy possesses efficacy as an initial operative intervention in cases of CRS where the patient is below the age of 12 years.
- The benefit that can be derived from adenoidectomy in children with CRS does not depend on the benefits that arise from endoscopic sinus surgery in general.
- Tonsillectomy does not possess efficacy in treating CRS unless it is performed as part of adenotonsillectomy.

9.4 Conclusion

Paediatricians should work with ENT specialists in a multidisciplinary way when treating infections of the head and neck area. Surgery may sometimes offer a definitive answer to cases where infection is recurrent due to bacterial biofilms acting as a reservoir of infection. Infections may be prevented from occurring in the head and neck if particular operations are performed, notably septoplasty, turbinoplasty and myringotomy (+/− insertion of grommets).

References

1. Mitchell RB, Archer SM, Ishman SL, Rosenfeld RM, Coles S, Finestone SA, Friedman NR, Giordano T, Hildrew DM, Kim TW, Lloyd RM, Parikh SR, Shulman ST, Walner DL, Walsh SA, Nnacheta LC. Clinical practice guideline: tonsillectomy in children (update)-executive summary. Otolaryngol Head Neck Surg. 2019;160(2):187–205. https://doi.org/10.1177/0194599818807917.
2. Rosenfeld RM, Green RP. Tonsillectomy and adenoidectomy: changing trends. Ann Otol Rhinol Laryngol. 1990;99:187–91.

3. Stewart MG, Friedman EM, Sulek M, et al. Quality of life and health status in pediatric tonsil and adenoid disease. Arch Otolaryngol Head Neck Surg. 2000;126:45–8.
4. Goldstein NA, Stewart MG, Witsell DL, et al. Quality of life after tonsillectomy in children with recurrent tonsillitis. Otolaryngol Head Neck Surg. 2008;138:S9–S16.
5. Wei JL, Mayo MS, Smith HJ, et al. Improved behavior and sleep after adenotonsillectomy in children with sleep-disordered breathing. Arch Otolaryngol Head Neck Surg. 2007;133:974–9.
6. Fujihara K, Koltai PJ, Hayashi M, et al. Cost-effectiveness of tonsillectomy for recurrent acute tonsillitis. Ann Otol Rhinol Laryngol. 2006;115:365–9.
7. Martens PJ, Fransoo R, Burchill C, Burland E. Health status and healthcare use patterns of rural, northern and urban Manitobans: is Romanow right? Health Policy. 2006;2:108–27.
8. Pickering AE, Bridge HS, Nolan J, et al. Double-blind, placebo controlled analgesic study of ibuprofen or rofecoxib in combination with paracetamol for tonsillectomy in children. Br J Anaesth. 2002;88:72–7.
9. Paradise JL, Bluestone CD, Colborn DK, et al. Tonsillectomy and adenotonsillectomy for recurrent throat infection in moderately affected children. Pediatrics. 2002;110:7–15.
10. Capper R, Canter RJ. Is there agreement among general practitioners, paediatricians and otolaryngologists about the management of children with recurrent tonsillitis? Clin Otolaryngol Allied Sci. 2001;26:371–8.
11. Richardson MA. Sore throat, tonsillitis, and adenoiditis. Med Clin North Am. 1999;83:75–83.
12. Jung KY, Lim HH, Choi G, et al. Age-related changes of IgA immunocytes and serum and salivary IgA after tonsillectomy. Acta Otolaryngol Suppl. 1996;523:115–9.
13. Brandtzaeg P. Immune functions and immunopathology of palatine and nasopharyngeal tonsils. In: Bernstein JM, Ogra PL, editors. Immunology of the ear. New York, NY: Raven Press; 1987. p. 63–106.
14. Brandtzaeg P. Immunology of tonsils and adenoids: everything the ENT surgeon needs to know. Int J Pediatr Otorhinolaryngol. 2003;67:S69–76.
15. Friday GA, Paradise JL, Rabin BS, et al. Serum immunoglobulin changes in relation to tonsil and adenoid surgery. Ann Allergy. 1992;69:225–30.
16. Bock A, Popp W, Herkner KR. Tonsillectomy and the immune system: a long-term follow up comparison between tonsillectomized and non-tonsillectomized children. Eur Arch Otorhinolaryngol. 1994;251:423–7.
17. Paulussen C, Claes J, Claes G, Jorissen M. Adenoids and tonsils, indications for surgery and immunological consequences of surgery. Acta Otorhinolaryngol Belg. 2000;54:403–8.
18. Kaygusuz I, Godekmerdan A, Karlidag T, et al. Early stage impacts of tonsillectomy on immune functions of children. Int J Pediatr Otorhinolaryngol. 2003;67:1311–5.
19. Brandtzaeg P. Immune function of the nasopharyngeal tissue. Adv Otorhinolaryngol. 2011;72:20–4.
20. Schupper AJ, Nation J, Pransky S. Adenoidectomy in children: what is the evidence and what is its role? Curr Otorhinolaryngol Rep. 2018;6(1):64–73. https://doi.org/10.1007/s40136-018-0190-8.
21. Ingram DG, Friedman NR. Toward adenotonsillectomy in children: a review for the general pediatrician. JAMA Pediatr. 2015;169(12):1155–61. https://doi.org/10.1001/jamapediatrics.2015.2016.
22. AAO/HNS Clinical Indicators: Adenoidectomy Available at: https://higherlogicdownload.s3-external1.amazonaws.com/ENTNET/Adenoidectomy-CIUpdated.pdf?AWSAccessKeyId=AKIAJH5D4I4FWRALBOUA&Expires=1504509869&Signature=8MwBTzIygBOHcHM6auKZO2CA6oo%3D.
23. Haapkyla J, Karevold G, Kvaerner KJ, Pitkaranta A. Trends in otitis media surgery: a decrease in adenoidectomy. Int J Pediatr Otorhinolaryngol. 2008;72(8):1207–13. https://doi.org/10.1016/j.ijporl.2008.04.012.

24. Schilder AG, Lok W, Rovers MM. International perspectives on management of acute otitis media: a qualitative review. Int J Pediatr Otorhinolaryngol. 2004;68(1):29–36. https://doi.org/10.1016/j.ijporl.2003.09.002.
25. Thomas K, Boeger D, Buentzel J, et al. Pediatric adenoidectomy: a population-based regional study on epidemiology and outcome. Int J Pediatr Otorhinolaryngol. 2013;77(10):1716–20. https://doi.org/10.1016/j.ijporl.2013.07.032.
26. Dearking AC, Lahr BD, Kuchena A, Orvidas LJ. Factors associated with revision adenoidectomy. Otolaryngol Head Neck Surg. 2012;146(6):984–90. https://doi.org/10.1177/0194599811435971.
27. van den Aardweg MT, Rovers MM, Kraal A, Schilder AG. Current indications for adenoidectomy in a sample of children in the Netherlands. B-ENT. 2010;6(1):15–8.
28. Lee CH, Chang WH, Ko JY, Yeh TH, Hsu WC, Kang KT. Revision adenoidectomy in children: a population-based cohort study in Taiwan. Eur Arch Otorhinolaryngol. 2017 Oct;274(10):3627–35. https://doi.org/10.1007/s00405-017-4655-z.
29. Bhattacharyya N, Lin HW. Changes and consistencies in the epidemiology of pediatric adenotonsillar surgery, 1996–2006. Otolaryngol Head Neck Surg. 2010;143(5):680–4. https://doi.org/10.1016/j.otohns.2010.06.918.
30. Gerhardsson H, Stalfors J, Odhagen E, Sunnergren O. Pediatric adenoid surgery in Sweden 2004–2013: incidence, indications and concomitant surgical procedures. Int J Pediatr Otorhinolaryngol. 2016;87:61–6. https://doi.org/10.1016/j.ijporl.2016.05.020.
31. Bitar MA, Birjawi G, Youssef M, Fuleihan N. How frequent is adenoid obstruction? Impact on the diagnostic approach. Pediatr Int. 2009;51(4):478–83. https://doi.org/10.1111/j.1442-200X.2008.02787.x.
32. Kubba H, Bingham BJ. Endoscopy in the assessment of children with nasal obstruction. J Laryngol Otol. 2001;115(5):380–4. https://doi.org/10.1258/0022215011907929.
33. Mlynarek A, Tewfik MA, Hagr A, et al. Lateral neck radiography versus direct video rhinoscopy in assessing adenoid size. J Otolaryngol. 2004;33(06):360–5. https://doi.org/10.2310/7070.2004.03074.
34. Feres MF, Hermann JS, Cappellette M Jr, Pignatari SS. Lateral X-ray view of the skull for the diagnosis of adenoid hypertrophy: a systematic review. Int J Pediatr Otorhinolaryngol. 2011;75(1):1–11. https://doi.org/10.1016/j.ijporl.2010.11.002.
35. Wallace IF, Berkman ND, Lohr KN, Harrison MF, Kimple AJ, Steiner MJ. Surgical treatments for otitis media with effusion: a systematic review. Pediatrics. 2014;133(2):296–311. https://doi.org/10.1542/peds.2013-3228.
36. Mikals SJ, Brigger MT. Adenoidectomy as an adjuvant to primary tympanostomy tube placement: a systematic review and meta-analysis. JAMA Otolaryngol Head Neck Surg. 2014;140:95–101. https://doi.org/10.1001/jamaoto.2013.5842.
37. Boonacker CW, Rovers MM, Browning GG, Hoes AW, Schilder AG, Burton MJ. Adenoidectomy with or without grommets for children with otitis media: an individual patient data meta-analysis. Health Technol Assess. 2014;18(5):1–118. https://doi.org/10.3310/hta18050.
38. Rosenfeld RM, Shin JJ, Schwartz SR, et al. Clinical practice guideline: otitis media with effusion executive summary (update). Otolaryngol Head Neck Surg. 2016;154(2):201–14. https://doi.org/10.1177/0194599815624407.
39. Brietzke SE, Shin JJ, Choi S, et al. Clinical consensus statement: pediatric chronic rhinosinusitis. Otolaryngol Head Neck Surg. 2014;151(4):542–53. https://doi.org/10.1177/0194599814549302.
40. Coticchia J, Zuliani G, Coleman C, et al. Biofilm surface area in the pediatric nasopharynx: chronic rhinosinusitis vs obstructive sleep apnea. Arch Otolaryngol Head Neck Surg. 2007;133(2):110–4. https://doi.org/10.1001/archotol.133.2.110.
41. Shin KS, Cho SH, Kim KR, et al. The role of adenoids in pediatric rhinosinusitis. Int J Pediatr Otorhinolaryngol. 2008;72(11):1643–50. https://doi.org/10.1016/j.ijporl.2008.07.016.
42. Brietzke SE, Brigger MT. Adenoidectomy outcomes in pediatric rhinosinusitis: a meta-analysis. Int J Pediatr Otorhinolaryngol. 2008;72(10):1541–5. https://doi.org/10.1016/j.ijporl.2008.07.008.

Communication with the Infected Child

10

Can Cemal Cingi, Erhan Eroğlu, and Gary L. Kreps

10.1 Introduction

Human development is divided by a number of different developmental psychology theories into "stages," which are non-repeatable phases in human mental development, each of which involves new behavioral and cognitive features in the child becoming apparent. While the speed with which an individual child passes from stage to stage differs according to genetic diathesis and environmental influences, according to researchers in this area, the order of completion of the stages is invariable [1].

To communicate effectively with children, the approach should give due regard to their age, be warm and approachable, consider the child as a whole, focus on strengths and accentuate positive characteristics and be adaptable to suit all children, including those at most disadvantage [1]. In addition, communicating with patients who are children inevitably involves the need to communicate effectively with parents, other family members (sometimes grandparents and siblings), and others who may have responsibility for the child's well-being [2, 3]. Sometimes consultations with these others occur in the presence of the child, and at other times communication with these others is conducted privately. It is important for the health care provider to enlist the cooperation of both the child patient, as well as with the significant others who are responsible for the child. This means building effective relationships with the child, as well as with the child's health significant

C. C. Cingi (✉) · E. Eroğlu
Department of Communication Design and Management, Faculty of Communication Sciences, Anadolu University, Eskişehir, Turkey
e-mail: ccc@anadolu.edu.tr

G. L. Kreps
Department of Communication, Center for Health and Risk Communication, George Mason University, Fairfax, VA, USA

 123
C. Cingi et al. (eds.), *Pediatric ENT Infections*,
https://doi.org/10.1007/978-3-030-80691-0_10

others for the effective delivery of care [2, 4]. The Relational Health Communication Competence Model (RHCCM) suggests that the more relationally competent health communication is between health care providers and patients, the better the outcomes of health care will be for patients [5–7]. Building meaningful interpersonal relationships with child patients and their health significant others is essential for providing effective treatments for children with infections.

Children understand and can-do different things at different points in their development, so communication needs to keep the child center stage and consider such age differences. In addition, personality and behavior differ according to genetic factors, social situation, and the environment. Communicating well is helpful in achieving other goals or targets in child development programs, such as the importance of hand hygiene, showing universal and mutual respect to others, stopping children being exploited or abused, preparing for school attendance, remaining healthy when HIV/AIDS positive, and being ready to cope with emergency situations [1].

10.2 Infectious Diseases in Children

Primary care services across the world are more often accessed due to an acute pediatric illness than for any other reason. Such illnesses are common, with coughing secondary to a respiratory tract infection (RTI) the most frequent of all. In the UK, more than a million appointments are made for this reason annually [8]. In spite of their being common, parents often see such encounters negatively [9, 10]. At the end of the appointment, they remain unsure, with the diagnosis insufficiently explained and ways to treat the condition unexplored in sufficient depth [10, 11]. Questions usually remain and the length of consultations is seen as inadequate. Health care professionals wish to help both patient and parent in the best way possible. Given the fact that the majority of acute illnesses resolve without clinical intervention, health providers see such appointments as wasteful and only adding to overuse of antimicrobials [12]. Primary care doctors account for 80% of antimicrobial use, with many antibiotics being used in spite of clear indications that they are ineffective (or less effective). Such use promotes microbial antibiotic resistance [13]. Parents, their offspring, health care providers and doctors all have a stake in improving the communication value of these encounters [14].

Doctor, patient, and parent form a triangle in clinical encounters with a child and this makes communication more complex, with parents telling the doctor what their child's needs are [15, 16]. Since the parents often talk on behalf of the child, the parents' wishes and fears may unconsciously dominate the consultation, rather than the child's actual needs [17]. The way parents communicate may cause the doctor to feel pressured (even if not) towards prescribing antibiotics [18, 19]. Likewise, how the doctor speaks and how the treatment options are presented (emphasizing the negative or accentuating the positive) may have an effect on parents' decisions to accept or decline options, hence on whether antibiotics are used or not [20]. The issue of antibiotic overusage has been approached through boosting communication skills via training programs, resulting in definite positive outcomes with adult patient encounters [21–23] and intimations of success in pediatric encounters, too [14, 24].

10.3 Communication with Parents

If parents and doctors failed to discuss in advance what they expect from consultations in terms of what needs to be communicated, how and by whom, misunderstandings occurred [25, 26]. Doctors characteristically used a "voice of medicine" in these appointments [25], by which is meant that the biomedical view of the problem was being privileged over the patients' usual ways of communicating, their focus on their own life and how they see the world around them, the "voice of the life-world" [27]. If the problem could not be framed straightforwardly in medical terms, the probability of communication failure increased. "Lifeworld"-framed parental explanations of concern about the diagnosis and the possible treatments (e.g., unwillingness for the child to miss school or the wish for the child to be healthy in time for a vacation) were viewed as refusal by doctors and taken to show the parent wished antibiotics to be given [28]. By doctors assuming that only a biomedical explanation is valid to understand the problem, they adversely affected the quality of communication within the encounter [14]. It is important to recognize and adapt communication efforts to the health literacy levels of parents (and pediatric patients) to make sure they understand relevant health information and feel that they are included in making relevant health care decisions [29–31].

Both doctors and parents virtually constantly saw diagnosis as the doctors' particular responsibility and area of expertise. For all types of diagnosis, the most frequently encountered way this was communicated was the following: the doctor stated what the diagnosis was and the parent agreed to it without replying very much at all [30, 32]. Stivers [30] and Ijas-Kallio [32] noted that parents might present the problem as just a description of symptoms ("symptoms only") or suggested a diagnosis ("candidate diagnosis") and this changed what happened in the encounter, with "symptoms only" leading directly to a diagnosis, but "candidate diagnosis" eliciting either agreement or refutation by the doctor. Ijas-Kallio [32] noted in addition that parents might sometimes give an extensive appraisal of the diagnosis, reasoning about factors which they considered to affect how acceptable a diagnosis was to them and might lead to them agreeing or disagreeing with the doctor's conclusion [14]. Most encounters led to the doctor's recommending washing out the patient's nostrils with saline to allow any nasal secretion to be removed [33].

10.4 Communication with Children

When talking with mothers, health care professionals, who were clearly very keen to ensure adherence to the therapeutic plan, focused solely on writing a prescription and reiterating the treatment regime in their attempts to improve adherence. Any other ways to increase parents' involvement, such as educating them about the absence of clear demarcations between healthy and unhealthy states in children, were simply not observed [33]. With regard to nonspecific communication techniques during clinical encounters, the majority of consultations were characterized by cordiality and a show of respect by professionals: they adopted a pleasant tone of voice and looked towards mothers while speaking, listened with due attention, and gave instructions in an amicable fashion, but they also failed to introduce themselves and did not utilize either the parent's or child's name [33].

10.4.1 Implications on Communication (Birth to 6 Years)

The following aspects of communication should be addressed when speaking to children of this age [1]:

- Adopt an affectionate tone of voice and simplify what you say.
- Show you are curious and want to learn.
- Demonstrate how we can explore safely, ask questions, and trust our new abilities.
- Consider how long a child can concentrate and how this lengthens with age.
- Treat it as a game and show how to learn by playing, repeating things frequently, singing, and making words rhyme. Alter your pace but keep within the limits of a child's abilities.
- Tell stories using familiar themes like other children, families, animals, and day-to-day things they do.
- Give scope for free play with the opportunity to pretend and imagine.
- Show and praise healthy things we can do to look after ourselves. Point out how children who are like or unlike them can play and work in unison. Demonstrate how relationships can be strong and adults nurturing.
- Reinforce singing, clapping, dancing, moving activities. Give opportunities to ask questions and provide replies and give encouragement to speaking.
- Give examples of enlightened views about gender and avoid clichéed ways of describing grown-ups and children.
- Provide easy-to-understand models of children who, with the help of adults who love them, can talk about many different feelings, conquer their fears, and approach problems healthily.
- Add stories about children who are self-reliant and able to cope, have a sense of fairness and look after their own interests and those of others.
- Show how children make choices about straightforward matters and give opinions of their own.
- Use clear language and vivid examples that children can understand and relate to.
- Encourage children to ask questions about anything they do not understand or are concerned about.

10.4.2 Implications of Communication for Middle Years (from 7 to 10 Years Old)

The middle years see the steady development of independence and individuation in children, who can now explore their surroundings. They employ more complex sentences; acquire vast quantities of information; develop novel skills such as how to read and write, how to undertake formal education, and learn a great deal about the Earth and other humans. By degrees they lose their egocentric orientation (where they are the center of the world) and develop some empathy towards others. Their inquisitiveness and growing social competence also leads to them accepting and tending to use ways to exclude others such as typecasting others by their ethnicity or gender, harassment and discrimination. They investigate the world in less constrained ways and still tend to have accidents. They are able to take ownership of their actions; little by little they learn to be patient in getting their needs met and master undertakings that bolster confidence in themselves and self-reliance. The examples they view or listen to at home, at school, among their community, and in the media shape how they act, what they think, and how they see the world. As the phase draws to its close, a few children, especially girls, are by then entering adolescence and will face the hurdles surrounding physical and emotional maturation [1].

Implications for how to communicate [1].

- Stories will need to last more time and contain greater drama.
- Put the child at the center of the tale and see characters from a child's perspective.
- Show doing well at school and learning as a chance to acquire and build on newfound abilities.
- Make the things students see and hear amusing and give them thought-provoking tasks (e.g., puzzles, mysteries to solve, sequences containing repeated sounds to say out loud).
- Let them interact to work out problems and think in ways that need judgment.
- Show how we can act to help others by kind actions, stopping disputes, and looking after others.
- Point out adults and other children who act in powerful and beneficial, ethical ways. Bring up subjects that are emotionally laden, such as children coping in a thoughtful and adaptive manner with unfair situations in society like bereavement, anger, handicap, and being abused.
- Present other children as believable role models for creating positive change in their own or others' lives, despite hardship.
- Tell tales with themes of being a friend, standing by others, and making correct moral choices.
- Use clear language and vivid examples that children can understand and relate to.
- Encourage children to ask questions about anything they do not understand or are concerned about.

10.4.3 Implications for Communication in Early Adolescent Years (11 Through 14 Years)

Many people see adolescence as a turbulent and trying time for those going through a multitude of changes all at the same time: in thinking and emotional style, in social relationships and body alterations. Adolescents are entering adult life and may often have difficulty controlling their emotions, bursting out with emotion or behaving threateningly. The disposition to behave in a reasoned way wars with wanting to be a dare devil; responsibility and irresponsibility collide.

Implications for Communication [1]:

- Show their peers (either as a group or individually) acting in laudable and adaptive ways.
- Showcase the wide range of opinions, ideas, and viewpoints that can exist.
- Show that children can become more independent at the same time as having a strong bond with their parents and show ways adults can still help children develop well.
- Talk about individuals who have a secure sense of their own worth. This is especially important when talking to female, handicapped, or minority ethnic adolescents.
- Show teenagers and grown-ups who have an enlightened view of how men and women can or should be.
- Give age-appropriate counseling (drug abuse, unsafe sex, violence, sexual love, bullying, and prejudicial treatment of others). Speak in a considerate way and without just telling them what to do or not do. Do not address them as inferiors. Show stories, which offer engaging topics even to children with a low reading age. Show thought-provoking tales that give clever ideas and show ingenious ways out of problems. Be amusing, witty, and inventive.
- Use clear language and vivid examples that children can understand and relate to.
- Encourage children to ask questions about anything they do not understand or are concerned about.

References

1. Kolucki B, Lemish D 2017. Communicating with children. Unicef. New York https://www.unicef.org/cwc/files/CwC_Final_Nov-2011.pdf. Accessed 28 Sept 2017.
2. Kreps GL. Commentary: communication and family health and wellness relationships. In: Socha T, Stamp G, editors. Parents and children communicating with society: exploring relationships outside of home. New York: Routledge Publishers; 2009. p. 207–12.
3. Levetown M. Communicating with children and families: from everyday interactions to skill in conveying distressing information. Pediatrics. 2008;121(5):e1441–60.
4. Kahana E, Kahana B. Patient proactivity enhancing doctor–patient–family communication in cancer prevention and care among the aged. Patient Educ Counsel. 2003;50(1):67–73.
5. Kreps GL. Relational health communication competence model. In: Thompson TL, editor. Encyclopedia of health communication, vol. III. Los Angeles, CA: Sage Publications; 2014. p. 1160–1.

6. Kreps GL. Relational communication in health care. Southern Commun J. 1988;53:344–59.
7. Query JL, Kreps GL. Testing a relational model of health communication competence among caregivers for individuals with Alzheimer's disease. J Health Psychol. 1996;1(3):335–52.
8. Hollinghurst S, Gorst C, Fahey T, Hay A. Measuring the financial burden of acute cough in pre-schoolchildren: a cost of illness study. BMC Fam Pract. 2008;9(1):10.
9. Francis NA, Crocker JC, Gamper A, Brookes-Howell L, Powell C, Butler CC. Missed opportunities for earlier treatment? A qualitative interview study with parents of children admitted to hospital with serious respiratory tract infections. Arch Dis Child. 2011;96(2):154–9.
10. Kai J. Parents' difficulties and information needs in coping with acute illness in preschool children: a qualitative study. BMJ. 1996;313(7063):987–90.
11. Akici A, Kalaca S, Ümit Ugurlu M, Oktay S. Prescribing habits of general practitioners in the treatment of childhood respiratory-tract infections. Eur J Clin Pharmacol. 2004;60(3):211–6.
12. Finkelstein J, Metlay JP, Davis RL, Rifas-Shiman SL, Dowell SF, Platt R. Antimicrobial use in defined populations of infants and young children. Arch Pediatr Adolesc Med. 2000;154(4):395–400.
13. Costelloe C, Metcalfe C, Lovering A, Mant D, Hay AD. Effect of antibiotic prescribing in primary care on antimicrobial resistance in individual patients: systematic review and meta-analysis. BMJ. 2010;340:c2096.
14. Cabral C, Horwood J, Hay AD, Lucas PJ. How communication affects prescription decisions in consultations for acute illness in children: a systematic review and meta-ethnography. BMC Fam Pract. 2014;15:63. https://doi.org/10.1186/1471-2296-15-63.
15. Cahill P, Papageorgiou A. Video analysis of communication in Paediatric consultations in primary care. Br J Gen Pract. 2007;57(544):866–71.
16. Mangione-Smith R, McGlynn EA, Elliott MN, McDonald L, Franz CE, Kravitz RL. Parent expectations for antibiotics, physician-parent communication, and satisfaction. Arch Pediatr Adolesc Med. 2001;155(7):800–6.
17. Tannen D, Wallat C. Interactive frames and knowledge schemas in interaction: examplesfrom a medical examination/interview. Soc Psychol Q. 1987;50(2):205–16.
18. Stivers T, Mangione-Smith R, Elliott MN, McDonald L, Heritage J. Why do physicians think parents expect antibiotics? what parents report vs what physicians believe. J Fam Pract. 2003;52(2):140–8.
19. Stivers T. Presenting the problem in pediatric encounters: "symptoms only" versus "candidate diagnosis" presentations. Health Commun. 2002;14(3):299–338.
20. Stivers T. Non-antibiotic treatment recommendations: Delivery formats and implications for parent resistance. Soc Sci Med. 2005;60(5):949–64.
21. Butler CC, Simpson SA, Dunstan F, Rollnick S, Cohen D, Gillespie D, et al. Effectiveness of multifaceted educational programme to reduce antibiotic dispensing in primary care: practice based randomised controlled trial. BMJ. 2012;344:d8173.
22. Cals JWL, Butler CC, Hopstaken RM, Hood K, Dinant G-J. Effect of point of care testing for C reactive protein and training in communication skills on antibiotic use in lower respiratory tract infections: cluster randomized trial. BMJ. 2009;338:b1374.
23. Little P, Stuart B, Francis NA, Douglas E, Tonkin-Crine S, Anthierens S, et al. Effects of internet-based training on antibiotic prescribing rates for acute respiratory-tract infections: a multinational, cluster, randomised, factorial, controlled trial. Lancet. 2013;382(9899):1175.
24. Harrington NG, Norling GR, Witte FM, Taylor J, Andrews JE. The effects of communication skills training on 'Pediatricians and Parents' communication during "sick child" visits. Health Commun. 2007;21(2):105–14.
25. Barry CA, Stevenson FA, Britten N, Barber N, Bradley CP. Giving voice to the life world. More humane, more effective medical care? a qualitative study of doctor–patient communication in general practice. Soc Sci Med. 2001;53(4):487–505.
26. Roberts C, Sarangi S. Theme-oriented discourse analysis of medical encounters. Med Educ. 2005;39(6):632–40.
27. Mishler EG. The discourse of medicine: dialectics of medical interviews. New York: Ablex Publication; 1984.

28. Stivers T. Negotiating antibiotic treatment in pediatric care: the communication of preferences in physician-parent interaction. Los Angeles, CA: University of California; 2000.
29. Kreps GL. Promoting patient comprehension of relevant health information. Israel J Health Policy Res. 2018;7:56. https://doi.org/10.1186/s13584-018-0250-z.
30. Kreps GL. One size does not fit all: Adapting communication to the needs and literacy levels of individuals. Ann Family Med. 2006;27(3):449–65.
31. Kreps GL, Sparks L. Meeting the health literacy needs of vulnerable populations. Patient Educ Couns. 2008;71(3):328–32.
32. Ijäs-Kallio T. Patient participation in decision making process in primary care. Tampere, Finland: University of Tampere; 2011.
33. de Carvalho AP, de Veríssimo ML. Communication and education in health consultations to children with acute respiratory infections. Rev Esc Enferm USP. 2011;45(4):847–54.

Part II

Symptoms and Signs

Fever: Pathogenesis and Treatment

Edhem Ünver, Nuray Bayar Muluk, and Oleg Khorov

11.1 Introduction

Pyrexia (fever) refers to an abnormal increase in temperature occurring under central nervous system control as a component of a co-ordinated biological response.

The average normal temperature is usually quoted as 37 °C (98.6 °F) [1, 2], a value arrived at following research conducted in the 1800s. Newer research involving oral measurement of temperature in young adults found the usual maximum average temperature reached 37.2 °C (98.9 °F) in the morning, and 37.7 °C (99.9 °F) during the day as a whole [3]. Patients' age, the time of day, how active they are and (for women) where within the menstrual cycle, and certain other variables, all affect the normal temperature [3, 4].

The average body temperature is higher in infants and young children than in other people, a situation attributable to infants' and young children's relatively higher ratio of surface area to mass and more active metabolism. In neonates (i.e. aged 28 days or less) the average normal temperature (via rectal thermometer) is 37.5 °C. The maximum normal temperature is 38 °C (100.4 °F), allowing for two standard deviations from the mean [5].

There is variation in the normal body temperature throughout the day. The temperature is lowest in the morning and highest in the afternoon or early evening. On average, this variation is 0.5 °C (0.9 °F) [6]. During a pyrexial illness, this variation

E. Ünver (✉)
Department of Pulmonology, Faculty of Medicine, Erzincan Binali Yıldırım University, Erzincan, Turkey

N. Bayar Muluk
Department of Otorhinolaryngology, Faculty of Medicine, Kırıkkale University, Kırıkkale, Turkey

O. Khorov
Department of Otorhinolaryngology, Grodno State Medical University, Grodno, Belarus

C. Cingi et al. (eds.), *Pediatric ENT Infections*,
https://doi.org/10.1007/978-3-030-80691-0_11

continues, although the baseline temperature is elevated. Diurnal temperature varies by up to 1 °C (1.8 °F) in certain cases where a pyrexial episode is resolving [1].

Since a raised body temperature may result from either pyrexia, in which the temperature rises in accordance with a change in hypothalamic thermoregulation, or hyperthermia, where the raised temperature is not accompanied by a hypothalamic thermostatic change, distinguishing between the two situations is key to understanding the pathophysiology and treating the cause [1].

11.2 Definition of Fever

Pyrexia (fever) refers to an abnormal increase in temperature occurring under central nervous system control as a component of a co-ordinated biological response. What constitutes an abnormal temperature varies according to age in children and where the temperature is recorded. The decision to search for an infective focus is informed by how old the child is and elements of the clinical presentation (such as immunodeficiency, sickle cell disorders and how grave the illness appears, amongst other factors). In the majority of cases, the degree of temperature elevation is less significant than other markers of disease severity such as irritability and meningismus [7–10].

11.2.1 Hyperthermia

Hyperthermia refers to an abnormally raised temperature that is not the result of resetting hypothalamic temperature regulation. This homeostatic dysequilibrium occurs because heat is generated more rapidly than it can be dissipated [11]. Anti-fever agents have no effect upon hyperthermia.

11.3 Pathogenesis

Pyrexia is the end result of an orchestrated physiological process initiated by production and secretion of the chemical mediators interleukin-1 (IL-1), IL-6, TNF, interferon-α, and other fever-promoting cytokines released by phagocytes, both in the circulation and within tissues [12]. Cytokines within the circulation reach the anterior hypothalamus, where they trigger a rapid elevation in the production of prostaglandins, notably PGE2 (prostaglandin E2). It is PGE2 which induces a higher set-point for thermoregulation.

Once the body thermostat has been reset to a higher temperature, the thermoregulatory centre sets off sequences of changes with the aim of raising body temperature to the desired level. The changes result in greater heat generation through raising metabolic activity, muscular tone and action, whilst reducing dissipation of heat by shunting blood from the skin to the deeper body structures. The temperature keeps on going up until the desired temperature is reached, after which a new equilibrium is established. Pyrexia does not appear to generate a maximal temperature exceeding 42 °C (107.6 °F), and indeed temperatures above 41 °C (106 °F) are seldom seen unless hyperthermia is also present [3, 13, 14].

Pyrogenic cytokines, as well as provoking pyrexia, cause increased hepatic production of acute phase proteins, lower the iron and zinc level of the blood, cause recruitment of leucocytes and speed up the degradation of protein within voluntary muscle. IL-1 can bring on the slow-wave phase of sleep, which may account for the tendency to sleepiness in patients who are pyrexial. Similarly, PGE2 may be responsible for muscular and joint pains which are a frequent accompaniment to pyrexia. The cardiac rate rises to accommodate the greater metabolic demands of pyrexia [1].

The hypothalamic thermoregulatory centre controls the body temperature. Heat is generally produced by hepatic and muscular metabolism, and lost via the skin and lungs. Typically, the hypothalamus keeps the body temperature within relatively strict limits if there are not extreme environmental influences to contend with. Once the temperature of the environment exceeds around 35 °C (95 °F), heat can no longer be lost and the body temperature inevitably increases [1].

11.4 Aetiology

Pyrexia indicates the presence of disease and the reason for it needs to be investigated, especially should a child appear unwell or the pyrexia persistent. The effectiveness of antipyretic treatment has no value in discriminating infection due to bacteria from those due to viruses [15–17].

11.4.1 Neonates

Neonates (i.e. below the age of 28 days) may present with pyrexia but without clear indications in the history or on examination as to likely cause. Despite this, 3% of such cases have a grave bacterial infection. It is vital to gain a clear patient account from the child's mother about the pregnancy, delivery and life up to then of the neonate. An infection within the first week of life is usually transmitted from the mother, whilst after that point, the infection is generally from either the community or hospital environments. To be sure of the details of a grave bacterial infection, laboratory assistance is needed. The patient must be fully investigated for sepsis, including blood culture, CSF +/− urine sampling. The peak occurrence of bacterial meningitis is at age 1 month or younger. It is thought that between 5% and 10% of neonates who test positive for Group B streptococci (GBS) also have meningitis [18, 19].

11.4.2 Young Infants

Managing pyrexia in an infant between 28 and 60 days old involves remaining highly alert to possible sources of infection, since physical examination often appears normal. In infants below the age of 3 months, a severe bacterial infection is seen in around 6–10% of cases, usually the result of urinary tract infection (UTI). Somewhat surprisingly, if a child aged below 3 months is found to have a definite viral infection, the chance that a severe bacterial infection is also present decreases compared to those without a viral infection [20]. However, infants suffering from bronchiolitis often have a UTI, too [18].

11.4.3 Children Aged Between 3 Months and 3 Years

The Agency of Health Care Policy and Research issued guidelines in 2012 [21], according to which, a rectal temperature of at least 38° in a child aged below 3 months is associated with a risk between 4.1% and 25.1% of a severe bacterial infection. These data were obtained in accident and emergency departments or primary care settings in North America.

In the past, 2–4% of patients aged between 3 and 36 months whose rectally recorded temperature was at least 38.5 °C were harbouring an occult blood-borne bacterial infection [22]. The principal pathogen was *Streptococcus pneumoniae*, with *Haemophilus influenzae* type b the second most likely cause. Vaccination has achieved great success against these organisms, with the result that only 0.5% (i.e. 1 in 200) children with pyrexia, who are otherwise immune competent, now harbour bacteria in the blood [23, 24].

Currently, occult bacterial infection of the blood is only seen in between 0.25 and 0.7% of such children, and two thirds of apparent bacteraemias are actually false positives, as a result of contamination [23–26]. The most frequent bacteria responsible (representing 2 out of 3 cases) are pneumococci or *Escherichia coli*. It is common that infants with a pneumococcal infection harbour bacterial strains of a type to which the conjugated vaccine, which targets seven different bacterial sugars, does not confer immunity [18].

Blood-borne infection by *S. pneumoniae* may appear as acute otitis media, pneumonia, sinusitis, meningitis, pyrexia-related convulsion, soft tissue infection (sometimes affecting the orbit or face), or have other features of pyrexia that do not point to a particular diagnosis. Infection with *E. coli* is usually seen in a child aged under one year and typically together with a urinary tract infection (UTI). 15% of blood-borne infections are secondary to *Staphylococcus aureus*, occurring in association with cellulitis, skin or musculoskeletal infection. The bulk of the other cases are due to Salmonella spp., *Neisseria meningitidis* or *Streptococcus pyogenes* [18].

11.5 History and Examination in Children

11.5.1 Neonates

It is vital to obtain a full history for any neonate suffering from pyrexia. The pattern of symptoms may point to an infective focus (e.g. diarrhoea, coughing) or be more general (e.g. not feeding, being irritable, lethargy). 20–50% of neonates with meningitis have a convulsion. It needs to be established if there is anyone in contact with the child who is already sick (either at home or elsewhere), if any illness has recently occurred, any vaccination has been administered and whether antibiotics have been prescribed around the time of birth or afterwards [18].

11.5.2 Prenatal History

The pregnancy history should be reviewed, encompassing any sexually transmitted infection, such as HIV, hepatitis B or C, treponemal infection, gonorrhoea, chlamydia or herpes simplex. The mother's GBS status should be reviewed, together with any precautions taken, how the delivery occurred, if the membranes were ruptured long before birth and whether the mother suffered from any pyrexial episode.

The following are risk factors for a severe bacterial infection: a neonate weighing below 2500 g at delivery, premature rupture of the membranes, sepsis or trauma during delivery, hypoxia in the foetus, the mother having an infection around the time of birth, and galactosaemia. Gestational age needs to be calculated, since prematurity heightens the risk of a severe bacterial infection [18].

11.5.3 Household Contacts

Any family members suffering from illness need to be recorded. If the patient has been in contact with animals at home or elsewhere (such as at a nursery), this should also be ascertained. The vaccination histories of others living in the house should be documented. If another pregnancy has been lost or a baby has previously died due to an infectious disease, then a congenital anomaly or primary immunodeficiency syndrome will need to be excluded as the cause [18].

11.5.4 Review of Systems and Physical Examination

All body systems need to be carefully reviewed for symptoms to pick up any clues about the origin of pyrexia. Patients should be completely examined and vital signs noted. Oximetry should be performed, and growth checked, with the various parameters assigned to the appropriate percentile. On general examination, note how active the child is, whether skin changes are present, muscular tone, and signs of irritability. Look for a focus of infection by checking the skin, mucosal membranes, ears and limbs.

If the umbilicus persists as a stump after 4 weeks age, this can indicate a white cell adhesive deficiency syndrome. Uncircumcised boys are at greater risk of a UTI. Aside from pyrexia, it is frequent for UTI in neonates to present as failure to thrive, icterus (usually a result of a conjugated hyperbilirubinaemia secondary to cholestasis), and vomiting. The following also may indicate a severe infective episode in a neonate: being irritability, not responding to soothing, inadequate skin perfusion, lack of tone, moving less than usual, and becoming lethargic [18].

11.5.5 History and Examination in Young Infants

As with a neonate, pyrexia in an infant may be reflected in symptoms pointing to an infective focus (diarrhoea or coughing) or be more general (e.g. not feeding, being irritable, lethargy). Identify if the infant has been in contact with anyone else suffering from illness at home or outside, such as at a nursery. Recent illness, vaccinations administered and any antimicrobial therapy all need to be noted [18].

11.5.5.1 Past Medical History and Household Contacts

In essence, the history to be obtained for an infant does not differ from that for a neonate. The history should include the pregnancy, delivery and early life. Note any other medical problems and any medication being used that might render an infection more likely. Additionally, note details of the diet and how well and long the child sleeps, as you would with any neonate. Eating less or sudden alterations in how sleep occurs may point towards a systemic infection.

If another pregnancy has been lost or a baby has previously died due to an infectious disease, then a congenital anomaly or primary immunodeficiency syndrome will need to be excluded as the cause, as is the case with neonates. It is important to establish who lives with the child and who is the main carer. Being in contact with new arrivals from overseas, and being homeless or poor are important factors to consider in assessing risk of infective illness and treating the case [18].

11.5.5.2 Review of Systems and Physical Examination

All body systems need to be carefully reviewed for symptoms to pick up any clues about the origin of pyrexia. Patients should be completely examined and vital signs noted. Oximetry should be performed, and growth checked, with the various parameters assigned to the appropriate percentile. Tachycardia (>160 bpm in infants) and tachypnoea ($>60.min^{-1}$) increase the risk of death occurring and are frequently associated with the onset of septic shock [18].

11.5.6 History and Examination in Children Aged Between 3 Months and 3 Years

History taking needs to concentrate on factors that put an infant or toddler at higher risk of severe bacterial infection.

11.5.6.1 History of Presenting Complaint

It is vital to record the patient's temperature and the measurement method employed. A rectally recorded temperature exceeding 38.5 °C (101 °F) indicates abnormality in a child of this age. As well as recording the temporal onset and duration of pyrexia, any other symptoms need to be carefully enquired after. The following is a non-exhaustive list of other symptoms to consider: loose stools, vomiting, nasal discharge, coughing, skin exanthem, and alteration in weight or eating habits [18].

11.5.6.2 Past Medical History

Search exhaustively for any evidence of prior infections and risk factors predisposing to severe infections by bacteria. Underlying chronic diseases, prior surgical operations, previous urinary tract infections (UTIs), and incomplete courses of pneumococcal or hib vaccinations should particularly be asked about. In patients aged under 9 months, the neonatal and perinatal history is of especial significance [18].

11.5.6.3 Family History

If siblings or first cousins are subject to recurrent infective episodes or the mother supplies a history of miscarriage, this should alert the clinician to the possibility of a primary immunodeficiency. It is vital to learn the human immunodeficiency virus (HIV) status of the parents. If immediate or more distant blood relatives are subject to chronic infections (such as hepatitis B or C, or tuberculosis), this is also of diagnostic significance. Acute infections in family members, e.g. croup or respiratory infections, is similarly an important point to consider [18].

11.5.6.4 Social History and Household Contacts

Assess whether the child has been exposed to animals, insects or woodland environments. Has the child been near dirty drinking water or sewage? Has he/she been travelling, especially if overseas? Does the child attend a nursery? This type of question will provide vital information which may say something about a possible epidemiological or environmental cause. Being in contact with ill individuals beyond the usual family members may also offer invaluable evidence [18].

11.5.6.5 Review of Systems and Physical Examination

Asking questions about all the body systems can reveal clues that point to the origin of pyrexia. The following are especially useful in pinpointing a focus: exanthems, conjunctivitis, otalgia and otorrhoea, swollen and tender lymph glands, symptoms related to breathing, alteration in appetite, weight loss, loose stools, vomiting, alteration in how often urine is passed and whether dysuria occurs, inability to bear weight, limbs that hurt when someone else moves them, and symptoms of clear neurological origin.

In a child between 3 and 36 months old with pyrexia, the following features of the physical examination are consistent with a severe bacterial infection: appearing ill, pyrexia, vomiting, abnormally raised respiratory rate with chest retraction and slow capillary refill. These appearances are seen in cases of bacterial infection in over 39.5% of those aged 2 to 3 years and in above 39% of those aged 3–24 months.

The cutaneous system, lymph glands, eyes, ears, nose, and pharynx all need to be carefully inspected, since a viral infection is associated with an exanthem or breathing difficulties in a great many infants. The chest must be inspected and auscultated as an invariable part of the physical examination. Inspect the abdomen to see if it is distended. Ileus or excessive intestinal activity may be apparent at auscultation. Check the capillary refill time in the fingers and toes. Check how far the joints move, look for signs of infection, and assess if there is tenderness in any particular area. Depending on the age of the patient, a neurological and developmental examination should be carried out [18].

11.6 Differential Diagnosis [18]

- Bacteraemia.
- Neonatal sepsis.
- Meningitis due to bacterial infection.
- Infection due to *E. coli.*
- Infection due to *H. influenzae.*
- Meningitis and Encephalitis.
- Bacteraemia due to *S. pneumoniae.*
- Urinary tract infection.
- Infection due to *S. aureus.*
- Infection due to Group B Streptococcus (GBS).

11.7 Diagnostic Studies

Markers of low risk are well established for a child older than 28 days. The reference range for leucocytes is 5000–15,000 cells/μL. There should be fewer than 1500 band cells/μL. Nonetheless, leucocyte count on its own is neither sensitive nor specific for bacteraemia or meningitis in young children and should not be relied on, without also carrying out a full sepsis screen [18].

11.7.1 Urine and Stool Studies

Given the fact that urinary tract infections (UTIs) are common in children of this age, urine should be collected for urinalysis and culture. In a single study, pyuria was evident in just 20% of infants with pyrexia who were found to have pyelonephritis. Urine for culture must be aspirated suprapubically or by inserting a catheter in the urethra, as urine from a collecting bag usually contains contaminating organisms [18].

11.7.2 Pulmonary Studies

If an infant presents with evidence of respiratory distress, for example, coughing, cold, abnormally raised respiratory rate, rales, rhonchi, chest retraction, grunting, flared nostrils, or wheeze, chest X-ray may be needed. At appropriate times of the year, an identification of the viral pathogen should be attempted via direct fluorescent antigen (DFA) testing or viral DNA polymerase chain reaction (PCR) and viral culture of nasal lavage fluid [18].

11.8 Treatment

Pyrexia represents an appropriate biological response rather than a pathological process. If a child has no other health problem, the majority of pyrexial illnesses are not severe, and require no intervention, as long as the aetiology is clear and fluid levels are maintained. Pyrexia alone is not responsible for brain insults. Clinical intervention is warranted if signs of a severe kind are present. It may be appropriate to initiate an antipyretic if a child is distressed (as indicated by reduced activity, a drop in volume of drinks consumed, etc). Whether an antipyretic drug lowers the body temperature or not reveals nothing about the likely bacterial or viral nature of an infection. There is no need to waken a sleeping child merely to administer an antipyretic [1].

The correct dose of an antipyretic agent depends on weight, not patient age. If prescribing an antipyretic for use with a child, the dose will be more accurate if written guidance is given and an accurately marked syringe supplied for liquid preparations. Relying on the instructions and equipment supplied with OTC preparations to ensure correct dosing is unwise given the wide margin of error using such equipment involves [27].

11.8.1 Antipyretic Agents

Anti-fever agents resolve pyrexia by resetting the hypothalamic set-point within normal bounds. The two most frequently encountered anti-fever agents in paediatric practice are paracetamol and ibuprofen. Since aspirin has an association with Reye syndrome, it is contraindicated in children [11].

11.8.1.1 Indications

Therapeutic interventions in children with pyrexia are individually tailored to suit the clinical presentation, in particular the likely cause, level of distress and need to investigate the pattern of pyrexia seen [1].

It is appropriate to treat pyrexia in the short term in cases such as the following [3, 14]:

- Shock.
- Underlying disease of the nervous, circulatory or respiratory system, or any disorder resulting in raised metabolic demand (e.g. following burns injury, or post-surgery).
- Fluid and electrolyte not in equilibrium.

- High fever (i.e. $\geq$40 °C (104 °F)).
- Distress.
- Significant cerebral injury.
- Following a cardiac arrest.

11.8.1.2 Paracetamol

The author recommends paracetamol in the majority of paediatric cases of pyrexia that require treatment. This is due to the agent's well-established safety, provided the dose is not exceeded [3].

It is not usually advisable to use paracetamol in children less than 3 months old, except under medical supervision, as pyrexia may be the sole indicator of a grave infection. The dosage of paracetamol is 10–15 mg/kg per dose (maximum dosage 1 g) by mouth every four to 6 h (with no more than five doses in any 24-hour period). The maximum daily dose is 75 mg/kg per day up to a total of 4 g/day. Some paracetamol preparations recommend lower amounts. The author does not suggest routine use of a loading dose (which would be 30 mg/kg), as it may complicate further dosing and lead to error [11].

The temperature falls by 1 or 2 degrees Celsius (1.8 to 3.6 Fahrenheit) in around 80% of paediatric cases of pyrexia [11, 28]. The onset of therapeutic action is within 30–60 min, with peak effect after 3 or 4 h. Therapeutic effects last between 4 and 6 h [1].

11.8.1.3 Ibuprofen

Ibuprofen is recommended as first-line treatment in any child aged over 6 months in whom an antipyretic and anti-inflammatory action is needed. Such is the case in, e.g. juvenile arthritis. Children receiving Ibuprofen should have adequate hydration [3].

The dosage of ibuprofen is 10 mg/kg per dose (with a maximum dose of 600 mg) by mouth every 6 h. Daily, the maximum daily dose is 40 mg/kg up to a total of 2.4 g [11]. The onset of therapeutic action is within 60 minutes, with the maximum effect (a fall in temperature of between 1 and 2 °C (1.8–3.6 °F)) occurring within 3 to 4 h. Therapeutic effects last 6–8 h [11, 28].

11.8.2 External Cooling

External cooling is the best way to counter heat stroke and other forms of heat-related illness, since lowering the body temperature swiftly is needed if end-organ damage is to be avoided. External cooling is not proposed to lower body temperature in infants and children with pyrexia but who are otherwise healthy. Studies where patients were randomised to receive either tepid sponging and antipyretic therapy together or antipyretic therapy only, the additional advantage of tepid sponging in lowering the body temperature was brief in duration, and sponging brought with it a higher degree of discomfort [29–31].

References

1. Ward MA. Fever in infants and children: pathophysiology and management. In: Edwards MS, Torchia MM (Eds.). UpToDate. Last updated: May 09, 2019.
2. Mackowiak PA, Wasserman SS. Physicians' perceptions regarding body temperature in health and disease. South Med J. 1995;88:934.
3. Ward MA, Hannemann NL. Fever: pathogenesis and treatment. In: Cherry JD, Harrison G, Kaplan SL, et al., editors. Feigin and Cherry's textbook of pediatric infectious diseases. 8th ed. Philadelphia: Elsevier; 2018. p. 52.
4. Schmitt BD. Fever in childhood. Pediatrics. 1984;74:929.
5. Herzog LW, Coyne LJ. What is fever? Normal temperature in infants less than 3 months old. Clin Pediatr (Phila). 1993;32:142.
6. Mackowiak PA, Wasserman SS, Levine MM. A critical appraisal of 98.6 degrees F, the upper limit of the normal body temperature, and other legacies of Carl Reinhold august Wunderlich. JAMA. 1992;268:1578.
7. Baraff LJ. Management of the febrile child: a survey of pediatric and emergency medicine residency directors. Pediatr Infect Dis J. 1991;10:795.
8. Dagan R, Sofer S, Phillip M, Shachak E. Ambulatory care of febrile infants younger than 2 months of age classified as being at low risk for having serious bacterial infections. J Pediatr. 1988;112:355.
9. Baraff LJ, Bass JW, Fleisher GR, et al. Practice guideline for the management of infants and children 0 to 36 months of age with fever without source. Agency for health care policy and research. Ann Emerg Med. 1993;22:1198.
10. Herzog L, Phillips SG. Addressing concerns about fever. Clin Pediatr (Phila). 2011;50:383.
11. Section on Clinical Pharmacology and Therapeutics, Committee on Drugs, Sullivan JE, Farrar HC. Fever and antipyretic use in children. Pediatrics. 2011;127:580.
12. Dinarello CA. Cytokines as endogenous pyrogens. J Infect Dis. 1999;179(Suppl 2):S294.
13. Trautner BW, Caviness AC, Gerlacher GR, et al. Prospective evaluation of the risk of serious bacterial infection in children who present to the emergency department with hyperpyrexia (temperature of 106 degrees F or higher). Pediatrics. 2006;118:34.
14. El-Radhi AS. Why is the evidence not affecting the practice of fever management? Arch Dis Child. 2008;93:918.
15. Weisse ME, Miller G, Brien JH. Fever response to acetaminophen in viral vs bacterial infections. Pediatr Infect Dis J. 1987;6:1091.
16. Baker MD, Fosarelli PD, Carpenter RO. Childhood fever: correlation of diagnosis with temperature response to acetaminophen. Pediatrics. 1987;80:315.
17. Bonadio WA, Bellomo T, Brady W, Smith D. Correlating changes in body temperature with infectious outcome in febrile children who receive acetaminophen. Clin Pediatr. 1993;32:343.
18. Gould JM. Fever in the infant and toddler follow-up. In: Steele RW. Medscape. Updated: Jan 08, 2019. https://emedicine.medscape.com/article/1834870-overview. Accessed 26 Nov 2019.
19. Edwards MS, Nizet V, Baker CJ. Group B streptococcal infections. In: Remington JS, Klein JO, Wilson CB, Baker CJ, editors. Infectious diseases of the fetus and newborn infant. 6th ed. Philadelphia, PA: Elsevier Saunders; 2006. p. 403.
20. Byington CL, Enriquez FR, Hoff C, et al. Serious bacterial infections in febrile infants 1 to 90 days old with and without viral infections. Pediatrics. 2004;113(6):1662–6.
21. Agency for Healthcare Research and Quality. Diagnosis and Management of Febrile Infants (0–3 months) Executive Summary. Agency for Healthcare Research and Quality. March 2012. Available at http://www.effectivehealthcare.ahrq.gov/reports/final.cfm.
22. Teele DW, Pelton SI, Grant MJ, et al. Bacteremia in febrile children under 2 years of age: results of cultures of blood of 600 consecutive febrile children seen in a "walk-in" clinic. J Pediatr. 1975 Aug.;87(2):227–30.
23. Herz AM, Greenhow TL, Alcantara J, et al. Changing epidemiology of outpatient bacteremia in 3- to 36-month-old children after the introduction of the heptavalent-conjugated pneumococcal vaccine. Pediatr Infect Dis J. 2006 Apr.;25(4):293–300.

24. Baraff LJ, Bass JW, Fleisher GR, et al. Practice guideline for the management of infants and children 0 to 36 months of age with fever without source. Agency for Health Care Policy and Research. Ann Emerg Med. 1993 Jul.;22(7):1198–210.
25. Wilkinson M, Bulloch B, Smith M. Prevalence of occult bacteremia in children aged 3 to 36 months presenting to the emergency department with fever in the postpneumococcal conjugate vaccine era. Acad Emerg Med. 2009;16:220–5.
26. Sard B, Bailey MC, Vinci R. An analysis of pediatric blood cultures in the postpneumococcal conjugate vaccine era in a community hospital emergency department. Pediatr Emerg Care. May 2006;22:295–300.
27. Yin HS, Wolf MS, Dreyer BP, et al. Evaluation of consistency in dosing directions and measuring devices for pediatric nonprescription liquid medications. JAMA. 2010;304:2595.
28. McIntyre J, Hull D. Comparing efficacy and tolerability of ibuprofen and paracetamol in fever. Arch Dis Child. 1996;74:164.
29. Thomas S, Vijaykumar C, Naik R, et al. Comparative effectiveness of tepid sponging and antipyretic drug versus only antipyretic drug in the management of fever among children: a randomized controlled trial. Indian Pediatr. 2009;46:133.
30. Alves JG, Almeida ND, Almeida CD. Tepid sponging plus dipyrone versus dipyrone alone for reducing body temperature in febrile children. Sao Paulo Med J. 2008;126:107.
31. Purssell E. Physical treatment of fever. Arch Dis Child. 2000;82:238.

Headache in Children

12

Hülya Maraş Genç, Bülent Kara, and Çiçek Wöber-Bingöl

12.1 Introduction

Headache is one of the most common symptoms in children and adolescents. Lifetime prevalence reaches 90%. In a review of 64 epidemiological studies, the mean prevalence of headache was 54.4% and the mean prevalence of migraine was 9.1% [1]. The World Health Organization included migraine among the top 10 health problems of children and adolescents in the 50 most populous countries of the world [2]. As an example, in Turkey, the one-year prevalence of headache was 73.7% and that of migraine was 26.7% (definite migraine 7.3%, probable migraine 19.4%) [3]. This nation-wide study applied for the first time a validated questionnaire intended to be used in different countries all over the world [3–8].

Headache originates from intracranial (dura, large blood vessels, and venous sinuses) and extracranial (periosteum, oropharynx, orbit, sinus, middle ear, teeth, facial and neck muscles) structures, but the brain itself does not have pain sensation [9]. In daily clinical practice, headache in children and adolescents requires an appropriate approach with respect to history, clinical examination, neuroimaging, and further diagnostic procedures. The prerequisite for adequate headache treatment is a correct diagnosis differentiating between primary and secondary headaches. Primary headaches, such as migraines and tension-type headaches, are

H. M. Genç (✉)
Section of Pediatric Neurology, Ümraniye Training and Research Hospital, University of Health Sciences, İstanbul, Turkey

B. Kara
Division of Pediatric Neurology, Department of Pediatrics, Faculty of Medicine, Kocaeli University, Kocaeli, Turkey

Ç. Wöber-Bingöl
Department of Child and Adolescent Psychiatry, Medical University of Vienna (former affiliation), Vienna, Austria

not attributed to another disorder whereas secondary headaches are caused by a specific disorder such as sinusitis, systemic infections, head or neck injuries, or brain tumors [10]. The co-existence of primary and secondary headaches is a particular diagnostic challenge [11]. Recurrent headaches are most often classified as migraine or tension-type headaches.

12.2 Temporal Pattern of Headaches

Headaches may be classified into five temporal patterns: acute, acute recurrent, chronic progressive, chronic non-progressive, and mixed [12, 13]. Classifying a headache to one of those groups may help in managing children and adolescents presenting with headache.

Acute headache represents a single episode of a headache without any history of previous events. This pattern is usually attributed to febrile illness related to upper respiratory tract infections, acute rhinosinusitis, otitis media, or the first attack of migraine. Rarely, it may be attributed to central nervous system infections (meningitis, encephalitis), increased intracranial pressure (hydrocephalus, brain tumor), arterial hypertension, vascular pathologies (subarachnoid hemorrhage, other intracranial hemorrhages, cerebral venous thrombosis), or exposure to a substance (non-headache medication, carbon monoxide).

Acute recurrent headache is characterized by recurring patterns of headache with symptom-free intervals. It is usually related to primary headaches, most importantly migraine and tension-type headache, and rarely trigeminal autonomic cephalalgias. Seizures, hypertension, metabolic disorders (electrolyte disturbances, hyperthyroidism), medications and mitochondrial encephalomyopathy, lactic acidosis, and stroke-like episodes (MELAS) may also cause an acute recurrent headache.

Chronic progressive headache stands out due to a gradual increase in the frequency and severity of the headache. This type of headache often suggests an underlying severe condition including hydrocephalus, expanding intracranial mass lesions (brain tumor, abscess), and symptomatic or idiopathic intracranial hypertension.

Chronic non-progressive headache represents a frequent or constant headache without a sustained increase in severity or other signs of progression. Chronic tension-type headache, chronic migraine, medication overuse headache, and chronic posttraumatic headache are included in this group.

In the mixed headache pattern, acute recurrent headache is superimposed on chronic non-progressive headache, e.g. migraine on a background of chronic tension-type headache.

12.3 History and Clinical Examination

Headache is very rarely the only and isolated symptom of a life-threatening disease. Usually, there are further symptoms not compatible with a primary headache disorder or the clinical examination shows abnormal findings. In pediatric emergency settings, headaches are most often attributed to viral diseases. In primary care, most patients presenting with headache suffer from primary headaches and headaches related to systemic infections [14].

Considering a large number of children and adolescents with primary or benign secondary headaches, it may be demanding to identify the few with a potentially life-threatening disorder. Red flags that require immediate medical attention include severe headaches that occur for the first time, headache onset during the night, occipital localization of the headache, progressive headaches, a marked change of pre-existing headaches, atypical associated symptoms, or headaches not responding to analgesics (Table 12.1) [11, 13].

Similarly, in children and adolescents with acute recurrent or chronic non-progressive headaches, a detailed history with the child and the parents is an essential prerequisite for adequate management (Table 12.2). In toddlers not yet able to verbalize pain, headaches may be inferred from behavior. The child may seclude oneself, stop playing, or may wish to lie down. A pale face and tearfulness can also indicate headache, especially if these symptoms are episodic. Older children can answer many questions about their headaches themselves, provided they are given appropriate attention [11, 13].

The physical and neurological examinations must be adopted to the age of the patient. They are generally normal in primary headaches [14]. Importantly, a normal clinical examination does not exclude a secondary headache. Symptoms and signs accompanying the headache may be crucial for the differential diagnosis, such as meningeal signs or a rash in meningitis; papilledema in increased intracranial pressure; focal neurological deficits in space-occupying lesions; altered mental status in encephalitis or increased intracranial pressure; fever in infections; a bruit on auscultation of the head, neck, and eyes in arteriovenous malformations; sinus tenderness in sinusitis; or temporomandibular joint (TMJ) tenderness in TMJ dysfunction.

12.4 Diagnostic Procedures

In children and adolescents presenting with headache, there is no "routine" diagnostic procedure. The decision about further investigations is based on history and the findings of the clinical examination. In patients with migraine and tension-type headache, the only examination, which can be recommended routinely is an ophthalmological consultation, as unrecognized refractive errors may have an impact on the frequency and severity of these headaches [11].

12.4.1 Neuroimaging

Neuroimaging is recommended if an intracranial disorder is suspected. Although magnetic resonance imaging (MRI) is a superior neuroimaging technique with respect to computed tomography (CT), in emergency management, CT offers fast recognition of most, but not all intracranial disorders causing acute or chronic

Table 12.1 Red flags in headache

History
• Headache occurring before the age of 5 years.
• Time since onset of headache less than six months.
• First or worst headache (thunderclap headache).
• Headache that awakens the child from sleep.
• Early morning headache.
• Occipital headaches.
• Headache onset during or shortly after exertion.
• Worsening of headache upon Valsalva maneuvers (coughing, straining, etc.)
• New-onset headache associated with.
o atypical or isolated symptoms,
■ e.g., exanthema or early morning vomiting,
o head trauma,
o infection,
o fever,
o increased blood pressure,
o polydipsia, polyuria,
o epileptic seizure,
o neurological symptoms,
■ except those which are consistent with typical migraine aura,
■ e.g., double vision, motor weakness, vertigo, unsteady stance or gait, disorders of consciousness, orientation or memory impairment,
o comorbid conditions,
■ e.g., immunosuppression, malignancy, coagulopathy, sickle cell disease, cyanotic heart disease, or neurocutaneous disorders,
o ventriculo-peritoneal or ventriculo-atrial shunt,
• Migrainous headache without a family history of migraine or its equivalents.
• Unusual headaches.
• Chronic progressive headache.
• A significant change in headache characteristics or associated symptoms.
Physical examination
• Sick appearance.
• Fever.
• Increased blood pressure.
• Impaired consciousness.
• Impaired orientation.
• New-onset cognitive impairment.
• Papilledema.
• Visual field defects.
• Cranial nerve palsies.
• Focal neurological deficits such as hemiparesis, dysphasia, or ataxia.
• Disorder of stance or gait.
• Increased head circumference.
• Precocious or delayed puberty

progressive headaches. Pathological findings in cranial CT usually require further evaluation by MRI and/or MR-angiography. Suspected cerebral venous thrombosis requires MRI and MR venography.

Elective cranial MRI may be indicated for re-assurance in patients with migraine or tension-type headache if the parents or the patient fear a brain tumor or another

Table 12.2 Questions for detailed history in children and adolescents with recurrent headaches[a]

1- When/how did the headache begin? (new-onset or chronic).
2- Do you have different types of headaches or are they always the same?
3- Has the headache worsened, has it improved, or has it stayed the same?
4- How many days a month do you have a headache?
5- How long does the headache typically last?
6- Do the headaches happen at any particular time?
7- Did you notice anything triggering the headache?
8- Do you notice any symptoms before the onset of headache (premonitory symptoms, aura)?
9- Where do you feel the pain?
10- What is the pain like? (throbbing, pressing or tightening, stabbing).
11- Do you notice any symptoms during the headache (nausea, vomiting, anorexia, photophobia, phonophobia, or other symptoms)?
12- What do you do during the headache? (interaction with daily activities).
13- What makes the headache worse or better (effect of physical activity, light, noise, smells, sleep, vomiting, analgesics)?
14- Are you taking pain killers for headache (substance, dosage).
15- When do you use the medication (at the onset of the headache or later during the attack)?
16- How many days a month do you use a pain killer?
17- Did you have any other therapies for your headache?
18- Do you have any problems at home, with friends or at school?
19- Do you have any other health problems or therapies?
20- Is there anybody in your family also having headaches?

[a]Adopted from Ref. 11 and 13.

serious disease [11, 15]. MRI may reveal incidental findings unrelated to headache or normal variants such as Virchow-Robin spaces, but the possibility of such findings does not outweigh the risk of doctor shopping when an expected referral for a cranial MRI is refused [16, 17]. If neuroimaging does not reveal a causative finding, regular follow-up visits are essential in persistent or recurrent headaches. There is no need to repeat neuroimaging if headache characteristics and physical examination do not change.

12.4.2 Laboratory Investigations

If history and physical examination are compatible with migraine or tension-type headache, laboratory investigations are not necessary. If a secondary headache is suspected, appropriate tests should be chosen.

12.4.3 Lumbar Puncture

Investigation of the cerebrospinal fluid (CSF) is indicated in patients with symptoms or signs of meningitis or encephalitis, in patients presenting with a thunderclap headache, if cranial CT is negative and for measuring the opening pressure in idiopathic intracranial hypertension (IIH). The latter must be performed in a lateral recumbent position. Lumbar puncture is contraindicated in patients with raised intracranial pressure (except IIH), anticoagulation or coagulopathies, and hemodynamically unstable.

12.4.4 Electroencephalography

Electroencephalography is only recommended when epileptic seizures are suspected. It has no place in the routine evaluation of headaches because it does not yield any information about the cause or type of headache.

12.5 Clinical Features

12.5.1 Migraine

A migraine attack may occur in any person. Recurrent attacks are related to genetic disposition (migraine history in first degree relatives), modulating factors such as the physiological decline in estrogen levels before menstruation and trigger factors [18, 19]. The number of potential migraine triggers mentioned in the literature is huge, but scientifically sound data on migraine triggers in children and adolescents are poor. Changes in the sleep-wake rhythm (too little or too much sleep), insufficient fluid intake, skipping meals, school stress, family conflicts, and fears are considered to be the most important triggers [15]. Foods or food additives are less important, except in the presence of food allergies. There is no trigger factor precipitating an attack in all migraine patients and the influence of a specific trigger may vary considerably in the individual patient [18–20]. Sensory stimuli such as light, noise, and smells may play a greater role in migraine with aura [15, 18].

As in adults, migraines in childhood and adolescence have a significant impact on activities of daily life. The unpredictable occurrence of attacks adversely affects school attendance, performance and concentration in school, homework and learning as well as leisure activities, and family life [3–5]. In a large study, the impairment of quality of life in adolescents with headaches was greater than that of asthma, diabetes, and cancer [21].

The onset of migraine headache may be preceded by premonitory and aura symptoms. A pale face, fatigue, and irritability are the most common premonitory symptoms. Aura symptoms are rare in children and become more common as adolescence progresses [11, 15].

The third edition of the International Classification of Headache Disorders (ICHD-3), the algorithmic system to define and classify all known headache disorders, of the Classification Committee of the International Headache Society, differentiates migraine without aura, migraine with aura, chronic migraine, and periodic syndromes of childhood.

Migraine without aura. Childhood migraine without aura is characterized by a significantly shorter duration than in adults, usually only a few hours (Table 12.3). The child appears sick, stops routine daily activities, wants to sleep, and frequently

Table 12.3 Diagnostic criteria for migraine without aura - ICHD-3[a]

A. At least five attacks fulfilling B through D.
B. Headache attacks lasting 4 to 72 hours (untreated or unsuccessfully treated, attacks may last 2 to 72 hours in children and adolescents).
C. Headache has at least two of the following characteristics:
   A- Unilateral location (headache is more often bilateral in children than adults).
   B- Pulsating quality.
   C- Moderate or severe pain intensity.
   D- Aggravation by or causing avoidance of routine physical activity.
D. During headache at least one of the following
   1- Nausea and/or vomiting.
   2- Photophobia and phonophobia (may be inferred from behavior in young children).
E. Not better accounted for by another ICHD-3 diagnosis.

[a]Adopted from Ref. [22].
ICHD-3 indicates The International Classification of Headache Disorders, third ed. Cephalalgia. 2018;38:1–211.

is migraine-free when waking up. The pain is most often localized in the forehead (in the middle or bilateral). Pain intensity is moderate to severe (typically more severe than tension-type headache) and pain may worsen with routine physical activity. The diagnosis of migraine without aura requires the presence of associated symptoms, nausea being the most common [22, 23]. Younger children may not verbalize sensitivity to light or noise, but photophobia and phonophobia may be understood from their preferring a darkened and quiet room.

Migraine with aura. Aura symptoms do not differ significantly from those in adults. Typical aura (Table 12.4) is differentiated from brainstem aura characterized by vertigo, tinnitus, hyperacusis, diplopia, dysarthria, ataxia, or decreased level of consciousness. Brainstem aura may be more common in children and adolescents than in adults. In few patients, a "confusional state" with disorientation and psychomotor restlessness may occur, for which, unlike epilepsy, there is usually no amnesia. Hemiplegic and retinal migraines are the least common [11, 22].

Chronic migraine is defined by headaches for 15 or more days per month including at least eight days with migraine for more than three months [22].

Periodic Syndromes of Childhood. Cyclic vomiting, abdominal migraine, and two rare conditions - benign paroxysmal vertigo and benign paroxysmal torticollis are included in this group. These disorders have in common the absence of an underlying cause and a (presumed) pathophysiological relation to migraine [22, 24].

12.5.2 Tension-Type Headache

Tension-type headache (TTH) is the most common of all headache types. ICHD-3 differentiates between infrequent and frequent episodic TTH depending on headache frequency (Table 12.5) [22]. Chronic TTH is defined by 15 or more headache days per month for more than 3 months. Pain is usually bilateral. Pain quality is most often described as pressing or tightening. Associated symptoms are absent or in the background [25, 26]. However, TTH may overlap with migraine or may be an

Table 12.4 Diagnostic criteria for migraine with typical aura - ICHD-3[a]

A. At least two attacks fulfilling criterion B and C.
B. One or more of the following fully reversible aura symptoms:
 1. Visual.
 2. Sensory.
 3. Speech and/or language.
C. At least three of the following six characteristics:
 1. At least one aura symptom spreads gradually over >5 min,
 2. Two or more symptoms occur in succession.
 3. Each individual aura symptom lasts 5–60 min.
 4. At least one aura symptom is unilateral.
 5. At least one aura symptom is positive.
 6. The aura is accompanied, or followed within 60 minutes, by headache.
D. Not better accounted for by another ICHD-3 diagnosis.

[a]Adopted from Ref. [22].
ICHD-3 indicates The International Classification of Headache Disorders, third ed. Cephalalgia. 2018;38:1-211.

Table 12.5 Diagnostic criteria for episodic tension-type headache (ETTH) - ICHD-3[a]

A. At least 10 episodes of headache [occurring on <12 days/year in infrequent ETTH and 1-14 days/month on average for >3 months in frequent ETTH] and fulfilling criteria B through D.
B. Headache lasting from 30 minutes to seven days.
C. At least two of the following four characteristics:
 1. Bilateral location.
 2. Pressing or tightening (non-pulsating) quality.
 3. Mild or moderate intensity.
 4. Not aggravated by routine physical activity such as walking or climbing stairs.
D. Both of the following.
 1. No nausea or vomiting.
 2. No more than one of photophobia or phonophobia.
E. Not better accounted for by another ICHD-3 diagnosis.

[a]Adopted from Ref. [22].
ICHD-3 indicates The International Classification of Headache Disorders, third ed. Cephalalgia. 2018;38:1–211.

evolution from TTH to migraine or contrariwise [23]. The characteristics of TTH in children and adolescents differ from those of adults only in a few aspects. In a clinic-based study, headache frequency was lower, headache duration was shorter and localization of the pain was more constant in children and adolescents as compared to adults. In addition, the use of analgesics increased significantly from childhood to adulthood [27].

12.5.3 Trigeminal Autonomic Cephalalgias

Cluster headache, characterized by severe painful attacks, is the most common form. Signs and symptoms include unilateral orbital, supraorbital, or temporal pain lasting in 15–180 min, associated with autonomic symptoms ipsilateral to the side of pain, such as lacrimation, conjunctival injection, miosis, ptosis, eyelid edema, nasal discharge, nasal congestion, forehead, and facial sweating. Contrary to migraine, attacks are often associated with restlessness or agitation [22].

12.5.4 Secondary Headaches

Secondary headaches are attributed to an underlying disorder. The principle diagnostic criteria for secondary headaches are shown in Table 12.6. Secondary headaches are mostly acute isolated or chronic progressive headaches. However, many children suffer from multiple headache types, and detailed history of different headache types is essential [12]. Here, only some of the secondary headaches will be discussed, namely potentially life-threatening, but rare ones; frequent and usually benign ones; and a few other important.

Rare, but potentially life-threatening disorders causing secondary headaches include intracranial infections such as meningitis and encephalitis, space-occupying lesions, and hemorrhages.

Central nervous system infections: Fever, toxic appearance, seizures, altered mental status, increased intracranial pressure, and meningeal irritation signs may be present requiring immediate evaluation.

Hydrocephalus and intracranial mass lesions: Chronic progressive headache, morning headache, vomiting, behavioral changes, nausea, developmental delay, vision impairment, increased intracranial pressure signs, increase in head circumference, focal neurologic signs, precocious or delayed puberty, seizures may be the presenting features of intracranial mass lesions and acute hydrocephalus. Neurocutaneous syndromes carry an increased risk of brain tumors.

Intracranial hemorrhage: Thunderclap headache is the hallmark of subarachnoid hemorrhage, but may also be seen in other disorders. Epidural, subdural, and

Table 12.6 General diagnostic criteria for secondary headaches - ICHD-3[a]

A. Any headache fulfilling criterion C.
B. Another disorder scientifically documented to be able to cause headache has been diagnosed.
C. Evidence of causation demonstrated by at least two of the following:
   1. headache has developed in temporal relation to the onset of the presumed causative disorder,
   2. either or both of the following:
      (a) headache has significantly worsened in parallel with worsening of the presumed causative disorder,
      (b) headache has significantly improved in parallel with the improvement of the presumed causative disorder,
   3. headache has characteristics typical for the causative disorder,
   4. other evidence exists of causation,
D. Not better accounted for by another ICHD-3 diagnosis.

[a]Adopted from Ref. 22.
ICHD-3 indicates The International Classification of Headache Disorders, third ed. Cephalalgia. 2018;38:1–211.

intracerebral hematoma may also be associated with acute headache. Chronic subdural hematoma may cause a chronic progressive headache. Urgent CT must be performed. In thunderclap headache, lumbar puncture is required for definitely ruling out subarachnoid hemorrhage, if CT is negative.

Systemic infections: Acute febrile illness, usually due to upper respiratory tract infections or influenza, is the most common cause of headache in children presenting to an emergency clinic [28].

Disorders of the paranasal sinuses and the ear: Given the subject of this book, headaches attributed to acute rhino-sinusitis and otitis media will be reviewed in more detail.

The headache related to acute rhino-sinusitis is usually located in the periorbital area, followed by the frontal, vertex, occipital and facial areas. Pain may be aggravated by pressure applied over the paranasal sinuses, but there is no significant correlation between the location of rhino-sinusitis and the site of pain [29]. Complicated rhino-sinusitis may extend to the orbit or intracranially and present with new onset of severe headache, vomiting, altered level of consciousness, signs of meningeal irritation, and focal neurologic deficits. Imaging studies are not usually necessary in uncomplicated cases, and findings should be interpreted in the context of clinical findings such as fever, cough, purulent nasal, or postnasal discharge.

As important as (or even more important than) diagnosing acute rhino-sinusitis it is essential to misdiagnose primary headaches for "sinus headache". In retrospective studies, sinus disease was incidentally found in 4.1–5.3% of children who underwent neuroimaging (MRI or CT) for headache [30, 31]. Sinus headache is one of the most frequent misdiagnoses given to children with headache [32]. In a prospective study including 214 children, approximately 40% of the children with migraine and 60% of the children with tension-type headache had been misdiagnosed as "sinus headache" [33]. An opacification of paranasal sinuses observed in neuroimaging should not preclude the diagnosis of migraine or other types of primary headache [32].

Acute otitis media is also a frequent diagnosis in pediatric emergency care. Headache attributed to ear disorders is aggravated by pressure applied to the affected ear or periauricular area. Headache in the absence of ear pain is unlikely a presentation of otological pathology. Complications of acute otitis media such as mastoiditis may also present with headache.

A frequent cause of facial pain is disorders of teeth usually causing localized toothache or more widespread facial pain. Periodontitis or pericoronitis is the most common cause of headache attributed to a disorder of the teeth or jaw [22].

Frequent secondary headaches related to systemic infections, acute rhinosinusitis, and otitis media, are usually benign. Further secondary headaches which are important in children and adolescents comprise posttraumatic headache, Chiari type 1 malformation, idiopathic intracranial hypertension, carbon monoxide intoxication, and last but not least medication overuse headache.

Headache attributed to trauma or injury is diagnosed, if a headache occurs in close temporal relation to head and/or neck trauma or injury [22]. Headache may be acute, usually resolving within seven-ten days, or persistent.

Chiari type 1 malformation may be an incidental finding in neuroimaging performed for headaches. Symptomatic Chiari malformation is characterized by a brief (<5 min) occipital or suboccipital headache worsened by neck flexion or Valsalva maneuvers. Sensory disturbance, upper extremity weakness, dizziness, and ataxia may accompany [7].

Idiopathic intracranial hypertension (*IIH*): Headache attributed to IIH typically occurs in obese girls or young women and is non-specific. Other symptoms include pulsating tinnitus, neck or back pain, diplopia, transient visual obscuration, and photopsia. Cerebral venous thrombosis and other causes of symptomatic intracranial hypertension must be excluded. Importantly IIH is usually associated with papilledema. The diagnosis should be confirmed by measuring the opening pressure of the cerebrospinal fluid [22].

In carbon monoxide poisoning, headache is the most common presenting symptom. Nausea, vomiting, altered consciousness may also be present. Usually, more than one member of a household is affected [34].

Medication overuse headache brings us back to primary headache disorders since this headache typically develops in patients with chronic migraine and chronic tension-type headache. It is diagnosed, if the headache is present on ≥15 days per month for more than three months and medication for acute headaches is used on ≥15 days (non-opioid analgesics) or ≥ 10 days per month (combination analgesics, triptans, ergotamines, or opioids). To prevent medication overuse headache, non-pharmacological and (rarely) pharmacological prophylaxis is important in children and adolescents with frequent headaches and the use of acute medication should be limited to 2 days per week on average.

12.6 Treatment

12.6.1 Secondary Headaches

The management of secondary headache depends on its cause. The headache usually resolves after successful treatment of the underlying disorder, such as antibiotics for bacterial infections; removal of a space-occupying intracranial lesion; implantation of a shunt for hydrocephalus; a few days of bed rest for acute headache after a mild head injury; weight loss, acetazolamide and repeated therapeutic lumbar punctures for IIH; or withdrawal of acute medication for medication overuse headache.

In addition, the child may require symptomatic pain management. Treatment of first choice is the oral administration of liquid paracetamol (10–15 mg/kg/dose) or liquid ibuprofen (7.5–10 mg/kg/dose). The dose may be repeated four to 6 h later.

12.6.2 Primary Headaches

In children and adolescents with primary headaches, a headache diary covering the duration, severity, quality, location of the pain, associated symptoms, and use of acute medication is very useful both for establishing the diagnosis (in particular for differentiating migraine and tension-type headache) and for monitoring the treatment.

In the following, the treatment of migraine and tension-type headache will be highlighted, and will not be discussed cluster headache and other primary headaches.

The mainstay in managing migraine and tension-type headache is the education of the patient and the parents. Education should cover the nature of the headache, trigger factors, coping with trigger factors, lifestyle, and specific non-pharmacological and, if necessary, pharmacological therapy including information about realistic treatment goals. Encouraging the child and the parents to adhere to acute and preventive therapies is essential. Lifestyle recommendations comprise regular and adequate sleep, a morning without stress, adequate hydration (with non-caffeinated fluids), regular meals, including breakfast, regular breaks when learning, regular exercise, and limited and careful use of electronic devices, avoiding the use of the mobile phone during thirty minutes before bedtime [11, 15, 35, 36].

During an acute migraine attack, parents should ensure that the child can rest in a quiet darkened room and that the atmosphere is relaxing and calming. Especially in (smaller) children, a few hours of sleep or an early night sleep often stops the attack and the children are migraine-free when they awake [11, 15, 36].

Analgesics should not be administered, if a migraine attack usually resolves within 2 h either spontaneously or after the child had vomited or with lying down and sleeping. If acute medication is necessary, the drug should be given as early as possible and the dose should be sufficient for the patient's age and weight. Liquid analgesics should be preferred in children. In general, evidence from randomized controlled studies is poor. Ibuprofen (7.5-10 mg/kg) is the first choice for treatment. Alternatively, paracetamol (10-15 mg/kg) can be used. None other non-opioid analgesics have been investigated in placebo-controlled studies for childhood and adolescence migraine. Acetylsalicylic acid should not be used until the age of 12 because of the risk of Reye's syndrome. There is no indication for opioids [37–39].

In migraine attacks refractory to non-opioid analgesics, triptans may be used. All triptans were examined in adolescents and some in children. Response rates, tolerability, and safety are comparable to adults, but many studies could not show superiority over placebo because of high placebo response rates [37]. In the European Union, triptans are not approved for use in children; sumatriptan nasal spray (20 mg) and zolmitriptan nasal spray (5 mg) are approved for adolescents from the age of 12. In the United States (US), almotriptan (6.25 mg or 12.5 mg), rizatriptan (5 mg or 10 mg), zolmitriptan nasal spray (20 mg), and the fixed combination of sumatriptan and naproxen are licensed for adolescents. Rizatriptan is also licensed for children aged 6–11. A fixed combination of sumatriptan and naproxen is not available outside the US, but in adolescents with migraine attacks unresponsive to both non-opioid analgesics and triptans, it may be useful to combine sumatriptan (or another triptan) with naproxen (or another non-opioid analgesic) [37, 40].

If the first triptan was ineffective or not tolerated, a different triptan should be tried. Triptans are contraindicated in disorders uncommon in children and adolescents, namely cerebral, coronary, and peripheral arterial disease, Raynaud syndrome, and uncontrolled hypertension. More importantly, triptans are contraindicated in the brainstem and hemiplegic migraine [40, 41].

Antiemetics should be used for refractory nausea or repeated vomiting, but not for one- or two-time vomiting, when the attack resolves immediately thereafter. Preferably, ondansetron should be used, even though its use is off-label (4 mg up to twice daily, if body weight is >10 kg) [42]. The European Medicines Agency (EMA) mentions migraine not at all as an indication for metoclopramide in children and adolescents, whereas they do in adults. EMA recommends that metoclopramide should be used in children (>1 year of age) only as a second-choice treatment (0.1–0.15 mg/kg up to three times daily) [43]. Regarding domperidone, EMA concludes that it may be used for nausea and vomiting in adolescents weighing ≥35 kg (oral dose: 10 mg up to three times daily; suppositories up to 30 mg twice daily). In children and adolescents weighing <35 kg, domperidone should be given by mouth at a dose of 0.25 mg per kg body weight (up to three times daily) [44].

If an acute migraine attack has been treated successfully and the attack recurs within 24 h, a second dose may be necessary, paying attention not to exceed the maximum daily dosage [40].

Use of acute medication should be limited to 2 days per week on average and additional prophylactic treatment is mandatory in patients with frequent migraine attacks to prevent medication overuse headache [36, 37].

Specific prophylactic treatment is required, if there are four or more days with burdensome migraine attacks per month (causing loss of school or leisure time activities) and if education about trigger factors and lifestyle modification alone does not sufficiently reduce the number of attacks. Prophylaxis should focus on non-pharmacological therapies and drugs should only be used if these therapies are not successful or the severity of migraine requires both non-pharmacological and pharmacological treatment.

Recommended therapies include on the one hand biofeedback, other relaxation techniques, cognitive behavioral therapy, and in adolescents possibly acupuncture and on the other hand flunarizine (5 mg daily) or propranolol (1–4 mg/kg/day) [36, 37, 39, 45]. Alternatively, topiramate or amitriptyline can be used. The choice of the drug is based on the patient's general history considering contraindications. Prophylactic medication should be used for 3–6 months. Due to its antidopaminergic effect flunarizine should not be used longer than 6 months [36, 37, 39]. It is important to inform the patient and the parents that it will take 4–6 weeks until the efficacy of the medication can be assessed.

Similar to migraine, treatment of tension-type headache consists of acute therapy and prophylaxis following the principles described above.

For acute therapy of tension headache in childhood, if possible, no medication, but relaxation and "distraction" should be used. If necessary, paracetamol or ibuprofen (see above) can be used. As in migraine, the use of acute medication does not exceed 2 days per week on average. Non-pharmacological prophylaxis is similar to migraine. For pharmaco-prophylaxis amitriptyline may be used [26, 35].

12.7 Conclusion

As a closing remark, we report a patient with co-existing primary and secondary headache seeking the attention of the doctor. A girl 6 years of age having migraine without aura since the age of 4, beginning 1 month ago in primary school. Migraine attacks usually occurring four times a year during the day and now in the first month of school, severe headaches occur four times a week awakening her from sleep. In this specific condition, one could say, this is the stress of school. Regarding to a specific concentrated case history, which should always be done it came out that this girl had 6 weeks ago a short viral infection. Since the headache characteristics changed markedly, immediate neuroimaging was mandatory, even though neurological examination was normal. MRI revealed occlusive hydrocephalus. She was operated on successfully within a few days and we are happy to close this chapter with the information that this girl is now a successful lawyer.

References

1. Wöber-Bingöl Ç. Epidemiology of migraine and headache in children and adolescents. Curr Pain Headache Rep. 2013;17:341.
2. Kyu HH, Pinho C, Wagner JA, et al. Global and national burden of diseases and injuries among children and adolescents between 1990 and 2013: findings from the global burden of disease 2013 study. JAMA Pediatr. 2016;170:267–87.
3. Wöber C, Wöber-Bingöl Ç, Uluduz D, et al. Undifferentiated headache: broadening the approach to headache in children and adolescents, with supporting evidence from a nationwide schoolbased cross-sectional survey in Turkey. J Headache Pain. 2018;19:18.
4. Wöber-Bingöl Ç, Wöber C, Uluduz D, et al. The global burden of headache in children and adolescents - developing a questionnaire and methodology for a global study. J Headache Pain. 2014;15:86.
5. Philipp J, Zeiler M, Wöber C, et al. Prevalence and burden of headache in children and adolescents in Austria – A nationwide study in a representative sample of pupils aged 10-18 years. J Headache Pain. 2019;20:101.
6. Jorgensen JE, McGirr KA, Korsgaard HO, et al. Translation and validation of the child and the adolescent hardship (Headache-attributed restriction, disability, social handicap and impaired participation) questionnaire into Danish language. Peer J. 2016;4:e1927.
7. Genc D, Zaborskis A, Vaičienė-Magistris N. Translation of the child and adolescent hardship (Headache-attributed restriction, disability, social handicap and impaired participation) questionnaire into the Lithuanian language and validation of its HRQoL (Headache-related quality of life) scale. Int J Environ Res Public Health. 2018;15:1579.
8. Al-Hashel JY, Ahmed SF, Alroughani R. Prevalence and burden of primary headache disorders in Kuwaiti children and adolescents: A community-based study. Front Neurol. 2019;10:793.
9. Lakshmikantha KM, Nallasamy K. Child with headache. Indian J Pediatr. 2018;85:66–70.
10. Özge A, Termine C, Antonaci F, Natriashvili S, Guidetti V, Wöber-Bingöl C. Overview of diagnosis and management of paediatric headache part I: diagnosis. J Headache Pain. 2011;12:13–23.

11. Wöber C, Wöber-Bingöl Ç. Clinical management of young patients presenting with headache. Funct Neurol. 2000;15(Suppl 3):89–105.

12. Langdon R, DiSabella MT. Pediatric headache: an overview. Curr Probl Pediatr Adolesc Health Care. 2017;47:44–65.

13. Rothner AD. The evaluation of headaches in children and adolescents. Semin Pediatr Neurol. 1995;2:109–18.

14. Bonthius DJ, Hershey AD. In: Drutz JE, Patterson MC, Swanson JW, Torchia MM, editors. Headache in children: approach to evaluation and general management strategies. Waltham, MA: UpToDate; 2020.

15. Wöber-Bingöl Ç. What does it mean to treat headache in children and adolescents? dealing with patients; dealing with parents; dealing with teachers. In: Guidetti V, Russell G, Sillanpää M, Winner P, editors. Headache and migraine in childhood and adolescence. London: Martin Dunitz; 2002. p. 459–66.

16. Schick S, Gahleitner A, Wöber-Bingöl Ç, et al. Virchow-Robin spaces in childhood migraine. Neuroradiology. 1999;41:283–7.

17. Wöber-Bingöl Ç, Wöber C, Prayer D, et al. Magnetic resonance imaging for recurrent headache in childhood and adolescence. Headache. 1996;36:83–90.

18. Wöber C, Wöber-Bingöl Ç. Triggers of migraine and tension-type headache. Handb Clin Neurol. 2010;97:161–72.

19. Wöber C, Brannath W, Schmidt K, et al. Prospective analysis of factors related to migraine attacks: the PAMINA study. Cephalalgia. 2007;27:304–14.

20. Peris F, Donoghue S, Torres F, et al. Towards improved migraine management: Determining potential trigger factors in individual patients. Cephalalgia. 2017;37:452–63.

21. Kernick D, Reinhold D, Campbell JL. Impact of headache on young people in a school population. Br J Gen Pract. 2009;59:678–81.

22. Headache Classification Committee of the International Headache Society (IHS). The international classification of headache disorders. Cephalalgia. 2018;38:1–211.

23. Kienbacher C, Wöber C, Zesch H, et al. Clinical features, classification and prognosis of migraine and tension-type headache in children and adolescents: a long-term follow-up study. Cephalalgia. 2006;26:820–30.

24. Lagman-Bartolome AM, Lay C. Pediatric migraine variants: a review of epidemiology, diagnosis, treatment, and outcome. Curr Neurol Neurosci Rep. 2015;15:34.

25. Anttila P, Metsähonkala L, Aromaa M, et al. Determinants of tension-type headache in children. Cephalalgia. 2002;22:401–8.

26. Wöber-Bingöl Ç, Hershey AD. Tension-type headache and other non-migraine primary headaches in the pediatric population. In: Olesen J, Goadsby PJ, Ramadan NM, Tfelt-Hansen P, KMA W, editors. The Headaches. 3rd ed. Philadelphia: Lippincott, Williams & Wilkins; 2006. p. 1079–81.

27. Wöber-Bingöl Ç, Wöber C, Karwautz A, et al. Tension-type headache in different age groups at two headache centers. Pain. 1996;67:53–8.

28. Kan L, Nagelberg J, Maytal J. Headaches in a pediatric emergency department: etiology, imaging, and treatment. Headache. 2000;40:25–9.

29. Yeo NK, Park WJ, Ryu IS, Lim HW, Song YJ. Is facial or head pain related to the location of lesion on computed tomography in chronic rhinosinusitis? Ann Otol Rhinol Laryngol. 2017;126:589–96.

30. Strauss LD, Cavanaugh BA, Yun ES, Evans RW. Incidental findings and normal anatomical variants on brain MRI in children for primary headaches. Headache. 2017;57:1601–9.

31. Gurkas E, Karalok ZS, Taskin BD, Aydogmus U, Yılmaz C, Bayram G. Brain magnetic resonance imaging findings in children with headache. Arch Argent Pediatr. 2017; 115:e349–55.

32. Neto RJV, Teixeira KCS, Guerreiro MM, Montenegro MA. Paranasal sinus disease in children with headache. J Child Neurol. 2017;32:1014–7.

33. Senbil N, Gürer YK, Uner C, Barut Y. Sinusitis in children and adolescents with chronic or recurrent headache: a case-control study. J Headache Pain. 2008;9:33–6.

34. Harper A, Croft-Baker J. Carbon monoxide poisoning: undetected by both patients and their doctors. Age Ageing. 2004;33:105–9.
35. Termine C, Özge A, Antonaci F, Natriashvili S, Guidetti V, Wöber-Bingöl C. Overview of diagnosis and management of paediatric headache. Part II: therapeutic management. J Headache Pain. 2011;12:25–34.
36. Wöber-Bingöl Ç, Hershey AD, Kabbouche MA. Managing headache in young people (What are the differences in the approach to management and in the use of drugs?). In: Martelletti P, Steiner TJ, editors. Handbook of headache. Cham, Switzerland: Springer; 2011. p. 1–15.
37. Wöber-Bingöl Ç. Pharmacological treatment of acute migraine in adolescents and children. Paediatr Drugs. 2013;15:235–46.
38. Richer L, Billinghurst L, Linsdell MA, et al. Drugs for the acute treatment of migraine in children and adolescents (Review). Cochrane Database of Systematic Reviews; 2018: cochranelibrary.com/cdsr/ https://doi.org/10.1002/14651858.CD005220.
39. Termine C, Özge A, Antonaci F, et al. Overview of diagnosis and management of paediatric headache. Part II: therapeutic management. J Headache Pain. 2011;12:25–34.
40. Oskoui M, Pringsheim T, Holler-Managan Y, et al. Practice guideline update summary: Acute treatment of migraine in children and adolescents: Report of the Guideline Development, Dissemination, and Implementation Subcommittee of the American Academy of Neurology and the American Headache Society. Neurology. 2019;93:487–99.
41. Hershey AD, Kabbouche MA, O'Brien HL, Kacperski J. Headaches. In: Kliegman RM, St Geme III JW, Blum NJ, Shah SS, Tasker RC, Wilson KM, editors. Nelson textbook of pediatrics. 21st ed. Philadelphia: Elsevier; 2020. p. 3128–40.
42. Talai A, Heilbrunn B. Ondansetron for acute migraine in the pediatric emergency department. Pediatr Neurol. 2020;103:52–6.
43. European Medicine Agency. Metoclopramide-containing medicines. 2020. https://www.ema.europa.eu/en/medicines/human/referrals/metoclopramide-containing-medicines. Accessed 5 Dec 2020.
44. European Medicines Agency. Domperidone-containing medicines. 2020. https://www.ema.europa.eu/en/medicines/human/referrals/domperidone-containing-medicines. Accessed 5 Dec 2020.
45. Oskoui M, Pringsheim T, Billinghurst L, et al. Practice guideline update summary: Pharmacologic treatment for pediatric migraine prevention. Report of the Guideline Development, Dissemination, and Implementation Subcommittee of the American Academy of Neurology and the American Headache Society. Neurology. 2019;93:500–9.

Otalgia: Pathogenesis, Diagnosis, and Treatment

13

Mümtaz Taner Torun, Nuray Bayar Muluk, and Ahmed El-Saggan

13.1 Introduction

Earache, which is also referred to as otalgia, is a regular sign as far as primary care is concerned with various likely causes. Normally, in situations where the causes emanate from the ear, the earn assessment ends up been anomalous resulting to an obvious diagnosis. On the other hand, in case of referred otalgia which could also be explained as secondary otalgia, the assessment of the ear tends to be normal with the ache been referred from various sites [1].

When it comes to primary otalgia, its cause is obvious from an assessment with the two most popular causes comprising otitis media and otitis externa. However, as far as the causes of secondary otalgia are concerned, it can be explained that it is most of the times challenging to determine due to the fact that the innervation of the ear is intricate while there are also other various likely sources of referred ache. However, some of the regular known causes of secondary otalgia comprise temporomandibular joint syndrome, sore throat, dental disease, and cervical spine arthritis. In cases where the examination is not apparent from the past and bodily assessment, selections comprise tests of suggestive intervention lacking a specific assessment, imaging trials, and reaching out to an expert in ear, nose, and throat [1].

M. T. Torun (✉)
Section of Otorhinolaryngology, Bandırma State Hospital, Bandırma, Balıkesir, Turkey

N. Bayar Muluk
Department of Otorhinolaryngology, Faculty of Medicine, Kırıkkale University, Kırıkkale, Turkey

A. El-Saggan
Department of Otolaryngology, Stavanger University Hospital, Stavanger, Norway

Normal causes of primary otalgia comprise otitis media, external otitis, mastoiditis, and auricular contaminations. Majority of doctors are sufficiently trained on how to identify these conditions. For example, when an ear happens to be draining and also experiencing tympanic membrane perforation, a diagnosis can be carried out by visually assessing the ear and taking note of pathology. Nevertheless, in situation where the tympanic membrane is perceived to be normal, diagnosis tends to be more challenging.

Referred otalgia is a subject on its own. Indeed, despite the fact that majority entities can be the cause of referred otalgia, their connection to the earache has to be established. A specific discussion of the diagnosis, intervention, prognosis, demographics, and other various aspects is not likely due to the fact that the different pathologies in charge of causing referred otalgia are quite varied [2].

13.2 Pathophysiology

Normally, the cranial nerves cervical nerves C2 and C3, VII (facial), V (trigeminal), IX (glossopharyngeal), and X (vagus) provides the ear with the consciousness fibers. These different nerves have lengthy courses in the chest, head, and the neck; hence various ailments tend to have ear pain. The inner ear structures tend to be innervated by the crania nerve VII that does not have any pain fibers. Thus, majority of the pathologic processes of the inner ear cannot have any ache [1, 3].

As far as the sensory intervention of the ear is concerned, it can be pointed out that it is served by the auriculotemporal part of the fifth cranial nerve, cervical nerves (I and II), Jacobson part of the glossopharyngeal nerve, and the Ramsey Hunt part of the facial nerve, and Arnold part of the vagus nerve. From a neurology perspective, the consciousness of otalgia is perceived to be centered on the spinal tract nucleus of fifth cranial nerve. As a result, various fibers such as different cranial nerve have been established to get into the spinal tract nucleus caudally next to the medulla. Therefore, noxious activation of any part of previously highlighted nerves might be considered as otalgia [2].

13.3 Epidemiology

From a study that was carried out by Kozin et al. and comprised 8,611,000 research subjects with the data been collected from the US emergency department, it was established that the most popular conditions were: Not Otherwise Specified (NOS) 60%, infected otitis external Not Otherwise Specified 11.8%, and Otalgia Not Otherwise Specified 6.8% [2, 4].

On the other hand, in a study carried out in Korea that involved 294 patients, it was found that when the prevalence rate of primary otalgia in children, men and women was contrasted, there was a high chance of referred otalgia to be identified in adults and in particular women. Moreover, the study also found that neuralgia was more regular in women [2, 5].

13.4 Causes

The causes of otalgia can be categorized into two categories, namely primary causes and secondary causes. The primary causes comprise the causes that emanate from the ear and directly cause the ache by stimulating the nociceptor fibers. In the case of the secondary causes, the aches that an individual feel emanate from the ear even though they are in reality coming from another source and need a higher extent of diagnosis so that the exact cause can be identified. Moreover, it can be noted that primary otalgia tends to be quite regular among kids while secondary otalgia is popular among grown-ups [6, 7].

13.4.1 The Primary Causes of Otalgia

Normally, there are various causes of otalgia that have been discussed by various scholars. From a review of the literature, scholars who have discussed the issue concur that the causes tend to be gentle and exist as upfront causes to a skilled physician. Contagion, shock, foreign bodies and obstructed cerumen are the regular situations normally identified with otoscopy. On the other hand, principal neoplasms of the ear tend to be infrequent and typically undoubtedly recognized when they exist on the earlobe and emanate in the peri-otic area. Moreover, even though cancers of the impermanent bone together with outer auditive canal are not common and normally identified when various advanced symptoms are experienced, it is important that they are also taken into consideration when one experiences otalgia and lingering ear discharge [8].

On a different perspective, it is crucial that skull-base osteomyelitis is always taken into consideration in patients who happen to be immunosuppressed or have been diagnosed with polyuria with serious ache and a background of labyrinthitis externa. The viruses normally accountable comprise *Pseudomonas* though might also be fungous. The ache is normally branded as serious and sore in character and exuding into the mandibula. As the condition advances, it leaves cranial synapse palsies, originally connecting facial synapse, then hypoglossal synapse and X vagus synapse. There is natural formation of tissue spotted in the base of the ear canal. This has to be examined by a surgeon focusing on ear, nose and throat due to the fact that variance urinalysis is squamous cell cancer of the temporal bone. Herpes zoster execrable viral infection exists with ache, blister entailing pinna/exterior aural meatus and facial nerve palsy [6].

13.4.2 Secondary Causes of Otalgia

In the event that the causes are not apparent, the secondary causes of ear pain have to then be taken into consideration. Mainly, odontogenic causes are a tremendously regular cause of referred otalgia. Indeed, these causes have been found to be present in 63% of cases [9, 10] and comprises swelling and contagion of dental structures, specifically those connected with the ulterior teeth. Another key cause of secondary otalgia comprises temporomandibular joint syndromes while patients with these symptoms also experience other different ontological symptoms, for instance tinnitus and vertigo [11]. The ache of temporomandibular joint syndromes replicates either the shared or muscles connected with motility of the jaw. In that perspective, exacerbation of pain related with chewing is likely to show where the pain is coming from [12]. A brief assessment of the teeth as well as the jaw might also permit beginning of elementary management and evade excess-examination. Trigeminal pain is also likely to exist with ache [13]. This specific analysis is normally straight; nevertheless, in situations the individual explains one-sided spells of ache which starts brusquely lasting for more than 60 s and are enormously agonizing [14]. It has been noted that pain could occur in additional cranial nerves and the present aspect is that the ache should succeed the spreading of the nerve.

The different tumors of the neck and head have to be perceived as the secondary causes of pain among the individuals with ordinary otology background and assessment [15]. What is of specific significance is the neoplasms that are in the oropharyngeal area and can exist with deep, unrelenting otalgia [15]. Moreover, patients that have to have cancer in this area might have other signs of upset, odynophagia and stinging throat, or might be symptomless. In view of the risk factors, they comprise exposure to tobacco, and taking alcohol for a long period of time. In order to identify these cancer, cervical lymphadenopathy is commonly used [6, 16].

Eagle's disease might be secondary to a calcified stylohyoid ligament that is likely to be intense in the tonsillar fossa [6, 17].

13.5 Diagnosis

13.5.1 Background

The gravity of otalgia is less likely to show the significance of the cause [18]. Thus, it is ideal to provide a detailed otology history in order to establish whether the cause is usually primary. Apart from that, a detailed review of ache, explore signs of otorrhea, loss of hearing, dizziness, aural ampleness and tinnitus. As far as some patients are concerned, the minimum history is what they need for a correct diagnosis to be carried out and effective treatment administered. In addition, the time course is also going to aid the probable cause of the ailment. Normally, lesser periods indicate a primary or gentle etiology while extended periods indicate a secondary cause. In situation where the cause is not practically swiftly evident, related signs have to be considered from various anatomical areas that are served by the similar nerves innervating the ear. Investigate on related signs including the oral cavity, comprising dental background, oropharyngeal signs comprising history of tonsil contaminations, and nasal and sinus passageway signs [6].

Significant questions to ask in the background of a patient with ear pain include [19]:

- *Age*—In infants and toddlers, most cases of ear pain result from middle ear disease. In older children and adolescents, a larger proportion of cases stem from otitis externa, throat infections, or temporomandibular joint disease.
- Blunt or penetrating.
- Fever.
- Nasal congestion [20, 21].
- Ear tenderness.
- Hearing loss.
- Ear drainage.
- Swimming.
- Minor trauma to the ear.
- Barotrauma.
- Environmental exposures.
- Past medical history [19].

13.5.2 Examination

Examinations need to be guided by the background even though they should commence with broader assessment of the outer ear comprising pre-auricular and postauricular areas together with otoscopic assessment of the hearing canal and observing the tympanic crust [22]. If there happens to be an anomalous discovery from the ear, the assessment has to then advance to assess the cranial nerves for infections [3]. An individual who happens to have a protuberant tympanic crust that is erythematous is a major discovery in acute otitis media (AOM). Infected expulsion in the hearing canal is likely to indicate otitis degree. Otherwise, it may signify a punctured suppurative otitis media that might be challenging to distinguish. Ache on inside of the otoscope is a likely indicator that the root is otitis externa. Severe mastoiditis comprises of an impediment of acute otitis media and a medical examination with major results comprising postauricular inflammation and erythema, soreness, and a lump of the auricle [23]. Elimination of the postauricular sulcus and likely inflammation comprising the postero–superior outer meatus is likely to spotted [6].

In case the ear and otoscopic assessments fail to identify a specific cause for otalgia, the next course of action would involve a complete assessment of head and neck with cranial nerve since there is a likelihood of referred pain. This section of the assessment has to entail examination and scrutiny of the oral cavity and oropharynx with main attention been on the soft palate, teeth, TMJ, tongue, posterior pharyngeal wall, and the tonsils. In order for the assessment to be effectively carried out, it will be important that any dentures are removed. Repeated opening and closing of the mouth might expose trismus, while audible or palpable crepitus would hint a TMJ anomaly. The front nasal cavities also need to be investigated using sufficient illumination. In addition, entire neck palpation in all areas for masses or lymphadenopathy is significant for analysis of metastatic ailment. Lateral palpation over the TMJ is likely to show dysfunction and pain present in the joints [6, 18].

13.5.3 Examination Tests

An examination of the ability of the ear through audiometry or even basic examination is designated for patients who realize loss in hearing. An examination of tympanic crust agility with inflatable otoscopy or tympanometry could be vital in case there happens to be doubts of middle ear ailment. In case the bodily assessment is ordinary and the aim is to exclude tumor, the individual needs to have naso-laryngoscopy and magnetic reverberation imaging of both the head and neck with gadolinium disparity carried out. In the event that the condition is obvious on inspection and the aim is to establish the degree of engrossment, calculated tomography with disparity media is normally shown. For instance, temporal bone trauma has to be examined through computerized tomography scanning [1].

13.6   Treatment

In most cases, in order to treat different types of infections, different types of antibiotics are used. However, in case the causative agent is assumed to have been viral, antivirals are used. On the other hand, when the cause is fungus, antifungals have to be used while in case the cause is esophagitis or gastroesophageal reflux disease, antiulcer/antacid medications can be used. After administering the medicine, the patient should be assessed again after 2 weeks.

Antibiotics
The antibiotic therapy needs to be inclusive and address all possible pathogens. However, in the event that the search for the cause of ache is ineffective, empiric antimicrobial therapy should be used.

Antivirals
Nucleoside analogs are primarily phosphorylated by viral thymidine kinase to ultimately establish a nucleoside triphosphate [2].

Acyclovir: Has exhibited inhibitory initiative against HSV-1 and HSV-2. Selectively combined into infected cells [2]. Famciclovir: This is a prodrug that when bio changed into lively metabolite, penciclovir, might impede viral DNA synthesis [2].

Valacyclovir: This is a prodrug swiftly changed to the active drug acyclovir. Even though quite costly, the drug has a more suitable dosing routine than acyclovir [2].

Analgesics

Ibuprofen could be used since it has inflammatory responses and ache by lessening prostaglandin replication [2]. In addition, Hydrocodone and acetaminophen could be used in combination to manage moderate to severe pain. Finally, Oxycodone and acetaminophen could both be used as a combination to relieve moderate to severe ache [2].

References

1. Ely JW, Hansen MR, Clark EC. Diagnosis of ear pain. Am Fam Physician. 2008;77(5):621–8.
2. Li JC. Otalgia. In: Meyers AD (Ed.). Medscape. Updated: May 03, 2017. http://emedicine.medscape.com/article/845173-overview. Accessed 8 Aug 2017.
3. Shah RK, Blevins NH. Otalgia. Otolaryngol Clin N Am. 2003;36(6):1137–51.
4. Kozin ED, Sethi RK, Remenschneider AK, et al. Epidemiology of otologic diagnoses in United States emergency departments. Laryngoscope. 2015;125(8):1926–33.
5. Kim SH, Kim TH, Byun JY, Park MS, Yeo SG. Clinical differences in types of otalgia. J Audiol Otol. 2015;19(1):34–8.
6. Harrison E, Cronin M. Otalgia. Aust Fam Physician. 2016 Jul;45(7):493–7.
7. Majumdar S, Wu K, Bateman ND, Ray J. Diagnosis and management of otalgia in children. Arch Dis Child Educ Pract Ed. 2009;94(2):33–6.
8. Yeung P, Bridger A, Smee R, Baldwin M, Bridger GP. Malignancies of the external auditory canal and temporal bone: a review. ANZ J Surg. 2002;72(2):114–20.
9. Taziki MH, Behnampour N. A study of the etiology of referred otalgia. Iran J Otorhinolaryngol. 2012;24(69):171–6.
10. Kim DS, Cheang P, Dover S, Drake-Lee AB. Dentalotalgia. J Laryngol Otol. 2007;121(12):1129–34.
11. Tuz HH, Onder EM, Kisnisci RS. Prevalence of otologic complaints in patients with temporomandibular disorder. Am J Orthod Dentofac Orthop. 2003;123(6):620–3.
12. Sharma S, Gupta DS, Pal US, Jurel SK. Etiological factors of temporomandibular joint disorders. Natl J Maxillofac Surg. 2011;2(2):116–9.
13. Weissman JL. A pain in the ear: the radiology of otalgia. AJNR Am J Neuroradiol. 1997;18(9):1641–51.
14. Türp JC, Gobetti JP. Trigeminal neuralgia versus atypical facial pain. Oral Surg Oral Med Oral Pathol Oral Radiol Endod. 1996;81(4):424–32.
15. Scarbrough TJ, Day TA, Williams TE, Hardin JH, Aguero EG, Thomas CR Jr. Referred otalgia in head and neck cancer: a unifying schema. Am J Clin Oncol. 2003;26(5):e157–62.
16. Cohan DM, Popat S, Kaplan SE, Rigual N, Loree T, Hicks WL Jr. Oropharyngeal cancer: current understanding and management. Curr Opin Otolaryngol Head Neck Surg. 2009;17(2):88–94.
17. Mayrink G, Figueiredo EP, Sato FR, Moreira RW. Cervicofacial pain associated with Eagle's syndrome misdiagnosed as trigeminal neuralgia. Oral Maxillofac Surg. 2011;16(2):207–10.
18. Charlett SD, Coatesworth AP. Referred otalgia: a structured approach to diagnosis and treatment. Int J Clin Pract. 2007;61(6):1015–21.
19. Greenes D. Evaluation of earache in children. In: Fleisher GR, Wiley JF (Eds.). UpToDate. Lastupdated: Jul 06, 2016. https://www.uptodate.com/contents/evaluation-of-earache-in-children?source=search_result&search=ear%20ache&selectedTitle=1~150. Accessed 8 Aug 2017.
20. Uitti JM, Laine MK, Tähtinen PA, et al. Symptoms and otoscopic signs in bilateral and unilateral acute otitis media. Pediatrics. 2013;131:e398.
21. McCormick DP, Jennings K, Ede LC, et al. Use of symptoms and risk factors to predict acute otitis media in infants. Int J Pediatr Otorhinolaryngol. 2016;81:55.
22. Neilan RE, Roland PS. Otalgia. Med Clin North Am. 2010;94(5):961–71.
23. van den Aardweg MT, Rovers MM, de Ru JA, Albers FW, Schilder AG. A systematic review of diagnostic criteria for acute mastoiditis in children. Otol Neurotol. 2008;29(6):751–7.

Otorrhea: Pathogenesis, Diagnosis, and Treatment

14

Fatma Ceyda Akın Öçal, Yavuz Fuat Yılmaz, and Kevin A. Peng

14.1 Introduction

Otorrhea is defined as drainage of aqueous material from the ear. Otorrhea has several causes, including disease of the middle ear, perforation of the tympanic membrane, or pathology of the outer ear canal [1]. Otorrhea [2] can be a sign as well as a symptom, and currently it is among the most frequent reasons for patients to seek medical treatment by an ear, nose, and throat (ENT) specialist. Many patients with otorrhea do not require hospital admission, but they do require several outpatient visits [3]. Otorrhea is typically seen in one of the following five forms: purulent (the most common), serous, mucoid, clear, or bloody. There are several known causes of otorrhea; inflammation is the major cause of purulent, serous, and mucoid otorrhea, while head and/or ear injury are among the most common reasons for clear and bloody otorrhea [4].

14.2 Etiopathogenesis

In the pediatric population, otorrhea is most likely due to some type of benign condition, which can be discerned via physical examination and analysis of the ear debris [1].

F. C. A. Öçal (✉) · Y. F. Yılmaz
Section of Otorhinolaryngology, Gülhane Training and Research Hospital, University of Health Sciences, Ankara, Turkey

K. A. Peng
Section of Otolaryngology and Neurotology, Burbank, Providence Saint Joseph Medical Center, Los Angeles, CA, USA

© The Author(s), under exclusive license to Springer Nature Switzerland AG 2022   169
C. Cingi et al. (eds.), *Pediatric ENT Infections*,
https://doi.org/10.1007/978-3-030-80691-0_14

14.2.1 Otorrhea of the Tympanostomy Tube

The most prevalent otorrhea is that of the tympanostomy tube. It has been reported that within 1 year of tube insertion, nearly 75% of patients experience tympanostomy tube otorrhea [5]. A current meta-analysis indicated that 16% of patients experienced otorrhea within 14 days of tube placement, and 26% experienced otorrhea later than 14 days; further, of these patients, 7.4% had more than one experience of otorrhea, while 4% had continuous otorrhea [6]. Otorrhea that occurs within 14 days of tube placement is most likely due to purulent or mucoid effusions during the operation; it is not typically caused by absent or serous effusions [7]. In addition, other studies have shown that tympanostomy tube otorrhea may be associated with the status of the middle ear during the procedure; however, it is not likely to be associated with the sterility of the ear canal [8–11].

Otorrhea of the tympanostomy tube is often seen in conjunction with acute infections of the upper respiratory tract, and is typically caused by the same bacteria seen in otitis media (e.g., *"Moraxella catarrhalis, Haemophilus influenzae, Streptococcus pneumonia"*). Nonetheless, *Pseudomonas aeruginosa* can develop into the most important bacteria in a short time-span (a few hours to a few days) [12]. Pediatric patients $\geq$4 years of age do not often receive ear cultures; however, when cultures are performed, most of them reveal Staphylococcus aureus [13, 14]. Causes of otorrhea can differ depending on the season. Summertime cases of otorrhea are likely due to extrinsic sources, with little to no relationship with pathogens of a nasopharyngeal source [13]. The majority of patients with tympanostomy tube otorrhea do not experience any discomfort, and the condition clears on its own in a couple days. In a study with pediatric patients $\leq$ age 6 who were given oral placebo and who had their tube cleaned daily, it was found that approximately 33% of them had their otorrhea cleared by day 4. However, patients with continuous otorrhea or those experiencing more symptoms may also need to be treated with antibiotics [15].

14.2.2 Foreign Body

Otorrhea may be caused by foreign bodies (FBs) in the ear if they are long-standing or if they consist of highly irritating substances. Patient history may or may not indicate their presence [1].

Typical FBs include the following [1]:

- Toys or small objects placed in the ear by toddlers themselves, or placed by older siblings into a younger sibling's ear.
- Insects, although they are often so irritating that removal occurs before the development of otorrhea.
- Food material, especially nuts with irritating oils that can cause a significant reaction.
- Button batteries (often used in small electronic devices such as hearing aids).
- Expelled tympanostomy tube with granulation tissue and bloody otorrhea.

Otoscopy is diagnostic. However, cerumen buildup or otorrhea may obscure the FB, and cleaning may be necessary to see the FB. Most ear FBs that do not cause otorrhea can be removed using simple techniques in the outpatient setting, without referral to an ENT specialist. However, complications do result from multiple manipulations, and an ENT consult should be called when in doubt or when necessary visualization and removal equipment are not available [1].

14.2.3 Otitis Externa

Infections located in the outer ear canal are known as otitis externa. This type of infection is often caused by damage (either chemical or mechanical) to the ear's protective barrier, which is composed of cerumen and skin. This damage and its subsequent secretions cause increases in pH, which are conducive to the survival of infection. Normally, *S. aureus* and *P. aeruginosa* cause these infections; however, *Candida albicans, Aspergilli, streptococci, and Escherichia coli* may also play a role. Otitis externa that is continuous or frequently reappears may be due to skin diseases (e.g., psoriasis, seborrhea, and eczema) or fungal infection. Those experiencing eczematous dermatitis localized to the ear canal may have moist vesicle and pustules (acutely) followed by scales and crusts (chronically) [8].

Acute bacterial external otitis, often called "swimmer's ear," is an infectious inflammation of the external auditory canal. Causes include water exposure or instrument damage to the outer ear canal (e.g., cleaning with cotton swabs or finger scratching). Common symptoms include pain, pruritus, and hearing loss. Minor trauma to the canal's protective skin barrier and protective cerumen layer can lead to bacterial overgrowth. *Pseudomonas aeruginosa* is the most common cause of otitis externa; however, it can also be caused by Staphylococcus epidermidis, Staphylococcus aureus, and both polymicrobial and anaerobic infections [1].

On physical examination, otitis externa presents with moderate to severe pain, and can include minor tragus manipulation or pulling on the auricle. An examination of the ear often reveals an erythematous, edematous ear canal with cellular debris. Since the middle ear is not necessarily involved in external otitis, there may be no middle ear effusion or purulent otitis media. When visible, the tympanic membrane (TM) itself is typically erythematous or covered with debris. In many cases, the membrane is difficult to see due to edematous narrowing of the canal. Otorrhea is purulent, white to yellow, and may dry to a crust [1].

14.2.4 Acute Otitis Media

Acute otitis media is not associated with otorrhea as a presenting sign; however, it is a complication of tympanic membrane perforation and may be associated with short-term hearing loss. In most cases, perforations will spontaneously heal within 2 months. A long-term perforation can be surgically treated via tympanoplasty. The affected ear must be protected from water [16].

Occasionally, acute otitis media can cause rupture of the tympanic membrane. Rupture is typically associated with a short duration of ear pain and fever, followed by pain relief with the onset of otorrhea (clear or white drainage). In most cases, the perforation will heal by the time the patient is seen by a physician, but the drainage may continue for some time, especially in cases that have developed otitis externa [1].

In many cases, the perforation may not be visible on otoscopy; this is because either (1) the otorrhea is obscuring visualization of the tympanic membrane (TM) or (2) the perforation has rapidly resealed. In cases when the perforation can be seen, the TM often has an abnormal appearance and a lack of mobility on pneumatic otoscopy. Perforations often heal spontaneously once the infection resolves [1].

14.2.5 Chronic Otitis Media

The chronic form of otitis media occurs when fluid persists behind the tympanic membrane. It is more common in children because "their Eustachian tubes are shorter, narrower, and more horizontal than those of adults." A unilateral chronic otitis media in adults may be indicative of a nasopharyngeal mass. Symptoms include thick otorrhea, a retracted or perforated tympanic membrane, or, less commonly, a bulging tympanic membrane [16].

Chronic suppurative otitis media (CSOM) is characterized by drainage in an ear that has experienced either (1) repeated acute otitis media, (2) TM perforation caused by trauma, or (3) tympanostomy tube insertion. A common presenting symptom of CSOM is hearing loss, without otalgia, in the affected ear. Other symptoms may include fever and vertigo. Otorrhea is fetid, purulent, and cheese-like. Granuloma tissue may be present in the middle ear space or in the medial canal [16].

Patients with CSOM experience drainage via a tear in the TM, which leads to diseased mucous in the mastoid and middle ear. This condition is deemed chronic if it lasts ≥6 weeks, at which time there may be osteitis, bone damage, and scarring [17–19]. The majority of patients do not experience pain, but in rare cases with bone involvement, there may be a rancid odor associated with extreme discomfort. Very severe cases of CSOM might also have intracranial complications. *P. aeruginosa* most commonly causes CSOM, but other causes include anaerobes, *Staphylococcus aureus*, and gram-negative bacilli [17, 18, 20]. *Mycobacteria* may be the cause of CSOM in cases with granulation of the middle ear [21]. CSOM is less often caused by conditions such as rhabdomyoscarcomas, tuberculosis, histiocytosis, and syphilis [8, 19].

14.2.6 Trauma to the External Ear Canal

Common traumatic causes of otorrhea include the presence of a foreign body, blunt trauma to the ear (due to physical violence, motor vehicle accident, or sports accident), recent head injury, perforated tympanic membrane, and barotrauma caused by recent flying or diving. A thorough ear examination is necessary in every case with bleeding from the ear. If the tympanic membrane cannot be visualized, immediate evaluation by an ENT specialist is mandatory to assess for mobility and perforation. In addition, patients should be warned that cotton-tipped swabs can be very dangerous to ear health and should never be inserted into the ear canal [16].

14.2.7 Polyps

Polyps in the external ear canal may be caused by a response to an inflammatory reaction or infection such as chronic otitis media, cholesteatoma, or retained foreign body (e.g., expelled tympanostomy tube) [22]. In rare cases, they may be due to a tumor (e.g., Langerhans Cell Histiocytosis, teratoma, or neoplasm). When manipulated, polyps create bloody or serous otorrhea, similar to that of granulomas. Ear polyps may resolve rapidly with topical antibiotics and/or anti-inflammatory therapy. However, if drainage persists for more than two to 3 weeks, the pediatric patient should be referred to an ENT specialist with pediatric expertise [1, 23].

14.2.8 Spontaneous Cerebral Spinal Fluid Otorrhea

While basilar skull fractures may result from head trauma, cerebrospinal fluid (CSF) otorrhea may also occur spontaneously via tegmen tympani defects in the floor of the temporal bone. These defects should be suspected in cases of persistent otorrhea, especially after the more common causes have already been excluded, or in any child with more than one episode of meningitis. High resolution computed tomography (CT) with thin cuts through the temporal bone provides a noninvasive means of diagnosis [1, 24].

14.3 Diagnosis

14.3.1 History

The following historical features should be sought in patients with otorrhea [1]:

- Features of drainage.
- Fever: Fever suggests the presence of an acute middle ear infection or necrotizing external otitis.
- Pain.
- Pruritus: Itching is a prominent feature of otitis externa (including otomycosis), allergic dermatitis, and foreign body in the ear.
- Swimming history.
- Trauma.
- Perforation.

14.3.2 Examination

A thorough examination requires inspection of the auricle and surrounding area, otoscopy of the external canal, tympanic membrane, and middle ear, and, in patients without obvious tympanic membrane perforation, assessment of tympanic membrane function by pneumatic otoscopy. In children with otorrhea, the external auditory canal is often filled with debris, which requires cleaning to allow proper visualization [1].

14.3.3 Culture of Ear Drainage

The majority of pediatricians recognize the type of environments conducive to infection by bacteria causing otitis media; however, many of them do not fully understand the reasons why Pseudomonas is often found in the ear. Pseudomonas is a type of gram-negative bacteria that is both motile and aerobic; it often localizes to moist areas, and can be found in soil, sewage, and areas with retained water. *P. aeruginosa* cannot be cultured from the ear without the presence of infection [25, 26]. Cases with *Pseudomonas*-induced otorrhea often have very damp ear canals caused by conditions such as an overabundance of cerumen or stenosis; further, a correlation has been reported between the amount of *Pseudomonas* in the ear canal and the amount of dampness in the ear [8, 25].

Otorrhea of the tympanostomy tube is typically caused by colonization of the upper respiratory tract or by bacteria causing otitis media (i.e., *M. catarrhalis, H. influenzae,* or *S. pneumoniae*), especially during the winter. In a relatively short period of time, the otorrhea causes excessive dampness, which causes the Pseudomonas to proliferate, making it the prevailing bacteria [12, 27]. In warmer weather, tympanostomy tube otorrhea in often caused by *Staphylococcus* or *Pseudomonas* coming from outside sources [8, 13, 28].

P. aeruginosa is the prevailing cause of otitis externa (61% of cases); however, these cases almost always show polymicrobial infection (44% of these cases) [8, 29].

14.3.4 Testing for Cerebrospinal Fluid Otorrhea

To test for cerebrospinal fluid (CSF) leakage, the clinician can perform a quick bedside test, which entails placing a drop of ear drainage on filter paper (coffee filter or paper towel). The test is considered to be positive if the drop quickly shows colorless liquid surrounding blood. It should be noted that this test cannot discern between clear fluids (e.g., saliva, saline, CSF) and has not been formally tested in a clinical setting [1].

Alternatively, the drainage can be tested for beta2 transferrin, which is a desialylated form of transferrin, a marker that is typically only expressed in CSF. However, this test is not available at many institutions [1].

Physicians can also check the urine, as glucose can be indicative of CSF. As blood also may contain glucose, this is not a trustworthy test, as it may present false positives [1].

14.3.5 Imaging

Potential imaging tests include "magnetic resonance imaging (MRI) or computed tomography (CT)" of the head, with thin cuts through the temporal bone, middle ear, and otic capsule [1].

When evaluating patients for the following diagnoses, imaging studies are necessary [1]:

- Basilar skull fracture with cerebrospinal fluid leakage.
- Spontaneous cerebrospinal fluid leakage.
- Necrotizing otitis externa.
- Cholesteatoma.
- External auditory canal mass or chronic polyps.

14.4 Treatment

The treatment of otorrhea depends on its etiology. In order to diagnose and manage otorrhea, the ear canal must be cleaned of any debris or foreign objects. If there is considerable drainage or swelling of the canal, the clinician may be unable to discern the root of the problem, and may not know if he/she should treat his client for otitis externa or otitis media. In addition, the ear must be completely cleared of any liquids so that any topically applied medications can reach the affected area. Prior to cleansing, the physician must thoroughly examine the ear canal so that he/she does not cause any injury to the canal wall or tympanic membrane. To do so, a small head lamp can be used so that the physician can use both hands to carefully examine the ear; this type of light is also important for throat and nose evaluations, and should be available in any pediatric office. Cleansing of the ear is accomplished via suction or with swabs. While suction is a better method, as it causes less injury to the ear, is more efficient at cleaning, and is much faster, some children may be afraid of the noise it makes [8].

Cases with otorrhea almost never need to undergo systemic therapy; the majority of patients are satisfied with topical ointments and cleansing. However, patients suffering from severe cases of cellulitis (caused by gram-positive bacteria) or those having long bouts of bacteria-induced upper respiratory infection may require systemic therapy. In addition, these patients should have their ear discharge cultured and analyzed [8].

A study by Venekamp et al. [30] including 331 pediatric participants reported that corticosteroid eardrops were less effective than antibiotic eardrops (±corticosteroid) with regard to number of days having discharge from the ear. Their results showed that the median number of days with ear discharge was five in the ciproflaxin group, seven in the ciprofloxacin-fluocinolone acetonide group, and 22 in the fluocinolone acetonide group. Another study including 48 pediatric patients indicated that with regard to rinsing the ear with antibiotic eardrops versus saline, the antibiotic eardrops (ciprofloxacin) were moderately more effective at resolving discharge from the ear after 1 week than the saline drops ("77% versus 46%; RR 1.67, 95% CI 1.04 to 2.69; moderate-quality evidence"); however, there was no difference between the two drops with regard to tube blockage [30].

Various treatments and combinations thereof are currently used in children who have been fitted with grommets and are experiencing discharge from the ear. Treatment preferences vary across countries and healthcare settings. The majority of the cases undergo observation, and if necessary, they are treated with antibiotics (orally or in eardrop form) ± corticosteroids. Less common treatments include systemic or ototopical corticosteroids and interventions such as cleansing the ear canal with microsuction equipment (in an ENT setting) and rinsing with saline (in a primary care or ENT setting) [30].

Most ENT surgeons prefer ototopical treatment with antibiotic eardrops (±corticosteroid) [31]. Aminoglycosides and chloramphenicol are potentially ototoxic; animal studies have shown that when applied locally onto the round window, they may penetrate into the inner ear and cause hair cell damage and sensorineural hearing loss. However, there is little evidence to suggest that similar processes occur in humans treated with these drops; middle ear secretions and thickened mucosa likely protect the round window and inner ear from their ototoxic effects [32, 33]. Quinolones are considered non-ototoxic [32], and they became widely available as eardrops in the 1990s. The recent clinical practice guidelines on tympanostomy tubes in children recommend quinolone drops as the first-line treatment for pediatric patients who have been fitted with grommets and who develop discharge from the ear [34]. However, in many countries, such as the UK, otic quinolone formulations are not widely available (in contrast to ophthalmic formulations). In this review, we will assess the safety and effectiveness of current therapies for pediatric patients who have been fitted with grommets and who develop long-term discharge from the ear, with a particular focus on oral versus ototopical antibiotics.

References

1. Strother CG, Sadow K. Evaluation of otorrhea (ear discharge) in children. In: Teach SJ, Wiley JF. UpToDate. Last updated: Aug 30, 2016. https://www.uptodate.com/contents/evaluation-of-otorrhea-ear-discharge-in-children. Accessed 8 Aug 2017.
2. Schloss M. Otorrhea. In: Bluestone CD, Stool SE, Scheetz MD, editors. Pediatric otolaryngology. 2nd ed. Philadelphia, PA: W.B. Saunders; 1990. p. 198–202.
3. Kimmelman CP. Office management of the draining ear. Otolaryngol Clin N Am. 1992;25:739–44.
4. Bardanis J, Batzakakis D, Mamatas S, Nasus A. Types and causes of otorrhea. Larynx. 2003;30:253–7.
5. Ah-Tye C, Paradise JL, Colborn DK. Otorrhea in young children after tympanostomytube placement for persistent middle-ear effusion: prevalence, incidence, and duration. Pediatrics. 2001;107(6):1251–8.

6. Rosenfeld RM. Surgical prevention of otitis media. Vaccine. 2001;19(Suppl 1):S134–9.
7. Balkany TH, Barkin RM, Suzuki BH, Watson WJ. A prospective study of infection following tympanostomy and tube insertion. Am J Otol. 1983;4(4):288–91.
8. Schroeder A, Darrow DH. Management of the draining ear in children. Pediatr Ann. 2004;33(12):843–53.
9. Kinsella JB, Fenton J, Donnelly MJ, McShane DP. Tympanostomy tubes and early postoperative otorrhea. Int J Pediatr Otorhinolaryngol. 1994;30(2):111–4.
10. Giebink GS, Daly K, Buran DJ, Satz M, Ayre T. Predictors for postoperative otorrhea following tympanostomy tube insertion. Arch Otolaryngol Head Neck Surg. 1992;118(5):491–4.
11. Scott BA, Strunk CL. Posttympanostomy otorrhea: the efficacy of canal preparation. Laryngoscope. 1992;102(10):1003–7.
12. Poole MD. Treatment of otorrhea associated with tubes or perforations. Ear Nose Throat J. 1993;72(3):225–6.
13. Mandel EM, Casselbrant ML, Kurs-Lasky M. Acute otorrhea: bacteriology of a common complication of tympanostomy tubes. Ann Otol Rhinol Laryngol. 1994;103(9):713–8.
14. Schneider ML. Bacteriology of otorrhea from tympanostomy tubes. Arch Otolaryngol Head Neck Surg. 1989;115(10):1225–6.
15. Ruohola A, Heikkinen T, Meurman O, et al. Antibiotic treatment of acute otorrhea through tympanostomy tube: randomized double-blind placebo-controlled study with daily follow-up. Pediatrics. 2003;111(5 pt 1):1061–7.
16. Lynch JS. How Should I Evaluate a Draining Ear? Medscape. 2012. http://www.medscape.com/viewarticle/766184_3. Accessed 8 Aug 2017.
17. Kenna MA, Bluestone CD, Reilly JS, Lusk RP. Medical management of chronic suppurative otitis media without cholesteatoma in children. Laryngoscope. 1986;96(2):146–51.
18. Fliss DM, Dagan R, Houri Z, Lieberman A. Medical management of chronic suppurative otitis media without cholesteatoma in children. J Pediatr. 1990;116(6):991–6.
19. Kimmelman CP. Office management of the draining ear. Otol Clin N Am. 1992;25(4):739–44.
20. Dagan R, Fliss DM, Einhorn M, Kraus M, Leiberman A. Outpatient management of chronic suppurative otitis media without cholesteatoma in children. Pediatr Infect Dis J. 1992;11(7):542–6.
21. Ma KH, Tang PS, Chan KW. Aural tuberculosis. Am J Otol. 1990;11(3):174–7.
22. Gliklich RE, Cunningham MJ, Eavey RD. The cause of aural polyps in children. Arch Otolaryngol Head Neck Surg. 1993;119:669.
23. Harris KC, Conley SF, Kerschner JE. Foreign body granuloma of the external auditory canal. Pediatrics. 2004;113:e371.
24. Rao AK, Merenda DM, Wetmore SJ. Diagnosis and management of spontaneous cerebrospinal fluid otorrhea. Otol Neurotol. 2005;26:1171.
25. Salit IE, Miller B, Wigmore M, Smith JA. Bacterial flora of the external canal in diabetics and non-diabetics. Laryngoscope. 1982;92(6 pt 1):672–3.
26. Stroman DW, Roland PS, Dohar J, Burt W. Microbiology of normal external auditory canal. Laryngoscope. 2001;111(11 pt 1):2054–9.
27. Brook I, Yocum P, Shah K. Aerobic and anaerobic bacteriology of otorrhea associated with tympanostomy tubes in children. Acta Otolaryngol. 1998;118(2):206–10.
28. Dohar J. Microbiology of otorrhea in children with tympanostomy tubes: implications for therapy. Int J Pediatr Otorhinolaryngol. 2003;67(12):1317–23.
29. Clark WB, Brook I, Bianki D, Thompson DH. Microbiology of otitis externa. Otolaryngol Head Neck Surg. 1997;116(1):23–5.
30. Venekamp RP, Javed F, van Dongen TM, Waddell A, Schilder AG. Interventions for children with ear discharge occurring at least two weeks following grommet (ventilation tube) insertion. Cochrane Database Syst Rev. 2016;11:CD011684.
31. Badalyan V, Schwartz RH, Scwhartz SL, Roland PS. Draining ears and tympanostomy tubes: a survey of pediatric otolaryngologists and pediatric emergency medicine physicians. Pediatr Emerg Care. 2013;29(2):203–8. https://doi.org/10.1097/PEC.0b013e318280d520.

32. Pappas S, Nikolopoulos TP, Korres S, Papacharalampous G, Tzangarulakis A, Ferekidis E. Topical antibiotic ear drops: are they safe? Int J Clin Pract. 2006;60(9):1115–9.
33. Phillips JS, Yung MW, Burton MJ, Swan IR. Evidence review and ENT-UK consensus report for the use of aminoglycoside-containing eardrops in the presence of an open middle ear. Clin Otolaryngol. 2007;32(5):330–6.
34. Rosenfeld RM, Schwartz SR, Pynnonen MA, Tunkel DE, Hussey HM, Fichera JS, Grimes AM, Hackell JM, Harrison MF, Haskell H, Haynes DS, Kim TW, Lafreniere DC, LeBlanc K, Mackey WL, Netterville JL, Pipan ME, Raol NP, Schellhase KG. Clinical practice guideline: tympanostomy tubes in children. Otolaryngol Head Neck Surg. 2013;149(1 Suppl):S1–35. https://doi.org/10.1177/0194599813487302.

Hearing Loss

15

Özlem Yüksel Coşar, Nuray Bayar Muluk, and Slobodan Spremo

15.1 Aetiology

15.1.1 Genetic Causes

According to the majority of authorities on the subject, a genetic aetiology is implicated in 50% or more of cases of auditory loss [1–5]. Hearing loss may occur as part of a syndrome or in isolation. Just as in every genetic disorder, the inheritance pattern may be autosomal dominant (AD) or recessive (AR), X-linked, mitochondrial or a spontaneous mutation [6].

Slightly over two in three cases of auditory loss of genetic type occur in isolation. Genetic causes are likely to account for the majority of seemingly unknown causes of deafness. A paediatric case of isolated deafness features complete or partial loss of auditory function in the absence of other indications of pathology. There is no specific risk that other abnormalities will occur, nor is a learning disability more likely. In certain cases, there will be a family history of auditory loss, in an immediate or a more distant relative. Some children carry a de novo mutation or an allele of AR type that is not known from any of the child's relatives. Other children later born to the same parents or to the patient him or herself may eventually reveal whether

Ö. Y. Coşar (✉)
Section of Otorhinolaryngology, Dr. Ersin Arslan Training and Research Hospital, Şahinbey, Gaziantep, Turkey

N. Bayar Muluk
Department of Otorhinolaryngology, Faculty of Medicine, Kırıkkale University, Kırıkkale, Turkey

S. Spremo
Department for Otorhinolaryngology, Faculty of Medicine, University of Banja Luka, University Clinic Center Banja Luka, Banja Luka, Bosnia and Herzegovina

C. Cingi et al. (eds.), *Pediatric ENT Infections*,
https://doi.org/10.1007/978-3-030-80691-0_15

the deafness was of genetic origin, a developmental anomaly or an event occurring in utero [6].

It has been shown through the use of genetic localisation techniques that around 20 or so genetic abnormalities may cause deafness. It has also been discovered that these genes may be inherited in a variety of different ways. The genes DFNA1 to DFNA48 are autosomal dominant. DFNB1 to DFNB67 are autosomal recessive. DFN1 to DFN8 are X-linked recessive, whilst mitochondrial inheritance occurs for mutations covering a minimum of five loci, amongst which are 12Sr RNA and tRNA-serine UCN [6].

Genetic mutations may result in abnormal function or structure of a protein. Examples might be defective collagen forming the basilar membrane or abnormal function of the gap junction beta-2 protein, which affects the permeability of the plasma membrane [7]. In certain genes, there is already knowledge of the one or several forms a mutation can take. The gene CCDC50 encodes the protein Ymer in DFNA44 hearing loss. Ymer is a protein found in the cytoplasm which prevents the epidermal growth factor receptor from being downregulated. Abnormality of the gene results in the Corti rods of the inner ear developing an abnormal structure [8, 9]. The various alleles are penetrant to varying degrees, so knowing that a particular allele is involved does not allow a straightforward prediction of how severe hearing loss may be [6].

Where deafness is not in isolation, it must be part of one of the above 300 syndromes known to cause hearing loss [10]. Amongst these genetic syndromes, some exhibit a specific mode of inheritance. Waardenburg and Gernet syndromes are inherited in an AD fashion, whilst Jervell Lange-Nielson and Winter syndromes are AR. The Alport and Rosenberg syndromes are X-linked. However, other syndromes are spontaneous, such as the cat-eye, Turner or Klinefelter syndromes [6].

There are typically signs of individual syndromes alongside deafness which help to narrow down the diagnostic possibilities. Nonetheless, some paediatric cases do not exhibit such signs before late childhood. Some cases appear in early childhood and present as hearing loss or with the consequences of metabolic or biochemical abnormalities [6].

As previously indicated, a syndrome may be confined to a particular organ or may be multi-systemic. Knowledge of those syndromes which cause hearing loss has come about at the same time as non-syndromic genetic hearing loss has been better understood. An example of this deeper understanding is Waardenburg-Shah syndrome. In this disorder, endothelin 3 is abnormal, causing abnormal ligand function on the intermediate striatum, the gut and skin melanocytes [6].

15.1.2 Prenatal Causes

In between 5% and 10% of cases, deafness is caused in utero. Sensorineural deafness may be caused by congenital infection by cytomegalovirus (CMV), herpesvirus, rubella, *Treponema pallidum*, *Toxoplasma gondii* or varicella [11]. Additionally, this type of deafness may arise through teratogenic toxicity by, for example, methyl mercury, retinoic acid, thalidomide or trimethadione. Usually, exposure to these teratogens gives rise to anatomical abnormalities and an examining paediatrician may use this as a clue to the underlying cause and thus prompt further investigation.

On occasion, however, any abnormality may be difficult to detect or may not appear until a later stage, such as Hutchinson teeth in congenital syphilis. In this situation, deafness may be the only warning sign of an underlying syndrome, or the first indication that developmental delay will eventually be seen. In a paediatric case where teratogenic exposure is certain, the failure to pick up a problem on neonatal screening should not be taken as the all clear and the child will need to be reassessed at a later date [1].

15.1.3 Perinatal Causes

Between 5% and 15% of deafness is caused by perinatal complications. If a child was born premature, had a low weight at birth, suffered anoxia or the Apgar score was concerning, had neonatal jaundice or sepsis, there is a risk of sensorineural deafness and so an audiological assessment is needed [1].

15.1.4 Postnatal Causes

Auditory loss occurs postnatally in between 10% and 20% of cases. Infective diseases of children, e.g. meningitis or mumps, carry a risk of auditory loss of sensorineural type. Furthermore, certain pharmacological agents, in particular aminoglycosides or furosemide, are toxic to the auditory system and thus may produce hearing loss. Middle ear infections or significant injury to the head have the potential to cause hearing loss, either sensorineural or conductive. Schieffer et al. carried out research that demonstrated an association of hearing loss of sensorineural type with iron deficiency anaemia, in both childhood and adolescence [12].

15.1.5 Unknown Causes

It is not possible to assign a definite aetiology for deafness in 20–30% of paediatric patients. In such individuals, the most probable explanation is that either the ear or central nervous system failed to develop normally. Thus, such events may be idiopathic or result from an infective episode or teratogenic event that passed undetected. It is probable that there are significant numbers of unknown de novo genetic mutations or unsuspected traits that are inherited recessively. There are even reports that deafness has occurred for psychological reasons [13].

15.2 Epidemiology

The prevalence of hearing loss in American children is around 5 to 10 per 1000. Profound deafness at birth is discovered in approximately 1–3 children out of every 1000, whilst between 3 and 5 children out of a 1000 have congenital mild or moderate deafness. In the latter situation, there may be problems acquiring language without audiological or speech therapy input [14]. Between 1% and 4% of infants discharged from neonatal intensive care (NICU) have deafness at a level calling for assistance. The prevalence of hearing loss may be increased by around 10–20% by cases where deafness is acquired [3].

There is an apparent rise in the numbers of adolescent Americans aged between 12 and 19 years with auditory problems [15]. Research dating from 2010 demonstrated an around 33% increase in the prevalence in 2005 to 2006, compared with the period 1988 to 1994. It is of especial note that significant hearing loss (at least 25 decibels loss) has risen most, such that this degree of auditory loss currently affects 5% of adolescents. The rising level of hearing loss in this age group is greatly affected by exposure to excessive noise.

The US Census reveals a rate of near to 3% of those employed experiencing a self-reported degree of deafness, whether conductive, sensorineural or of mixed type.

The global incidence of sensorineural hearing loss is between 9 and 27 children in every thousand [1].

15.2.1 Age- and Sex-Related Demographics

Most cases of deafness in childhood are present from birth or acquired around the time of birth [4]. Nonetheless, deafness may begin at any stage in life. Between around 10% and 20% of patients have non-congenital deafness, albeit this figure includes cases where a genetic disorder does not result in immediately apparent hearing loss, instead being gradually revealed during childhood and adolescence.

It is thought that deafness affects both males and females in equal numbers. There may be particular reasons for hearing loss, whether congenital or acquired, that are more common in boys or girls, but the overall rates of hearing loss do not differ between the sexes [1].

15.3 High-Risk Criteria for Hearing Loss in Neonates and Infants

During the neonatal period (i.e. up to 28 days postpartum), the following are risk factors for hearing loss [1]:

- Congenital or early-onset deafness in a family member.

- Congenital infections with pathogens capable of causing sensorineural deafness.
- Abnormal craniofacial development.
- A weight at birth less than 1.5 kg (3.3 pounds).
- Jaundice at a level sufficient to require an exchange transfusion.
- Having been exposed to drugs that cause ototoxicity.
- Meningitis of bacterial origin.
- Apgar score concerning at birth.
- Lengthy period when assisted ventilation was required.
- Diagnosis of a syndrome known to cause sensorineural deafness.

In a child aged over 28 days but less than 2 years, the following are risk factors [1]:

- History of difficulties involving hearing, speaking, language development or delayed milestones.
- Meningitis secondary to bacterial infection.
- Any of the risk factors in neonates if they previously applied.
- Injury to the head, particularly a fractured temporal bone.
- Diagnosis of a syndrome known to cause sensorineural deafness.
- Having been exposed to drugs that cause ototoxicity.
- Diseases causing neurodegeneration.
- Infections with an association with sensorineural deafness.

15.4 Indications for Auditory Assessment and Findings

If a parent or someone who cares for a child voices concerns that a child may be deaf, an audiological evaluation should occur without delay. Since it is possible to detect hearing loss from birth onwards, there are no grounds to postpone evaluation from a belief that a diagnosis at an early age is less reliable. An evaluation should consider other conditions that retard language development or produce behavioural issues, whilst acknowledging that deafness may also produce such a picture. An assessment of hearing loss can give a concrete outcome, in contrast to the essentially subjective nature of behavioural or linguistic investigations, which rely on the experience of the assessor to give an answer.

If a child has profound sensorineural deafness (i.e. a loss of greater than 90 decibels) congenitally or acquired perinatally, they may not coo as expected when aged between 6 and 9 months and language development may be clearly delayed. If the magnitude of auditory impairment is below this level, the child may have slightly abnormal speech, acquire new language late, exhibit problem behaviours or do badly in education. The extent to which the child is impaired in speaking and acquiring language has a correlation with the magnitude of auditory loss.

A child may present with problematic behaviour of a mild or severe kind but such problems are mostly related to the child's own character and how the parents address the issue. It is wise to perform an audiological assessment on a child prior to diagnosing defective speech, learning disability, autistic spectrum disorders, ADHD or an adjustment disorder [1].

15.5 Types of Auditory Impairment

Auditory loss of conductive type covers any disorder in which there is impairment of transmitted sound from the air to the cochlea. The following are all examples of conditions that cause conductive loss: anomalous anatomy of the helix or pinna, wax blocking the external auditory meatus, middle ear effusion, and ossicles which function abnormally, such as when they become immobile. A key condition responsible for conductive deafness is otosclerosis.

Another significant condition responsible for conductive deafness is cholesteatoma. This is a growth that destroys surrounding tissues but is not malignant. There are also neoplastic lesions affecting the middle ear, such as glomus tumours (tympanicum or jugulare), cranial nerve VII schwannomas and haemangiomata. Conductive loss also occurs if the bony roof of the mastoid cells is dehiscent, as may occur with an encephalocoele. Conductive defects cause sounds usually to be perceived by the patient as much quieter than usual, but otherwise not subject to distortion [1].

By contrast, sensorineural deafness is caused by disrupted transmission of the sound from the cochlea onwards, resulting from loss of the cochlear hair cells or injury to the vestibulocochlear nerve. The patient's auditory perception is of sounds being far quieter and of distortion occurring. Distortion of the sound occurs separately from the severity of deafness overall. Thus, hearing loss may be no greater than mild, but the patient may be unable to pick out speech with any accuracy.

In situations where there is no auditory response from the brainstem, an absent middle ear muscle reflex, the otoacoustic emissions are normal or the cochlear microphonics are normal, there is a suspicion of auditory dyssynchrony.

Auditory impairment of mixed type features elements of both conductive and sensorineural deafness [1].

15.6 Tests for Hearing Loss

15.6.1 Auditory Brainstem Response (ABR) and Brainstem Auditory Evoked Response (BAER) Testing

ABR tests rely on the same physical principles as electroencephalographic recordings. If a functioning ear is stimulated auditorily, the signal can be followed electroencephalographically as it passes onwards towards central areas within the nervous system. When BAER is used formally in tests, use is made of clicks or tones at particular pitches and varying volume levels [1].

15.6.2 Otoacoustic Emission (OAE) Testing

OAE tests rely on the principle that the inner ear itself generates particular sounds, which can themselves be recorded. Otoacoustic emissions come from functioning ears and are probably generated by activity of the hearing apparatus itself. These emissions may occur spontaneously or in response to a stimulus. The exact mechanism by which they occur and the reason they are absent in sensorineural deafness is not fully known. Nonetheless, the absence of OAEs correlates very accurately with auditory impairment.

OAE testing is relatively swift and has low associated cost. The operator does not require extensive training. This method is employed in neonatal screening for deafness. The subject (a neonate) lies down and an earphone is laid over one ear. The device produces a sound and any otoacoustic emission subsequently recorded. Evoked OAE testing is 100% sensitive and 82% specific.

OAE testing is limited by an inherent inability to differentiate between hearing loss of a conductive or sensorineural type. It also lacks the ability to identify a retrocochlear problem. The majority of studies evaluating OAE testing found there to be a small number of false positives generated. This is likely to be due to the need for sounds to both enter and exit the ear canal for OAEs to be detected, which may not occur if the canal is blocked. By contrast, it is sufficient for sounds used in ABR just to pass into the canal. Furthermore, OAE employed in NICU appears to be unsuccessful in many cases. Auditory testing in normal neonates born at term employs a second step to confirm the result, which may consist of a second OAE test or use of ABR tests [1].

15.6.3 Audiometry

Routine audiometric testing can be employed in a child who has reached the development level of a normal 4 or 5 years old. The child wears a headset and is told to lift the hand on the side where they hear a tone. The use of pure tones, with a particular pitch and volume, allows responses to be noted. This type of audiometry permits conductive auditory impairment to be distinguished from sensorineural defects. The ability to recognise speech may likewise be assessed.

Audiometry is gold standard practice where a patient is of normal intellect and is able to carry out the instructions given. The sensitivity and specificity of the procedure are influenced by how well the test subjects comprehend the instructions and how willing they are to comply with them [1].

15.7   Screening Programme for Neonatal Hearing Loss

Auditory impairments are amongst the most frequently occurring of congenital anomalies. They occur in between two to four infants out of a thousand. Before neonatal hearing loss screening was carried out on all newborns, only neonates who were considered high-risk and were on the appropriate register (HRR) were tested. The inadequacy of this practice was demonstrated by the realisation that up to half of those with congenital auditory impairments did not fall into any risk category. There are now accessible screening programmes in place that are appropriately sensitive and specific and lead to few inappropriate referrals [16].

The key to prevention of grave impairments to a child's psychosocial, educational and language development is to detect hearing problems at an early stage and intervene without delay. In cases where hearing loss is not picked up by the age of 6 months, speech and language acquisition are retarded. However, as long as the condition is detected and interventions put in place by no later than the age of 6 months, there is the possibility for a child to speak normally and understand language at the level of a child of the same age without hearing loss [16].

A study conducted by the US Centres for Disease Control and Prevention examined the growth in hearing loss diagnoses between 2006 and 2012. This research found that the rate of neonates detected with hearing loss following a second test increased from 4.8% to 10.3% within this period. There was also an accompanying rise in patients enrolled in early intervention services for hearing loss, from 55.4% to 61.7%. The study did, nonetheless, note discrepancies in how diagnoses of hearing loss (but not screening results) and involvement with remedial services was reported [17].

15.7.1 Prevalence of Hearing Loss

Hearing in childhood plays an absolutely key role in how speech, language and cognitive ability develop.

Research conducted retrospectively on data gathered from large-scale screening programmes aiming to screen all neonates for hearing loss indicates that irreversible auditory impairment has one of the highest frequencies amongst congenital anomalies. The American Academy of Paediatrics Task Force on Newborn and Infant Hearing commented in 1999 that, "significant bilateral hearing loss has been shown to be present in approximately 1 to 3 per 1000 newborns in the well-baby nursery population, and in approximately 2 to 4 per 1000 infants in the intensive care unit population" [10]. The neonatal screening programmes for hearing loss in the states of Rhode Island, Colorado and Texas registered between two and four cases out of every 1000 infants screened [18–20]. Connolly et al. discovered, in their 2005 study based on retrospective review, that the rate of hearing loss in infants identified as possessing risk factors was 1 in 75, whereas the rate when risk factors were absent was 1 in 811 [21]. It is possible that estimates of how prevalent deafness is will keep varying with the increasingly complete picture that universal neonatal screening is providing [16].

15.7.2 Risk Factors

Before neonatal screening for deafness was universally implemented, the usual practice was only to screen those infants who fulfilled the criteria for high risk and were placed on the high-risk register (HRR). The Joint Committee on Infant Hearing (JCIH) 2000 Position Statement identifies the following as risk factors for neonatal hearing loss [22]:

- A history of irreversible auditory impairment beginning in childhood in a family member.
- Prenatal exposure to the following infective agents: CMV, rubella, *T. gondii* or herpesvirus.
- Abnormal craniofacial development, including anatomical anomalies affecting the auricle and the external auditory meatus.
- Markers of neonatal risk, such as jaundice of sufficient severity to warrant an exchange transfusion, persistent pulmonary hypertension of the newborn (PPHN) requiring the neonate to be artificially ventilated, and any reason for extracorporeal membrane oxygenation (ECMO) to be employed.
- Postnatal infective episode of a type known to cause sensorineural deafness, such as bacterial meningitis.
- Physical findings consistent with any of the syndromes which may result in deafness (sensorineural or conductive) or abnormal function of the eustachian tubes.
- Any of the syndromes which may cause continuously deteriorating deafness, e.g. neurofibromatosis, osteopetrosis or Usher syndrome.
- Diseases characterised by neurodegeneration, e.g. Hunter syndrome. Neuropathy affecting sensorimotor system, e.g. Charcot-Marie-Tooth syndrome.
- A parent or other caregiver expresses concern about the child's ability to hear, speak, use language or develop appropriately.
- Cranial injury.
- Recurrent or chronic middle ear infection with an effusion that has gone on for a minimum of 3 months.

15.7.3 Early Identification and Intervention

Thanks to the introduction of universal neonatal screening for auditory impairment, the age at first diagnosis is starting to fall. Connolly et al. performed a study in 2005 that calculated the average age when deafness was first diagnosed had fallen to 3.9 months after screening began and that patients were on average 6.1 months when intervention began [21].

Children who are hard-of-hearing usually acquire language and reach academic milestones late. It is especially evident how severe or profound deafness affects children, but there are problems of various degrees in the speech and language acquisition even of children whose hearing is only mildly or moderately impaired.

Research findings indicate that the reading ability of deaf children graduating from high school is significantly below that of those whose hearing is normal. Children with hearing impairment had reading scores at graduation that were equal to the normal level of children aged between 9 and 11 years [16].

15.7.4 Methods of Screening

There have been neonatal screening programmes utilising ABR, OAE and automated ABR (AABR). ABR tests have been used for the last two decades to evaluate the auditory system pathways from the vestibulocochlear nerve onwards as far as the auditory brainstem. These tests are manual or diagnostic, but there is also a modification of ABR, the AABR, which has been utilised in screening since around 1987. David Kemp was the scientist responsible for discovering that OAEs exist. This discovery paved the way for a different type of device, the OAE test, which is now widespread in use [23]. The majority of neonatal auditory impairment screening programmes that are offered to all newborns employ OAEs or AABR. Classic audiometry lacks sufficient sensitivity or specificity to be utilised as a screening tool.

15.7.5 Otoacoustic Emissions

OAEs are of value in assessment of whether the cochlear is diseased. They reflect the sounds that are produced as a normal physiological response by the outer hair cells when sound is being perceived. OAEs can be swiftly detected and their presence indicates that the cochlear is working normally, at any rate. The measuring apparatus consists of a probe located in the external auditory meatus from which a pulse of sound (a tone or click) is emitted and by which the OAEs can be picked up by a microphone.

At present, neonatal auditory impairment screening utilises two different measures of otoacoustic emission—transient evoked otoacoustic emissions (TEOAEs) and distortion product otoacoustic emissions (DPOAEs). If the middle ear is working healthily, these two measures permit assessment of the cochlear response to sounds ranging in frequency from 500 to 6000 Hz. If OAEs are detected, this demonstrates that the auditory mechanism is working within the normal range, or nearly so [24].

The advantages of OAE testing are speed, efficiency and the ability to sensitively measure the peripheral auditory response at particular frequencies. The disadvantage is that the test is less effective if the testing environment is noisy and there is low frequency noise emanating from the surroundings, if vernix is present in the external auditory meatus or if the middle ear is diseased.

OAEs are inadequate for screening neonates with risk factors for the development of neural auditory impairment, such as auditory neuropathy/dyssynchrony. If a child has been admitted to NICU or remained longer than 5 days in hospital, ABR testing is called for, to prevent a missed diagnosis of auditory neuropathy. The inadequacy of OAE testing is due to the fact that this particular pathology does not impair the way the cochlear works and thus OAEs will generally appear normal [16].

AABR utilises electrophysiological techniques to evaluate the integrity of the auditory pathway from the vestibulocochlear nerve up to the auditory brainstem. Typical placement of the electrodes for the test is over the superior frontal bone, the mastoid process and the nucha. The electrodes are single use. A tiny single use earpiece is fitted to the neonate's ear and a click of 35 dB intensity is given via the earpiece. The earpiece masks background noise. For the majority of AABR devices, the result of testing is compared to a template based on pooled data from normal neonates. The device calculates whether the test has been passed or failed on the basis of how well the subject-generated waveform fits to the ideal. The majority of OAE measuring devices on the market are suitable for use in screening babies aged below 6 months [16].

15.7.6 Diagnostic Auditory Brainstem Response

It is unusual to employ diagnostic ABR tests in neonatal screening programmes offered to all neonates, since the test takes too long, is too expensive and an audiologist must carry out the test and perform the interpretation of the results. As with AABRs, diagnostic ABRs employ electrophysiological techniques to evaluate the integrity of the auditory pathways from the vestibulocochlear nerve to the auditory brainstem [16].

Typically, ABRs are recorded with single-use electrodes located on the forehead plus one on each mastoid process. Usually measurement involves the forehead electrode plus the mastoid electrode on the same side as the stimulus. A series of brief clicks is presented to each ear via an earpiece placed in the ear canal.

In contrast to the procedure used in AABR testing, whereby the response is measured to a single click of 35 decibels hearing level, in manual ABR testing, clicks of varying intensities are provided so that it can be established what the minimum intensity is which can give a reproducible auditory response. ABR tests in this format can provide information on both how severely hearing is impaired and whether the impairment is sensorineural, conductive or neural. It does this by comparing conduction through both air and bone. Clicks can elicit an ABR in the range around 1000 to 4000 Hz, providing information on how sensitive hearing is. Tone bursts may also be employed when required to ascertain how hearing loss is configured [16].

References

1. Shah RK. Hearing Impairment Workup. In: Elluru RG (Ed). Medscape. Updated: Sep 24, 2019. https://emedicine.medscape.com/article/994159-workup#c8. Accessed 14 Oct 2020.
2. Morton NE. Genetic epidemiology of hearing impairment. Ann N Y Acad Sci. 1991;630:16–31.

3. Roizen NJ. Etiology of hearing loss in children. Nongenetic causes. Pediatr Clin North Am. 1999;46(1):49–64.

4. McGee J, Walsh EJ. Cochlear transduction and the molecular basis of auditory pathology. In: Cummings otolaryngology: head & neck surgery. 5th ed. St. Louis: Mosby; 2010.

5. Hildebrand MS, Husein M, Smith RJH. Cochlear genetic sensorineural hearing loss. In: Cummings otolaryngology: head & neck surgery. 5th ed. St. Louis: Mosby; 2010.

6. Bondurand N, Pingault V, Goerich DE, Lemort N, Sock E, Le Caignec C, et al. Interaction among SOX10, PAX3 and MITF, three genes altered in Waardenburg syndrome. Hum Mol Genet. 2000;9(13):1907–17.

7. Marlin S, Garabédian EN, Roger G, Moatti L, Matha N, Lewin P, et al. Connexin 26 gene mutations in congenitally deaf children: pitfalls for genetic counseling. Arch Otolaryngol Head Neck Surg. 2001;127(8):927–33.

8. Tashiro K, Konishi H, Sano E, Nabeshi H, Yamauchi E, Taniguchi H. Suppression of the ligand-mediated down-regulation of epidermal growth factor receptor by Ymer, a novel tyrosine-phosphorylated and ubiquitinated protein. J Biol Chem. 2006;281(34):24612–22.

9. Modamio-Hoybjor S, Mencia A, Goodyear R, del Castillo I, Richardson G, Moreno F, et al. A mutation in CCDC50, a gene encoding an effector of epidermal growth factor-mediated cell signaling, causes progressive hearing loss. Am J Hum Genet. 2007;80(6):1076–89.

10. Erenberg A, Lemons J, Sia C, Trunkel D, Ziring P. Newborn and infant hearing loss: detection and intervention. American Academy of Pediatrics. Task force on newborn and infant hearing, 1998–1999. Pediatrics. 1999;103(2):527–30.

11. Richardson SO. The child with "delayed speech". Contemp Pediatr. 1992;9(9):55.

12. Schieffer KM, Connor JR, Pawelczyk JA, Sekhar DL. The relationship between Iron deficiency Anemia and sensorineural hearing loss in the pediatric and adolescent population. Am J Audiol. 2017;26(2):155–62.

13. Parodi M, Rouillon I, Rebours C, Denoyelle F, Loundon N. Childhood psychogenic hearing loss: identification and diagnosis. Eur Ann Otorhinolaryngol Head Neck Dis. 2017;134(6):415–8.

14. Kerschner JE. Neonatal hearing screening: to do or not to do. Pediatr Clin N Am. 2004;51(3):725–36.

15. Shargorodsky J, Curhan SG, Curhan GC, Eavey R. Change in prevalence of hearing loss in US adolescents. JAMA. 2010;304(7):772–8.

16. Delaney AM. Newborn Hearing Screening. In: Meyers AD (Ed). Medscape. Updated: 2020. https://emedicine.medscape.com/article/836646-overview#a4. Accessed 14 Oct 2020.

17. Williams TR, Alam S, Gaffney M, Centers for Disease Control and Prevention (CDC). Progress in identifying infants with hearing loss—United States, 2006–2012. Morb Mortal Wkly Rep. 2015;64(13):351–6.

18. Vohr BR, Carty LM, Moore PE, Letourneau K. The Rhode Island hearing assessment program: experience with statewide hearing screening (1993-1996). J Pediatr. 1998;133(3):353–7.

19. Downs MP. Universal newborn hearing screening--the Colorado story. Int J Pediatr Otorhinolaryngol. 1995;32(3):257–9.

20. Finitzo T, Albright K, O'Neal J. The newborn with hearing loss: detection in the nursery. Pediatrics. 1998;102(6):1452–60.

21. Connolly JL, Carron JD, Roark SD. Universal newborn hearing screening: are we achieving the joint committee on Infant hearing (JCIH) objectives? Laryngoscope. 2005;115(2):232–6.

22. JCIH. Position statement: principles and guidelines for early hearing detection and intervention programs. Joint committee on infant hearing, American Academy of Audiology, American Academy of Pediatrics, American speech-language-hearing association, and directors of speech and hearing programs in state health and welfare agencies. Pediatrics. 2000;106(4):798–817.

23. Kemp DT. Stimulated acoustic emissions from within the human auditory system. J Acoust Soc Am. 1978;64(5):1386–91.

24. Jedrzejczak WW, Konopka W, Kochanek K, Skarzynski H. Otoacoustic emissions in newborns evoked by 0.5kHz tone bursts. Int J Pediatr Otorhinolaryngol. 2015;79(9):1522–6.

Vertigo and Dizziness in Children

16

Utku Mete, Nuray Bayar Muluk, and Claudio Vicini

16.1 Introduction

It is unusual for a child or adolescent patient to complain of vertigo. However, in adults it is more commonly seen. Research conducted using a survey methodology has found a yearly incidence of 23% for dizziness in general and 5% for vestibular vertigo, in particular [1]. A study which recently assessed the frequency of diagnoses coded using ICD-9 and relating to problems with balance and the vestibular apparatus considered records from more than 560,000 consultations with paediatricians stretching over 4 years. These showed that unspecified dizziness occurred in a mere 0.4%, peripheral symptoms in 0.03% and central vestibulopathy in 0.02% of encounters [2, 3].

Harrison was the first researcher in recent times to discuss vertigo in children, in 1962 [4]. Even though there has been substantial progress in diagnostic investigative technology since the 1960s, the account given by the patient and the physical examination remain the cornerstone of diagnosis. Children or adolescents who complain of feeling dizzy generally present initially to a paediatrician, following assessment by whom a number receive the diagnosis of true vertigo. Since feeling dizzy or suffering from vertigo may be the sign of a serious underlying disorder, onward referral for extra investigations and assessment by a specialist in ENT or neurology is often undertaken [3, 5–7].

U. Mete (✉)
Section of Otorhinolaryngology, Bursa City Hospital, Bursa, Turkey

N. Bayar Muluk
Department of Otorhinolaryngology, Faculty of Medicine, Kırıkkale University, Kırıkkale, Turkey

C. Vicini
Unit of Otolaryngology, Ferrara, and Hospital Morgagni Pierantoni, Unit of Otolaryngology, University of Ferrara, Forli, Italy

C. Cingi et al. (eds.), *Pediatric ENT Infections*,
https://doi.org/10.1007/978-3-030-80691-0_16

The most valuable diagnostic information in cases of vertigo comes from detailed and focused history taking. Taking a history in paediatric cases suffers from various limitations, notably the child's ability to communicate effectively, limited words to describe the experience and difficulty in remaining focused. Because of these inherent limitations, the history may misdirect the clinician towards diagnosing coordination difficulties or a behavioural issue [8]. In such a situation, there is all the more need for a meticulously performed physical examination and appropriate laboratory investigations. Unfortunately, here too, the child may not comply fully with examination of the ears and nervous system. Yet one more complication relates to the fact that paediatric patients are frequently highly successful in adapting themselves to static vestibular impairment. A lesion to the vestibular system that would, in an adult, cause loss of balance and great disruption to the activities of daily living may produce no signs at all in a child [3].

Vertigo in children and adolescents is frequently ascribed to vestibular neuritis or labyrinthitis, but it may also be psychological in origin in up to 22% of cases. The majority of authorities do not list a psychological origin as a possible cause of paediatric vertigo, but where it is acknowledged to occur, the frequency usually ranges between 5% and 17% [8–10]. Of particular note may be recently published research into apparently inexplicable neurological symptoms in children, such as vertigo, dizziness, cephalgia and syncope, where the rate of mental health problems of at least one type was above 90% [11].

Whilst the majority of researchers consider benign paroxysmal vertigo of childhood (BPVC) to frequently underlie vertigo in a child, one study put its frequency at only 8% of cases. BPVC is classified as part of the migraine spectrum and originates centrally. Some sufferers from BPVC have headaches and as the disease progresses, may move onto migraine-associated vertigo [12].

16.2 Definitions

Dizziness is "a disturbed sense of relationship to space" [13]. Patients suffering from many different disorders have dizziness as their presenting complaint. Dizziness may be present as the only symptom, or in conjunction with vertigo. Vertigo refers to feeling unbalanced and the sensation that the surroundings are spinning around the patient, or vice versa. It is usual to treat vertigo in a different category from other conditions resulting in feeling dizzy or off-balance [14–15].

Vertigo arises due to an abnormally functioning vestibular system. The vestibular system consists of both a peripheral and central portion. The former is made up of the vestibule and the semicircular canals, whilst the latter consists of elements within the brainstem, cerebellum and vestibulospinal tract. Vertigo is frequently triggered by migraine spectrum conditions, BPVC, cranial injury, travel sickness or disorders affecting the middle ear (such as an effusion or an infection).

There are also numerous disorders which cause patients to feel dizzy, but do not affect the vestibular system. These are described as pseudovertigo. Some of the frequently occurring causes of pseudovertigo are anaemia, orthostatic hypotension, a presyncopal episode, being pregnant, hyperventilating, anxiety and depression.

16.3   Dizziness with Vertigo

In cases of vertigo, the patient may talk of feeling they are spinning around. Nystagmus is often elicited when the patient is examined. When the symptom begins abruptly, the underlying aetiology may be an acute problem or represent the beginning of a chronic condition [14].

The most probable underlying aetiologies in a child with vertigo are migraine, BPVC and disorders of the middle ear resulting in labyrinthitis of bacterial or serous type [16–21]. The conditions causing vertigo that bring the greatest risk to life are grave cerebral injury or infection of the central nervous system.

Consideration of how old a patient with vertigo is also of benefit in reducing the number of diagnostic possibilities to consider. A patient less than 5 years old is most likely to be suffering from the complications of middle ear inflammation or benign paroxysmal vertigo. A remoter possibility is paroxysmal torticollis of infancy. It is unusual for a patient who is less than 10 years old to be suffering from Meniere's disease, multiple sclerosis or benign paroxysmal positional vertigo (BPPV). One study looked at the most frequent diagnoses within particular age ranges. The three groups were pre-schoolers, junior school students and children aged 13 years and above. In the first two groups, the most frequent diagnosis was benign paroxysmal vertigo, whereas the oldest group typically were suffering from vestibular migraine [22].

16.4   Aetiology

16.4.1 Central Nervous System Infection

If there is a viral or bacterial infection affecting the central nervous system, dizziness or vertigo may develop when there is involvement of the vestibular system. In such cases, it is usual for other indications of infection to be present, e.g. pyrexia, cephalgia, nuchal rigidity or alteration in mental state. A number of studies that retrospectively examined diagnoses given to children attending as outpatients with complaints of vertigo with or without dizziness noted that there was no instance of meningitis or encephalitis [23–25]. Nonetheless, if a paediatric patient complaining of these symptoms is pyrexial or exhibits an alteration in mental state, it is vital to ensure that there is no underlying central nervous infection, in view of its seriousness.

16.4.2 Intracranial Tumour or Abscess

Whilst intracranial space-occupying lesions seldom present as vertigo, a mass lesion in the vicinity of the fourth ventricle or the central vestibular nuclei can potentially result in the patient feeling dizzy, vertiginous or exhibit nystagmus since the lesion may press on or displace adjacent structures or produce a localised inflammatory reaction. In such cases, moving the head usually causes a worsening in symptoms [14].

16.4.3   Drug Overdose and Other Poisons

Illicit drug use (e.g. barbiturates, alcohol, ketamine or phenylcyclohexyl piperidine) can also produce vertigo and provoke nystagmus. When these agents are used, the patient usually presents with an alteration in mental state and behaves differently from usual. It is possible to confirm rapidly and objectively the presence of these drugs, other than ketamine. The diagnosis is then straightforward. Ketamine intoxication is confirmed clinically, on the basis of presentation and observation in hospital. In all cases of vertigo or dizziness secondary to substance-misuse, treatment consists of support alone [14].

16.4.4   Otitis Media

The most frequently occurring paediatric condition producing vestibular problems is otitis media [15]. By the time a child is 1 year old, he or she has a 60–80% chance of having had acute otitis media on at least one occasion, and this figure rises to between 80% and 90% by the age of 2–3 years. Acute otitis media (whether suppurative or serous) may lead to labyrinthitis, which may cause the child to feel dizzy, experience vertigo or become deaf. Acute otitis media is associated with typical signs at otoscopy, such as reddening of the ear drum and tympanic bulging, alongside other signs of a middle ear effusion. These findings are diagnostic.

16.4.5   Migraine Syndromes

Migrainous vertigo is the label used for a condition in which vertigo occurs episodically in an individual who has previously suffered from migraine or who presents with features suggestive of migraine. Whereas adult migraine sufferers typically experience cephalgia in migraine, children with migraines may not complain of headache at all, but do experience vertigo and exhibit nystagmus or other signs of migraine. Furthermore, the proportion of paediatric cases of classic migraine in which the aura produces vertigo may be as high as 19%. Basilar arterial migraine manifests as at least two symptoms during the aura related to areas supplied by the basilar artery. Thus vertigo is seen in this condition, which occurs in the majority of cases in patients aged under 20 years. There is symptomatic resolution within 2 h, after which throbbing cephalgia is experienced [14].

16.4.6   Vestibular Neuritis

Vestibular neuritis (vestibular neuronitis or labyrinthitis) is a condition affecting the peripheral vestibular system. It begins abruptly without clear trigger and presents as rapidly developing, severe symptoms of vertigo, nausea, vomiting and being unable to walk steadily. The condition occurs frequently amongst adults but is seldom found in a child. Sufferers exhibit a preference for lying motionless on the unaffected side. Auditory impairment does not occur as part of the condition. The aetiology is believed to be an inflammatory response in the vestibular nerve following an infection with mumps, measles, Epstein-Barr virus or herpes or the viral infection itself. Despite this putative aetiology, under half of those affected give an account indicating a probable viral episode. The condition has a duration of either several weeks or months [14].

16.4.7   Benign Paroxysmal Vertigo of Childhood (BPVC)

Patients with BPPV present with repeated brief episodes of vertigo, generally triggered by movement of the head. There are several alternative terms used to refer to BPPV, e.g. "positional nystagmus of the benign paroxysmal type" [26] or "benign recurrent vertigo" [27], which reflect the fact that abrupt alteration in the position of the head is key to understanding how attacks begin and that the condition can be reversed [28]. BPPV may also on occasion be termed "cupulolithiasis" [28] or "canalithiasis" [29], by reference to the supposed aetiology [28, 30].

The first mention of paediatric cases of BPPV was by Basser in 1964 [31]. He noted the occurrence of BPPV in 17 patients (male and female) who were all younger than 4 years old. The symptomatic presentation was of an abrupt onset of episodes in which the child complained of vertigo, not accompanied by deafness or tinnitus, lost his or her balance, had an unsteady gait, became fearful, turned pale, sweated profusely and sometimes vomited. This pattern repeated itself on a number of occasions each month extending over a number of years. The episodes would usually resolve before the child reached his or her eighth birthday. Whilst the pathogenic mechanism was unknown, it seemed probable that alteration in the posterior vascular supply to the CNS was involved.

16.4.7.1   Pathophysiology

Whilst the precise pathogenic mechanism of BPPV (as well as BPVC, the condition when it occurs in a child) remains unclear, there is a general consensus amongst researchers that vestibular symptoms arise from widespread injury to the neuroepithelium of the vestibular apparatus [32]. Symptoms may arise due to debris from damaged cells (such as otoconial crystal fragments) floating around in the endolymph or may be the result of otoconial fragmentation from the utricle, with the pieces ending up deposited in the cupula [29, 32, 33]. Schuknecht coined the terms "cupolithiasis" or "canalithiasis" [29] to refer to this situation. He argued that debris mainly accumulated in the posterior semicircular canal. However, histology of the temporal bone indicates that debris may also accumulate within the lateral or superior canals [34]. The fact that debris can accumulate in this way indicates the possibility that the condition reflects degeneration due to injury or age-related change [32, 35].

The fact that temporal bone samples from children do not show evidence of accumulated debris is taken as evidence favouring the explanation of BPVC as a migrainous condition [34]. Bachor et al. [34] examined 121 sections of temporal bone from children aged up to the age of 10 years and noted that accumulated debris was rarely seen. Ischaemic injury, furthermore, occurred focussed on the otoconia of the utricle, which may support the theory that BPVC is related to arterial supply.

In fact, the theory that BPVC is in reality a paediatric migraine syndrome has much to commend it. Migrainous cephalgia is found across the entire age range in childhood, with cases noted even from the age of 18 months [37]. Bille [37] noted that migraine occurred in 4% of children in a sample consisting of 8993 children aged between 7 and 15 years old and attending school. Russell and Abu-Arafeh's research involved a survey of 2165 schoolchildren [36]. Some 314 replied that they had experienced feeling dizzy at least once within the preceding 12 months. From the children reporting dizziness, 57 reported three episodes of dizziness associated with migraine or without an obvious association. This last group had symptoms of benign paroxysmal vertigo occurring in isolation in 47% of cases.

16.4.7.2 Diagnosis

To examine the vestibular system calls for both direct and indirect testing. To examine a young child's second, third and eighth cranial nerves as well as the vestibulo-ocular reflex, play peek-a-boo with the child whilst checking gaze fixation and gaze shift [38]. To examine dynamic visual acuity, which provides indirect information on how the vestibular system is working, the child can be asked to shake his or head to indicate "no" as rapidly as possible, whilst the doctor checks for nystagmus [38]. In an older child, Frenzel goggles may also be used [35, 38].

Weber Rinne testing, finger-nose pointing and asking the child to hop, skip and jump, whilst keeping the eyes open or closed act as useful screening examinations [39]. The vestibular system can be specifically tested via the Hallpike-Dix positioning manoeuvre, before and after wearing Frenzel goggles (ICS Medical, USA) [26, 38]. Non-specific testing may be done with Fukuda stepping, which confirms the vestibular system is involved and does not call for specialised apparatus [38–40]. Peabody and Bruininks-Oseretsky testing similarly provide valuable diagnostic information.

16.4.7.3 Treatment

Whilst there are detailed protocols available to use to treat BPPV in adults, e.g. the University of Michigan Vestibular Rehabilitation Program [41], there are no such guidelines in existence for paediatric cases. There are some protocols which may be employed to teach paediatric patients to achieve balance, but most suffer from inadequate reliability and validity [42].

16.4.8 Motion Sickness

Motion sickness occurs when the input from the visual, vestibular and somatosensory systems do not match, such as when a person sitting in a cabin on board a seagoing vessel has somatosensory input indicating that the body is stationary, but the movement of the ship is registered by the vestibular system. This mismatch results in a feeling of nausea. If the vestibular apparatus itself generates signals that are mismatched with input from the somatosensory system, this also leads to motion sickness, whether the mismatch is caused by motion or not. A child suffering from motion sickness may appear pale, sweat profusely, complain of feeling dizzy and nauseous and may vomit. This condition is generally seen on journeys by boat, car or aeroplane. The incidence is greatly raised in paediatric migraine sufferers. Motion sickness is seldom associated with vertigo [14].

16.4.9 Meniere's Disease

Meniere's disease presents clinically as feeling the ear is full on the affected side, ringing in the ears, vertigo, and varying degrees of auditory impairment of sensorineural type in one ear. Autonomic involvement may also occur, with the patient appearing pale, feeling nauseous and vomiting. In this condition, there is hydrops of the endolymphatic system, such that the parts of the labyrinth which contain endolymph become distorted and distended. Although Meniere's disease is known to occur at all ages, the peak incidence is in an adult older than 20 but younger than 40. Where the condition occurs in paediatric patients, the most frequent association is with congenitally anomalous inner ear anatomy [14].

16.4.10 Perilymphatic Fistula

A perilymphatic fistula refers to an anomalous communication connecting the inner and middle ear. The condition may be present from birth, in which case it results in irreversible sensorineural deafness, or may be acquired. Acquired cases may result from pressure injury (in divers, flight descent when the cabin pressure is not properly regulated, sneezing, coughing or other situation where the middle ear is subject to abrupt alteration in pressure), cranial trauma, and injury to, or infection of, the middle ear. Perilymphatic fistula is a diagnostic possibility where the problem has an abrupt onset or is variable and the patient complains of feeling dizzy or the head spinning. Symptomatic deterioration occurs if the middle ear pressure alters and this can be shown clinically by employing pneumatic otoscopy, getting the patient to perform the Valsalva manoeuvre (giving positivity of Hennebert's sign) or demonstrating that vertigo and nystagmus occur when a loud stimulus is given (Tullio phenomenon).

16.5 Dizziness Without Vertigo (Pseudovertigo)

There are a number of different conditions which cause the symptom of feeling dizzy but lack head spinning (i.e. vertigo). These symptoms are those of presyncope or match the feeling of being "lightheaded". Clues in the history, physical examination and simple extra tests are frequently sufficient for diagnostic purposes. Paediatric cases of presyncope or ataxia typically present in this way.

Individuals who feel dizzy because of being unable to maintain balance, rather than due to vertigo, need to be meticulously assessed for a potentially serious ataxic disorder. The various syndromes causing ataxia occur at different ages. Involvement of a paediatric neurology specialist to undertake extra tests and provide advice is frequently advisable.

Ear wax impacted in the canal is a potential reason for feeling dizzy and becoming deaf on one side. The consistency of ear wax ranges from semi-liquid to a hard solid. The consistency is a result of varying composition, length of time present in the external auditory meatus (cerumen has a tendency to harden over time) and volume of desquamated keratinocytes. The range of possible colours extends from very dark red to black to not-quite white. If impacted wax is the cause, removing it will solve the problem [14].

References

1. Neuhauser HK, Radtke A, Von Brevern M, Lezius F, Feldmann M, Lempert T. Burden of dizziness and vertigo in the community. Arch Intern Med. 2008;168(19):2118–24.
2. O'Reilly RC, Morlet T, Nicholas BD, et al. Prevalence of vestibular and balance disorders in children. Otol Neurotol. 2010;31(9):1441–4.
3. Gruber M, Cohen-Kerem R, Kaminer M, Shupak A. Vertigo in children and adolescents: characteristics and outcome. Sci World J. 2012;2012:109624. https://doi.org/10.1100/2012/109624.
4. Harrison MS. Vertigo in childhood. J Laryngol Otol. 1962;76:601–16.
5. Fried MP. The evaluation of dizziness in children. Laryngoscope. 1980;90(9):1548–60.
6. Uneri A, Turkdogan D. Evaluation of vestibular functions in children with vertigo attacks. Arch Dis Child. 2003;88(6):510–1.
7. Erbek SH, Erbek SS, Yilmaz I, et al. Vertigo in childhood: a clinical experience. Int J Pediatr Otorhinolaryngol. 2006;70(9):1547–54.
8. Tusa RJ, Saada AA, Niparko JK. Dizziness in childhood. J Child Neurol. 1994;9(3):261–74.
9. Szirmai A. Vestibular disorders in childhood and adolescents. Eur Arch Otorhinolaryngol. 2010;267:1801–4.
10. Riina N, Ilmari P, Kentala E. Vertigo and imbalance in children: a retrospective study in a Helsinki University otorhinolaryngology clinic. Arch Otolaryngol. 2005;131(11):996–1000.
11. Inal Emiroğlu FN, Kurul S, Miral S, Dirik E. Assessment of child neurology outpatients with headache, dizziness, and fainting. J Child Neurol. 2004;19(5):332–6.
12. Krams B, Echenne B, Leydet J, Rivier F, Roubertie A. Benign paroxysmal vertigo of childhood: long-term outcome. Cephalalgia. 2011;31:439–43.
13. Dizziness. In: Dorland's medical dictionary. 29th ed. Philadelphia, PA: WB Saunders; 2000. p. 538. ISBN-10: 0721694934, ISBN-13: 978-0721694931.
14. Walls T, Teach SJ. Causes of dizziness and vertigo in children and adolescents. In: Nordli DR Jr, Isaacson GC, Fleisher GR, Wiley JF II, Wilterdink JL (Eds). Uptodate. 2020.
15. Casselbrant ML, Mandel EM. Balance disorders in children. Neurol Clin. 2005;23:807.
16. Ravid S, Bienkowski R, Eviatar L. A simplified diagnostic approach to dizziness in children. Pediatr Neurol. 2003;29:317.
17. Gioacchini FM, Alicandri-Ciufelli M, Kaleci S, et al. Prevalence and diagnosis of vestibular disorders in children: a review. Int J Pediatr Otorhinolaryngol. 2014;78:718.
18. Raucci U, Vanacore N, Paolino MC, et al. Vertigo/dizziness in pediatric emergency department: five years' experience. Cephalalgia. 2016;36:593.

19. Sommerfleck PA, González Macchi ME, Weinschelbaum R, et al. Balance disorders in childhood: Main etiologies according to age. Usefulness of the video head impulse test. Int J Pediatr Otorhinolaryngol. 2016;87:148.
20. Humphriss RL, Hall AJ. Dizziness in 10 year old children: an epidemiological study. Int J Pediatr Otorhinolaryngol. 2011;75:395.
21. Jahn K, Langhagen T, Heinen F. Vertigo and dizziness in children. Curr Opin Neurol. 2015;28:78.
22. Lee JD, Kim CH, Hong SM, et al. Prevalence of vestibular and balance disorders in children and adolescents according to age: a multi-center study. Int J Pediatr Otorhinolaryngol. 2017;94:36.
23. Bower CM, Cotton RT. The spectrum of vertigo in children. Arch Otolaryngol Head Neck Surg. 1995;121:911.
24. Choung YH, Park K, Moon SK, et al. Various causes and clinical characteristics in vertigo in children with normal eardrums. Int J Pediatr Otorhinolaryngol. 2003;67:889.
25. Riina N, Ilmari P, Kentala E. Vertigo and imbalance in children: a retrospective study in a Helsinki University otorhinolaryngology clinic. Arch Otolaryngol Head Neck Surg. 2005;131:996.
26. Dix MR, Hallpike CS. The pathology, symptomatology and diagnosis of certain common disorders of the vestibular system. Ann Otol Rhinol Laryngol. 1952;61:987–1016.
27. Slater R. Benign recurrent vertigo. J Neurol Neurosurg Psychiatry. 1979;42:363–7.
28. Katsarkas A, Kirkham TH. Paroxysmal positional vertigo – a study of 255 cases. J Otolaryngol. 1978;7:320–8.
29. Schuknecht HF. Positional nystagmus of the benign paroxysmal type. In: Nauton RF, editor. The vestibular system. San Diego, CA: Academic Press; 1975. p. 421–8.
30. Batson G. Benign paroxysmal vertigo of childhood: a review of the literature. Paediatr Child Health. 2004;9(1):31–4. https://doi.org/10.1093/pch/9.1.31.
31. Seyed RA. Can the determination of salivary cotinine level be a new method in diagnosis and follow-up of childhood tinnitus? Iran Red Crescent Med J. 2020;22(2):1–7. https://doi.org/10.5812/ircmj.95472.
32. Fife TD, Tusa RJ, Furman JM, et al. Assessment: vestibular testing techniques in adults and children. Report of the therapeutics and technology assessment subcommittee of the American Academy of Neurology. Neurology. 2000;55:1431–41.
33. Hall SF, Ruby RRF, McClure JA. The mechanics of benign paroxsysmal vertigo. J Otolaryngol. 1976;8:151–8.
34. Bachor E, Wright CG, Karmody CS. The incidence and distribution of copular deposits in the pediatric vestibular labyrinth. Laryngoscope. 2002;112:147–51.
35. Tusa RJ, Saada AA, Niparko JK. Dizziness in childhood. J Child Neurology. 1994;9:261–74.
36. Russell G, Abu-Arafeh I. Paroxysmal vertigo in children – an epidemiological study. Intl J Pediatr Otorhinolaryngol. 1999;49:S105–7.
37. Bille B. Migraine in school children. Acta Paediatr. 1962;51(Suppl 136):14–151.
38. Phillips JO, Backous DD. Evaluation of vestibular function in young children. Otolaryngol Clin N Am. 2002;35:765–90.
39. Eviatar L, Eviatar A. Neurovestibular examination of infants and children. Adv Otorhinolaryngol. 1978;23:169–91.
40. Goebel JA. Practical management of the dizzy patient. Philadelphia: Lippincott Williams & Wilkins; 2001. p. 289–310.
41. Telian SA, Shepard NT. Update on vestibular rehabilitation therapy. Otolaryngol Clin N Am. 1996;29:359–71.
42. Westcott SL, Lowes LP, Richardson PK. Evaluation of postural stability in children: current theories and assessment tools. Phys Ther. 1997;77:629–45.

Nasal Obstruction in Childhood

Sinem Gökçe Kütük, Sema Başak, and Gordon Soo

17.1 Introduction

Nasal obstruction is the most common symptom in the field of rhinology. Its aetiology is based on similar reasons in adulthood and childhood. The nose may become blocked when the blood vessels supplying the mucosa become dilated in response to histamine release triggered by exposure to a pathogen or allergen. Sinusitis causes inflammation which may also involve the nose, as may secretions draining from the lesion, and these may worsen blockage. A deviated septum frequently blocks the nose. Hypertrophied turbinates may play a major role in nasal obstruction, given that half of the air passing through the nose goes through the middle passage. If the septum becomes perforated, the nasal airflow becomes turbulent, and this may cause reactive hypertrophy of the turbinates, causing even greater constriction to airflow. The nasal valve may also collapse if its framework of cartilage is inadequate, and this, too, can obstruct the nose. Rhinoplasty potentially plays a key role amongst iatrogenic causes of a blocked nose.

A list of potential aetiologies for nasal obstruction may be drawn up as follows [1]:

- Deviated septum.
- Hypertrophied turbinates.

S. G. Kütük (✉)
Section of Otorhinolaryngology, Aydın State Hospital, Aydın, Turkey

S. Başak
Department of Otorhinolaryngology, Faculty of Medicine, Aydın Adnan Menderes University, Aydın, Turkey
e-mail: hsbasak@adu.edu.tr

G. Soo
Department of Otorhinolaryngology, Head and Neck Surgery, Hong Kong Special Administrative Region, The Chinese University of Hong Kong, Hong Kong, People's Republic of China

C. Cingi et al. (eds.), *Pediatric ENT Infections*,
https://doi.org/10.1007/978-3-030-80691-0_17

- Rhinoplasty.
- Perforated septum.
- A collapsed nasal valve.
- Choanal atresia.
- Neoplastic lesions.
- Polyp formation [2].
- Allergic rhinitis.
- Haematoma on the septum.
- Rhinitis medicamentosa.
- Vasomotor rhinitis.
- Sinusitis [3].

17.2 Deviation of the Septum

The septum may deviate in the course of development. In some cases, trauma is sustained to the cartilaginous septum either neonatally or at birth, but this trauma passes unnoticed until the septum develops in a markedly deviated fashion. Microfractures to the foetal nose may occur at a late stage of pregnancy or during parturition, resulting in the cartilaginous framework being weakened on the affected side. Consequently, the developing cartilage deviates in the direction of the fracture and the unaffected side gradually becomes stronger. There is evidence showing a correlation between the side to which the septum deviates and the way the foetus presented at delivery [4].

Injury sustained by a child or adult may result in a deviated septum. An injury occurring whilst the patient was a child may lead to a severely obstructed nose in adulthood since, once the septum begins to deviate, the degree of deviation tends to become more severe over time [4].

A blow to the nose may occur in any direction and with varying degrees of force, and the pattern of cartilaginous injury is similarly varied. Fractures may be horizontal or vertical. A single fracture or several fractures may be produced. The adjacent nasal bones or the ethmoidal perpendicular plate are also at risk of being fractured. The septal cartilage may undergo subluxation under the vomeral groove. Where the septal cartilage articulates with the osseous septum is typically the region where the septum is maximally deviated by any injury [4].

17.2.1 Pathophysiology

The cartilaginous septum supports the dorsum of the nose in a way that permits a sufficient degree of shock absorption to prevent the nose being deformed by all but very forceful blows. However, if the applied pressure goes beyond the biomechanical elastic limit, cartilage fails by fracturing [4].

If no injury occurs, the cartilaginous septum grows in a straight direction, with each side exerting an equal stress on the cartilage. When traumatic damage is sustained by the septum, one side becomes weaker and this careful balance is lost. The stronger (dominant) side grows more vigorously than the other side and the septum begins to deviate. The convex face of the deviated septum is where overgrowth occurs and usually corresponds to the side contralateral to the site of trauma [4].

As patients age, the degree of trauma necessary to cause the septum to deviate increases, such that a child (or, more particularly, an adolescent undergoing rapid growth) who undergoes a relatively minor nasal injury may sustain microfracture on one side that ultimately results in a severely deformed pattern of nasal septal cartilaginous development [4].

17.3 Nasal Polyps

A broad definition of a nasal polyp is of any pathological lesion growing out of the mucosal lining of the nose or adjacent sinuses. A number of different pathogenic processes occurring in the interior of the nose may result in polyposis. The type of polyp that is usually referred to is non-malignant, partially transparent and grows out of the internal nasal mucosal lining or within the adjacent sinusal cavities, especially in the region where the sinuses normally drain.

Chronic sinusitis, allergic rhinitis, cystic fibrosis (CF) and allergic fungal sinusitis (AFS) often cause the formation of several polyps in a child's nose. The differential diagnosis for a solitary polyp includes an antrochoanal polyp, a benign massive polyp, or tumorous growth, both cancerous and non-cancerous, such as an encephalocoele, glioma, haemangioma, papilloma, juvenile nasopharyngeal angiofibroma, rhabdomyosarcoma, lymphoma, neuroblastoma, sarcoma, chordoma, nasopharyngeal carcinoma or inverted papilloma. Any child who develops several polyps in the nasal lining that are non-malignant in origin needs to be assessed for potentially underlying cystic fibrosis or asthma. Patients should be told that polyposis is a chronic condition and thus the polyps tend to recur after surgical removal.

The first-line treatment for polyposis of the nose uses steroids, either by mouth or intranasally. In paediatric cases where pharmacotherapy at the highest permissible dose does not alleviate the situation and polyposis is secondary to chronic rhinosinusitis, or multiple benign polyposis is the diagnosis, operative removal is called for [5].

17.3.1 Pathophysiology

The pathogenetic basis of nasal polyp formation remains unclear. There are hypotheses that polyposis is a result of persistent inflammatory responses, abnormal action by the autonomic nervous system or is genetically determined. The majority of explanations of nasal polyposis agree that the condition is the end-stage of a persistent inflammatory response. Accordingly, we would expect to see polyposis occurring in disorders that involve chronic inflammation within the interior of the nose [5].

In fact, there are a number of such conditions known, where numerous polyps of a non-malignant type are produced, namely [5]:

- Bronchial asthma. Polyposis occurs in between 20% and 50% of cases.
- Cystic fibrosis. Polyposis occurs in between 6% and 44% of cases [6].
- Allergic rhinitis.
- Allergic fungal sinusitis. Polyposis occurs in 85% of cases.
- Chronic rhinosinusitis.
- Primary ciliary dyskinesia.
- Aspirin hypersensitivity. Polyposis occurs in between 8% and 26% of cases.
- Alcohol intolerance. Polyposis occurs in 50% of cases.
- Churg-Strauss syndrome. Polyposis occurs in 50% of cases.
- Young syndrome (which consists of chronic sinusitis, polyp formation in the nose and azoospermia).
- Non-allergic rhinitis with eosinophilia syndrome (NARES). Polyposis occurs in 20% of cases.

The majority of researchers have concluded that there is a greater association of nasal polyposis with non-atopic than atopic disorders. There is a statistically significant difference between the rate of polyp formation in atopic vs. non-atopic asthma, the rates being 5% and 13%, respectively, and thus higher in non-atopic asthma. Indeed, one study involving 3000 allergy sufferers found polyposis in a mere 0.5% [3, 5].

17.3.2 Aetiology

It appears that a chronic inflammatory response is key to the way polyps form in the nose, at least at the beginning. Numerous polyps are seen in paediatric cases of chronic rhinosinusitis, allergic rhinitis, cystic fibrosis or allergic fungal sinusitis. The differential diagnosis of a polyp occurring singly is an antrochoanal polyp, a benign massive polyp, a cyst affecting the tear duct or one of a number of other conditions, congenital, benign or malignant, namely [5]:

- Cyst within the tear duct.
- Encephalocoele.
- Glioma.
- Dermoid tumour.
- Haemangioma.
- Papilloma.
- Juvenile angiofibroma of the nasopharynx.
- Rhabdomyosarcoma.
- Lymphoma.
- Neuroblastoma.
- Sarcoma.

- Chordoma.
- Carcinoma of the nasopharynx.
- Inverted papilloma.

Any paediatric case where polyps of benign type are found within the nose requires exclusion of cystic fibrosis or asthma as an underlying cause [5].

17.4 Prognosis

It is frequently noted that polyps reform after pharmacological or operative treatment, unless the polyp occurred singly, such as with antrochoanal polyps. For more details, see the section on operative removal.

There seems to be an improvement in the ability to smell and the quality of life of patients with nasal polyposis occurring in the context of chronic rhinosinusitis who undergo an endoscopic sinus surgical procedure [7, 8]. Pagella et al. [9] reported that polyposis recurred in 20.5% of children aged under 18 years who had an antrochoanal polyp removed endoscopically (i.e. functional endoscopic sinus surgery, FESS). The sample consisted of 58 individuals.

The evidence base on which to judge the comparative effectiveness of therapy is slender. There is a systematic review undertaken by Galluzzi et al. [10], which gathered data on 285 cases and looked at how effective particular operative interventions were in paediatric cases of antrochoanal polyp. The review covers the following interventions: FESS, FESS in combination with transcanine sinusoscopy (i.e. mini Caldwell-Luc procedure), Caldwell-Luc itself, or simple polypectomy. The results obtained were that, overall, polyps recurred in 15% of cases. FESS had a recurrence rate of 17.7%. There were no recurrences with a combined approach, but Caldwell-Luc alone had a recurrence rate of 9.1%. Simple polypectomy was associated with 50% recurrence.

17.5 Pharmacological Management

17.5.1 Corticosteroids

The mainstay of pharmacotherapy for nasal polyposis is the use of steroids either by mouth or intranasal application [11–13]. There is minimal advantage from the use of histamine blockers, decongestant agents or cromolyn sodium. Whilst allergic rhinitis is treatable by immunotherapy, monotherapy of this type rarely causes polyps to disappear. In cases where opportunistic bacterial invasion has occurred, antimicrobial chemotherapy is indicated.

Thus, corticosteroid therapy, by mouth or intranasally, is the first-line therapy. The US FDA has not granted a licence for corticosteroid injection into the polyp directly following reported loss of sight on one side in three individuals who had this treatment using Kenalog. It seems likely that the exact size of the agent components plays a role in how safe this procedure is, with the likelihood that agents of greater molecular mass (e.g. Triamcinolone) have a lower propensity to be inadvertently injected intracranially. In any case, the clinician must avoid the needle entering a vessel.

The pharmacotherapy with the highest efficacy in nasal polyposis is corticosteroids by mouth. Experts generally recommend an adult prednisone dose of 30–60 mg daily over 4 days to 1 week, tapering off over the following 7–21 days. The recommended dose in paediatric cases is more variable, although the upper limit is typically 1 mg/kg/day for between 5 and 7 days, tapering off over the following 7–21 days. Patients who respond best to prednisone therapy are those with a raised eosinophil count; therefore this treatment is liable to be most effective in cases where polyposis complicates allergic rhinitis or asthma [5].

17.6 Allergic Rhinitis

Allergic rhinitis generally has its onset in young children. The pathogenetic mechanism occurs via binding of IgE (immunoglobulin E) to a variety of allergens which come into contact with the mucosal lining of the nose. From the age of 2 years onwards, some children develop allergic rhinitis in response to allergens present outside, but the peak incidence occurs between the ages of 4 and 6 years. On the other hand, even before age 2 years, some children already have a hypersensitivity to allergens found indoors that results in clinically apparent signs of allergic rhinitis (AR). The usual allergenic triggers are house dust mites, pet dander, cockroaches, moulds or pollen spores [14].

Specific IgE to these allergens (dust mites etc) is present in the mucosal lining of the nose, attached to the plasma membrane of mast cells through the Fcε receptor. An allergen, such as tree pollen, is bound by IgE. If two IgE molecules both attach themselves to the same allergen, this event triggers a cascade of pro-inflammatory signals to be released, in particular histamine. The familiar presentation of allergic rhinitis is caused by this cascade of signals. Patients with AR sneeze have a blocked nose, suffer from nasal discharge, may cough and experience nasal, ocular and pharyngeal pruritus. They may have pressure over the sinuses, cephalgia and nose bleeds [14].

The prevalence of outdoor allergens depends on the location and the season. A knowledge of allergenic prevalence at particular periods is of value in identifying AR and offering treatment. It may also assist with deciding if a specific allergy is the cause of symptoms. An illustration of applying this knowledge would be to know that a case of blocked nose occurring in November in the area of Boston, Massachusetts, USA, cannot represent AR secondary to hypersensitivity to tree pollen, since the relevant allergen is not prevalent until the spring [14].

Coming into contact with an allergen tends to trigger an inflammatory reaction in the lower as well as upper airways. Thus both the nose and lungs react to the antigenic stimulation. There is a growing consensus to treat both the upper and lower airway as a unified whole, rather than as discrete entities. Research findings indicate that the majority of asthmatic individuals also suffer from AR. There have been guidelines issued regarding how AR can affect asthma [15]. Allergic inflammation in the upper airway sets off lower airway responses, as well as the other way round. The risk of requiring hospital admission for a flare-up of asthma is three times elevated in an asthmatic patient whose AR is uncontrolled, whilst the risk of attending Accident and Emergency doubled [16]. It has been shown that effective management of AR improves asthma outcomes and vice versa.

Children suffering from AR may present with the following symptoms [14]:

- Nasal discharge, stuffiness, postnasal drip.
- Pallor of the nasal turbinates, potentially accompanied by watery rhinorrhoea.
- Repeated urge to sneeze.
- Palatal, nasal, ocular or otic pruritus.
- Snoring.
- Frequently occurring pharyngitis.
- Persistent need to clear the throat or cough.
- Cephalgia.

The physical examination of paediatric cases of AR includes examination of the head, eyes, ears, nose and pharynx. The following are signs to look for [14]:

- When examining the head, darkened, swollen inferior blepharae are termed "allergic shiners". There may be a line below the eyelid, termed a Morgan-Dennie line. Since atopic individuals frequently rub their nose (the so-called "allergic salute"), this may leave a visible crease running transversely across the inferior third of the nasal skin.
- The eyes also show characteristic signs. The palpebral conjunctivae may be noticeably reddened and the papillae of the tarsal conjunctivae may become hypertrophied. There may be conjunctival oedema, which typically weeps clear fluid. If the pruritus has led to repeated excoriation, cataracts may develop in extreme cases.
- There may be signs of persistent ear infection or an effusion of the middle ear.
- The nasal interior reveals larger than usual turbinates covered with mucosa that has a slightly blue tinge as a result of mucosal oedema. There may be a discharge, often clear or white in colour, although occasionally yellowish green. Persistent wiping of the nose may cause bleeding, so dried blood may be apparent. Polyps are infrequently seen. If a polyp is seen, it is essential to be able to exclude cystic fibrosis as an underlying cause in paediatric cases.
- Pharynx: The front teeth may be a different colour and the palate arched higher than usual as a result of long-term mouth-breathing. There may be malocclusion. The rear throat may have cobble stoning apparent resulting from persistent blockage of the nose and postnasal drip.

17.7 Investigations

Where the presentation is typical of AR, there may be no call for laboratory investigations. However, if the presentation is unclear, there are a number of investigations which have value in diagnosis, namely [14]:

- Skin prick testing. This test benefits from a high sensitivity to and specificity for airborne allergens.
- Specific IgE to particular allergens is of value if a putative allergic culprit is identified.
- Serological IgE titre is helpful in that a raised titre may indicate AR, but it lacks the sensitivity of cutaneous tests.
- Nasal smear.

17.7.1 Radiological investigations

Generally speaking, there is little role for radiological investigations in a child with AR, provided there is no suspicion of rhinosinusitis. If such a suspicion does exist, plain CT scanning of the sinuses is warranted [14].

17.7.2 Procedures

Cutaneous allergy testing is valuable in confirming an allergen is responsible for symptoms. Two methods are available: skin pricking or intradermal.

Spirometric analysis is potentially of value since up to 70% of paediatric asthma cases have comorbid AR.

Direct rhinoscopy can assist in differentiating between an obstruction or an infection as the cause of AR, and to assess whether polyps have formed.

17.7.3 Therapy

There are three key elements involved in treating AR [14]:

- Avoiding allergenic or environmental triggers.
- Pharmacotherapy.
- Immunotherapy to induce tolerance to a specific antigen. This may be delivered subcutaneously or sublingually.

17.7.4 Drug Treatment

There are numerous pharmacological agents which find use in AR, such as histamine blockers, steroids, decongestants, saline, sodium cromolyn, and leukotriene receptor antagonists. Some agents are given by mouth, whilst others are topical.

The following is a list of the agents which may be employed in children suffering from AR [14]:

- Second-generation histamine blockers (such as cetirizine, levocetirizine, loratadine, desloratadine or fexofenadine).
- Topical histamine blockers (such as azelastine or intranasal olopatadine).
- Topical steroids administered intranasally such as beclometasone, budesonide, ciclesonide, flunisolide, fluticasone, mometasone and triamcinolone.
- Combined histamine blocker and steroid preparations (such as azelastine/fluticasone administered intranasally).
- Topical decongestants such as ipratropium.
- Topical mast cell stabilising agents (such as cromolyn sodium administered intranasally).
- Anti-leukotrienes, such as montelukast.

17.7.5 Non-pharmacological Treatment

There are also some treatment modalities other than drug treatment [14]:

- Immunotherapy targeting a specific allergen. This is the sole curative treatment. It must be matched with the particular allergen to which an individual is sensitive.
- Irrigating the nose with saline is beneficial in around half of individuals with AR.
- Where the allergen is known, eradication of exposure.

References

1. Lin SJ. What causes of nasal obstruction? In: Meyers AD (Ed). Medscape. Updated: Nov 04, 2019. https://www.medscape.com/answers/874822-177608/what-causes-of-nasal-obstruction (Accessed online at October 15, 2020).
2. Nishijima H, Kondo K, Yamamoto T, et al. Influence of the location of nasal polyps on olfactory airflow and olfaction. Int Forum Allergy Rhinol. 2018 8(6):695–706.
3. Battisti AS, Pangia J. Sinusitis. Hosp Pract. 2018 Jan.;14(12):12.
4. Watson D. Septoplasty. In: Meyers AD (Ed). Medscape. Updated: Mar 27, 2019. https://emedicine.medscape.com/article/877677-overview#a8. Accessed 15 Oct 2020.
5. McClay JE. Pediatric Nasal Polyps Treatment & Management. In: Elluru RG (Ed). Medscape. Updated: Oct 25, 2019. https://emedicine.medscape.com/article/994274-treatment#d5. Accessed 15 Oct 2020.

6. Babinski D, Trawinska-Bartnicka M. Rhinosinusitis in cystic fibrosis: not a simple story. Int J Pediatr Otorhinolaryngol. 2008;72(5):619–24.
7. Lind H, Joergensen G, Lange B, Svendstrup F, Kjeldsen AD. Efficacy of ESS in chronic rhinosinusitis with and without nasal polyposis: a Danish cohort study. Eur Arch Otorhinolaryngol. 2016;273(4):911–9.
8. Andrews PJ, Poirrier AL, Lund VJ, Choi D. Outcomes in endoscopic sinus surgery: olfaction, nose scale and quality of life in a prospective cohort study. Clin Otolaryngol. 2016;41(6):798–803.
9. Pagella F, Emanuelli E, Pusateri A, Borsetto D, Cazzador D, Marangoni R, et al. Clinical features and management of antrochoanal polyps in children: cues from a clinical series of 58 patients. Int J Pediatr Otorhinolaryngol. 2018;114:87–91.
10. Galluzzi F, Pignataro L, Maddalone M, Garavello W. Recurrences of surgery for antrochoanal polyps in children: a systematic review. Int J Pediatr Otorhinolaryngol. 2018;106:26–30.
11. Kirtsreesakul V, Wongsritrang K, Ruttanaphol S. Clinical efficacy of a short course of systemic steroids in nasal polyposis. Rhinology. 2011;49(5):525–32.
12. Naclerio RM, Pinto J, Baroody F. Evidence-based approach to medical and surgical treatment of nasal polyposis. J Allergy Clin Immunol. 2013;132(6):1461–2.
13. Bachert C, Zhang L, Gevaert P. Current and future treatment options for adult chronic rhinosinusitis: focus on nasal polyposis. J Allergy Clin Immunol. 2015;136(6):1431–40.
14. Becker JM. Pediatric Allergic Rhinitis. In: Jyonouchi H (Ed). Medscape. Updated: Jul 17, 2018. https://emedicine.medscape.com/article/889259-overview#a5. Accessed 15 Oct 2020.
15. [Guideline] World Health Organization (WHO). Allergic rhinitis and its impact on asthma. 2008.
16. Crystal-Peters J, Neslusan C, Crown WH, Torres A. Treating allergic rhinitis in patients with comorbid asthma: the risk of asthma-related hospitalizations and emergency department visits. J Allergy Clin Immunol. 2002;109(1):57–62.

Rhinorrhea: Pathogenesis, Diagnosis, and Treatment

18

Murat Koçyiğit, Cemal Cingi, and Ali Arslantaş

18.1 Introduction

Nasal discharge or rhinorrhea is a very common problem, especially in children [1]. Rhinorrhea occurs when excess fluid drains from the nose. The fluid is mucus that is thin or thick, clear or opaque, and can be intermittent or constant. The nose and sinuses normally produce mucus that keeps the nose moist and is typically swept back into the throat and swallowed [2].

During airflow through the nose, several components including turbinates, septum, and the ostiomeatal complex contribute to natural turbulence of the air column. This turbulence is physiologically important, because alteration of any of these internal structures can affect the perception of airflow. For example, a person with a large septal perforation will have a constant sensation of nasal obstruction due to disruption of the normal turbulence patterns, even though the nasal passage itself is widely patent [3].

There is also airflow around the turbinates and into the natural ostia of the sinuses during normal respiration. Therefore, particles or allergens in the air can potentially affect both the nasal and sinus mucosa, resulting in inflammation within the upper airway [3].

M. Koçyiğit (✉)
Section of Otorhinolaryngology, Kanuni Sultan Süleyman Training and Research Hospital, University of Health Sciences, İstanbul, Turkey

C. Cingi
Department of Otorhinolaryngology, Faculty of Medicine, Eskişehir Osmangazi University, Eskişehir, Turkey

A. Arslantaş
Department of Neurosurgery, Faculty of Medicine, Eskişehir Osmangazi University, Eskişehir, Turkey

C. Cingi et al. (eds.), *Pediatric ENT Infections*,
https://doi.org/10.1007/978-3-030-80691-0_18

18.2 Etiology of the Rhinorrhea

There are many conditions that can cause the nose to discharge, including:

18.2.1 Allergic Rhinitis (AR)

AR commonly affects pre-pubescent adolescence and results from an immunoglobulin E (IgE) response to multiple allergens in the sinus. Outdoor allergen sensitization for AR can be associated with children over the age 2 years. Yet, the most common age of sensitization is found in children over the age of 4 years. On the other hand, indoor allergen sensitization is more common in children under the age of two years. Common allergens are pet dander, mold, pollen, dust mites, and cockroaches [4].

Pediatric AR signs and symptoms [4]:

- Runny nose, congestion, and postnasal drip.
- Pale or swollen sinus cavity, clear nasal discharge.
- Itchy, watery eyes, nose and/or ears.
- Sneezing, snoring, sore throat, cough, and pressure behind eyes and nose.

18.2.1.1 Diagnosis

History

Patients with AR may have a straightforward medical history or multiple symptom complex nature. In a patient with seasonal allergies or a new family pet, the diagnosis can be easier to determine. On the other hand, adolescent patients may have multiple signs or symptoms, which are not taken seriously by family members that are unfamiliar of AR. Often, seasonal allergies in young children may be mistaken for pet allergies in the spring when pet dander is at its peak. In addition, older children may become desensitized to allergies over the years and appear less severe [4].

Examination

A typical child examination includes all the orifices of the head, the throat, and may involve specific evaluation of the following [4]:

- Head: Allergic shiners, Morgan-Dennie lines, and a crosswise crease on the nose.
- Eyes: Erythema of palpebral conjunctivae and hypertrophy of tarsal conjunctivae; chemosis of the conjunctivae, or severe rubbing causing cataracts.
- Ears: Chronic infection or oozing of the middle ear.
- Nose: Swollen turbinate with pale-bluish mucosa; clear or white nasal discharge; dried blood.
- Throat: Frontal incisors discoloration, high arched palate, and malocclusion; cobblestoning of the posterior pharynx [4].

Testing

Patients with AR and a straightforward medical history do not need laboratory tests. When the medical history is complex, a more specific medical workup may be necessary [4]:

- Skin-prick and/or allergy skin testing.
- Allergen-specific or Serum IgE.
- Nasal swab.

Imaging

Generally, imaging for pediatric AR is only necessary if there is suspicion of sinusitis [4].

18.2.1.2 Treatment

Three categories for AR therapies [4]:

- Isolation from allergens.
- Over the counter or prescribed medicine.
- Immunotherapy to build immunity.

Pharmacotherapy

Various types of treatments have been used for AR and can be categorized as intranasal and oral therapies [4].

Children with AR are routinely administered the following medications [4]:

- Antihistamines (oral/intranasal).
- Corticosteroids (intranasal).
- Antihistamine/corticosteroid combination (intranasal).
- Decongestants (intranasal).
- Mast cell stabilizers (intranasal).
- Leukotriene receptor antagonists.

Nonpharmacotherapy

Management opportunities for AR do not include medication [4]:

- Immunotherapy (allergen-specific): personalized therapy.
- Saline nasal irrigation.
- Stimulus removal.

Surgical Option

Surgery is typically not needed for pediatric AR. If needed, the following surgery can be done [4]:

- Turbinectomies.
- Nasal polypectomy.

18.2.2 Chronic Non-allergic Rhinitis (NAR)

Chronic NAR is characterized by the incidence of one or more of the cardinal symptoms of rhinitis with no known etiology [5]:

- Sneezing.
- Stuffy nose.
- Congestion.
- Postnasal drip.

NAR occurs mostly after the age of 20 as compared to AR that occurs in adolescence [5–7].

The most frequent and prominent clinical manifestations are nasal blockage and postnasal drip [8]. In contrast, patients with AR report prominent eye symptoms, sneezing, and rhinorrhea [5]. Patients with NAR often cannot readily identify triggers, such as times of year when specific pollens are prevalent or exposure to animals. In contrast, most patients with AR can identify one or more triggers [5]. Symptoms most commonly occur throughout the year (e.g., perennial), although the condition may be exacerbated by weather conditions, particularly during the spring and fall [9]. Symptoms in allergic patients usually show seasonal patterns, although some have perennial symptoms [5].

18.2.2.1 Pathogenesis
Chronic (NAR) characterizes a group with no known pathogenesis [10–12], and can be categorized as non-inflammatory and inflammatory [5].

18.2.2.2 Diagnosis
History
The diagnosis of chronic NAR is characterized by an examination of both the patient history and physical assessment combined with the absence of evidence for clinical allergy to aeroallergens. It is therefore a diagnosis of exclusion. However, in practical terms, allergy testing is not essential to making a presumptive initial diagnosis of NAR and beginning therapy. In addition, AR and NAR can coexist, and in such cases, it may only become clear that the patient has both disorders in retrospect once an effective combination of medications is found [5].

Examination
The nasal turbinates can appear boggy and edematous in both AR and NAR. The mucosal tissue is more often erythematous in the non-allergic disease in comparison with the pale bluish hue or pallor observed with AR [5].

Testing
In evaluating patients for allergy, clinicians should be mindful that a positive skin test for allergy or a positive in vitro test by itself does not prove that the patient is

allergic to that substance. The result must be consistent with the clinical history, with symptoms occurring during the appropriate season, or upon exposure [5].

18.2.2.3 Treatment

Patients with chronic NAR are not as pharmacologically responsive as AR [13, 14]. Specifically, most find oral antihistamines unhelpful [15, 16]. However, there are two classes of medications for the treatment of chronic NAR [5, 7, 17, 18]:

- Topical intranasal glucocorticoids (INGCs).
- Topical antihistamine azelastine.
- Additionally, ipratropium can be used for chronic NAR [19, 20].

18.2.3 Sinusitis

Pediatric sinusitis (PS) is a very common complication that is treated routinely by physicians. Even though PS has been examined for centuries, full appreciation for PS has not been realized until recently. Routinely, antibiotic therapy has been used to treat acute PS, which has had good results. Unfortunately, chronic and recurrent sinusitis has been more of challenge with very little success. The current goal is for the physician to treat with an antibiotic in combination with treatment options that target a partially identifiable problem [21].

18.2.3.1 Pathogenesis

The ostiomeatal complex (OMC) is a very important anatomic structure found in the sinus. Interestingly, OMC obstruction has not been shown as a main basis for PS. However, alterations in the anterior ethmoids have been shown to exacerbate OMC drainage, which results in CMS and FS [21].

Normal mucous movement to the sinus natural ostia can be interrupted by infection. This is secondary to viral URTIs or nasal allergies. Additionally, there are other factors to contribute to chronic disease, such as AR, immune deficiency, disorders of ciliary function, structural abnormalities, and GER [21].

18.2.3.2 Classification

Any complication which effects mucociliary clearance, reduces ventilation, or alters local or systemic defense results in recurrent sinusitis, which is very difficult to treat [21].

Acute Sinusitis (AS)
- Usually subsides over a 30-day period.
- Can associate with URTI.
- Symptoms include daytime cough and rhinorrhea.
- Other signs/symptoms:
  - Congestion.
  - Can associate with low-grade fever.

- Middle ear infection.
- Moodiness/Headache.
- Signs/symptoms of severe infection:
  - Oozing nasal drainage.
  - High fever.
  - Puffy eyes.

Recurrent AS

Episodes that last less than 30 days and are intermittent at least 10 days [22].

Subacute Sinusitis

Characterized by signs/symptoms that last 30–90 days [22].

Chronic Sinusitis

- Characterized by continual signs and/or symptoms that extend longer than 90 days with no getting better.
- Six or more persistent incidents throughout the year.
- Acute exacerbations short of being entirely healthy.
- More prevalent nighttime cough [22].

18.2.3.3 Etiology

Microbiological agents and associated conditions constitute the main causes of sinusitis [22].

Acute pathogens [22]:

- *S. pneumoniae.*
- Non-typeable *H. influenzae.*
- *M. catarrhalis-S. pyogenes.*

Chronic pathogens [22]:

- No determined bacteria.
- Chronic sinusitis—polymicrobial infection.
- Commonly cultured bacteria.
  - *S. aureus.*
  - Non-typeable *H. influenzae.*
  - *M. catarrhalis.*
  - *Peptostreptococcus, Prevotella, Bacteroides,* and *Fusobacterium* species.
  - Pseudomonas.

18.2.3.4 Diagnosis

Examination

Execute a detailed head and neck inspection on patients with sinusitis using the following methods [23]:

Anterior Rhinoscopy

- Difficult to perform in young children.
- Great for determining purulence or sinus drainage.
- Vasoconstrictive agents (oxymetazoline and lidocaine) may be additive.
- Observation of polyps prompts cystic fibrosis evaluation [22].

Nasal Endoscopy

- Most accurate intranasal assessment other than the OR.
- Difficult to complete in young children [22].

Testing and Imaging
For sinusitis diagnosis, laboratory exams are not useful. Nevertheless, these exams can be useful to determine AR, CF, or immunodeficiency.

CT scans:

- CT scans are the gold standard for assessment of the paranasal sinuses. CT gives a robust image of the OMC [22].
- Demonstrate excellent precision in diagnosis of PS.
- Mandatory requirement before endoscopic sinus surgery.

  Plain radiography/sinus series [22]:

- Poor association with CT.
- Moderately accurate for screening of maxillary sinus disease.

  MRI [22]: Helpful when intracranial problems are suspected.
  Multiple techniques for the patient workup include [22]:

- Nasal endoscopy.
- Maxillary sinus puncture.
- Swab of the middle meatal.

18.2.3.5 Treatment
Antibiotics
Signs for antibiotic treatment for AS are [22]:

- Recurrent AS.
- Severe AS.
- Toxic child.

  Treatment with antibiotics should not be administered longer than 10–14 days [22].

Steroids

- Nasal steroids are necessary for concurrent AR [22].
- Decongestants and antihistamines
- The effectiveness of nasal decongestants is variable. Topical solutions may increase the comfort level of the patient. Patients with atopy respond better to antihistamines [22].

Endoscopic Surgery

Should only be considered as a last resort [22].

18.3 Nasal Foreign Body (NFBs)

NFBs are routinely observed in the ER. NFBs are mostly encountered in children; however, adults can be affected as well [23]. Children are known to explore their bodies and are prone to lodge things into their nose or other orifices. One can see a scenario where a child may lodge a foreign body to block nasal irritation or drainage [23]. These NFBs may require surgery or end up in death if the object makes its way into the airway [24].

Interestingly, unilateral NFBs are observed in the right side more often than the left side, which may be indicative of handedness [25]. To determine whether NFB is the specific cause, physical inspection is routinely used, and relies heavily on patient cooperation [26]. Objects can be observed in any part of the nose cavity; however, most are found predictably below the inferior turbinate or anterior to the middle turbinate [27].

Complications arise upon repeated efforts to remove the NFB in which the NFB may become more lodged. Thus, removal of the NFB is essential on the first attempt and often requires strategic planning. Moreover, specific instrumentation may be helpful in the planning and accuracy of first attempt removal. Reducing edema of the nasal mucosa may also contribute to a successful NFB removal [23].

18.4 Diagnosis and Treatment of Rhinorrhea

18.4.1 Diagnosis

The patient history can be useful in determining the discharge type and its chronic or recurrent state. If recurrent, the association with patient geographic location, season, or other exposures should be investigated. The review of systems should analyze symptom causation [28].

A full examination is needed to rule out the possibility of other diseases that may occur in children with AR or other diseases causing nasal discharge [5].

For imaging, plain graphs, a CT scan, or a MRI can be used.

18.4.2 Treatment

Treatment of the rhinorrhea depends on the underlying diseases. For each of the etiology, the treatment modalities should be considered according to the current guidelines.

References

1. No authors listed. Nasal Discharge.Patient. https://patient.info/doctor/nasal-discharge (Accessed online at August 9, 2017).
2. No authors listed. Chronic rhinorrhea (Runny nose). Stanford Children's Health. http://www.stanfordchildrens.org/en/service/ear-nose-throat/conditions/chronic-rhinorrhea (Accessed online at August 9, 2017).
3. Wang MB. Etiologies of nasal symptoms: An overview. Corren J, Feldweg AM (Eds.). UpToDate. Last updated: May 10, 2016. https://www.uptodate.com/contents/etiologies-of-nasal-symptoms-an-overview?source=search_result&search=nasal%20discharge&selectedTitle=1~150. Accessed 9 Aug 2017.
4. Becker JM. Pediatric Allergic Rhinitis. In: Jyonouchi H (Ed.). Medscape. Updated: May 05, 2017. http://emedicine.medscape.com/article/889259-overview. Accessed 9 Aug 2017.
5. Lieberman PL. Chronic nonallergic rhinitis. Corren J, Feldweg AM (Eds.). UpToDate. Last updated: Aug 10, 2015. Literature review current through: Jul 2017.| This topic last updated: Aug 10, 2015. https://www.uptodate.com/contents/chronic-nonallergicrhinitis?source=see_link. Accessed 9 Aug 2017.
6. Togias A. Age relationships and clinical features of nonallergic rhinitis. J Allergy Clin Immunol. 1990;85:182.
7. Settipane RA. Rhinitis: a dose of epidemiological reality. Allergy Asthma Proc. 2003;24:147.
8. Lindberg S, Malm L. Comparison of allergic rhinitis and vasomotor rhinitis patients on the basis of a computer questionnaire. Allergy. 1993;48:602.
9. Sibbald B, Rink E. Epidemiology of seasonal and perennial rhinitis: clinical presentation and medical history. Thorax. 1991;46:895.
10. Bousquet J, Fokkens W, Burney P, et al. Important research questions in allergy and related diseases: nonallergic rhinitis: a GA2LEN paper. Allergy. 2008;63:842.
11. Wallace DV, Dykewicz MS, Bernstein DI, et al. The diagnosis and management of rhinitis: an updated practice parameter. J Allergy Clin Immunol. 2008;122:S1.
12. van Rijswijk JB, Blom HM, Fokkens WJ. Idiopathic rhinitis, the ongoing quest. Allergy. 2005;60:1471.
13. Blom HM, Godthelp T, Fokkens WJ, et al. The effect of nasal steroid aqueous spray on nasal complaint scores and cellular infiltrates in the nasal mucosa of patients with nonallergic, non-infectious perennial rhinitis. J Allergy Clin Immunol. 1997;100:739.
14. Lacrois JS, Pochon N, Lundberg JM. Increased concentration of sensory neuropeptide in the nasal mucosa from patients with nonallergic chronic rhinitis. In: Passall D, editor. The new frontier of otorhinolaryngology in Europe. Sorrento, Italy: Monduzzi Editore; 1992. p. 59.
15. Mullarkey MF. Eosinophilic nonallergic rhinitis. J Allergy Clin Immunol. 1988;82:941.
16. Rinne J, Simola M, Malmberg H, Haahtela T. Early treatment of perennial rhinitis with budesonide or cetirizine and its effect on long-term outcome. J Allergy Clin Immunol. 2002;109:426.
17. Kondo H, Nachtigal D, Frenkiel S, et al. Effect of steroids on nasal inflammatory cells and cytokine profile. Laryngoscope. 1999;109:91.
18. Tamaoki J, Yamawaki I, Tagaya E, et al. Effect of azelastine on platelet-activating factor-induced microvascular leakage in rat airways. Am J Phys. 1999;276:L351.

19. Grossman J, Banov C, Boggs P, et al. Use of ipratropium bromide nasal spray in chronic treatment of nonallergic perennial rhinitis, alone and in combination with other perennial rhinitis medications. J Allergy Clin Immunol. 1995;95:1123.
20. Bronsky EA, Druce H, Findlay SR, et al. A clinical trial of ipratropium bromide nasal spray in patients with perennial nonallergic rhinitis. J Allergy Clin Immunol. 1995;95:1117.
21. Ramadan HS. Medical treatment of pediatric sinusitis. In: Meyers AD (Ed.). Medscape. Updated: Jan 25, 2017. http://emedicine.medscape.com/article/873149-overview. Accessed 9 Aug 2017.
22. Shin KS, Cho SH, Kim KR, et al. The role of adenoids in pediatric rhinosinusitis. Int J Pediatr Otorhinolaryngol. 2008;72(11):1643–50.
23. Baluyot ST. Foreign bodies in the nasal cavity. In: Paparella MM, Shumrick DA, editors. Otolaryngology. Philadelphia: W.B. Saunders; 1980. p. 2009–16.
24. Patil PM, Anand R. Nasal foreign bodies: a review of management strategies and a clinical scenario presentation. Craniomaxillofac Trauma Reconstr. 2011;4(1):53–8. https://doi.org/10.1055/s-0031-1272902.
25. Fischer JI. Nasal foreign bodies. In: Dronen SC (Ed.). Medscape. Updated: Jul 24, 2017. http://emedicine.medscape.com/article/763767-overview. Accessed 9 Aug 2017.
26. DeWeese DD, Saunders AH. Acute and chronic diseases of the nose. In: DD DW, Saunders AH, editors. Textbook of otolaryngology. St. Louis: Mosby; 1982.
27. Fried MP. Nasal congestion and rhinorrhea. Merck Manual Professional Version. http://www.merckmanuals.com/professional/ear,-nose,-and-throat-disorders/approach-to-the-patient-with-nasal-and-pharyngealsymptoms/nasal-congestion-and-rhinorrhea (Accessed online at August 9, 2017)
28. Kalan A, Tariq M. Foreign bodies in the nasal cavities: a comprehensive review of the aetiology, diagnostic pointers, and therapeutic measures. Postgrad Med J. 2000;76:484–7.

Dysphonia

19

Yücel Kurt, Cemal Cingi, and Bert Schmelzer

19.1 Introduction

Dysphonia or hoarseness is the terminology employed in describing alterations in how the voice sounds. A changed voice may be harsh-sounding, breathy, laboured, exhausted, abrasive, shaky or lacking strength. The frequency of the voice may alter, the range be more limited, voice cracks occur, its strength may lessen and its resonant quality may be abnormal. Vocal disorder does not refer to a diagnosis per se, but instead is a manifestation of some underlying condition. There are limitations on clinical understanding of dysphonia in children imposed by the practical difficulties in performing a fibreoptic laryngoscopic examination on a child, who may not understand why the procedure is required and thus fail to comply. Despite these difficulties, flexible naso-laryngoscopy is able to furnish dynamic visualisation of the larynx and how it works in children [1].

In patients between the ages of 4 and 12 years, the frequency of voice-related complaints is 6–23%. There are various aetiologies, including inflammation, infection, trauma, congenitally acquired lesions and neurological, iatrogenic or

Y. Kurt (✉)
Section of Otorhinolaryngology, Finike State Hospital, Finike, Antalya, Turkey

C. Cingi
Department of Otorhinolaryngology, Faculty of Medicine, Eskişehir Osmangazi University, Eskişehir, Turkey

B. Schmelzer
Section of Otorhinolaryngology, Head and Neck Surgery, Ziekenhuis Netwerk Antwerpen (ZNA), Antwerpen, Belgium

functional causes [2–4]. Injury to the voice may be caused by psychological or social issues, e.g. hyperactive or impulsive behaviour, in addition to prolonged crying. Such factors are often present in paediatric patients [5, 6]. Whilst children are playing, they often raise their voice and shout, which may lead to stress on the voice and tightening of muscles in the neck. Behaving in this way is typical of patients suffering from hyperfunctional or musculoskeletal dysphonia and may lead to the development of nodules on the vocal cords [7].

Laryngoscopic examination is a key element in diagnosing a number of conditions affecting the larynx and in ensuring appropriate therapy is offered. Vocal nodule is the most common diagnosis in paediatric patients with dysphonia. The lesion arises due to the vocal cords suddenly colliding with each other repeatedly whilst the child uses his or her voice [7, 8], which produces traumatic injury extending to the submucosal capillary vessels. This trauma leads to oedema and the beginning stages of a nodular lesion. The histopathological appearances of a vocal nodule are proliferative epithelium, a thickened basal lamina and profuse fibronectin deposition within the lamina propria [9–11].

19.2 Definition

The central feature of dysphonia is hoarseness. At any one time, approximately 1% of the general population suffers from dysphonia [12], and an individual has a 30% risk of developing dysphonia at some point during their life [13]. Any condition which impairs vocal production may be referred to as dysphonia, and thus any situation where the voice sounds hoarser than usual, the voice cannot perform as expected or there is strain when speaking. The key element in the pathogenic mechanism is abnormal muscular tone, resulting in the vocal folds oscillating abnormally, as occurs in hypertonic dysphonia. The glottis may be unable to close completely when the patient uses his or her voice. Additionally, the vocal folds may become bulkier, as occurs with tumours [14].

There are multiple aetiologies which may underlie a diagnosis of dysphonia, namely [14]:

- Laryngitis, both acute and chronic.
- Functional dysphonia.
- Tumour formation, benign or cancerous.
- Posttraumatic, e.g. after intubation.
- Neurological causes, e.g. paralysis of the vocal folds.
- Normal age-related change.
- Psychological conditions.

As well as voice nodules, there are a number of other potential diagnoses in paediatric patients with dysphonia, notably vocal cysts, sulcus vocalis, mucosal bridge, a paralysed cord and papilloma formation. Ten ways visible on videolaryngostroboscopy in which the mucosa within the larynx may be anatomically anomalous were described. Amongst the anomalies they describe are vocal cysts, bridging mucosal elements, glottic microweb and sulcus vocalis. The voice may become symptomatic in early childhood or later. Misusing the voice may cause the condition to manifest symptomatically [11].

19.3 Vocal Cord Nodules

Nodules of the vocal cord are recognised to occur in both childhood and adulthood as so-called screamer's or singer's nodules. The pathological alterations to the vocal folds arise when hyperkinetic dysphonia remains untreated. The initial stage features hyperplastic growth of the vocal cord along its medial margin. The cord undergoes maximum stress at the point where the anterior third abuts the middle third, which is where hyperplasia develops. The cord swells from resulting oedema, but the condition may still regress. However, if oedema persists, a fibrotic reaction occurs and tough nodules are formed [15, 16], which means that the vocal folds are no longer able to fully close in the nodular region. The preferred method of treating vocal nodules is voice therapy [17–19].

19.4 Acute Laryngitis

Laryngitis (i.e. laryngeal inflammation) is amongst the most highly prevalent of disorders to affect the larynx. Both acute laryngitis and chronic laryngitis occur [20, 21]. It begins abruptly and typically does not require intervention. However, where laryngitis persists longer than 3 weeks, a diagnosis of chronic laryngitis may be made. The risk factors for acute laryngitis are misusing the voice, being exposed to harmful substances or an infection causing an infective episode of the upper airway. The usual pathogens responsible for acute laryngitis are viruses, although bacteria are also occasionally responsible [20].

It is rare for misuse of the voice to provoke acute laryngitis, but patients with acute laryngitis do frequently misuse their voices. Either the infective agent itself or the inflammatory reaction produces dysphonia. The usual problem arises when an individual attempts to overcome hoarseness during an episode of acute laryngitis and by doing so inadvertently damages their voice [20].

Acute laryngitis consists of an inflammatory process involving the larynx and the mucosal covering of the vocal folds, with a duration not exceeding 3 weeks. Acute laryngitis secondary to infection resolves through leucocytic action, which eradicates the pathogen. The oedema associated with inflammation affects the vocal cord oscillation. The pressure needed to set the cords in motion may rise to a point where the patient has difficulty phonating, and thus sounds hoarse. If the requisite pressure to cause vocal fold oscillation exceeds that which the patient is capable of producing, the patient becomes frankly aphonic [20].

The typical appearance of the vocal cords in acute laryngitis is erythematous and oedematous. Patients suffering from laryngitis speak at a lower pitch than usual because of the uneven, swollen vocal cords. An alternative theory is that it is increased rigidity rather than increased thickness that accounts for the change in pitch. In most cases, supportive therapy suffices to allow the inflammatory reaction to subside and the vocal cords to recover their usual oscillatory characteristics [20].

19.4.1 Causes

There are a number of infectious agents which can provoke acute laryngitis. The majority are viruses responsible for infective episodes affecting the upper airway, such as [22]:

- Rhinovirus.
- Parainfluenza virus.
- Respiratory syncytial virus.
- Adenovirus.
- Influenza virus.
- Measles virus.
- Mumps virus.
- Bordetella pertussis.
- Varicella-zoster virus.

There are also a number of other potential causes, e.g. [20]:

- Gastro-oesophageal reflux disorder (GORD).
- Toxins in the environment (such as polluted air).
- Injury to the voice.
- Inhaled anti-asthmatic agents.

19.4.1.1 Signs and Symptoms of Acute Laryngitis

Patients with acute laryngitis have symptoms of both an upper airway infective episode (coughing, pyrexia, rhinitis) and dysphonia (hoarseness). They may also have the following symptoms [22]:

- Pain in speaking.
- Difficulty swallowing.
- Painful swallowing.
- Shortness of breath.
- Nasal discharge.
- Postnasal drip.
- Pharyngitis.
- Blocked nose and sinuses.
- Excessive tiredness.
- A general feeling of being unwell.

19.5   Vocal Cord Polyps/Vocal Cord Cysts

Polyps may develop on a vocal cord adjacent to the free edge. They are unilateral and impair the use of the voice [23]. The pathogenic mechanisms responsible for vocal cord polyposis are chronic laryngitis or phonation trauma, a condition affecting the capillary vessels supplying the mucosa, which leads to localised oedema and remodelling, in the context of an inflammatory response. The condition is triggered by patients abusing their voice [24]. If the mucosal excretory glands become blocked, this can cause formation of a retention cyst. Retention cysts lead to dysphonia and the patient speaks more quietly and is readily tired by speaking. Polyps are ideally treated by surgically excising them at their pedestal [14].

19.6   Recurring Papillomatosis

There are two types of recurrent papillomatosis—recurrent juvenile papillomatosis (RJP) and recurrent adult papillomatosis (RAP). RJP typically occurs in patients aged between 2 and 4 years old. It is one of the key paediatric conditions producing dysphonia or shortness of breath [25–27]. Human papillomavirus (HPV) has more than 100 variants, the key ones being types 6, 11, 16 and 18 [25, 28]. Paediatric cases of HPV11 are associated with high-grade lesions which can potentially block the airway [27].

19.7   Gastro-oesophageal Reflux Disease (GORD)

Gastro-oesophageal reflux disease (GORD) in children occurs through the mechanism of repeated, brief periods when the inferior sphincter of the oesophagus opens and allows material within the stomach to be refluxed into the oesophagus. It occurs because the sphincter has not yet fully developed [29].

19.7.1 Signs and Symptoms

GORD usually produces symptoms linked either to vomiting, such as failure to gain sufficient weight, or to the corrosive effect of stomach acid on the epithelial lining of the oesophagus. It is challenging to evaluate in a child the characteristic symptoms that adults with GORD report [29].

Children suffering from GORD often cry and do not sleep properly. They show reduced interest in eating. Some further features of the presentation in an infant or younger child are as follows [29]:

- Crying (in a usual or unusual way) and behaving irritably.
- Apnoeic episodes with or without cardiac slowing.

- Anorexia. Loss of weight, retarded growth or failure to thrive.
- An episode where the child's life appears at risk.
- Emesis.
- Wheeze or stridor.
- Abdominodynia or sternalgia.
- Recurrent pneumonitis.
- Pharyngitis, dysphonia with or without laryngitis.
- Persistent cough.
- Water brash.
- Sandifer syndrome (consisting of posturing plus opisthotonus or torticollis).

Older paediatric patients may exhibit any of the features listed here, but in addition may complain of dyspepsia and give an account of emesis, regurgitation, carious dentition and bad breath [29].

19.7.2 Diagnosis

In the majority of cases, GORD in a child is a clinical diagnosis. A trial of conservative treatment may be commenced to assess the response. Where the case presents in an unclear way or where there is little benefit from starting treatment, ongoing assessment, including imaging, will be indicated [29].

In children, no particular physical sign of GORD may be considered archetypal; however the following might be observed [29]:

- Young children before the age of speaking may cry and exhibit irritability, fail to grow, suffer from hiccoughing, sleep poorly or exhibit features of Sandifer syndrome (such as arching).
- A toddler or child over toddling age may have severe tooth decay resulting from refluxed gastric juices attacking the dental enamel.

19.7.3 Procedures

There are techniques available which permit the evaluation and visualisation of the oesophagogastric region, namely [29]:

- Oesophageal manometry.
- Oesophagogastroduodenoscopy.

The latter may also be coupled with biopsy to allow a histopathological examination of the stomach or oesophagus.

19.7.4 Imaging Studies

There are also radiological methods available for investigation of a child with GORD, such as [29]:

- Upper gastrointestinal imaging series.
- Gastric scintigraphy.
- Oesophagographic study.

19.7.5 (Electro)Physiological Studies

There are also physiological investigations which can confirm the presence of GORD, i.e. [29]:

- Acidity (pH) measurement within the oesophagus. This technique represents the Gold Standard in diagnosis.
- Measurement of impedance to current flow in the lumen of the oesophagus. This technique can distinguish between reflux of acid or non-acid type. It detects flow passing in a reverse direction from normal. Unfortunately, normal ranges are not yet available for use with children.

19.8 Management

The therapeutic aims in treating GORD are to reduce gastric acidity and, where possible, to shorten the time the bolus remains within the stomach [29].

19.8.1 Non-pharmacological Treatment

The following are techniques not involving drugs that may be of value in paediatric patients [30]:

- Meals should be low volume, occur often and cereal should be used to render a more viscous feed material.
- The child should not lie down following the feed.
- The head end of the bed should be raised.
- In an infant above the age of 6 months, they should be placed on their front.

Older paediatric patients with GORD may, in addition, find the following measures beneficial [29]:

- Dietary avoidance of tomatoes, citrus fruits, fruit juice, peppermint, chocolate or caffeinated drinks.
- Meals should be smaller and occur more often than usual.
- A diet which contains less fat allows for swifter movement of a bolus through the stomach.
- Eating regularly and healthily.
- Losing weight.
- Where a child already uses alcohol or smokes, this should be discouraged.

In cases which are treatment resistant to pharmacotherapy, one alternative to a surgical intervention is continuous intragastric feeding via a nasogastric tube [31].

19.8.2 Drug Treatment

Pharmacotherapy in children with GORD consists of the following [29]:
Antacid agents (such as aluminium hydroxide or magnesium hydroxide)

- Histamine blockers with action on the H2 receptor, such as nizatidine, cimetidine, ranitidine or famotidine.
- Proton pump inhibition using lansoprazole, omeprazole, esomeprazole [32], dexlansoprazole, rabeprazole sodium or pantoprazole.

None of the prokinetic agents which are licensed at present, including metoclopramide, have proven efficacy in reducing how often or how many reflux events occur.

19.8.3 Surgery

It is rare for a case of GORD to progress to a stage necessitating surgery, such as gastrostomy or fundoplication, although this may occur should optimal pharmacological therapy fail despite stepping up sequentially. Another situation where surgery is indicated is where GORD is potentially life-threatening, either in the short or long term. Operative interventions aim to increase the tension around the inferior oesophageal sphincter and, where feasible, decrease the tendency for the stomach to herniate through the diaphragm, a phenomenon which sometimes occurs in cases of GORD [29].

19.9　Vocal Cord Paralysis

The vocal cords may be partially or totally paralysed following trauma to the recurrent laryngeal nerve. If the glottis cannot completely close, or the vocal cords oscillate abnormally, the patient becomes dysphonic. In most cases (between 24% and 79%), vocal cord paralysis is due to iatrogenic injury, as may occur in operations in the vicinity of the Xth cranial nerve or the recurrent laryngeal nerve [33–36]. A particular risk arises from thyroid surgery, which is associated with irreversible vocal cord paresis in between 0.5% and 2.3% of cases [37, 38]. There have also been associations reported between vocal cord paralysis and other surgical interventions, notably cervical spine or thoracic surgery [36].

References

1. Sood S, Street I, Donne A. Hoarseness in children. Br J Hosp Med. 2017;78(12):678–83.
2. Carding PN, Roulstone S, Northstone K. The prevalence of childhood dysphonia: a cross-sectional study. J Voice. 2006;20:623–30.
3. Fuchs M, Meuret S, Stuhrmann NC, Schade G. Dysphonia in children and adolescents. HNO. 2009;57:603–14.
4. Tavares ELM, Brasolotto A, Santana MF, Padovan CA, Martins RHG. Epidemiological study of dysphonia in 4–12 year-old children. Braz J Otorhinolaryngol. 2011;77:736–46.
5. Connelly A, Clemente WA, Kubba H. Management of dysphonia in children. J Laryngol Otol. 2009;123:642–7.
6. Angelillo N, Di Costanzo B, Angelillo M, Costa G, Barillari MR, Barillari U. Epidemiological study on vocal disorders in pediatric age. J Prev Med Hyg. 2008;49:1–5.
7. Behlau MS, Goncalves MIR. Consideration on the infantile dysphonia. In: Ferreira LP, editor. Trabalhando a voz. Sao Paulo, Brazil: Summus Editorial; 1987. p. 99–107.
8. Mackiewicz-Nartowicz H, Sinkiewicz A, Bielecka A. Laryngovideostroboscopy in children: diagnostic possibilities and constraints. Int J Pediatr Otorhinolaryngol. 2011;75:1015–7.
9. Karkos PD, McCormick M. The etiology of vocal fold nodules in adults. Curr Opin Otolaryngol Head Neck Surg. 2009;17:420–3.
10. Martins RH, Defaveri J, Custodio Domingues MA, de Albuquerque E Silva R, Fabro A. Vocal fold nodules: morphological and immunohistochemical investigations. J Voice. 2010;24:531–9.
11. Martins RH, Hidalgo Ribeiro CB, Fernandes de Mello BM, Branco A, Tavares EL. Dysphonia in children. J Voice. 2012;26(5):674. https://doi.org/10.1016/j.jvoice.2012.03.004.
12. Cohen SM, Kim J, Roy N, Asche C, Courey M. Prevalence and causes of dysphonia in a large treatment seeking population. Laryngoscope. 2012;122:343–8.
13. Roy N, Merrill RM, Gray SD, Smith EM. Voice disorders in the general population: prevalence, risk factors, and occupational impact. Laryngoscope. 2005;115:1988–95.
14. Reiter, R., Hoffmann, T.K., Pickhard, A., Brosch, S., 2015. Hoarseness. Deutsches Ärzteblatt Online. https://doi.org/10.3238/arztebl.2015.0329.
15. Johns MM. Update on the etiology, diagnosis, and treatment of vocal fold nodules, polyps, and cysts. Curr Opin Otolaryngol Head Neck Surg. 2003;11:456–61.
16. Kunduk M, McWhorter AJ. True vocal fold nodules: the role of differential diagnosis. Curr Opin Otolaryngol Head Neck Surg. 2009;17:449–52.
17. Schwartz SR, Cohen SM, Dailey SH, et al. Clinical practice guideline: hoarseness (dysphonia). Otolaryngol Head Neck Surg. 2009;141:1–31.

18. Syed I, Daniels E, Bleach NR. Hoarse voice in adults: an evidence-based approach to the 12 minute consultation. Clin Otolaryngol. 2009;34:54–8.
19. Sulica L, Behrman A. Management of benign vocal fold lesions: a survey of current opinion and practice. Ann Otol Rhinol Laryngol. 2003;112:827–33.
20. Shah RK. Acute laryngitis. In: Meyers AD (Ed). Medscape. Updated: Sep 11, 2020. https://emedicine.medscape.com/article/864671-overview. Accessed 15 Oct 2020.
21. Gupta G, Mahajan K. Acute laryngitis. Treasure Island, FL: StatPearls; 2020.
22. Postma GN, Koufman JA. Laryngitis. In: Bailey BJ, editor. Head and neck surgery-otolaryngology. 2nd ed. Philadelphia, PA: Lippincott-Raven; 1998. p. 731–9.
23. Martins RH, Defaveri J, Domingues MA, de Albuquerque Silva R. Vocal polyps: clinical, morphological, and immunohistochemical aspects. J Voice. 2011;25:98–106.
24. Bohlender J. Diagnostic and therapeutic pitfalls in benign vocal fold diseases. Laryngorhinootologie. 2013;92:239–57.
25. Venkatesan NN, Pine HS, Underbrink MP. Recurrent respiratory papillomatosis. Otolaryngol Clin N Am. 2012;45:671–94.
26. Derkay CS, Wiatrak B. Recurrent respiratory papillomatosis: a review. Laryngoscope. 2008;118:1236–47.
27. Mauz PS, Zago M, Kurth R, et al. A case of recurrent respiratory papillomatosis with malignant transformation, HPV11 DNAemia, high L1 antibody titre and a fatal papillary endocardial lesion. Virol J. 2014;11:114–20.
28. Malagón T, Drolet M, Boily MC, et al. Cross protective efficacy of two human papillomavirus vaccines: a systematic review and meta-analysis. Lancet Infect Dis. 2012;12:781–9.
29. Schwarz SM. Paediatric gastroesophageal reflux. In: Cuffari C (Ed). Medscape. Updated: Mar 14, 2019. Accessed 15 Oct 2020.
30. Chao HC, Vandenplas Y. Effect of cereal-thickened formula and upright positioning on regurgitation, gastric emptying, and weight gain in infants with regurgitation. Nutrition. 2007;23:23–8.
31. Orenstein SR. Management of supraesophageal complications of gastroesophageal reflux disease in infants and children. Am J Med. 2000;108(4A):139S–43S.
32. Tolia V, Gilger MA, Barker PN, Illueca M. Healing of erosive esophagitis and improvement of symptoms of gastroesophageal reflux disease after esomeprazole treatment in children 12 to 36 months old. J Pediatr Gastroenterol Nutr. 2015;60(Suppl 1):S31–6.
33. Reiter R, Pickhard A, Smith E, et al. Vocal cord paralysis analysis of a cohort of 400 patients. Laryngorhinootologie. 2015;94:91–6.
34. Takano S, Nito T, Tamaruya N, Kimura M, Tayama N. Single institutional analysis of trends over 45 years in etiology of vocal fold paralysis. Auris Nasus Larynx. 2012;39:597–600.
35. Loughran S, Alves C, Mac Gregor FB. Current aetiology of unilateral vocal fold paralysis in a teaching hospital in the west of Scotland. J Laryngol Otol. 2002;116:907–10.
36. Sielska-Badurek E, Domeracka-Kołodziej A, Zawadzka R, Debowska-Jarzebska E. Vocal fold paralysis in the Medical University of Warsaw's ambulatory of Phoniatry in years 2000–2011. Oto laryngol Pol. 2012;66:313–7.
37. Rayes N, Seehofere D, Neuhaus P. The surgical treatment of bilateral benign nodular goiter: balancing invasiveness with complications. Dtsch Ärztebl Int. 2014;111:171–8.
38. Jeannon JP, Orabi AA, Bruch GA, Abdalsalam IIA, Simo R. Diagnosis of recurrent laryngeal nerve palsy after thyroidectomy: a systematic review. Int J Clin Pract. 2009;63:624–9.

Bülent Saat, Cemal Cingi, and Glenis Scadding

20.1   Introduction

Sore throat is the most common complaint seen by primary care physicians and pediatricians. The main causes of sore throat are viral or bacterial pharyngitis/tonsillitis, but also laryngitis, acute laryngo-tracheitis, sinusitis, allergic rhinitis, reflux, and lung infections, and sometimes tumors cause symptoms of a sore throat. Viral pharyngitis accounts for the vast majority of patients, only 20–30% of them are due to bacterial infection, most commonly group A beta-hemolytic streptococcus (AGBHS) [1].

Antimicrobial agents do not provide benefit in the treatment of acute viral pharyngitis, only in bacterial infections It is very important to diagnose accurately the cause of pharyngitis in order to prevent unnecessary antimicrobial therapy, which increases antibiotic resistance, healthcare costs, and the likelihood of side effects [2].

Because the symptoms of viral and bacterial sore throat are similar, differential diagnosis may not be possible on clinical examination alone [3]. A scoring system has been established by researchers to determine when a culture should be taken for the correct diagnosis. This system requires further evaluation [4].

B. Saat (✉)
Section of Otorhinolaryngology, Ankara Occupational and Environmental Diseases Hospital, Ankara, Turkey

C. Cingi
Department of Otorhinolaryngology, Faculty of Medicine, Eskişehir Osmangazi University, Eskişehir, Turkey

G. Scadding
University College London, Royal National Throat, Nose, and Ear Hospital (Honorary Consultant Physician in Allergy and Rhinology), London, UK

© The Author(s), under exclusive license to Springer Nature Switzerland AG 2022   231
C. Cingi et al. (eds.), *Pediatric ENT Infections*,
https://doi.org/10.1007/978-3-030-80691-0_20

20.2   Definition

In infants and children, sore throat caused by pharyngitis and tonsillitis increases markedly in winter and is more commonly due to viral infections rather than bacteria. AGBHS is responsible for 20–30% of pediatric bacterial pharyngitis [1]. In general, they are mild to moderate infections with no serious mortality but can lead to major complications and sequelae such as scarlet fever, toxic shock syndrome, acute glomerulonephritis, and acute rheumatic fever when not properly treated [5, 6].

Viral pharyngitis is treated symptomatically; on the other hand, bacterial pharyngitis, especially caused by AGBHS, requires antimicrobial treatment due to the risk of possible complications.

20.3   Epidemiology and Risk Factors

In children under 5 years of age, viruses cause 85–95% of throat infections; bacterial pharyngitis being very rare [7]. However, for children aged 5–15 years, viruses cause about 70% of throat infections, the rest are bacterial, commonly due to AGBHS.

The epidemiology of viral infections varies according to the age of the patient and the season. Parainfluenza, influenza, respiratory syncytial virus (RSV), and Rhinovirus are more common in autumn and winter months. Most viruses cause infection in younger children; however Influenza can be seen in all age groups and should come to mind in epidemic periods. Epstein-Barr virus (EBV) and herpes simplex virus (HSV) cause pharyngitis in young adults. Adenovirus infections are infectious agents related to swimming pool exposure and do not show seasonal characteristics [8].

AGBHS can be transmitted via the airway with close contact, and also through skin lesions. In addition to familial spread, contamination is common in public places such as nurseries. The frequency of incidence among genders is not different, but uncommon in children younger than 5 and older than 15 [7]. Incidence of AGBHS tonsillopharyngitis is higher in winter and in low socioeconomic areas [9]. Foods such as milk, eggs, and ice cream contaminated with groups C and G streptococci cause epidemics in the form of streptococcal food poisoning or pharyngitis [10]. Neisseria gonorrhea usually follows oro-genital contact; therefore a careful history must be taken [10].

20.4   Etiology

The most common viral etiological agents are Rhinovirus and Adenovirus, less common ones are EBV, HSV, Influenza virus, Parainfluenza virus, and Coronavirus, and uncommon etiological factors are Enterovirus (e.g., poliovirus, coxsackievirus, echovirus), RSV, CMV, Rotavirus, Reovirus, Rubella virus, Varicella-zoster virus, Measles, and HIV-1 [11].

GABHS is the most common cause of bacterial pharyngitis. Therefore sometimes "bacterial" or "streptococcal" pharyngitis is used for this disease [2]. A small percentage of sore throats will be caused by a variety of other bacterial organisms (e.g., Group C and G streptococcus), and also rarely Corynebacterium diphtheriae, Neisseria gonorrhoeae, Mycoplasma pneumoniae, Yersinia species, Francisella tularensis, Chlamydia trachomatis, Chlamydophila pneumoniae, Treponema pallidum, and Arcanobacterium haemolyticum [12].

20.5 Clinical Findings

Nasal symptoms (such as sneezing, discharge, congestion), pharyngeal irritation, dry cough, diarrhea, hoarseness, and eye symptoms are usually present in viral pharyngitis. Describe the throat findings in routine viral and bacterial pharyngitis and what might indicate Strep here please. Although pharyngitis may look like a streptococcal throat initially, if fever and fatigue last longer than 7 days, infectious mononucleosis should be kept in mind. In these patients, the spleen and liver are generally enlarged in addition to generalized tender lymphadenopathy. Blood count with the presence of $\geq 20\%$ atypical lymphocytes and other serological tests- which/specify them are helpful for diagnosis of infectious mononucleosis [1]. Patients given ampicillin develop a diffuse, pruritic maculopapular eruption indicating infectious mononucleosis [12]. "Pharyngoconjunctival fever" (consisting of red eye due to conjunctivitis and fever) can be seen in adenoviral pharyngitis [3, 8]. Oropharyngeal ulceration or vesicles suggest Herpes virus or Coxsackie virus [8].

However symptoms can be more serious in AGBHS pharyngitis. Fever (temperature $\geq$ 100.4 °F or 38 °C), bodily aches, headache, tonsillar exudates, abdominal pain, enlarged and hyperemic tonsils, and swollen and tender lymph nodes are usually seen [3, 11, 13]. In contrast to streptococcal pharyngitis, cough is present in 75% of patients with pharyngitis due to Mycoplasma pneumonia [10]. If foul-smelling gray-white pharyngeal membrane is present, Corynebacterium diphtheriae must be considered. This carries the risk of airway obstruction [10].

20.6 Diagnosis

Viral tonsillopharyngitis cannot be clearly distinguished on clinical findings; although some symptoms such as hepatosplenomegaly, red eye, and foul-smelling gray-white pharyngeal membrane may give some idea about causation, clinical findings may be insufficient to make definite distinction between viral and bacterial pharyngitis. Several clinical scoring systems have been developed that are capable of making this distinction possible; the most common one is "Centor Scoring" as defined by Centor [14, 15]. Tonsillar exudate, swollen tender anterior cervical nodes, the lack of cough and fever are used as Centor criteria, score of 3–4 suggests a 40–60% likelihood of AGBHS indicating further laboratory test and score < 3 suggests unlikely AGBHS (Table 20.1) [14, 16–18]. The Centor score was later modified by adding age, also called as McIsaac score, and adapted for children [10, 19].

Without laboratory tests, viral or AGBHS tonsillopharyngitis cannot be clearly distinguished from clinical findings. However, the implementation of these laboratory tests is not always possible in rural areas. If AGBHS tonsillopharyngitis is considered with clinical scoring, laboratory tests should be requested. However if patient has very severe general condition or suspected peritonsillar infiltrate, abscess or scarlatiniform rash antibiotic should be prescribed, if possible after a swab has been taken for culture [18].

The patient needs to be admitted to hospital quickly for further examination and treatment in the following circumstances [8, 13, 16] (Box 20.1).

Table 20.1 Patients with variables and probability of positive culture according to Centor [14]

Patients with variables[a]	Probability of positive culture
4 variables	56%
3 variables	32%
2 variables	15%
1 variable	6.5%
0 variables	2.5%

[a]Variables: tonsillar exudates, swollen tender anterior cervical nodes, lack of a cough, and history of fever [14]

Box 20.1 Circumstances in which the patient needs to be admitted to hospital quickly for further examination and treatment [8, 13, 16]

Circumstances	Oral intake is limited due to high fever
	Difficulty in swallowing
	Severe fatigue
	Characteristic tonsillar or pharyngeal membrane
	Systemic symptoms such as stridor
	Respiratory distress
	Muffled voice
	Trismus or difficulty in opening mouth
	Asymmetric pharyngeal swelling
	Suspicion of serious complications such as parapharyngeal, retropharyngeal, or peritonsillar abscess
	Immunosuppression

20.6.1 Laboratory Evaluation

20.6.1.1 Throat Swabs

Microbiological diagnosis is not required if the clinical findings of the patient are strongly suggestive of viral etiology [4]. But if bacterial pharyngitis is considered, center score is 3–4, rapid antigen detection testing (RADT) and / or culture can be used to confirm the diagnosis [1, 8, 20]. RADT is easy and gives quick results. The specificity of the test is high, 90% [3, 18, 21]. If the rapid test is positive, throat culture is not necessary. The diagnostic sensitivity of the rapid test is 70–80% [4, 22, 23]. If clinical AGBHS is considered but RADT is negative, throat culture should be done.

20.6.1.2 Throat Culture

Single swab throat culture in blood agar if done by correct technique is the gold standard for AGBHS diagnosis and diagnostic accuracy is 90–95% [1, 4, 16, 18, 21, 24]. Throat culture is recommended for children with suspicion of AGBHS or modified Centor score of 3–4 [1, 13, 15, 19]. Although microbiological diagnosis of throat culture is accepted as the gold standard in the diagnosis, 24–48 hours is required for the result, leading to delayed treatment, increased infection, and unnecessary antibiotic usage. Also the results vary according to culture technique, which is more difficult in children. Negative culture may result because the swab may not have been taken correctly or the patient may have used antibiotics prior to culture [1, 16, 21].

20.6.1.3 Other Laboratory Tests

Laboratory techniques such as complete blood count, C-reactive protein (CRP), ASO, and erythrocyte sedimentation rate (ESR) are not recommended for diagnosis of AGBHS tonsillopharyngitis. A complete blood count may be required if EBV infection is being considered. Since the high level of the ASO indicates the past infection, ASO also should not play role in diagnosis of acute infection; therefore it is unnecessary. ASO and Anti-DNase-B begins to increase after 3–8 weeks of acute infections [1, 4]. They are used to show previous AGBHS infection in those with suspicion of rheumatoid fever or glomerulonephritis [20, 25].

20.7 Treatment

20.7.1 Symptomatic Treatment

Paracetamol is first choice for acute sore throat pain in pediatric patients. Ibuprofen is an alternative but can cause renal complications in dehydrated children. Aspirin should not be used in children because of the danger of Reye's syndrome.

Oral corticosteroids are preferred in case of infectious mononucleosis since pain and swelling can cause severe dysphagia and life-threatening airway obstruction [16]. Otherwise they are not advised for sore throats [13, 20].

20.7.2 Antimicrobial Treatment

First-line antimicrobial treatment for AGBHS is oral phenoxymethylpenicillin (penicillin V) for 10 days, second line is ampicillin [1, 8, 16, 18, 20]. If the patient is penicillin allergic, consider a macrolide (azithromycin, clarithromycin, or clindamycin) or first-generation cephalosporin [16, 25].

References

1. Stanford T, Bisno A, et al. Clinical Practice Guideline for the Diagnosis and Management of Group A Streptococcal Pharyngitis:2012 Update by the Infectious Disease Society of America-ISDA Guidelines. Clinical Infectious Diseases.2012: September 9, 91–17.
2. Guidelines&Protocols. Advisory Committee. Diagnosis and Management of Sore Throat, 2003. http://iskra.bfm.hr/upload/sore-throat-british-colombia.pdf. Accessed 27 Aug 2020.
3. Aung K. Viral pharyngitis clinical presentation. In: Bronze MS. Medscape. Updated: Jul 24, 2017. http://emedicine.medscape.com/article/225362-clinical. Accessed 27 Aug 2020.
4. Pelucchi C, Ginoryan L, Galeone ES, Huovinen P, Little P, Verheij T. ESMID: guidelines for the management of acute sore throat. Clin Microbiol Infect. 2012;18(Suppl 1):1–28.
5. Australian Institute of Health and Welfare. Rheumatic Heart Disease: all but forgotten in Australia except among Aboriginal and Torres Strait Islander peoples. Canberra. Australian Institute of Health and Welfare Bulletin 2004 (August). Issue 16.
6. McCormick A, Fleming D, Charlton C. Morbidity statistics from general practice, fourth national survey 1991–92. HMSO, Office for National Statistics: London, UK; 1995.
7. Worrall G. Acute sore throat. Can Fam Physician. 2011 Jul;57(7):791–4.
8. Infants and Children Acute Management of Sore Throat. 3rd Ed. Clinical Practice Guideline. NSW Government. 2014. http://www1.health.nsw.gov.au/pds/ActivePDSDocuments/GL2014_021.pdf. Accessed 27 Aug 2020.
9. Bisno AL, Gerber MA, Gwaltney JM, Kaplan EL, Schwartz RH. Practice guidelines for the diagnosis and management of group a streptococcal pharyngitis. Clin Infect Dis. 2002;35:113–25.
10. Acerra JR: Pharyngitis clinical presentation. In: Talevera FMedscape updated: Apr 17, 2017. http://emedicine.medscape.com/article/64304-clinical.
11. Carillo-Marquez MA: Bacterial pharyngitis clinical presentation. In: Bronze MS Medscape updated 17, 2016. http://emedicine.medscape.com/article/225243-overview.
12. Balfour HH, Dunmire SK, Hogquist KA. Infectious mononucleosis. Clin Transl Immunology. 2015;4(2):e33. https://doi.org/10.1038/cti.2015.1.
13. Wald ER. Patient education: sore throat in children (Beyond the Basics). In: Edwards MS, Torchia MM. Uptodate. http://www.uptodate.com/contents/sore-throat-in-children-beyond-the-basics. Accessed 28 Aug 2020.
14. Centor RM, Witherspoon JM, Dalton HP, Brody CE, Link K. The diagnosis of strep throat in adults in the emergency room. Med Decis Mak. 1981,1(3).239–46.
15. Aalbers J, O'Brien KK, Chan WS, et al. Predicting streptococcal pharyngitis in adults in primary care: a systematic review of the diagnostic accuracy of symptoms and signs and validation of the Centor score. BMC Med. 2011;9:67.
16. Al-Katheeri HA, et al. The diagnosis and management of tonsillitis in adults and children. Clinical Guidelines for the State of Qatar.Date issiued: December 2016.
17. Ebell MH, Smith MA, Barry HC, Ives K, Carey M. The rational clinical examination. Does this patient have strep throat? JAMA. 2000;284(22):2912–8.
18. Andrasević AT, Baudoin T, Vukelić D, Matanović SM, Bejuk D, Puzevski D, Abram M, Tesović G, Grgurev Z, Tomac G, Pristas I. ISKRA guidelines on sore throat: diagnostic and therapeutic approach--Croatian national guidelines. Lijec Vjesn. 2009;131(7–8):181–91.

19. McIsaac WJ, Goel V, To T, Low DE. The validity of a sore throat score in family practice. CMAJ. 2000;163(7):811–5.
20. Shah UK. Tonsillitis and Peritonsillar abscess guidelines clinical presentation. In: Meyers A medscape updated: Jan 19, 2017. http://emedicine.medscape.com/article/871977-guidelines.
21. Somro A, Akram A, Khan MI, et al. Pharyngitis and sore throat: a review. Afr J Biotechnol. 2011;10(33):6190–7.
22. Cohen JF, Bertille N, Cohen R, Chalumeau M. Rapid antigen detection test for group a streptococcus in children with pharyngitis. Cochrane Database Syst Rev. 2016 Jul 4;7:CD010502. https://doi.org/10.1002/14651858.CD010502.pub2.
23. Simon HK. Pediatric pharyngitis clinical presentation. In: Steele RW Medscape Updated: 23 Aug 2017. http://emedicine.medscape.com/article/967384-clinical
24. Murphy TP, Harrison RV, Hammoud AJ, Yen G: Pharyngitis. Guidelines for Clinical Care Ambulatory. © Regents of the University of Michigan. http://www.med.umich.edu/1info/FHP/practiceguides/pharyngitis/pharyn.pdf. (Initial Release November, 1996 Most Recent Major Update May, 2013).
25. Choby BA. Diagnosis and treatment of streptococcal pharyngitis. Am Family Phys. 2009;79(5):383–90.

Sertaç Düzer, Nihat Susaman, and Andrew A. Winkler

21.1 Introduction

The subepithelial and submucosal lymphatic tissues extend from the Eustachian tube to the tongue root. These coalesce into individual masses in the oropharynx to form the tonsils. Waldeyer's Lymphatic Ring is a collection of other pharyngeal lymphatic structures, including the anterior lingual tonsil (tonsilla lingualis), the upper lateral tubarian tonsils (tonsilla tubaria), the upper posterior pharyngeal tonsil (tonsilla pharyngea), and the lateral palatine tonsils (tonsilla palatina). Waldeyer first described this organization of lymphatics in 1884 [1–3].

The palatine tonsils, which are the largest component of Waldeyer's Ring, begin to appear in the third intrauterine month. They originate from the endoderm of the second pharyngeal pouch between the second and third pharyngeal arches. Active mesenchymal development of the palatine tonsils occurs at the 14th week of fetal life with invasion of the tissued by monocular cells. The mesenchymal community differentiates into tonsillar lymphoid tissue. The invagination of the surface epithelium forms fissures in the buds' center. These subsequently form lymphocytes from the thymus infiltrate, and tonsillar crypts develop [3–5].

Tonsillar follicles comprised of lymph nodes form beneath the tonsil mucosa. The tonsils are situated within the tonsillar fossa, formed by palatoglossal and palatopharyngeal arches or pillars. The tonsils do not entirely fill the fossa. The space not occupied by tonsil tissue at the superior aspect of the fossa is larger and is called

S. Düzer (✉) · N. Susaman
Section of Otorhinolaryngology, Elazığ Fethi Sekin City Hospital, Elazığ, Turkey

A. A. Winkler
Department of Otolaryngology, University of Colorado School of Medicine, Aurora, CO, USA

the fossa supratonsillaris. Folds of mucosa within the tonsillar fossa are also described. A half-moon-shaped mucosal fold extending between the superior aspect of the two arches covering the tonsillar fossa is called plica semilunaris. The fold between the palatoglossal arch and the tonsil is called plica triangularis [6]. The plica triangularis itself also contains lymphoid tissue [1].

The palatine tonsils are active immunological organs and strengthen the upper airway mucosal immunity. They have a structure that allows antigens from inhaled air to be transported directly to lymphoid cells within the tonsil. The specialized epithelium of these tissues plays a vital role in antigen presentation and antibody formation. T cell lymphocytes' dominance in the peripheral blood gives way to B cell predominance in tonsil tissue. B lymphocytes constitute 50–65% of all lymphocytes in tonsillar tissue whereas T cells comprise 40% and mature plasma cells 3% [1, 7].

The growth of palatine tonsils is generally limited to the oropharynx. However, due to excessive and/or asymmetrical growth, they may extend to the nasopharynx and may cause velopharyngeal obstruction, while hypopharyngeal direction of growth may lead to obstructive symptoms even if there is no prominent finding in the mouth [8].

The medial side of the tonsil is free and lined with stratified squamous epithelium. As described above, crypts or tonsillar fossula are present on the tonsil surface and end blindly within the tonsil [1, 6]. Its lateral face tightly adheres to the pharyngo-bacillary fascia by dense elastic fibers [1]. The capsule itself sits on the medial superior pharyngeal constructor and palatopharyngeus muscles [6]. Trabeculae, through which blood vessels, nerves, and efferent lymphatics pass, extend from the capsule towards the tonsil [1]. Close proximity of the facial artery and glossopharyngeal nerve is an important consideration for tonsillectomy operations, as the lateral side of the muscle should not be violated. Temporary loss of taste and pain in the ear are commonplace following tonsillectomy due to injury to the glossopharyngeal nerve during surgery or postoperative edema [2, 6]. Another important structure in the neighborhood of the tonsillar fossa is the carotid artery. It passes approximately 2–2.5 cm on posterolateral side of the tonsils. It should be kept in mind that carotid injuries may occur if the dissection is performed extensively or by passing a needle too deeply during suturing [9].

Potential spaces surrounding the tonsillar fossa are important as they can be avenues for spread of infection. Most proximate to Waldeyer's ring are the peritonsillar and parapharyngeal spaces. The peritonsillar space is bound by the palatoglossal pillar anteriorly, the palatopharyngeal pillar posteriorly, the capsule of the palatine tonsil medially, and the superior pharyngeal constrictor muscle laterally. The loose areolar connective tissue of the peritonsillar space communicates with the parapharyngeal space. The parapharyngeal space is an inverted pyramid lateral to the peritonsillar space bound superiorly by the base of the skull, inferiorly by the greater cornu of the hyoid bone, anteriorly by the pterygomandibular raphe and medial pterygoid, posteriorly by the cervical vertebrae, and laterally by the parotid gland. Furthermore, the parapharyngeal space is adjacent to other deep neck spaces, including the retropharyngeal space and the prevertebral "danger" space providing pathways for infection and tumor spread from the tonsil to distant areas including the mediastinum [10].

21.2 Symptoms and Findings

The term tonsillar hypertrophy is often used to describe abnormally large tonsils. A standard size, weight, and volume of tonsils does not exist. A tonsil may be hypertrophic if the tonsillar tissue produces airway obstructive symptoms even if they are relatively small [11]. Tonsil hypertrophy, often together with other elements of Waldeyer's Ring, is relatively common in infants and children. The exact cause is unclear, although it is sometimes accepted as a genetic trait.

Tonsils grow from early childhood to puberty. They may undergo physiological hypertrophy due to dietary, genetic, and hormonal factors. After puberty, they undergo slow atrophy or involution. Growth is due to a general increase in parenchymal cells, and specific cellular activity is detected in germinal centers. When tonsillar hypertrophy follows inflammatory activity, the increase in size occurs primarily in the tonsil's connective tissue stroma. The tonsil size is of no clinical significance unless it grows large enough to cause mechanical airway obstruction or causes difficulty in swallowing [12].

Tonsillar hypertrophy causes varying degrees of airway obstruction. The duration of airway obstruction symptoms and signs may not be obvious to the patient or parents. Frequently obstructive symptoms occur only at night during sleep. Pediatric specialists, allergists, neonatologists, chest specialists, and otolaryngologists can evaluate these symptoms differently with their disciplinary approaches. Often parents perceive snoring and breathing problems in a child to be simple social problems. For these reasons, the incidence of patients with tonsillar hypertrophy with obstructive symptoms is unknown [11]. One indication of underlying obstructive breathing problems in children is synchronous eating difficulties. They usually prefer soft foods that require little chewing. Due to nutritional problems, their growth and development percentiles may fall below 25 [13, 14].

21.3 Classification

Various classifications are used for tonsillar hypertrophy and the degree of airway obstruction. Brodsky [15] developed a system that defines the degree of tonsillar hypertrophy on exam to facilitate communication between physicians.

In this system

- Grade 0: The tonsils are located in the fossa and have no extension to the airway (Fig. 21.1).
- Grade 1: The tonsils protrude slightly beyond the fossa, and less than 25% of the airway is obstructed (Fig. 21.2).

Fig. 21.1 The tonsils are located in the fossa and have no extension to the airway. Grade 0

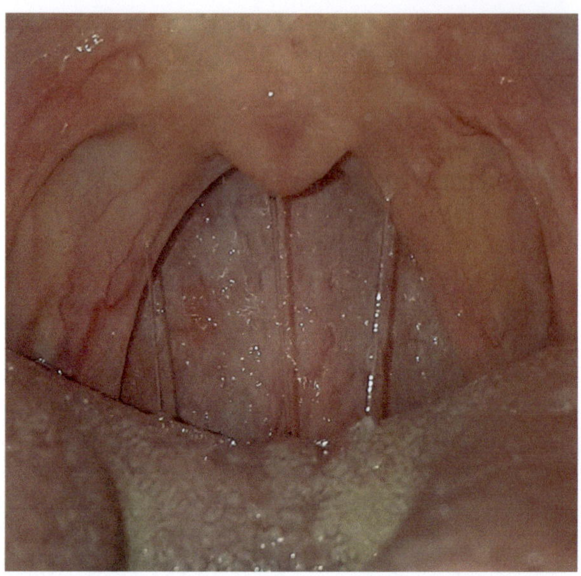

Fig. 21.2 The tonsils protrude slightly beyond the fossa, and less than 25% of the airway is obstructed, Grade 1

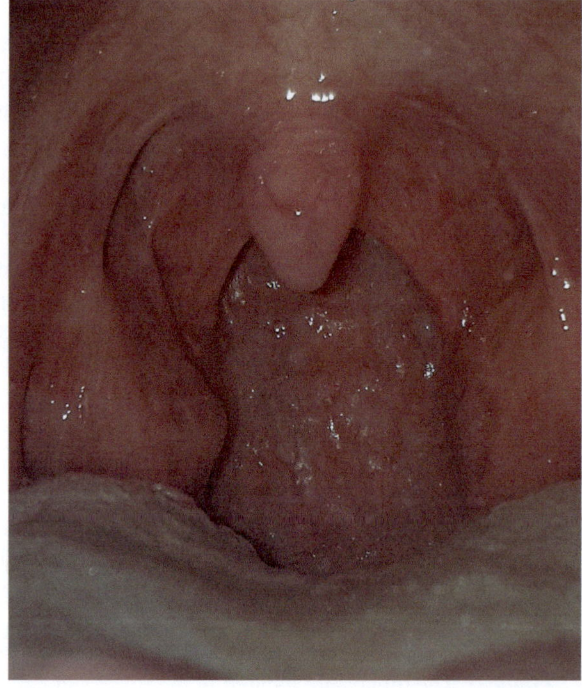

- Grade 2: The tonsils can be seen more clearly, and 25–50% of the airway is blocked (Fig. 21.3).
- Grade 3: Tonsils are prominently large, and 50–75% of the airway is obstructed (Fig. 21.4).
- Grade 4: The tonsils are full, and more than 75% of the airway is obstructed; It was evaluated (Fig. 21.5a, b).

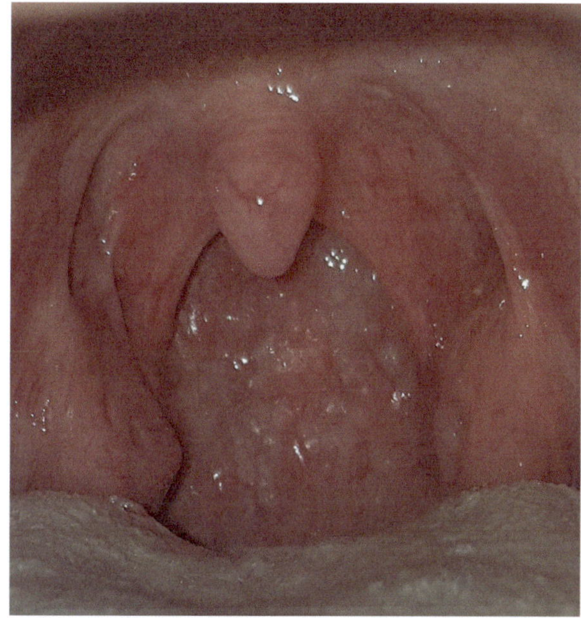

Fig. 21.3 The tonsils can be seen more clearly, and 25–50% of the airway is blocked, Grade 2

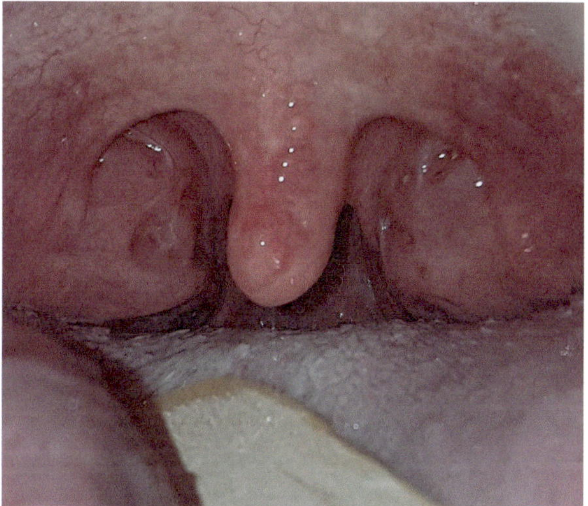

Fig. 21.4 Tonsils are prominently large, and 50–75% of the airway is obstructed, Grade 3

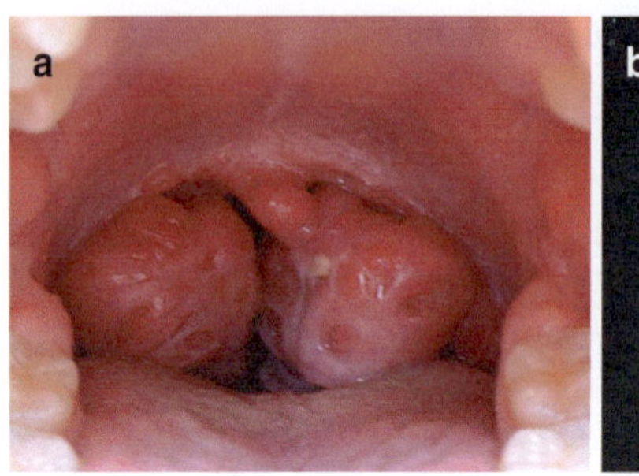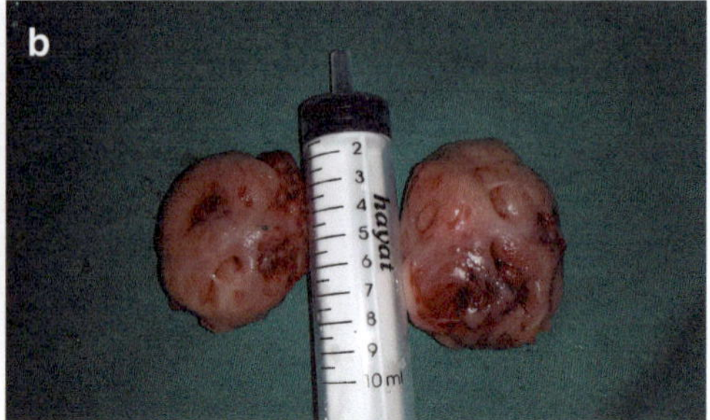

Fig. 21.5 (**a**) and (**b**): The tonsils are full, and more than 75% of the airway is obstructed; It was evaluated, Grade 4

21.4 Diagnosis and Clinical Importance

Tonsillar hypertrophy with airway obstruction is diagnosed by history and physical examination findings obtained from the patient's parent or primary caregiver. The family often reports observed irregular breathing, loud snoring, and restless sleep patterns. Similarly, it is not unusual to observe unusual sleeping positions and chest retractions. On physical examination, pharyngeal obstruction is frequently detected. Tonsillar hypertrophy that cannot be detected directly during the regular examination should be considered as well. Airway pathologies without pharyngeal tonsil or palatine tonsil hypertrophy and sleep-disordered breathing are rare [11].

Pathological tonsils that cannot be detected by direct examination can be evaluated more readily with fiberoptic endoscopy, especially in the pediatric group. Nasopharyngeal pathologies can be quickly evaluated in endoscopic examination of a child who is cooperative. Additional pathological conditions in this region can also be evaluated for pharyngeal obstruction during sleep under controlled deep sedation. In healthy children with tonsillar hypertrophy without craniofacial anomaly, the benefit of only fiberoptic endoscopy is minimal [16].

In children with signs and symptoms of tonsillar hypertrophy, lateral neck radiography has been used for initial evaluation. The size of the pharyngeal tonsil lymphoid tissue may not be sufficient to predict obstruction [17]. However, lateral X-rays are a simple way to help assess the condition of the nasopharynx and oral airway. Cephalometric analyses may help detect obstruction compatible with overnight evaluation, but this is more useful in patients with craniofacial anomalies undergoing craniofacial surgery [18].

Chronic tonsillar hypertrophy is the most common cause of upper airway obstruction in children. In severe cases, cor pulmonale and pulmonary vascular hypertension may be encountered. The etiology of cor pulmonale and pulmonary ventilation-perfusion abnormalities are associated with chronic upper airway obstruction leading to chronic alveolar hypoventilation. This results in chronic hypercapnia and hypoxia, leading to respiratory acidosis, pulmonary artery vasoconstriction, and right ventricular enlargement. In turn, this may eventually result in cardiac failure [2].

Obstructive sleep apnea is a common finding in children with a history of tonsillar hypertrophy, and tonsillar hypertrophy is the most common cause of sleep apnea in children [19]. Obtaining a complete health history from the child's caregiver is essential to reveal symptom severity. Findings that support significant sleep disturbances include witnessed apnea attacks, excessive snoring, chronic mouth breathing, frequent awakening while asleep, excessive sleepiness, enuresis, decreased school performance, dysphasia, and hyponasal and hypernasal speech originating from enlarged tonsils affecting regular palate movements [20]. In adults, obstructive sleep apnea is often associated with classic obesity-related Pickwickian syndrome. Describing the polysomnographic findings, Leach et al. [20] stated that obesity is not a factor in children with obstructive sleep apnea caused by tonsillar hypertrophy. Most children with airway obstruction associated with tonsillar hypertrophy have a snoring history at night [20, 21]. Excessive snoring in children is an essential indicator of obstructive sleep apnea. Apneas may be observed directly by parents and care givers is best or via polysomnography [22]. Enuresis is another indicator of severe underlying airway obstruction in children. Enuresis is the low night-time release of the antidiuretic hormone associated with rapid eye movement (REM) sleep period diseases. Weider et al. [23] described the treatment of enuresis-associated chronic tonsillar hypertrophy and airway obstruction with adenotonsillectomy. In their study, patients who developed secondary enuresis after childhood responded to this treatment. Conversely, 24 patients with primary enuresis (congenitally present) did not respond to surgery, possibly as a result of other neurological factors. Chronic tonsillar hypertrophy and airway obstruction trigger enuresis as a result of impaired growth hormone release. Polysomnographic testing is indicated to determine the severity of sleep disturbance in patients with concern for sleep apnea or significant sleep disturbance without significant adenotonsillar hypertrophy on examination [20].

The primary causes of obstructive sleep apnea in non-syndromic children are anatomical factors such as tonsillar hypertrophy, obesity, and craniofacial anomalies that can cause narrowing of the upper airway. The presence of obstructive sleep apnea without anatomical abnormalities may suggest an underlying change in the neuromotor tone of the upper airway [24]. An obstructed airway can alter craniofacial growth and development. Furthermore, an underlying abnormal craniofacial skeleton can lead to additional airway obstruction. Pathophysiology related to skeletal changes, for example, may cause midline hypoplasias, a shallow and narrow nasopharynx and oropharynx [25, 26]. Over the past decade, pediatric sleep medicine studies have evaluated behavioral and neurocognitive changes that may occur even in mild sleep disorders. Behavioral problems related to sleep-disordered breathing include hyperactivity, attention deficit syndromes, aggression, and inability to socialize. Neurocognitive disorders include failure in school and deficiency in learning and problem-solving skills [27]. In children, sleep changes, snoring, suffocation, panting, restless sleep, intermittent sleep, sweating neck, hyperextension, witnessed apneas, and parasomnia [27]. Polysomnography is the gold standard for diagnosing obstructive sleep apnea in children. In polysomnography, it records simultaneous cardiorespiratory, electromyographic, and electroencephalographic data during sleep and gives information about the degree of airway obstruction during sleep [28].

The relationship between sleep and growth hormone secretion was first reported by Quabbe et al. [29]. It has been reported that after the correction of obstructive sleep apnea in children, an increase in growth was observed, and an increase in serum insulin-like growth factor-1 level was also observed. The physiological release of growth hormone is closely related to the sleep-wake cycle [30].

Stradling et al. looked at the effect of tonsillectomy on growth. They found that children's heights increased significantly during the 6 months following surgery compared to a control group. On average, the patients' weight increased from the 43rd percentile prior to surgery to the 63rd percentile after surgery, compared to a control group that was unchanged over the same time period. The 6-month height increase in the patient group was 9.7 cm/year versus 7.5 cm/year in the control group [31]. Another study demonstrated that adenotonsillar hypertrophy causing obstructive sleep disorder disrupts the secretion of growth hormone by disrupting the sleep pattern and structure and may cause growth and development delay. This was especially concerning between the age of 3 and 5, when growth hormones are very active [32].

Unlike the palatine tonsil, the other elements of Waldeyer's ring are not readily visible but possess anatomical relationships to the ear and paranasal sinuses, which can lead to pathology [33]. It has been hypothesized that facial growth abnormalities may occur with obstructive tonsillar hypertrophy or with the forward displacement of the tongue that develops as a result. Older measurement studies have demonstrated changes in the dimensions of the soft palate and oropharynx in children with the tonsillar's obstructive growth compared to controls [34, 35].

Chronic infection is a cause tonsillar hypertrophy. Chronic antigenic stimulation of tonsillar lymphocytes has been identified as the most common underlying cause of tonsillar hyperplasia. H. Influenza, S. Aureus, and Bacteroides melaninogenicus are among the most common bacterial agents present in hypertrophied tonsils [36, 37]. A similar conclusion was found in a study of previous Epstein Barr virus infection and tonsillar hypertrophy [38].

Acute tonsillitis is the most common acute disease of the palatine tonsil. There are three types of tonsillitis: acute, recurrent, and chronic. Fever, dysphagia, sore throat, exudate, and redness of the tonsils, and painful swelling in the neck lymph nodes are the prominent symptoms of the acute tonsillar disease [39]. For the diagnosis of recurrent tonsillitis, the frequency of attacks should be at least seven times in the last year, at least five attacks each year in the last 2 years, or at least three attacks each year in the last 3 years. At least one or more of the following findings should be detected to diagnose acute tonsillitis: Fever>38.3 °C, cervical lymphadenopathy, exudate, or positive group A beta streptococcal culture from a tonsil swab, and antimicrobial treatment of streptococcal infection [40]. Episodes of tonsillitis must be documented in the medical record, though streptococcal throat culture need not be positive during each infection event.

Chronic tonsillitis is a clinical diagnosis. It is based on a history of tonsillitis and sore throat that recurs three to four times a year and does not respond to adequate antibiotic treatment [41]. Peritonsillar abscess is a suppurative infection of the tonsils that penetrates the tonsillar capsule from the upper pole into the peritonsillar space. The infection then becomes purulent and coalesces between the capsule and the posterior wall of the tonsillar fossa. Any agent that causes acute and chronic tonsillitis, especially anaerobic bacteria, can progress to peritonsillar abscess. As noted above, peritonsillar infection can also spread to the retropharyngeal space and beyond. Peritonsillar abscess is usually one-sided with fever, difficulty swallowing, speech disorder, and trismus. The "hot potato" voice in which the mouth is moved as little as possible is typical to relieve the pain during mouth opening. On examination, the soft palate near the tonsil on the affected side is edematous. The uvula is edematous and will often be shifted towards the opposite side [4, 42].

Tonsillar hypertrophy causes a wide variety of signs and symptoms and is associated with several different disease processes. Consequently, there is no standard guide to the management and follow-up of children with tonsillar hypertrophy. When evaluating these children, with comprehensive interview of family and pediatrician are tantamount, followed by physical examination with or without nasal endoscopy. The data collected will provide the best chance for obtaining an accurate diagnosis [34, 35].

References

1. Wiatrak BJ, Woolley AL. Pharyngitis and adenotonsillar disease. In: Cummings CW, Flint PW, Harker LA, Haugey BH, Richardson MA, editors. Otolaryngology head and neck surgery. 3rd ed. St.Louis, MO: Mosby Year Book; 1998.
2. Resuli AS. A comparison of lucigenin-free oxygen radicals in reactive hyperplasia and recurrent tonsillitis. Phnx Med J. 2019;1(1):15–9.
3. Georinger GC, Vidic B. The embryogenesis and anatomy of waldeyer's ring. Otolaryngol Clin N Am. 1987;20(2):207–17.
4. Kornblut AD. Non-neoplastic diseases of the tonsils and adenoids. In: Paparella MM, Shumich DA, editors. Otolaryngology. 3rd ed. Philadelphia, PA: WB Saunders; 1991.
5. Brodsky L. Tonsillitis, tonsillectomy and adenoidectomy. In: Byron JB, editor. Head and neck surgery otolaryngology. 2nd ed. Philadelphia, PA: Lippincott; 1998.
6. Arıncı K, Elhan A. Throat anatomy. In: Arıncı K, Elhan A, editors. Anatomy. 2nd ed. Ankara, Turkey: Güneş Book House; 1987.
7. Richtsmeier WJ, Shikhani AH. The physiology and immunology of the pharyngeal lymphoid tissue. Otolaryngol Clin N Am. 1987;20(2):219–28.
8. Abdel-aziz M, El-Fouly M, Nassar AR, Kamel A. The effect of hypertrophied tonsils on the velopharyngeal function in children with normal palate. Int J Pediatr Otorhinolaryngol. 2019;119:59–62. https://doi.org/10.1016/j.ijporl.2019.01.017.
9. Sapcı T, İspir F, Saydam B, Karavuş A, Ozbilen G, Akyol H, et al. Measurement of the distance between the tonsillar fossa and the arteria carotis interna by computed tomography. PTT Hospital Medical J. 2000;22(1):14–7.
10. Karatas E, Sapmaz E, Kurnaz B. Surgical anatomy of the Waldeyer lymphoid tissue. Turkey Clinics J ENT-Special Topics. 2012;5(4):43–7.
11. Potsic WP. Assessment and treatment of Adenotonsillar hypertrophy in children. Am J Otolaryngol. 1992;13:259–64. https://doi.org/10.1016/0196-0709(92)90046-V.
12. Ballenger JJ. Oropharynx diseases. In: Ballenger JJ, Snow JB, editors. Otorhinolaryngology head and neck surgery. 16th ed. Shelton, CT: PMPH; 2002.

13. Bandyopadhyay A, Muston H, Slaven JE, et al. Endoscopic airway findings in infants with obstructive sleep apnea. J Pulm Respir Med. 2018;8:1–5. https://doi.org/10.417 2/2161-105X.1000448.
14. Lind MG, Lundell BP. Tonsillar hyperplasia in children. A cause of obstructive sleep apneas, CO, retention, and retarded growth. Arch Otolaryngol. 1982;108:650–8. https://doi.org/10.1001/archotol.1982.00790580044015.
15. Brodsky L. Modern assessment of tonsils and adenoids. Pediatr Clin North America. 1989;36:1551–69. https://doi.org/10.1016/S0031-3955(16)36806-7.
16. Scher AE, Shprintzen RJ, Thorpy MJ. Endoscopic observations of obstructive sleep apnea in children with anomalous upper airways: predictive and therapeutic value. Int J Pediatr Otorhinolaryngol. 1986;11:135–46. https://doi.org/10.1016/s0165-5876(86)80008-8.
17. Mlynarek A, Tewfik MA, Hagr A, et al. Lateral neck radiography versus direct video Rhinoscopy in assessing adenoid size. J Otolaryngol. 2004;33(6):360–5. https://doi.org/10.2310/7070.2004.03074.
18. Shigemoto S, Shigeta Y, Nejima J, et al. Diagnosis and treatment for obstructive sleep apnea: fundamental and clinical knowledge in obstructive sleep apnea. J Prosthodont Res. 2015;59(3:161–71.
19. Frank Y, Kravath RE, Pollak CP. Obstructive sleep apnea and its therapy: clinical and polysomnographic manifestations. Pediatrics. 1983;71:737–42.
20. Leach JL, Olson J, Hermann J, Manning S. Polysomnographic and clinical findings in children with obstructive sleep apnea. Arch Otolaryngol Head Neck Surg. 1992;118:741–4. https://doi.org/10.1001/archotol.1992.01880070071013.
21. Gislason T, Benediktsdóttir B. Snoring, apneic episodes, and nocturnal hipoxemia among children 6 months to 6 years old: an epidemiologic study of lower limit of prevalence. Chest. 1995;107:963–6. https://doi.org/10.1378/chest.107.4.963.
22. Carrol JL, others. Inability of clinical history to distinguish primary snoring from obstructive sleep apnea syndrome in children. Chest. 1995;108:610–8. https://doi.org/10.1378/chest.108.3.610.
23. Weider DJ, Sateia MJ, West RP. Nocturnal enurezis in children with upper airway obstruction. Otolaryngol Head Neck Surg. 1991;105:427–32. https://doi.org/10.1177/019459989110500314.
24. Arens R, Marcus CL. Pathophysiology of upper airway obstruction: a developmental perspective. Sleep. 2004;27(5):997–1019. https://doi.org/10.1093/sleep/27.5.997.
25. Harding SM. Prediction formulae for sleep-disordered breathing. Curr Opin Pulm Med. 2001;15(4):670–4. https://doi.org/10.1097/00063198-200111000-00003.
26. Parinen M, Telakivi T. Epidemiology of obstructive sleep apnea syndrome. Sleep. 1992;15(6):S1–4. https://doi.org/10.1093/sleep/15.suppl_6.S1.
27. Mitchell RB. Sleep-disordered breathing in children: are we underestimating the problem? Eur Respir J. 2005;25(2):216–7. https://doi.org/10.1183/09031936.05.00124704.
28. Kotagal S. Childhood obstructive sleep apnea. BMJ. 2005;330:978–9.
29. Quabbe H, Schilling E, Helge H. Patern of growth hormone secretion during 24 hour fast in normal adults. J Clin Endocrinol Metab. 1996;26:1173–7. https://doi.org/10.1210/jcem-26-10-1173.
30. Bar A, Tarasuik A, Segev Y, Philip M, Tal A. The effect of adenotonsillectomy on serum insu- lin-like growth factor-I and growth in children with obstructive sleep apnea syndrome. J Pediatr. 1999;135(1):76–80. https://doi.org/10.1016/s0022-3476(99)70331-8.
31. Stradling JR, Thomas G, Warley ARH, Williams P, Freeland A. Effect of adenotonsillectomy on nocturnal hypoxaemia, sleep disturbance, and symptons in snoring children. Lancet. 1990;335:249–53. https://doi.org/10.1016/0140-6736(90)90068-g.
32. Gorur K, Unal M, Ozcan C, Vayısoglu Y. The effects of chronic adenotonsillar hypertrophy on height and weight development in children. Turkish Otol and Head Neck Surg J. 2000;8(3):182–6.
33. Sridhar MR. A clinical study to determine the effects of adenoidectomy in cases of secretory otitis media in school going children. Int J Otorhinolaryngol Head Neck Surg. 2018;4(6):1–4. https://doi.org/10.18203/issn.2454-5929.ijohns20184180.

34. Brodsky L, Adler E, Stanievich JF. Naso- and oropharyngeal dimensions in children with obstructive sleep apnea. Int J Pediatr Otorhinolaryngol. 1989;17:1–11. https://doi.org/10.1016/0165-5876(89)90288-7.
35. Brodsky L, Moore L, Stanievich JF. A comparison of tonsillar size and oropharyngeal dimensions in children with obstructive adenotonsillar hypertrophy. Int J Ped Otorhinolaryngol. 1987;13:149–56. https://doi.org/10.1016/0165-5876(87)90091-7.
36. Brodsky L, Moore L, Stanievich JF, Ogra PL. The immunology of tonsils in children: the effect of bacterial load on the presence of B- and T-cell subsets. Laryngoscope. 1988;98:93–8. https://doi.org/10.1288/00005537-198801000-00019.
37. Brodsky L, Moore L, Stanievich JF. The role of Haemophilus infiuenzae in the pathogenesis of tonsillar hypertrophy in children. Laryngoscope. 1988;98:1055.
38. Aka S, Ozker BY, Demiralay E, Canbay İE. Role of Ebstein-Barr virus in children with tonsillar hypertrophy. Turk Arch Ped. 2013;48:30–4. https://doi.org/10.4274/tpa.963.
39. Paradise JL, Bluestone CD, Bachman RZ, et al. Efficacy of tonsillectomy for recurrent throat infection in severely affected children. New Engl J Med. 1984;310:674–83.
40. Mitchell R, Archer SM, Ishman SL, et al. Clinical practice guideline: tonsillectomy in children (update). Otolaryngol Head Neck Surg. 2019;160(1S):S1–S42. https://doi.org/10.1177/0194599818801757.
41. Yazkan FO. Approach to Tonsilla palatine and its nonneoplastic diseases. Med J SDU. 2017;24(4):198–208. https://doi.org/10.17343/sdutfd.298817.
42. Klug ET. Peritonsillar abscess: clinical aspects of microbiology, risk factors, and the association with parapharyngeal abscess. Dan Med J. 2017;64(3):B5333.

Cervical Lymphadenopathy in Children

22

Nazan Sarper and Giulio Cesare Passali

22.1 Introduction

Cervical lymphadenopathy (cLAP) is the enlargement of the lymph nodes (>1 cm diameter) of the neck, including preauricular, parotid, jugulodigastric (at the angle of the jaw), submental, submandibular, posterior cervical, superficial cervical, deep cervical, occipital and posterior auricular (mastoid) lymph nodes (Fig. 22.1).

Cervical lymphadenitis describes the inflamed lymph node(s) of the neck. They may be tender, hyperemic and cellulitis of the subcutaneous tissue may also develop. Nodes are fluctuant when filled with pus (abscess). Acute or chronic infection or injury to the proximal tissues causes inflammatory response and drainage to the nodes by lymphatic channels occurs. Submaxillary and deep cervical nodes are frequently enlarged because most of the lymphatic drainage of the head and neck go to these lymph node sites [1].

In the differential diagnosis of the childhood cervical masses, it must be remembered that midline congenital neck masses are generally benign and patients with midline masses must be referred to pediatric surgeons. Local and systemic infections must be screened initially by a family physician, a pediatrician, or a pediatric infectious diseases specialist. Ear, nose, and throat (ENT) infections associated with cLAP also may be evaluated by an ENT specialist. Needle aspiration of cervical lymphadenitis at presentation is controversial.

In many quite healthy children, cervical lymph nodes are frequently palpated by sensitive parents. In children, mobile cervical lymph nodes <1.5 cm without any

N. Sarper (✉)
Division of Pediatric Hematology, Department of Pediatrics, Faculty of Medicine, Kocaeli University, Kocaeli, Turkey
e-mail: nazan.sarper@kocaeli.edu.tr

G. C. Passali
Department of Otorhinolaryngology, Catholic University of Sacred Heart, Roma, Italy

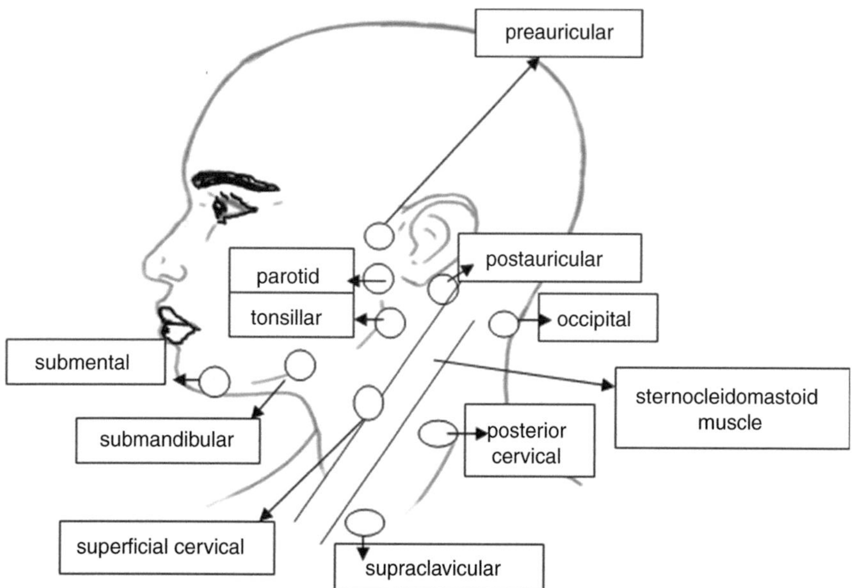

Fig. 22.1 Location of cervical lymph nodes

other symptoms and with normal blood counts are rarely malignant. Etiology is generally infection in cLAPs of children; malignancy is rare even in children referred to pediatric hematologists and oncologists. Lymphoma is the most common malignancy in the cervical area.

Pediatric hematologists and oncologists must decide which cLAP deserves excision for histological examination; this will lessen unnecessary invasive interventions for reactive cLAPs. Surgeons should never aspirate these lymph nodes for diagnosis of malignancy without consultation of a pediatric hematologist or oncologist. Excisional biopsies will provide adequate tissue for pathologic examinations. Peripheral blood smears and bone marrow smears must be examined in the first step, because in malignancies infiltrating bone marrow (leukemia, lymphoma, sometimes neuroblastoma) diagnosis may be confirmed with a less invasive intervention. This review aims to help family physicians, pediatricians, and ENT surgeons for a better approach to cLAPs of children and to prevent unnecessary anxiety of sensitive parents.

22.2 Anamnesis

The course of the disease, associating fever, malaise, rash, upper respiratory symptoms, sore throat, earache, toothache, night sweats, and weight loss must be questioned. Acute lymphadenopathy that subsides within 2 weeks is generally of infectious origin. Viral upper respiratory tract infections and group A streptococcal infection (tonsillitis, tonsillopharyngitis) usually cause cLAP. Membranous tonsillitis and cLAP may be due to infectious mononucleosis. In patients with a history of ingestion of unpasteurized milk, contact with cattle, suffering from fever and night sweats, and having hepatosplenomegaly, brucellosis should be considered. Persisting fever for more than 5 days, strawberry tongue, non-exudative conjunctivitis, dry and red lips, peeling skin, and cLAP are symptoms of Kawasaki disease. In the presence of B symptoms (night sweats, weight loss more than 10% of body weight in 6 months) lymphomas or infectious diseases such as tuberculosis and human immune deficiency virus (HIV) infection should be considered [2]. History of exposure to an adult with tuberculosis may support tuberculosis lymphadenitis.

The syndrome of periodic fever, aphthous stomatitis, pharyngitis, and cervical adenitis (PFAPA syndrome) must be considered in children with a history of frequent febrile attacks.

Exposure to hens was found to be a risk factor for non-tuberculous mycobacteria [3]. *Mycobacterium chelonae* was reported to involve the submandibular glands following dental pathology [4].

In a child with cLAP, any pain in the extremities or back pain may be due to leukemia or bone marrow involvement of malignancy like neuroblastoma or associating arthritis and fever may be due to juvenile idiopathic arthritis.

The following questions must be asked to every patient with cLAP. When the cLAP appeared? Is the course progressive, regressive, or intermittent? Is there any associating symptom?

After the regression of symptoms of acute infections, cLAP may be palpable for some months. In otherwise asymptomatic, immunocompetent children there is no need for serial ultrasonographic examinations or antimicrobial administrations. Physicians and families should observe these cLAPs to follow any progression. Serological studies for cytomegalovirus (CMV) and Epstein Barr virus (EBV) also have no contribution to the management of such children except increasing expenses.

22.3 Clinical Examination

The patient must incline the head forward and relax the neck muscles during the examination. All cervical lymph node regions must be palpated. In infections of the scalp and outer ear, in rubella and toxoplasmosis, suboccipital nodes are enlarged. Enlargement of the pre-auricular lymph nodes may indicate eye-lid infections, conjunctivitis, or infections of the ears, teeth, or the parotid glands. Enlargement of the submental/submandibular lymph nodes is often due to infections of the oral cavity, the nose, the maxillary sinus, or the face. Jugulodigastric lymph nodes are enlarged in patients with palatine tonsil infections [5].

cLAP in the lateral neck can be inflammatory or neoplastic. Masses in the posterior triangle (behind or lateral to the sternocleidomastoid muscle) are generally malignant, most of which are lymphomas [1].

Similar to location, characteristics of the lymph node may help diagnosis. Painful, hot, mobile nodes not larger than 1.5 cm in diameter are generally due to local infections of the head and neck region. A fluctuant, painful, and swollen node refers to lymphadenitis. Firm, non-tender nodes with low mobility and larger than 2–2.5 cm may be malignant (lymphoma and rarely carcinoma). Lymphomas also involve nodes along the jugular vein.

Large cLAP and supraclavicular nodes should be biopsied. Fine needle aspiration is not reliable to exclude malignancy in children [6].

Axillary, inguinal lymph nodes, liver, and spleen must be also palpated to evaluate systemic disease as lymphoma/leukemia or systemic infection or metabolic disease. Asymmetric tonsils and cLAP should raise suspicion for lymphoma [7]. Right supraclavicular lymph nodes are enlarged during thoracic carcinomas, lymphomas, tuberculosis, and sarcoidosis. Left supraclavicular nodes enlarge during retroperitoneal malignancies. In a study, patients with cLAP referred to a university hospital were evaluated retrospectively. The mean age of the patients was 79.4 ± 46.7 months. It was reported that predictive factors for malignancy were having cLAP larger than 30 mm, rubbery lymph node, high serum C-reactive protein (CRP) and lactate dehydrogenase (LDH) values, no hilum in ultrasonography, and progressive enlargement of a lymph node. Only 2.7% of the patients had malignancy which was lymphomas [8].

Mycobacterium tuberculosis or atypical mycobacteria may also involve cervical nodes. During the infection, the skin overlying the node may develop a pinkish or violaceous discoloration caused by increased vascularity. It is a cold abscess and in the course of the disease, adherence of the skin to the underlying mass is observed. If left untreated, fluctuance and spontaneously draining sinus tracts may develop.

Other masses of the region, which are located in the midline, are of congenital origin. These are thyroglossal cysts, branchial cleft cysts, cystic hygromas, lipoma, and ectopic thyroid tissue. Cysts are solitary, non-tender, round masses with well-defined borders if they are not secondarily infected. Thyroglossal duct cysts are the most common congenital masses of the midline [9]. These cysts move on protrusion of the tongue. They may have an associated sinus tract and mucus drainage. Thyroglossal duct cysts must be differentiated from other midline masses, including epidermoid cysts, lipomas, thyroid tumors, and the rare midline lymph node.

The second most common benign congenital neck mass is the branchial cleft cyst that lies at the anterior border of the sternocleidomastoid muscle. When they are not infected only a skin dimple may be observed. These cysts usually appear in school-aged children [1].

Cystic hygromas are the third most frequent cause of congenital neck masses. These arise from lymphatics derived from the jugular vein or the mesenchymal tissue. They can occur elsewhere but usually are found posterior to the sternocleidomastoid muscle in the supraclavicular fossa. They are soft and transilluminate well. They may cause compression symptoms to the surrounding structures when an increase in size is associated with an upper respiratory tract infection. Hygroma persists while other lymph nodes decrease in size after the resolution of the infection [1].

Midline masses located anterior to the sternocleidomastoid muscle are benign except thyroid tumors [10].

Differential diagnosis in cLAP with associated characteristic history and/or clinical findings is listed below in Sects. 22.4–22.7 [2].

22.4 Infections

- Streptococcal infections (sore throat, skin infections).
- Staphylococcal infections (skin infections, other local infections).
- Tuberculosis disease (exposure to adults with tuberculosis).
- Non-tuberculosis mycobacterial infections.
- Brucellosis (contact with cattle, ingestion of unpasteurized milk, fever, night sweats, splenomegaly).
- Bartonellosis (cat-scratch disease; contact with cats).
- Tularemia (contact with rodents, tick bite, often purulent lymph nodes).
- Borreliosis (tick bite history, erythema chronicum migrans).
- Epstein-Barr virus (EBV) infection (malaise, membranous tonsillitis, splenomegaly, rash).
- HIV infection/AIDS (risk of contact with this infection).
- Measles (fever, coryza, characteristic rash, and no vaccination history).
- Rubella (retro-auricular, suboccipital lymphadenopathy and rash).
- Toxoplasmosis (contact with cats, consumption of raw meat, generally without other symptoms).
- Leishmaniasis (fever, hepatosplenomegaly, and pancytopenia).
- Yersiniosis (intestinal symptoms).
- Fungal infections (histoplasmosis, coccidioidomycosis, blastomycosis, tinea, skin or respiratory tract manifestations).

22.5 Immunological Diseases

- Kawasaki disease (fever, conjunctivitis, strawberry tongue, red dry lips, exanthema).
- The lupus erythematosus (skin manifestations, hematological and other organ involvements).
- Sarcoidosis (fever and dyspnea).
- Dermatomyositis (characteristic skin findings and proximal muscle weakness).
- Juvenile idiopathic arthritis (chronic arthritis, fever, and rash in systemic forms).
- Autoimmune lymphoproliferative syndrome (cytopenias, splenomegaly).
- PFAPA syndrome (periodic fever, aphthous stomatitis, pharyngitis, and cervical adenitis).
- Chronic granulomatous disease (frequent bacterial and fungal infections, purulent lymph node inflammation).
- Castleman's disease (±splenomegaly ± hepatomegaly).

22.6 Metabolic Diseases

- Gaucher's disease (splenomegaly and neurological symptoms).
- Niemann-Pick disease (splenomegaly and neurological symptoms).

22.7 Neoplastic Diseases

- Malignant lymphoma (hard, non-tender, immobile lymph nodes ± B symptoms).
- Leukemia (indolent lymph nodes, pain in the extremities, increased bruising, malaise, and changes in blood counts).

22.8 Laboratory Investigations

In patients with an obvious local infection (tonsillitis, otitis, scalp infection, dental abscess) and an acute cLAP, an antimicrobial drug is started after performing a local culture. When there are symptoms of acute viral upper respiratory infection as sore throat, rhinitis, there is no need for laboratory investigation and treatment. But when the cause of cLAP is uncertain, although their elevation is non-specific, erythrocyte sedimentation rate (ESR), CRP, and LDH are studied. A blood count and microscopic examination of the peripheral blood smear is essential. Blood culture should be obtained if the patient is severely ill and febrile. Blasts in the peripheral smear are diagnostic for acute leukemia. In the presentation of acute leukemia, thrombocytopenia, neutropenia, and anemia are generally present but white blood cell (WBC) count may be high, low, or within normal limits for age. When blood counts are abnormal or there are blasts in the peripheral smear and/or any pain in the extremities, bone marrow aspiration and biopsy should be performed at once. Because this procedure can be performed with sedo-analgesia outside the operation room, it is minimally invasive, and it gives the chance of diagnosis on the same day. Reactive lymphocytes (Downey cells) on peripheral smear may confirm the diagnosis of infectious mononucleosis. An increase in the bands or neutrophils confirms bacterial infections.

In patients with a family history of tuberculosis, tuberculin skin test (TST) and interferon-gamma (IFN-γ) release assays (IGRAs) are performed. When a fluctuating and painful lymph node is present and sonography also confirms lymphadenitis, antimicrobial treatment must be started at once without further investigation.

Needle aspiration of the affected node in acute cervical lymphadenitis generally reveals an etiologic agent. Inflamed nodes may be aspirated. A local anesthetic cream should be applied and aspiration is performed after 45 min using an 18- or 20 -gauge needle attached to a 20 mL syringes. If no material is aspirated, sterile saline is injected into the node and re-aspirated. The aspirate should be inoculated directly from the syringe onto aerobic (including chocolate agar) and anaerobic media, onto Sabouraud agar (for fungi), and into a broth medium suitable for the early detection of mycobacteria, such as the BACTEC radiometric assay [1]. Gram and acid-fast stains must be performed as a guide to initial antimicrobial therapy before culture results are obtained. Cultures of the infected skin lesions and exudates on the tonsils must be performed.

Staphylococcus aureus, Staphylococcus epidermidis, Streptococcus pneumoniae, group A streptococci, *Streptococcus pyogenes,* viridians group streptococci, and rarely methicillin-resistant *S. aureus* (MRSA) and clindamycin-resistant *S. aureus* are isolated from suppurative lymphadenitis in children [11, 12]. In children with poor dental hygiene or periodontal disease causing cLAP, anaerobic bacteria may be isolated.

If cat-scratch or cat exposure and fever are present in history, serologic tests for the detection of immunoglobulin (Ig) G antibodies to *Bartonella* spp. should be performed, but high positivity for IgG against *Bartonella henselae* in children with cLAP and fever is shown due to the high number of kittens living in private houses [13]. Cat scratch disease is generally a benign and self-limiting disease.

In persistent cLAP, further investigations are required. Serology for EBV, CMV, human herpesvirus (HHV) -6, HIV, histoplasmosis, coccidioidomycosis, toxoplasmosis, tularemia, and *Brucella* should be performed.

Nontuberculous mycobacteria (NTM) may be isolated from lymph nodes. They are found in food, water, animals, and soil and may cause cervical adenitis. The tuberculin skin test (TST) is positive but IFN-γ release assays (IGRAs) are generally negative in NTM infections. Genetic tests are used for their identification.

22.9 Imaging

Ultrasonography is performed when neck mass is large or increasing in size, or has not responded to initial antibiotic therapy. It is useful in diagnosing suppuration. Abscess forming lymph nodes and tuberculous lymphadenitis are characterized by central cystic changes with loss of the echogenic hilum [14]. In children, the etiology of cLAP is frequently infectious or reactive and ultrasonography is less helpful in differential diagnosis compared to adult patients. In addition to sonographic examination of the cLAP, sonography of the abdomen and chest X-ray is performed to evaluate systemic involvement of the lymph nodes or other organ involvements. Computerized tomography (CT) of the chest and CT or magnetic resonance imaging (MRI) of the abdomen is also performed for the identification of the malignancies.

22.10 Histological Examination

If the cLAP persists, enlarges, is hard, or is fixed to the adjacent structures, biopsy should be performed. Biopsy material should be delivered to the microbiology laboratory also for cultures and dyes as Giemsa, periodic acid–Schiff, and methenamine silver stains (for fungus). If a child has a history of a cat-scratch or cat exposure and histological examination reveals noncaseating granulomas, diagnosis is often cat-scratch disease [15].

Excision of the lymph nodes in suspicion of tuberculosis helps both diagnosis and treatment [16]. *Mycobacterium avium* complex (MAC) is the predominant isolate of the cLAP and for satisfactory aesthetic results, total excision within 1 month after its onset is recommended [17].

Tuberculosis and sarcoidosis are granulomatous diseases but sarcoidosis involving cervical lymph nodes is very rare in children [18].

In older children, indication for excisional lymph node biopsy is more frequent because they are more likely to have lymphomas. The selection of the enlarged lymph node for the biopsy is important. Biopsy specimens from the lower neck and supraclavicular area should be preferred. Upper cervical, submandibular, axillary, and parotid lymph nodes are much more likely to be affected by reactive hyperplasia, which may not be related to the underlying disease process. If lymphoma is suspected, for optimal histological examination and immunohistochemistry, excisional lymph node biopsy is always preferred to fine-needle aspiration and through-cut biopsies.

In childhood, 80% of cLAPs is due to benign diseases. Under 6 years of age if there is malignancy the most frequent causes are acute leukemia, neuroblastoma, rhabdomyosarcoma, and non-Hodgkin lymphoma. Between the ages of 7 and 13, non-Hodgkin and Hodgkin lymphoma, and rarely rhabdomyosarcoma and thyroid cancer are diagnosed. After age 13, Hodgkin's disease is the most frequent cause of malignant cLAP [19].

22.11 Etiological Differentiation in Pediatric Cervical Lymphadenopathy

Although there are plenty of diseases associated with cLAP in children, about two-thirds of the cLAP is benign and self-limited. In a meta-analysis of 2687 subjects of children and adolescents 0–21 years, 67.8% had benign etiology and only about 4% had malignancy. The most common malignancy was non-Hodgkin's lymphoma [20]. If the general condition of the child is good, cLAP is <1.5 cm diameter, mobile and non-tender and there is no associating pathological physical examination signs or symptoms and blood counts are also normal, more than 95% is benign and self-limited.

22.12 Treatment of Common Bacterial Lymphadenitis

When a fluctuating and painful lymph node is present and sonography also confirms lymphadenitis, antimicrobial treatment is started. In suppurative lymphadenitis of children, it is shown that surgical drainage has no benefits to medical treatment [21]. If there is no clinical improvement despite antibiotics, image-guided aspiration should be considered.

Empirical antimicrobial therapy should be directed against *S. aureus* or *S. pyogenes.* Penicillinase-resistant penicillins or some cephalosporins should be used. Oxacillin or nafcillin 150 mg/kg/day iv, q6h or cefazolin 75–100 mg/kg/day iv, q8h may be used if MRSA is uncommon and parenteral therapy is required. For oral treatment cephalexin 50–75 mg/kg/day q8h, or amoxicillin-clavulanate are also recommended against methicillin-susceptible *S. aureus* (MSSA), streptococci, and oral anaerobic organisms. In penicillin-allergy, cephalosporins are good alternatives. Azithromycin 10 mg/kg/day on day 1, then 5 mg/kg/day on days 2–5 is another alternative. Ceftriaxone 50–100 mg/kg/day iv may also be used and has the advantage of the long half-life. Daptomycin is another alternative for children older than 1 year. Recommended dosages are 1–<2 y, 10 mg/kg, iv, qd; 2–6 y, 9 mg/kg, iv, qd; 7–11 y, 7 mg/kg, qd; 12–17 y, 5 mg/kg, qd [21, 22].

For community-acquired (CA) MRSA, clindamycin 30–40 mg/kg/day q8h, for parenteral or oral use is an empirical or alternative therapy. It also has good activity against anaerobic infections. Cloxacillin 50 mg/kg/day, dicloxacillin 25 mg/kg/day, or cephalexin 25 to 50 mg/kg/day are other alternatives for oral route. Ceftaroline is a fifth-generation beta-lactam cephalosporin antibiotic that is active against MRSA and some gram-negative organisms. Recommended dosage is 2 mo–<2 y, 24 mg/kg/day, iv, q8h; ≥2 y, 36 mg/kg/day, iv, q8h (max. Single dose 400 mg); >33 kg, 400 mg/dose, iv, q8h or 600 mg/dose, iv, q12h. Daptomycin is also active against MRSA but is not used in infants due to potential toxicity. In a severely ill child needing hospitalization, vancomycin 60 mg/kg/day, iv, q6h may be combined with another agent as empirical antimicrobial until culture results are obtained. Linezolid is active against MRSA and group A streptococci (*S. pyogenes*) but should be a second-line therapy for patients, following clinical failure or a microbiological need has been confirmed [1, 22].

In a patient with periodontal or dental disease, antibiotics with anaerobic coverage, penicillin V 50 mg/kg/day, amoxicillin-clavulanate 40 mg/kg/day, or clindamycin 30 mg/kg/day should be initiated [1].

Patients with moderate to severe systemic symptoms and cellulitis in addition to cervical lymphadenitis frequently require parenteral therapy for the first few days. Treatment should be continued for at least 10 days or approximately 5 days after signs of local inflammation and systemic toxicity have disappeared. Analgesics should be also given in infants and children. If abscess formation occurs, drainage is indicated and therapy should be continued until resolution [1].

In cervical lymphadenitis of NTM, surgical excision is the treatment of choice. Antimicrobial therapy alone is less effective [1].

In PFAPA syndrome, fever and pharyngitis subside with corticosteroids.

22.13 Conclusion

In children, cLAP is generally benign and self-limited. The etiology of cLAP may be found by history (exposures, travel) and physical examination in most of the cases. Upper respiratory infections cause bilateral, multiple, mobile, cLAP. A child with lymph nodes smaller than 20 mm diameter, without any other signs and symptoms, is observed for 2 weeks. If lymph nodes regress at the end of 2 weeks, no treatment is required. If there is fever and/or hot, tender lymph nodes and whole blood counts, peripheral smear (leukocytosis, increase in band forms and neutrophils), ESR and CRP support acute infection, antibiotics against *S. aureus* and *S. pyogenes* should be started. Inflammation of the tonsils and infected teeth must not be overlooked because they might be the focus of infection. Some worrisome features suggesting malignancy are firm, rubbery, non-tender, fixed, unilateral cLAP larger than 20 mm; supraclavicular LAP; fever lasting more than 1 week; night sweats, weight loss (>10% of body weight); associating enlarged mediastinal lymph nodes and nodes not responding to 2 weeks of antibiotic therapy. In the presence of worrisome features, early evaluation of bone marrow smear and/or excisional biopsy of the most abnormal node (if multiple nodes are involved) should be performed and consulted with a pediatric hematology-oncology specialist. Associating symptoms and signs (skin rash, hepatosplenomegaly, arthritis, conjunctivitis) will help to diagnose systemic diseases. Treatment with glucocorticoids must be avoided before diagnostic evaluation is completed because this approach will mask the disease [23].

References

1. Healy CM, Baker CJ. Cervical lymphadenitis. In: Cherry JD, Harrison GJ, Kaplan SL, Steinbach WJ, Hotez PJ, editors. Feigen and Cherry's textbook of pediatric infectious diseases, vol. 1. 8th ed. Philadelphia, PA: Saunders Elsevier; 2019. p. 124–33.
2. Lang S, Kansy B. Cervical lymph node diseases in children. GMS Curr Top Otorhinolaryngol Head Neck Surg. 2014;13:1–27.
3. Garcia-Marcos PW, Plaza-Fornieles M, Menasalvas-Ruiz A, Ruiz-Pruneda R, Paredes-Reyes P, Miguelez SA. Risk factors of non-tuberculous mycobacterial lymphadenitis in children: a case-control study. Eur J Pediatr. 2017;176:607–13.
4. Alvi A, Myssiorek D. *Mycobacterium chelonae* causing recurrent neck abscess. Pediatr Infect Dis J. 1993; 12: 617–9.
5. Ghirardelli ML, Jemos V, Gobbi PG. Diagnostic approach to lymph node enlargement. Haematologica. 1999;84:242–7.
6. Locke R, Comfort R, Kubba H. When does an enlarged cervical lymph node in a child need excision? a systematic review. Int J Pediatr Otorhinolaryngol. 2014;78:393–401.
7. Guimarães AC, de Carvalho GM, Bento LR, Correa C, Gusmão RJ. Clinical manifestations in children with tonsillar lymphoma: a systematic review. Crit Rev Oncol Hematol. 2014;90:146–51.
8. Bozlak S, Varkal MA, Yıldız I, et al. Cervical lymphadenopathies in children: a prospective clinical cohort study. Int J Pediatr Otorhinolaryngol. 2016;82:81–7.
9. Kepertis C, Anastasiadis K, Lambropoulos V, Mouravas V, Spyridakis I. Diagnostic and surgical approach of thyroglossal duct cyst in children: Ten years data review. J Clin Diagn Res. 2015;9:PC13–5.
10. Vassilatou E, Proikas K, Margari N, Papadimitriou N, Hadjidakis D, Dimitriadis G. An adolescent with a rare midline neck tumor: thyroid carcinoma in a thyroglossal duct cyst. J Pediatr Hematol Oncol. 2014;36:407–9.
11. Cengiz AB, Kara A, Kanra G, Seçmeer G, Ceyhan M, Ozen M. Acute neck infections in children. Turk J Pediatr. 2004;46:153–8.
12. Fellner A, Marom T, Muallem-Kalmovich L, et al. Pediatric neck abscesses: no increase in methicillin-resistant Staphylococcus aureus. Int J Pediatr Otorhinolaryngol. 2017; 101:112–6.

13. Asano T, Ichiki K, Koizumi S, Kaizu K, Hatori T, Fujino O. High prevalence of antibodies against *Bartonella henselae* with cervical lymphadenopathy in children. Pediatr Int. 2010;52:533–5.
14. Ahuja A, Ying M, Yuen YH, Metreweli C. Power Doppler sonography of cervical lymphadenopathy. Clin Radiol. 2001;56:965–9.
15. Özkan EA, Göret CC, Özdemir ZT, et al. Evaluation of peripheral lymphadenopathy with excisional biopsy: six-year experience. Int J Clin Exp Pathol. 2015;8:15234–9.
16. Xu JJ, Peer S, Papsin BC, Kitai I, Propst EJ. Tuberculous lymphadenitis of the head and neck in Canadian children: experience from a low-burden region. Int J Pediatr Otorhinolaryngol. 2016;91:11–4.
17. Maltezou HC, Spyridis P, Kafetzis DA. Nontuberculous mycobacterial lymphadenitis in children. Pediatr Infect Dis J. 1999;18:968–70.
18. Welter SM, DeLuca-Johnson J, Thompson K. Histologic review of sarcoidosis in a neck lymph node. Head Neck Pathol. 2018;12:255–8.
19. Brown RL, Azizkhan RG. Pediatric head and neck lesions. Pediatr Clin N Am. 1998;45:889–905.
20. Deosthali A, Donches K, DelVecchio M, Aronoff S. Etiologies of Pediatric Cervical Lymphadenopathy: A Systematic Review of 2687 Subjects. Glob Pediatr Health. 2019;6:2333794X19865440.
21. Kwon M, Seo JH, Cho KJ, et al. Suggested protocol for managing acute suppurative cervical lymphadenitis in children to reduce unnecessary surgical interventions. Ann Otol Rhinol Laryngol. 2016;125:953–8.
22. Bradley JS. Antimicrobial therapy according to clinical syndromes. In: Bradley JS, Nelson JD, Barnett ED, Cantey JB, Kimberlin DW, Palumbo PE, Sauberan J, Smart JH, Steinbach WJ, editors. Nelson's pediatric antimicrobial therapy. 26th ed. Itasca, IL: American Academy of Pediatrics; 2020. p. 63–123.
23. McClain KL Peripheral lymphadenopathy in children: evaluation and diagnostic approach. Kaplan SL, Mahoney DH, Drutz JE, Torchia MM (eds). Uptodate. 2020, https://www.uptodate.com/contents/peripheral-lymphadenopathy-in-children-evaluation-and-diagnostic-pproach?topicRef=5982&source=see_link#H17. Accessed 1 Nov 2020.

Halitosis in Children Secondary to ENT Infections

Tuğçe Küçükoğlu Çiçek, Nuray Bayar Muluk, and William Reisacher

23.1 Introduction

Halitosis refers to malodour emanating from the mouth. It is derived etymologically from the Latin word "halitus", signifying "breath", and the Greek suffix (−osis) indicating a pathological process. The common lay term is "bad breath" [1, 2]. Halitosis is especially concerning for a child, as it may lead to exclusion, awkwardness in social situations and a degree of stigma. Studies have confirmed the negative impact that halitosis has on a person's quality of life, particularly with respect to interpersonal relationships [3]. Sometimes the sufferer and his/her relatives have not noticed the condition, which comes to light following a visit to the dentist or general practitioner [2].

It is important to distinguish between cases where halitosis is genuine (objective) and where it is delusional (subjective).

Pseudohalitosis occurs where a patient has a subjective awareness of bad breath that is not shared by anyone else, including the examining healthcare professional [4]. It has been noted that pseudohalitosis is rising in children. One explanation is that there is an increasingly intense marketing focus on products designed to improve mouth hygiene and the general appearance of the teeth [4, 5].

Halitophobia is an abnormal fear of others perceiving the patient to have halitosis, whether or not the condition is present. It is a psychological condition that may

T. K. Çiçek (✉)
Section of Otorhinolaryngology, Adana City Training and Research Hospital, University of Health Sciences, Adana, Turkey

N. Bayar Muluk
Department of Otorhinolaryngology, Faculty of Medicine, Kırıkkale University, Kırıkkale, Turkey

W. Reisacher
Department of Otolaryngology, Head and Neck Surgery, Weill Cornell Medical College, New York, NY, USA

call for psychotherapy once an organic aetiology has been excluded. Halitophobia may be viewed as a special instance of the olfactory reference syndrome [6, 7].

23.2 Aetiology

Halitosis is a problem affecting both males and females and is multifactorial in origin. The key component in the aetiology is the breakdown of sulphur-containing organic matter within the mouth by proteolytic, anaerobic Gram-negative bacterial species. The principal site in the mouth where malodorous volatile sulphur compounds (VSC) arise is a coated tongue [1]. A relationship between the consumption of alcohol or spices and halitosis has also been suggested [8].

23.2.1 Intraoral Causes

In between 80% and 85% of cases of paediatric halitosis, the root cause lies in the oral cavity. Conditions affecting the gums and periodontal disorders are causes of halitosis, namely acute necrotising ulcerative gingivitis, herpetic gingivitis, periodontitis, pericoronitis, periodontal abscess and tonsillitis. A recent systematic review with meta-regression analysis estimated the prevalence of halitosis in adolescents and adults to be 31.8% [9]. Moreover, the prevalence seems to be increasing over time, particularly in countries with low-medium income where the prevalence of periodontal disease is also higher [10].

A further set of problems may also cause halitosis, in particular severe tooth decay with extensive gaps between teeth allowing food remnants to accumulate, teeth in malalignment, exposed dental pulp with necrosis, prosthetic or orthodontic devices that are poorly fitting, coated tongue and oral candida infection [11]. Mouth cancers, such as lingual or buccal malignant neoplasms, as well as conditions that affect the mucosa, such as tuberculosis or infection with *Treponema pallidum*, may alter the microbial flora and cause malodour [12].

23.2.2 Extraoral Causes

The halitotic focus may be located in the nasal cavity, sinuses, tonsils or within the upper airway (intra-pharyngeal or intralaryngeal). A foreign body within the nasal cavity may form a focus for bacterial infection [4]. Atrophic rhinitis may result from *Klebsiella ozaenae* infection, whereas acute infection of the pharynx and sinuses is frequently the result of Streptococci. An abscess within the nasopharynx or a malignancy of the larynx both have the potential to produce halitosis as well. The tonsils possess deep crypts which may harbour the bacterial species responsible for malodorous VLCs, especially in cases of tonsillitis (both acute and chronic) and tonsilith formation [13]. Halitosis can also have a pulmonary origin, as in cases of chronic bronchitis, pulmonary abscess, cystic fibrosis or bronchiectasis. A number of respiratory pathologies are linked to the presence of *Pseudomonas aeruginosa*, a bacterium that produces the foul-smelling 2-amino-acetophenone [6]. Other causes of extraoral halitosis include gastroesophageal reflux disease (GERD) and less commonly diabetic ketoacidosis [4, 7].

23.3 Distinguishing Between Halitosis of Intra-oral and Extra-oral Origin

It is straightforward for a trained observer to distinguish between halitosis of intra- and extra-oral origin by comparing the smell of breath via the nose with that coming from the oral cavity. Intra-oral halitosis will only render breath coming from the mouth objectionable. There is a theoretical possibility that an oral halitotic focus may contaminate the nasal breath since the oral and nasal cavities are in communication via the nasopharynx, but this does not appear to occur. Intra-oral halitosis may also be characterised by exhalation of VSCs, notably hydrogen sulphide and methyl-mercaptan. These compounds have not been isolated from nasal breath samples in individuals whose halitotic focus was outside the mouth [14].

23.4 ENT Infections and Halitosis

ENT infections causing halitosis can be classified depending on the region involved: intraoral (such as tonsillitis), nasal or nasopharyngeal (adenoiditis and rhinosinusitis) and hypopharyngeal.

23.4.1 Tonsillitis

The faucial tonsils contribute to Waldeyer's ring, a ring of immune defences encircling the naso- and oro-pharynx and guarding the entrance to the aerodigestive tract. This location permits the tonsils to encounter antigenic material in the form of airborne particles, food and drink and microbes entering the tract. In paediatric tonsillitis, the appearance of the tonsils resembles a cauliflower. There may also be deep grooves resulting from entrapped food particles. As the food is degraded, an unpleasant odour is released. Individuals whose tonsils feature large grooves may experience halitosis when they eat particular foods (such as pistachio nuts, other nuts or dried fruits) as these foods are liable to become lodged in the grooves. The grooves, formed by the intersecting tonsillar crypts, form a very suitable environment for anaerobes to thrive in the upper airways [15, 16]. The tonsil is the site of continuous immune activity, including a low-grade inflammatory response, due to the presence of these bacteria. There may, however, be no symptoms and thus the case fails to come to clinical attention. The ongoing inflammation within the tonsil can result in halitosis in a similar way to the bacterial tongue coating [15–17].

There are multiple reports in the literature which conclude that removal of the tonsils is beneficial in treating halitosis caused by chronic tonsillitis [18, 19]. Tonsillar radio-frequency ablation has been shown to reduce halitosis [18]. A different study examined how severe doctors, patients, partners or other relatives considered bad breath. This study also made use of Finkelstein's test where the tonsils are massaged and any discharge smelled. The values were then compared with those obtained 4 and 8 weeks after surgery. Prior to surgery, Finkelstein test was positive for 86.3% of cases, and 100% when the test was subsequently repeated. At baseline, 95.5% of patients had an awareness of bad breath, and in 40.9% of cases, there was a caseous discharge noted from time to time. At a point 8 weeks after tonsillectomy, 79.5% of patients felt their bad breath had completely resolved and 20.4% felt it had somewhat reduced. Every patient in the trial reported that the Finkelstein test was negative [19].

23.4.2 Gingivitis and Inadequate Mouth Hygiene

There exists a number of points within the oral cavity where particles of food may remain stuck. Microbial degradation of these particles may produce halitosis. Examples of such points are the dental surfaces, the dental fissures and the interdental spaces and periodontal spaces. The tongue also contains pores which may be plugged by debris. Inadequate attention to mouth hygiene in paediatric patients is a matter of grave concern. Poor hygiene may cause dental caries, including areas lying underneath a filling or crown. Halitosis may occur in children whose parents neglect their oral health, in children who do not brush their teeth frequently enough or in those children whose diet consists of sticky and sugar-laden food [20, 21].

23.4.3 Sinus Infection

It is very common for the sinuses to be infected in children. Sinusitis results in discharge into the nasal cavity and pharynx, which provides suitable conditions for microbial overgrowth to occur. This results in halitosis that fails to resolve, even with exemplary oral hygiene, such as daily brushing and mouthwash [22]. One study which evaluated the benefit in functional endoscopic surgery in 52 paediatric cases (average age 7.4 years) of chronic sinusitis noted that 90% (47 children) had purulent rhinorrhoea, while 63% (33 children) suffered from postnasal discharge. Two-thirds of the cases (67%, 35 children) suffered from offensive-smelling breath. Following operative intervention, halitosis ceased altogether in 34 cases (66%) and was less noticeable in 5 cases (9%). Ascribing causality in this study was complicated by the fact that antimicrobials were administered post-operatively, and thus either intervention or both interventions may be responsible.

23.4.4 Nasal Foreign Body

Children frequently insert small objects (beads, toys, food) into their nasal cavity out of curiosity. These foreign bodies, if they become lodged in the nasal cavity, may form a focus for bacterial infection and result in halitosis. A key presenting feature of a nasal foreign body is unilateral purulent rhinorrhoea. Foreign body insertion by a child is particularly common in younger children [20].

23.4.5 Mouth Breathing

Mouth breathing causes the oral cavity to become dry. Saliva can no longer perform its normal function of washing the cavity. This situation leads to microbial overgrowth and production of unpleasant odours. Thus, snoring or mouth breathing during sleep are frequently associated with halitosis [20].

23.4.6 Malocclusion

If teeth are not contained within the dental arch, suffer from crowding or malposition, or are crooked, they have an increased risk of undergoing premature decay and may contribute to halitosis. Accordingly, even in the absence of carious disease, the dentition may contribute to halitosis if teeth have an abnormal shape or there are gaps between the teeth [23].

23.4.7 Poor-Quality Dental Fillings and Dentures

Unless a dental restoration (whether an amalgam filling or composite-type) conforms properly to the dental anatomy, it will be impossible to keep clean either by brushing or flossing between the teeth and food will tend to be impacted, leading to halitosis. The only cure in this situation is replacement of the restoration [23].

23.5 Assessment of Halitosis

The first consideration is to exclude potential pseudo-halitosis and halitophobia, for which the treatment is psychological. There are a variety of ways to screen for genuine halitosis, including organoleptic assessment by the clinician, gas chromatographic measurement, sulphide detection, BANA testing, quantification of activity by beta-galactosidase, the saliva incubation test, measurement of ammonia and ninhydrin testing.

23.5.1 Direct Methods Used to Detect Halitosis

23.5.1.1 Organoleptic Detection

Organoleptic detection is the most straightforward method and the most frequently employed. It simply calls for the placement of a plastic tube in the oral cavity of the patient. The doctor then smells the breath coming out of the tube, and grades it according to a scale ranging from zero to five:

- Grade 0 indicates the clinician cannot detect any malodour.
- Grade 1 indicates a barely detectable malodour.
- Grade 2 indicates a slight but definitely detectable malodour.
- Grade 3 indicates the malodour is clearly noticeable.
- Grade 4 malodour is powerful.
- Grade 5 malodour is somewhat overpowering [24].

The advantages of the organoleptic test are its low cost and ability to be performed without specialist equipment. However, it may be unpleasant for the examining physician.

23.5.1.2 Gas Chromatographic Analysis

Gas chromatographic analysis permits an estimation of the levels of VSCs present, even where their level is extremely low. Saliva, tongue coating or any oral sample are suitable. The VSCs detected include dimethyl sulphide, methyl mercaptan, and hydrogen sulphide. This method enjoys considerable reliability, but it is unfortunately costly to perform, not portable and can only be carried out by staff with appropriate training. These limitations mean it is confined to academic or research settings. One further drawback is that it cannot detect molecules of types other than VSCs, which may be responsible for halitosis [25, 26].

23.5.1.3 Portable Monitoring of Sulphides

There are portable detectors available which test for sulphides. To perform the test, have the patient keep a disposable tube within the mouth for 5 min and breathe only via the nose. The detector can identify VSCs in exhaled air and gives an appropriate reading. Like gas chromatography, though, it is limited by the inability to detect molecules causing halitosis that are not VSCs [27, 28].

23.5.2 Indirect Methods Used to Detect Halitosis

23.5.2.1 Benzoyl-DL-Arginine-Alpha-Naphthylamide (BANA)

The BANA test is an easily performed and rapid way to identify the presence of certain pathogenic bacteria. If proteolytic, obligatorily anaerobic species such as *Porphyromonas gingivalis*, *Treponema denticola*, and *Tannerella forsythia*, which can cause halitosis, are present, bacterial trypsin turns BANA red. In this way,

BANA can demonstrate that such microbes are present, particularly on the lingual dorsum or in plaque form under the tongue [29].

23.5.2.2 Ammonia Monitoring

To monitor ammonia levels, a significant contributor to halitosis, a single-use tube is used, connected to a pump. The equipment used can measure the quantity of ammonia within the sample [30, 31].

23.5.2.3 Ninhydrin Technique

The ninhydrin technique is an easily performed and rapid way to identify amines and polyamines present in halitosis. Isopropanol is needed to perform the test [32].

23.5.2.4 Salivary Incubation Test

Salivary incubation allows for greater sensitivity in detecting halitosis, but cannot be performed instantly in clinic. A sample of saliva from the patient is anaerobically incubated at body temperature for several hours, which allows any malodour present to increase to more easily detectable levels [25].

23.5.2.5 Quantification of Beta-Galactosidase Activity

Beta-galactosidase activity is strongly implicated in causing halitosis. A sample of saliva is added to a paper disc and the colour change in the paper indicates the level of enzymatic activity [25, 33].

23.5.2.6 Polymerase Chain Reaction

Increasingly, bacterial PCR testing is replacing methods which rely on the detection of VSCs. It is a rapid technique with a high level of both sensitivity and specificity [34].

23.6 Conclusion

Halitosis may be a problem of which a person is unaware. Therefore, it usually depends on family, friends and caregivers noticing it. While the majority of cases are relatively benign, long-term damage can accrue due to halitosis; hence prompt diagnosis and appropriate treatment are essential to ensure minimal harm to a person's health [18].

References

1. Guedes CC, Bussadori SK, CostadaMota AC, Amancio OMS. Halitosis: prevalence and association with oral etiological factors in children and adolescents. J Breath Res. 2019;13:026002. https://doi.org/10.1088/1752-7163/aafc6f.
2. Tungare S, Zafar N, Paranjpe AG. Halitosis. Treasure Island, FL: StatPearls Publishing; 2020.

3. De Geest S, Laleman I, Teughels W, Dekeyser C, Quirynen M. Periodontal diseases as a source of halitosis: a review of the evidence and treatment approaches for dentists and dental hygienists. Periodontol. 2016;71:213–27. https://doi.org/10.1111/prd.12111.

4. Struch F, Schwahn C, Wallaschofski H, Grabe HJ, Völzke H, Lerch MM, Meisel P, Kocher T. Self-reported halitosis and gastro-esophageal reflux disease in the general population. J Gen Intern Med. 2008;23(3):260–6.

5. Porter SR, Scully C. Oral malodour (halitosis). BMJ. 2006;333(7569):632–5.

6. Yaegaki K, Coil JM. Examination, classification, and treatment of halitosis; clinical perspectives. J Can Dent Assoc. 2000;66(5):257–61.

7. Scully C, Greenman J. Halitology (breath odour: aetiopathogenesis and management). Oral Dis. 2012;18(4):333–45.

8. Porter SR. Diet and halitosis. Curr Opin Clin Nutr Metab Care. 2011;14:463–8. https://doi.org/10.1097/MCO.0b013e328348c054.

9. Silva MF, Leite FRM, Ferreira LB, et al. Estimated prevalence of halitosis: a systematic review and meta-regression analysis. Clin Oral Invest. 2018;22:47–55. https://doi.org/10.1007/s00784-017-2164-5.

10. Petersen PE, Ogawa H. The global burden of periodontal disease: towards integration with chronic disease prevention and control. Periodontol. 2012;60:15–39.

11. Tulupov DA, Bakhmutov DN, Karpova EP. Halitosis concomitant with chronic ENT pathology in children. Vestn Otorinolaringol. 2013;5:59–61.

12. Aylıkcı BU, Colak H. Halitosis: from diagnosis to management. J Nat Sci Biol Med. 2013;4(1):14–23.

13. Fletcher SM, Blair PA. Chronic halitosis from tonsilloliths: a common etiology. J La State Med Soc. 1988 Jun;140(6):7–9.

14. Tangerman A, Winkel EG. Extra-oral halitosis: an overview. J Breath Res. 2010;4:017003.

15. Ferguson M, Aydın M, Mickel J. Halitosis and the tonsils: a review of management. Otolaryngol Head Neck Surg. 2014;151(4):567–74.

16. Rio AC, Franchi-Teixeira AR, Nicola EM. Relationship between the presence of tonsilloliths and halitosis in patients with chronic caseous tonsillitis. Br Dent J. 2008;204:E4.

17. Myers NE, Compliment JM, Post JC, Buchinsky FD. Tonsilloliths a common finding in pediatric patients. Nurse Pract. 2006;31:53–4.

18. Tanyeri HM, Polat S. Temperature-controlled radiofrequency tonsil ablation for the treatment of halitosis. Eur Arch Otorhinolaryngol. 2011;268:267–72.

19. Al-Abbasi AM. Tonsillectomy for the treatment of halitosis. Niger J Med. 2009;18:295–8.

20. Karimi M. The causes of Holitosis in children. Pediatr Dent Care. 2016;2:1. https://doi.org/10.4172/2573-444X.1000132.

21. Ferguson M, Aydin M, Mickel J. Halitosis and the tonsils: a review of management. Otolaryngol Head Neck Surg. 2014;151:567–74.

22. Vandenberg SJ, Heatley DG. Efficacy of adenoidectomy in relieving symptoms of chronic sinusitis in children. Arch Otolaryngol Head Neck Surg. 1997 Jul;123(7):675–8.

23. Froum SJ, Rodriguez Salaverry K. The dentists role in diagnosis and treatment of halitosis. Compend Contin Educ Dent. 2013;34:670–5.

24. Greenman J, Duffield J, Spencer P, Rosenberg M, Corry D, Saad S, Lenton P, Majerus G, Nachmani S, El-Maaytah M. Study on the organoleptic intensity scale for measuring oral malodor. J Dent Res. 2004;83(1):81–5.

25. van den Broek AM, Feenstra L, de Baat C. A review of the current literature on aetiology and measurement methods of halitosis. J Dent. 2007;35(8):627–35.

26. Salako NO, Philip L. Comparison of the use of the Halimeter and the Oral Chroma™ in the assessment of the ability of common cultivable oral anaerobic bacteria to produce malodorous volatile sulfur compounds from cysteine and methionine. Med Princ Pract. 2011;20(1):75–9.

27. Rosenberg M, McCulloch CA. Measurement of oral malodor: current methods and future prospects. J Periodontol. 1992;63(9):776–82.

28. Kozlovsky A, Goldberg S, Natour I, Rogatky-Gat A, Gelernter I, Rosenberg M. Efficacy of a 2-phase oil: water mouthrinse in controlling oral malodor, gingivitis, and plaque. J Periodontol. 1996;67(6):577–82.
29. Shimura M, Yasuno Y, Iwakura M, Shimada Y, Sakai S, Suzuki K, Sakamoto S. A new monitor with a zinc-oxide thin film semiconductor sensor for the measurement of volatile sulfur compounds in mouth air. J Periodontol. 1996;67(4):396–402.
30. Toda K, Li J, Dasgupta PK. Measurement of ammonia in human breath with a liquid-film conductivity sensor. Anal Chem. 2006;78(20):7284–91.
31. Amano A, Yoshida Y, Oho T, Koga T. Monitoring ammonia to assess halitosis. Oral Surg Oral Med Oral Pathol Oral Radiol Endod. 2002;94(6):692–6.
32. Iwanicka-Grzegorek K, Lipkowska E, Kepa J, Michalik J, Wierzbicka M. Comparison of ninhydrin method of detecting amine compounds with other methods of halitosis detection. Oral Dis. 2005;11(Suppl 1):37–9.
33. Yoneda M, Masuo Y, Suzuki N, Iwamoto T, Hirofuji T. Relationship between the β-galactosidase activity in saliva and parameters associated with oral malodor. J Breath Res. 2010;4(1):017108.
34. Kamaraj RD, Bhushan KS, Vandana KL. An evaluation of microbial profile in halitosis with tongue coating using PCR (polymerase chain reaction)- a clinical and microbiological study. J Clin Diagn Res. 2014 Jan;8(1):263–7.

Facial Paralysis in Children

24

Sena Genç Elden, Deniz Demir, and Chae-Seo Rhee

24.1 Introduction

Facial paralysis in children is a condition that requires urgent intervention in otorhinolaryngology practice and appropriate treatment should be initiated as soon as possible. The incidence of acquired peripheral facial paralysis in children is between 5 and 21 per 100,000 per year [1]. Facial paralysis is divided into peripheral and central according to the nerve damage regions [2]. Facial paralysis in children can occur due to congenital or acquired causes and may be a sign of a serious underlying disease. The quality of life of the child is generally negatively affected by its aesthetic and functional effects.

Scottish scientist Sir Charles Bell defined the "weakness" of the facial nerve in 1821 [1]. Since then, there has been controversy over the causes and treatment of facial paralysis.

24.2 Etiology and Epidemiology

Facial paralysis in children can occur due to idiopathic causes, congenital causes, infection, neoplasia, metabolic causes, traumatic events, or inflammation (Table 24.1) [3, 4].

S. G. Elden (✉)
Section of Otorhinolaryngology, Hendek State Hospital, Hendek, Sakarya, Turkey

D. Demir
Department of Otorhinolaryngology, Faculty of Medicine, Sakarya University, Sakarya, Turkey

C.-S. Rhee
Department of Otorhinolaryngology, Head and Neck Surgery, College of Medicine, Seoul National University, Seoul, Korea

© The Author(s), under exclusive license to Springer Nature Switzerland AG 2022
C. Cingi et al. (eds.), *Pediatric ENT Infections*,
https://doi.org/10.1007/978-3-030-80691-0_24

Table 24.1 Etiology of facial paralysis

	Infectious:
Idiopathic	• Acute otitis media.
• Bell's palsy.	• Chronic otitis media/ cholesteatoma.
Congenital	• Ramsay Hunt syndrome.
• Birth trauma.	• Epstein-Barr virus.
• Melkersson-Rosenthal syndrome.	• Haemophilus influenzae.
• Albers-Schönberg disease (Osteopetrosis).	• Lyme disease.
• Möbius syndrome.	• Cytomegalovirus.
• Goldenhar syndrome (Oculoauriculovertebral dysplasia).	• Adenovirus.
• Syringobulbia.	• Rubella.
• Arnold-Chiari syndrome.	• Mumps.
• Hereditary congenital facial paresis 1.	• Mycoplasma pneumoniae.
• Hereditary congenital facial paresis 2.	• Human immunodeficiency virus.
• Branchio-Oto-renal syndrome.	• Cat scratch.
• Hereditary myopathies.	
• Teratogenesis.	
Traumatic	Inflammatory
• Temporal bone fractures.	• Henoch-Schönlein purpura.
• Iatrogenic.	• Kawasaki syndrome.
Hypertension associated	• Temporal arteritis.
	• Periarteritis Nodosa.
	• Guillain-Barre syndrome.
	• Sarcoidosis.

24.2.1 Idiopathic (Bell's Palsy)

Paralysis is idiopathic in approximately 50% of cases and is described as Bell Palsy [4]. In children between the ages of 1 and 15, Bell's Palsy is seen with a frequency of 6.1 per 100,000 per year [5]. Herpes simplex 1 virus (HSV) is thought to be involved in the etiology, but the definite cause is unknown [4]. In patients with facial paralysis, HSV has been detected in the geniculate ganglion and postauricular muscle [6]. It is thought that the nerve is damaged due to compression caused by HSV reactivation in the geniculate ganglion and associated neuronal inflammation and edema [6, 7].

24.2.2 Congenital Causes

Congenital facial paralysis may occur due to birth trauma or developmental defects. The most common cause is birth trauma [4]. Birth weight of more than 3500 grams, use of forceps, or prematurity increase the risk of traumatic facial paralysis [8]. It usually has a favorable prognosis and the facial nerve is completely recovered within a few months without any sequelae.

Due to possible vascular or genetic factors, developmental abnormalities include aplasia or hypoplasia of nerve nuclei, abnormalities in facial nerve, and primary myopathy [9]. Facial paralysis can be seen with other organ pathologies and the recovery rate is very low [10].

24.2.3 Melkersson-Rosenthal Syndrome

Typical features of this disease are peripheral facial paralysis, episodic facial edema, and fissured tongue. It mostly starts in childhood and can be familial and sporadic [11]. Patients may show all the features, suffer the symptoms sequentially, or have only one part of the syndrome [3].

24.2.4 Moebius Syndrome

The prevalence of Moebius syndrome is approximately 1 /150,000 [4]. Moebius syndrome is a clinical condition caused by unilateral or bilateral congenital facial paralysis with abducens (cranial nerve VI) function abnormalities. Other cranial nerve anomalies may accompany [9].

24.2.5 Albers-Schönberg Disease (Osteopetrosis)

Due to hereditary defect in osteoclastic activity, the balance in bone formation is disturbed in favor of osteoblastic activity, and therefore the nerve foramina is compressed and facial paralysis occurs [3].

24.2.6 Goldenhar Syndrome

Facial development anomalies such as facial paralysis, maxillary–mandibular hypoplasia, and hemifacial microsomia are seen in Goldenhar syndrome [3].

24.2.7 Hereditary Congenital Facial Paresis

Hereditary congenital facial paresis is an isolated dysfunction of the facial nerve [9]. It is a rare clinical condition with autosomal dominant inheritance and characterized by ptosis and facial asymmetry [12].

24.2.8 Infectious Causes

In a study conducted in the USA, it was determined that 1/3 of children with facial paralysis were due to infectious causes [3].

24.2.8.1 Herpes Simplex Virus (HSV)

Herpes simplex virus (HSV) activation is the likely cause of Bell's Palsy. The findings obtained from studies conducted show that HSV-1 DNA ratios in saliva and tears of patients with Bell's Palsy are increased compared to controls [13].

In another study, while HSV-1 genomes were identified in the facial nerve and postauricular muscle in 11 of 14 patients who underwent decompression surgery for Bell's Palsy, HSV-1 genomes were not found in the control group [14].

24.2.8.2 Ramsay Hunt Syndrome

This syndrome is caused by the reactivation of the varicella zoster virus (VZV) latent in the geniculate ganglion [15]. It is typically characterized by ipsilateral facial paralysis, ear pain, and vesicles in the external auditory canal or auricle, while vestibulocochlear signs such as taste disturbance, tinnitus, hearing loss, hyperacusis, and vertigo can be seen [6]. The prevalence of this syndrome 10 years of age is reported as 2,7/100000 [4].

Primary infection of VZV causes chickenpox. VZV in the auricle or vesicles on the tongue then migrates to the geniculate ganglion, where the facial nerve remains latent with its sensory branches [16].

If a woman becomes infected with chickenpox during pregnancy, the fetus may become infected in the uterus and Ramsay Hunt syndrome may develop in the infant period [16]. Balatsouras et al. reported Ramsay Hunt syndrome in a 3-month-old baby whose mother was infected with chickenpox in the second trimester of pregnancy, who recovered without medical treatment [16, 17]. Chickenpox in infancy is considered as one of the important risk factors for childhood zoster [15].

24.2.8.3 Lyme Disease

Lyme is a spirochetal disease caused by Borrelia Burgdorferi. The disease is known to cause erythema chronicum migrans, meningopolyneuritis, myocardial conduction abnormalities, and Lyme arthritis [11]. Lyme disease is a major cause of facial paralysis in children in areas where this tick-borne spirochete infection is common [4]. The annual incidence of Lyme disease in the USA is about 300000 people, with most cases originating in the Northeast and Upper Midwest of the country [18]. Facial paralysis is the most common neurological symptom of Lyme disease [19]. Children with Lyme disease show bilateral facial paralysis more frequently than adults [20]. Since Lyme disease is the most common known cause of pediatric bilateral facial paralysis, a patient presenting with such clinical signs should be considered to have Lyme disease, especially in endemic areas, until proven otherwise [18].

Lyme disease diagnosis is based on at least one of the following findings:

1. Positive serum or CSF antibody levels against Borrelia burgdorferi.
2. Erythema migrans in the patient's history or concurrent with facial paralysis.
3. A positive PCR test.

Erythema migrans is defined as an enlarging erythematous lesion that is at least 5 cm in diameter [19]. However, if a history of previous systemic or dermatological findings is consistent with Lyme disease, serology testing should not delay initiation of the appropriate empirical antibiotic [18].

24.2.8.4 Human Immunodeficiency Virus (HIV) Infection

Acute peripheral facial paralysis, similar to Bell Palsy, may occur as the first and only symptom of asymptomatic HIV infection. The incidence of peripheral facial paralysis in people with HIV infection is 100 times higher than in the normal population [21].

The pathogenesis of facial paralysis in HIV infection has remained unclear [21]. HIV is usually neurotrophic and can cause edema of the nerve fibers in the facial nerve or geniculate ganglion, resulting in an increase in the brain MRI signal of the affected facial nerve [22]. While Bell Palsy or Guillain Barre syndrome may develop in the early stages of HIV, cellular immunity decreases in the late period and herpes zoster-associated facial paralysis, facial nerve involvement secondary to meningeal lymphomatosis, and various chronic peripheral neuropathies may also occur [22].

24.2.8.5 Facial Paralysis from Bacterial Infection

Facial paralysis can be caused by acute otitis media, chronic otitis media, or necrotizing otitis externa [11]. Only 0.005% of otitis media patients develop facial paralysis [3]. There are three theories explaining facial paralysis in otitis media. First, infection retrograde from the tympanic cavity to the fallopian canal or chorda tympani in the early stage can cause viral reactivation. Second, bacterial inflammatory toxins cause demyelination of the facial nerve. In the advanced stage, inflammation can cause inflammation and compression of the facial nerve in the fallopian canal [3]. In chronic otitis media, a cholesteatoma can give rise to erosion of the fallopian canal with the direct spread of the infection [3, 11]. Cholesteatoma should be suspected, especially if the onset of paralysis is progressive [11]. Bacterial infection in the middle ear is usually easily diagnosed by simple examination of the external auditory canal and tympanic membrane. Computed tomography (CT) scanning may allow better visualization of the anatomy of the facial nerve along the petrous part of the temporal bone.

In immunocompromised patients with otitis externa, a necrotizing chronic infection that spreads through the vascular and facial planes may occur and cause skull base cellulitis and facial paralysis [11].

Studies have revealed that it may be complicated by facial paralysis in children with tuberculous meningitis, Salmonella typhi meningitis, and meningococcal meningitis [1].

24.2.8.6 Cat Scratch Disease

Cat scratch disease is a common reason of lymphadenitis caused by infection with the pleomorphic gram-negative bacillus Bartonella henselae. The cause of facial paralysis in this disease is due to inflammation in the parotid gland and compression of the facial nerve by lymphadenitis developing in the preauricular region [23].

Other infectious agents that may cause facial paralysis in children are cytomegalovirus, Epstein-Barr virus, adenovirus, Human Herpes Virus-6, rubella, mumps, echovirus, coxsackievirus, and Mycoplasma pneumoniae [24, 25].

24.2.9 Neoplastic Causes

Facial paralysis lasting more than 3 weeks and progressing gradually, failure to improve within 6 months, ipsilateral recurrence, hemifacial spasm, other accompanying associated cranial neuropathies, and clinical features such as pain and single branch involvement should raise suspicion of neoplastic etiology.

In 1990, malignancy was found in 12% of the patients admitted to a pediatric hospital with idiopathic facial nerve palsy [3]. Rare primary tumors of the facial nerve include neurinoma and hemangioma. More often, facial paralysis emerges as a symptom in patients with central nervous system tumors, head and neck tumors, rhabdomyosarcoma, Burkitt's lymphoma, middle ear primary lymphoma, and more [6]. In a small number of cases in children it may present as a symptom of leukemia [26].

24.2.10 Other Conditions

- Facial paralysis can be seen in inflammatory pathologies such as Henoch-Schönlein purpura, Kawasaki syndrome, Temporal Arteritis, Periarteritis Nodosa, Guillain-Barre syndrome, and Sarcoidosis [4, 7].
- Temporal region, facial or skull trauma may cause facial paralysis in children. In addition, iatrogenic paralysis may occur after parotid gland surgery or otologic procedures. Approximately 20% of peripheral facial paralysis cases are caused by trauma [3, 4].
- Facial paralysis due to hypertension is rarely seen in children. When this reason is ignored, steroids used in treatment cause the progression of hypertension and delay the diagnosis. Facial paralysis was observed as the first symptom in an infant with hypertension due to aortic stenosis [6]. According to autopsy studies, hypertension causes facial paralysis by causing bleeding in the facial nerve canal [3].
- When neonatal asymmetric crying faces are present, they can be caused by congenital unilateral lower lip paralysis due to congenital hypoplasia of the depressor angularis oris muscle, and this can mimic congenital facial paralysis [9].

24.3 Diagnosis

24.3.1 History and Physical Examination

A detailed history should be taken, and a systemic and neurological examination should be performed for every patient presenting with facial paralysis. In the history, when the complaint started, the rate of development, associated symptoms, presence of systemic disease, signs of infection, travel to areas endemic for Lyme and trauma should be questioned.

Facial paralysis is usually characterized by a sudden onset of paralysis or weakness in the facial muscles. In peripheral facial paralysis, facial movement is evaluated by observing the response to commands to close the eyes, raise eyebrows, frown, show teeth, wrinkle lips, and stretch the soft tissues of the neck. In physical examination, flattening of the forehead and nasolabial fold, eyebrow sagging, inability to close the eye, and a pulled mouth on the unaffected side are observed [6]. The degree of paralysis is classified according to the House-Brackmann grading system [27]. (Table 24.2) In young children, this examination is difficult, and it is necessary to follow the child spontaneously and while crying. In crying babies, there is a disability to close the eyelid on the affected side and the mouth angle is seen to be pulled towards the unaffected side. Additional symptoms such as hyperacusis, reduced tears, or reduced taste may aid in the localization of the lesion [3]. During eye closure, the eye turns up and in on the affected side, and this is called the Bell phenomenon [6].

Peripheral facial paralysis is usually unilateral and less than 2% is seen bilaterally [18]. The most common causes of bilateral facial paralysis in adults and children are Lyme disease, trauma, and Bell Palsy [18]. Forehead muscle movements are preserved in central facial paralysis. This indicates a central lesion, and an evaluation of intracranial pathology is required.

Bell Palsy is an exclusion diagnosis, so a diagnosis is made after other possible causes have been ruled out [5]. Therefore, neurological signs and symptoms suggesting that other structures of the central or peripheral nervous system are involved,

Table 24.2 House-Brackmann facial nerve grading system

Grade 1. Normal	Normal facial function
Grade 2. Mild	Mild weakness noticed only on close inspection; eyes can be closed with minimal effort; slight asymmetry with laughing at maximal effort.
Grade 3. Moderate	Apparent weakness that does not lead to disfiguration; may not be able to raise an eyebrow; the eye can be completely closed with maximal effort; there is a strong but asymmetrical mouth movement; synkinesis, which is obvious but does not lead to disfiguration; there is a mass movement or spasm.
Grade 4. Moderately severe	Apparent and disfigurable weakness; can not be raised eyebrows; the eye cannot be completely closed with maximal effort and mouth movements are asymmetrical; severe synkinesis, mass movement or spasm.
Grade 5. Severe	Barely noticeable movement; the eye cannot be completely closed, there is slight movement in the corner of the mouth; Synkinesis, contracture and spasm are generally absent.
Grade 6. Total paralysis	No movement

the presence of systemic disease, signs of systemic infection, findings suggesting the presence of otitis media, an examination of the external auditory canal, membranes, and oropharyngeal cavities, especially herpes zoster vesicles, are other factors that need to be measured. If facial paralysis is noticed immediately after birth, questions should be asked about prolonged labor, use of forceps, or a history of facial and periauricular ecchymosis. The patient should be examined for signs of craniofacial dysmorphism or other syndromes.

24.3.2　Laboratory Testing

Diagnosis is made primarily based on anamnesis and physical examination. Laboratory tests and imaging methods are not routinely required in every case. Those who have a specific treatment, such as for Lyme disease, and who live or have a history of travel to the area where Lyme disease is endemic, should be confirmed by serological testing and Western blot for anti-Borrelial antibodies [18]. We can diagnose the patient we suspect of Ramsay Hunt syndrome with an enzyme-linked immunosorbent test (ELISA) that looks for the antibody titer against Herpes Varicella-Zoster. Likewise, we can use ELISA and western blot methods if we suspect HIV infection.

24.3.3　Topographic Tests

The Schirmer test, stapes reflex, taste test, and saliva secretion test, which are topographic tests used in facial paralysis, are intended to determine the level of facial nerve damage [9].

24.3.4　Audiological Evaluation

We evaluate the eighth cranial nerve function with an audiogram. Unilateral sensorineural hearing loss raises the suspicion of a pontocerebellar corner tumor, while conductive hearing loss raises suspicion of middle ear disease. The stapedial reflex test is helpful for stapedius muscle function to determine the lesion site [11].

24.3.5　Lumbar Puncture

Lumbar puncture is recommended in children with cranial nerve palsy if clinical meningitis such as severe or prolonged headache, fever, papilledema, or neck stiffness is suspected. In cases of facial paralysis associated with meningitis, analysis of cerebrospinal fluid may reveal an increased white blood cell count or protein. In the cerebrospinal fluid analysis in Lyme disease, lymphocytic pleocytosis, protein elevation, or association is seen. Antibody level in CSF is more specific than serum antibody level [3].

24.3.6 Electrodiagnostic Studies

These tests are important in determining the neurophysiological status of the facial nerve, the prognosis of paralysis, or the indication for further interventions, including surgical decompression [11, 28].

- Nerve Excitability Test (NET): This is the simplest test to show facial nerve damage. The difference between both sides is evaluated. The difference between the two sides in this test is important in determining the prognosis. A difference of more than 3.5 mA indicates a poor prognosis. However, the most important disadvantages of this test are that the results may vary depending on the person who performs it and that it is not useful for bilateral lesions [28, 29].
- Maximal Stimulation Test (MST): Maximal current is measured instead of the threshold value used in NET. The aim is to stimulate all fibrils. A comparison is made between the two sides and differences in muscle contraction are expressed as equal, decreased, or no response. Patients with a reduced response or no response are considered to have advanced degeneration. Although this test is a subjective test, it has a high prognostic value and is frequently used due to its low cost [29].
- Electroneurography (ENoG): Same as MST. Unlike this test, muscle movements are evaluated not visually, but with the bipolar electrode placed in the nasolabial sulcus, and the combined action potentials are recorded. In this way, both quantitative and objective data are obtained. Normally, the difference between the two measurements is expected to be 3%. If the decrease in the amplitude level is more than 10% on the paralyzed side compared to the healthy side, 90% of these patients are considered to have degeneration, indicating a poor prognosis [29]. It is known that ENoG is the most useful test for evaluating the early diagnosis of facial paralysis. Despite this, ENOG is an expensive test [28].
- Electromyography (EMG): In this test, the action potentials that occur during muscle contraction are recorded through the electrodes. Denervated muscles produce unintentional, spontaneous electrical potentials with lower amplitude than normal. These are called "fibrillation potential." This situation indicates degeneration in the nerve leading to the muscle. However, in axonal degeneration, 14–21 days must pass for this fibrillation to occur. Therefore, it is not meaningful to perform EMG before this period. This feature is an important disadvantage of EMG. NET and ENoG do not benefit after the loss of excitability. If fibrillation potentials that show fibers with degeneration are seen, complete recovery is not expected in most patients. Appearance of polyphasic reinnervation potentials 4–6 weeks after paralysis is a finding in favor of recovery [29, 30].

24.3.7 Imaging

Imaging should be requested for patients with Bell Palsy who do not show clinical remission and progress, in traumatic cases, in patients with acute mastoiditis, with chronic otitis media or with other neurological symptoms. MRI with gadolinium is very useful in intracranial facial nerve evaluation. Gadolinium involvement increases in the labyrinthine segment in Bell Palsy. With this technique, cerebellopontine angle (CPA) tumors and parotid tumors can be diagnosed. A high-resolution CT is particularly useful for evaluating the facial nerve in patients with chronic otitis media, undergoing mastoid surgery, and post-trauma [11, 31, 32].

24.4 Treatment

The treatment of peripheral facial paralysis, especially grade and probable cause determined [32]. Multidisciplinary approach is required in the treatment.

24.4.1 Drug Therapy

Spontaneous recovery is common in idiopathic cases. The aim of treatment is to minimize the possibility of inadequate recovery and decrease the rate of complications [4]. Steroid use early in the onset of a paralysis significantly increases the chances of a full recovery [6]. In children, it is recommended that oral corticosteroids be used within 3 days of the onset of symptoms. Many centers give a combination of steroid and antiviral therapy for idiopathic peripheral facial paralysis in adults [33]. However, there is no definitive evidence for treatment. Though there are studies showing that combined therapy is more effective [34, 35], there are also studies showing that it is not superior to steroid therapy alone [36]. The recommended treatment regimen is 1–2 mg/kg of prednisone per day for 10 days, gradually reducing the dose [4]. Theoretically, it is thought that steroids can prevent nerve damage with their antiedematous properties [33].

In Ramsay Hunt syndrome, antivirals should be added to the treatment and treatment should be started as soon as possible from 2 years old. In treatment, 80 mg/kg acyclovir is given every 6 h for 5 days or 20 mg/kg valaciclovir three times a day in children older than 12 years, up to a maximum of 1000 mg three times a day [4]. When treatment is started in the first 72 h after the onset of symptoms, the complete recovery rate is 75% [4, 16].

In children whose eyes cannot be fully closed, application of artificial eye drops is required many times and eyelid closure at night. Once the eyelid patch is made, make sure the eyelid is closed under the patch [3, 32].

Antibiotic or antiviral treatment should be started immediately if facial paralysis is thought to be caused by infectious diseases. For example, an empirical oral therapy for Borrelia should be strongly considered while awaiting results of titers if the patient has come from or visited a Lyme endemic area, even if there are no associated signs or symptoms. It is recommended to use doxycycline or amoxicillin for 21–28 days [3].

In children with acute otitis media, wide-spectrum intravenous antibiotic therapy is given along with a wide myringotomy or ventilation tube application. CT is the best method to determine the effect of middle ear pathologies on the facial nerve. These findings may require immediate surgical evaluation [32].

24.4.2 Surgery

Decompression of the labyrinthine segment of the facial nerve in patients with Bell palsy is not recommended due to the lack of systematic clinical studies and the risk of sensorineural hearing loss [4].

In children with a permanent facial paralysis, surgical techniques of dynamic facial reanimation may be considered to temporarily restore facial symmetry. Among these, the most common ones are locoregional muscle transfers and muscle and nerve grafts [4]. Although these techniques can help the child psychologically, they do not completely restore normal physiological function.

24.5 Prognosis

The prognosis may vary according to the underlying cause, the grade of paralysis, and the time of initiation of treatment [4, 33]. Since the volume of the facial nerve in the canal is smaller in children, it is less affected by the pressure caused by edema and the effect of treatment is observed faster, so the prognosis is better than for adults [33].

Bell Palsy's prognosis is very good, approximately 70%, with spontaneous recovery within 3 months, without sequelae [4]. Complete paralysis, no improvement within 3 weeks, severe pain, or reduction of >50% of compound muscle action potential has a poor prognosis [37].

The prognosis in Ramsay Hunt syndrome is worse than in Bell Palsy. In order to increase the recovery rate of facial nerve function, treatment should be started as soon as possible, and therefore early diagnosis is very important [16]. If the treatment is started within the first 3 days, there is a 75% improvement, 48% improvement within 4–7 days, and 30% improvement after 7 days [14, 16].

Congenital facial paralysis has a poor prognosis for recovery of function due to inadequate development of the facial nerve or canal. During the perinatal period, traumatic facial paralysis has an excellent prognosis. Recovery without sequelae is seen within a few months [4].

In patients with severe axon damage, recovery can be both delayed and there can be sequelae. In approximately 5% of cases, sequelae such as contracture, spasm, and synkinesis may occur [4, 37]. The sequelae that occur during the healing process of facial nerve palsy are thought to be caused by the misdirection of regenerated axons during the regeneration process of the facial nerve innervating muscles other than the mimic muscles they originally innervated. Therefore, there is twitching around the mouth when blinking, and the eye may close or blink when smiling [38]. Likewise, crocodile tear syndrome occurs as a result of misdirection between the secretory nerve fibers that innervate the salivary and tear glands [39].

References

1. Özkale Y, Erol I, Saygı S, Yılmaz İ. Overview of pediatric peripheral facial nerve paralysis: analysis of 40 patients. J Child Neurol. 2015;30(2):193–9.
2. Wang L, Wang Z, Wan C, Cai X, Zhang G, Lai C. Facial paralysis as a presenting symptom of infant leukemia: a case report and literature review. Medicine. 2018;97(51):e13673.
3. Lorch M, Teach SJ. Facial nerve palsy: etiology and approach to diagnosis and treatment. Pediatr Emerg Care. 2010;26(10):763–9.
4. Ciorba A, Corazzi V, Conz V, Bianchini C, Aimoni C. Facial nerve paralysis in children. World J Clin Cases. 2015;3(12):973.
5. Lunan R, Nagarajan L. Bell's palsy: a guideline proposal following a review of practice. J Paediatr Child Health. 2008;44(4):219–20.
6. Pavlou E, Gkampeta A, Arampatzi M. Facial nerve palsy in childhood. Brain Dev. 2011;33(8):644–50.
7. Öge AE, Kocasoy Orhan E. Çocukta Periferik Yüz Felci. In: Dervent A, Ayta S, Çokar Ö, Uludüz D, editors. Çocuk Ve Ergende Nörolojik Hastalıklara Yaklaşım Rehber Kitabı 2015. 1st ed. Ankara, Turkey: Turkish Neurological Society; 2015.
8. Laing JH, Harrison DH, Jones BM, Laing GJ. Is permanent congenital facial palsy caused by birth trauma? Arch Dis Child. 1996;74(1):56–8.
9. Terzis JK, Anesti K. Developmental facial paralysis: a review. J Plast Reconstr Aesthet Surg. 2011;64(10):1318–33.
10. Yetiser S. Non-traumatic congenital facial nerve paralysis; electroneurophysiologic evaluation of four cases. Int J Pediatr Otorhinolaryngol. 2005;69(10):1419–27.
11. Jackson CG, von Doersten PG. The facial nerve: current trends in diagnosis, treatment, and rehabilitation. Med Clin N Am. 1999;83(1):179–95.
12. Alrashdi IS, Rich P, Patton MA. A family with hereditary congenital facial paresis and a brief review of the literature. Clin Dysmorphol. 2010;19(4):198–201.
13. Khine H, Mayers M, Avner JR, Fox A, Herold B, Goldman DL. Association between herpes simplex virus-1 infection and idiopathic unilateral facial paralysis in children and adolescents. Pediatr Infect Dis J. 2008;27(5):468–9.
14. Murakami S, Mizobuchi M, Nakashiro Y, Doi T, Hato N, Yanagihara N. Bell palsy and herpes simplex virus: identification of viral DNA in endoneurial fluid and muscle. Ann Int Med. 1996;124(1_Part_1):27–30.
15. Hato N, Kisaki H, Honda N, Gyo K, Murakami S, Yanagihara N. Ramsay Hunt syndrome in children. Ann Neurol. 2000;48(2):254–6.
16. Kansu L, Yilmaz I. Herpes zoster oticus (Ramsay Hunt syndrome) in children: case report and literature review. Int J Pediatr Otorhinolaryngol. 2012;76(6):772–6.
17. Balatsouras DG, Rallis E, Homsioglou E, Fiska A, Korres SG. Ramsay Hunt syndrome in a 3-month-old infant. Pediatr Dermatol. 2007;24(1):34–7.
18. Wong K, Sequeira S, Bechtel K. Pediatric bilateral facial paralysis: an unusual presentation of Lyme disease. Pediatr Emerg Care. 2020;36(11):e651–3.
19. Peltomaa M, Saxen H, Seppälä I, Viljanen M, Pyykkö I. Paediatric facial paralysis caused by Lyme borreliosis: a prospective and retrospective analysis. Scand J Infect Dis. 1998;30(3):269–75.
20. Cook SP, Macartney KK, Rose CD, Hunt PG, Eppes SC, Reilly JS. Lyme disease and seventh nerve paralysis in children. Am J Otolaryngol. 1997;18(5):320–3.
21. Sathirapanya P, Fujitnirun C, Setthawatcharawanich S, Phabphal K, Limapichat K, Chayakul P, Silpapojakul K, Jaruratanasirikul S, Siripaitoon P, Chusri S, Kositpantawong N. Peripheral facial paralysis associated with HIV infection: a case series and literature review. Clin Neurol Neurosurg. 2018;172:124–9.
22. Kim MS, Yoon HJ, Kim HJ, Nam JS, Choi SH, Kim JM, Song YG. Bilateral peripheral facial palsy in a patient with human immunodeficiency virus (HIV) infection. Yonsei Med J. 2006;47(5):745–7.

23. Valor C, Huber K. Atypical presentation of cat scratch disease: Parinaud's oculo glandular syndrome with facial nerve paresis. Case reports 2018:bcr-2018.
24. Morgan M, Nathwani D. Facial palsy and infection: the unfolding story. Clin Infect Dis. 1992;14(1):263–71.
25. Papan C, Kremp L, Weiß C, Petzold A, Schroten H, Tenenbaum T. Infectious causes of peripheral facial nerve palsy in children—a retrospective cohort study with long-term follow-up. Eur J Clin Microbiol Infect Dis. 2019;38(11):2177–84.
26. Buyukavci M, Tan H, Akdag R. An alarming sign for serious diseases in children: bilateral facial paralysis. Pediatr Neurol. 2002;27(4):312–3.
27. House J W. Facial nerve grading systems. Laryngoscope. 1983;93(8):1056–69.
28. Ikeda M, Abiko Y, Kukimoto N, Omori H, Nakazato H, Ikeda K. Clinical factors that influence the prognosis of facial nerve paralysis and the magnitudes of influence. Laryngoscope. 2005;115(5):855–60.
29. Basut O. Fasiyal Sinir Hastalıkları. In: Koç C, editor. Kulak Burun Boğaz Hastalıkları Ve Baş Boyun Cerrahisi. 3rd ed. Ankara, Turkey: Turkish Neurological Society; 2019.
30. Sittel C, Stennert E. Prognostic value of electromyography in acute peripheral facial nerve palsy. Otol Neurotol. 2001;22(1):100–4.
31. Swartz JD, Harnsberger RH, Mukherji SK. The temporal bone: contemporary diagnostic dilemmas. Radiol Clin N Am. 1998;36(5):819–53.
32. Shargorodsky J, Lin HW, Gopen Q. Facial nerve palsy in the pediatric population. Clin Pediatr. 2010;49(5):411–7.
33. Lee Y, SooYoon H, Yeo SG, Lee EH. Factors associated with fast recovery of bell palsy in children. J Child Neurol. 2020;35(1):71–6.
34. Lee HY, Byun JY, Park MS, Yeo SG. Steroid-antiviral treatment improves the recovery rate in patients with severe Bell's palsy. Am J Med. 2013;126(4):336–41.
35. Adour KK, Ruboyianes JM, Trent CS, Von Doersten PG, Quesenberry CP Jr, Byl FM, Hitchcock T. Bell's palsy treatment with acyclovir and prednisone compared with prednisone alone: a double-blind, randomized, controlled trial. Ann Otol Rhinol Laryngol. 1996;105(5):371–8.
36. Sullivan FM, Swan IR, Donnan PT, Morrison JM, Smith BH, McKinstry B, Davenport RJ, Vale LD, Clarkson JE, Hammersley V, Hayavi S, McAteer A, Stewart K, Daly F. Early treatment with prednisolone or acyclovir in Bell's palsy. N Engl J Med. 2007;357(16):1598–607.
37. Finsterer J. Management of peripheral facial nerve palsy. Eur Arch Otorhinolaryngol. 2008;265(7):743–52.
38. Husseman J, Mehta RP. Management of synkinesis. Facial Plast Surg. 2008;24(02):242–9.
39. Yamamoto E, Nishimura H, Hirono Y. Occurrence of sequelae in Bell's palsy. Acta Oto-Laryngologica. 1987;104(Sup 446):93–6.

Snoring in Children

Taşkın Tokat, Deniz Demir, and Refika Ersu

25.1 Introduction

Snoring is a common symptom of upper airway obstruction with a prevalence varying between 3% and 12% [1, 2]. The most common risk factors for upper airway obstruction in children are hyperplasia of adenoid and/or tonsillar tissue, nasal obstruction, and obesity [3–5]. These risk factors are related to sleep-disordered breathing (SDB), which has a wide range of disease spectrum from primary snoring (PS) and upper airway resistance syndrome (UARS) to obstructive sleep apnea (OSA) [6]. Although primary snoring is considered the most benign form of SDB and is not generally treated, recent studies suggested that PS may not as benign as it was considered before [7]. Snoring children have higher oxygen saturation dip rates than those in the control group [8]. Children with PS had a tendency for hyperactivity and behavior disorders and had poor school performance which are adverse consequences of SDB in children [9]. In another study, it was observed that 37% of the children with PS developed OSA in 4 years, and 7% of them had OSA varying between mild and severe [10].

T. Tokat (✉) · D. Demir
Department of Otorhinolaryngology, Faculty of Medicine, Sakarya University, Sakarya, Turkey

R. Ersu
Section of Pediatric Sleep Medicine, Children's Hospital of Eastern Ontario, University of Ottawa, Ottawa, ON, Canada

25.2 Obstructive Sleep-Disordered Breathing and Clinical Entities

Obstructive SDB is a general definition, and SDB in childhood is defined as "a syndrome of upper airway dysfunction during sleep, characterized by snoring and/or increased respiratory effort secondary to increased upper airway resistance and pharyngeal collapsibility" [11]. The spectrum of pediatric obstructive sleep-disordered breathing varying from mild to severe includes the following:

1. Snoring is defined as making a noisy sound secondary to the vibration of the soft palate during sleep.
2. Primary snoring is defined as the presence of snoring at least three nights a week without apnea, hypopnea, frequent arousals, or gas exchange abnormalities [12].
3. Upper airway resistance syndrome is defined as sleep disturbance and frequent awakenings secondary to negative intrathoracic pressure increase during inspiration without apnea, hypopnea, or oxygen desaturation.
4. Obstructive hypoventilation is characterized by snoring and increased end-expiratory carbon dioxide partial pressure without any apnea or hypopneas.
5. Obstructive sleep apnea is described as increased obstructive apnea and hypopnea events during sleep in the presence of snoring, increased breathing effort during sleep or daytime symptoms of sleep-disordered breathing.

25.3 Epidemiology of Snoring in Children

A recent meta-analysis showed that prevalence of habitual snoring in children is 7.45% (95% confidence intervals, 5.75–9.61) [13]. The previous studies indicated that the prevalence of sleep disorders is higher in males. Obesity is a significant risk factor for SDB and having a body mass index higher than 28 kg/m^2, increased the risk of OSA 4 to 5 times in a group composed of 399 children whose ages varied between 2 and 18 of years old. The incidence of OSA determined objectively ranges between 2.2% and 3.8% [14, 15]. In two different studies evaluating the prevalence of SDB with face-to-face interviews with parents and on several symptoms during the examination, the incidence of SDB was 4.1% and 6% [16, 17].

25.4 Etiology of Snoring in Children

Pediatric snoring is caused by an increase in upper airway narrowing and upper airway collapsibility. Adenotonsillar hypertrophy is the most common reason for upper airway narrowing in the pediatric age group (Table 25.1) [18]. Obesity, dental malocclusion, frequent exposure to respiratory infections, recurrent otitis media, allergic rhinitis, and lower socioeconomic status are risk factors for snoring [19–21]. Children with micrognathia, macroglossia, craniofacial syndromes (e.g., Treacher Collins syndrome, Crouzon syndrome, Apert syndrome, Pierre Robin sequence), Down syndrome, and Mucopolysaccharidoses are also at increased risk of snoring and OSA [22].

Table 25.1 Common causes of snoring in children [65]

Adenotonsillar hypertrophy.

Rhinological causes (allergic rhinitis, vasomotor rhinitis, chronic rhinosinusitis, upper respiratory tract viral infections, polyps, turbinate hypertrophy, and deviated septum).

Obesity.

Abnormal craniofacial morphology (syndromes, dental malocclusion, retrognathia, and hypognathia).

Neuromuscular disorders (e.g., muscular dystrophy).

25.5 Pathogenesis and Mechanisms of Snoring

Upper airway patency is associated with the interaction between respiration dynamics, anatomic structures, and neuromuscular connections. Furthermore, the extent of patency is determined by the balance between the forces that narrow the airway (e.g., negative pressure during inspiration; the size, form, and relaxation of pharyngeal structures) and that supports the airway patency (e.g., pharyngeal dilator muscle tone, stiffness of pharyngeal structures) [23].

The researchers developed an upper airway resistance model to define upper airway collapsibility better by considering the airway as a stiff tube, where the collapsible part is the pharynx. Depending on this model, when there are conditions of flow limitation, maximum inspiratory airflow is identified by the pressure changes of the collapsible segment (nasal passages) rather than the trachea's pressure through the diaphragm [24]. Collapse occurs when the pressure outside the collapsible component is higher than the one inside of it. OSA occurs when there is an imbalance between collapsible airway and resisting neuromuscular compensation in children. Increased upper airway collapsibility may develop due to the conditions leading to a low muscle tone like cerebral palsy and neuromuscular disorders and inflammatory conditions like allergic rhinitis affecting upper airways [25]. The imbalance, composed of the airway forces, leads to an increase in upper airway obstruction. Upper airway obstruction in OSA disappears through awakening. Therefore the patients with OSA are characterized by the recurrent attacks of upper airway obstruction, which are recovered by awakening and increased by sleeping.

While 80% of the obstructive events in children with OSA occurs during rapid eye movement sleep (REM), 80% of the obstructive events in adults with OSA appears during non-REM sleep [26]. It is thought that the body position during sleep plays a role on obstructive events. Sleeping on the back is associated with more severe upper airway obstruction than sleeping on one side or in the prone position. The prevalence and severity of OSA are higher in children with obesity and adults, and the severity of OSA increases in parallel with increasing obesity [27]. Obese patients experience changes in their respiratory dynamics caused by a reduced functional residual capacity, airway narrowing due to an unusual tissue mass and high pressure on the neck and pharynx. To cope with the upper airway resistance due to reduced functional residual capacity and narrowing of the pharynx, respiratory effort is increased and further results in more negative pressure in the pharynx and upper airway.

Mandibular retrognathia, micrognathia and/or adenotonsillar hypertrophy, craniofacial malformations, obesity, and prematurity are the other predisposing factors in the development of OSA [28]. The children with Down syndrome develop upper airway obstruction as a result of midface hypoplasia and macroglossia. In these children, adenotonsillectomy commonly alleviates the upper airway obstruction; however, obstruction may be persistent due to the obstruction at other levels [29]. These patients may need more complicated and aggressive airway surgery methods such as tongue reduction or lingual tonsillectomy [30] or respiratory support with positive airway pressure.

25.6 Evaluation of the Snoring Children

The clinical findings of sleep-disordered breathing in children are quite different from those of adults. Snoring and mouth breathing in children are observed less compared to adults. Daytime sleepiness in children with sleep apnea is not a rule but an exception, and hypopnea are common during sleep. In contrast, hypersomnolence during the daytime due to obstructive sleep apnea in adults is more common [31]. Children with sleep-disordered breathing may present with hyperactivity, developmental retardation, and aggressive behavior instead of being sleepy [32].

Children with primary snoring do not have apneas, hypopneas, or gas exchange abnormalities due to the compensatory neuromuscular mechanisms that prevent significant airway obstruction while sleeping [33]. In UARS, there is upper airway obstruction, frequent awakenings, as well as snoring. These patients can have daytime behavior changes and hypersomnolence; however, there are no significant abnormalities in the polysomnography [34]. Obstructive sleep apnea is characterized by obstructive events on polysomnography and children with OSA can experience hypersomnolence, behavioral disorders, and hyperactivity during daytime. While the significant structural factor contributing to OSA pathogenesis in small children is adenotonsillar hypertrophy, it is considered as obesity during adolescence [35].

25.7 Diagnostic Approach to Snoring

In the snoring child's assessment, the first step is to obtain a detailed sleep history and history of daytime symptoms. The frequency of snoring by any specific triggers such as upper airway infection should be questioned. Furthermore, sleep and wake up time, sleep duration, abnormal positions during sleep, parasomnias, nocturnal enuresis, and presence of observed apneas, gasping and cyanosis should be evaluated.

Daytime symptoms including poor school performance, hyperactivity, aggressive behavior should also be investigated as they may not always be attributed to an upper airway obstruction. Daytime somnolence is a rare symptom of childhood sleep apnea but maybe seen in older children with obesity.

During physical examination, in addition to a head and neck examination, the measurements of height and weight should also be obtained. In the snoring children, mouth breathing and "hot-potato" voice occur because of tonsillar hypertrophy. Hypernasal speech and adenoid face may be observed due to adenoid hypertrophy. Examination with a flexible endoscope allows evaluation of adenoids, nasopharynx, and nasal cavity. On the other hand, tonsillar hypertrophy, macroglossia, and micrognathia are evaluated by clinical examination [36]. Nevertheless, the tongue's position, lack of child collaboration, and the factors depending on the examiner restrict these examinations' benefit for estimating the extent and location of obstruction during sleep. Atrophy in the nasal examination in inferior turbinate based on lack of airflow or inferior turbinate hypertrophy depending on turbulent flow can also be identified. Lateral naso-pharyngeal X-ray can be used as an alternative method to nasopharyngoscopy. Adenoid tissue can be detected through lateral naso-pharyngeal X-ray in children as young as 6 months of age. During naso-pharyngeal graphy, the mouth should be closed, and the head and neck should be in parallel with the vertical axis. Otherwise, retropharyngeal "pseudo mass" can develop owing to the flexion of the airway [37].

The third edition of the *International Classification of Sleep Disorders* (the American Academy of Sleep Medicine) published a clinical practice guideline that addressed the diagnosis and management of obstructive sleep apnea syndrome [38]. The guideline states that history and physical examination are insufficient in distinguishing primary snoring from OSA, and polysomnography (PSG) is a golden standard for specific diagnosis (Table 25.2). Performance of PSG in pediatric patients has similar technical properties to that of adults. However, monitoring children during PSG and interpreting PSG are different from those of adults. One of the parents

Table 25.2 OSA criteria in Children based on third edition of the International Classification of Sleep

Disorders (ICSD) (The American Academy of Sleep Medicine) [66].
A-One of these findings.
1. Snoring.
2. Labored/obstructed breathing.
3. Daytime consequences [sleepiness, hyperactivity, and so forth].
B- The PSG criterion for diagnosis requires either one or more obstructive events.
1. AHI > 1 (obstructive or mixed apnea or obstructive hypopnea).
2. Obstructive hypoventilation, manifested by. $Paco_2$. 50 mm Hg for. 25% of sleep time and the one or more of parameters of following.
Snoring.
Paradoxical thoracoabdominal movement.
Flattening of the nasal airway pressure waveform.
For diagnosis OSA must be A + B.

should also stay with the child, and an experienced sleep technician is needed. Children can be more active during sleep compared to adults. Since partial airway obstruction and obstructive hypoventilation without apnea in OSA can be observed in children, it is recommended that CO_2 pressure measurements should be performed. In adults with OSA, apnea episodes are usually followed by cortical awakening and sleep interruption, while in children with OSA, only 20%of obstructive events are associated with cortical awakening [39].

The data related to an electrocardiogram, electromyogram, electroencephalography electrooculogram, limb movements, and breathing measurements during sleep are recorded in PSG. The breathing measurements generally recorded are airflow, respiratory effort, pulse oximetry, end-tidal carbon dioxide, and rarely esophageal pressure measurements. The terms central, obstructive, and mixed apnea are also valid for children and infants. However, the prevalent criteria useful for adult patients cannot be applied to this population. Obstructive apnea is generally defined as the interruption of airflow despite chest-wall and abdomen's continual movement for at least two breathing cycles in children [40].

In childhood OSA, apnea-hypopnea periods are observed mostly during the REM period of sleep. Adult apnea is defined as the interruption of airflow for 10 s or more. During this period, adults have 2 or 3 breathing cycles. In the childhood age group, much shorter periods of apnea (during at least two breathing cycles) are scored due to the high number of physiological breathing for a minute than adults [41]. Apnea index (AI) is the number of the obstructive, central, and mixed apneas that are observed per hour of sleep (Table 25.3). Obstructive hypopnea is defined as a decrease of 30% in airflow, a decrease of more than 3% in oxygen saturation, or an arousal. Obstructive apnea-Hypopnea Index (oAHI) is the total number of obstructive apnea, mixed apnea, and hypopnea per one-hour of sleep. In childhood OSA is defined when oAHI is greater than 1/h. The patients whose oAHI ranges from 1 to 5 are considered to have a mild OSA, while those having oAHI varying between 5 and 9 are regarded to have a moderate OSA. The ones with oAHI over 10 are considered to have severe OSA [42]. Hypoventilation is diagnosed when end-tidal CO_2 pressure is >50 mmHg for more than 25% of total sleep time [43]. Alternative diagnosis methods are also used in childhood as PSG is time-consuming and costly study and the need for a trained technician, and the small number of centers limit the availability.

Obstructive apnea and hypopnea events may lead to desaturation. Pulse oximetry, measuring oxygen saturation during sleep, is an effective method for screening OSA as it is an affordable, portable, and easily applied device. However, obstructive events in children do not often lead to significant desaturation. Therefore, negative

Table 25.3 Obstructive sleep apnea severity defined by polysomnography in children

OSA severity oAHI.
None 0.
Mild 1–5.
Moderate 6–10.
Severe >10.

pulse oximetry study does not rule out obstructive sleep apnea. Movement artifacts can cause wrong desaturation measurements. The positive predictive value of pulse oximetry is 97%. Sonographic recording of snoring is the other way of evaluation, and it can be used alone or together with another method like pulse oximetry [44]. Nonetheless, the sonographic recording is inefficient for distinguishing central apnea and obstructive apnea. It is suggested that sonographic recordings should be evaluated by using pulse oximetry in adults. However, they are not commonly used during childhood. Home video recordings is another alternative method; however studies showed that they are not specific and require the intensive attention of parents [45]. Daytime nap sleep studies can be done in adults as daytime sleepiness is observed frequently. These studies are not preferred in children because apnea and hypoxia episodes are more common during REM episodes, which is rarely observed during daytime sleep [46]. As alternative diagnostic methods have limited diagnostic value for children with SDB, PSG remains as the gold standard method [47].

25.8 Treatment of Snoring

American Academy of Pediatrics (AAP) has recommended adenotonsillectomy as the first step of treatment for children with OSA and adenotonsillar hypertrophy [48]. Besides improving the results of PSG, adenotonsillectomy relieves the symptoms and improves the quality of life in these children [49]. Additionally, it is usually regarded as primary treatment option for children with SDB and complex medical conditions such as Down syndrome, obesity, and cerebral palsy, where upper airway muscles are poorly controlled [50–53]. However, in such conditions, persistent SDB is quite common following adenotonsillectomy. There is an increase in sleep quality, improvement in voice quality, improvement in growth, the disappearance of nocturnal enuresis, and improvement in the quality of life as well as behavioral and cognitive functions following adenotonsillectomy [54].

Many techniques have been developed for tonsillar excision. Cold knife, monopolar or bipolar diathermy, ligasure, and coblation are among the most commonly used ones [55]. Bleeding, pain, laryngospasm, vomiting, and dehydration are the most common and significant postoperative tonsillectomy problems. Tonsillotomy or partial tonsillectomy, or intracapsular tonsillectomy are the methods successfully applied among children with tonsillar hypertrophy. With these methods, frequency of postoperative pain is low, and therefore the operation is more comfortable for children. However, they have a high rate of recurrence than that of tonsillectomy [56]. Also, in children with recurrent tonsillitis, tonsillotomy should be avoided.

Nasal septal surgery can be taken into consideration for a severe septal deviation. While every case is evaluated individually, it is more rational to wait until the adolescent's developmental period is completed. Polyposis and inferior concha hypertrophy can obstruct the nasal airway. Thus intervention may be necessary.

For obstructive sleep apnea in children with craniofacial abnormalities (Apert's or Crouzon's syndromes), craniofacial surgery would be successful [57]. Operations like mandibular or maxillomandibular advancement and other craniofacial operations are delayed until puberty or, if possible, until adulthood due to potential complications. In patients with isolated micrognathia, the success rate has been reported to be 95.6% while success rates are lower in syndromic children [58]. Rapid maxillary expansion is another technique applied by orthodontists. The procedure is based on the principle of providing an increase in palatal transverse diameters by releasing mid-palatal suture gradually for 10–20 days after the fixation period lasting between 6 and 12 months. It has been indicated that this orthodontic treatment reduces the symptoms of USB and improves the polysomnography parameters [59].

The operations such as uvulopalatopharyngoplasty, volume reduction of soft palate via radiofrequency, hypopharyngeal and tongue-base surgery, and hyoid suspension are rarely used in snoring surgery of children, and the studies related to their benefits are insufficient.

In clinical practice, tracheostomy is mostly assigned for significant cases and syndromes in which all other treatment choices are unsuccessful. On the other hand, it can be the last resort for children with severe neurological dysfunction and severe multisystem disease. Tracheostomy has high efficiency in treating obstructive sleep apnea, but it is related to impaired quality of life [60].

25.8.1 Non-surgical Treatment Options

25.8.1.1 Corticosteroids/Leukotriene Receptor Antagonists
Intranasal steroid and leukotriene receptor antagonist seem promising in children with obstructed SDB. Children with OSA have increased expression of leukotriene C4 synthase and leukotriene receptors 1 and 2 in the upper airway. Previous studies showed a reduction in the size of adenoids with nasal steroid treatment for 6–12 weeks and/or montelukast treatment [61, 62].

25.8.2 Weight Management

The data related to the effects of weight loss on snoring in children and adolescents are insufficient. Symptoms of OSA and PSG improved through weight loss in a group of 61 adolescents followed during a treatment program of weight loss [63]. In obese children with mild adenotonsillar hypertrophy, snoring continues after adenotonsillectomy. Thus, reducing the body weight, possibly with a dietician's help, should be considered primarily for these children.

25.8.3 Continuous Positive Airway Pressure (CPAP)

CPAP is a successful method preferred in children with residual OSA after adenotonsillectomy, OSA caused by obesity, craniofacial abnormalities, neuromuscular disorders, and children who did not benefit from other treatments. The primary purpose is to prevent upper airway collapse during the respiratory cycle, improve functional residual lung capacity, and reduce respiratory effort. On the other hand, lack of equipment suitable for little children, difficulty adapting to equipment, and increasing cost may limit the benefit of CPAP [64].

References

1. Gislason T, Benediktsdottir B. Snoring, apneic episodes, and nocturnal hypoxemia among children 6 months to 6 years old. Chest. 1995;107:963–6.
2. Royal Australasian College of Physicians. Indications for tonsillectomy and adenotonsillectomy in children. A joint position paper of the Pediatrics and Child Health Division of the Royal Australasian College of Physicians and The Australian Society of Otolaryngology, Head and Neck Surgery. Sydney, RACP. 2008.
3. Guilleminault C, Pelayo R. Sleep-disordered breathing in children. Ann Med. 1998;30:350–6.
4. Olsen K, Kern EB. Nasal influences on snoring and obstructive sleep apnea. Mayo Clin Proc. 1995;65:1095–105.
5. Brooks LJ, Stephens BM, Bacevice AM. Adenoid size is related to severity but not to the number of obstructive apnea in children. J Pediatr. 1998;132:682–6.
6. Marcus CL, Brooks LJ, Draper KA, et al. Diagnosis and management of childhood obstructive sleep apnea syndrome. Pediatrics. 2012;130:e714–55.
7. Loughlin GM. Primary snoring in children – no longer benign. J Pediatr. 2009;155:306–7.
8. Ali NJ, Pitson DJ, Stradling JR. Natural history of snoring and related behaviour problems between the ages of 4 and 7 years. Arch Dis Child. 1994;71:74–6.
9. Brockmann PE, Urschitz MS, Schlaud M, et al. Primary snoring in school children: prevalence and neurocognitive impairments. Sleep Breath. 2012;16:23–9.
10. Li AM, Zhu Y, Au CT, et al. Natural history of primary snoring in school-aged children. A 4-year follow-up study. Chest. 2013;143:729–35.
11. Kaditis AG, Alonso Alvarez ML, Boudewyns A, et al. Obstructive sleep disordered breathing in 2- to 18-year-old children: diagnosis and management. Eur Respir J. 2016;47:69–94.
12. Young T, Palta M, Dempsey J, Peppard PE, Nieto FJ, Hla KM. Burden of sleep apnea: rationale, design, and major findings of the Wisconsin sleep cohort study. WMJ. 2009;108:246–9.
13. Lumeng JC, Chervin RD. Epidemiology of pediatric obstructive sleep apnea. Proc Am Thorac Soc. 2008;5:242–52.
14. Rosen CL, Larkin EK, Kirchner HL, et al. Preva- lence and risk factors for sleep-disordered breathing in 8- to 11-year-old children: associa- tion with race and prematurity. J Pediatr. 2003;142:383–9.
15. Schlaud M, Urschitz MS, Urschitz-Duprat PM, et al. The German study on sleep-disordered breathing in primary school children: epidemiological approach, representativeness of study sample, and preliminary screening results. Paediatr Perinat Epidemiol. 2004;18:431–40.
16. Spruyt K, O'Brien LM, Macmillan Coxon AP, Cluydts R, Verieye G, Ferri R. Multidimensional scaling of pediatric sleep breathing problems and bio-behavioral correlates. Sleep Med. 2006;7:269–80.
17. Johnson EO, Roth T. An epidemiologic study of sleep-disordered breathing symptoms among adolescents. Sleep. 2006;29:13–42.
18. Dayyat E, Kheirandish-Gozal L, Sans Capdevila O, Maarafeya MM, Gozal D. Obstructive sleep apnea in children: relative contributions of body mass index and adenotonsillar hypertrophy. Chest. 2009;136:137–44.
19. Gozal D, Kheirandish-Gozal L, Sans Capdevila O, Dayyat E, Kheirandish E. Prevalence of recurrent otitis media in habitually snoring school-aged children. Sleep Med. 2008;9:549–54.
20. Montgomery-Downs HE, Gozal D. Snore-associated sleep fragmentation in infancy: mental development effects and contribution of secondhand cigarette smoke exposure. Pediatrics. 2006;117:496–502.

21. Kuehni CE, Strippoli MP, Chauliac ES, Silverman M. Snoring in preschool children: prevalence, severity and risk factors. Eur Respir J. 2008;31:326–33.
22. Pham LV, Schwartz AR. The pathogenesis of obstructive sleep apnea. J Thorac Dis. 2015;7:1358–72.
23. White DP. Pathogenesis of obstructive and central sleep apnea. Am J Respir Crit Care Med. 2005;172:1363–70.
24. Jordan AS, Eckert DJ, Wellman A, Trinder JA, Malhotra A, White DP. Termination of respiratory events with and without cortical arousal in obstructive sleep apnea. Am J Respir Crit Care Med. 2011;184:1183–91.
25. Dempsey JA, Veasey SC, Morgan BJ, O'Donnell CP. Pathophysiology of sleep apnea. Physiol Rev. 2010;90:47–112.
26. Spruyt K, Gozal D. REM and NREM sleep-state distribution of respiratory events in habitually snoring school-aged community children. Sleep Med. 2012;13:178–84.
27. Trang H. Sleep-disordered breathing in obese children. Mecanisms, diagnosis and management. In: Frelut ML, editor. The ECOG's eBook on child and adolescent obesity; 2015.
28. Cielo CM, Marcus CL. Obstructive sleep apnoea in children with craniofacial syndromes. Paediatr Respir Rev. 2015;16(3):189–96.
29. Prosser JD, Shott SR, Rodriguez O, Simakajornboon N, Meinzen-Derr J, Ishman SL. Polysomnographic outcomes following lingual tonsillectomy for persistent obstructive sleep apnea in down syndrome. Laryngoscope. 2017;127(2):520–4.
30. Eskiizmir G. Lingual tonsillectomy for the management of persistent obstructive sleep apnea after adenotonsillectomy in children. Otolaryngol Head Neck Surg. 2010;142(2):301.
31. Gozal D, Wang M, Pope DW Jr. Objective sleepiness measures in pediatric obstructive sleep apnea. Pediatrics. 2001;108:693–7.
32. Messner AH. Treating pediatric patients with obstructive sleep disorders: an update. Otolaryngol Clin N Am. 2003;36:519–30.
33. Zucconi M, Bruni O. Sleep disorders in children with neurologic diseases. Semin Pediatr Neurol. 2001;8:258–70.
34. Owens JA, Spirito A, McGuinn M. The Children's sleep habits questionnaire (CSHQ): psychometric properties of a survey instrument for school-aged children. Sleep. 2000;15(23):1043–51.
35. Marcus CL, Curtis S, Koerner CB, Joffe A, Serwint JR, Loughlin GM. Evaluation of pulmonary function and polysomnography in obese children and adolescents. Pediatr Pulmonol. 1996;21:176–83.
36. Major MP, Flores-Mir C, Major PW. Assessment of lateral cephalometric diagnosis of adenoid hypertrophy and posterior upper airway obstruction: a systematic review. Am J Orthod Dentofac Orthop. 2006;130:700–8.
37. Fernbach SK, Brouillette RT, Riggs TW, Hunt CE. Radiologic evaluation of adenoids and tonsils in children with obstructive sleep apnea: plain films and fluoroscopy. Pediatr Radiol. 1983;13:258–65.
38. Sateia MJ. International classification of sleep disorders-third edition: highlights and modifications. Chest. 2014;146:1387–94.
39. Rosen CL, D'Andrea L, Haddad GG. Adult criteria for obs- tructive sleep apnea do not identify children with serious obstruction. Am Rev Respir Dis. 1992;146:1231–4.
40. Marcus CL, Omlin KJ, Basinki DJ, et al. Normal polysomnographic values for children and adolescents. Am Rev Respir Dis. 1992;146:1235–9.
41. Balbani AP, Weber SA, Montovani JC. Update in obstructive sleep apnea syndrome in children. Rev Bras Otorrinolaringol. 2005;71:74–80.
42. Esteller E, Santos P, Segarra F, Estivill E, Lopez R, Matiñó E, Ade-mà JM. Clinical and polysomnographic correlation in sleep-related breathing disorders in children. Acta Otorrinolaringol Esp. 2013;64:108–14.
43. Seyed RA, Samur H. The results of uvulopalatopharyngoplasty in patients with moderate obstructive sleep apnea syndrome having cardiac arrhythmias. Multidiscip Cardiovasc Ann. 2020;11(2):1–7. https://doi.org/10.5812/mca.103810.

44. Brouillette RT, Lavergne J, Leimanis A, et al. Differences in pulse oximetry technology can affect detection of sleep-disorderd breathing in children. Anesth Analg. 2002;94:47–53.
45. Sivan Y, Kornecki A, Schonfeld T. Screening obstructive sleep apnoea syndrome by home videotape recording in children. Eur Respir J. 1996;9:2127–31.
46. Saeed MM, Keens TG, Stabile MW, et al. Should children with suspected obstructive sleep apnea syndrome and normal nap sleep studies have overnight sleep studies? Chest. 2000;118:360–5.
47. Nixon GM, Brouillette RT. Diagnostic techniques for obstructive sleep apnoea: is polysomnography necessary? Paediatr Respir Rev. 2002;3:18–24.
48. Marcus CL, Brooks LJ, Draper KA. Et al; American Academy of Pediatrics. Diagnosis and management of childhood obstructive sleep apnea syndrome. Pediatrics. 2012;130(3):576–84.
49. Mitchell RB. Adenotonsillectomy for obstructive sleep apnea in children: outcome evaluated by pre- and postoperative polysomnography. Laryngoscope. 2007;117:1844–54.
50. Magardino TM, Tom LW. Surgical management of obstruc- tive sleep apnea in children with cerebral palsy. Laryngoscope. 1999;109:1611–5.
51. Merrell JA, Shott SR. OSAS in down syndrome: T & a versus T & a plus lateral pharyngoplasty. Int J Pediatr Otorhinolaryngol. 2007;71:1197–203.
52. Mitchell RB, Kelly J. Outcome of adenotonsillectomy for obstructive sleep apnea in obese and normal-weight children. Otolaryngol Head Neck Surg. 2007;137:43–8.
53. Praud JP, Dorion D. Obstructive sleep disordered breathing in children: beyond adenotonsillectomy. Pediatr Pulmonol. 2008;43:837–43.
54. Waters KA, Cheng AT. Adenotonsillectomy in the context of obstructive sleep apnoea. Paediatr Respir Rev. 2009;10:25–31.
55. Lachanas VA, Hajiioannou JK, Karatzias GT, et al. Comparison of Liga sure vessel sealing system, harmonic scalpel, and cold knife tonsillectomy. Otolaryngol Head Neck Surg. 2007;137:385–9.
56. Vlastos IM, Parpounas K, Economides J, et al. Tonsillectomy versus tonsillotomy performed with scissors in children with tonsillar hypertrophy. Int J Pediatr Otorhinolaryngol. 2008;72:857–63.
57. Mixter RC, David DJ, Perloff WH, et al. Obstructive sleep apnea in Apert's and Pfeiffer's syndromes: more than a craniofacial abnormality. Plast Reconstr Surg. 1990;86:457–63.
58. Tahiri Y, Viezel-Mathieu A, Aldekhayel S, et al. The effectiveness of mandibular distraction in improving airway obstruction in the pediatric population. Plast Reconstr Surg. 2014;133:352–9.
59. Villa MP, Malagola C, Pagani J, et al. Rapid maxillary expansion in children with obstructive sleep apnea syndrome: 12-month follow-up. Sleep Med. 2007;8:128–34.
60. Cohen SR, Suzman K, Simms C, et al. Sleep apnea surgery versus tracheostomy in children: an exploratory study of the comparative effects on quality of life. Plast Reconstr Surg. 1998;102:1855–64.
61. Goldbart AD, Goldman JL, Veling MC, et al. Leukotriene modifier therapy for mild sleep-disordered breathing in children. Am J Respir Crit Care Med. 2005;172:364–70.
62. Kheirandish-Gozal L, Gozal D. Intranasal budesonide treatment for children with mild obstructive sleep apnea syndrome. Pediatrics. 2008;122:e149–55.
63. Verhulst SL, Franckx H, Van Gaal L, De Backer W, Desager K. The effect of weight loss on sleep-disordered breathing in obese teenagers. Obesity (Silver Spring). 2009;17(6):1178–83.
64. Manickam PV, Shott SR, Boss EF, et al. Systematic review of site of obstruction identification and non-CPAP treatment options for children with persistent pediatric obstructive sleep apnea. Laryngoscope. 2016;126(2):491–50.
65. Vlastos IM, Hajiioannou JK. Clinical practice. Diagnosis and treatment of childhood snoring. Eur J Pediatr. 2010;169:261–7.
66. American Academy of Sleep Medicine. International Classification of Sleep Disorders. 3rd ed. Darien, IL: American Academy of Sleep Medicine; 2014. p. 52–60.

Dysphagia in Children

26

Bilal Sizer, Nuray Bayar Muluk, and Nitin R. Ankle

26.1 Introduction

Dysphagia refers to discomfort experienced during deglutition. The process of deglutition involves transfer of a solid or liquid bolus from the oral cavity into the pharynx, thence to the oesophagus and finally to the stomach. Problems affecting any of these stages may lead to dysphagia. There are multiple causes for difficulty in feeding or deglutition, anatomical and physiological, in children, and they affect individuals whose development is in other respects abnormal as well as those whose development is otherwise healthy. If there is an anomalous anatomical configuration of the mouth, throat or oesophagus, this may interfere with feeding normally [1, 2].

26.2 Dysphagia in Children

Deglutition involves a complex sequence of muscular contractions co-ordinated by several different nerves, both cranial and cervical, and located in the labial, lingual, palatal, oropharyngeal, pharyngeal, laryngeal, oesophageal and retrosternal regions.

B. Sizer (✉)
Section of Otorhinolaryngology, Memorial Diyarbakır Hospital, Diyarbakır, Turkey

N. Bayar Muluk
Department of Otorhinolaryngology, Faculty of Medicine, Kırıkkale University, Kırıkkale, Turkey

N. R. Ankle (✉)
Department of Otorhinolaryngology, Head and Neck Surgery, Jawaharlal Nehru Medical College, KLE Academy of Higher Education and Research (KAHER), Belagavi, Karnataka, India

Dysphagia may result from any disorder which has the potential to disturb the coordination between these different actors in the process of deglutition [3–5].

The upper aerodigestive tract of a child, unlike that of an adult, undergoes a series of alterations as the child grows and matures, which means that the pathogenesis of disorders causing dysphagia and feeding difficulty is distinctly different between children and adults. In early childhood, the mouth, throat and larynx are continuously undergoing alterations in their anatomical configuration. The physiological control of deglutition also matures step by step to allow for a change from the reflex actions of suckling to the movements involved in chewing and to address the need to permit both breathing and swallowing of food. Where the child lacks the ability to adapt to the alterations in anatomy or where neurological control mechanisms are impaired, deglutition may be hindered, with the result that chronic lung disorders or malnutrition develop.

The number of cases of dysphagia seen in children is rising, which may be attributed to higher numbers of infants born prematurely or with low birth weight who survive and then go on to develop complicated disorders which may impinge on the anatomical integrity of the structures involved in deglutition or their physiological actions [6–8].

26.3 The Physiology of Healthy Deglutition

The neurological control mechanisms involved in deglutition are somewhat complex. There is integration of sensory information carried by afferent fibres at the level of the brainstem. The efferent outflow involves the generation of a pattern of impulses that allow deglutition to occur efficiently and safely. Neural control coordinates the actions of the pharyngeal, laryngeal and oesophageal musculature.

There are four elements of this neurological control mechanism which have been extensively characterised:

1. The cranial nerves carry the afferent sensory input required.
2. Motor efferent fibres within the cranial nerves and the ansa-cervicalis.
3. The cerebrum, midbrain and cerebellum have projections which form synaptic connections at the level of the midbrain.
4. The brainstem contains twin deglutition centres.

When the child swallows, a bolus (whether solid or liquid) moves in succession from the oral cavity to the pharynx, then descends through the oesophagus before entry into the stomach. This movement depends upon synchronisation by the nervous system of the action of muscles lying under voluntary as well as involuntary control. Descriptions of deglutition usually consider the process to consist of three separate stages, involving the mouth, pharynx and oesophagus in turn. The stages each accomplish a specific goal. Dysphagia arises when there is an abnormality affecting at least one of these stages [6, 8].

26.3.1 Mouth (Oral) Stage

The mouth stage involves the action of muscles that are controlled voluntarily. It starts with food entering the oral cavity. The tongue and the muscles of mastication act in a co-ordinated fashion to form the chewed food into bolus form. Mechanoreceptors provide the necessary feedback to achieve this objective. The bolus is gathered in the middle of the lingual upper surface, which rises, propelling the bolus towards the pharynx in a manner resembling gut peristalsis. As the bolus is propelled towards the throat, an involuntary reflex is activated to swallow the bolus. This is the swallowing reflex [6, 8].

The mouth stage of swallowing calls for a high degree of co-ordination between the sensory input and motor output. The muscles of facial expression are supplied by the seventh cranial nerve, whereas the muscles that move the mandible are supplied by the trigeminal nerve. For the tongue to move in a co-ordinated way, there needs to be co-ordinated action by the four intrinsic muscles of the tongue and four extrinsic muscles. The former are supplied by the twelfth cranial nerve, the latter being supplied by branches of the ansa-cervicalis. The palatal, pharyngeal and laryngeal musculatures are supplied by the ninth and tenth cranial nerves. There is sensory supply from the second division of the fifth and the seventh, ninth and tenth cranial nerves. In infants, deglutition is almost entirely co-ordinated through reflexes controlled at brainstem level. However, with the introduction of solids and development of the cerebral cortex, voluntary control over swallowing begins gradually to increase [6, 9].

26.3.2 Pharyngeal Stage

For the most part, the pharyngeal stage in deglutition does not call for voluntary control. This stage is triggered to occur by the presence of food or saliva within the pharynx, and involves a number of responses occurring one after the other. The pharyngeal mechanoreceptors supply sensory input to the deglutition centre located within the medulla oblongata. This sensory input is carried by the fifth, ninth and tenth cranial nerves [10]. The deglutition centre within the medulla relays the signal to begin the motor sequence of swallowing to the nucleus ambiguus and the dorsomedial nucleus of Cranial Nerve X. The velum takes up position against the rear wall of the pharynx, separating the oropharynx from the nasopharynx and ensuring the bolus descends rather than entering the nasal cavity. The oropharyngeal musculature contracts against the lingual base and thus the bolus is conveyed onward. There is some adjustment to the exact muscular movements that depends on proprioceptors, which is needed to accommodate the variation in bolus volume and consistency expected during eating [6, 9, 11].

Since the pharynx forms part of the aerodigestive tract, it fulfils a dual purpose as an airway and a passage for food. This situation necessitates reciprocal inhibition of the respiratory and gastrointestinal systems. At the beginning of the pharyngeal stage, breathing halts and the larynx undergoes traction upwards and forwards, preventing it from obstructing the bolus on its descent. Both pairs of vocal cords shut and the epiglottis bends backwards, closing off the entrance to the laryngeal lumen, as the larynx moves superiorly. This action of raising the larynx widens the entrance to the oesophagus, and the constrictor muscles within the pharynx constrict to produce a peristaltic wave that carries the bolus towards the oesophageal entrance [6, 12]. Beyond this stage onwards, deglutition enters involuntary phase.

If food does perchance enter the larynx, its presence will be detected by mechano- and chemoreceptors, which trigger the vocal folds to snap shut and produces a halt in breathing. This failure to carry on breathing persists whilst the food remains lodged in the larynx. In neonates, there is inadequate respiratory reserve, so this protective reflex may make the child hypoxic. At the same time, coughing may also be triggered by food entering the larynx. Coughing may be initiated by sensory input originating in the larynx itself or from tracheal receptors. Nonetheless, this extra layer of protection is not found in three quarters of babies born prematurely, nor in half of those born at term. Furthermore, infants who sustain impairment to the nervous system may also lack the coughing reflex [6, 12].

26.3.3 Oesophageal Stage

The oesophagus acts as a tube connecting the pharynx with the stomach which is closed at both ends by default. Muscular sphincters keep the ends closed except when deglutition occurs. The upper muscular ring of the oesophagus opens to permit deglutition and this opening is further assisted by the upwards movement of the larynx. A peristaltic wave actively moves the bolus in the direction of the gastric entrance. The lower muscular ring needs to remain contracted at times other than swallowing, otherwise the stomach contents risk being refluxed back up the oesophagus. Peristalsis is orchestrated by the myenteric plexus of the oesophagus acting with impulses provided by the tenth cranial nerve [6, 12].

The term oral dysphagia is applied to a variety of different problems affecting the oral stage. Such problems include over- and under-sensitivity to the taste or texture of food, losing food out of the mouth or being impaired in the ability to form food into a bolus and move it within the oral cavity. Pharyngeal dysphagia results from weak muscular action by the musculature of this region, misjudged initiation of deglutition, inadequate repositioning of the larynx and failure to protect the airway and a reduced ability to sense the passage of bolus. The consequences of pharyngeal dysphagia may include the passage of bolus upwards into the nasal cavity, food remaining in the pharynx when swallowing has finished, penetrative injury to the pharynx, aspirated bolus and choking. Oesophageal dysphagia encompasses a number of issues including cricopharyngeal achalasia, in which the upper oesophageal muscular ring does not open to let the bolus pass and the oesophagus suffers from abnormal motility.

Dysphagia may be noticed in the following circumstances: the child cannot retain food in the oral cavity, food and saliva are inadequately under the child's control, the voice sounds wet, the child coughs when eating or there are attempts to clear the throat at any point prior to, during or post deglutition [1–3].

For most cases, a thorough and precise history should allow the correct diagnosis to become obvious. Some important specific items to enquire about when taking the history include whether the child has been seen swallowing non-food matter, or if some items of small size appear missing (such as watch batteries), if the child may have swallowed a corrosive substance, loss of voice, pyrexia (particularly if there are lesions within the mouth), excessive salivation, pharyngitis, jaw muscle spasm or nuchal rigidity. Some causes of paediatric dysphagia are detailed in Table 26.1 [8].

Table 26.1 Causes of dysphagia in children [8]

Life-threatening	Foreign body within oesophagus
	Stevens-Johnson syndrome
	Corrosive substance ingestion
	Retropharyngeal abscess
	Epiglottitis
	Central nervous system infection (e.g. meningitis, encephalitis, cerebral abscess)
	Impairment of deglutition(e.g. cerebral palsy, myasthenia gravis, botulism, Miller Fisher syndrome)
	Tetanus
	Diphtheria
	Poliomyelitis
	Central nervous system tumours
	Perforation of the oesophagus
Common	Stomatitis
	Infectious pharyngitis
	Quinsy
	Dystonic reaction
	Injury to the oropharynx
Oesophageal causes	Oesophagitis
	Megaoesophagus
	Diverticula,
	Membranes,
	Rings,
	Dysphagia lusoria,
	Stenosis,
	Tracheo-oesophageal fistula
Other	Achalasia
	Rheumatic disease (e.g. juvenile systemic sclerosis, dermatomyositis)
	Myasthenia gravis
	Crohn's disease
	Thyroid enlargement (e.g. acute suppurative thyroiditis)
	Tumour of the oesophagus
	Vascular ring
	Globus sensation
	Macroglossia
	Cleft anomalies
	Lingual goitre
	Cervical cysts
	Ranula
	Soft palate palsy in diphtheria
	Acromegaly
	CNS diseases like bulbar paralysis
	Cerebral ischaemia
	Amyotrophic lateral sclerosis

Frequently occurring infections of the upper respiratory tract may be responsible for cases of paediatric dysphagia. Although it has been known since the 1970s that tonsillitis may worsen dysphagia through alteration to the action of muscles involved in swallowing, there is minimal research available that has focused on the pharyngeal musculature in cases of tonsillitis [6, 8, 13].

26.4 Stomatitis

Stomatitis refers to an inflammatory process involving the mucosae found within the oral cavity and oropharynx. It is amongst the most frequently occurring reasons for paediatric dysphagia and is characteristically found in association with a viral infective episode. Hand, foot and mouth disease is a disorder caused by Coxsackie A virus, one of the enteroviridae. It presents as pyrexia, vesicular lesions on the lining of the cheeks and the tongue, and tiny, painful skin lesions distributed over the hands, feet and buttocks. The same pathogen is also responsible for herpangina, a rash with vesicles found on the palatal tonsils and the velum, seen mainly in paediatric patients between the ages of 3 and 10 years. Herpangina produces a painful throat, pyrexia and pain on swallowing. It generally occurs as part of an outbreak in the summer months. Herpes simplex virus type 1 is the pathogen responsible for herpetic gingivostomatitis. The usual age range is from 6 months to 5 years old. This disorder presents with a prodromal pyrexia and systemic symptoms, after which lesions develop in the mouth and elsewhere. The lesions are initially vesicular, but then join together, producing areas of sore ulceration. The presentation often includes pyrexia, halitosis, painful swallowing, loss of appetite and swollen lymph nodes under the chin or in the neck.

Viral stomatitis secondary to enteroviruses may be treated by supporting the patient to drink enough liquid and providing analgesics to be given by mouth. For a subset of such cases, topical treatments may be efficacious. Where pain is of marked severity, consider using opiate pain killers. Sometimes a child may decline oral fluids and it may be necessary to supply fluids intravenously [14, 15].

26.5 Infectious Pharyngitis

In a case of paediatric dysphagia where there are signs and symptoms of pharyngitis due to an infection, treatment depends on the most likely pathogen involved. Infectious agents that frequently occur include the enteroviruses, adenovirus, Epstein-Barr virus, Group A Streptococci or *Neisseria gonorrhoeae*. Some paediatric patients experience such severe odynophagia that oral fluid intake becomes inadequate to maintain hydration. How to go about diagnosing pharyngitis secondary to infection and the management of the dehydrated child is reported elsewhere in the literature. See, for example, Ref. [16].

26.6 Quinsy

Paediatric cases of quinsy are typically associated with marked pharyngitis, generally one-sided, and pyrexia. Patients are said to speak as if they were eating a hot potato. There may be excessive salivation, which may drip from the mouth. The symptom of muscular spasm, resulting from irritation to the internal pterygoid muscle, is seen in approaching 2 out of 3 cases of quinsy and is thus a useful sign diagnostically. The peak age at which this lesion occurs is during adolescence, but it does occur even in younger paediatric patients. Distinguishing between peritonsillar abscess and a retropharyngeal abscess or epiglottitis is sometimes challenging, since these conditions may also be associated with sialorrhoea and muscular spasm of the jaw [17, 18].

Physical examination of children with quinsy may reveal a highly oedematous tonsil that exhibits fluctuance and a uvula deviating away from the lesion. The posterior velum may be visibly swollen or bulging in the vicinity of the tonsil. It may feel full on palpation, and may be fluctuant.

The treatment for quinsy depends principally on surgically draining the abscess, supplying antibiotic pharmacotherapy and instigating supportive measures [17, 18].

26.7 Epiglottitis

Cases where the clinician suspects epiglottitis need to be treated as medical emergencies. It is seldom seen amongst children who have received the Hib vaccination. Early diagnosis and rapid intervention are the only ways to prevent the high morbidity and mortality associated with the condition. Epiglottitis in paediatric patients classically presents as dysphagia that comes on suddenly and worsens in a matter of hours, coupled with hypersalivation in a distressed child. An abruptly beginning marked pyrexia (above 38.8 deg, but below 40 °C), painful swallowing and pharyngitis of marked severity are also common in cases of epiglottitis secondary to infection. Epiglottitis can also be triggered if a child drinks some corrosive liquid or very hot drinks [18, 19].

The usual appearance of a paediatric case of epiglottitis is toxic, possibly sitting down with the trunk bent forwards, neck sticking out and chin protruded, a manoeuvre that helps to make the airway as free from obstruction as possible. Such patients may refuse to lie flat. Whilst in some cases there is a history of a mild upper respiratory tract infection, generally the patient has only appeared sick for at most 24 h, sometimes even less than 12 h [8, 10, 19].

26.8 Retropharyngeal Abscess

The peak age of occurrence for a retropharyngeal abscess is between 2 and 4 years old. This lesion is frequently the result of multiple pathogens. The main bacteria responsible are *Streptococcus pyogenes* (group A streptococcus), *Staphylococcus aureus* (including methicillin-resistant *S. aureus*), and anaerobic bacteria found in the respiratory tract, such as *Fusobacteria, Prevotella* or *Veillonella* spp. [8, 10].

In the first stages of a retropharyngeal abscess, there may be no features that differ from a simple sore throat. However, as the lesion matures, the upper aerodigestive tract becomes inflamed and obstructed, which produces more symptoms. Paediatric cases of this lesion start to appear unwell and a moderate pyrexia may be noted. They may have difficulty swallowing, pain when swallowing, hypersalivation, extending the neck may be painful, torticollis may be seen and they may speak as if eating a hot potato. Furthermore, such children may present with respiratory distress, stridor, cervical oedema or a mass lesion, and the lymph nodes may be swollen [8, 10].

26.9 Diphtheria

Diphtheria is no longer common in developed countries, but remains common in less developed nations globally. This disease is an acute, transmissible condition resulting from infection with *Corynebacterium diphtheriae*, a Gram-positive bacillary pathogen. Respiratory diphtheria begins slowly, presenting as pharyngitis, painful swallowing, malaise and a pyrexia, which is not high. In a considerable number of cases, the bacterial toxin secreted by the pathogen leads to the development of a pseudomembranous covering, which may be found anywhere along the respiratory airways, from proximal to distal. It results in pain upon swallowing. Signs of associated neurological impairment, such as uncoordinated swallowing, difficulty in swallowing, blockage of the upper airways, with or without aspiration in the lungs rarely complicates this disorder when mild. However, in severe cases there is a risk of up to 75% that such complications will occur [8, 20, 21].

26.10 Stevens-Johnson Syndrome

The precise pathogenic mechanism behind Stevens-Johnson syndrome (SJS) and toxic epidermal necrolysis (TEN) has not been established, but both disorders involve significant desquamation of skin or mucosa. Dysphagia and sialorrhoea are frequently seen when there is severe loss of mucosa within the oropharynx. If less than one tenth of the skin area is affected, such desquamation is termed Stevens-Johnson syndrome, whilst if at least three tenths of the skin is affected, toxic epidermal necrolysis is diagnosable. If between 10% and 30% of the skin is affected, there is said to be overlap between these two syndromes.

In virtually every case, TEN is linkable to a drug exposure, whereas SJS is both drug-associated as well as a possible consequence of infection. In both conditions there is a prodromal syndrome lasting between 1 and 3 days up to when the lesions appear on the mucosae or epidermis. During the prodrome, patients are pyrexial and have symptoms resembling an influenza episode. The lesions feature vesicles and bullae, which worsen over the course of a few days. It is possible for the disorder to involve multiple organ systems and the trachea and bronchi may also be affected [8, 22, 23].

26.11 Tetanus

The anaerobic bacterium, *Clostridium tetani*, synthesises a toxin that results in severe muscular spasm through its action on nervous tissue. Tetanus is currently seldom seen in developed countries, but is still present in developing nations. A frequent presentation in a child with systemic tetanus is dysphagia and spasm of the jaw muscles. It may also present with nuchal rigidity, opisthotonus and the so-called *risus sardonicus*.

Children suffering from generalised tetanus typically experience a prolonged contraction of the voluntary muscles, with severe muscle spasms occurring from time to time. Tetanus has no effect on how awake or aware patients are, and the prolonged contraction and muscular spasms generate a severe level of pain. These muscular spasms may be set off by a high noise level or intense sensory stimulation of other kinds, such as tactile or photic [8, 24, 25].

26.12 Cornelia de Lange Syndrome (CdLS)

CdLS is an infrequently occurring congenital disorder that produces disease of the auditory system and the aerodigestive tract. Its manifestations may be seen in a variety of organ systems, which then necessitate the involvement of a number of paediatric disciplines. ENT opinion is often required.

The initial description of this disorder was published in 1933 by the Dutch paediatrician and neuropathologist, Cornelia Catharina de Lange. She supplied a description of two children with a very specific dysmorphic facial appearance, delayed development and abnormal arms and legs. She used the term typhus degenerative Amstel Damensis, but it is today referred to as Cornelia de Lange Syndrome, in her honour. The incidence is 1 in 10,000 live births. It is equally common in both males and females [26, 27]. CdLS has a varied phenotype.

The multi-systemic nature of CdLS calls for multi-disciplinary management. Paediatric ENT specialists may treat auditory impairment, ensure a patent airway and address craniofacial anomalies. The long-term and multi-disciplinary nature of management imposes a considerable task on those caring for such children. There are, however, a number of centres where expertise has developed and an American foundation for CdLS also exists. This infrastructure helps to facilitate research and to offer social services to the affected families. The centres of expertise are valuable as models on which to base planning a service for patients affected by CdLS [28, 29].

References

1. Duffy KL. Dysphagia in Children. Curr Probl Pediatr Adolesc Health Care. 2018;48(3):71–3. https://doi.org/10.1016/j.cppeds.2018.01.003.
2. Raol N, Schrepfer T, Hartnick C. Aspiration and dysphagia in the neonatal patient. Clin Perinatol. 2018;45(4):645–60. https://doi.org/10.1016/j.clp.2018.07.005.Epub.
3. Arvedson JC. Assessment of pediatric dysphagia and feeding disorders: clinical and instrumental approaches. Dev Disabil Res Rev. 2008;14(2):118–27.

4. Hawdon JM, Beauregard N, Slattery J, Kennedy G. Identification of neonates at risk of developing feeding problems in infancy. Dev Med Child Neurol. 2000;42(4):235–9.

5. Lefton-Greif MA. Pediatric dysphagia. Phys Med Rehabil Clin N Am. 2008;19(4):837–51.

6. Willging JP. Pediatric esophageal and swallowing disorders. In: Licameli GR, Tunkel DE, editors. Pediatric otorhinolaryngology: diagnosis and treatment. New York, NY: Thieme Medical and Scientific Publishers; 2013. p. 100–8.

7. Newman LA, Keckley C, Petersen MC, Hamner A. Swallowing function and medical diagnoses in infants suspected of dysphagia. Pediatrics. 2001;108(6):E106.

8. Furnival RA, Woodward GA. Evaluation of dysphagia in children. In: Fleisher GR editor, UpToDate. Last updated Aug 14, 2019.

9. Dodds WJ, Stewart ET, Logemann JA. Physiology and radiology of the normal oral and pharyngeal phases of swallowing. AJR Am J Roentgenol. 1990;154(5):953–63.

10. Vinckenbosch P, Guilcher P, Lambercy K, Richard C. Abcèsrétropharyngé de l'enfant [Retropharyngeal abscess in children]. Rev Med Suisse. 2017;13(577):1698–702.

11. Miller AJ. The search for the central swallowing pathway: the quest for clarity. Dysphagia. 1993;8(3):185–94.

12. Loughlin GM, Lefton-Greif MA. Dysfunctional swallowing and respiratory disease in children. Adv Pediatr Infect Dis. 1994;41:135–62.

13. Vaiman M. The influence of tonsillitis on Oral and throat muscles in adults. Otolaryngol Head Neck Surg. 2007;136(5):832–7. https://doi.org/10.1016/j.otohns.2006.11.026.

14. Mantegazza C, Angiero F, Zuccotti GV. Oral manifestations of gastrointestinal diseases in children. Part 3: Ulcerative colitis and gastro-oesophageal reflux disease. Eur J Paediatr dent. 2016;17(3):248–50.

15. Montgomery-Cranny JA, Wallace A, Rogers HJ, Hughes SC, Hegarty AM, Zaitoun H. Management of recurrent aphthous stomatitis in children. Dent Update. 2015;42(6):564–6. https://doi.org/10.12968/denu.2015.42.6.564.

16. Weber R. Pharyngitis. Prim Care. 2014;41(1):91–8. https://doi.org/10.1016/j.pop.2013.10.010.

17. Mitchell RB, Archer SM, Ishman SL, Rosenfeld RM, Coles S, Finestone SA, Friedman NR, Giordano T, Hildrew DM, Kim TW, Lloyd RM, Parikh SR, Shulman ST, Walner DL, Walsh SA, Nnacheta LC. Clinical practice guideline: tonsillectomy in children (update)-executive summary. Otolaryngol Head Neck Surg. 2019;160(2):187–205. https://doi.org/10.1177/0194599818807917.

18. Lee CH, Hsu WC, Ko JY, Yeh TH, Kang KT. Trends in the management of peritonsillar abscess in children: A nationwide population-based study in Taiwan. Int J Pediatr Otorhinolaryngol. 2019;125:32–7. https://doi.org/10.1016/j.ijporl.2019.06.016.

19. Baiu I, Melendez E. Epiglottitis. JAMA. 2019;321(19):1946. https://doi.org/10.1001/jama.2019.3468.

20. Muhamad Ramdan I, Susanti R, Ifroh RH, Noviasty R. Risk factors for diphtheria outbreak in children aged 1-10 years in East Kalimantan Province, Indonesia. F1000Res. 2018;7:1625. https://doi.org/10.12688/f1000research.16433.1.

21. Exavier MM, Paul Hanna M, Muscadin E, Freishstat RJ, Brisma JP, Canarie MF. Diphtheria in Children in Northern Haiti. J Trop Pediatr. 2019;65(2):183–7. https://doi.org/10.1093/tropej/fmy021.

22. Liotti L, Caimmi S, Bottau P, Bernardini R, Cardinale F, Saretta F, Mori F, Crisafulli G, Franceschini F, Caffarelli C. Clinical features, outcomes and treatment in children with drug induced Stevens-Johnson syndrome and toxic epidermal necrolysis. Acta Biomed. 2019;90(3-S):52–60. https://doi.org/10.23750/abm.v90i3-S.8165.

23. Miliszewski MA, Kirchhof MG, Sikora S, Papp A, Dutz JP. Stevens-Johnson syndrome and toxic epidermal necrolysis: an analysis of triggers and implications for improving prevention. Am J Med. 2016;129(11):1221–5. https://doi.org/10.1016/j.amjmed.2016.03.022.

24. Brook I. Tetanus in children. Pediatr Emerg Care. 2004;20(1):48–51. https://doi.org/10.1097/01.pec.0000106245.72265.71.

25. Rhinesmith E, Fu L. Tetanus disease, treatment, management. Pediatr Rev. 2018;39(8):430–2. https://doi.org/10.1542/pir.2017-0238.

26. Eliason MJ, Melzer JM, Gallagher TQ. Cornelia de Lange syndrome: what every otolaryngologist should know. Ear Nose Throat J. 2017;96(8):E6–9. https://doi.org/10.1177/014556131709600802.
27. Cornelia de Lange Foundation. www.CdLSusa.org. Last accessed June 20, 2017.
28. Sataloff RT, Spiegel JR, Hawkshaw M, et al. Cornelia de Lange syndrome. Otolaryngologic manifestations. Arch Otolaryngol Head Neck Surg. 1990;116(9):1044–6.
29. Mikołajewska E. Interdisciplinary therapy in Cornelia de Lange syndrome—review of the literature. Adv Clin Exp Med. 2013;22(4):571–7.

Cough in Children

Emine Atağ, Zeynep Seda Uyan, and Refika Ersu

27.1 Introduction

Cough is one of the most common causes of physician referrals in children. The prevalence of cough varies depending on many factors. There is little accurate data about cough epidemiology among children. A community-based study found the prevalence of cough as 5–10% in primary school children [1], and it is estimated to be more frequent in preschool children according to the prospective and retrospective studies [2]. Cough can lead to impaired quality of life, absence from school, and increased health costs due to increased doctor visits and excessive medication use. Cough is also associated with concerns and stress of parents related to its etiology, fear of choking, and chronic respiratory involvement [3, 4].

27.2 Pathophysiology

Coughing is a normal reflex activity caused by airway irritants, infections, or aspirated contents. In healthy children, approximately 11 cough episodes per day are considered normal and the mean value may range between 1 and 34 [5].

E. Atağ (✉)
Division of Pediatric Pulmonology, Department of Pediatrics, Faculty of Medicine, Medipol University, İstanbul, Turkey
e-mail: emine.atag@medipol.com.tr

Z. S. Uyan
Division of Pediatric Pulmonology, Department of Pediatrics, Faculty of Medicine, Koç University, İstanbul, Turkey

R. Ersu
Section of Pediatric Sleep Medicine, Children's Hospital of Eastern Ontario, University of Ottawa, Ottawa, ON, Canada

C. Cingi et al. (eds.), *Pediatric ENT Infections*,
https://doi.org/10.1007/978-3-030-80691-0_27

The cough starts either with the stimulation of cough receptors of the cough reflex arc or by voluntary initiation. The cough receptors are found in the upper and lower airways, as well as in the sinuses, nose, external ear, tympanic membrane, pericardium, pleura, and diaphragm. There are two types of cough receptors, namely chemosensitive and mechanosensitive. The alignment and relative abundance of these receptors vary in the airways. Large airways are more sensitive to mechanical stimuli [6]. Signals from cough receptors are transferred to the cough center which is further transmitted to efferent pathways consisting of the larynx, trachea, bronchi, and respiratory muscles. The motor component of coughing has 3 phases. It starts with an inspiration, continues with forced breathing against the closed glottis, and results in the opening of the glottis which allows the expulsion of mucus by a rapid expiration [7].

Abnormalities of the cough mechanism can result in an ineffective cough. For example, conditions affecting the central nervous system can lead to suppression of cough reflex. A different pathophysiological event occurs in microaspiration syndromes, where a decrease in cough response occurs due to recurrent stimulation of receptors caused by tachyphylaxis. The weakness of respiratory muscles can also reduce coughing efficiency through impaired motor action or force of coughing. In patients with airway malacia, the airway diameter and adequate flow rates cannot be maintained, and cough efficiency is reduced. The inability to close the upper airways due to laryngeal disorders is also associated with decreased cough efficiency. Lastly, altered mucus rheology such as a thick and sticky mucus that occurs in cystic fibrosis may cause insufficient clearance of secretions [8].

The respiratory system and the efficiency of coughing mature with age from infancy to adulthood. Although there is no gender difference in prepubertal children, post-pubertal girls have an increased cough susceptibility that is similar to adults [2]. As the cough reflex does not completely mature before the age of 5, foreign body aspiration usually occurs before this age. Children have a predisposition to developing atelectasis due to the paucity of collateral ventilation and smaller airways compared to adults [9].

Changes in the sensitivity of the afferent nerves of the cough reflex pathway may affect the density of the cough which usually results in an increased cough response to the environmental stimuli. This condition is named plasticity. Chronic inflammation caused by allergies, infections, and cigarette smoke may result in an increased cough response via plasticity [7].

27.3 Definition of Cough

The definition of cough is necessary to identify its cause and appropriate management. Pediatric cough can be defined according to the duration of the symptoms, etiology, and characteristics:

- Acute, subacute, chronic cough: based on the duration.
- Specific, nonspecific cough: based on underlying primary etiology of chronic cough.
- Moist, dry, or classically recognizable cough: according to its characteristics/quality [10].

27.3.1 Acute Cough

A cough lasting less than 2 weeks is called acute cough. Acute respiratory infections (ARI) are the most common causes of acute cough in children. A birth cohort study evaluating the incidence and symptoms of ARI showed that during the first 2 years of life, healthy Australian children had a mean incidence rate of 0.56 ARI per child-month. The rates of upper respiratory infections (URTI) and lower respiratory infections (LRTI) among all episodes were 83% and 17%, respectively. Dry coughs comprised 42.6% of URTI coughs [11]. The acute cough usually develops following URTIs in children; however, a detailed medical history and systemic physical examination for underlying causes are required for all children with acute cough. Cough is the main symptom in children with foreign body aspiration but decreased respiratory sounds and wheezing may also occur. Although acute cough is usually seen in foreign body aspiration, some undiagnosed cases of aspiration may also present with chronic cough. An acute cough may also be the reason for a referral to a doctor in many respiratory and non-respiratory diseases [2].

Common etiologies of acute cough include:

- Upper respiratory tract infection.
- Lower respiratory tract infection.
- Exacerbation of preexisting conditions: Asthma, bronchiectasis.
- Foreign body inhalation.
- Exposure to environmental pollutants.
- Cardiac diseases: Pulmonary embolism, heart failure.
- Thoracic or extrathoracic malignancy.

Specific pointers in a child with cough can indicate the presence of the specific cough and careful assessment is required to detect a possible underlying problem. Specific pointers include the following [10]:

- Auscultatory findings (wheeze, crepitations, differential breath sounds, stridor).
- Cough characteristics (e.g., cough with choking, neonatal-onset).
- Cardiac abnormalities.
- Chest pain.
- Chest wall deformity.
- Daily productive cough.
- Digital clubbing.
- Dyspnea.
- Exposure to pertussis, tuberculosis.
- Failure to thrive.
- Feeding difficulties or dysphagia.
- Hemoptysis.
- Immune deficiency.
- Medications or drugs.
- Neurodevelopmental abnormality.

27.3.1.1 Diagnostic Evaluation of Acute Cough

Further testing is usually not necessary for children with acute cough, because it is usually a self-limiting event. The most important part of the diagnosis of acute cough is to identify whether it is a life-threatening illness such as foreign body inhalation or pulmonary embolism, or a non-life-threatening disease such as respiratory tract infections. It is also important to detect the presence of specific pointers. A chest X-ray is required in cases of suspected pneumonia. Expiratory chest radiographs are necessary for the diagnosis of patients with a history of foreign body aspiration. Normal radiography does not exclude aspiration, so rigid bronchoscopy should be done in cases with high clinical suspicion even if the chest X-ray is normal.

The characteristics of cough sound may vary depending on the underlying cause. The presence of wheezing may suggest asthma. A metallic cough may occur in patients with airway malacia and viral croup. While a paroxysmal cough is representative of pertussoid syndromes, an intermittent staccato cough is seen in patients with *Chlamydia trachomatis* or *Mycoplasma pneumoniae* infections. Psychogenic conditions should be considered in cases with a croaking, honking cough (Table 27.1) [10, 12].

27.3.2 Subacute Cough

If the cough lasts 2–4 weeks, it is defined as a subacute cough. Subacute cough often occurs due to recurrent and persistent respiratory infections. The patient's defense factors are important in children presenting with subacute cough. It is suggested to observe the patient for 4 weeks and to perform further examination in cases where the cough persists.

27.3.3 Chronic Cough

Chronic cough in children is different from adults in many aspects (Table 27.2). While the duration for chronic cough definition in adults is 8 weeks, cough persisting longer than 4 weeks is called a chronic cough in children. The time interval accepted for the definition of chronic cough is similar in many guidelines and allows early diagnosis of serious underlying diseases such as foreign body aspiration and bronchiectasis to prevent late respiratory complications. However, these guidelines

Table 27.1 Etiology of cough according to its characteristics in children

Cough Characteristics	Possible Etiology
Barking, brassy or metallic cough	Croup, airway malacia, habit cough
Productive cough with casts	Plastic bronchitis
Honking, croaking, absence in the night	Psychogenic
Paroxysmal	Pertussis and parapertussis
Dry, staccato	Chlamydia in infants

Table 27.2 Common etiologies of chronic cough according to the age of the child

Children younger than 5 years of age	Children older than 5 years of age
Respiratory tract infections	Asthma
Gastroesophageal reflux	Respiratory tract infections
Congenital airway lesions	Upper airway cough syndrome
Asthma	Protracted bacterial bronchitis
Protracted bacterial bronchitis	Environmental factors
Environmental factors	Bronchiectasis
Foreign body inhalation	Psychogenic cough

also suggest watchful waiting for certain patients with chronic cough when specific symptoms and/or signs are absent. Chronic cough is further sub-classified into two groups as specific and nonspecific cough [10].

27.3.3.1 Specific Cough

If the medical history, associated symptoms, and physical examination findings indicate a primary respiratory or systemic disease, then the chronic cough is considered as a specific cough. Patients with the abovementioned specific pointers should be further examined according to the potential cause.

27.3.3.2 Nonspecific Cough

A nonspecific chronic cough describes the cough in the absence of specific signs in the medical history and physical examination. Chronic cough is more likely to be nonspecific if it is dry, and there are no signs or symptoms suggestive of any chronic diseases on physical examination or with diagnostic tests (spirometry, chest radiography). The chronic cough usually develops following URTI. In this case, cough occurs because of increased receptor sensitivity and usually resolves spontaneously. Environmental factors may cause chronic nonspecific cough. Exposures to specific allergens, pulmonary irritants, and cigarette smoke should be questioned. As children usually recover spontaneously in this group, the "watch, wait, and review" approach is suggested for nonspecific cough [9].

27.3.3.3 Wet-Moist-Productive Cough and Dry Cough

It is very important to define the characteristics of the cough and distinguish whether the cough is dry or moist in the differential diagnosis.

It is more appropriate to use the term "wet cough" instead of "productive cough" in young children because they are not able to expectorate sputum. A wet cough may occur secondary to excessive mucus secretions or defective mucociliary clearance. On the other hand, dry cough may occur due to hypersensitization of the cough reflex pathway regardless of the etiology, and thus may suggest respiratory or non-respiratory conditions characterized by chronic inflammation. It should also be known that a dry cough can turn into a wet cough when airway secretions increase. In patients with a wet cough lasting for more than 4 weeks, and in patients with signs of respiratory or systemic disease, further investigations are necessary [9].

27.4 Common Etiologies of Chronic Cough

A practical approach to a child with chronic cough is shown in Fig. 27.1 [10].

27.4.1 Asthma

Asthma is a common chronic inflammatory disease of the airways and is characterized by reversible airflow obstruction, bronchial hyperresponsiveness, and varying and recurring symptoms. Both symptoms and the degree of airflow obstruction are typically temporary and reversible. Some factors, such as exposure to environmental allergens, change in climatic conditions, viral respiratory infections, and exercise may cause asthma symptoms by triggering bronchoconstriction.

The cough may be an initial symptom in asthmatic children. Although studies evaluating chronic cough etiologies in children showed that asthma is the most common cause of chronic cough, the isolated cough does not always represent asthma. In a child with typical episodic symptoms, meticulously obtained medical and familial history, detailed physical examination and the confirmation of reversible airflow obstruction support the diagnosis of asthma. Supportive evidence for asthma includes wheezing, and a chronic dry, nocturnal, and paroxysmal cough that is triggered by exercise, cold air, sleep, or allergens [10]. A study about the association of nocturnal dry cough at ages 1–7 years with doctor-diagnosed asthma at 8 years of age showed that nocturnal dry cough in early childhood is associated with the presence of doctor-diagnosed asthma at age 8, independent of the presence of wheeze [13]. Exacerbation with exercise is nonspecific and may be found in many respiratory diseases. A history of eczema or bronchiolitis or a family history of the atopic disease may also support the possibility of asthma. Asthma may also present with recurrent right middle lobe atelectasis.

Asthmatic patients may have an obstructive pattern on spirometry, which is reversible with bronchodilator agents. Spirometry can also indicate an exaggerated bronchoconstrictive response to specific triggers [10].

27.4.2 Upper Airways Disorders

Upper airway cough syndrome (postnasal drip syndrome) has been consistently found as a major cause of chronic cough in different patient groups. Children with upper airway cough syndrome have induced cough due to the stimulation of cough receptors due to postnasal drainage. Cough receptors may also be activated by inflammatory mediators. Changes in environmental temperature and humidity can also activate cough receptors in the upper airway [14].

Any event in the hypopharynx and larynx that causes mechanical or chemical stimulation of the afferent nerves of cough reflex may cause chronic cough, as they are located in this area.

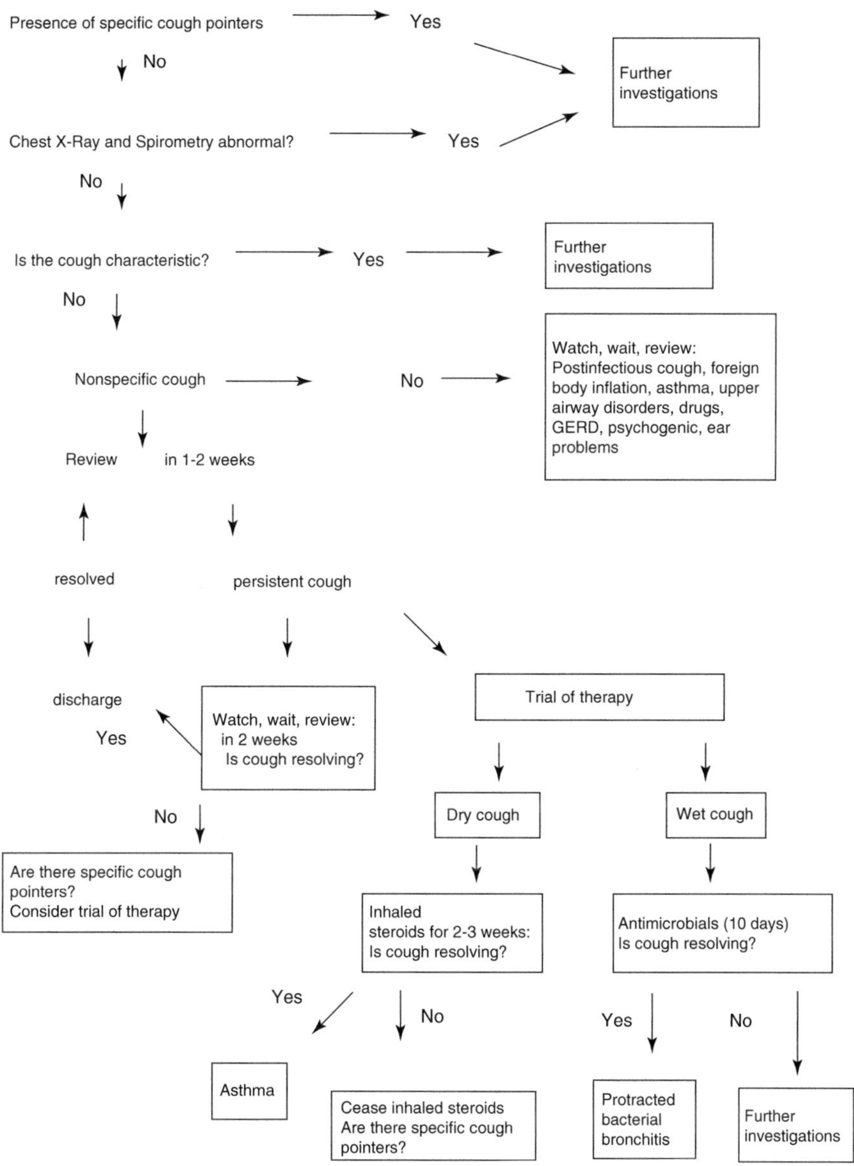

Fig. 27.1 Evaluation of a child with chronic cough; adopted from Ref. [10]

The most common clinical conditions of this syndrome are allergic rhinitis, postinfectious rhinitis, vasomotor rhinitis, acute nasopharyngitis, and bacterial sinusitis.

A previous history of upper respiratory illness and triggering factors of cough should be obtained from medical history. On physical examination, nasal quality of voice should be noted. Oropharynx examination may reveal the presence of secretions in the nasopharynx and a cobblestone appearance of the oropharyngeal mucosa. Symptoms of upper airway cough syndrome include throat clearing, a feeling of postnasal dripping into the back of the throat, and persistent nasal congestion or discharge [14].

27.4.3 Gastroesophageal Reflux Disease and Laryngopharyngeal Reflux

Gastroesophageal reflux (GER) develops due to lower esophageal sphincter dysfunction and results in involuntary movement of gastric contents to the esophagus. It is considered a disease if it causes morbidity. Laryngopharyngeal reflux is characterized by upper esophageal sphincter malfunction and results from the passing of the esophageal content beyond the upper esophageal sphincter into the oropharynx and nasopharynx. Both conditions can be seen normally, with the incidence rising to 40–50% at 4 months of age and gradually decreases after 12 months [14].

It is generally accepted that cough develops with two main mechanisms in gastroesophageal and laryngopharyngeal reflux. The first involves microaspirations of the gastric contents in the bronchial system directly inducing the cough reflex, and the second involves vagal nerves in the esophagus stimulated with reflux [15]. A comprehensively obtained medical history and physical examination are often sufficient for the diagnosis of reflux. Additional tests are required for patients who have complications due to reflux. Diagnostic tools including fluoroscopic examination of the upper gastrointestinal system, esophageal pH and impedance monitoring, manometry, endoscopy, scintigraphy reflux studies, and rhinolaryngoscopy can be used for diagnosis. Increased secretions, edema, and irregularities in the upper airways and vocal cords can be seen as the bronchoscopic and laryngoscopic findings [16]. Unlike the data in adults where GER is a common cause of chronic cough, GER is detected more rarely as a source of chronic cough in children [17]. A retrospective study found GER as a cause in only 5 of 156 children with chronic cough aged between 5 and 16 years [18]. The association between reflux and cough and response to antisecretory therapy has not been proven by controlled studies. As there is no clear evidence that GER is a common cause of isolated chronic cough in children, empirical GER therapy is not recommended in children with chronic cough according to pediatric guidelines [19].

27.4.4 Airway Lesions

Airway lesions are well-known causes of chronic cough in children. A study among children with congenital tracheomalacia secondary to congenital vascular anomaly revealed that 75%
of children had a persistent cough at presentation [10]. In another study where children with chronic cough and/or recurrent croup were examined, airway anomalies were found in 53% of patients. The most common diagnosis was

tracheomalacia in this study [20]. Airway malacia leads to decreased mucociliary clearance, which causes chronic cough due to chronic bronchial inflammation and infections. Children with airway malacia may have recurrent infections and pneumonia and may sometimes be diagnosed incorrectly as asthma. As bronchoscopy is required for the diagnosis of the airway lesions, it should be performed in children with unexplained chronic cough.

Vocal cord dysfunction (VCD) is a functional disorder characterized by the paradoxical movement of the vocal cords, causing abnormal adduction of vocal cords particularly during inspiration. VCD creates an obstructed airway and mimics asthma. The degree of vocal cord adduction can be variable. The underlying pathophysiology of VCD involves a hyper-functional and inappropriate laryngeal closure reflex.

Transient VCD can be seen following URTIs that cause prolonged postnasal discharge. The clinical presentation is variable, patients may be asymptomatic or have periodic mild symptoms, or they can suffer from severe asthmatic symptoms. On spirometry, flow-volume loops reveal a limitation of inspiratory flow which is characteristic for variable extrathoracic obstruction (inspiratory loop flattening) during symptomatic periods. Laryngoscopy is helpful for symptomatic patients, and paradoxical vocal cord movement can be seen on laryngoscopy [16, 21].

27.4.5 Recurrent Respiratory Tract Infections and Postinfectious Cough

Chronic cough in preschool children may occur as a result of recurrent episodes of URTI and infections such as pertussis. A prolonged cough may also be seen if the child is re-infected with another virus before recovering from a URTI. Upper respiratory tract infections are seen episodically, and their frequency increases in winter. Living in crowded places, exposure to air pollution, and attending kindergarten increase the occurrence of recurrent URTI risk. A mean annual incidence for URTI can be 5–8 episodes in children younger than 4 years of age, and 2.4–5 episodes in children between the ages of 10 and 14 years [10]. While cough typically resolves within 1–3 weeks following URTI in some children, it may be persistent and may lead to chronic cough. In a cohort study investigating the relationship between persistent cough and respiratory pathogens, the persistent cough rate was 20% and *Moraxella catarrhalis* was found to be associated with cough persistence [22]. Pertussis, pertussis-like, and mycoplasma infections may also cause a persistent cough. Mycoplasma infections occur more commonly in children older than 10 years of age, and pertussis should be considered in children with a history of spasmodic cough and pertussis contact.

The pathogenesis of postinfectious cough is unknown, but it is generally accepted that epithelial inflammation by neutrophils and lymphocytes is responsible for chronic cough. Inflammation of the mucosa generates hypersecretion of the mucus, inducing the cough reflex. The postinfectious cough usually resolves spontaneously and does not require treatment. Antibiotic therapy should only be given to patients who are considered to have a bacterial infection [14].

27.4.6 Protracted Bacterial Bronchitis

Protracted bacterial bronchitis (PBB) is one of the major causes of chronic wet cough in children. PBB is defined as the presence of all of the three following clinical criteria: (1) a chronic wet or productive cough lasting longer than 4 weeks in children; (2) absence of the signs suggesting other causes of wet or productive cough (specific pointers); and (3) resolving of the cough after 2 weeks of antibiotic therapy [23].

The prevalence of PBB varies between 11% and 40% according to studies conducted in Turkey and Australia evaluating chronic cough etiologies in children admitted to pediatric pulmonology clinics with chronic wet cough [24, 25]. However, while the actual prevalence of PBB is not known, it is more common, especially in young children. It is mostly misdiagnosed as asthma. PBB develops due to excessive neutrophilic airway inflammation due to bacterial infections. Persistent colonization and inflammation of the airways may cause an increase in mucus secretion and airway inflammation, which may result in airway damage and bronchiectasis. *Streptococcus pneumoniae, Haemophilus influenzae,* and *M. catarrhalis* are the most common bacteria responsible for the etiology of bronchitis. The diagnosis is made clinically, and with the exclusion of other possible diagnoses such as cystic fibrosis and immunodeficiencies. Chest radiographs in PBB may be normal or may reveal only peribronchiolar changes such as bronchial wall thickening. Purulence of the bronchoalveolar lavage fluid and malacia of proximal airways are common bronchoscopic findings in children with PBB. A prolonged course of antibiotic therapy is suggested for children with a chronic wet cough without any specific finding of respiratory or systemic disease. Bronchoscopy should be performed in non-responders and cases with specific findings pointing to an underlying disease [14, 26].

27.4.7 Bronchiectasis

Bronchiectasis is a chronic pulmonary disease characterized by irreversible enlargement of damaged bronchi. The main clinical complaint is a chronic wet or productive cough associated with recurrent pulmonary exacerbations. Many clinical etiological conditions are leading to bronchiectasis. Cystic fibrosis, primary ciliary dyskinesia, impaired immune function, previous pneumonia, recurrent aspiration, including an aspirated foreign body may cause bronchiectasis. In about 40% of cases, however, the cause of bronchiectasis is unknown. These cases are called idiopathic bronchiectasis. In addition to the chronic and recurrent infections and inflammation, decreased mucociliary activity results in increased sputum and dilatation and distortion of the airways [27]. The most common symptom in children with bronchiectasis is chronic wet cough, but children may not be able to expectorate sputum. Therefore, the absence of sputum expectoration does not exclude bronchiectasis.

Bronchiectasis should be considered in children with a chronic wet cough who do not respond to treatment, especially those with findings of underlying chronic diseases such as hemoptysis, digital clubbing, failure to thrive, and/or chest wall deformity. The evaluation requires a detailed medical history and physical examination, as well as laboratory and radiographic investigations, and lung function testing in older children. High-resolution computed tomography (HRCT) is the most sensitive diagnostic modality to confirm bronchiectasis and should be performed when the chest radiograph is normal or nonspecific in a patient with clinically suspected bronchiectasis. An increased broncho-arterial ratio on HRCT scans is the typical finding for bronchiectasis. The mainstay of therapy involves treating the underlying cause, improving mucociliary clearance, treating, and preventing infections. However, for the minority of patients with localized disease, surgery may be considered [28].

27.4.8 Primary Ciliary Dyskinesia

Primary ciliary dyskinesia (PCD) is a rare genetic disorder of mucociliary function. PCD is characterized by the abnormal ciliary structure and/or function resulting in chronic URTIs and LRTIs, male infertility, and laterality defects in nearly 50% of cases [29].

The symptoms and signs of PCD depend on the age of the patient. Most children have a history of respiratory problems in the neonatal period despite a full-term gestation. Nasal congestion is common, affecting >90% of the patients with PCD, appearing in early infancy. Nasal polyps and chronic sinusitis can occur in PCD. Recurrent ear infections are frequently reported in preschool children years and can cause conductive hearing loss. Almost all patients have chronic wet cough from the early infancy period. In patients with PCD, the cough persists almost every day without a seasonal difference. Most of the patients of preschool age have a history of recurrent lower respiratory tract infections. However, frequent antibiotic use for the treatment of otitis and nasal congestion may decrease the occurrence of pneumonia or bronchitis in young children with PCD. Older children may present with bronchiectasis, which occurs in approximately 50% of patients by 8 years of age [30]. Left-right laterality defects may occur in PCD, and nearly half of the patients have situs inversus totalis. Complex congenital heart disease can also be seen in patients with left-right laterality defects. The diagnosis of PCD is difficult and requires evaluation of clinical data, nasal nitric oxide levels, electron microscopy, videomicroscopic analysis of ciliary function, immunofluorescence staining, and genetic investigations [31].

27.4.9 Cystic Fibrosis

Cystic fibrosis (CF) is a multi-systemic, autosomal recessively inherited disorder due to mutations in the cystic fibrosis transmembrane conductance regulator (CFTR) gene. CF affects primarily the respiratory tract, gastrointestinal system, and sweat glands. CFTR dysfunction causes dehydration of cell surface liquid. Altered airway secretions inhibit normal ciliary function and cough clearance, and lead to susceptibility to respiratory tract infections. Pancreatic dysfunction develops due to obstruction of intra-pancreatic ducts with thickened secretions [32].

The onset and progression of clinical manifestations are variable. The main clinical findings are fatty stools, failure to thrive, and recurrent respiratory tract infections. Meconium ileus may occur in the neonatal period. Persistent and recurrent LRTIs with resistant bacterial species can cause bronchiectasis. Cough is a prominent symptom and is frequently productive. With the progression of lung disease, dyspnea may occur. Atelectasis may develop as a result of the accumulation of purulent secretions. CF patients have chronic upper respiratory tract disease, clinically revealed as nasal congestion and rhinorrhea. Chronic sinusitis and nasal polyposis are common among CF patients. Digital clubbing develops in virtually all patients in time. Hemoptysis may occur in older patients during exacerbations, and massive hemoptysis can be fatal.

Clinical suspicion of CF, positive results in newborn screening, and a family history of CF require further investigations. The sweat test remains the most available and useful approach for the diagnosis of CF. CFTR mutation analysis has become important in infants with positive CF newborn screening results, in older patients with inconclusive diagnosis, and for genetic counseling. Effective airway clearance and treatment of exacerbations are critical components of CF therapy. Novel approaches to therapy targeting CFTR mutations have the potential to halt the disease process [32, 33].

27.4.10 Foreign Body Aspiration

Foreign body aspiration (FBA) should be taken into account in children with sudden onset of cough, particularly if the child's age is less than 5 years. The absence of a choking episode does not rule out FBA and may be a risk factor for the diagnostic delay. In a retrospective review of children who were admitted with suspected FBA, the most common symptom was cough (100%). Twenty percent of children out of 48 who presented late had no history of choking in this study. In another study, cough frequency was 88%, and a caregiver witnessed an acute symptomatic event such as choking in 67% of children [34]. Patients often present with acute cough, but the chronic cough can also be the presenting symptom in a missed FBA diagnosis. Associated symptoms may include wheezing and the cough may be either wet or dry. The chest radiograph may show signs of unilateral hyperinflation or atelectasis. However, a normal chest radiograph does not exclude FBA. Bronchoscopy is essential for the diagnosis and removal of the foreign body [35].

27.4.11 Environmental Pulmonary Toxins

It is well known that exposure to inhaled toxic fumes can lead to respiratory system problems characterized by an acute or chronic cough. Cigarette smoke exposure has been associated with chronic cough compared to children without cough [10].

Mallol, et al. [36] investigated the effect of cigarette smoking on the prevalence of asthma symptoms among 4738 adolescents. Symptoms suggestive of asthma including cough were notably higher in the persistent smoker group compared to non-smokers. The number of cases with asthmatic symptoms associated with active tobacco smoking was 223 (27%). They concluded that active tobacco smoking increases asthma symptoms. The indoor use of biomass for cooking is common in developing countries. Several studies showed that indoor biomass smoke has an important impact on global respiratory health. Exposure to indoor biomass smoke in children is significantly associated with respiratory infections that increase the prevalence of cough. Several studies revealed that inhalation of other ambient pollutants (e.g., particulate matter and nitrogen dioxide) may also cause increased cough in children, especially in the presence of other pulmonary diseases [10].

27.4.12 Psychogenic Cough

The psychogenic cough should be considered in children with chronic cough if any etiology of cough is not detected via systematic investigation. A barking or honking quality of cough and absence of cough during sleep are typical features of psychogenic cough. Psychogenic cough is associated with sudden, brief, intermittent, involuntary, or semivoluntary movements or sounds. Phonic tics such as cough, throat clearing, sniffing, and grunting are more common in older children. Symptoms persist throughout the day and children with psychogenic cough seem to be unconcerned. Stress and secondary gains exacerbate symptoms. Viral infections may also trigger a psychogenic cough [37]. It resolves with activities that distract the child and disappears during sleep. The psychogenic cough can be frequently confused with asthma. Other causes of chronic cough in cases with a psychogenic cough should be excluded, as there are no specific clinical features as well as diagnostic tests. Consultation with a psychologist or a psychiatrist is also necessary, as the trials of non-pharmacological therapy including behavioral modification techniques and psychotherapy are more successful than pharmacological methods [14].

27.4.13 Drug-Induced Cough

Adverse effects of drug therapy may cause bronchopulmonary disorders. Nonspecific isolated cough, bronchial obstruction, or alveolitis due to parenchymal involvement may occur because of the adverse effects of drug therapy.

The best known of these drugs are angiotensin-converting enzyme (ACE) inhibitors, which cause a chronic cough in up to 35% of the users [38]. The increase in bradykinin levels due to the inhibition of ACE is responsible for the cough. While beta-blockers and nonsteroidal anti-inflammatory drugs (NSAIDs) produce cough as a result of drug-related bronchoconstriction especially in asthmatic children, calcium channel antagonists are known to induce reflux cough by lowering the lower esophageal sphincter pressure and by a dose-dependent impairment of esophageal clearance [38]. Cytotoxic and biological agents such as tumor necrosis factor (TNF)-blocking agents or rituximab may induce interstitial lung disease. Chronic cough may occur as a side effect of cytoreductive therapy for hematopoietic cell transplantation [39]. Meticulous evaluation of drug history and ruling out other causes of cough can help in the differential diagnosis of drug-induced cough. The discontinuation of the drug is the mainstay of management [40].

27.4.14　Cardiac Causes

The cough may be an initial finding of heart failure due to pulmonary congestion and airway compression. In patients with chronic heart failure, a dry irritating cough may occur, especially during sleep. It is often confused with asthma, bronchitis, or ACE inhibitor-induced cough. A nonproductive cough with shortness of breath may be indicative for the patients with acute pericarditis; however, a cough may be a symptom of pulmonary embolism. Moreover, cough can also develop as a side effect of medications, such as ACE inhibitors or beta (β)-blockers. Therefore, a targeted diagnostic evaluation and treatment approaches are required for relieving cough in such patients [41].

27.4.15　Otogenic Causes: Stimulation of Arnold Nerve

The stimulation of the vagus nerve causes cough. Excitation of the auricular branch of the vagus nerve which nerves the external auditory canal can cause coughing and it is called as Arnold nerve reflex. Wax impaction, foreign body in the auditory canal, inflammation, and exposure to cold air may induct Arnold nerve reflex and result in coughing. In a study investigating the prevalence of Arnold reflex among adults and children with chronic cough, Arnold reflex was found rarer in children compared to adults as an underlying etiology of chronic cough (3% vs. 25%) [42].

27.4.16　Thoracic Tumors

Pediatric pulmonary neoplastic disorders are uncommon and may present at any age. Space-occupying lesions should be considered for patients in whom respiratory symptoms do not regress with appropriate treatment. Thoracic tumors are classified according to their anatomical location, i.e., airway, mediastinum, lung parenchyma, and the chest wall [43]. Thoracic tumors may be congenital or acquired, benign, or malignant. The most prominent symptoms of airway tumors are chronic cough and wheezing due to bronchial obstruction. Mediastinal tumors remain mostly asymptomatic. Symptoms are the result of direct pressure on structures, specifically narrowing of the trachea or bronchi and compression of the lung parenchyma. The mediastinum is divided into anterior, middle, and posterior compartments. Most of the mediastinal masses arise from the anterior and posterior compartments. Parenchymal and chest wall tumors are very rare and usually asymptomatic until masses become large to cause pressure symptoms [44].

27.5 Diagnostic Evaluation of Chronic Cough

Chronic cough can be caused by many respiratory and non-respiratory disorders (Table 27.3). The main strategy should be to determine the main cause for chronic cough and treatment should be planned according to the etiology. A detailed history is essential, with attention to time and clinical setting of onset, exacerbating factors, associated symptoms, prior history suggestive of atopic disease, a complete medical, smoking, drug and exposure history, family history, previous treatments, and their effects. The evaluation of the characteristics of the cough is essential since chronic wet cough is consistently pathological and further evaluations are necessary to investigate the presence of bronchiectasis.

If the cough is associated with wheezing or dyspnea, many clinical conditions including asthma, FBA, recurrent aspirations, tracheobronchomalacia, bronchiolitis obliterans, interstitial lung diseases, and cardiac diseases should be considered in the differential diagnosis. Clinicians must investigate possible aggravating environmental factors and triggers, diurnal patterns, and also family history regardless of the underlying etiology [12].

In cases accompanied by atopic dermatitis or allergic rhinitis, family history of asthma, presence of specific triggers such as exercise, irritants, or allergens, a

Table 27.3 Etiology of chronic cough in children

Pulmonary causes	Extrapulmonary causes
Asthma	Upper airway disorders
Recurrent aspirations	Ear disease
Recurrent infections of the respiratory tract	Esophageal disorders
Protracted bacterial bronchitis	Psychogenic cough
Bronchiectasis	Cardiac disease
Foreign body aspiration	Drugs
Airway lesions	–
Space-occupying lesions	–
Environmental pollution, passive smoking	–

diagnosis of asthma should be considered. The presence of hemoptysis can lead to a differential diagnosis of pneumonia, pulmonary abscess, bronchiectasis, cystic fibrosis, FBA, tuberculosis, or tumors. Frequent throat clearing, postnasal drip, nasal discharge, nasal obstruction, and halitosis would suggest upper airway cough syndrome. In patients with the chronic oto-sino-pulmonary disease and situs abnormalities or cardiac defects, PCD should be considered. The presence of nasal polyposis, fatty stools, failure to thrive, and history of meconium ileus in the neonatal period suggests CF. Tuberculosis should be considered in a patient with nocturnal sweating, fever, general malaise, weight loss, constitutional symptoms, and a persistent wet cough despite empiric antibiotic treatment. Cough with food-related regurgitation and choking suggests aspiration syndromes. Psychogenic cough is dry, barking, repetitive, occurs during the day, and resolves during sleep. It is aggravated by stress and diminishes with distraction. Finally, it is also important for the diagnostic approach to examine the environmental factors and to investigate the specific findings in the patient. A detailed physical examination including all systems should be performed in patients [12].

Chronic cough may have significant consequences; therefore children with chronic cough should be meticulously evaluated, and if required, appropriate further investigations should be done. Diagnostic tests should be determined according to a detailed history and a complete physical examination. Chest radiographs and lung function tests with a bronchodilator reversibility test are baseline diagnostic procedures to evaluate the etiology of chronic cough. The extent of investigations should be chosen according to patients' characteristics and local possibilities.

Feeding and swallowing assessment for aspiration, pH monitoring and impedance testing for GER, diagnostic tests for immunodeficiency, sweat chloride test for CF, HRCT scan for bronchiectasis, bronchoscopy for aspirated foreign bodies, and/or to obtain bronchoalveolar lavage can be performed. For productive cough, sputum culture should be obtained. Allergy testing may be helpful for the investigation of atopy [45]. Since asthma is difficult to diagnose and exclude in children, treatment response can be used for the diagnosis of asthma. For this reason, asthma medications are used for 2–3 weeks, and if there is no response, medications should be discontinued. According to guidelines, empirical therapy for GER is not recommended in children with chronic dry cough with no other systemic disease findings [19, 46].

27.6 Treatment

The main objectives of the treatment of cough are the definition and treatment of the specific underlying cause, detection, and prevention of environmental toxins such as smoking and the triggering factors, determination of the effects of cough on the patient and family, and definition of expectations. Periodic evaluation of the patient is crucial for both confirming the diagnosis and determining the optimal treatment. It should be kept in mind that some children with specific cough may have more than one cause at the same time. Since the etiologies and treatment approaches of cough in children are different from adults, the use of specific algorithms developed for children improves the outcomes [47, 48]. Specific cough treatment should be tailored according to the underlying cause. There are different treatment options for children with nonspecific cough. It is very important to choose the most appropriate treatment according to the patient's age and cough characteristics and to closely monitor the patient's response to treatment [10].

27.6.1 Treatment of Nonspecific Cough

27.6.1.1 Watchful Observation

In most children with nonspecific cough, the first step in treatment is the follow-up of patients for a time frame without medication. Increased receptor sensitivity during viral infections in most cases leads to chronic cough and this situation resolves within 2–3 weeks. In children with an acute cough following a URTI and with normal physical examination findings, further examination is not necessary [46]. In a study, it was found that a watchful observation approach without treatment could be applied safely in children with nonspecific dry cough [47].

27.6.1.2 Drugs Used for Cough

Over the Counter Cough Medications

Over the counter (OTC) cough medications are used in the symptomatic treatment of URTIs. They consist of antihistamines, decongestants, antitussives, expectorants, mucolytics, and antipyretics and analgesics and their combinations. Studies conducted among children showed that OTC cough medications are not more effective than placebo. As age-related drug metabolism causes toxicity, they are not recommended in children younger than 2 years. The use of drugs containing codeine also should not be used in children <12 years of age due to the risk of depression of the respiratory system [49].

Asthma Treatment

Bronchodilators are not recommended for acute and chronic cough unless there is evidence of bronchial obstruction. There are no randomized controlled studies regarding the use of nedocromil, cromoglycate, and theophylline in children with chronic cough [10, 50]. Montelukast is widely used in the treatment of asthma, but its efficacy in chronic nonspecific cough is controversial. Concerns about mental side effects limit its clinical use [51]. In a meta-analysis evaluating the efficacy of montelukast in prolonged nonspecific cough, no significant difference was found between the use of montelukast and placebo [52, 53].

Short-term inhaled steroids are recommended in patients with chronic nonspecific cough. In a meta-analysis in which two randomized controlled trials were assessed, no difference was observed between the use of low-dose beclomethasone and placebo in the first study, but the second study indicated that the use of high-dose fluticasone for 2 weeks led to significant improvement in children with persistent nocturnal cough. In both studies, it was stated that prolonged use was not appropriate due to steroid-related side effects, and the evidence was found weak to recommend the use of inhaled steroids [54]. The use of budesonide (or beclomethasone) equivalent to 400 µg/day inhaled steroids is recommended. The patient's response to the treatment should be evaluated after 2–3 weeks. In cases that do not respond to treatment, the patient should be investigated for other causes. The cessation of cough with inhaled steroid therapy may suggest the diagnosis of asthma or spontaneous resolution [10].

Antibiotics

Antibiotics are recommended especially in patients with a chronic wet cough who are suspected to have persistent bacterial bronchitis (PBB). In a randomized controlled study among children with a chronic wet cough, half of the patients received oral amoxicillin-clavulanate treatment for 2 weeks and the other half received placebo. While cough resolved in 48% of the patients in the first group, this rate was found to be 16% in the placebo group [55]. In a meta-analysis evaluating the effects of antibiotics in children with a chronic wet cough, it was reported that 2-week antibiotic treatment used against the most common pathogens in children with chronic wet cough was effective. The recommended duration of the treatment for PBB is usually 2 weeks, but in a small number of cases, the treatment may need to be extended to 4 weeks. Although the most commonly used antibiotic treatment is amoxicillin-clavulanate, antibiotic selection should be made according to the most common pathogens [56, 57].

Antibiotics are also recommended for chronic sinusitis patients with worsening clinical findings and persistent nasal discharge lasting more than 10 days [58]. In a Cochrane analysis, it has been shown that the risk of chronic cough can be reduced by giving antibiotic therapy for 10 days. Moreover, in a consensus report it was stated that extending the antibiotic duration to 20 days, antibiotic selection according to culture results in cases not responding to empirical therapy, adding daily nasal saline and steroids improved the results [59, 60].

Gastroesophageal Reflux Treatment

Although uncontrolled studies are addressing the efficacy of empirical GER treatment in chronic cough, this has not been demonstrated in a Cochrane analysis evaluating GER treatment including thickeners and prokinetic drugs [10]. The results of the studies evaluating antiacid drugs were similar. In a study conducted in children with uncontrolled asthma and GER symptoms, adding proton pump inhibitors to the asthma treatment did not improve the outcomes [61, 62]. In a meta-analysis evaluating 19 studies, it was shown that the use of proton pump inhibitors in children and adults with GER symptoms and chronic cough was not beneficial [63]. The fact that patients do not benefit from acid suppression indicates that respiratory complaints are less associated with acid reflux. In a study investigating the relationship between 24 h of pH-meter analysis and reflux in children with chronic cough, 84% of cough episodes were found to be unrelated to acid reflux [64]. In a prospective study comparing children over the age of 1 with respiratory and gastrointestinal symptoms due to GER, it was observed that weak alkaline reflux was higher than acid reflux in the group with respiratory symptoms [65]. Empirical antireflux therapy is not recommended for children without GER symptoms in guidelines. Medical treatment, diet, and lifestyle changes are recommended for patients with typical reflux symptoms [10, 46].

Treatments for Nasal Symptoms

Chronic cough may occur in upper airway cough syndrome due to postnasal discharge and larynx irritation. Topical decongestants are very effective in the treatment of nasal obstruction. The prolonged use should be avoided, as rebound effects may occur. Topical decongestants are not suitable for use in children under 2 years of age due to the narrow therapeutic and toxic dose range [66, 67]. Topical steroids are effective in the treatment of cough due to allergic rhinitis due to their local anti-inflammatory effects. In a study evaluating the use of intranasal mometasone, it was shown that mometasone was more effective than placebo for cough and other symptoms associated with adenoid hypertrophy [68]. In a study comparing the use of intranasal saline and fluticasone with the use of antibiotics and nasal decongestants, it was observed that cough and nasal symptoms improved faster in the saline and fluticasone group [69].

27.7 Conclusion

Cough is one of the most common causes of physician referrals in children. Cough is also of great importance due to probable underlying diseases, its impacts on quality of life, and health costs. Etiologic factors and management are different than adults and pediatric guidelines are required for improved outcomes.

References

1. Faniran AO, Peat JK, Woolcock AJ. Persistent cough: is it asthma? Arch Dis Child. 1998;79:411–4.
2. Chang AB. Pediatric cough: children are not miniature adults. Lung. 2010;188:33–40.
3. Marchant JM, Newcombe PA, Juniper EF, Sheffield JK, Stathis SL, Chang AB. What is the burden of chronic cough for families? Chest. 2008;134:303–9.
4. Vernacchio L, Kelly JP, Kaufman DW, Mitchell AA. Cough and cold medication use by US children, 1999-2006: results from the slone survey. Pediatrics. 2008;122:e323–9.
5. Munyard P, Bush A. How much coughing is normal? Arch Dis Child. 1996;74:531–4.
6. Chang AB. Cough. Pediatr Clin N Am. 2009;56:19–31.
7. Ioan I, Poussel M, Coutier L, et al. What is chronic cough in children? Front Physiol. 2014;28(5):322.
8. Smith KG, Kamdar AA, Stark JM. Lung defenses: intrinsic, innate, and adaptive. In: Wilmott RW, Deterding R, Li A, et al., editors. Kendig's disorders of the respiratory tract in children. 9th ed. Philadelphia, PA: Elsevier; 2018. p. 120–33.
9. Chang AB, Berkowitz RG. Cough in the pediatric population. Otolaryngol Clin N Am. 2010;43:181–98.

10. Chang AB, Glomb WB. Guidelines for evaluating chronic cough in pediatrics: ACCP evidence-based clinical practice guidelines. Chest. 2006;129(1 Suppl):s260–83.

11. Sarna M, Ware RS, Sloots TP, Nissen MD, Grimwood K, Lambert SB. The burden of community-managed acute respiratory infections in the first 2-years of life. Pediatr Pulmonol. 2016;51:1336–46.

12. Lamas A, Ruiz de Valbuena M, Máiz L. Cough in children. Arch Bronconeumol. 2014;50:294–300.

13. Boudewijn IM, Savenije OE, Koppelman GH, et al. Nocturnal dry cough in the first 7 years of life is associated with asthma at school age. Pediatr Pulmonol. 2015;50:848–55.

14. Wagner JB, Pine HS. Chronic cough in children. Pediatr Clin N Am. 2013;60:951–67.

15. de Benedictis FM, Bush A. Respiratory manifestations of gastro-oesophageal reflux in children. Arch Dis Child. 2018;103:292–6.

16. Ramanuja S, Kelkar PS. The approach to pediatric cough. Ann Allergy Asthma Immunol. 2010;105:3–8.

17. Chang AB, Oppenheimer JJ, Weinberger MM, et al. Etiologies of chronic cough in pediatric cohorts: chest guideline and expert panel report. Chest. 2017;152:607–17.

18. Usta Guc B, Asilsoy S, Durmaz C. The assessment and management of chronic cough in children according to the british thoracic society guidelines: descriptive, prospective, clinical trial. Clin Respir J. 2014;8:330–7.

19. Chang AB, Oppenheimer JJ, Kahrilas PJ, et al. Chronic cough and gastroesophageal reflux in children: chest guideline and expert panel report. Chest. 2019;156:131–40.

20. Greifer M, Santiago MT, Tsirilakis K, Cheng JC, Smith LP. Pediatric patients with chronic cough and recurrent croup: the case for a multidisciplinary approach. Int J Pediatr Otorhinolaryngol. 2015;79:749–52.

21. Mueller GA, Wolf S, Bacon E, Forbis S, Langdon L, Lemming C. Contemporary topics in pediatric pulmonology for the primary care clinician. Curr Probl Pediatr Adolesc Health Care. 2013;43:130–56.

22. O'Grady KF, Grimwood K, Sloots TP, et al. Upper airway viruses and bacteria and clinical outcomes in children with cough. Pediatr Pulmonol. 2017;52:373–81.

23. Kantar A, Chang AB, Shields MD, et al. ERS statement on protracted bacterial bronchitis in children. Eur Respir J. 2017;50(2):1602139.

24. Marchant JM, Masters IB, Taylor SM, Cox NC, Seymour GJ, Chang AB. Evaluation and outcome of young children with chronic cough. Chest. 2006;129:1132–41.

25. Gedik AH, Cakir E, Torun E, et al. Evaluation of 563 children with chronic cough accompanied by a new clinical algorithm. Ital J Pediatr. 2015;41:73.

26. Gallucci M, Pedretti M, Giannetti A, et al. When the cough does not improve: a review on protracted bacterial bronchitis in children. Front Pediatr. 2020;8:433.

27. Goyal V, Grimwood K, Marchant J, Masters IB, Chang AB. Pediatric bronchiectasis: no longer an orphan disease. Pediatr Pulmonol. 2016;51:450–69.

28. Wurzel DF, Chang AB. An update on pediatric bronchiectasis. Expert Rev Respir Med. 2017;11:517–32.

29. Knowles MR, Zariwala M, Leigh M. Primary ciliary dyskinesia. Clin Chest Med. 2016;37:449–61.

30. Shapiro AJ, Zariwala MA, Ferkol T, et al. Genetic disorders of Mucociliary clearance consortium. Diagnosis, monitoring, and treatment of primary ciliary dyskinesia: PCD foundation consensus recommendations based on state of the art review. Pediatr Pulmonol. 2016;51:115–32.

31. Ferkol T. Movement. Paediatr Respir Rev. 2017;24:19–20.

32. Michelson P, Faro A, Ferkol T. Pulmonary disease in cystic fibrosis. In: Wilmott RW, Deterding R, Li A, et al., editors. Kendig's disorders of the respiratory tract in children. 9th ed. Philadelphia, PA: Elsevier; 2018. p. 777–87.

33. Wallis C. Diagnosis and presentation of cystic fibrosis. In: Wilmott RW, Deterding R, Li A, et al., editors. Kendig's disorders of the respiratory tract in children. 9th ed. Philadelphia, PA: Elsevier; 2018. p. 769–76.

34. Sink JR, Kitsko DJ, Georg MW, Winger DG, Simons JP. Predictors of foreign body aspiration in children. Otolaryngol Head Neck Surg. 2016;155:501–7.
35. Karakoç F, Karadağ B, Akbenlioğlu C, et al. Foreign body aspiration: what is the outcome? Pediatr Pulmonol. 2002;34:30–6.
36. Mallol J, Castro-Rodriguez JA, Cortez E. Effects of active tobacco smoking on the prevalence of asthma-like symptoms in adolescents. Int J Chron Obstruct Pulmon Dis. 2007;2:65–9.
37. Haydour Q, Alahdab F, Farah M, et al. Management and diagnosis of psychogenic cough, habit cough, and tic cough: a systematic review. Chest. 2014;146:355–72.
38. Yılmaz İ. Angiotensin-converting enzyme inhibitors induce cough. Turk Thorac J. 2019;20:36–42.
39. Atzeni F, Boiardi L, Sallì S, Benucci M, Sarzi-Puttini P. Lung involvement and drug-induced lung disease in patients with rheumatoid arthritis. Expert Rev Clin Immunol. 2013;9:649–57.
40. Schreiber J. Drug-induced lung diseases. Dtsch Med Wochenschr. 2011;136:631–4.
41. Rao KNM. Diagnosis and management of chronic cough due to extrapulmonary etiologies. Indian J Clin Pract. 2014;25:437–42.
42. Dicpinigaitis PV, Kantar A, Enilari O, Paravati F. Prevalence of Arnold nerve reflex in adults and children with chronic cough. Chest. 2018;153:675–9.
43. Hyun JS, Chao SD. Tumors of the chest. In: Wilmott RW, Deterding R, Li A, et al., editors. Kendig's disorders of the respiratory tract in children. 9th ed. Philadelphia: Elsevier; 2018. p. 1072–92.
44. Pattugalan TD, Dovey ME. Pulmonary manifestations of oncologic disease and treatment. In: Light MJ, Blaisdell CJ, Homnick DN, Schechter MS, Wienberger MM, editors. Pediatric pulmonology. Itasca, IL: American Academy of Pediatrics; 2011. p. 833–42.
45. Alsubaie H, Al-Shamrani A, Alharbi AS, Alhaider S. Clinical practice guidelines: approach to cough in children: the official statement endorsed by the Saudi pediatric pulmonology association (SPPA). Int J Pediatr Adolesc Med. 2015;2:38–43.
46. Shields MD, Bush A, Everard ML, McKenzie S, Primhak R, British Thoracic Society Cough Guideline Group. BTS guidelines: recommendations for the assessment and management of cough in children. Thorax. 2008;63(Suppl 3):iii1–iii15.
47. Chang AB, Van Asperen PP, Glasgow N, et al. Children with chronic cough: when is watchful waiting appropriate? Development of likelihood ratios for assessing children with chronic cough. Chest. 2015;147:745–53.
48. Chang AB, Robertson CF, van Asperen PP, et al. A cough algorithm for chronic cough in children: a multicenter, randomized controlled study. Pediatrics. 2013;131:e1576–83.
49. Tobias JD, Green TP, Coté CJ. American Academy of Pediatrics section on anesthesiology and pain medicine, AAP Committee on drugs. Codeine: time to say "no". Pediatrics. 2016;138:e20162396.
50. Chang A, Marchant JM, McKean M, Morris P. Inhaled cromones for prolonged non-specific cough in children. Cochrane Database Syst Rev. 2004;2:CD004436.
51. Ernst P, Ernst G. Neuropsychiatric adverse effects of montelukast in children. Eur Respir J. 2017;50(2):1701020.
52. Chang AB, Winter D, Acworth JP. Leukotriene receptor antagonist for prolonged non-specific cough in children. Cochrane Database Syst Rev. 2006;2:CD005602.
53. Dong S, Zhong Y, Lu W, Jaing H, Mao B. Montelukast for postinfectious cough: a systematic review of randomized controlled trials. West Indian Med J. 2015;65:350–7.
54. Tomerak AA, McGlashan JJ, Vyas HH, McKean MC. Inhaled corticosteroids for non-specific chronic cough in children. Cochrane Database Syst Rev. 2005;4:CD004231.
55. Marchant J, Masters IB, Champion A, Petsky H, Chang AB. Randomised controlled trial of amoxycillin clavulanate in children with chronic wet cough. Thorax. 2012;67:689–93.
56. Chang AB, Oppenheimer JJ, Weinberger M, Rubin BK, Irwin RS. Children with chronic wet or productive cough--treatment and investigations: a systematic review. Chest. 2016;149:120–42.
57. Chang AB, Oppenheimer JJ, Weinberger MM, et al. CHEST expert cough panel management of children with chronic wet cough and protracted bacterial bronchitis: chest guideline and expert panel report. Chest. 2017;151:884–90.

58. Hersh AL, Jackson MA. Hicks LA; American Academy of Pediatrics Committee on infectious diseases. Principles of judicious antibiotic prescribing for upper respiratory tract infections in pediatrics. Pediatrics. 2013;132:1146–54.
59. McCallum GB, Plumb EJ, Morris PS, Chang AB. Antibiotics for persistent cough or wheeze following acute bronchiolitis in children. Cochrane Database Syst Rev. 2017;8(8):CD009834.
60. Brietzke SE, Shin JJ, Choi S, et al. Clinical consensus statement: pediatric chronic rhinosinusitis. Otolaryngol Head Neck Surg. 2014;151:542–53.
61. Størdal K, Johannesdottir GB, Bentsen BS, et al. Acid suppression does not change respiratory symptoms in children with asthma and gastro-oesophageal reflux disease. Arch Dis Child. 2005;90:956–60.
62. Holbrook JT, Wise RA, Gold BD, et al. Lansoprazole for children with poorly controlled asthma: a randomized controlled trial. JAMA. 2012;307:373–81.
63. Chang AB, Lasserson TJ, Gaffney J, Connor FL, Garske LA. Gastro-oesophageal reflux treatment for prolonged non-specific cough in children and adults. Cochrane Database Syst Rev. 2006;4:CD004823.
64. Chang AB, Connor FL, Petsky HL, et al. An objective study of acid reflux and cough in children using an ambulatory pHmetry-cough logger. Arch Dis Child. 2011;96:468–72.
65. Zenzeri L, Quitadamo P, Tambucci R, et al. Role of non-acid gastro-esophageal reflux in children with respiratory symptoms. Pediatr Pulmonol. 2017;52:669–74.
66. Woo T. Pharmacology of cough and cold medicines. J Pediatr Health Care. 2008;22:73–9.
67. Schenkel EJ. Paediatric issues relating to the pharmacotherapy of allergic rhinitis. Expert Opin Pharmacother. 2000;1:1289–306.
68. Yilmaz HB, Celebi S, Sahin-Yilmaz A, Oysu C. The role of mometasone furoate nasal spray in the treatment of adenoidal hypertrophy in the adolescents: a prospective, randomized, crossover study. Eur Arch Otorhinolaryngol. 2013;270:2657–61.
69. Tugrul S, Dogan R, Eren SB, Meric A, Ozturan O. The use of large volume low pressure nasal saline with fluticasone propionate for the treatment of pediatric acute rhinosinusitis. Int J Pediatr Otorhinolaryngol. 2014;78:1393–9.

Chronic Cough in Children

Feride Marim and Kostas Priftis

28.1 Introduction

Coughing is an extremely important reflex action that protects the airway by preventing food being aspirated and by clearing accumulated debris from the airway. Paediatric patients may present with a chronic or persistent cough that arises in response to multiple disease processes. Parents frequently seek out a specialist opinion if their child has a chronic cough. Indeed, persistent coughing erodes the child's quality of life, leads to repeated attendance in clinics and may expose the patient to unnecessary side effects if an ineffective treatment regime is instigated [1–4]. The latest research on chronic cough, both individual studies and systematic reviews, indicates that the use of treatment protocols tailored to this condition allows a diagnosis to be reached without delay and leads to more favourable clinical outcomes, e.g. a briefer symptomatic period and a better quality of life [5–8].

A cough that has lasted at least 4 weeks is typically categorised as "chronic"; however some experts consider that a cough in paediatric patients with a duration between 3 and 8 weeks is a "prolonged acute cough". Whatever the precise definition of a chronic cough, one indisputable fact is that this condition differs considerably in the paediatric age range from in adults, as a result of the different form of the airways, the extra susceptibility of children to harm from exposure to noxious substances, a lesser degree of ability to prevent the coughing reflex in children and the dynamic nature of the developing nervous and immune systems in children as they

F. Marim (✉)
Section of Pulmonology, Evliya Çelebi Training and Research Hospital, Kütahya Dumlupınar University, Kütahya, Turkey

K. Priftis
Third Pediatric Department of Athens, Respiratory and Allergy Unit, National and the Kapodistrian University of Athens, University General Hospital "Attikon", Athens, Greece
e-mail: kpriftis@otenet.gr

C. Cingi et al. (eds.), *Pediatric ENT Infections*,
https://doi.org/10.1007/978-3-030-80691-0_28

grow up. It is advisable to regard a chronic cough in childhood as indicating some underlying disorder [1].

Coughing involves a complicated series of actions affecting the respiratory system initiated by a neural reflex. The coughing reflex may have evolved as a way to stop material from the gut entering into the lower respiratory tract, and to keep infections and irritant substances away from the lungs. The reflex involves activation of a number of nervous pathways in the peripheral and central nervous systems and the contraction of both muscles of respiration and other muscle groups. There has been an increased research focus over the last decade in the physiological and clinical aspects of coughing, leading to a significant alteration in the way cough is understood neurophysiologically, and an appreciation of several novel causes for the symptom. The pathophysiology of persistent cough in childhood and in adulthood has been the focus of an important research effort [9].

28.2 Epidemiology

The monthly prevalence of coughing in preschoolers is around 35% overall, although how this rate may vary from country to country has so far not yet been subjected to systematic evaluation. The prevalence of chronic coughing does certainly differ in different geographical locations, from a reported rate of 1% in India, 9% in Eastern Europe and between 5% and 12% in China. Where there is a greater level of air pollution, the frequency of chronic cough also rises. These estimates are influenced by subjective judgements about coughing and whether parents report their child's symptoms or not. There is a need for a systematic investigation into how rates of chronic cough vary globally [1].

28.3 Differences Between Chronic Cough in Children and in Adults

Clinical research indicates that coughing is a symptom which resolves slowly in paediatric patients once the trigger is no longer present. Treating the underlying cause of a cough succeeds in virtually every paediatric case of chronic cough. For children, the likelihood of persistent coughing is affected by the maturational development of the respiratory system, both in form and in function. Many studies have been undertaken into the anatomical alterations occurring in children's respiratory tracts. One consistent finding from this research is that paediatric cases of persistent cough are likely to have tracheobronchomalacia. Coughing in the first few months of life has been linked to the physiological maturation of the trachea [10].

For a child to be able to cough, the various parts of the cough reflex need to be in working order. To understand the cough reflex in young children is complex, since there are many different neural maturational processes occurring. The central nervous system (CNS) develops very rapidly over the initial years of childhood, but once this rapid phase of development comes to an end, the brain continues to mature at a slower rate [10]. Lebel et al. studied the central nervous system white and grey matter development by means of diffusion-weighted magnetic resonance imaging (DWI). This research indicated that some CNS structures were incomplete until adolescence, whilst others developed even into early adulthood [11]. There were also different rates of maturation for different pathways in the CNS. The form the CNS takes ultimately depends on the interplay of genetics, epigenetic modifications and the environment. As neuroimaging techniques have become more sophisticated, it has increasingly become possible to track the results of these factors on how the CNS matures [12].

28.4 Initial Assessment of a Chronic Cough in Children

The first steps in assessing a persistent cough in a child is to obtain a thorough history and perform a detailed physical examination with the aim of detecting the pathological cause. If a cough begins abruptly, but there are no other indications of disease in a preschooler, the clinician should suspect a foreign body has been aspirated and thus arrange for bronchoscopy. A plain thoracic film and spirometrical analysis are vital, as long as the child cooperates with the investigation. Other investigations may be required, as suggested by the differential diagnosis. If there remains doubt about the underlying disorder and where no abnormality is detectable on spirometry or imaging, watchful waiting for a maximum of four more weeks is clinically justifiable. In cases of chronic cough, it is important to distinguish between a productive and non-productive cough. Non-productive cough may often be the result of being exposed to polluted air (smoking, fires or traffic pollution), an allergy or sequela of an infection. In a patient with productive cough, sputum culture is recommended [1, 13–15].

Children may also be prone to a habitual (tic) cough. As with any other tic-like behaviour, the child may be able to suppress the cough, the cough may disappear when the child concentrates on something else, coughing may change character when the child is questioned about it and it may differ from day to day. The child may be aware of a growing urge to cough, as occurs with other tics. Such a cough used to be termed a psychosomatic cough, but the current diagnostic terminology is somatic cough disorder. This diagnosis can only be applied once all other causes of cough, including rarer ones, and a tic disorder have been excluded [1, 13–15].

28.5 Phenotypes of Chronic Cough in Children

28.5.1 Postnasal Drip Syndrome/Upper Airways Cough Syndrome

Persistent cough may also arise due to postnasal drip. This phenomenon occurs in rhinitis or infective sinusitis. The child generally has other symptoms, although it is possible for the sole presenting complaint to be a cough.

Some diagnostic terms which were previously in use, such as postnasal drip syndrome, rhinitis and rhinosinusitis, are subsumed under the term upper airways cough syndrome, in the guidelines issued by the American College of Chest Physicians (ACCP) for the diagnosis and treatment of coughing. So far, however, there remains debate about whether UACS is a distinct nosological entity and what its pathogenetic mechanism may be. The guidelines advocate use of a histamine blocker from the first generation combined with a decongestant agent, but there is no randomised control trial which has actually investigated this course of action. It is believed that these older anti-histamines exert a suppressant effect on coughing by centrally acting cholinergic antagonism. There may be a set of patients in whom the label UACS is appropriate, the syndrome perhaps representing a greater tendency to have the coughing reflex triggered, but precisely how this might occur is unknown. The fact that local therapy to the upper airways does not seem to prevent coughing may be taken to show that there is an inflammatory process affecting the whole length of the respiratory tract, set off by asthma or GORD [1, 13, 14].

28.5.2 Cough in Asthma

Asthma is diagnosed based on clinical features. The use of a particular test to rule asthma in or out is not universally accepted. Asthma demonstrates considerable heterogeneity and the role of asthma in persistent coughing is not fully decided. If the presence of inflammation with eosinophilia is established, this acts as a valuable biomarker in asthma grading and to guide pharmacotherapy. The majority of paediatric cases of asthma are distinguished by inflammation and oedema of the airways, a frequent cause of wheeze. On occasion, however, these features are absent and asthma is only apparent when the child has a persistent cough that is exacerbated by viral infective episodes, occurs during sleep or is set off by exertion or breathing in cold air [15, 16].

There are three types of coughing which may occur in a patient with asthma. The classic presentation of asthma is with reversible airway obstruction and hyper responsiveness of the bronchi. Spirometry is essential to identify these features. The diagnosis of cough variant asthma (CVA) as initially used referred to a case where asthma was present, but where the only symptom noted was coughing, which recovered somewhat following bronchodilator therapy. Any paediatric or adult case where cough persists should be investigated for eosinophil-dominated inflammation. Possibly the test with the highest sensitivity and specificity for the detection of eosinophilic inflammation is quantification of eosinophils in sputum, but this test is not usually offered, takes up time and can only be performed by staff with relevant expertise. The measurement of nitric oxide in exhaled air is a reliable marker of eosinophilic activity in the airways and predicts treatment response to corticosteroids. The easiest and most widely offered test is a blood eosinophil count, but this normally varies depending on the time of day and the season, so it needs to be repeated. The value of 0.3 cells/microlitre is a convenient cut-off when diagnosing eosinophilic inflammation in the airways [17, 18].

28.5.3 Gastro-oesophageal Reflux Disease (GORD) and Cough in Children

In some paediatric cases of chronic cough, the cause is the regurgitation of gastric contents into the pharynx, in other words, GORD. Although GORD is often associated with heartburn, this does not always occur. In certain cases, dysphonia and a tendency to choke may be amongst the presenting symptoms. Diagnosis of GORD calls for measurement of pH within the oesophagus. It is hard to establish a definite relationship between chronic cough and GORD. Symptoms of cough due to GORD may not always respond to treatment of the underlying condition. Accordingly, it is still a moot point whether pharmacotherapy for GORD also offers benefit for paediatric persistent cough. In any case, if a child presents with persistent cough and has a symptomatic presentation consistent with GORD, management should address the GORD via appropriate changes in diet and lifestyle and initiation of pharmacotherapy to suppress gastric acid production. The following three-stage approach to management should be attempted prior to assigning a diagnosis of reflux-related cough:

- Unequivocal benefit from a course of proton pump inhibitor therapy lasting between 1 and 2 months.
- Symptoms reappear when treatment is withdrawn.
- Benefit reappears when treatment begins afresh. The dosage should be titrated against the child's symptoms [18, 19].

28.5.4 Post-viral Cough

Following a viral infective episode of the respiratory tract, a child may recover in every respect other than being left with a cough that persists for several weeks. There are no targeted treatments for a post-viral cough and spontaneous resolution should occur. School children may be offered anti-tussive agents, but not all cases benefit. Around one in three cases of chronic cough in a child no younger than 5 years old represent whooping cough and the median length of symptomatic period is close to 4 months. In younger children, fits of coughing in pertussis usually precede a sharp breath in, the "whoop" in whooping cough. However, whooping sometimes fails to occur during early infancy or in later childhood. Other potential pathogens implicated in post-viral cough are *Mycoplasma*, rhinovirus or respiratory syncytial virus. For virtually all such cases spontaneous resolution is the norm. However, such cases require follow-up to ensure that resolution actually occurs. The probable pathogenetic mechanism is delayed healing of the mucosal lining of the airways following an infection, with concomitant over-sensitivity of the cough reflex sensory arm. Treating these patients with medications used in asthma has no apparent benefit [20].

28.5.5 Productive (Moist or Wet) Cough

A wet-sounding or productive cough indicates that the airways contain pooled secretions, either from excessive production or because clearance cannot occur. In all cases of paediatric cough that are chronic and productive, the clinician should order investigations that allow exclusion of a suppurative pulmonary lesion causing chronic infection of the bronchi and which cause bronchiectasis in the long term.

Persistent bacterial bronchitis (PBB) appears to occur frequently and there is growing recognition that it causes a persistent productive cough in early childhood. It frequently affects those with mild asthma and may sometimes actually have been mistaken for asthma [21]. Seear et al. studied a group of paediatric patients with a persistent wet cough and where the presenting features differed from most key diagnoses to be expected in such cases. They used the term "chronic bronchitis" to refer to such cases, despite this term having generally fallen into disuse. In a number of individuals, there was a previous history of invasive treatment, such as mechanical ventilation for a lengthy period, or heart surgery, whilst others were from families of low socioeconomic status, particularly from native American Indian families. In all cases, the patient was suffering from persistent productive cough. The isolated pathogens included *Streptococcus pneumoniae*, *Haemophilus influenzae* and *Moraxella*. A raised neutrophil count was seen in samples of sputum or bronchoalveolar lavage fluid. Older paediatric patients in this situation typically exhibit no abnormality on spirometrical analysis, although they may cough during the investigation. Plain thoracic films exhibit normal appearances or thickening of the walls of the bronchi of a non-specific type. The symptoms improved following treatment with antibiotics, possibly for a lengthy period of between a fortnight and 1 month. One agent used was amoxicillin with clavulanic acid. Seear et al. suggest the condition arose after earlier damage to the respiratory system, as might occur following infection, or could be iatrogenic. This injury then provoked an ongoing inflammatory response and formation of a biofilm by bacteria, which resisted normal treatment.

A recent study conducted by Kompare and Weinberger has examined a cohort of paediatric patients who suffered from bronchitis caused by bacterial infection. In most cases, bronchitis dated from infancy. Nearly three in four of these patients had accompanying broncho- or tracheomalacia. There was a good treatment response to antibiotic pharmacotherapy, albeit many cases then recurred, necessitating retreatment. If a child's cough disappears and appears fully healthy following suitable antibiotic pharmacotherapy, this confirms the diagnosis of persistent bacterial bronchitis, with no need to further investigate the child [20–22].

28.5.6 "Habitual" Cough

A habitual cough refers to a cough with no apparent objectively demonstrable cause. It may occur as a post-viral phenomenon following an otherwise uncomplicated viral episode. Usually such a cough is non-productive and keeps coming back or involves a honking noise. A habitual cough should disappear when the child sleeps. Habitual cough may occur in the context of a tic disorder. All cases of habitual cough are linked to psychological disturbance and treatment of underlying psychological issues typically improves the coughing [23]. Diagnosis of a psychogenic (i.e. somatic) cough is according to specific diagnostic criteria, but these criteria do not solely occur in this type of cough [15]. Many clinicians use the term "somatic cough disorder" fairly indiscriminately to refer to a cough with no clear cause. Nonetheless, recently it has become apparent that psychogenic coughing is linked to specific neurobiological alterations. It is inappropriate to use the existence of mental disturbance, i.e. depression or an anxiety state, to justify a diagnosis of psychogenic cough. In children, as in adults, persistent cough that resists treatment may itself be the reason for the psychological disturbance. A number of treatment strategies that involve non-drug modalities, such as hypnotherapy, hypnotic suggestion, reassurance, counselling or referral to mental health specialists have been recommended by some authorities. There is, however, no evidence base on which to assess such recommendations.

28.5.7 Irritant Cough

Children who breathe in cigarette fumes or other air pollution (such as from wood fires or traffic fumes) are at risk of developing a new cough or of exacerbation of a cough linked to asthma or nasal inflammation.

28.6 Treatment

Therapy in cases of chronic cough is guided by the underlying aetiology. The various treatment options, including choice of medication, are outlined in the preceding chapter.

References

1. Morice AH, Millqvist E, Bieksiene K, Birring SS, Dicpinigaitis P, Domingo Ribas C, Hilton Boon M, Kantar A, Lai K, McGarvey L, Rigau D, Satia I, Smith J, Song WJ, Tonia T, van den Berg JWK, van Manen MJG, Zacharasiewicz A. ERS guidelines on the diagnosis and treatment of chronic cough in adults and children. Eur Respir J. 2020;55(1):1901136. https://doi.org/10.1183/13993003.01136-2019.
2. Chang AB, Oppenheimer JJ, Weinberger M, Grant CC, Rubin BK. Irwin RS; CHEST expert cough panel. Etiologies of chronic cough in pediatric cohorts: CHEST guideline and expert panel report. Chest. 2017;152(3):607–17. https://doi.org/10.1016/j.chest.2017.06.006.
3. Marchant JM, Newcombe PA, Juniper EF, et al. What is the burden of chronic cough for families? Chest. 2008;134(2):303–9.
4. Thomson F, Masters IB, Chang AB. Persistent cough in children— overuse of medications. J Paediatr Child Health. 2002;38(6):578–81.

5. Chang AB, Robertson CF, van Asperen PP, et al. A cough algorithm for chronic cough in children: a multicentre, randomized controlled study. Pediatrics. 2013;131(5):e1576–83.

6. Karabel M, Kelekci S, Karabel D, et al. The evaluation of children with prolonged cough accompanied by American College of Chest Physicians guidelines. Clin Respir J. 2014;8(2):152–9.

7. Chang AB, Oppenheimer JJ, Weinberger MM, et al. Use of management pathways or algorithms in children with chronic cough: systematic reviews. Chest. 2016;149(1):106–19.

8. McCallum GB, Bailey EJ, Morris PS, et al. Clinical pathways for chronic cough in children. Cochrane Database Syst Rev. 2014;9:CD006595.

9. Kantar A, Seminara M. Why chronic cough in children is different. Pulm Pharmacol Ther. 2019;56:51–5. https://doi.org/10.1016/j.pupt.2019.03.001.

10. Schmitt JE, Neale MC, Fassassi B, Perez J, Lenroot RK, Wells EM, Giedd JN. The dynamic role of genetics on cortical patterning during childhood and adoles-cence. Proc Natl Acad Sci U S A. 2014;111:6774–9.

11. Lebel C, Walker L, Leemans A, Phillips L, Beaulieu C. Microstructural maturationof the human brain from childhood to adulthood. Neuroimage. 2008;40:1044–155.

12. Khundrakpam BS, Lewis JD, Zhao L, Chouinard-Decorte F, Evans AC. Brainconnectivity in normally developing children and adolescents. NeuroImage. 2016;134:192–203.

13. Irwin RS, Baumann MH, Bolser DC, Boulet LP, Braman SS, Brightling CE, Brown KK, Canning BJ, Chang AB, Dicpinigaitis PV, Eccles R, et al. Diagnosis and management of cough executive summary: ACCP evidence-based clinical practice guidelines. Chest. 2006;129(1 Suppl):1S–23S.

14. Dicpinigaitis PV, Morice AH, Birring SS, McGarvey L, Smith JA, Canning BJ, Page CP. Antitussive drugs--past, present, and future. PharmacolRev. 2014;66(2):468–512.

15. Haydour Q, Alahdab F, Farah M, Barrionuevo P, Vertigan AE, Newcombe PA, Pringsheim T, Chang AB, Rubin BK, McGarvey L, Weir KA, et al. Management and diagnosis of psychogenic cough, habit cough, and tic cough: a systematic review. Chest. 2014;146(2):355–72.

16. Ando A, Smallwood D, McMahon M, Irving L, Mazzone SB, Farrell MJ. Neural correlates of cough hypersensitivity in humans: evidence for central sensitisation and dysfunctional inhibitory control. Thorax. 2016.

17. Chung KF, McGarvey LP, Mazzone SB. Chronic cough as a neuropathic disorder. Lancet Respir Med. 2013;1(5):412–22.

18. Spring PJ, Kok C, Nicholson GA, Ing AJ, Spies JM, Bassett ML, Cameron J, Kerlin P, Bowler S, Tuck R, Pollard JD. Autosomal dominant hereditary sensory neuropathy with chronic cough and gastro-oesophageal reflux: clinical features in two families linked to chromosome 3p22-p24. Brain. 2005;128(Pt 12):2797–810.

19. Chang AB, Oppenheimer JJ, Kahrilas PJ, Kantar A, Rubin BK, Weinberger M. Irwin RS; CHEST expert cough panel. Chronic cough and gastroesophageal reflux in children: CHEST guideline and expert panel report. Chest. 2019;156(1):131–40. https://doi.org/10.1016/j.chest.2019.03.035.

20. de Benedictis FM, Bush A. Respiratory manifestations of gastro-oesophageal reflux in children. Arch Dis Child. 2018;103(3):292–6.

21. Kompare M, Weinberger M. Protracted bacterial bronchitis in young children: association with airway malacia. J Pediatr. 2012;160:88–92.

22. Shields MD, Doherty GM. Chronic cough in children. Paediatr Respir Rev. 2013;14(2):100–5. https://doi.org/10.1016/j.prrv.2012.05.002.

23. Vertigan AE. Somatic cough syndrome or psychogenic cough-what is the difference? J Thorac Dis. 2017;9(3):831–8.

Gülru Polat and Kamil Janeczek

29.1 Introduction

Wheezes are sounds auscultated during examination of the lungs. They have a musical character and a duration of at least a quarter of a second. Wheezes are generated by vibrations of the wall of an airway which has almost completely collapsed, leaving the walls virtually touching. The pitch ranges from low to high, and the wheeze may involve just one note or several. They are possible throughout the respiratory cycle. Infants and other paediatric patients frequently exhibit wheeze at presentation. A third of children under the age of 3 years have suffered from an acute wheeze on one or more occasions [1–3].

Table 29.1 Aetiology of paediatric wheeze [2]

Acute
Asthma
Bronchiolitis
Laryngotracheobronchitis
Atypical bacterial infection (*Mycoplasma pneumoniae*)
Tracheitis secondary to bacterial infection
Aspirated foreign bodies
Foreign bodies within the oesophagus

G. Polat (✉)
Dr. Suat Seren Chest Diseases and Chest Surgery Training and Research Hospital, University of Health Sciences, İzmir, Turkey

K. Janeczek
Department of Lung Diseases and Rheumatology, Medical University of Lublin, Lublin, Poland

Wheezes are sometimes distinguished from rhonchi on the basis of the pitch of the main note involved, with wheezes having a frequency in excess of 400 Hz, whilst rhonchi are deeper pitched. Despite some experts' use of the distinction, what precise benefit this offers clinicians remains debateable [4, 5].

Wheeze may be generated in any of the conductive airways forming the proximal portion of the respiratory tract. However, for wheezing to occur, there must not only be significant constriction of the air passages, but also enough air passing to provide the energy dissipated as vibration of the walls of the airway. Accordingly, if a patient who is experiencing an acute attack of asthma is not wheezing, this is an alarming finding that may herald the onset of respiratory failure. If the lesion setting up the conditions for wheeze to occur is a large, immotile blockage, one affecting the central airways or tracheomalacia, the note is usually of lower pitch and has the same quality wherever it is auscultated (i.e. it is homophonous), although the intensity of the wheeze diminishes as the stethoscope is placed further from the origin of the sound. This differs from the heterophonous nature of wheeze produced when the underlying lesion produces varying degrees of constriction in the narrower airways. In a heterophonous wheeze, the wheeze sounds quite different over different auscultation areas [5, 6].

Stridor is a sound of unvarying character which may be most easily auscultated over the front of the neck. Stridor may occupy any portion or all of the respiratory cycle, according to where an obstruction to airflow occurs and how severe the obstruction is. Typically, stridor is most evident when the patient breathes in if the cause lies outside the thorax, whilst a cause within the thorax leads to stridor that is most pronounced on expiration [2].

There have been numerous studies, both European and American, examining how frequently wheeze occurs in children up to the age of five. When repeated episodes of cough, wheezing and being out of breath are considered together, 32% of children in the age range are affected in the colder half of the year. The frequency reported in the North of Europe is 29%, whilst in the South of the continent, 48% are affected. In the USA as a whole, 27% of children were affected. The significance of wheeze varies somewhat, with some cases reflecting no serious underlying condition and resolving spontaneously, whilst other cases have a serious underlying respiratory pathology. Doctors encountering children with wheeze need to diagnose the most probable underlying condition as straightforwardly and swiftly as is feasible and instigate any treatment required, whilst setting the parents' minds at rest [3, 5, 7].

29.2 Aetiology

Asthma is the likeliest cause for a child to wheeze recurrently, whatever age this begins and independent of whether there are other indications of an allergic disposition, a trigger can be identified or how often wheezing occurs [1]. Despite the prominence of asthma as a cause of wheeze, not every child with asthma does in fact wheeze, and there are several other disorders affecting infants and children that may also result in wheeze. A differential diagnosis for a child with wheeze encompasses several potential causes, both congenital and acquired.

Wheezes may be categorised clinically on the basis of the onset and how the airway is being narrowed. Wheeze that begins abruptly de novo may be due to asthma, an infective episode or be due to a sudden blockage to an air passage. Wheeze that is persistent or tends to recur suggests a congenital anomaly, a cardiac cause, a consequence of aspiration, immunodeficiency or lung disorders. The child's age when the wheeze started may also provide diagnostic clues. There are some disorders causing a wheeze that are most likely in an infant, whereas some others are more probable in an older child [8, 9].

29.2.1 Infection

The most frequent aetiology for a child below the age of 2 years who develops an acute wheeze is viral bronchiolitis. This condition is generally caused by respiratory syncytial virus (RSV). A number of other viral infections may also make children wheeze, namely rhinovirus and other paramyxoviruses, such as parainfluenza virus and metapneumovirus. The usual presentation involves onset of nasal discharge, coughing and intermittent pyrexia which precedes the development of a wheeze and a raised respiratory rate. When the patient is examined, there will be evidence of a blocked nose, tachypnoea, extra respiratory effort and wheeze auscultated in all areas and with a polyphonic character. Laryngotracheobronchitis may also account for a paediatric case of wheezing. Rather less frequently, and mainly in an older child, wheezing may result from pneumonia due to atypical bacteria, e.g. *Mycoplasma*. Although a child suffering from tracheitis secondary to bacterial infection may also have a wheeze, there are typically other indications to point in that direction, such as a markedly high pyrexia, severe level of discomfort and a toxic appearance [2, 9].

29.2.2 Foreign Body (FB) Aspiration

It is important for clinicians to be alert to the possibility a child has aspirated a foreign body, irrespective of whether there is an accompanying account showing choking occurred. Aspirated FBs are especially likely if wheeze is only on one side of the child's lungs or the sounds of breathing differ between the sides. For anatomic reasons, the foreign body most often locates in right main bronchi. The right bronchi is an extension of the trachea, it runs more vertically, it is wider and shorter compared to the left bronchi. Where an aspirated FB remains undiagnosed at acute presentation, more persistent symptoms may be observed at a later date. An FB lodged in the oesophagus may also cause a child to wheeze acutely, if it causes the airways to be compressed. In such cases, problems with feeding and swallowing help to narrow down the likely cause [2, 10, 11].

29.2.3 Structural Causes

Anomalous anatomical structures, such as those within the trachea and bronchi, vascular rings and vascular slings constitute some of the most frequent reasons for very young children to present with wheeze, especially in the first month or two following birth. The cases do not gain any benefit from treatment with asthma pharmacotherapy [2, 10, 11]. The following chapter in this collection goes into greater detail.

29.2.4 Functional (Nonstructural) Causes

Besides asthma, there also exist a number of functional disorders capable of producing wheezing, e.g. aspiration syndrome, paradoxical vocal fold function, bronchopulmonary dysplasia and infrequently occurring diseases, including primary ciliary dyskinesia and bronchiolitis obliterans [2, 10, 11]. More details can be found in the following chapter.

29.3 Evaluation and Differential Diagnosis

It is frequently possible to diagnose the cause of wheeze in children accurately on the basis of the history and physical examination alone. If the clinical suspicion is that the airways are reversibly obstructed, bronchodilator treatment may be tried empirically. The majority of those who benefit from such a treatment are asthmatic, although there is also some benefit in other inflammatory disorders where the bronchi undergo constriction, namely bronchopulmonary dysplasia (BPD), cystic fibrosis (CF) and aspiration. Investigations of value in particular cases where the diagnosis is unclear include X-ray, lung function tests, bronchoscopic examination, sweat test and certain laboratory-based tests. The diagnostic criteria and initial management of asthma receive a separate detailed discussion elsewhere in this volume. However, the key points for clinicians to consider are the need for the correct medication to be administered without delay, the child and parents to be taught about asthma and ways to prevent further deterioration in the child's asthma to be put in place [10, 12].

When taking the history, it needs to be established precisely what "wheezing" consists of (in other words, whether wheezing is an appropriate characterisation), when symptoms began, if it is continuing and what other symptoms are also present. In any paediatric case of wheezing, the child or carers should give as much detail as possible about the wheeze. Often nowadays a parent may have videoed such an episode and can show the clip. Frequently members of the public use "wheezing" in a loose sense to refer to any kind of audible breathing, especially originating in the upper airways. This might include snoring, nasal blockage, rattles, gurgling sounds or stridor [13, 14]. If the child currently exhibits no wheeze when examined and the history from the parents needs to be relied upon, the clinician needs to check exactly what the nature of the audible breathing was. Wheezing that suddenly comes on, especially if preceded by choking, suggests a foreign body as the cause. Wheezing that continues and starts in the first few months of life points to congenital, possibly anatomical anomalies. The wheezing of an asthmatic child is usually paroxysmal and appears at intervals. Where wheezing has been gradually worsening, the situation may be the result of a mass (tumour or lymph node enlargement) pressing on a bronchus from outside. Children suffering from interstitial pulmonary disease may also exhibit wheezing that persists, although this is not a common situation [14, 15].

Wheezing is often caused by a viral infection in very young children. Around 30% of children below the age of 2 years wheeze as a result of a respiratory infection. The peak incidence is from the age of 2–6 months. The usual presentation in an infant involves the usual symptoms of a cold followed by development of a cough and wheeze. From time to time, respiratory distress may develop in the next 3–5 days. These symptoms typically improve within a fortnight. There is variable benefit from bronchodilator treatment and systemic steroids. No benefit, however, comes from administering antibiotics, cough medicines or histamine blockers. Usually the infant then appears quite healthy for a time, after which point up to half of such cases then begin wheezing again when a subsequent viral infection occurs. Although persistent wheezing linked to a viral infection usually resolves by the age of 3 years, asthma may develop in a number of these children [16, 17].

Coughing and wheezing frequently co-occur. It is advantageous to ascertain whether the cough is productive or not in attempting to ascertain the likely diagnosis. Productive coughs are generally related to high levels of mucous secretion, usually in response to a pathogen or an inflammatory process, such as bronchiectasis, CF, primary ciliary dyskinesia or persistent episodes of aspiration. A dry cough, on the other hand, is generally related to constriction of the bronchi per se or an anatomical anomaly, such as airway malacia, external compression or vascular rings. Since the mechanism responsible for a non-productive cough may result in secondary complications, however, such as the accumulation of mucus due to a structural blockage and subsequent infection, and thus begin to be productive, this clinical distinction may not always be of much diagnostic value. Asthmatic children may have a productive or non-productive cough when they present. This variability is due to different levels of obstructed air passages and varying degrees of mucous secretion, both intra- and inter-individually [18].

29.4   Physical Examination

When physically examining a child who is wheezing, note the child's weight and height, check the oxygen saturation level, pulse and blood pressure, perform a detailed thoracic examination and inspect the hands for indications of cyanosis and clubbed fingers. Cyanosis or clubbing are not usual in asthmatic children.

When examining the chest, the clinicians should especially note the following [2, 19]:

- Inspect for signs of respiratory distress, increased respiratory rate, retracted muscles and chest wall deformity. Examples of potential abnormalities are an increased antero-posterior measurement, which may develop following prolonged hyperinflation of the chest, pectus excavatum due to longstanding obstructed air passages, which exacerbate the alterations in pressure within the thorax, and scoliosis, which may result in the airways becoming compressed.
- Palpate the trachea to check whether it is deviated, as well as the supratracheal nodes for enlargement and tenderness.
- Percuss to ascertain where the diaphragm is. Percussion also reveals variable resonance in different pulmonary areas. Many clinicians omit percussion, but it is a vital part of examining a child's chest.
- Auscultate the chest to find out where the wheeze comes from and identify its nature. Listen for differences in air entry over the lung fields. If expiration lasts longer than usual, the airways are probably narrower than normal. Wheeze generated by a large blockage or one which affects a central air passage sounds the same in each part of the lung, although it will be quieter in areas far away from the origin. A wheeze of this kind occurs with a vascular ring, narrowing below the glottis and in tracheomalacia. In disorders leading to obstruction of small bore air passages, such as in asthma, cystic fibrosis, primary ciliary dyskinesia or an aspiration syndrome, there is a non-uniform distribution of airway narrowing. If wheeze is concentrated in a specific location, the underlying lesion is likely to be structural in nature. In such a case, imaging studies with or without bronchoscopic examination is appropriate [2, 19].

29.5 Imaging

A thoracic film is needed in a paediatric patient with a de novo wheeze, for which no cause has been identified, or in whom wheeze is longstanding and treatment has so far failed. In paediatric asthma attacks, thoracic films are not routinely ordered, although they may sometimes be required. In the majority of children, a film without contrast is sufficient to visualise the large bore air passages, including the air within the trachea and the bronchi forming the main stem, and is of value in distinguishing between a localised and a widespread lesion. An overall hyperinflated chest is an indication of widespread trapped air and diseased air passages, as occurs in asthma, cystic fibrosis, primary ciliary dyskinesia and aspiration syndromes. Abnormality with a specific focus is consistent with anomalous lung architecture or an aspirated foreign body. Thoracic films allow the identification of disorders affecting the pulmonary parenchyma, atelectasis and a subset of cases where bronchiectatic pathology is evident.

Thoracic films may bring to light enlargement of the heart or pulmonary vasculature, oedematous lungs and further indications of heart failure. Plain chest x-ray is of benefit in identifying a mass within the mediastinum, hypertrophy of the lymph nodes and sometimes reveals a likely vascular ring.

Computed tomographic (CT), magnetic resonance imaging (MRI), magnetic resonance angiography (MRA), and multidetector computed tomography (MDCT) of the thoracic cavity allows for a detailed structural assessment of the mediastinum, great vessels and pulmonary parenchyma. These investigations may be extremely beneficial in narrowing down the diagnostic possibilities.

29.6 Laboratory Investigations of Value in Establishing a Differential Diagnosis

Laboratory investigations are of limited value in the first stages of assessing a child who is wheezing, since, generally speaking, the most likely diagnosis is identified from the history and physical examination. Laboratory testing therefore carries out a confirmatory role in diagnosis or can assist with excluding competing diagnoses. A full blood count is valuable if the child has been wheezing persistently or has indications of systemic illness. Potential abnormalities include anaemia, raised white cell count or leukopenia. A raised eosinophil count is consistent with allergy or infection by a parasite. Further investigations are ordered as indicated by the diagnosis under consideration. Viruses are a significant reason for children to wheeze, due to a variety of different pathological processes. Paramyxoviruses (such as the respiratory syncytial and parainfluenza viruses) and picornaviruses are major pathogens causing wheeze in young children. Recently a new member of the paramyxovirus family has been discovered, metapneumovirus. This virus infects both upper and lower portions of the respiratory tract and can trigger wheeze. Virological investigations are thus sometimes beneficial when it is suspected that an infant is wheezing due to a viral bronchiolitis. Routine virological investigations are, however, unnecessary. There is a more detailed discussion of testing later in this chapter [2, 9, 20, 21].

29.6.1 Sputum Staining and Culture

It is advantageous to perform staining and culture of sputum in paediatric cases where there is a high likelihood of a bacterial infection underlying a wheeze. A fungal infection or an atypical bacterial infection (such as *Mycobacterium*) may also be detected in this way. If such a cause is deemed possible, tuberculin cutaneous testing and specific immunoglobulin titres may be requested. It is reasonable to request anti-*Mycoplasma* immunoglobulin titres if an atypical infection is suspected, given the ever more prominent role of *Mycoplasma* as a trigger for wheeze. *Mycoplasma*, moreover, may increase the likelihood of a child becoming asthmatic in the future [2, 9, 22, 23].

29.6.2 Sweat Chloride Test

Sweat chloride testing detects abnormality of chloride transport as found in cystic fibrosis cases. It is an appropriate test in children with persistent pulmonary disease, such as chronic wheeze. Although the introduction of universal neonatal screening programmes for CF means most cases are picked up in the neonatal period, some CF cases may be screened negatively. This is the rationale for requesting a sweat test, if the clinical picture is consistent with cystic fibrosis. A positive sweat test triggers both a repeat test and DNA sequencing for confirmation [24].

29.6.3 Endoscopy

Endoscopic examination is valuable where the child is thought to have aspirated a foreign body, there is persistence of the symptoms, or treatment resistance occurs. The rigid bronchoscope can be used for cases where wheezing comes on abruptly and an aspirated foreign body is thought possible. The flexible bronchoscope provides visualisation of structural anomalies in the airways. If the patient is sedated but awake, and breathing spontaneously, this technique also allows assessment of airway malacia. In a child where the putative diagnosis is abnormal structure or function of the vocal folds, nasopharyngoscopy is of value, since it provides views of the vocal folds and larynx. Bronchoalveolar lavage may be performed using a bronchoscope, if the differential diagnosis is an infection or an aspiration syndrome [25].

29.7　Treatment

The approach to managing a case depends on the confirmed diagnosis. Although there are many different underlying reasons for children of preschool age to wheeze and considerable associated morbidity, there is only limited knowledge of what influences how wheezing presents and how these factors impinge upon the prognosis. If wheezes are widespread in the lungs, an empirical bronchodilator therapy by inhalation is helpful, since a positive response indicates probable airway obstruction of a reversible kind. Despite this general situation, no response or a limited response does not definitively exclude a diagnosis of asthma. Wheezing, particularly in babies and young children, is affected by inflammatory oedema within the airways as much as by airway narrowing. Hence, in a case where the clinical suspicion of asthma persists despite initial bronchodilator treatment failure, it is wise to persevere with steroids by inhalation alongside bronchodilator agents for a minimum of 14 days (with a 5–7 day course of oral steroids in severe cases), so that there is a possibility for treatment response to be seen and the diagnosis thereby confirmed. Further investigations will be needed if there is still minimal response to such treatment, or if there is a suspicion that asthma co-exists with another disorder. It is beneficial to evaluate sensitivity in patients and evaluate likely exposure to triggers when predicting the likelihood of further attacks. This may also help clarify which patients stand to gain most from a regular daily dose of an inhaled steroid [26].

References

1. Martinati LC, Boner AL. Clinical diagnosis of wheezing in early childhood. Allergy. 1995;50:701.
2. Fakhoury K. Evaluation of wheezing in infants and children, in Redding G. Editor, UpToDate, Last updated Jun 7, 2019.
3. Bisgaard H, Szefler S. Prevalence of asthma-like symptoms in young children. Pediatr Pulmonol. 2007;42:723.
4. Dorkin HL. Noisy breathing. In: Loughlin GM, Eigen H, editors. Respiratory disease in children: diagnosis and mangement. Philadelphia, PA: Williams and Wilkins; 1994. p. 167.
5. Loudon R, Murphy RL Jr. Lung sounds. Am Rev Respir Dis. 1984;130:663.
6. Le Souëf P. Viral infections in wheezing disorders. Eur Respir Rev. 2018;27(147):170133. https://doi.org/10.1183/16000617.0133-2017.
7. Eldeirawi K, Persky VW. History of ear infections and prevalence of asthma in a national sample of children aged 2 to 11 years: the third National Health and nutrition examination survey, 1988 to 1994. Chest. 2004;125:1685.
8. Ferreira SM, Ferreira AG Jr, Meguins LC, Neto DB. Asthma as a clinical presentation of cor triatriatum sinister in a Brazilian Amazon child: a case report. J Cardiovasc Med (Hagerstown). 2009;10:795.
9. Chipps BE. Evaluation of infants and children with refractory lower respiratory tract symptoms. Ann Allergy Asthma Immunol. 2010;104:279.
10. Sink JR, Kitsko DJ, Georg MW, Winger DG, Simons JP. Predictors of foreign body aspiration in children. Otolaryngol Head Neck Surg. 2016;155(3):501–7. https://doi.org/10.1177/0194599816644410.
11. Sink JR, Kitsko DJ, Mehta DK, Georg MW, Simons JP. Diagnosis of pediatric foreign body ingestion: clinical presentation, physical examination, and radiologic findings. Ann Otol Rhinol Laryngol. 2016;125(4):342–50. https://doi.org/10.1177/0003489415611128.
12. Pearce N, Aït-Khaled N, Beasley R, et al. Worldwide trends in the prevalence of asthma symptoms: phase III of the International Study of Asthma and Allergies in Childhood (ISAAC). Thorax. 2007;62:758.
13. Bloomberg GR. Recurrent wheezing illness in preschool-aged children: assessment and management in primary care practice. Postgrad Med. 2009;121:48.
14. Official American Thoracic Society Clinical Practice Guidelines: Diagnostic Evaluation of Infants with Recurrent or Persistent Wheezing. http://www.thoracic.org/about/newsroom/press-releases/journal/wheezing-in-infants.pdf.
15. Griese M. Chronic interstitial lung disease in children. Eur Respir Rev. 2018;27(147):170100. https://doi.org/10.1183/16000617.0100-2017.
16. Konstantinou GN, Papadopoulos NG, Manousakis E, Xepapadaki P. Virus-induced asthma/wheeze in preschool children: longitudinal assessment of airflow limitation using impulse Oscillometry. J Clin Med. 2019;8(9):1475. https://doi.org/10.3390/jcm8091475.
17. Nicolai A, Frassanito A, Nenna R, Cangiano G, Petrarca L, Papoff P, Pierangeli A, Scagnolari C, Moretti C, Midulla F. Risk factors for virus-induced acute respiratory tract infections in children younger than 3 years and recurrent wheezing at 36 months follow-up after discharge. Pediatr Infect Dis J. 2017;36(2):179–83. https://doi.org/10.1097/INF.0000000000001385.
18. Koehler U, Hildebrandt O, Fischer P, Gross V, Sohrabi K, Timmesfeld N, Peter S, Urban C, Steiß JO, Koelsch S, Kerzel S, Weissflog A. Time course of nocturnal cough and wheezing in children with acute bronchitis monitored by lung sound analysis. Eur J Pediatr. 2019;178(9):1385–94. https://doi.org/10.1007/s00431-019-03426-4.

19. Martinez FD, Wright AL, Taussig LM, Holberg CJ, Halonen M, Morgan WJ. Asthma and wheezing in the first six years of life. The group health medical associates. N Engl J Med. 1995;332(3):133–8. https://doi.org/10.1056/NEJM199501193320301.
20. Valdivieso Castro M, Tuduri Limousin I, Cardenal Alonso-Allende TM, Álvarez Martínez L, Oliver Llinares FJ. Protocolo probabilístico para el manejo del cuerpo extraño en la vía aérea [Probabilistic algorithm for management of suspected foreign body aspiration in children]. Cir Pediatr. 2018;31(4):162–5.
21. Asilsoy S, Yazici N, Demir S, Erbay A, Koçer E, Sarıalioğlu F. A different cause for respiratory disorder in children: cases with pulmonary Langerhans cell histiocytosis. Clin Respir J. 2017;11(2):193–9. https://doi.org/10.1111/crj.12324.
22. Zar HJ, Hanslo D, Apolles P, Swingler G, Hussey G. Induced sputum versus gastric lavage for microbiological confirmation of pulmonary tuberculosis in infants and young children: a prospective study. Lancet. 2005;365(9454):130–4. https://doi.org/10.1016/S0140-6736(05)17702-2.
23. Guo Y, Zou Y, Zhai J, Li J, Liu J, Ma C, Jin X, Zhao L. Phenotypes of the inflammatory cells in the induced sputum from young children or infants with recurrent wheezing. Pediatr Res. 2019;85(4):489–93. https://doi.org/10.1038/s41390-018-0268-5.
24. Aziz DA, Billoo AG, Qureshi A, Khalid M, Kirmani S. Clinical and laboratory profile of children with cystic fibrosis: experience of a tertiary care center in Pakistan. Pak J Med Sci. 2017;33(3):554–9. https://doi.org/10.12669/pjms.333.12188.
25. Rosen R, Amirault J, Johnston N, Haver K, Khatwa U, Rubinstein E, Nurko S. The utility of endoscopy and multichannel intraluminal impedance testing in children with cough and wheezing. Pediatr Pulmonol. 2014;49(11):1090–6. https://doi.org/10.1002/ppul.22949.
26. Fitzpatrick AM, Bacharier LB, Guilbert TW, Jackson DJ, Szefler SJ, Beigelman A, Cabana MD, Covar R, Holguin F, Lemanske RF Jr, Martinez FD, Morgan W, Phipatanakul W, Pongracic JA, Zeiger RS, Mauger DT, NIH/NHLBI AsthmaNet. Phenotypes of recurrent wheezing in preschool children: identification by latent class analysis and utility in prediction of future exacerbation. J Allergy Clin Immunol Pract. 2019;7(3):915–24. https://doi.org/10.1016/j.jaip.2018.09.016.

Pelin Duru Çetinkaya, Zeynep Arıkan Ayyıldız, and Demet Can

30.1 Introduction

Infants and very young children frequently experience wheezing. One third of school age children manifest recurrent wheezing during the first 5 years of life [1]. Wheezing is a common health problem and either transient or persistent, it causes significant morbidity, poor quality of life, frequent utilization of the health care system and high economic costs [1, 2].Wheezing has a broad age specific differential diagnosis. Asthma is the most prevalent diagnosis in all age groups and as it is not clearly documented in preschool ages, there have been attempts to classify preschool wheezing into different phenotypes to aid diagnosis, follow-up, and treatment. Our level of knowledge on phenotypes and their prognosis has strongly improved especially after the availability of the advanced age results of birth cohorts. The earliest classification scheme was proposed by Martinez in the Tucson Children's Respiratory Study [3]. This scheme allowed us to recognize four phenotypes, as follows: never wheezed, early transient wheezers, persistent wheezers, and late-onset wheezers. Later schemes divided the persistent wheezers into those with and without allergy, with invariable involvement of immunoglobulin E [4, 5]. More practical approach was proposed by the European Respiratory Society Task Force to use the terms episodic wheezing to describe children who wheeze intermittently and

P. D. Çetinkaya (✉)
Section of Pulmonology, Adana City Training and Research Hospital, University of Health Sciences, Adana, Turkey

Z. A. Ayyıldız
Section of Pediatric Allergy and Immunology, Medical Park Hospital, İzmir Economy University, İzmir, Turkey

D. Can
Division of Allergy and Immunology, Department of Pediatrics, Faculty of Medicine, Balıkesir University, Balıkesir, Turkey

are well between episodes, and multiple trigger wheezing for children who wheeze both during and outside discrete episodes [2]. Multiple trigger wheezing has been suggested that it may be an early indication of later allergic asthma and may be more likely to respond asthma treatment than episodic wheezing. In order to simplify etiologies in childhood wheezing, it is preferred to classify wheezing as acute and chronic (recurrent and persistent) wheezing and causes of chronic wheezing are outlined in Table 30.1 [6].

Table 30.1 Differential diagnosis of chronic (persistent and recurrent) wheezing in children

Structural abnormality
Central airway abnormalities
Tracheomalacia, laryngomalacia, bronchomalacia
Laryngeal clefts
Tracheal stenosis/webs
Compression of an airway
Extrinsic
Vascular ring, vascular compression
Lymphadenopathy/tumors
Mediastinal masses
Intrinsic
Bronchial cysts
Bronchial tumors
Hemangiomas
Mixed
Congenital bronchopulmonary malformations
Endobronchial tuberculosis
Cardiac abnormalities
Non-structural abnormality
Asthma
Aspiration syndromes
Gastroesophageal reflux
Swallowing disorders
Retained foreign body aspiration
Bronchopulmonary dysplasia
Bronchiolitis obliterans
Bronchiectasis
Pulmonary hemosiderosis
Parasitic infestations
Vocal cord dysfunction
Pulmonary edema
Interstitial lung disease
Inherited diseases
Cystic fibrosis
Primary ciliary dyskinesia
Primary immunodeficiency disorders
Alpha 1 antitrypsin deficiency

30.2 Etiology

There are wide ranging underlying causes for persistent or recurrent wheeze, depending on the specific age group. Differential diagnosis includes both structural (anatomical) and functional etiologies. Among the functional etiologies for persistent wheeze, asthma, aspiration syndromes, and vocal cord dysfunction must be noted. Structural causes often lead to persistent wheezing, while functional causes such as asthma, gastroesophageal reflux disease, and vocal cord dysfunction lead to recurrent wheezing. Structural abnormalities include abnormal conformation of the trachea and bronchus or a vascular sling or ring. These conditions are some of the most frequent causes of wheezing in infants. Asthma medications offer no benefit in these structural lesions [6, 7].

30.2.1 Abnormalities of the Tracheobronchial Tree

Abnormalities of tracheobronchial tree generally manifest with noisy breathing in infants. Although an infant may begin to wheeze since birth, it is also possible for wheezing to appear around the age of two or 3 months. This kind of wheezing consists of a single note and is louder when the child has an infection affecting the upper respiratory tract. Cough that resembles croup or stridor also accompany wheezing. In mild cases, child may breathe noisily but otherwise appear very healthy, but at the severe end of the spectrum child may experience marked respiratory distress.

Vascular slings and rings can cause obstruction of the airways and cause a wheeze or a stridor [8–12]. Examples of such vascular anomalies are complete rings, as occur with a duplicated or right-facing aorta, or incomplete rings and slings looping around the pulmonary arteries. Symptoms and signs of vascular rings present since birth especially if an obstruction of airways is present. The usual presenting feature in children affected by such a condition is stridor during both inspiration and expiration, but they may also exhibit wheeze, respiratory distress, and recurrent respiratory infections. The abnormal vessel may also compress the esophagus causing feeding difficulties and vomiting. A wheeze may also be caused by a fistula between the trachea/bronchus and other hollow structures, most frequently in the form of a fistula connection between the trachea and the esophagus. These children may develop a persistent cough and repeated episodes of pneumonia, alongside with a tendency to wheeze. Feeding may trigger coughing or choking in these children [13].

30.2.2 Mediastinal Masses

A mediastinal mass, such as a tumor, a lesion of the thymus, a cyst arising from the bronchus, an angioma or hypertrophy of the lymph nodes may compress the tracheobronchial tree, leading to persistent coughing and wheeze that is chronic and may worsen over time. Location of the mediastinal lesion is helpful in deciding the most likely diagnosis [14].

30.2.3 Retained Foreign Body Aspiration

Foreign body aspiration is generally one of the causes of acute wheezing, whereas up to 10% of the children with aspiration events have negative or doubtful histories [15]. In cases where the foreign body is not recognized, wheezing and coughing may be detected because of post-obstructive pneumonia [16].

30.2.4 Cardiovascular Disease

Cardiovascular disorders in children may cause wheezing. Disorders which result enlargement of pulmonary arteries, as occurs when there is a significant left-to-right shunt may cause compression of the large airways, resulting in wheezing. However, the most common cardiac cause of wheezing is overcirculation and congestion of pulmonary veins. Congestive heart failure, pulmonary flow obstruction, and left ventricular insufficiency can cause congestion of pulmonary veins. Wheezing occurs because of the stretching of pulmonary capillaries and edema around the bronchioles. Clinicians need to maintain a high degree of suspicion for this condition in order not to miss the diagnosis. It has been recorded that the sole symptom in certain cases of cor triatriatum was wheezing [17–20].

30.2.5 Asthma

Asthma is one of the most common causes of persistent wheezing. Asthma presents with recurrent cough, wheezing attacks, and chest tightness in children. Approximately 80% of asthmatic patients start to have symptoms during the first 5 years of life [21]. Recurrent wheezing seen in preschool children are commonly triggered by upper respiratory infections and only 40% of these initial wheezers continue to wheeze at older age and have, or develop, asthma [22]. Allergic sensitization is commonly seen in childhood asthma, so identification of a sensitization during early years increases the likelihood that wheezing will persist during early school years and diagnosis of asthma ensues.

Asthma predictive index (API) is a tool for identification for high-risk children for development of asthma developed in the Tucson Children's Respiratory Study [23–25]. To have a positive API, children must have wheezing attacks before 3 years of age and have either one in two major criteria (parental asthma or personal atopic dermatitis) or two of three minor criteria (allergic rhinitis, eosinophilia ≥4% or wheezing unrelated to colds). A modified version is developed afterwards, requiring at least 4 wheezing episodes before the age of 3 and incorporating aeroallergen sensitization as major criteria and food sensitization as a minor criteria replacing the allergic rhinitis [26]. These indexes are successful in predicting risks of children for asthma, they are simple and noninvasive and used widely in decision-making.

30.2.6 Aspiration Syndromes

The various syndromes resulting from aspiration play an important role in childhood wheezing. It is possible for a child with an aspiration syndrome to receive the incorrect diagnosis of treatment-resistant asthma. Aspiration syndromes occur in association with a number of other conditions, both structural and non-structural. Of the non-structural conditions which are linked to aspiration, the most prevalent is the gastroesophageal reflux disorder (GORD). Because of the chronic microaspiration noted in GORD, the respiratory mucosa becomes inflamed and swollen, resulting persistent coughing and wheezing. Feeding bottle use in infants while lying increase the risk of asthma and wheezing before the age of 5. Pediatric cases of GORD may not show the classical symptoms, namely heartburn or vomiting, instead exhibit less obvious manifestations, such as nocturnal cough, dysphonia, or recurrent croup [27, 28].

30.2.7 Swallowing Disorders

Swallowing disorders involve abnormal activity by the muscles or nerves of the pharyngeal and laryngeal regions. This can lead to ineffective muscle contraction and dysphagia. The glottis may not close completely, the normal coughing reflex may fail to function, and the child may aspirate on repeated occasions. Dysphagia may also result from anomalous anatomy, e.g., laryngeal clefts, or paralysis of the vocal folds. Infants with swallowing problems are unable to suck effectively or swallow, they drip saliva from their mouths, are excessively tired, apathetic and may have a raised respiratory rate or stop breathing during feeding. A child with swallowing disorder generally coughs during feeding, but this may be absent when the laryngeal and tracheal cough reflexes have been overstimulated [29].

30.2.8 Bronchopulmonary Dysplasia

Bronchopulmonary dysplasia (BPD) is a chronic lung disease that develops in preterm neonates treated with oxygen and positive pressure ventilation. The etiology of BPD is multifactorial and involves disruption of lung development and injury due to antenatal (intrauterine growth restriction, maternal smoking) and/or postnatal factors (e.g., mechanical ventilation, oxygen toxicity, and infection). The diagnosis of BPD is based on fulfilling criteria based on a standardized definition which is a single entity of oxygen requirement either at 28 postnatal days or 36 weeks postmenstrual age. Depending upon the extent of pulmonary edema / atelectasis, infants may have mild to severe retractions, rales and wheezing which may also be audible. The long-term complications that can arise from BPD include repeated episodes of respiratory system infection, wheezing episodes, and pulmonary hypertension [13].

30.2.9 Vocal Cord Dysfunction (VCD)

Vocal cord dysfunction (VCD) which is a functional disorder of vocal cords that mimics attacks of asthma and/or upper airway obstruction [30, 31]. It generally occurs towards the end of childhood, but may also be seen in young children when there is an underlying stress factors [32, 33]. When a healthy individual breathes in and out, the vocal folds abduct and they adduct while swallowing, coughing, and speaking. In patients with VCD, this healthy pattern is partially inverted, so that the folds abduct when the individual breathes out and they adduct while the individual breathes in. This abnormal vocal cord movement results respiratory distress and stridor. The clinical picture may be similar to asthma, croup, and upper airway obstruction. The diagnosis is confirmed by laryngoscopy results which shows paradoxical movement of vocal cords. Treatment of VCD is based on speech therapy associated with psychotherapy in selected cases [30].

30.2.10 Bronchiolitis Obliterans

Bronchiolitis obliterans is a rare form of chronic obstructive lung disease resulting in fibrosis of the smaller airways that follows a severe insult to the lower respiratory tract. This may be triggered by chemical exposure, infections, or immunological injury. In some cases, no cause can be identified. Adenovirus is the most common viral pathogen in bronchiolitis obliterans. Patients are presented with hypoxemia, dyspnea, persistent cough, and wheezing [34, 35]. The correct diagnosis is suggested by the lack of significant reversal of the airway obstruction with bronchodilators and or corticosteroids and computed tomography findings.

30.2.11 Cystic Fibrosis (CF)

CF is one of the most common autosomal recessive disorders among Caucasians with an incidence of 1: 2000-3000 live births. It is characterized with chronic sinopulmonary infections, pancreatic insufficiency, and failure to thrive. Infants with cystic fibrosis frequently present with recurrent wheezing. Besides this, pulmonary function tests performed in children with CF also showed that these children had bronchial hyperreactivity [36].

30.2.12 Primary Ciliary Dyskinesia (PCD)

Primary ciliary dyskinesia is a rare disease with an incidence of 1: 10,000–30,000 in the general population. PCD is inherited as an autosomal recessive trait and characterized by chronic/recurrent upper and lower respiratory infections that begin at an early age. Laterality such as situs-in versus or heterotaxy and complex congenital heart disease are noted in half of the cases. Primary ciliary dyskinesia should be included in the differential diagnosis of a child who suffers from repeated, severe infective episodes affecting the upper respiratory tract, suppurative ear disease or persistent sinusitis [37].

30.2.13 Primary Immunodeficiencies

Wheezing is generally noted with viral respiratory infections in childhood. Children with primary immunodeficiency disorders may suffer from persistent or chronic pulmonary infections, which are complicated by bronchiectasis and irreversible damage to lung tissues, if the diagnosis is missed or the treatment is suboptimal. Humoral immunodeficiencies are the most common type of immunodeficiencies that lead to recurrent upper and lower respiratory infections but complement deficiencies, T-lymphocytic dysfunction and phagocytosis and chemotaxis defects can also lead to similar clinical findings [13].

30.3 Evaluation of a Child with Persistent/Recurrent Wheezing

Detailed history of wheezing, especially age of onset and presence of other symptoms with physical examination findings, generally provides clues to the diagnosis. In young children differential diagnosis is broad and anatomical anomalies should be kept in mind. Noisy breathing, postural effects on wheezing and poor response to bronchodilators and corticosteroids are the common features of structural abnormalities.

Gastroesophageal reflux is common in infancy and might be associated with recurrent and persistent wheezing. Wheezing related to feeding and postural increase in symptoms are important features in the history. Foreign body aspiration history should be asked carefully in all infants and young children because many of the parents do not remember the event or they need to ask the caregivers.

Family and consanguinity history for inherited diseases like cystic fibrosis, immunodeficiency and PCD is very important in evaluating infants with persistent wheezing.

Investigations should be ordered according to the positive findings. But a chest radiography should be taken to evaluate mass, infiltrations, great vessel abnormalities, congenital bronchopulmonary malformations or possible foreign body aspiration. Barium studies may show a filling defect caused by a vascular ring as well as gastroesophageal reflux. Echocardiography, computed tomography or magnetic resonance imaging helps definitive diagnosis of vascular rings. Direct visualization of airways by laryngoscopy and bronchoscopy helps detection of airway malacia, foreign body, vocal cord dysfunction, and any lesions compressing the airway.

Persistent wheezing and frequent respiratory infections also should raise suspicion for inherited causes of persistent wheezing and sweat chloride test and immune profile should be investigated. Bronchiectasis may also present with wheezing, and secondary causes like PCD, CF, and primary immunodeficiency disorders should be in differential diagnosis.

In preschool aged children with recurrent wheezing, family history for atopy and allergic history including food allergy, atopic dermatitis, and allergic rhinitis is extremely important in predicting the risk of asthma. Thus assessment of evidence of sensitization to inhalant and food allergens by skin prick testing or by determination of allergen specific IgE should be a part of an investigation in these children.

Congenital conditions become less likely to present in older ages and asthma becomes the most common cause of persistent/chronic wheezing in school age group and adolescents. Spirometry is helpful in demonstrating reversible airway obstruction being highly suggestive of asthma. Bronchodilator response and inspiratory and expiratory flow volume loops is important in diagnosis of asthma while the latter also helps diagnosing vocal cord dysfunction. Bronchoprovocation tests shows bronchial hyperreactivity and may be needed in selected cases.

30.4 Conclusion

Persistent wheezing in children needs carefully consideration of broad differential diagnosis especially in infancy. Appropriate identification of underlying conditions may lead to surgical correction, discontinuation of unnecessary treatment, symptom resolution and early effective treatment if possible.

Identification of high-risk children for asthma is also important because it improves the prognosis by means of treatment and preventive measures.

References

1. Mallol J, García-Marcos L, Solé D, Brand P, EISL Study Group. International prevalence of recurrent wheezing during the first year of life: variability, treatment patterns and use of health resources. Thorax. 2010;65(11):1004–9.
2. Ducharme FM, Tse SM, Chauhan B. Diagnosis, management and prognosis of preschool wheeze. Lancet. 2014;383:1593.
3. Martinez FD. What have we learned from the Tucson Children's respiratory study? Paediatr Respir Rev. 2002;3:193–7.
4. Brand PL, Baraldi E, Bisgaard H, et al. Definition, assessment and treatment of wheezing disorders in preschool children: an evidence-based approach. Eur Respir J. 2008;32(4):1096–10110.
5. Can D. Can phenotypes in preschool wheezing be recognized? Journal Dr. Behçet Uz Children's Hospital. 2019;9(3):167–74.

6. Tenero L, Piazza M, Piacentini G. Recurrent wheezing in children. Transl Pediatr. 2016;5(1):31–6.
7. Bacharier LB. Evaluation of the child with recurrent wheezing. J Allergy Clin Immunol. 2011;128(3):690.
8. Lee SL, Cheung YF, Leung MP, et al. Airway obstruction in children with congenital heart disease: assessment by flexible bronchoscopy. Pediatr Pulmonol. 2002;34:304.
9. McLaren CA, Elliott MJ, Roebuck DJ. Vascular compression of the airway in children. Paediatr Respir Rev. 2008;9:85.
10. Turner A, Gavel G, Coutts J. Vascular rings--presentation, investigation and outcome. Eur J Pediatr. 2005;164:266.
11. Bakker DA, Berger RM, Witsenburg M, et al. Vascular rings: a rare cause of common respiratory symptoms. Acta Paediatr. 1999;88:947.
12. Ruzmetov M, Vijay P, Rodefeld MD, et al. Follow-up of surgical correction of aortic arch anomalies causing tracheoesophageal compression: a 38-year single institution experience. J Pediatr Surg. 2009;44:1328.
13. Fakhoury K. Evaluation of wheezing in infants and children in: post T, ed. UpToDate. Waltham, MA: UpToDate; 2019. https://www.uptodate.com/contents/evaluation-of-wheezing-in-infants-and-children. Accessed 07 June 2019.
14. Simpson I, Campbell PE. Mediastinal masses in childhood: a review from a paediatric pathologist's point of view. Prog Pediatr Surg. 1991;27:92–126.
15. Even L, Heno N, Talmon Y, et al. Diagnostic evaluation of a foreign body aspiration in children: a prospective study. J Pediatr Surg. 2005;40:1122–7.
16. Sink JR, Kitsko DJ, Georg MW, et al. Predictors of foreign body aspiration in children. Otolaryngol Head Neck Surg. 2016;155(3):501–7.
17. Moss AJ, McDonald LV. Cardiac disease in the wheezing child. Chest. 1977;71:187.
18. Rabinovitch M, Grady S, David I, et al. Compression of intrapulmonary bronchi by abnormally branching pulmonary arteries associated with absent pulmonary valves. Am J Cardiol. 1982;50:804.
19. Tanabe T, Rozycki HJ, Kanoh S, et al. Cardiac asthma: new insights into an old disease. Expert Rev Respir Med. 2012;6:705.
20. Pisanti A, Vitiello R. Wheezing as the sole clinical manifestation of cor triatriatum. Pediatr Pulmonol. 2000;30:346.
21. Yunginger JW, Reed CE, OÇonnel EJ, et al. A community based study of theepidemiology of asthma. Incidence rates, 1964-1983. Am Rev Respir Dis. 1992;146:888–94.
22. Martnez FD, Wright AL, Taussig LM, et al. Asthma and wheezing in the first six years of life. The group health medical associates. N Engl J Med. 1995;332(3):133–8.
23. Castro-Rodriguez JA, Holberg CJ, Wright AL, et al. A clinical index to define risk of asthma in young children with recurrent wheezing. Am J Respir Crit Care Med. 2000;162:1403–6.
24. Castro-Rodriguez JA. The asthma predictive index: early diagnosis of asthma. Curr Opin Allergy Clin Immunol. 2011;11:157–61.
25. Leonardi NA, Spycher BD, Stripolli MP, et al. Validation ofthe asthma predictive index and comparison with simple clinical prediction rules. J allergy Clin Immunol. 2011;127:2466–72.
26. AminP LL, Epstein T. Optimum predictors of childhood asthma: persistent wheeze or the asthma predictive index? J Allergy Clin Immunol Prect. 2014;2:709–15.
27. Sheikh S, Stephen T, Howell L, et al. Gastroesophageal reflux in infants with wheezing. Pediatr Pulmonol. 1999;28:181–6.
28. Patra S, Singh V, Chandra J, et al. Gastro-esophageal reflux in early childhood wheezers. Pediatr Pulmonol. 2011;46:272–7.
29. Bhatt J, Prager JD. Neonatal stridor: diagnosis and management. Clin Perinatol. 2018;45(4):817–31.
30. Christopher KL, Wood RP, Eckert C, et al. Vocal cord dysfunctionpresenting as asthma. N Engl J Med. 1983;308:566–70.
31. David RS, Brugman SM, Larsen GL. Use of videography in the diagnosis of vocal cord dysfunction: a case report with video clips. J Allergy Clin Immunol. 2007;119:1329–31.

32. O'Connell MA, Sklarew PR, Goodman DL. Spectrum of presentation of paradoxical vocal cord motion in ambulatory patients. Ann Allergy Asthma Immunol. 1995;74:341–4.
33. Powell DM, Karanfilov BI, Beechler KB, et al. Paradoxical vocal cord dysfunction in juveniles. Arch Otolaryngol Head Neck Surg. 2000;126:29–34.
34. Zhang XM, Lu AZ, Yang HW, et al. Clinical features of postinfectious bronchiolitis obliterans in children undergoing long-term nebulization treatment. World J Pediatr. 2018;14(5):498–503.
35. Jang YY, Park HJ, Chung HL. Serum YKL-40 levels may help distinguish exacerbation of post-infectious bronchiolitis obliterans from acute bronchiolitis in young children. Eur J Pediatr. 2017;176(7):971–8.
36. Hiatt P, Eigen H, Yu P, et al. Bronchodilator responsiveness in infants and young children with cystic fibrosis. Am Rev Respir Dis. 1988;137:119.
37. Turnbull A, Balfour-Lynn IM. Recent advances in paediatric respiratory medicine. Arch Dis Child. 2016;101(2):193–7.

Part III

Infections

Pediatric Otitis Externa 31

İbrahim Aladağ, Abdulkadir İmre,
and Sergei Karpischenko

31.1　Introduction

The most common form of otitis externa (OE) is acute. Acute OE (swimmer's ear) is defined as an diffuse inflammatory condition of the external ear canal with or without involvement of pinna. It is usually associated with swimming in children over 2 years of age. Deterioration of local defence mechanism of external ear by prolonged ear canal wetness, maceration, local trauma, external devices, dermatitides or canal obstruction make the canal epithelium vulnerable to infections. Three clinical stages of OE have been described: preinflammatory; acute inflammatory; and chronic. Bacterial organisms are primarily responsible pathogens in acute OE. However, chronic OE is defined as lasting 3 months or longer is usually caused by underlying inflammatory dermatologic disease or inadequately treated acute OE.

31.2　Anatomy

The external ear canal is composed of two parts; cartilaginous (outer) and osseous (inner) part. The outer cartilaginous part includes a thin layer of subcutaneous tissue between the skin and cartilage. Anterior and inferior part of the cartilaginous structure involve fissures of Santorini that allow spread of infection to

İ. Aladağ (✉) · A. İmre
Department of Otorhinolaryngology, Faculty of Medicine, Katip Çelebi University, İzmir, Turkey

S. Karpischenko
Department of Otorhinolaryngology, The First Pavlov State Medical University of Saint Petersburg, Saint Petersburg, Russia

C. Cingi et al. (eds.), *Pediatric ENT Infections*,
https://doi.org/10.1007/978-3-030-80691-0_31

preauricular soft tissue and parotid gland. The inner osseous part formed by tympanic bone, periosteum and skin. Narrowest part of the external ear canal at the junction of cartilaginous and bony part is called isthmus. In contrast to skin of bony canal, cartilaginous part contains many sebaceous and apocrine glands and hair cells. These three structures constitute the apopilosebaceous unit of the external ear canal and serve as a protective function. Glandular secretions form an acidic cerumen which is a local defensive barrier to bacterial infections. Excessive cleaning of the ear canal may harm to this local defensive mechanism and may cause infection. The ear canal normally self-cleansing structure, however, individual anatomic variation of the canal may predispose some patients to cerumen accumulation.

Ear canal infection can be spread to associated lymph nodes via lymphatic channels. Anterior and superior part of the ear canal lymphatics drain into prearicular and superior deep cervical nodes. Posterior part, drain into postauricular and superior deep cervical nodes. Inferior part, drain into infra-auricular lymph nodes [1].

31.3 Pathogenesis and Definition

OE have been categorized into three clinical stages: preinflammatory stage; acute inflammatory stage, including mild, moderate, and severe forms; and chronic stage [2]. Acute OE is inflammation of the external ear canal skin with variable edema that may extend to pinna. Diagnosis is clinically based on symptoms and signs of ear canal inflammation. Presentation of the disease varies between minimal discomfort and necrotising OE. In early period, disease often begins with itching of the ear canal and minimal edema. As the disease progresses, severe pain occur with swallowing of the canal skin. Purulent discharge occurs and surrounding skin may become involved. Ear pain which can be intensified by jaw motion is the symptom that best correlates with the severity of disease. The tenderness of the tragus or the pinna is frequently severe and that may be disproportionate with physical examination findings of the ear canal.

Diagnostic criteria include; rapid onset (usually within 48 h) in the past 3 weeks ofsymptomsand signs of ear canal inflammation (Table 31.1). Acute OE can be classified according to duration of infection: acute, subacute, and chronic.

Table 31.1 Diagnostic criteria of acute otitis externa

Symptoms of ear cana linflammation	Signs of ear cana linflammation
Otalgia (often severe) with or without jaw pain	Tenderness of the tragus, pinna, or both
Itching	Diffuse ear canal erythema, edema or both
Aural fullness with or without hearing loss	Otorrhea, cellulitis of the pinna and surrounding skin or regional lymphadenitis

Adapted from Rosenfeld RM, Brown L, Cannon CR, et al. Clinical practice guideline: acute otitis externa. OtolaryngolHeadNeckSurg 2006; 134(Suppl 4): S4–23

31.4 Epidemiology

Diagnoses of acute OE display a obvious seasonality. Incidence peaked during summer months (44% occured in June through August), and reached their lowest rate in the winter. Most patients with otologic complaints visit emergency departments and cause a significant burden. However, a greatmajority of these patientsdo not need emergent care. In the paediatric age group, 6.79% of all emergency department visits is associated with otologic diagnosis. Although the paediatric patients mostly present with otitis media (82.1%), external ear disesases (9%) is the second common diagnoses in the emergency department [3]. Data from ambulatory care centers show that estimated annual rates of outpatient visits in US is highest among children aged 5–14 years. Approximately, 34% of all visits were for these children. Lifetime prevelance is up to 10%. Direct health-care payments are estimated at approximately half a billion dollars per year in US [4].

31.5 Etiology-Predisposing Factors

The etiology of the disease is multifactorial. Various factors that results in removal of the protective lipid layer from the ear canal and permitting bacteries to invade the apopilosebaceous unit may cause acute OE. However, the most common predisposing factor is swimming. Risk factors for acute OE include following [5]:

- Lack of cerumen.
- Swimming or diving.
- Trauma from external devices (hearing aids, foreign body, ear plugs).
- Hot and humid climates.
- Coexistence of skin disease (eczema, atopic dermatitis and other inflamatory dermatoses).
- Ear canal obstruction secondary to exostoses or stenosis.
- Comorbidites such as diabetes mellitus and immunsuppression.

A number of preventive measures is recommended to avoid recurrent infections, including water precautions (use of ear plug while swimming, using hair dryer after swimming), avoidance of straching the canal skin (traumatic self-cleaning, cotton swabs, sharp objects), treatment of underlying dermatitis, or use of prophylactic acidifying drop such as asetic acid 2% otic solutions after swimming.

31.6 Microbiology

The most common pathogens for acute otitis externa are pseudomonas aeruginosa and staphylococcus aureus (Table 31.2). Normally, external ear canal have polymicrobial bacterial flora as the part of normal flora including aerobic (staphylococcus epidermidis, pseudomonas aeruginosa) and anaerobic (proprionibacterium acnes,

Table 31.2 Organisms isolated from ear canal in otitis externa

Aerobicbacteria	Aerobicbacteria
Pseudomonasaeruginosa	Bacteroidesfragilis
Staphylococcusaureus	Peptostreptococcusmagnus
Staphylococcusepidermidis	
Proteusmirabilis	
Acinetobactercalcoacetius	
Enterobacteraerogenes	

Adapted from Clark WB, Brook I, Bianki D, et al. Microbiology of otitisexterna. OtolaryngolHead-NeckSurg. 1997; 116(1): 23–5

peptococcus sp) bacteria. However, Bacteroides sp. is not part of the normal external ear canal flora. Fungal infection such as Aspergillus species and Candida speciesare distinctly very rare in primary acute otitis externa but may be more common after treatment with topical antibiotics [6]. Routine ear canal sample collection for culture is not necessary in primary uncomplicated acute OE. Culture results should be assessed with caution because they may reflect normal flora. However, in patients with recalcitrant infections, uncontrolled diabetes, immunocompromise, and a history of temporal radiotherapy culture may identify the responsible pathogen and assist in the choice of appropriate antibotic therapy [7].

31.7 Diagnosis and Staging

Diagnosis is clinically based on symptoms and signs of ear canal inflammation. Senturia et al. classified the clinical progress of OEas the following clinical stages: preinflammatory, acute inflammatory and chronic inflammatory. Acute inflammatory stage is also divided into three form including mild, moderate and severe [8].

*Preinflammatory stage*begins with the removal of protective lipid layer of the ear canal resulting in obstruction of the apopilosebaceous unit. Local trauma and wetness remove the protective lipid layer of the canal skin. The skin then becomes edematous which resulting in obstruction of the glands. Consequently, sense of aural fullness and itching begins.

Acute inflammatory stage begins with the distruption of epithelial layer and invasion of the bacterial organisms. In mild acute inflammatory stage, pain and tenderness of the tragus or pinna occur. On examination, otoscopy will reveal mild erythema and minimal edema in the ear canal. Minimal odorlessand blurry secretion with or without debris may be seen. As the disease progress to moderate stage, pain and itching will increase, canal edema worsen, and more thicker seropurulent secretion occur. In the severe inflammatory stage, further progression of the inflammation result in complete obliteration of the ear canal. Severe pain, abundant purulent secretion and severe canal edema are predominant symptoms and findings in this stage. Involvement of the surrounding skin and soft tissues are also frequently seen in this stage. Drooping of the superior canal, auricular edema and regional adenopathy may occur. If the disease progress, infection can spread to anterior adjacent structures including parotid gland and temporomandibular joint via fissures of Santorini, posterior connective tissue overlying mastoid region.

Chronic inflammatory stage is presented with noticeable thickening of the ear canal skin secondary to existing of infection for a long time. The longstanding itching is the main symptom in this stage. Patients feel less pain in this stage. Edema of the ear canal skin and secondary dermatological lesions adjacent to auricle such as eczematization or superficial ulceration can be seen on physical examination. Finally, advanced form of this stage marked with thick ear canal skin is called hypertrophic chronic OE.

Recalcitrant otitis externa can be defined as the clinical condition that fail to respond meticulous local care and topical therapy. Treatment of uncomplicated acute OE should be followed by relief of symptoms including otalgia, itching and aural fullness within 48–72 h. However, complete improvement may take a week or more. Therefore re-evaluation is recommended for those patients without findings of early resolution. In such a case, patients should be reassesed for the patency of the ear canal for any obstruction and need of aural toilet or wick placement. If the obstruction fail to respond topical therapy, systemic oral antibiotic treatment that covers P. aeruginosa should be kept in mind. Topical treatment failure related to various factors including; ear canal blockage with marked edema, inadequate canal cleaning, resistant microorganisms, noncompliance of patients to therapy, contact dermatitis secondary to ear drops or accompanying dermatologic disorders such as dermatitis and psoriasis. Recalcitrant infections usually occur due to poor adherence to treatment and chronic instrumentation of the ear canal skin. However, patients with longstanding recalcitrant infections should be reassessed for malignant OE [9].

Necrotising (malignant) otitis externa (NEC) is described almost exclusively in elderly diabetics. NEC is very rare in children and fewer than 20 cases are reported in the literature. In those children reported host factors include anemia, diabetes mellitus, diabetes insipitus, malignancy (leukemia and neuroblastoma) and chemotherapy. Although higher mortality rates (40 to 50%) reported in adults with accompanying multiple cranial nerve palsies, there is no reported mortality in children regardless of cranial nerve complications. Therefore, a greater overall response to appropriate treatment is suspected in children [10, 11].

31.8 Differential Diagnosis

Diffuse acute OE often present with severe otalgia and tenderness of the tragus or pinna, or both. The characteristic sign of diffuse acute otitis externa is the tenderness of the tragus or pinna. The other diseases causing otalgia, otorrhea, and ear canal inflammation should be distinguished from acute OE. Accurate diagnosis enables clinican to treat the condition appropriately. Dermatoses of the ear canal such as eczema, irritant contact dermatitis, allergic contact dermatitis and seborrheic dermatitis are slightly common and can mimic acute otitis externa. The diseases that may may be confused with OE is listed in Table 31.3.

Table 31.3 Differentialdiagnosis of otitis externa

Disease	Clinicalfeatures	Treatment/Comment
Acuteotitismedia	Presence of ertythemainvolvingtympanicmembranewithouttragaltenderness	Pneumaticotoscopy/tympanometry
Eczema (atopicdermatitis)	Presence of chronicpruritiswithhistory of atopy. Lesionsareusuallyoccur in childhoodwithother skin lesions	Topicalsteroid
Seborrheicdermatitis	Presentwithgreasyyellowishscalingaffectingtheears, scalp, hairline, centralface.	Lubricatingormoisturizing of theearcanalandtopical anti-inflammatorymedications.
Contactdermatitis (irritant/contact)	Occurwhenpatientscomes in contactwithanyagentthat can produce skin responseincludingmetals,chemicalsoroticpreperations. Presentwitherythema,weepingandvesiculationaccompaniedwithpruritis.	Avoidfromcausativeagent. Topicalsteroidtreatmentorotherantinflammatoryagentsuch as calcineurininhibitors (tacrolimus 0.1% oinment)
Furunculosis/ carbunculosis	Localizedotitisexternaresultingfrom an infectedhairfollicle. S. aureus is themostcommoncausativeagent. Focalswellingand pustular lesion is thepredominantlesion.	Treatmentincludelocalheat, incisionanddrainage, andantibiotictreatment.
Herpeszosteroticus	Presentwithvesicles on theearcanalandauricle, severe otalgia, facialparesis/paralysis	Treatmentincludesantiviralsandsystemicsteroids
Perichondritis	The skin overtheaffectedareabecomescrustedandserous/ purulentexudateweepsfrominvolvedcartilage. Affectedareainduratedandearcanalmayswellsandobliterated	Debridementandtreatmentwithtopicalorsystemicantibiotics
Relapsingpolychondritis	Episodicinflammatorydestructionof cartilagesincludingear, larynx, trachea, ornose.	Diagnosis is made on thebasis of thehistory, physicalexaminationwithelevatedsedimentation rate andcartilagebiopsy. Treatmentinclude oral steroids.
Referred otalgia	Normal otoscopy/earexamination	Complete headandneckexaminationincludingtemporomandibularjoint

Physical examination should include each ear grossly, surrounding skin and lymph nodes, and then in detail with an otoscope or microscope. Manipulation of the canal is often cause discomfort and pain. If the examination becomes painful, physican should stop. However, gentle cleaning of the canal using smaller ear speculum with suction ease the use of topical agents [12].

31.9 Medical Treatment

31.9.1 Pain Management

Pain can be severe and intense. Pain management is the main part of the treatment of acute otitis externa. Appropriate use of analgesics is necessary to accomplish patient comfort. Nonsteroidal anti-inflammatory medication (with or without opioid combination) or acetaminophen are usually sufficient for pain relief. Early pain treatment is indicated, beacuse preventing of pain easier than treat. Therefore, administration at fixed intervals is better than on a pro re nata basis [13].

31.9.2 Topical Therapy

Topical treatmentsalone is the main initial treatment of uncomplicated acute otitis externa. Topical low-pH antiseptic solutions, antibiotics (quinolone, aminoglycoside) and steroids (dexamethasone, hydrocortisone) are used for the initial treatment of acute OE. In general, no clinically significant differences were found in clinical therapeutic outcomes among the various topical agents [14]. Patient education is significant to increase adherence to therapy, especially if patients insist on oral antiotics. Aural canal cleaning by removing the debris from the ear canal enhance the penetration of eardrops into theear canal. However, this procedureis painful and can not be performed easily due to tenderness of the ear, especially in pediatric patients. Acute analgesia provided by analgesic cream or benzocaine otic solution may be required to perform adequate aural canal cleaning. However, topical anesthetic drops (eg, benzocaine otic solution) should not be prescribed in patients with nonintact tympanic membrane or tympanostomy tube [15]. Ear drops should be applied to the affected ear upward until the canal filled when patient lying down for about 3–5 min. If the ear canal blocked by significant skin edema, an ear wick can be placed into the canal to facilitate the penetration of ear drops.

In patients treated with antibiotic/steroid topical agents, symptoms usually last nearly 6 days after drops has begun. Nevertheless, if symptoms persist, patients should continue to ear drops further seven daysuntil their symptoms resolve. If the symptoms persist beyond 2 weeks, patients should be reassessed for therapy failure and alternative treatment [16].

31.9.3 Topical Therapy in Nonintact Tympanic Membrane

Prescription of topical drops in patients with perforated tympanic membrane or tympanostomy tubes required special consideration forpotential ototoxicity. Agents can reach the round window membrane and penetrate into the inner ear. Clinical experience show that hearing loss does not develop after a short course of treatment; however, severe hearing loss has been reported following prolonged application of ear drops [17, 18].

If the tympanic membrane is non intact, ear drops containing alchol, low pH antiseptic/ acidifying solutions, or both should not be used due to ototoxicity and pain. Amynoglicoside ear drops also should not be prescribed in patients with perforated tympanic membrane. Particularly, neomycin can cause permanent sensorineural hearing loss and manufacturer apperently warned that neomycin/polymyxin B/hyrocortisone not be used with nonintact tympanic membrane [18]. Quinolones are the solely topical antimicrobial drugs approved by the FDA for the middle ear use. Quinolones are safe and well-tolerated agents with broad antimicrobial spectrum [19]. Common topical otic preperations are listed in Table 31.4. However, Rosenfeld and colleagues reported no significant differences in clinical cure rates of acute otitis externa between antiseptic versus antimicrobial or antimicrobial-steroid combination versus antimicrobial alone [16]. No matter what topical medication used, approximately 65% to 90% of patients had improved within 7–10 days.

Table 31.4 Common topical agents for acute otitis externa

Agents	Dosages	Use in non intact Tympani cmembrane	Comments
Boricacid 4%	Three to four times daily	No	May causepainandirritation
Boricacid 4% /ethylalchol 25%	Three to four times daily	No	May causepainandirritation
Aceticasid 2%	Four to six times daily	No	May causepainandirritation
Alumininumacetate13% (Burow'ssolution)	Once to twice daily	No	Ototoxic
Ciprofloxacin 0.3%	Two to three times daily	Yes	Safe, well-tolerated agent
Ofloxacin 0.3%	Once to twice daily	Yes	Low risk of sensitization
Gentamicin	Two to three times daily	No	Vestibulotoxic
Ciprofloxacin 0.3%, dexamethasone 0.1%	Twotothreetimesdaily	Yes	Safe, well-tolerated agent
Neomycin/polymyxin B/ hydrocortisone	Three to four times daily	No	Ototoxic, high risk of contact sensitization

31.9.4 Systemic Antimicrobials

Clinical guideline on acute OE strongly recommended that clincans should not use systemic antimicrobials as initial treatment for acute otitis externa, unless there is involvement of the anatomic regions outside the ear canal or the presence host factors such as diabetes mellitus or immunosuppression [14, 20]. An argument opposed the prescribing oral antibiotics for acute OE is the effectiveness of topical agents that do not contain antibiotics. Boric acid, acetic acid, and aluminum acetate are effective topical solutions as a single agent [21, 22]. A randomized multicenter trial also found no significant differences in bacteriologic efficacy or pain duration between topical treatment and topical treatment combined with oral amoxicilin [20].

Systemic therapy should be initiated in patients with diabetes, AIDS with immune deficiency, malign OE or infection that extended outside the ear canal such as auricle, pinna and skin of the face. In this situation, systemic antibiotics should cover P aeruginosa and S aureus.

31.10 Surgical Treatment

Surgical management is very rarely required for hypertrophic chronic OE. Very thick ear canal skin can permanently obliterates the ear canal. In such a case, if topical or systemic treatment can not recanalize the lumen of the ear canal surgical management may be required. Surgical management includes; enlargement of the bony canal by canaloplasty using drill, resurfacing of the canal with split-thickness skin graft and performing a wide meatoplasty by removing sufficient amount of conchal cartilage.

References

1. Linstrom CJ, Lucente FE, Joseph EM. Infections of the external ear. 3th ed. Philadelphia: Lippincott Williams and Wilkins; 2001.
2. Hughes E, Lee JH. Otitis externa. Pediatr Rev. 2001;22(6):191–7.
3. Kozin ED, Sethi RK, Remenschneider AK, Kaplan AB, Del Portal DA, Gray ST, Shrime MG, Lee DJ. Epidemiology of otologic diagnoses in United States emergency departments. Laryngoscope. 2015;125(8):1926–33.
4. Piercefield EW, Collier SA, Hlavsa MC, Beach MJ. Estimated burden of acute otitis externa-United States, 2003-2007. MMVR Morb Mortal Wkly Rep. 2011;60(19):605–9.
5. Russell JD, Donnelly M, McShane DP, Alun-Jones T, Walsh M. What cuases acute otitis externa? J Laryngol Otol. 1993;107(10):898–901.
6. Martin TJ, Kerschner JE, Flanary VA. Fungal causes of otitis externa and tympanostomy tube otorrhea. Int J Pediatr Otorhinolaryngol. 2005;69(11):1503–8.
7. Clark WB, Brook I, Bianki D, Thompson DH. Microbiology of otitis externa. Otolaryngol Head Neck Surg. 1997;116:23–5.
8. Senturia BA, Marcus MD, Lucente FE. Diseases of the external ear. 2nd ed. New York: Grune and Stratton; 1980.
9. Selesnick SH. Otitis externa: management of the recalcitrant case. Am J Otol. 1994;15(3):408–12.

10. Sobie S, Brodsky L, Stanievich JF. Necrotising external otitis in children: report of two cases and review of the literature. Laryngoscope. 1987;97(5):598–601.
11. Franco-Vidal V, Blanchet H, Bebear C, Dutronc H, Darrouzet V. Necrotising external otitis: a report of 46 cases. Otol Neurotol. 2007;28(6):771–3.
12. Fischer M, Dietz A. Acute external otitis and its differential diagnosis. Laryngorhinootologie. 2015;94(2):113–25.
13. American Academy of Pediatrics. Committee on Psychosocial Aspects of Child and Family Health; Task Force on Pain in Infants, Children, and Adolescents. The assessment and manegement of acute pain in infants, children, and adolescents. Pediatrics. 2001;108(3):793–7.
14. Kaushik V, Malik T, Saeed SR. Interventions for acute otitis externa. Conchrane Database Syst Rev. 2010;1:CD004740.
15. Rosenfeld RM, Schwartz SR, Cannon CR, Roland PS, Simon GR, Kumar KA, et al. Clinical practice guideline: acute otitis externa. Otolaryngol Head Neck Surg. 2014;150(1):S1–24.
16. Rosenfeld RM, Singer M, Wasserman JM, Stinnett SS. Systematic review of topical antimicrobial therapy for acute otitis externa. Otolaryngol Head Neck Surg. 2006;134(4 suppl):S24–48.
17. Rakover Y, Keywan K, Rosen G. Safety of topical ear drops containing ototoxic antibiotics. J Otolaryngol. 1997;26(3):194–6.
18. Winterstein AG, Liu W, Xu D, Antonelli PJ. Sensorineural hearing loss associated with neomycin eardrops and nonintact tympanic membranes. Otolaryngol Head Neck Surg. 2013;148(2):277–83.
19. Mösges R, Nematian-Samani M, Hellmich M, Shah-Hosseini K. A meta-analysis of the efficacy of quinolone containing otics in comparison to antibiotic-steroid combination drugs in the local treatment of otitis externa. Curr Med Res Opin. 2011;27(10):2053–60.
20. Roland PS, Belcher BP, Bettis R, et al. A single topical agent is clinically equivalent to the combination of topical and oral antibiotic treatment for otitis externa. Am J Otolaryngol. 2008;29(4):255–61.
21. Amamni S, Moeini M. Comparison of boric acid and combination drug of Polymyxin, neomycin and hydrocortisone (polymyxin NH) in the treatment of acute otitis externa. J Clin Diagn Res. 2016;10(7):MC01–4.
22. Jinnouchi O, Kuwahara T, Ishida S, Okano Y, Kasei Y, Kunimoto K, et al. Anti-microbial and therapeutic effects of modified Burow's solution on refractory otorrhea. Auris Nasus Larynx. 2012;39(4):374–7.

Otitis Media in Infants

32

Özlem Naciye Atan Şahin, Nuray Bayar Muluk,
and Ayşe Engin Arısoy

32.1 Introduction

Acute otitis media (AOM) is one of the most frequent infections in children. It is a burden due to its increased associated doctor visits, antibiotic needs, increased surgery, and potential contribution to hearing and speech complications. Acute otitis media has been shown in all ages but is mostly found in infants and young children. The attack rate for AOM peaks between 6 and 18 months of age. In the United States (US), nearly 80% of children less than 2 years of age have at least one episode of AOM annually, and most continue to have episodes through age 5 years [1].

However, in the USA, the incidence of AOM decreased after starting universal immunization of infants with the 7-valent pneumococcal conjugate vaccine (PCV7) in 2000, and in 2010 further declined following with the 13-valent pneumococcal conjugate vaccine (PCV13). Before immunization, in 1989, the cumulative incidence of more than an episode of AOM identified 62% at ≤ 1 year old and 83% at ≤ 3 years old. After universal immunization of infants with the PCV in a prospective longitudinal cohort (2006–2016) of 615 children, the cumulative incidence of more than an episode of AOM was 23% at ≤ 1 year old, 42% at ≤ 2 years old, and 60% at ≤ 4 years old [1].

Ö. N. Atan Şahin (✉)
Department of Pediatrics, Faculty of Medicine, Acıbadem Mehmet Ali Aydınlar University, İstanbul, Turkey

N. Bayar Muluk
Department of Otorhinolaryngology, Faculty of Medicine, Kırıkkale University, Kırıkkale, Turkey

A. E. Arısoy
Division of Neonatology, Department of Pediatrics, Faculty of Medicine, Kocaeli University, Kocaeli, Turkey

© The Author(s), under exclusive license to Springer Nature Switzerland AG 2022

C. Cingi et al. (eds.), *Pediatric ENT Infections*,
https://doi.org/10.1007/978-3-030-80691-0_32

Several factors (immature immunity, craniofacial abnormalities, low birth weight (LBW), gastroesophageal reflux, decreasing maternal antibodies, shorter and hypofunctional eustachian tubes, early nasopharyngeal colonization with bacterial pathogens, etc.) give rise to an enhanced occurrence in infants [2–4]. Acute otitis media has a high risk of recurrence and continued middle ear effusion (MEE). The use of tympanograms and acoustic reflectometry (AR) is precise in diagnosing AOM in infants less than 5 months old [5].

32.2 Risk Factors

Acute otitis media frequency in neonates and infants younger than 3 months old is unknown [6, 7]. However, it is reported to be between 2% and 9% in some studies [8].

32.2.1 Race and Ethnicity

Race and ethnic inequalities among otitis media (OM) diagnoses were prospectively studied in a well-controlled cohort, including greater than 11,000 infants of 1–6 months old in the USA [9, 10]. Non-Hispanic Caucasian children had higher OM rates following adjustments for gender, maternal age, marital status, parity, number of siblings, breastfeeding, and daycare size and attendance. Non-Hispanic African American children had lower OM rates, similar to non-Hispanic Asian children. All groups of children showed increased OM rates following multivariable adjustment. After stratifying race and ethnicity, the attendance at daycare among Hispanics was not a risk factor [10].

32.2.2 Respiratory Infections and Exposure to Other Children

Koch et al. [11] executed a prospective analysis of Greenland Inuit children 0–2 years of age. Several risk factors have been linked with upper respiratory tract infections (URTIs), including AOM. In a systematic international review, OM prevalence in children was linked to parental smoking and lack of breastfeeding [12]. Amusa et al. [13] documented that exposure to wood-burning smoke and multiple children in a single room were risk factors for OM in Nigeria. Interestingly, in other studies, child-to-child exposure was not a risk factor for distinguishing recurrent AOM (RAOM) from chronic otitis media (COM) with effusion (COME) [10, 14, 15].

32.2.3 Lack of Breastfeeding

Previous studies demonstrated that exclusive breastfeeding lowers the occurrence of AOM before 6 months [16]. As the duration of breastfeeding increases, it provides better protection for children younger than 2 years old.

32.2.4 Exposure to Passive Smoke and Pollutants

There is increasing evidence supporting an association between air pollution exposure and a higher risk of OM in children. Young children are more vulnerable to OM. Previous studies were mainly conducted in high or middle-income countries; evidence from low-income countries is limited.

A study in Mozambique examined the OM risk factors of 750 children under 6 years of age [17]. Exposure to tobacco, wood and charcoal smoke, short-term breastfeeding, and overcrowding were associated with OM. In a recent systematic review that included 24 studies, NO_2 exposure showed the most consistent OM relationship; other specific pollutants showed inconsistent associations [18].

There are studies with contradicting results regarding susceptibility to COM and RAOM in children. Predictive factors for RAOM and COME were examined in 210 children diagnosed with AOM less than 2 years of age [15]. Male gender, winter season, and persistent symptoms enhanced the risk of subsequent OM. Breastfeeding was not associated with COME, but winter, bilateral AOM, family history of RAOM, and AOM history were found associated [15].

32.2.5 Genetics

The OM heritability was shown in a study that included more than 9000 twins [19]. This report demonstrated that the same genes are linked to OM risk in both males and females. In a 5-year follow-up study, MEE heritability diminished after the third year [20]. However, the cumulative effect remained significant after 5 years [10]. Common variants and a rare variant of the FUT2 gene were associated with recurrent middle ear infections in European-American children. FUT2 gene modifies the microbiome of the middle ear making individuals more susceptible to infections. In this study, the authors concluded that the frequency of population-specific FUT2 variants makes the gene a potential target for preventive screening and future treatments for OM, including the middle ear microbiome.

32.2.6 Prenatal and Perinatal Factors

Daly et al. [10] showed a relationship between very low birth weight (VLBW, <1500 g) and frequent OM.

32.2.7 Laterality

McCormick et al. [20] classified risk factors for 566 bilateral versus unilateral AOM in children. Children with bilateral AOM were younger and had increased susceptibility to *Haemophilus influenzae* infection and severe tympanic membrane inflammation than unilateral diseased children. These results explain the persistent symptoms observed in bilateral AOM children [10].

32.2.8 Atopy and Allergic Disease

Nafstad et al. [21] demonstrated that OM in infancy was a risk factor for asthma at age 10. This finding does not validate the notion for early infection as protective against atopy and allergy much later in life.

32.2.9 Pacifier Use

A pooled analysis of two studies with 4110 children who used pacifiers had a slightly higher incidence of AOM than children who did not [22].

32.3 Microbiology

Streptococcus pneumoniae, non-typeable *H. influenzae,* and *Moraxella catarrhalis* were detected as most bacterial isolates from middle ear fluid in children with AOM. Respiratory syncytial virus (RSV), rhinoviruses, influenza viruses, and adenoviruses were the most common viral pathogens. In a series, bacteria (with or without viruses) were detected in 92%, viruses (with or without bacteria) in 70%, and both bacteria and viruses in 66% [23].

32.4 Diagnosis

Ear examination complications of the external auditory canal and the tympanic membrane can cause misdiagnosis of AOM in infants. An oto-microscopic examination may be necessary [24]. Consequently, severe stages of ear disease may be accompanied by acute mastoiditis. In neonates and infants younger than 12 weeks, the infection may spread, causing bacteremia, sepsis, and/or meningitis [7, 25].

In several national guidelines, tympanocentesis is a procedure recommended in patients not responding to antimicrobial treatment. Tympanocentesis may be useful for the correct diagnosis in selected patients. It is an indispensable method to track microbiologic shifts in AOM and allow clinicians to treat AOM better [26].

Acute suppurative otitis media (ASOM) is associated with MEE and inflammation in the presence or absence of an intact tympanic membrane. Tympanocentesis is also the most common technique to diagnose ASOM, relieve pain, identify the responsible microorganism, determine appropriate antibiotics [26], and predict and prevent severe complications in infants [27].

Ilia et al. [4] determined that AOM indicates clinical complications and prognostic factors if frequently occurring within the first 2 months of life. The 147 of the total 160 infants followed-up, the youngest patients with AOM had more siblings and did not use pacifiers as frequently. Besides, purulent otorrhea and irritability were most commonly found in the early AOM group. AOM was accompanied by meningitis and mastoiditis in two infants each.

32.4.1 History

Children with AOM often have rapid onset otalgia, irritability, otorrhea, and/or fever. These symptoms are nonspecific and often correspond with viral respiratory infection [28, 29]. In a prospective survey, 354 children were admitted to a pediatrician for acute respiratory illness, fever, earache, and excessive crying. Ninety percent were found to have AOM. Interestingly, 72% of children without AOM in another study had these same symptoms. Other URTI symptoms frequently come before or associate with AOM. For this reason, clinical history alone is not a good predictor of AOM in infants [27, 28].

32.4.2 Otoscopic Examination and Tympanometry

MEE is usually established with pneumatic otoscopy [30]. However, it may be accompanied by tympanometry or acoustic reflectometry (AR) [31–32]. The otoscopy findings indicating MEE and inflammation with AOM have been characterized. AOM diagnosis can be made with a level of uncertainty because of the failure to clear the external auditory canal's cerumen, ear canal narrowing, or inability to generate a satisfactory seal for otoscopy or tympanometry [33].

32.4.3 Acoustic Reflectometry

Acoustic reflectometry (AR) does not require a seal of the canal and can be useful to determine MEE [31, 32]. When MEE is uncertain, the AOM diagnosis cannot be fully confirmed [27].

Diagnosis of AOM must meet all three criteria, which include 1- rapid onset, 2- MEE confirmation, and 3- middle-ear inflammation. Clinicians may discuss AOM certainty's level upon establishing these three criteria for AOM diagnosis [27].

32.5 Antibiotic Therapy

There are two strategies for antibiotic therapy of AOM: (1) Immediate treatment with antibiotics and (2) observation with the initiation of antibiotic treatment if the symptoms and signs worsen or fail to improve after 48–72 h.

Immediate antimicrobial treatment is recommended for children ≤6 months of age, children with severe symptoms or signs (mild or severe ear pain, over 48 h of pain, or fever ≥39 °C), for all children with otorrhea, intracranial complications, and/or a history of recurrence, and bilateral AOM of children under 24 months of age.

Immediate antimicrobial treatment or observation is recommended for children between 6 and 24 months of age with unilateral non-severe AOM and children ≥24 months of age with unilateral or bilateral non-severe AOM [16].

According to the latest epidemiologic data and guidelines, amoxicillin is the first choice antibiotic for its efficacy, safety, cost, effectiveness, taste, and antimicrobial spectrum [34–36]. If treatment failure occurs and the initial treatment was amoxicillin, the second option should be amoxicillin-clavulanic acid (80–90 mg/kg/day). Amoxicillin-clavulanate is also recommended if concurrent purulent conjunctivitis is present, amoxicillin was taken within the last 30 days, or the child has a RAOM history not responding to amoxicillin, and in children with a high risk of antibiotic resistance (daycare attendance, not vaccinated against pneumococci, living in an area with a high prevalence of resistance isolates) [37–39].

Macrolides should be used in children with a history of recent and/or severe allergy to penicillin. For children with non-type1 penicillin hypersensitivity, cefdinir, cefuroxime, or ceftriaxone may be the appropriate option [37–39].

32.6 Conclusion

Acute otitis media diagnosis and management in infants may be complicated. Inflammation and MEE linked to AOM have been well described. Tympanic membrane bulging is the robust predictor of AOM and MEE. Tympanograms and AR are the most precise diagnostics for OM in infants less than 5 months. Acoustic reflectometry is a useful tool not requiring ear canal sealing, and it can define the MEE presence by a single slight opening in the cerumen. Antibiotic treatment is recommended in appropriate cases.

References

1. Pelton S, Tähtinen P. Acute otitis media in children: epidemiology, microbiology, clinical manifestations, and complications. In: Kaplan SL, Isaacson GC, Torchia MM (eds.). UpToDate https://www.uptodate.com/contents/acute-otitis-media-in-children-epidemiology-microbiology-clinical-manifestations-and-complications. Accessed 30 Dec 2020.
2. Gaddey HL, Wright MT, Nelson TN. Otitis media: rapid evidence review. Am Fam Phys. 2019;100:350–6.
3. De Antonio R, Yarzabal JP, Cruz JP, Schmidt JE, Kleijnen J. Epidemiology of otitis media in children from developing countries. A systematic review. Int J Pediatr Otorhinolaryngol. 2016;85:65–74.
4. Ilia S, Galanakis E. Clinical features and outcome of acute otitis media in early infancy. Int J Infect Dis. 2013;17:e317–20.
5. Venekamp RD, Damoiseaux RAMJ, Schilder AGM. Acute otitis media in children. Am Fam Physician. 2017;95:109–10.

6. Sakran W, Makary H, Colodner R, et al. Acute otitis media in infants less than three months of age: clinical presentation, etiology, and concomitant diseases. Int J Pediatr Otorhinolaryngol. 2006;70:613–7.

7. Sommerfleck P, González Macchi ME, Pellegrini S, et al. Acute otitis media in infants younger than three months not vaccinated against Streptococcus pneumoniae. Int J Pediatr Otorhinolaryngol. 2013;77:976–80.

8. Megged O, Abdulgany S, Bar-Meir MB. Does acute otitis in the first month of life increase the risk for recurrent otitis? Clin Pediatr. 2018;57:89–92.

9. Vernacchio L, Lesko SM, Vezina RM, et al. Racial/ethnic disparities in the diagnosis of otitis media in infancy. Int J Pediatr Otorhinolaryngol. 2004;68:795–804.

10. Daly KA, Hoffman HJ, Kvaerner KJ, et al. Epidemiology, natural history, and risk factors: panel report from the ninth international research conference on otitis media. Int J Pediatr Otorhinolaryngol. 2010;74:231–40.

11. Koch A, Mølbak K, Homøe P, et al. Risk factors for acute respiratory tract infections in young Greenlandic children. Am J Epidemiol. 2003;158:374–84.

12. Gunasekera H, Haysom L, Morris P, Craig J. The global burden of childhood otitis media and hearing impairment: a systematic review. Pediatrics. 2008;121:S107.

13. Amusa YB, Ijadunola IK, Onayade OO. Epidemiology of otitis media in a local tropical African population. West Afr J Med. 2005;24:227–30.

14. Hammarén-Malmi S, Tarkkanen J, Mattila PS. Analysis of risk factors for childhood persistent middle ear effusion. Acta Otolaryngol. 2005;125:1051–4.

15. Damoiseaux RA, Rovers MM, Van Balen FA, Hoes AW, de Melker RA. Long-term prognosis of acute otitis media in infancy: determinants of recurrent acute otitis media and persistent middle ear effusion. Fam Pract. 2006;23:40–5.

16. Lieberthal AS, Carrol AE, Chonmaitree T, et al. The diagnosis and management of acute otitis media. Pediatrics. 2013;131:e964–e99.

17. da Costa JL, Navarro A, Neves JB, Martin M. Household wood and charcoal smoke increase the risk of otitis media in childhood in Maputo. Int J Epidemiol. 2004;33:573–8.

18. Bowatte G, Tham R, Perret JL, et al. Air pollution and otitis media in children: a systematic review of literature. Int J Environ Res Public Health. 2018;15(2):257.

19. Kvestad E, Kvaerner KJ, Røysamb E, Tambs K, Harris JR, Magnus P. Otitis media: genetic factors and sex differences. Twin Res. 2004;7:239–44.

20. McCormick DP, Chandler SM, Chonmaitree T. Laterality of acute otitis media: different clinical and microbiologic characteristics. Pediatr Infect Dis J. 2007;26:583–8.

21. Nafstad P, Brunekreef B, Skrondal A, Nystad W. Early respiratory infections, asthma, and allergy: 10-year follow-up of the Oslo birth cohort. Pediatrics. 2005;116:e255–62.

22. Rovers MM, Numans ME, Langebach E, Grobbe DE, Verjejj TJ, Schilder AG. Is pacifier use a risk factor for otitis media? A dynamic control study. Fam Pract. 2008;25:233–6.

23. Ruohola A, Meurman O, Nikkari S, et al. Microbiology of acute otitis media in children with tympanostomy tubes: prevalence of bacteria and viruses. Clin Infect Dis. 2006;43:1417–22.

24. Tarantino V, D'Agostino R, Taborelli G, Melagrana A, Porcu A, Stura M. Acute mastoiditis: a 10 year retrospective study. Int J Pediatr Otorhinolaryngol. 2002;66:143–8.

25. Turner D, Leibovitz E, Aran A, et al. Acute otitis media in infants younger than two months of age: microbiology, clinical presentation, and therapeutic approach. Pediatr Infect Dis J. 2002;21:669–74.

26. Pichicero ME, Wright T. The use of tympanocentesis in the diagnosis and management of acute otitis media. Curr Infect Report. 2006;8:189–95.

27. American Academy of Pediatrics. Subcommittee on Management of Acute Otitis Media. Diagnosis and management of acute otitis media. Pediatrics. 2004;113:1451–65.

28. Niemela M, Uhari M, Jounio-Ervasti K, Luotonen J, Alho OP, Vierimaa E. Lack of specific symptomatology in children with acute otitis media. Pediatr Infect Dis J. 1994;13:765–8.

29. Kontiokari T, Koivunen P, Niemela M, Pokka T, Uhari M. Symptoms of acute otitis media. Pediatr Infect Dis J. 1998;17:676–9.
30. Harmes KM, Blackwood RA, Burrows HL, et al. Otitis media diagnosis and treatment. Am Fam Physician. 2013;88:435–40.
31. Puhakka T, Pulkkinen J, Silvennoinen H, Heikkinen T. Comparison of spectral gradient acoustic reflectometry and tympanometry for detection of middle-ear effusion in children. Pediatr Infect Dis J. 2014;33:e183–6.
32. Linden H, Teppo H, Revonta M. Spectral gradient acoustic reflectometry in the diagnosis of middle-ear fluid in children. Eur Arc Otorhinolaryngol. 2007;264:477–81.
33. Rosenfeld RM. Diagnostic certainty for acute otitis media. Int J Pediatr Otorhinolaryngol. 2002;64:89–95.
34. Ovnat Tamir S, Shemesh S, Oron Y, et al. Acute otitis media guidelines in selected developed and developing countries: uniformity and diversity. Arch Dis Child. 2017;102:450–7.
35. Suaya YA, Gessner BD, Fung S, et al. Acute otitis media, antimicrobial prescriptions, and medical expenses among children in the United States during 2011-2016. Vaccine. 2018;36:7479–86.
36. Ryabak A, Levy C, Bonacorsi S, et al. Antibiotic resistance of potential otopathogens isolated from nasopharyngeal flora of children with acute otitis media before, during and after pneumococcal conjugate vaccines implementation. Pediatr Infect Dis J. 2018;37:e72–8.
37. Marchisio P, Galli L, Bortone B, et al. Updated guidelines for the management of acute otitis media in children by the Italian Society of Pediatrics: treatment. Ped Infect Dis J. 2019;38:10–21.
38. Hersh AL, Jackson MA, Hicks LA, et al. Principles of judicious antibiotic prescribing for upper respiratory tract infections in pediatrics. Pediatrics. 2013;132:1146–54.
39. Coker TR, Chan LS, Newberry SJ, et al. Diagnosis, microbial epidemiology, and antibiotic treatment of acute otitis media in children: a systematic review. JAMA. 2010;304:2161–9.

Acute Otitis Media

Erdem Atalay Cetinkaya and Vedat Topsakal

33.1 Introduction

Middle ear infections comprise infection and inflammation of the tympanic cavity, which starts medial of the tympanic membrane. The middle ear comprises not only a cavity containing the auditory ossicles and their muscles but also inner layers of the tympanic membrane, air filled cavities of the mastoid part of the temporal bone and the Eustachian tube that communicates with the nasopharynx. Acute otitis media (AOM) originates here and within 21 days a process of acute inflammation occurs in the tympanic cavity [1]. It is the most frequent infection requiring medical care in children under 5 years of age. Every year, the cost to society of treating this disease amounts to billions of euros. Despite studies on prevention and treatment of AOM, the costs of this disease continue to increase and its prevalence remains high. The increase in antimicrobial-resistant bacteria has prompted a reevaluation of the conventional management of AOM. There is an overwhelming consensus, however, that antibiotics are the ideal initial therapy for AOM, for valid reasons [2, 3]. Surgical management can be categorized into three methods: tympanocentesis, and myringotomy with or without ventilation tube insertion. Especially when children fail to improve or worsen while receiving antibiotics surgical intervention can be required [4, 5].

E. A. Cetinkaya (✉)
Section of Otorhinolaryngology, Antalya Training and Research Hospital, University of Health Sciences, Antalya, Turkey

V. Topsakal
Department of Otorhinolaryngology, Head and Neck Surgery, Vrije Universiteit Brussel (VUB), University Hospital UZ Brussel, Brussels Health Campus, Brussels, Belgium

33.2   Pathophysiology

Otitis media in mankind is associated with evolutionary changes (adaptations to bipedalism, a large brain, and speech) and other inheritance and dietary influences. Normally human middle ear cavity contains ambient air consisting of oxygen, carbon dioxide, nitrogen, argon, and water vapor (at various partial pressure). Since the middle ear is a closed compartment with the volume of gas, it is likely to depend on external pressure changes, and in abrupt changes the Eustachian tube functions as a safety valve. Normally when we swallow this tube opens to equalize pressure changes to avoid malfunction and discomfort. Volume changes due to processes like inflammation causing gas exchange with venous capillary vessels of mucosal cell layers are usually not abrupt but rather chronic. In comparison to atmospheric pressure, carbon dioxide and oxygen readily pass through the venous capillary membranes producing a net vacuum of pressure [6]. The Eustachian tube demonstrates a two-stage postnatal development, according to Mulder's animal model. First, as the animal begins breathing and swallowing, the mucociliary system matures, providing defense/clearance. The dorsal segment subsequently reaches maturity. Aeration of the middle ear indicates that this part provides ventilation. In that case, various purposes are fulfilled by various sections of the Eustachian tube: clearance, defense, and ventilation [7].

Eustachian tube dysfunction and abnormal middle ear gas exchange seems to be the principal causes of AOM. Two major etiologies, irritant and infectious reactions, are inflammation within the lumen. The response to allergens and chemicals, such as smoke, involves irritant reactions, whereas infectious reactions usually include a viral or bacterial infection. Both processes result in the release of pro-inflammatory cytokines that, in response to injury, promote edema of the epithelium. Inflammation of the nasopharynx can spread to the nasopharyngeal opening of the Eustachian tube, which affects middle ear pressure. The resulting acute inflammatory response in the tympanic cavity is characterized by normal vasodilatation, invasion of leukocytes, phagocytosis, exudation, and local immunological responses, which together constitute the clinical profile of AOM. The higher the degree of impairment of the transmucosal gas exchange, the greater the decrease in the middle ear total pressure leading to gradually a retraction of the ear drum and perhaps eventually cholesteatoma [6–8].

33.2.1 Microbiology

33.2.1.1   Viral Origin

Upper respiratory tract infections (URTIs) involving the nasopharynx are responsible for most of the AOM cases. The pathology is typically of viral origin, but allergic reactions may produce a similar result [9]. Viruses, such as respiratory syncytial virus (RSV), rhinovirus, influenza (types A and B) coronavirus, enterovirus, adenovirus, and parainfluenza (types 1–3), are the causative agents in 90% of AOM cases [10]. It has been reported that RSVs have the strongest association with AOM. In at least one quarter of all pediatric cases of AOM, concurrent or antecedent URTIs are detected, but the virus itself rarely seems to be the causative pathogen in the tympanic cavity. In addition somebody with HIV can die from complications of AOM. According to some previous study, during the influenza season, trivalent influenza A vaccine administration has been shown to decrease the rate of AOM [11]. Whereas, Influenza vaccination for prevention of AOM is not recommended by Dutch guidelines because it is insufficiently effective [12].

33.2.1.2 Bacterial Origin

The most common bacterial pathogens causing AOM are *Streptococcus pneumoniae*, *Haemophilus influenzae*, and *Moraxella* (*Branhamella*) *catarrhalis* [13]. *S. pneumoniae* is the pathogen most frequently associated with AOM. Being present in about 40% of all cases; children with this pathogen appear to have more serious disease. Serotypes 19 (23%), 23 (12.5%), 6 (12%), 14 (10%), 3 (8.5%), and 18 (6%) are frequently isolated in ear aspirates from AOM patients. The serotypes responsible for AOM changed after 7-valent pneumococcal conjugate vaccine (PCV7) was introduced [14]. Because vaccination at a young age with a pneumococcal conjugate vaccine AOM seems to prevent, the working group endorses the importance of pneumococcal vaccination in the national vaccination program [12]. All three mentioned bacteria are capable of forming biofilms that are thought to be responsible for drug resistance. *Staphylococcus aureus*, group A *Streptococcus*, group B *Streptococcus*, and gram-negative bacilli can be isolated in about 15% of AOM and in about 5% of OAM multiple causative pathogens can be isolated. Patients with compromised immune systems encounter opportunistic infections, such as *Mycobacterium* or *Chlamydia*. During the perinatal period, the organisms most frequently responsible for sepsis and meningitis are *Escherichia coli*, *Enterococcus* bacteria, and group B streptococci. Such agents are often retrieved from the middle ear, although the proportion of neonates with AOM is likely to be less than 10% [9, 13].

33.2.2 Risk Factors

Factors that increase the chance of developing AOM include an URTI (such as the common cold or sinusitis), attending a daycare center, anatomic or functional defects of the Eustachian tube (such as Down syndrome or cleft palate), gastroesophageal reflux, history of allergy (such as environmental or food allergies), genetic predisposition, and exposure to smoke from cigarettes (including passive smoking). Children whose mothers drank alcohol during pregnancy and those who are formula-fed are also at higher risk of AOM, which typically onsets in the winter [15].

33.2.2.1 Age, Gender, and Daycare Attendance

While adults can suffer from ear infections, children aged 6–72 months are the most vulnerable to AOM. Nearly 75% of children will have experienced an AOM episode by their third birthday, and almost half of these will have three or more AOM episodes by that time. Boys are more likely to have otitis media than girls, particularly chronic otitis media. While daycare is part of life for many children, it is also one of the most significant risk factors for AOM. Toddlers in nursery schools or daycare are more likely to develop AOM as they are exposed to more URTIs [16].

33.2.2.2 Immune System and Anatomy

During childhood, the immune system progressively matures. The passive IgG antibody transplacentally transferred from maternal blood circulation and in breast milk provides vital early defense against many infectious diseases such as AOM. Young children become more vulnerable to infections as maternal protection fades away. Gradually maturing innate and adaptive immune systems kick in. Children will also, however, develop viral, bacterial, and parasitic infections that need to be fought off and controlled by immune responses. Such antigen activation result in immunological memory, in addition to facilitating recovery [17].

Children have a higher risk to encounter AOM because their immune systems have had less exposure to common viruses. Viral infections are usually the direct or indirect cause of AOM. Children with immune disorders or immunosuppressive therapy are even at greater risk. Much attention has been paid to the role of immunoglobulins; in particular, immunoglobulin G2 and immunoglobulin G4 are responsible for immunity to polysaccharide antigens; deficiencies in their formation can lead to AOM [18].

Anatomically the Eustachian tube is a complex structure and not just a static pipe with a lumen, skeleton, mucosal lining, and soft tissue and muscles surrounding it. In its inferior and medial two-thirds, the skeleton of the tube is composed of cartilage, and in the superior and lateral one-third of the bone. Within the petrous part of the temporal bone lies the bony portion, while the cartilaginous portion is tightly attached to the sphenoid bone superiorly. The bony part is normally patented and, like the cartilaginous section, does not open and close dynamically. The four muscles connected to the Eustachian tube feature are inside the bone and cartilage: tensor veli palatini, levator veli palatini, tensor tympani, and salpingopharyngeus. The tensor veli palatini is the most important muscle for dilation [19].

In infants, the Eustachian tube is anatomically shorter even more horizontal and more floppy, than in adults, enabling the movement of pathogen from the nasopharynx to the middle ear and raising the risk of AOM. Additionally, the bony and cartilaginous portions of the tube are arranged in a straight line between the pharyngeal and tympanic orifices. The dominantly supine positioning of infants can also increase the risk of infection. The skull base expands downward as children develop, steadily raising the angle of the Eustachian tube from about 10 degrees at birth to 45 degrees in adults; at the same time, the length of the Eustachian tube increases from 13 mm to 35 mm. Eustachian tube and surrounding defects, such as cleft palate, Down syndrome, and craniofacial abnormalities, increase the risk of ear infections [6, 19]. Moreover, Ozturk et al. found that the length of the mucosal surface of the Eustachian tube's posterior wall is longer than that of the anterior wall. Also pediatric specimens were shown to have more mucosal folds (microturbinates) on the posterior wall than in adult specimens. They concluded that these microturbinates can provide essential safety and clearance [20].

Children deprived to healthcare tend to have more prolonged and frequent AOM episodes. Children are more likely to develop an AOM if they have an eye infection, sore throat, or cold, and URTIs are readily transmitted from person to person. Larger adenoids can also contribute to the development of AOM in some children since they can hinder Eustachian tube function [8].

33.2.2.3 Allergy and Gastroesophageal Reflux Disease

AOM is more likely to develop in children with allergies or asthma. An allergic reaction at the nasopharyngeal opening of the Eustachian tube mucosa promotes stasis and, eventually, middle ear effusion. Bernstein described the hyperimmune effects of immunoglobulin E on the Eustachian tube mucosa [21]. Gastroesophageal reflux disease is seen in 62.9% of AOM cases. In 85.3% of AOM patients, pepsin and pepsinogen are found in the middle ear cavity, which can be explained by reflux; however, a clear cause-and-effect connection has not been established [22].

33.2.2.4 Genetics

Genetics predisposition plays role in an individual's susceptibility to AOM. A family history of AOM, particularly in an older sibling, also increases the risk of AOM. Certain cytokine polymorphisms are correlated with an individual's susceptibility to AOM and the seriousness of the inflammation; interleukin-1, interleukin-6, and tumor necrosis factor alpha were found in pharyngeal secretions during URTI, and increased levels of interleukin-1 were associated with the transition to AOM [23]. It is believed that the Fc gamma receptor, interleukin-10, Toll-like receptor 4, transmembrane protein CD14, surfactant, and interferon gamma are all associated with the risk of AOM [24]. Bhutta et al. stated that upregulation of hypoxia signaling, reaction to hypoxia, Toll-Like Receptor signaling, the complement and the RANK-RANKL pathways were shown by microarray analysis of middle ear effusions. RTqPCR showed that hypoxia signaling genes were upregulated and VEGF protein titers were elevated. In the microarray study, mucoid and serous effusions had distinct cytological profiles parallel to variations in T-lymphocyte, NK cell, and myeloid cell signatures [25].

33.2.2.5 Feeding and Exposure to Smoking

Babies who are breastfed, particularly for 6 months or longer, have fewer and briefer AOM episodes than infants fed with artificial milk. Breast milk is believed to provide many immune benefits; bottle-fed babies have fewer antibodies to immunoglobulin G and a higher prevalence of *Haemophilus influenzae* [8]. Infants and toddlers who continuously use pacifiers may be at higher risk of developing AOM than those who use them less often. Also, babies fed from a bottle while lying on their backs are more prone to AOM, probably because this position permits fluid to accumulate in the Eustachian tubes. Many dietary deficiencies have been found in AOM cases, including of vitamin A, zinc, selenium, and omega-3 fatty acids [26].

Paternal smoking and exposure to smoking through other routes are among the major risk factors for AOM; exposure to smoke induces mucosal inflammation, goblet hyperplasia, and increased mucus production, thus impairing the immune response of the respiratory epithelium and increasing pathogen bacterial colonization via increased bacterial binding [27].

33.3   Clinical Manifestations of AOM and Examinations

Otalgia is a significant symptom of AOM, as reflected in its high positive predictive value; however, alone, it is not sufficient for a diagnosis of AOM. In addition to otalgia (or infant irritability), a history of fever, nausea, and lethargy may also be seen in AOM cases. Otorrhea as A clear or bloody fluid can be present. In addition, pus or a dry crust on the outside of the ear canal may be seen [8]. Patients with AOM may also have hearing loss.

Otoscopic examination can be performed with several instruments. These include the traditional hand-held otoscope, pneumatic otoscopy, otomicroscope and video endoscope (Fig. 33.1a, b, c). In routine daily practice, the hand-held otoscope is more often available and used than others, but in some situations it fails to reveal information. Video otoscopy is now readily accessible and enables video images to be viewed.

Pneumatic otoscopy assists in assessing the tympanic membrane 's mobility. Air reaches the EAC with an appropriate seal and boosts pressure. Via concaving into the middle ear cavity, a normal tympanic membrane will respond. Middle ear effusion is the most common cause of reduced tympanic membrane mobility. Consequently, pneumatic otoscopy is essential in the diagnosis of acute otitis media and otitis media with effusion.

On examination (Fig. 33.2), and when inflammation is present, the tympanic membrane is generally immobilized due to the presence of liquid behind it. As the liquid behind the tympanic membrane is pressurized, the tympanic membrane may also show redness and vascularization, and bulge outward. A red, bulging and immobile tympanic membrane with an air bubble is a good indicator of the presence of AOM. Other signs are loss of tympanic membrane landmarks and light reflex on otoscopic inspection, particularly in the malleus [28]. The bulging is usually on the posterior upper quadrant but the absent view of in the malleus handle demands some experience to diagnose this.

Pneumatic otoscopy is the standard method for diagnosing AOM and provides the clearest route to visualization of tympanic cavity effusion and immobility of the membrane. Furthermore, pneumatic otoscopy has high sensitivity of and specificity of 90% and 80%, respectively [8, 9]. If the presence of effusion is not obvious tympanometry, could help to make the diagnosis. Tympanometry can be used for examining uncooperative children and has a predictive value of 90%. However, alone, it is not sufficient for diagnosing AOM [8, 9].

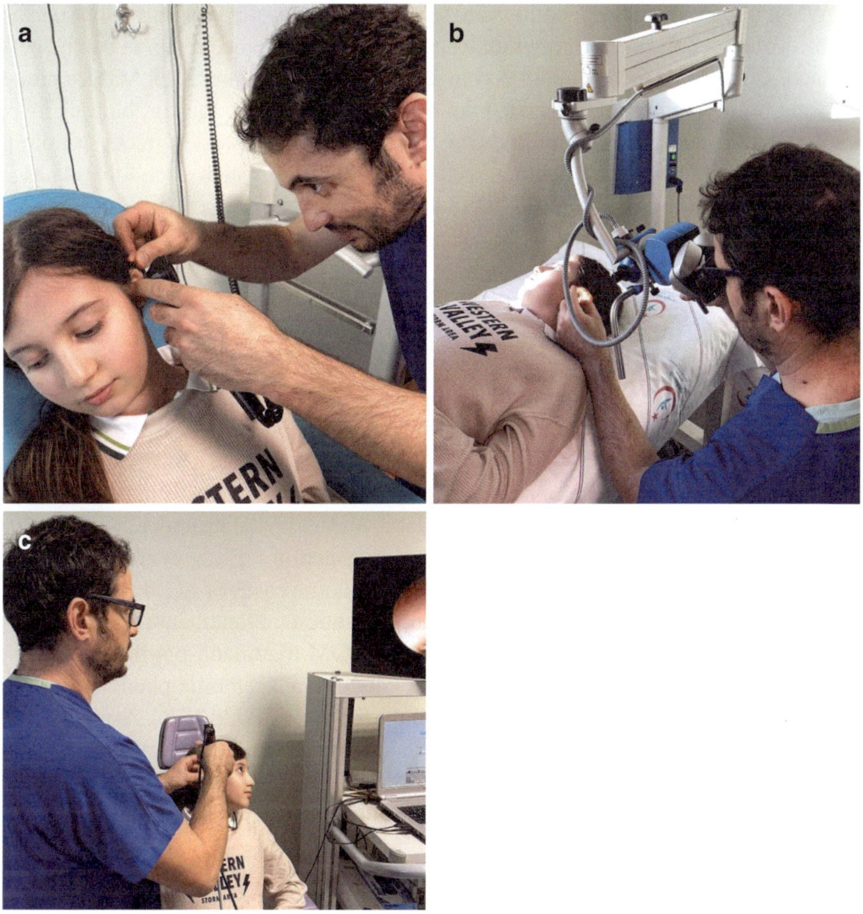

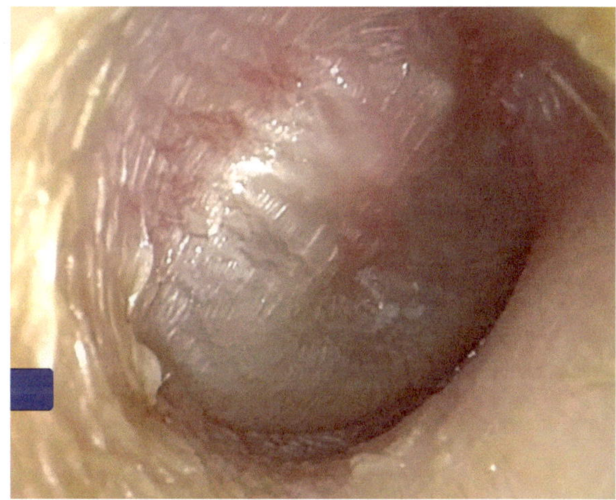

Fig. 33.1 Pediatric ear examination with (**a**) otoscope, (**b**) microscope and (**c**) endoscope. (© Dr. Erdem Atalay Cetinkaya)

Fig. 33.2 AOM: Otoscopic appearance of the tympanic membrane; bulging, complete effusion, opacification and marked erythema. (© *Dr. Erdem Atalay Cetinkaya*)

When intracranial complications are suspected, diagnostic imaging tests, such as high-resolution computed tomography and magnetic resonance imaging can be performed. Conditions to be considered in the differential diagnosis of AOM include external otitis, temporomandibular joint arthralgia, trauma to the ear, bullous myringitis, and acute viral pharyngitis. Otalgia may also be caused by teeth grinding, wisdom tooth pain, or other dental issues. The rarer reasons such as childhood nasopharyngeal carcinoma, chronic otitis media w/o cholesteatoma should not be forgotten [4, 8, 9].

33.4 Treatment

The cornerstone of the treatment of AOM consists of appropriate analgesics since in essence it is a self-limiting disease. Nevertheless, Antibiotics are also widely used in the treatment of AOM [29]. The American Academy of Pediatrics guidelines state that prescribing antibiotics is appropriate in extreme cases of AOM, as well as in bilateral and non-serious cases and in those aged under 2 years. In patients under 24 months of age with unilateral disease, and in older children, watchful waiting or antibiotic treatment represent the management choices. Many pediatric cases of AOM resolve spontaneously and it is important to avoid daily use of antibiotic treatment [9].

Analgesia remains a major consideration in AOM treatment, but the guidelines also mention local anesthesia [8]. Pain killers, including acetaminophen, ibuprofen, and aspirin, can help reduce pain, nausea, and irritability (Table 33.1). Aspirin is not recommended because of the risk of Reye's syndrome which is in children with a current viral infection. Treating an ear infection with decongestants and antihistamines is not recommended, these can only be administered as supportive symptoms management [4, 30].

A beta-lactamase inhibitor (i.e., clavulanate) should be used if there is a history of amoxicillin use in the last 4 weeks, or if the patient has conjunctivitis. Given their distinct chemical structures, it is highly unlikely that cefdinir, cefuroxime, cefpodoxime, and ceftriaxone will show cross-reactivity in cases with penicillin allergy (Table 33.2) [9, 14, 16].

Table 33.1 Treatments for otalgia in cases of AOM

Acetaminophen, ibuprofen	*Mild to moderate pain*
Narcotic analgesia with codeine or analogs	*Moderate to severe pain (risks: Respiratory depression, alteration of consciousness, gastrointestinal tract disorder, and constipation)*
Myringotomy or tympanocentesis	*Needs experience and has potential risks*
Topical applications • *Benzocaine, procaine, lidocaine.* • *Naturopathic agents.*	*In children older than 5 years of age* *In patients over 6 years of age, amethocaine/phenazone show comparable efficacy*
Home remedies (e.g., external application of heat or cold, oil drops in the external auditory canal)	*No controlled studies performed; may have limited efficacy*
Homeopathic agents	*No controlled studies performed*

Table 33.2 Initial antibiotic treatment

Recommended first-line antibiotic treatment	Alternative antibiotic treatment
Amoxicillin BID 80–90 mg/kg/day	*Cefdinir*, 14 mg/kg/day
Amoxicillin-clavulanate BID (*amoxicillin,* 90 mg/kg/day *with clavulanate,* 6.4 mg/kg/day)	*Cefuroxime*, 30 mg/kg/day
	Cefpodoxime, 10 mg/kg/day
	Ceftriaxone, 50 mg IM/IV

If there is no response to initial antibiotic treatment after 48–72 h, clindamycin 30–40 mg/kg/day and tympanocentesis, with or without a third-generation cephalosporin, is recommended. When tympanocentesis indicates multidrug-resistant bacteria, clinical assistance from an infectious disease specialist is needed [8, 30]. Neonates younger than 6 weeks of age with invasive or unusual pathogens, as well as immunosuppressed or immunocompromised patients, should be managed with tympanocentesis. Tympanocentesis is also used in some other situations, such as when second-line antibiotic treatment fails, or when antibiotic treatment in culture guidance is needed [5, 31].

Reduced period of antimicrobial therapy resulted in less desirable results for children aged 6 to 23 months with acute otitis media than for standard duration; in addition, neither the rate of adverse effects nor the rate of development of antimicrobial resistance was lower with the shorter protocol [32].

33.5 Complications

AOM complications are categorized by location as the disease spreads beyond the mucosal structures in the middle ear cleft. Signs of possible imminent problems include swelling of postauricular areas causing loss of skin crease, lowering of the posterior canal wall, or puckering of the attic. The potential complications of AOM are as follows:

(a) Intra temporal: tympanic membrane perforation, acute coalescent mastoiditis, purulent mastoiditis (Fig. 33.3), paralysis of the seventh cranial nerve, acute labyrinthitis (SNHL+/−vertigo), petrous apicitis (Gradenigo Syndrome), a necrotic form of acute otitis, and pathological change in chronic otitis media.
(b) Extracranial: Bezold abscess, Citelli abscess.
(c) Intracranial: meningitis, subarachnoid abscess, brain abscess, encephalitis, subdural abscess, otitis hydrocephalus, and thrombosis of the sigmoid sinus.
(d) Systemic: bacteremia, bacterial endocarditis, and septic arthritis [1, 8].

33.6 Prevention

Precautionary measures to prevent occurrence of AOM mainly consist of predisposing factors include treating for allergies and adenoids hypertrophy, gastroesophageal reflux. Ensuring good hygiene habits, and up-to-date vaccines for infants.

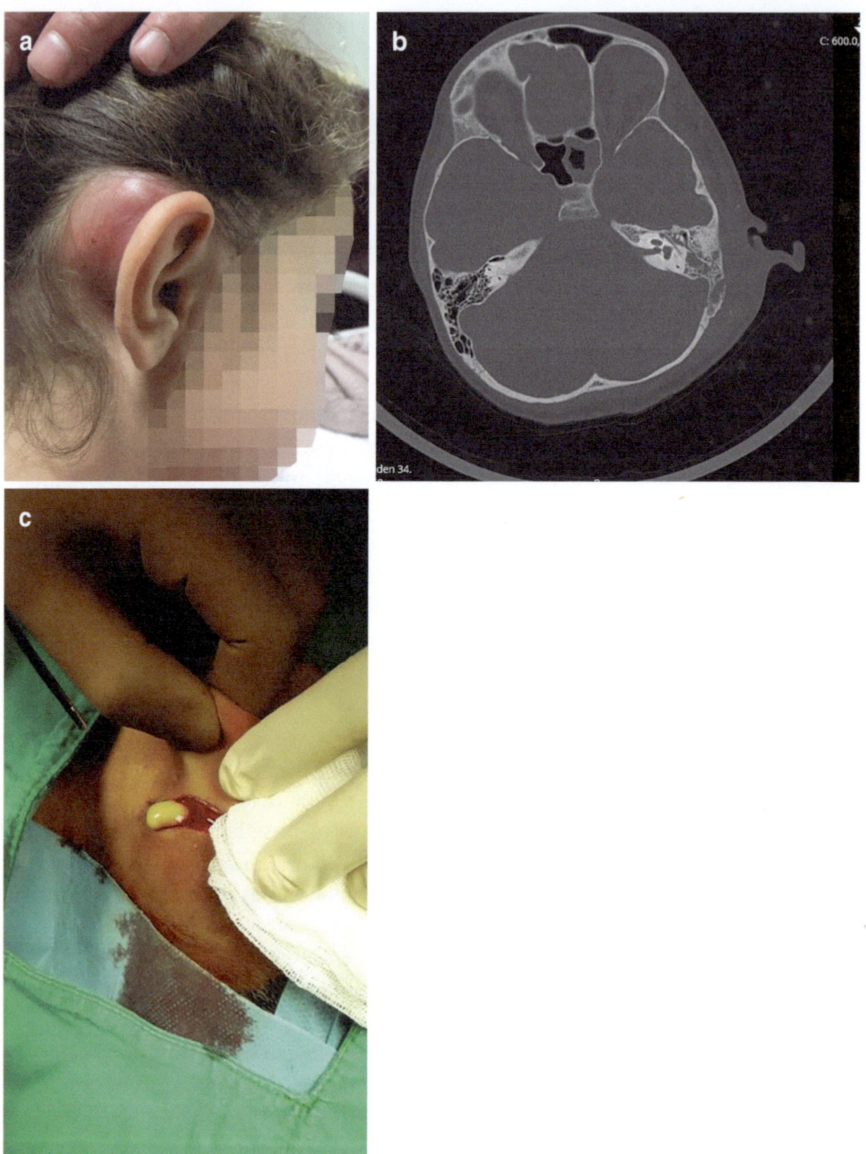

Fig. 33.3 (**a**) Pediatric mastoiditis with subperiosteal abscess. Note the loss of the skin crease, (**b**) Axial view temporal bone computed tomography; radiolucency representing abscess cavity is shown overlying left mastoid cortex and note the erosion of the mastoid cortex. (**c**) The abscess cavity is entered with a scalpel (© *Dr. Erdem Atalay Cetinkaya*)

Pneumococcal conjugate vaccine has been shown to decrease AOM incidence, and myringotomy with ventilation tube insertion can be used in cases for recurrent disease [33]. Pneumococcal conjugate vaccine is more effective if administered during infancy. To reduce the likelihood of an AOM, smoking should be avoided and infants should be breastfed for the first 6 months of life; pacifiers should be avoided after the age of 3 years and best minimized where possible. If the baby is bottle-fed, the head should be elevated [15]. Early training for a child to learn how to blow the nose is a general advice. Some bioflavonoid and *Echinacea pallidum* have shown some efficacy for preventing the common cold. Similarly, xylitol (a natural sugar) that has been found to prevent AOM, by reducing gene expression of the pneumococcal capsular locus that induces ultrastructural changes in the pneumococcal capsule. It is usually found in chewing gum. Evidence regarding the potential for probiotics to prevent AOM is equivocal [26, 34].

References

1. Rettig E, Tunkel DE. Contemporary concepts in management of acute otitis media in children. Otolaryngol Clin N Am. 2014;47(5):651–72.
2. Tahtinen PA, Laine MK, Ruohola A. Prognostic factors for treatment failure in acute otitis media. Pediatrics. 2017;140(3):e20170072.
3. Basco WT. Predicting treatment failure in kids with AOM. Medscape. 2017;
4. Chi DH, Kitsko DJ. Otitis media. In: Licameli GR, Tunkel DE, editors. Pediatric otorhinolaryngology: diagnosis and treatment. New York: Thieme; 2013.
5. Bluestone CD. Role of surgery for otitis media in the era of resistant bacteria. Pediatr Infect Dis J. 1998;17(11):1090–8.
6. Alper CM, Luntz M, Takahashi H, et al. Panel 2: Anatomy (Eustachian Tube, Middle Ear, and Mastoid-Anatomy, Physiology, Pathophysiology, and Pathogenesis). Otolaryngol Head Neck Surg. 2017;156(4_suppl):S22–40.
7. Mulder JJ, Kuijpers W, Peters TA, et al. Development of the tubotympanum in the rat. Laryngoscope. 1998;108(12):1846–52.
8. Graham JM, Scadding GK, Bull PD. Pediatric ENT. Berlin: Springer; 2007.
9. Siddiq S, Grainger J. The diagnosis and management of acute otitis media: American Academy of Pediatrics guidelines. Arch Dis Child Educ Pract Ed. 2015;100(4):193–7.
10. Nokso-Koivisto J, Marom T, Chonmaitree T. Importance of viruses in acute otitis media. Curr Opin Pediatr. 2015;27(1):110–5.
11. Heikkinen T, Chonmaitree T. Importance of respiratory viruses in acute otitis media. Clin Microbiol Rev. 2003;16(2):230–41.
12. Richtlijn Otitis Media bij kinderen in de tweede lijn, 2012.
13. Vergison A. Microbiology of otitis media: a moving target. Vaccine. 2008;26:G5–G10. https://doi.org/10.1016/j.vaccine.2008.11.006.
14. Cunningham M, Guardiani E, Kim HJ, et al. Otitis media. Future Microbiol. 2012;7(6):733–53.
15. van Ingen G, Le Clercq CMP, Touw CE, et al. Environmental determinants associated with acute otitis media in children: a longitudinal study. Pediatr Res. 2019;87(1):163–8. https://doi.org/10.1038/s41390-019-0540-3.

16. Toll EC, Nunez DA. Diagnosis and treatment of acute otitis media: review. J Laryngol Otol. 2012;126(10):976–83.
17. Simon AK, Hollander GA, McMichael A. Evolution of the immune system in humans from infancy to old age. Proc Biol Sci. 2015;282(1821):20143085.
18. McCormick DP, Grady JJ, Diego A, et al. Acute otitis media severity: association with cytokine gene polymorphisms and other risk factors. Int J Pediatr Otorhinolaryngol. 2011;75(5):708–12.
19. Swarts JD, Alper CM, Luntz M, Bluestone CD, et al. Panel 2: Eustachian tube, middle ear, and mastoid--anatomy, physiology, pathophysiology, and pathogenesis. Otolaryngol Head Neck Surg. 2013;148(4 Suppl):E26–36.
20. Ozturk K, Snyderman CH, Sando I. Do mucosal folds in the eustachian tube function as micro-turbinates? Laryngoscope. 2011;121(4):801–4.
21. Bernstein JM. The role of IgE-mediated hypersensitivity in the development of otitis media with effusion. Otolaryngol Clin N Am. 1992;25(1):197–211.
22. Miura MS, Mascaro M, Rosenfeld RM. Association between otitis media and gastroesopha-geal reflux: a systematic review. Otolaryngol Head Neck Surg. 2012;146(3):345–52.
23. Post C. Genetics of otitis media. Adv Otorhinolaryngol. 2011;70:135–40.
24. Hafrén L, Kentala E, Järvinen TM, et al. Genetic background and the risk of otitis media. Int J Pediatr Otorhinolaryngol. 2012;76(1):41–4.
25. Bhutta MF, Lambie J, Hobson L, et al. Transcript analysis reveals a hypoxic inflammatory environment in human chronic otitis media with effusion. Front Genet. 2020;10:1327. https://doi.org/10.3389/fgene.2019.01327.
26. Levi JR, Brody RM, McKee-Cole K, Pribitkin E, O'Reilly R. Complementary and alternative medicine for pediatric otitis media. Int J Pediatr Otorhinolaryngol. 2013;77(6):926–31.
27. Shawabka MA, Haidar H, Larem A, et al. Acute otitis media-an update. J Otolaryngol ENT res. 2017;86(11):1055–61. https://doi.org/10.15406/joentr.2017.08.00252.
28. Lieberthal AS, Carroll AE, Chonmaitree T, et al. The diagnosis and management of acute otitis media. Pediatrics. 2013;131(3):e964–99.
29. Venekamp RP, Sanders SL, Glasziou PP, et al. Antibiotics for acute otitis media in children. Cochrane Database Syst Rev. 2015;6:CD000219.
30. Barclay L. Pediatric ear infection: updated AAP treatment guidelines. Medscape Medical News. 2013. http://www.medscape.com/viewarticle/779817. Accessed January 3, 2020.
31. Blomgren K, Pitkäranta A. Current challenges in diagnosis of acute otitismedia. Int J Pediatr Otorhinolaryngol. 2005;69(3):295–9.
32. Hoberman A, Paradise JL, Rockette HE, et al. Shortened antimicrobial treatment for acute otitis Media in Young Children. N Engl J Med. 2016;375(25):2446–56.
33. Dagan R, Pelton S, Bakaletz L, et al. Prevention of early episodes of otitismedia by pneu-mococcal vaccines might reduce progression to complex disease. Lancet Infect Dis. 2016;16(4):480–92.
34. Cetinkaya EA, Ciftci O, Alan S, et al. The efficacy of hesperidin for treatment of acute otitis media. Auris Nasus Larynx. 2019;6(2):172–7.

Mastoiditis

34

Emel Tahir, Senem Çengel Kurnaz,
and Georg Mathias Sprinzl

34.1 Introduction

Acute mastoiditis is a destructive inflammatory disease of the mastoid bone, and is the most common intratemporal complication of acute otitis media (AOM) [1]. Prior to the widespread use of antibiotics, approximately 20% of AOM cases were complicated with mastoiditis [2]. Recent studies reveal a change in the incidence of acute mastoiditis, as there have been increases in the incidence of unconventional pathogens such as Actinomyces, Pseudomonas, and penicillin-resistant pneumococci [3, 4].

Until recently, the incidence of mastoiditis had been decreasing since the 1980s. Therefore, the cause of this recent increase has been a subject of interest in the current literature. In addition, some studies have shown an increase in the number of cases with complicated AOM. It has been reported that these increases are due to an increased number of antibiotic-resistant microorganisms [5].

Over time, the introduction of antibiotics and advances in microbiology have led to changes in treatment approaches for acute mastoiditis. Previously, mastoidectomy was the treatment of choice, especially for childhood mastoiditis. However, in recent years, more conservative interventions have gained popularity. Currently, well-accepted first-line treatments for mastoiditis include antibiotherapy, placement of tympanostomy tube, or paracentesis [6].

E. Tahir (✉) · S. Ç. Kurnaz
Department of Otorhinolaryngology, Faculty of Medicine, Ondokuz Mayıs University, Samsun, Turkey

G. M. Sprinzl
Department of Otorhinolaryngology, Head and Neck Surgery, University Clinic Saint Poelten, Saint Poelten, Austria

© The Author(s), under exclusive license to Springer Nature Switzerland AG 2022   393
C. Cingi et al. (eds.), *Pediatric ENT Infections*,
https://doi.org/10.1007/978-3-030-80691-0_34

34.2 Pathogenesis

At birth, the mastoid is composed of a single cell (antrum) that is connected to the middle ear via the aditus ad antrum. Mastoid pneumatization begins after birth and is complete around 2 years of age. Because their mastoid cells are not yet completely developed, younger children are more commonly affected by mastoiditis. During infection, the middle ear mucosa becomes edematous and obstructs the aditus ad antrum, leading to mastoiditis. This obstruction causes serous and purulent material to accumulate in the mastoid cells. The resulting increase in pressure causes the destruction of the thin osseous septa between the mastoid air cells, leading to cavity formation. Another important contributing factor to mastoiditis is that the Eustachian tube of newborns and young children has a narrower angle, making them more susceptible to AOM [7].

Especially in childhood cases of AOM, despite apparent clinical improvements, the inappropriate selection or dosage of antibiotics can result in a failure to eradicate the bacteria. In such cases, histopathological changes (e.g., inflammatory reaction in the mastoid mucosa, granulation tissue, and "osteitis") are partially reduced, but continue to exist. Progression of unresolved AOM can lead to "osteolysis." Further, recurrent infections can stimulate the infection process and can lead to intratemporal or intracranial complications [8].

34.3 Signs and Symptoms

Clinical findings of acute mastoiditis depend on the patient's age and his/her clinical picture. An uncomplicated infection in a patient younger than 2 years can manifest with fever, ear pain, irritability, retroauricular pain, swelling, erythema, and a downwards or outwards deviation of the auricle. Most of these patients either have otorrhea or a swollen, immobile, and opaque tympanic membrane. In children older than 2 years, the inflammatory process is limited to the mastoid tissue, and the auricle is often displaced upwards and outwards. In all age groups, the development of subperiosteal abscess manifests with an erythematous and fluctuating tender mass over the mastoid bone [9].

"Bezold abscess" can develop during the course of mastoiditis if the infection spreads vertically from the air cells in the mastoid apex. However, due to the widespread use of antibiotics, subperiosteal abscess is rarely seen nowadays, and the only signs of suppressed mastoiditis may be retroauricular swelling and tenderness [10].

34.4 Microbiology

The most common bacterial agent in AOM is Streptococcus pneumoniae (35%), followed by Haemophilus influenzae (25%) and Moraxella catarrhalis (15%). These three microorganisms are responsible for more than 75% of all AOM cases with a bacterial etiology. The remaining 25% of cases are due to either Group A beta hemolytic Streptococci, Staphylococci, or other bacteria and viruses. S. pneumoniae and H. influenzae are the most common pathogens in newborns younger than 6 weeks; however, Gram-negative bacilli (e.g., Escherichia coli, Klebsiella strains, and Pseudomonas aeruginosa) are also commonly observed (20%) etiological agents in this age group. Among AOM agents, S. pneumoniae has the highest pathogenicity, and usually does not heal without treatment. However, otitis caused by H. influenzae and M. catarrhalis can heal spontaneously [11].

It is often difficult to identify the causative agents of infection. To avoid contamination from the outer ear canal, microbiological samples should be obtained from the middle ear via tympanosynthesis or aspiration through an ear tube. Culture of cerebrospinal fluid (CSF) is of utmost importance in cases of bacterial meningitis, as blood culture is rarely productive. While cases of AOM are often caused by commonly encountered pathogens in AOM, the causative agents in acute mastoiditis include *Streptococcus pneumoniae, Streptococcus pyogenes, Pseudomonas aeruginosa,* and *Staphylococcus aureus* [11].

Some studies have shown that cases of mastoiditis caused by Pseudomonas have less fever and milder leukocytosis than those caused by other pathogens. Cases of mastoiditis caused by Pseudomonas often have perforation in the tympanic membrane or have a history of parasynthesis/tympanostomy tube placement [12]. Even in some cases in which Pseudomonas is not the primary pathogen, Pseudomonas may be isolated in culture due to contamination from the outer ear canal through the perforated tympanic membrane.

Penicillin-resistant pneumococcus is extremely rare. However, there is controversy in the literature regarding the expansion of the spectrum for AOM empirical antibiotherapy [13].

The introduction of the conjugated pneumococcus vaccine has reduced the incidences of meningitis and septicemia due to pneumococcus. In addition, the incidence of AOM and the frequency of tympanostomy have also decreased. It has been observed that the pneumococcus vaccination caused a shift in AOM pathogenesis from pneumococci to H. influenza. Studies investigating the effect of this vaccination on the incidence of acute mastoiditis did not find a reduction in the postvaccination period, which the authors attributed to the rise of antibiotic-resistant microorganisms [14].

34.5 Diagnosis

In general, mastoiditis is diagnosed clinically. However, computed tomography (CT) is the first choice among imaging modalities in patients with acute mastoiditis.

In cases with acute mastoiditis, direct X-ray reveals the coalescence of mastoid air cells, loss of aeration, bone destruction, and surrounding hyperostotic areas. While the loss of aeration in mastoid tissue has no diagnostic value, it can be detected in 50% of cases with AOM. On the other hand, while the coalescence of air cells is a diagnostic sign, it is seen in a small minority of patients. Moreover, direct X-ray can be normal in patients with acute or complicated mastoiditis [15].

A computed tomography (CT) scan of temporal bone can reveal mastoiditis and the destruction of the mastoid bone much better than conventional radiograms. CT is helpful in detecting cranial complications and in diagnosing subacute mastoiditis. CT signs of mastoiditis include destruction and blurring in the mastoid main line and loss of bone septa surrounding the mastoid air cells [16]. (Fig. 34.1) CT can also detect lytic lesions in the temporal bone and abscess formation in the soft tissue. However, it should be kept in mind that even in the absence of bone destruction, there may be facial paralysis, meningitis, lateral sinus thrombophlebitis, extradural abscess, and/or brain abscess in patients with mastoiditis.

While technetium-99 bone scintigraphy can be used to detect osteolytic lesions, it is not preferred in children. Magnetic resonance imaging (MRI) has the highest sensitivity for revealing vascular thrombosis, a complication of mastoiditis. In addition, Gadolinium-enhanced MRI is quite sensitive for detecting extra-axial fluid collections and other vascular complications [17].

If possible, all patients should undergo a complete blood count and be tested for inflammation markers such as CRP and ESR. High fever and profound elevation of

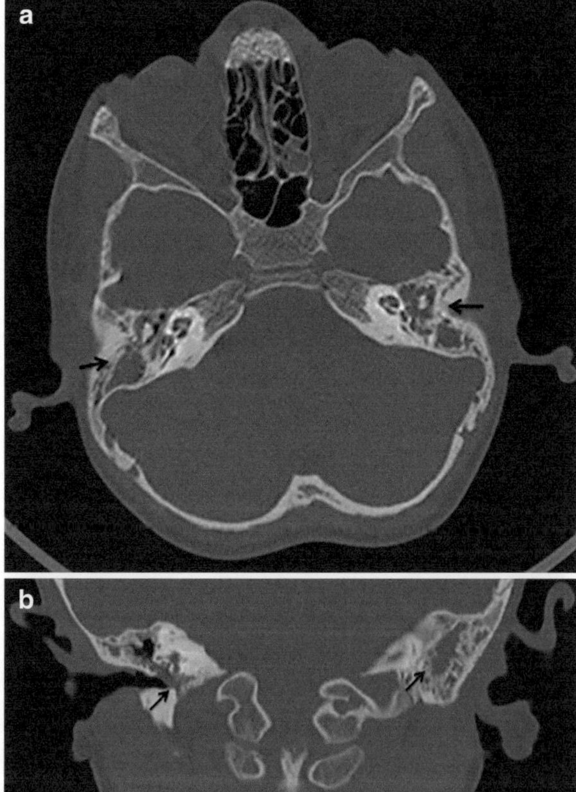

Fig. 34.1 Acute bilateral otomastoiditis in a 7-year-old boy with fever and bilateral otalgia. Axial (**a**) and coronal (**b**) temporal bone CT images reveal right-sided partial opacification and left-sided complete opacification of both middle ear and mastoid air cells (arrows) with intact tympanic membranes. Note no evidence of ossicular chain or bony destruction (Courtesy of Saffet Ozturk, MD)

infection markers (e.g., neutrophil count and CRP) should prompt investigation for complicated infection [18].

34.6 Complications

Complications of mastoiditis are similar to those of AOM. Of the mastoiditis cases, 7–16% have complications, which can be potentially life-threatening conditions requiring emergency intervention. In acute mastoiditis, the direction of the spread of infection determines the site of and the type of the complications. Rarely, erosion of the medial part of the mastoid can lead to the development of "Bezold's abscess" between the sternocleidomastoid and digastric muscles [19]. Additionally, the inflammatory process can spread to the petrous air cells and cause "Gradenigo" syndrome, which is characterized by palsy of cranial nerve 6, pain along the trigeminal nerve trace, and otorrhea. Posterior spreading of inflammation towards the occipital bone results in calvarium osteomyelitis known as "Citelli's abscess." In addition, patients may develop labyrinthitis, which can lead to the involvement of the chorda tympani and the facial nerve, causing hearing loss. Finally, erosion of the inner cortical bone can cause suppurative complications of the central nervous system including epidural, subdural, temporal lobar, or cerebellar abscesses, meningitis, and venous sinus thrombosis [20, 21].

The complications of mastoiditis can be classified into two categories as extracranial (intratemporal) or intracranial (extratemporal) (Table 34.1) [22].

34.6.1 Infratemporal (Extracranial) Complications

34.6.1.1 Labyrinthitis
Labyrinthitis caused by otitis media is a life-threatening complication that can cause meningitis. Symptoms during the course of otitis media that should raise suspicion for labyrinthitis include acute vertigo, nausea-vomiting, and sensorineural hearing loss. Serous labyrinthitis is more common that purulent labyrinthitis and is caused by the toxic and metabolic products of the invading bacteria or the host's inflammatory cells. Serous labyrinthitis may lead to mild vestibular or cochlear damage that can be cured with treatment. On the other hand, in purulent labyrinthitis, bacteria

Table 34.1 Complications of the mastoiditis [22, 23]

Intratemporal (extracranial) complications	Intracranial (extratemporal) complications
• Labyrinthitis.	• Extradural abscess.
• Petrositis.	• Meningitis.
• Facial paresis/paralysis.	• Subdural abscess.
	• Brain abscess/Otitic hydrocephalus.
	• Lateral (sigmoid) sinus thrombophlebitis.
	• Bezold's abscess.
	• Zygomatic abscess.

are present in the inner ear fluids, and therefore, the patient often has advanced stage and/or permanent hearing loss and vestibular damage. Further, patients with purulent labyrinthitis also have a high risk of meningitis and other intracranial complications. Antibiotics are the first line of treatment in labyrinthitis caused by acute otitis media. In addition, patients should also undergo paracentesis to drain the pus in the middle ear [24].

34.6.1.2 Petrositis

Petrositis is a rare complication. In its classical form, known as Gradenigo syndrome, there is retro-orbital pain, in-turning of the eye due to abducens paralysis, and ipsilateral otitis media. The diagnosis of petrositis is similar to that of mastoiditis. However, CT has higher diagnostic value for petrositis.

The treatment of petrositis includes radical mastoidectomy (i.e., opening the pneumatized spaces of the petrous bone) to drain the infection. Patients who do not show regression of symptoms despite this surgical treatment may require exploration of the petrous apex via the middle fossa approach [25].

34.6.1.3 Facial Paresis/Paralysis

Facial paralysis occurring during the course of acute suppurative otitis media does not typically lead to permanent nerve damage. Further, the lesion in the facial nerve is limited to neuropraxia, mild compression, and edema [25]. Appropriate treatment (including antibiotics and paracentesis performed at the suppurative phase to drain the pus in the middle ear) can lead to improvement within days. No further treatment is required if the infection is under control and if there is no sign of nerve degeneration [26]. However, in many cases mastoidectomy and VT insertion is recommended to shorten the duration of facial palsy and the course of the disease.

34.6.2 Intracranial (Extratemporal) Complications

34.6.2.1 Extradural Abscess

Extradural abscesses or granulation tissues that lead to abscess may remain clinically occult until detection during mastoidectomy. However, extradural abscesses may go unrecognized, even during mastoidectomy, unless the dura of the middle and the posterior fossa are opened and inspected. Treatment of extradural abscess requires elevation of the bone plane above the dura for proper drainage. If present, granulation tissue over the dura should also be cleaned to prevent penetration into the dura [27].

34.6.2.2 Meningitis

It is easy to suspect bacterial meningitis in otitis cases presenting with headache, fever, nuchal rigidity, and Kernig's and Brudzinski's signs. The major challenges in the diagnosis of meningitis are (1) to determine the route by which the infection caused the meningitis and (2) to determine whether the meningitis was caused by the same microorganism that caused the otitis [27]. Children who develop meningitis during the course of acute otitis media often have the hematogenous spread of H. influenza type B. If the causative agent responsible for meningitis during acute otitis is S. pneumoniae or H. influenza of an undetermined type, the patient should undergo CT to determine whether he/she has any congenital anomalies of the inner ear that may facilitate the transfer of the infectious agent from the middle ear to the CSF [28].

Patients with acute otitis media and meningitis should undergo treatment with antibiotics and paracentesis to drain the pus in the middle ear. Since H. influenzae type B is a common agent in meningitis, the antibiotic should account for beta lactamase inhibition [28].

34.6.2.3 Subdural Abscess

Because of their close proximity to the cerebral cortex and their mass effect, subdural abscesses can cause local compression symptoms such as convulsions and altered consciousness. The diagnosis of subdural abscess can easily be made with CT, while MRI is helpful for distinguishing subdural lesion from chronic hematoma or non-suppurative effusion [29].

Treatment of subdural abscesses that develop as a result of acute otitis media includes antibiotics, paracentesis to drain the pus inside the middle ear, and surgery. For subdural abscesses that develop due to *chronic* otitis media, the infection should be eradicated with mastoidectomy, the granulations on the dura should be cleaned, and the subdural abscess should be surgically drained [30].

34.6.2.4 Brain Abscess

Intracranial abscesses develop clinically in four stages. In the first stage (onset of cerebritis), there is mild fever, and the patient may have difficulty concentrating, fatigue, and headache. These symptoms are usually disregarded, and they may regress within a couple of days. The second stage (latent phase) is when the abscess is localized. Clinically, this stage is completely silent, and may last a couple of weeks. In the third stage (manifested abscess), the abscess develops at the site where the cerebritis first occurred, leading to focal neurological signs, convulsions, and loss of consciousness due to compression. In the terminal fourth stage (abscess rupture), the abscess ruptures into the ventricle or subarachnoid space, quickly resulting in mortality [31].

Intracranial abscesses associated with otitis media are mostly seen in the middle fossa, and to a lesser extent, in the posterior fossa. Before they become manifest at the third stage, the diagnosis of intracranial abscesses is only possible by CT or contrast enhanced MRI scans, which may be requested due to suspicion. However, it should be kept in mind that abscesses may not present any radiological signs in the early stage, and therefore, the examinations should be repeated every 2–3 weeks [32].

The surgical treatment of brain abscess should aim to eradicate both the primary infection site in the middle ear as well as the abscess itself. Preferably, both surgical procedures should be applied in a single session. However, if the brain abscess poses a life-threatening risk, the first surgical intervention should aim to remove the brain abscess and reduce intracranial pressure, while the second intervention should target the temporal bone [22].

34.6.2.5 Lateral Sinus Thrombophlebitis

Lateral sinus thrombophlebitis may be completely asymptomatic, or it can manifest with fulminant sepsis and intermittent fever. It is caused by a cholesteatoma or by granulation tissue, which is often located on the lateral sinus wall. The thrombus can advance distally towards the internal jugular vein, or proximally towards the transverse sinus. Thrombophlebitis of the internal jugular vein can cause disseminated deep vein infection, and it may also lead to jugular foramen syndrome, which involves paralysis of the cranial nerves 9–10–11. Thrombophlebitis of the lateral and transverse sinuses can lead to intracranial hypertension (otitic hydrocephalus) and to multiple brain abscesses caused by septic venous thrombi. Lateral sinus thrombosis can be diagnosed clinically with the Tobey-Ayer test, the Queckenstedt test, or MRI. In the Tobey-Ayer test, lateral sinus thrombophlebitis is identified by a sudden increase in cerebrospinal fluid (CSF) pressure as measured by lumbar puncture during compression of the contralateral internal jugular vein. Further, there should be a lack of pressure change when the ipsilateral internal jugular vein is compressed, in favor of thrombus. In the Queckenstedt test, lateral sinus thrombophlebitis is identified by a failure to observe a sudden increase or decrease in CSF pressure as measured by lumbar puncture when both internal jugular veins are compressed and decompressed, respectively. This favors impaired circulation between the ventricular system and the subarachnoid space [33, 34].

In cases where lateral sinus thrombophlebitis causes an obstruction, the main goal of surgical treatment is to clean the granulation tissue over the dura. If there is accompanying otitic hydrocephalus, treatment should be aimed at reducing the intracranial pressure, and vision monitoring is required. In cases where lateral sinus thrombophlebitis causes septic or aseptic thromboemboli, the thrombus should be surgically excised, and then the distal internal jugular vein and the proximal lateral sinus should be ligated [35].

34.6.2.6 Otitic Hydrocephalus

Otitic hydrocephalus refers to increased intracranial pressure. This increased pressure can be a result of lateral sinus thrombosis caused by otitis media in the absence of meningitis, subdural abscess, or intracranial abscess. Cases with otitis who experience headache and lethargy should be checked for otitic hydrocephalus. The increased intracranial pressure can cause papilledema, which can be diagnosed using MRI to show lateral sinus thrombosis. Acetazolamide, corticosteroids, diuretics, mannitol, and large volume lumbar puncture can be used to reduce the intracranial pressure [35, 36].

34.7 Follow-Up and Treatment

Several publications have defined treatment algorithms for complicated and uncomplicated acute mastoiditis. In the past, simple mastoidectomy was a first line treatment; now, it is obsolete, and many clinics are using more conservative methods.

However, despite years of accumulated knowledge, there is no standard treatment algorithm for acute mastoiditis [37–40].

Proper antibiotic treatment of acute suppurative otitis media should cause symptoms to subside within 2–5 days. Physical examination signs favoring acute infection should disappear within the first week, and the middle ear should show signs of aeration both clinically and radiologically after 8 weeks of treatment. In cases with acute otitis media, suspicion should be raised about mastoiditis if the patient has a lack of symptomatic response to antibiotherapy within 1 week, has recurrence of symptoms within 2–3 weeks, has edema in the skin of the posterior wall of the external ear canal, and has tenderness during palpation of the auricle and retroauricular area. In such cases, the middle ear should be drained with paracentesis, and if possible, the sampled purulent material should be cultured for aerobic and anaerobic bacteria. Further, the patient should undergo weekly follow-up examinations during 2–3 weeks of antibiotherapy tailored to the antibiogram. Although it is theoretically recommended to follow-up with the patient until aeration is observed in the mastoid radiograms, one should be cautious about exposure to radiation, especially in the pediatric age group [39, 40].

Uncomplicated acute mastoiditis is typically treated with intravenous antimicrobial therapy and myringotomy. Additionally, tympanostomy tubes can be placed when necessary. The same treatment can be applied to patients with isolated facial paralysis. If there are no improvements in local and systemic signs within 48 h of treatment, simple mastoidectomy is indicated. In the presence of subperiosteal abscess, the patient should undergo simple mastoidectomy, tympanostomy tube placement, and antimicrobial therapy [41].

Mastoidectomy is recommended for complicated cases. However, there is a consensus in the literature that, based on the clinical picture, the initial treatment should include myringotomy and/or tympanostomy tube placement, intravenous antibiotherapy, as well as incision and drainage in cases with abscess. Mastoidectomy should definitely be performed in cases with intracranial complications or in those with intratemporal complications such as petrositis or labyrinthitis. Radical mastoidectomy should only be considered in the presence of otorrhea that is refractory to simple mastoidectomy [42].

Antibiotherapy in acute mastoiditis should begin empirically, and should cover the common bacterial pathogens. Appropriate treatment options include Cefepime 3×50 mg/kg, ceftazidime 3×50 mg/kg, or four doses of piperacillin-tazobactam 240–300 mg/kg/day. In cases with penicillin allergy, four doses of clindamycin 40 mg/kg/day and three doses of aztreonam 120 mg/kg provide both Gram-positive and -negative efficacy. Patients with a severe clinical course who are suspected to have secondary meningitis or patients with a high risk for resistant pneumococcal infections and methicillin-resistant *S. aureus* infections should have four doses of vancomycin 60 mg/kg/day added to their treatment. The most commonly used combination for intracranial complications is ceftriaxone, vancomycin, and metronidazole. The antibiotherapy can be modified based on culture results in cases where a drainage procedure is performed. The patient's vaccination status and the hospital's resistance status should be considered and accounted for when choosing the appropriate antibiotic. Treatment that is started empirically should be modified according to the culture and antibiotic sensitivity results [43, 44]. In patients that are allergic to penicillin, glycopeptides (e.g., vancomycin or teicoplanin) can be administered in combination with metronidazole, or linezolid can be combined with metronidazole.

The duration of intravenous antibiotherapy should be 7–10 days in uncomplicated cases, while cases on oral antibiotics should undergo treatment for 4 weeks. Failure to observe mastoid aeration after 2–3 months of treatment despite improvement in symptoms and physical examination findings suggests the development of "masked mastoiditis." It should be kept in mind that signs and symptoms of acute mastoiditis are suppressed with antibiotherapy or paracentesis in approximately 70% of cases. In addition, failure to treat masked mastoiditis with mastoidectomy in a timely manner has been shown to lead to intracranial complications in 20% of cases [45].

In cases without mastoid aeration despite 3 months of treatment, it may be necessary to use CT to investigate for bone destruction, and MRI may be needed to determine extradural abscess or lateral sinus thrombophlebitis. In cases where mastoid bone aeration does not return to normal, surgical treatment (mastoidectomy) is indicated due to the risk of developing serious intracranial complications. In otogenic sigmoid sinus thrombosis, anticoagulants may be added, and in the presence of intracranial complications, steroid and mannitol can be added to the treatment regimen [46].

Although there is no definitive consensus on the treatment algorithm for mastoiditis, the most widely accepted approach in the literature is as follows:

- For uncomplicated cases: Intravenous antibiotherapy, and if necessary, myringotomy.
- For cases with subperiosteal abscess: Drainage of abscess, myringotomy, and antibiotherapy.
- In all cases: Microbiological examination of sample obtained during myringotomy, if performed.
- For complicated cases: Following imaging studies, myringotomy, simple mastoidectomy, and intravenous therapy.
- For complicated cases with subperiosteal abscess who were not cured with aforementioned treatments: Mastoidectomy.
- For all cases: Samples obtained during mastoidectomy should be sent for microbiological examination.
- For all cases: Following discharge, all patients should continue oral antibiotic treatment and be closely followed clinically for at least 10 days.

Patients with chronic otitis may develop acute mastoiditis during infection exacerbations. In such cases, mastoidectomy is obligatory, and CT and MRI can be used for investigating bone destruction and other complications, respectively. Acute mastoiditis superimposing chronic otitis media should be treated surgically as soon as

Table 34.2 Mastoidectomy indications for the treatment of acute mastoiditis

Mastoidectomy indications for the treatment of acute mastoiditis
• Lack of response (48 h) to intravenous antibiotherapy.
• Development of complication(s): Facial palsy, meningitis with and without sigmoid thrombosis, meningitis with cerebrellar abscess.
• Recurrent subcutaneous abscess.

there is a response to parenteral antibiotic treatment. Mastoidectomy indications for the treatment of acute mastoiditis are shown on Table 34.2.

34.8 Subacute (Masked) Mastoiditis

Subacute (masked) mastoiditis was recently identified. This condition is characterized by low grade infection in the middle ear and mastoid bone. This condition is often characterized by permanent or recurrent middle ear effusion in patients with acute otitis media who did not receive sufficient antimicrobial treatment. Patients with subacute mastoiditis may have fever, otalgia, abnormal tympanic membrane appearance, and cranial complications [46].

In the literature, masked mastoiditis (also known as "latent" or "silent" mastoiditis) refers to a subclinical infectious inflammatory process occurring in the bone structures and in the mucosal lining of mastoid cells despite an intact tympanic membrane. The widespread use of broad-spectrum antibiotics has decreased the incidence of classical mastoiditis; however, it has increased the incidence of masked mastoiditis. This is an unfortunate clinical problem, as masked mastoiditis has a chronic and subclinical course and has the potential to cause life-threatening situations [47, 48].

Patients with masked mastoiditis typically do not have any clinical symptoms. However, some cases may experience mild or moderate recurrent fever, tenderness over the mastoid bone, and headache. AOM is considered to be healed in nearly all masked mastoiditis patients, and therefore no clinical signs may be detected until the emergence of intratemporal or intracranial complications. However, masked mastoiditis should be suspected in patients that develop perforation and discharge. Other signs suggestive of a continuing occult infection in the mastoid region include pulsation, granulation tissue, or localized hyperemia over the pars flaccida, over the posterior upper quadrant of the pars tensa, and/or the neighboring outer ear canal [45–47].

34.9 Mastoiditis in Patients with Cochlear Implant

The increased application of cochlear implants has led to an increase in associated (directly or indirectly) complications, including electrode problems, facial paralysis, flap problems, and infection. Since young children typically suffer from acute mastoiditis and are the recipients of cochlear implants, there has been an increased incidence in mastoiditis due to cochlear implant. Among patients with cochlear implant, the prevalence of otogenic infections, such as mastoiditis, is around 1% [49].

Cortical mastoidectomy is also recognized as a risk factor for acute mastoiditis (Osborn, acute mastoiditis). When the septa is removed during mastoidectomy, the natural barriers that protect against the spread of infection are destroyed, and as a result, AOM can progress to mastoiditis within a short time. In addition, implants can trigger a foreign body reaction, leading to infectious complications. In these cases, the foreign body should be removed as soon as possible, as it can cause important social, economic, and psychological issues. It is especially important to remove the implant in children who have begun their auditory/verbal development [50]. However, many clinicians may have a serious dilemma regarding the best way to remove the implant and control the infection. Acute mastoiditis often develops within the first 2 years following cochlear implant placement, and the symptoms are the same as those in children without implant. Intravenous antibiotic treatment should be initiated promptly, and the patient should be closely monitored for intra-temporal/intracranial complications. In such patients, meningitis can progress rapidly via direct dissemination from the implant. Intravenous ceftriaxone is the first option in antibiotherapy, and the treatment can last up to 6 weeks. In patients who are refractory to medical treatment, or in complicated cases, surgical treatment options include placement of tympanostomy tube, abscess drainage, and mastoidectomy. Removal of the implant should be considered in patients who have persistent infections refractory to surgical treatment [51].

References

1. Gliklich RE, Eavey RD, Iannuzzi RA, et al. A contem- porary analysis of acute mastoiditis. Arch Otolaryngol Head Neck Surg. 1996;122:135–9.
2. Pritchett CV, Thorne MC. Incidence of pediatric acute mastoiditis: 1997-2006. Arch Otolaryngol Head Neck Surg. 2012;138:451–5.
3. BilavskyE Y-BH, Samra Z, et al. Clinical, laboratory, and microbiological differences between children with simple or complicated mastoiditis. Int J Pediatr Otorhinolaryngol. 2009;73:1270–3.
4. Spratley J, Silveira H, Alvarez I, et al. Acute mastoiditis in children: review of the current status. Int J Pediatr Otorhinolaryngol. 2000;56:33–40.
5. Choi SS, Lander L. Pediatric acute mastoiditis in the post-pneumococcal conjugate vaccine era. Laryngoscope. 2011;121:1072–80.
6. Tawfik KO, Ishman SL, Altaye M, et al. Pediatric Acute Otitis Media in the Era of Pneumococcal Vaccination. Otolaryngol Head Neck Surg. 2017;156:938–45.
7. Attlmayr B, Zaman S, Scott J, et al. Paediatric acute mastoiditis, then and now: is it more of a problem now? J Laryngol Otol. 2015;129:955–9.
8. Nadol JB Jr, Eavey RD. Acute and chronic mastoiditis: clinical presentation, diagnosis, and management. Curr Clin Top Infect Dis. 1995;15:204–29.
9. van den Aardweg MT, Rovers MM, de Ru JA, et al. A systematic review of diagnostic criteria for acute mastoiditis in children. Otol Neurotol. 2008;29:751–7.
10. Glynn F, Osman L, Colreavy M, et al. Acute mastoiditis in children: presentation and long term consequences. J Laryngol Otol. 2008;122:233–7.

11. Tamir SO, Roth Y, Dalal I, et al. Acute mastoiditis in the pneumococcal conjugate vaccine era. Clin Vaccine Immunol. 2014;21:1189–91.
12. Nussinovitch M, Yoeli R, Elishkevitz K, et al. Acute mastoiditis in children: epidemiologic, clinical, microbiologic, and therapeutic aspects over past years. Clin Pediatr. 2004;43:261–7.
13. Van Zuijlen DA, Schilder AG, Van Balen FA, et al. National differences in incidence of acute mastoiditis: relationship to prescribing patterns of antibiotics for acute otitis media? Pediatr Infect Dis J. 2001;20:140–4.
14. Koutouzis EI, Michos A, Koutouzi FI, et al. Pneumococcal Mastoiditis in Children Before and After the Introduction of Conjugate Pneumococcal Vaccines. Pediatr Infect Dis J. 2016;35:292–6.
15. Burakgazi G, Bayaroğullari H, Öztürk F, et al. Radiological imaging of rare intracranial complications secondary to otitis media and mastoiditis. J Craniofac Surg. 2017;28:620–4.
16. Marom T, Roth Y, Boaz M, et al. Acute mastoiditis in children: necessity and timing of imaging. Pediatr Infect Dis J. 2016;35:30–4.
17. Saat R, Laulajainen-Hongisto AH, Mahmood G, et al. MR imaging features of acute mastoiditis and their clinical relevance. Am J Neuroradiol. 2015;36:361–7.
18. Laulajainen-Hongisto A, Saat R, Lempinen L, et al. Bacteriology in relation to clinical findings and treatment of acutemastoiditis in children. Int J Pediatr Otorhinolaryngol. 2014;78:2072–8.
19. Lin YH, Lin MY. Bezold abscess. Ear Nose Throat J. 2015;94:45–6.
20. Valles JM, Fekete R. Gradenigo syndrome: unusual consequence of otitis media. Case Rep Neurol. 2014;6:197–201.
21. Sahoo AK, Preetam C, Samal DK, et al. Citelli's abscess following otitis media: a case report. Iran J Otorhinolaryngol. 2017;29:161–3.
22. Mattos JL, Colman KL, Casselbrant ML, et al. Intratemporal and intracranial complications of acute otitis media in a pediatric population. Int J Pediatr Otorhinolaryngol. 2014;78:2161–4.
23. Raveh E, Ulanovski D, Attias J, et al. Acute mastoiditis in children with a cochlear implant. Int J Pediatr Otorhinolaryngol. 2016;81:80–3.
24. Oestreicher-Kedem Y, Raveh E, Kornreich L, et al. Complications of mastoiditis in children at the onset of a new millennium. Ann Otol Rhinol Laryngol. 2005;114:147–52.
25. Lavin JM, Rusher T, Shah RK. Complications of pediatric otitis media. Otolaryngol Head Neck Surg. 2016;154:366–70.
26. Maranhão AS, Andrade JS, Godofredo VR, et al. Intratemporal complications of otitis media. Braz J Otorhinolaryngol. 2013;79:141–9.
27. Quesnel S, Nguyen M, Pierrot S, et al. Acute mastoiditis in children: a retrospective study of 188 patients. Int J Pediatr Otorhinolaryngol. 2010;74:1388–92.
28. Horowitz G, Fishman G, Brenner A, et al. A novel radiographic sign and a new classifying system in mastoiditis-related epidural abscess. Otol Neurotol. 2015;36:1378–82.
29. Heran NS, Steinbok P, Cochrane DD. Conservative neurosurgical management of intracranial epidural abscesses in children. Neurosurgery. 2003;53:893–7.
30. Enoksson F, Groth A, Hultcrantz M, et al. Subperiosteal abscesses in acute mastoiditis in 115 Swedish children. Int J Pediatr Otorhinolaryngol. 2015;79:1115–20.
31. Ghaffar FA, Wördemann M, McCracken GH Jr. Acute mastoiditis in children: a seventeen-year experience in Dallas, Texas. Pediatr Infect Dis J. 2001;20:376–80.
32. Isaacson B, Mirabal C, Kutz JW Jr, et al. Pediatric otogenic intracranial abscesses. Otolaryngol Head Neck Surg. 2010;142:434–7.
33. Kuczkowski J, Dubaniewicz-Wybieralska M, Przewoźny T, et al. Otitic hydrocephalus associated with lateral sinus thrombosis and acute mastoiditis in children. Int J Pediatr Otorhinolaryngol. 2006;70:1817–23.
34. Koitschev A, Simon C, Löwenheim H, et al. Delayed otogenic hydrocephalus after acute otitis media in pediatric patients: the changing presentation of a serious otologic complication. Acta Otolaryngol. 2005;125:1230–5.
35. Omer Unal F, Sennaroğlu L, Saatçi I. Otitic hydrocephalus: role of radiology for diagnosis. Int J Pediatr Otorhinolaryngol. 2005;69:897–901.
36. Kuczkowski J, Narozny W, Mikaszewski B. Otitic hydrocephalus. Arch Neurol. 2005;62:1940.

37. Marchisio P, Bianchini S, Villani A, et al. Diagnosis and management of acute mastoiditis in a cohort of Italian children. Expert Rev Anti-Infect Ther. 2014;12:1541–8.
38. Psarommatis IM, Voudouris C, Douros K, et al. Algorithmic management of pediatric acute mastoiditis. Int J Pediatr Otorhinolaryngol. 2012;76:791–6.
39. Lin HW, Shargorodsky J, Gopen Q. Clinical strategies for the management of acute mastoiditis in the pediatric population. Clin Pediatr (Phila). 2010;49:110–5.
40. Loh R, Phua M, Shaw CL. Management of paediatric acute mastoiditis: systematic review. J Laryngol Otol. 2017;7:1–9.
41. Ghadersohi S, Young NM, Smith-Bronstein V, et al. Management of acute complicated mastoiditis at an urban, tertiary care pediatric hospital. Laryngoscope. 2017;127:2321–7.
42. Kordeluk S, Kraus M, Leibovitz E, et al. Challenges in the management of acute mastoiditis in children. Curr Infect Dis Rep. 2015;17:479.
43. Voudouris C, Psarommatis I, Nikas I, et al. Pediatric masked mastoiditis associated with multiple intracranial complications. Case Rep Otolaryngol. 2015;2015:897239.
44. Atzeni M, Iozzi C, Pinna M, et al. A case of complicated otomastoiditis. Pediatr Med Chir. 2015;37:108.
45. Migirov L, Kronenberg J. Mastoidectomy for acute otomastoiditis: our experience. Ear Nose Throat J. 2005;84:219–22.
46. Tarantino V, D'Agostino R, Taborelli G. Acute mastoiditis: a 10 year retrospective study. Int J Pediatr Otorhinolaryngol. 2002;66:143–8.
47. Zawawi F, Cardona I, Akinpelu OV, et al. Acute mastoiditis in children with cochlear implants: is explantation required?Otolaryngol. Head Neck Surg. 2014;151:394–8.
48. Migirov L, Yakirevitch A, Henkin Y, et al. Acute otitis media and mastoiditis following cochlear implantation. Int J Pediatr Otorhinolaryngol. 2006;70:899–903.
49. Go C, Bernstein JM, de Jong AL, et al. Intracranial complications of acute mastoiditis. Int J Pediatr Otorhinolaryngol. 2000;52:143–8.
50. Grossman Z, Zehavi Y, Leibovitz E, et al. (2016) severe acute mastoiditis admission is not related to delayed antibiotic treatment for antecedent acute otitis media. Pediatr Infect Dis J. 2016;35(2):162–5.
51. Zanetti D, Nassif N. Indications for surgery in acute mastoiditis and their complications in children. Int J Pediatr Otorhinolaryngol. 2006;70:1175–82.

Labyrinthitis

35

Mustafa Acar, Cemal Cingi, and Jacques Magnan

35.1 Introduction

Labyrinthitis refers to a condition wherein the inner ear (i.e. labyrinth) becomes inflamed. Labyrinthitis presents clinically as disordered balance or impaired hearing, the severity of which may vary, and may be uni- or bilateral. The labyrinth may become acutely inflamed as a result of either viral or bacterial infections, whether of the ear or systemic. The condition can also result from an autoimmune disorder. If the labyrinth becomes ischaemic, it may function abnormally, in a way resembling the pathology seen in labyrinthitis [1].

The usual age of onset for labyrinthitis secondary to viral infection is between the ages of 35 and 60 years. It seldom affects children. Suppurative labyrinthitis is found in paediatric patients below the age of 2 years and is secondary to meningitis. The highest risk for meningitis is below the age of 2 years. Suppurative inflammation of the labyrinth may also occur secondary to middle ear infection when not treated or in patients with cholesteatoma, an event which may occur at all ages [2]. Since most cases of acute or chronic middle ear inflammation by far occur in children, this is the group at highest risk of developing serous labyrinthitis [1].

M. Acar (✉)
The Acar Ear, Nose, and Throat Diseases and Surgery Clinic, Eskişehir, Turkey

C. Cingi
Department of Otorhinolaryngology, Faculty of Medicine, Eskişehir Osmangazi University, Eskişehir, Turkey

J. Magnan
Department of Otolaryngology, Head and Neck Surgery, Aix-Marseille University and NORD Hospital, Marseille, France

35.2 Anatomy

A clear picture of the anatomy of the inner ear, middle ear, mastoid and subarachnoid space is a prerequisite for a full appreciation of the pathogenic processes involved in inner ear inflammation. The inner ear consists of a bony covering that envelops a fragile system of membranes within which exist the organs of sense responsible for hearing and the perception of balance.

The inner ear contains the following sensory organs: the utricle, saccule, semicircular canals, and cochlea. The clinical presentation of labyrinthitis is produced by injury to these organs resulting from invasion by a pathogen or by the inflammatory response itself.

The inner ear is located inside the petrous temporal bone in the vicinity of the mastoid cavity. The oval and round windows are the interface between the inner and middle ear, whilst the inner ear communicates with the central nervous system and the subarachnoid cavity via the internal auditory canal and the cochlear aqueduct. Bacterial pathogens may invade the inner ear through these communicating routes, or may gain entry if the osseous portion of the inner ear is congenitally defective or later becomes defective. Viral pathogenic entry may be blood-borne or through the anatomical communications listed above. Since labyrinthitis secondary to a virus and that caused by bacteria differ considerably, they will be addressed here as distinct disease entities [1].

35.3 Viral and Bacterial Pathogens Responsible for Labyrinthitis

There is a dearth of direct evidential support for viruses as an aetiology, but plentiful indirect evidence comes from epidemiological studies indicating associations between viral pathogens and inflammation of the inner ear. A bout of viral labyrinthitis often follows an infective episode affecting the upper airways and may be observed during epidemics. There is degeneration of the axons within the vestibular nerve observable on histopathological examination, a finding consistent with a viral cause in vestibular neuritis [3].

The bacterial pathogens responsible for labyrinthitis are identical with those causing meningitis or ear infection. Where cholesteatoma formation has triggered an infection, the pathogen is more likely to be Gram-negative.

The following viruses are capable of provoking inner ear inflammation [1]:

- Cytomegalovirus (CMV)
- Mumps virus
- Varicella-zoster virus (VZV)
- Measles virus
- Influenza virus
- Parainfluenza virus
- Rubella virus

- Herpes simplex virus
- Adenovirus
- Coxsackievirus
- Respiratory syncytial virus

The following bacteria are capable of provoking inner ear inflammation [1]:

- *Streptococcus pneumoniae*
- *Haemophilus influenzae*
- *Moraxella catarrhalis*
- *Neisseria meningitidis*
- *Streptococci generally*
- *Staphylococci*
- *Proteus* spp
- *Bacteroides* spp
- *Escherichia coli*
- *Mycobacterium tuberculosis*

35.4 Classification

35.4.1 Viral Labyrinthitis

Auditory impairment due to a virus may be present from birth or occur later. Deafness that occurs prior to birth and is considered viral in origin is most frequently associated with rubella or cytomegalovirus. Deafness of viral origin arising after birth and due to a virus typically follows a bout of mumps or rubeola virus. Abrupt sensorineural hearing loss (SNHL) of idiopathic origin is also suspected to be due to a virus. Auditory impairment secondary to CMV has been demonstrated experimentally to be linked crucially to proteins involved in inflammation [4].

One particular type of virally induced inner ear inflammation is worthy of separate consideration, herpes zoster oticus, i.e. Ramsay-Hunt syndrome. This syndrome occurs several years after a primary episode of VZV infection, when the pathogen is reawakened from dormancy. It appears the pathogen targets both the spiral and vestibular ganglia as well as the eighth cranial nerve [5]. Around a quarter of those affected by herpes oticus have problems with hearing or balance alongside the characteristic features of the Ramsay-Hunt syndrome, i.e. paralysed muscles of the face and a rash consisting of vesicles [6].

35.4.2 Bacterial Labyrinthitis

Bacterial labyrinthitis may be a complication in both meningitis and middle ear infections, the result of pathogenic entry into the inner ear, as occurs in the suppurative form, or by spread of toxins produced by the pathogen into the labyrinth, alongside pro-inflammatory molecular signals, as occurs in the serous form. The most frequently occurring complication in middle ear infections is inner ear inflammation. One study noted that labyrinthitis was the diagnosis in 32% of cases where a complication occurred, either intra- or extra-cranially [7].

Whilst bacterial labyrinthitis has become infrequent since antibiotics have been widely available, deafness secondary to bacterial meningeal infection is still a major reason for deafness to develop [8]. Up to 20% of paediatric cases of meningitis feature symptoms related to hearing or balance [9]. Deafness secondary to meningitis is generally bilateral, in contrast to cases where deafness follows an ear infection, most of which affect only one side.

35.4.3 Suppurative Labyrinthitis

Bacterial pathogens that cause meningitis and are within the cerebrospinal fluid may invade the inner ear membranes via the internal acoustic meatus or the cochlear aqueduct, whereas pathogenic spread from otitis media or mastoiditis to the inner ear generally occurs when the horizontal semicircular canal becomes dehiscent [10]. This situation may arise when cholesteatoma erodes the structure. It has become unusual for otitis media to be complicated by suppurative inner ear infection now that antibiotics are available. Where suppurative inner ear infections are seen, virtually invariably cholesteatoma is noted to be present. Bacterial labyrinthitis frequently results in profound deafness, vertigo of a severe degree, ataxia and nausea with emesis.

Labyrinthitis ossificans is a frequent consequence of a suppurative inner ear infection. This condition results in bone being laid down, replacing the membranous labyrinth. It is important to decide early on about whether to implant a cochlear device. Deafness may progressively deteriorate following meningitis if the membranous portions of the cochlea and inner ear become necrotic and scarred [11].

35.4.4 Serous Labyrinthitis

Serous labyrinthitis may develop without bacteria actually invading the inner ear spaces. This condition results from inflammation produced by the diffusion of pathogenic toxins as well as molecules involved in the inflammatory response across the round window membranous covering. Some of the molecules involved are cytokines and complement proteins [9]. Disorders of the middle ear, both acute and chronic, can provoke serous labyrinthitis, especially otitis media, where it is amongst the most frequent of complications.

These mediators of inflammation are deposited within the tympanic duct, precipitating lightly near the inner face of the round window. Inflammatory cells effect entry into the duct in the vicinity of the basal turn of the cochlea. This in turn causes sensorineural auditory impairment of up to moderate severity, affecting perception of high-pitched sounds.

Patients with an effusion of the middle ear have auditory impairment of a mixed type when assessed audiometrically. There may be symptoms related to vestibular dysfunction, albeit less frequently. The therapeutic goal is to eradicate the pathogen and allow the middle ear to be drained of its fluid build-up. Auditory impairment is generally temporary, although risks becoming chronic unless therapeutic intervention is undertaken [1].

35.4.5 Autoimmune Labyrinthitis

SNHL may rarely be caused by autoimmune labyrinthitis. The autoimmune pathology may be localised or a manifestation of a systemic autoimmune disorder, e.g. granulomatosis with polyangiitis or polyarteritis nodosa [12, 13].

35.5 Prognosis

Labyrinthitis, in particular the bacterial form, imposes high morbidity on patients. Indeed, bacterial labyrinthitis of all types, is the cause of one in three cases of non-congenital deafness.

Following an episode of meningitis, there is a 10-20% risk in children of developing irreversible deafness [9, 14]. Dizziness occurred at a frequency of 23% in cases of meningitis secondary to infection with *S. pneumoniae* [15].

A patient with Ramsay-Hunt syndrome with auditory impairment has a 6% chance this will become permanent sensorineural deafness [10]. The pathogen that has the greatest association with deafness after meningitis is *S. pneumoniae* [16].

Both suppurative and serous inner ear infections run the risk of producing Ménière syndrome in patients. The probable pathogenetic mechanism is fibrotic scarring of the endolymphatic duct and perturbation of the exchange of sodium and potassium ions [1].

35.6 Diagnosis

35.6.1 History

A detailed and complete patient account of symptomatology, previous illnesses and drug history is vital in cases of vertigo and auditory impairment where there is a suspicion of labyrinthitis. The following are symptoms which should be specifically enquired after [1]:

- Vertigo. When it happens and how long it lasts. What effect movement, especially of the head, produces and any other features.
- Auditory loss. Is it one- or two-sided, slight or severe? How long has it been a problem? Any other features should also be noted.

- Does the ear feel full?
- Ringing in the ears.
- Discharge from the ear.
- Earache.
- Nausea and vomiting.
- Pyrexia.
- Weakness of muscles in the face. Asymmetrical appearance.
- Nuchal pain or rigidity.
- Infections affecting the upper airway, either currently or recently.
- Changes in vision.

Furthermore, there are specific features to look for in the previous medical history, in particular [1]:

- Periods of feeling dizzy or auditory impairment
- Any infective episodes
- Contact with infected individuals
- Otosurgery
- Raised or low blood pressure
- Diabetes mellitus
- Cerebrovascular accident
- Migraine
- Injury (cranial or neck trauma)
- A history of deafness or ear problems in a blood relative

The drug history must also be gathered carefully. In particular, note if any of the following medications have been prescribed [1]:

- Aminoglycoside antibiotics or other drugs with known ototoxicity
- Beta-blockers or other blood pressure agents
- Sedatives, such as benzodiazepines
- Anticonvulsants

The patient should also be questioned about their use of alcohol or any recreational drugs.

35.6.2 Physical Examination

The head and neck need to be meticulously examined, with special attention paid to testing the cranial nerves, doing an ophthalmic examination and performing otoscopy. The nervous system should be examined briefly. Where meningitis is suspected, check for the presence of physical signs indicating meningeal irritation.

Examination of the ears involves the following steps [1]:

- Inspect externally, noting evidence of mastoid inflammation, cellulitis or previous otosurgical interventions.
- Examine the external auditory meatus, checking for otitis externa, ear discharge or vesicles.
- Inspect the ear drum, checking to see if it is perforated, if cholesteatoma, a middle ear effusion or acute middle ear infection is present.

Ophthalmic examination involves the following steps [1]:

- Check for the full range of eye movement and that the pupils respond appropriately.
- Check for papilloedema by means of fundoscopy.
- Check whether nystagmus occurs spontaneously, can be evoked by gaze or change of position.
- As long as the patient is willing to co-operate, carry out a Dix-Hallpike manoeuvre.
- Where vision has altered, refer for an ophthalmic specialist opinion.

When examining the nervous system, the following steps are needed [1]:

- Assess cranial nerves I to XII inclusive.
- Perform the Romberg test to check balance and ask the patient to walk heel-to-toe.
- Test for abnormality of the cerebellum by the finger-nose pointing test and getting patients to run their heel along the opposite shin.

35.6.3 Imaging Studies

35.6.3.1 CT Scanning

If there is a danger that the patient is suffering from meningitis, CT scanning should be contemplated prior to performing a spinal tap. CT imaging is also beneficial in cases of suspected mastoiditis. Studies of the temporal bone have value in managing cases of cholesteatoma and labyrinthitis.

Plain CT is optimal to observe the presence of fibrotic scarring and calcification within the inner ear in cases of persistent inner ear inflammation and labyrinthitis ossificans [1].

35.6.3.2 Magnetic Resonance Imaging (MRI)

MRI is useful to exclude acoustic neuroma, cerebrovascular accident, cerebral abscess, or epidural haematoma as a reason for vertigo and auditory impairment.

In cases of acute or subacute labyrinthitis, T1-weighted MRI studies show enhancement of the cochlea, vestibule and semicircular canals [17], an appearance with a high specificity for labyrinthitis. The appearances also have a correlation with other evaluations of the patient, both objective and subjective. It is probable that recent advances in MRI technology have now made a T1 enhanced study the preferred investigation where a clinical suspicion of labyrinthitis exists [18]. Use of a gadolinium-based contrast agent helps to differentiate a neoplasm occurring within the cochlea from other labyrinthine lesions, e.g. labyrinthitis [19].

35.6.3.3 Audiological Test

In every case of potential labyrinthitis, audiography should be undertaken. In cases where illness is critical or the degree of vertigo very severe, wait until the patient's condition is stable and testing will not be distressing. Different causes of inner ear inflammation can produce different features on the audiogram. Thus, labyrinthitis secondary to middle ear infection typically results in auditory impairment of mixed type, whilst labyrinthitis secondary to viral infection is more likely to produce a sensorineural auditory deficit. In a patient whose level of co-operation is insufficient for routine audiography, it may be better to measure otoacoustic emissions or the auditory brainstem response [1].

Viral labyrinthitis typically produces a pattern of hearing loss of at most moderate severity and mainly the higher pitches in the diseased ear. This is not always the case, and losses may affect any range of frequencies.

Bacterial labyrinthitis of suppurative type produces auditory impairment that may be profound or slightly less so in the affected ear. If labyrinthitis follows meningitis, both sides may well be affected. Serous labyrinthitis secondary to bacterial infections results in auditory impairment, with loss of the higher frequencies and is unilateral. Where an effusion develops, there may also be conductive deafness [1].

35.6.3.4 Vestibular Testing

In unclear presentations to narrow down the diagnosis or to inform the predicted degree of recovery, vestibular caloric testing or electronystagmography are of potential benefit. There is evidence to support the contention that detailed study of the vestibulo-ocular reflex may reveal the cause in cases of labyrinthitis.

Cases of viral labyrinthitis lead to nystagmus accompanied by unilateral caloric vestibular paresis/hypofunction.

Cases of suppurative (bacterial) labyrinthitis lead to nystagmus but no caloric response on the affected side.

Electronystagmography is generally normal in cases of serous labyrinthitis secondary to bacterial infection, although the caloric response may be attenuated on the diseased side. Nonetheless, caution must be exercised in interpreting a decreased caloric response, since this may also occur if there is an effusion in the middle ear [1].

35.7 Treatment

35.7.1 Viral Labyrinthitis

Patients with viral labyrinthitis should be treated at first supportively, encouraging them to rest in bed and take adequate fluids. The majority of cases do not require hospitalisation. It is important to advise such patients of the need to consult a physician if there is any deterioration, in particular signs of nervous system involvement such as double vision, dysarthria, difficulty walking and muscular weakness or absent sensation in particular areas. If patients are profoundly nauseous or vomit a great deal, there may be a need to supply fluids intravenously and supply an anti-emetic drug.

35.7.2 Bacterial Labyrinthitis

The choice of a suitable antibiotic in cases of bacterial labyrinthitis depends on microbial culture and susceptibility testing. Suppurative inner ear infections are treated by eradication of the pathogen, supporting the patient, ensuring drainage from the middle ear or mastoid, and containing further extension of the infection.

35.7.3 Surgical Care

Labyrinthitis secondary to middle ear infection is treated by myringotomy and aspiration of the effusion. It may be necessary to site a tube to ventilate the ear. Aspirated fluid is sent for microscopy, microbial culture and susceptibility testing.

The optimal surgical management of mastoid infection and cholesteatoma involves draining the lesion and carrying out a mastoidectomy.

References

1. Boston ME. Labyrinthitis. In: Egan RA (Ed). Medscape. Updated: Sep 02, 2020. https://emedicine.medscape.com/article/856215-overview (Accessed online at October 15, 2020).
2. Jang CH, Park SY, Wang PC. A case of tympanogenic labyrinthitis complicated by acute otitis media. Yonsei Med J. 2005;46(1):161–5.
3. Schuknecht HF, Kitamura K II, Louis H. Clerf Lecture. Vestibular neuritis. Ann Otol Rhinol Laryngol Suppl. 1981;90(1 Pt 2):1–19.
4. Schraff SA, Schleiss MR, Brown DK, Meinzen-Derr J, Choi KY, Greinwald JH, et al. Macrophage inflammatory proteins in cytomegalovirus-related inner ear injury. Otolaryngol Head Neck Surg. 2007;137(4):612–8.
5. Kuhweide R, Van de Steene V, Vlaminck S, Casselman JW. Ramsay hunt syndrome: pathophysiology of cochleovestibular symptoms. J Laryngol Otol. 2002;116(10):844–8.
6. Hato N, Kisaki H, Honda N, Gyo K, Murakami S, Yanagihara N. Ramsay hunt syndrome in children. Ann Neurol. 2000;48(2):254–6.

7. Wu JF, Jin Z, Yang JM, Liu YH, Duan ML. Extracranial and intracranial complications of otitis media: 22-year clinical experience and analysis. Acta Otolaryngol. 2012;132(3):261–5.
8. Wu JF, Jin Z, Yang JM, Liu YH, Duan ML. Extracranial and intracranial complications of otitis media: 22-year clinical experience and analysis. Acta Otolaryngol. 2012;132(3):261–5.
9. Nadol JB Jr. Hearing loss as a sequela of meningitis. Laryngoscope. 1978;88(5):739–55.
10. Gulya AJ. Infections of the labyrinth. In: Bailey BJ, Johnson JT, Pillsbury HC, Tardy ME, Kohut RI, editors. Head and neck surgery-otolaryngology, vol. 2. Philadelphia, Pa: JB Lippincott; 1993. p. 1769–81.
11. Berlow SJ, Caldarelli DD, Matz GJ, Meyer DH, Harsch GG. Bacterial meningitis and sensorineural hearing loss: a prospective investigation. Laryngoscope. 1980 Sep.;90(9):1445–52.
12. Harris JP, Ryan AF. Fundamental immune mechanisms of the brain and inner ear. Otolaryngol Head Neck Surg. 1995;112(6):639–53.
13. Broughton SS, Meyerhoff WE, Cohen SB. Immune-mediated inner ear disease: 10-year experience. Semin Arthritis Rheum. 2004;34(2):544–8.
14. Woolley AL, Kirk KA, Neumann AM Jr, McWilliams SM, Murray J, Freind D. Risk factors for hearing loss from meningitis in children: the Children's hospital experience. Arch Otolaryngol Head Neck Surg. 1999;125(5):509–14.
15. Bohr V, Paulson OB, Rasmussen N. Pneumococcal meningitis. Late neurologic sequelae and features of prognostic impact. Arch Neurol. 1984;41(10):1045–9.
16. Kutz JW, Simon LM, Chennupati SK, Giannoni CM, Manolidis S. Clinical predictors for hearing loss in children with bacterial meningitis. Arch Otolaryngol Head Neck Surg. 2006;132(9):941–5.
17. Mark AS, Seltzer S, Nelson-Drake J, Chapman JC, Fitzgerald DC, Gulya AJ. Labyrinthine enhancement on gadolinium-enhanced magnetic resonance imaging in sudden deafness and vertigo: correlation with audiologic and electronystagmographic studies. Ann Otol Rhinol Laryngol. 1992;101(6):459–64.
18. Kopelovich JC, Germiller JA, Laury AM, Shah SS, Pollock AN. Early prediction of postmeningitic hearing loss in children using magnetic resonance imaging. Arch Otolaryngol Head Neck Surg. 2011;137(5):441–7.
19. Peng R, Chow D, De Seta D, Lalwani AK. Intensity of gadolinium enhancement on MRI is useful in differentiation of intracochlear inflammation from tumor. Otol Neurotol. 2014;35(5):905–10.

Common Cold in Children

36

Nihat Susaman, Nuray Bayar Muluk, and Suela Sallavaci

36.1 Introduction

Upper respiratory tract infection (URI) represents the most common acute illness evaluated in the outpatient setting. URIs range from the common cold—typically a mild, self-limited, catarrhal syndrome of the nasopharynx—to life-threatening illnesses such as epiglottitis [1].

The common cold is the most frequent human illness. An estimated 25 million individuals seek medical care for uncomplicated upper respiratory tract infections (URI) annually in the United States [2, 3]. Infants and children are affected more often and experience more prolonged symptoms than adults. The common cold accounts for approximately 22 million missed days of school and 20 million absences from work, including parents' time away from work while caring for ill children [3, 4].

36.2 Definition

The common cold (nasopharyngitis or the rhinopharyngitis): Inflammation of the nares, pharynx, hypopharynx, uvula, and tonsils [1].

The common cold is an acute, self-limiting viral infection of the upper respiratory tract, involving, to variable degrees, sneezing, nasal congestion and discharge

N. Susaman (✉)
Section of Otorhinolaryngology, Elazığ Fethi Sekin City Hospital, Elazığ, Turkey

N. Bayar Muluk
Department of Otorhinolaryngology, Faculty of Medicine, Kırıkkale University, Kırıkkale, Turkey

S. Sallavaci
Department of Otorhinolaryngology, University Hospital Centre "Mother Teresa", Tirana, Albania

(rhinorrhoea), sore throat, cough, low grade fever, headache, and malaise. It can be caused by members of several families of viruses; the most common are the more than 100 serotypes of rhinoviruses [5].

36.3   Pathogenesis

URIs involve direct invasion of the mucosa lining the upper airway. Inoculation of bacteria or viruses occurs when a person's hand comes in contact with pathogens and the person then touches the nose or mouth or when a person directly inhales respiratory droplets from an infected person who is coughing or sneezing [1].

After inoculation, viruses and bacteria encounter several barriers, including physical, mechanical, humoral, and cellular immune defences. Physical and mechanical barriers include the following [1]:

- Hair lining the nose filters and traps some pathogens.
- Mucus coats much of the upper respiratory tract, trapping potential invaders.
- The angle resulting from the junction of the posterior nose to the pharynx causes large particles to impinge on the back of the throat.
- Ciliated cells lower in the respiratory tract trap and transport pathogens up to the pharynx; from there they are swallowed into the stomach.

Viruses that cause colds are spread by three mechanisms [6]:

- Hand contact: Self-inoculation of one's own conjunctivae or nasal mucosa after touching a person or object contaminated with cold virus.
- Inhalation of small particle droplets that become airborne from coughing (droplet transmission).
- Deposition of large particle droplets that are expelled during sneezing and land on nasal or conjunctival mucosa (typically requires close contact with an infected person).

36.4   Aetiology

Viral agents occurring in URIs include a vast number of serotypes, which undergo frequent changes in antigenicity, posing challenges to immune defence. Pathogens resist destruction by a variety of mechanisms, including the production of toxins, proteases, and bacterial adherence factors, as well as the formation of capsules that resist phagocytosis [1].

"Common cold" and "flu" are syndromes of familiar symptoms caused by viral infection of the upper respiratory tract. It is difficult to define the syndromes exactly because of great variation in the severity, duration, and types of symptoms. Rhinoviruses account for 30–50% of all colds, and coronaviruses are the second most common agent, accounting for 10–15% of colds [3]. Influenza viruses account for 5–15% of colds, and cold viruses such as respiratory syncytial virus are responsible for much flu-like illness [7], demonstrating that there is much overlap in aetiology and symptomatology of common cold and flu syndromes [8].

Of the more than 200 viruses known to cause the symptoms of the common cold, the principal ones are as follows [1]:

- Rhinoviruses: These cause approximately 30-50% of colds in adults; they grow optimally at temperatures near 32.8 °C (91 °F), which is the temperature inside the human nares.
- Coronaviruses: While they are a significant cause of colds, exact case numbers are difficult to determine because, unlike rhinoviruses, coronaviruses are difficult to culture in the laboratory.
- Enteroviruses, including coxsackieviruses, echoviruses, and others.
- Other viruses that account for many URIs include the following:
- Adenoviruses.
- Orthomyxo viruses (including influenza A and B viruses).
- Paramyxo viruses (e.g. parainfluenza virus [PIV]).
- RSV.
- EBV.
- Human metapneumovirus (hMPV).
- Bocavirus: Commonly associated with nasopharyngeal symptoms in children [9].

The incubation period (time between contact with infectious material until the onset of symptoms) for most common cold viruses is 24 to 72 hours [5].

36.5 Epidemiology

The incidence of the common cold varies by age. Rates are highest in children younger than 5 years. Children who attend school or day care are a large reservoir for URIs, and they transfer infection to the adults who care for them. In the first year after starting at a new school or day care, children experience more infections, as do their family members. Children have about 3-8 viral respiratory illnesses per year, adolescents and adults have approximately 2-4 colds annually, and people older than 60 years have fewer than 1 cold per year [1].

Cold weather results in more time spent indoors (e.g. at work, home, school) and close exposure to others who may be infected. Humidity may also affect the prevalence of colds, because most viral URI agents thrive in the low humidity that is characteristic of winter months. Low indoor air moisture may increase friability of the nasal mucosa, increasing a person's susceptibility to infection [1].

36.6 Symptoms

Most symptoms of URIs—including local swelling, erythema, oedema, secretions, and fever—result from the inflammatory response of the immune system to invading pathogens and from toxins produced by pathogens [1].

An initial nasopharyngeal infection may spread to adjacent structures, resulting in the following [1]:

- Sinusitis
- Otitis media
- Epiglottitis
- Laryngitis
- Tracheobronchitis
- Pneumonia

The symptoms of the common cold generally appear in a well-recognised order, usually starting with a sore throat which then progresses to nasal discharge or blockage, headache, fever, body aches and pains. This is sometimes followed by a cough, which can be persistent, and sinus problems can also be present. Influenza is a more serious illness with a rapid onset of fever, shivering, headache, sweating, body aches and generalised malaise, and effective management depends on early recognition in the community and rapid diagnosis [10, 11].

In infants, fever and nasal discharge are common manifestations. Additional manifestations may include fussiness, difficulty feeding, decreased appetite, and difficulty sleeping [5].

In school-aged children, nasal congestion, nasal discharge and cough are the predominant symptoms. In a prospective study of 81 colds in school-aged children (5 to 12 years), parents recorded signs and symptoms during the first 10 days of illness [12]. Signs and symptoms included cough, sneeze, feverish (defined as ill-appearing, flushed, warm to touch), congestion, nasal discharge, and headache; sore throat and hoarseness were not evaluated. Rhinovirus RNA was detected in 46 percent of episodes [5].

Approximately three-quarters of children remained symptomatic on day 10 of illness [5]:

- *Fever*: Fever may be the predominant manifestation of the common cold during the early phase of infection in young children.
- *Nasal symptoms*: Nasal congestion, nasal discharge, and sneezing are usually present.
- *Cough*: Cough occurs in more than two-thirds of children with the common cold and may be the most bothersome symptom for the child's caregivers [12, 13]. Cough may affect the child's sleep, school performance, and ability to play; it also may disturb the sleep of other family members and be disruptive in the classroom [14]. The cough may linger for an additional week or two after other symptoms have resolved, but should gradually improve [5].

- *Sore throat*: A scratchy sensation of throat irritation is often the first symptom of an URTI. This symptom may be related to early viral infection of the nasopharynx rather than the nasal epithelium [15]. The sensation of throat irritation may be caused by the formation of bradykinin in the airway in response to infection, since intranasal administration of bradykinin causes symptoms of rhinitis and a sore throat [16, 17].

- *Rhinorrhoea*: The nasal discharge associated with URTIs is a complex mix of elements derived from glands, goblet cells, plasma cells, and plasma exudates from capillaries, with the relative contributions from these different sources varying with the time course of the infection and the severity of the inflammatory response [18]. A watery nasal secretion is an early URTI symptom and is often accompanied by sneezing. This early phase of nasal secretion is a reflex glandular secretion that is caused by stimulation of trigeminal nerves in the airway, similar to sneezing [8].

- *Nasal congestion*: Nasal congestion is a later symptom of URTIs that increases in severity over the first week of symptoms [19]. Nasal congestion is caused by the dilation of large veins in the nasal epithelium (venous sinuses) in response to the generation of vasodilator mediators of inflammation such as bradykinin [8, 20, 21].

- *Sinus pain*: The paranasal sinuses surround the nasal airway and any infection of the airway usually involves the sinuses, causing inflammation and the accumulation of secretions in the sinuses [22]. The origin of sinus pain may be related to several factors—e.g. pressure changes in the sinus air space and pressure changes in the blood vessels draining the sinus [23]. The ostia of the paranasal sinuses are often occluded because the nasal epithelium becomes inflamed and congested with an URTI; this may result in gas absorption from the sinus and "vacuum maxillary sinusitis" [24]. However, sinuses with patent ostia may also be painful, indicating that the generation of inflammatory mediators within the sinus may be sufficient to trigger the sensation of pain either by direct stimulation of pain nerve fibres or via distension of blood vessels that are also served by sensory nerves [8, 23].

- *Watery eyes*: Watery eyes (epiphora) is a common symptom associated with allergic and infectious rhinitis [25, 26]. In children aged 7 years, 70% of cases of epiphora are related to allergic disease or URTIs [27]. The nasolacrimal duct may be obstructed at its opening into the nose by inflammation and congestion of blood vessels in the nasal epithelium around the opening of the duct, causing an accumulation of tears and the symptom of watery eyes. The nasolacrimal duct has been shown to have a vascular plexus of veins (cavernous tissue) similar to the venous sinuses of the nasal epithelium, and congestion of this plexus causes obstruction of the duct [8, 28].

- *Muscle aches and pains*: Muscle aches and pains (myalgia) are a common symptom of URTIs, with around 50% of patients with common cold experiencing these symptoms [29]. Myalgia is a symptom of the acute phase response to infection and there is evidence that the symptom is caused by the effects of cytokines on skeletal muscle [30]. Proinflammatory cytokines have been implicated as inducing the breakdown of muscle proteins, and tumour necrosis factor was initially referred to as cachetin because of its role in causing muscle wasting or cachexia [8, 31].

- Other symptoms and signs of the common cold may include sore hoarseness, headache, irritability, difficulty sleeping, decreased appetite, anterior cervical adenopathy, and conjunctival injection. Vomiting and diarrhoea are uncommon [3, 6, 12].

36.7 Diagnosis

Common cold has no specific diagnostic laboratory test. Nasal eosinophilia may be used to exclude allergic rhinitis while polymorphonuclear (PMN) predominance indicate noncomplicated common cold rather than bacterial infection. The identification of the pathogens responsible for common cold can be made by culture tests, antigen tests and serology. The patients' eligibility for antiviral therapy should first be evaluated by these tests. Bacterial cultures should be performed when group A Streptococcus, Bordetella pertussis or nasal diphtheria are suspected. Other pathogens identified from nasal mucosa does not indicate that they are the responsible microorganisms [32, 33].

36.8 Treatment

Supportive therapy is the only recommended treatment of the common cold since the main reason for common cold are viruses [33].

Nasal and sinus symptoms are most often treated with sympathomimetic agents, which act by direct and/or indirect stimulation of α- and β-adrenergic receptors, resulting in the contraction of swollen nasal and sinus blood vessels and leading to a reduction in both congestion and mucus outflow. Local or systemic agents are available and probably the most characterised oral agent in terms of clinical evidence is pseudoephedrine. Pain and fever can be controlled by simple analgesics, such as paracetamol, aspirin and ibuprofen. However, the inflammatory nature of rhinovirus infection, coupled with the generalised and sometimes severe body aching seen in influenza, suggests that, in terms of efficacy and safety, ibuprofen would be one of the agents of choice, particularly in influenza [11].

Using the aforementioned arguments, a logical and powerful combination for treatment would be ibuprofen and pseudoephedrine, which has been shown to be effective in the relief of the symptoms of heavy colds and flu [34, 35] with combinations being more effective than either agent alone [34]. This combination should of course be given in sufficient dosage to significantly reduce symptoms and ideally be presented as a slow-release (SR) combination, which would require only twice-daily dosing to provide continuous symptom relief and aid patient compliance [11].

Supportive treatment is the main treatment method in common cold. Antihistamines, decongestants, antitussives, and expectorants, singly and in combinations, are all marketed for symptomatic relief in children. However, there have been few clinical trials of these products in infants and children and none that demonstrate benefit for treatment of the symptoms of the common cold [36]. In addition, for children younger than 2 years of age, prescription and over-the-counter cough and cold medications have been associated with fatal overdose. Common cold and cough medications are among the first twenty chemicals that cause death below age 5 [32, 37].

36.8.1 Antiviral Treatment

There is no specific antiviral treatment for rhinovirus infections. Ribavirin can be used in RSV infections but it is not recommended in treatment of the common cold. Oseltamivir and Zanamivir which are neuro-aminidase inhibitors are known to have mild effect on influenza virus infection. Oseltamivir can prevent otitis media during the course of influenza virus infection. Drug is most effective when used in first 48 hours of the disease so the differential diagnosis must be made very carefully [32].

36.8.2 Symptomatic Therapy

Symptomatic therapy may include antipyretics, saline nasal irrigation, adequate hydration, and use of a humidifier. In children with reactive airway disease or asthma beta-agonist medications should be used to relieve associated bronchospasm [32].

- Antipyretics: Acetaminophen or ibuprofen may be used to alleviate fever during the first few days [32].
- Antihistamines: The anticholinergic effects of the first-generation antihistamines may help reduce the secretions associated with the common cold. However, in controlled trials, antihistamines have been ineffective in relieving the symptoms of children with URI, weather administered in combination with decongestants or as monotherapy [32, 38–40].
- Decongestants: Decongestants are sympathomimetic medications that cause vasoconstriction of the nasal mucosa. They are available in oral and topical formulations. Commonly used decongestants include pseudoephedrine hydrochloride, and phenylephrine hydrochloride, and oxymetazoline. In adults, such medications have been shown to decrease nasal congestion and increase patency, but there are no studies demonstrating the effectiveness of these medications in children. Side effects of decongestants may include tachycardia, elevated diastolic blood pressure, palpitations [32, 41].

References

1. Meneghetti A. Upper Respiratory Tract Infection. In: Mosenifar Z (Ed.). Medscape. Updated: Feb 17, 2017. http://emedicine.medscape.com/article/302460-overview#a2 (Accessed online at August 10, 2020).
2. Gonzales R, Malone DC, Maselli JH, Sande MA. Excessive antibiotic use for acute respiratory infections in the United States. Clin Infect Dis. 2001;33:757.
3. Heikkinen T, Järvinen A. The common cold. Lancet. 2003;361:51–9.
4. Bramley TJ, Lerner D, Sames M. Productivity losses related to the common cold. J Occup Environ Med. 2002;44:822.
5. Pappas DE. The common cold in children: Clinical features and diagnosis. In: Edwards MS, Torchia MM (Eds.). UpToDate. Last updated: Sep 25, 2015. https://www.uptodate.com/contents/the-common-cold-in-children-clinical-features-and-diagnosis?source=search_result&search=Nasopharyngitis&selectedTitle=1~150 (Accessed online at August 10, 2020).
6. Pappas DE, Hendley JO. The common cold and decongestant therapy. Pediatr Rev. 2011;32:47.
7. Zambon MC, Stockton JD, Clewley JP, Fleming DM. Contribution of influenza and respiratory syncytial virus to community cases of influenza-like illness: an observational study. Lancet. 2001;358:1410–6.
8. Eccles R. Understanding the symptoms of the common cold and influenza. Lancet Infect Dis. 2005;5:718–25.
9. Meriluoto M, Hedman L, Tanner L, Simell V, Mäkinen M, Simell S, et al. Association of human bocavirus 1 infection with respiratory disease in childhood follow-up study. Finland Emerg Infect Dis. 2012;18(2):264–71.
10. Fleming D, Wood M. The clinical diagnosis of influenza. Curr Med Res Opin. 2003;18:338–41.
11. Stillings M, Little S, Sykes J. Common cold and influenza symptom management: the use of pharmacokineticconsiderations to predict the efficacy of a twice-daily treatment for colds and flu. Curr Med Res Opin. 2003;19(8):791–9.
12. Pappas DE, Hendley JO, Hayden FG, Winther B. Symptom profile of common colds in school-aged children. Pediatr Infect Dis J. 2008;27:8.
13. Kelly LF. Pediatric cough and cold preparations. Pediatr Rev. 2004;25:115.
14. Shields MD, Bush A, Everard ML, et al. BTS guidelines: Recommendations for the assessment and management of cough in children. Thorax. 2008;63(Suppl 3):iii1.
15. Winther B, Gwaltney JM, Mygind N, Turner RB, Hendley O. Sites of rhinovirus recovery after point innoculation of the upper airway. JAMA. 1986;256:1763–7.
16. Rees GL, Eccles R. Sore throat following nasal and oropharyngeal bradykinin challenge. Acta Otolaryngol. 1994;114:361–14.
17. Proud D, Reynolds CJ, Lacapra S, Kagey-Sobotka A, Lichenstein LM, Naclerio RM. Nasal provocation with bradykinin induces symptoms of rhinitis and a sore throat. Am Rev Respir Dis. 1988;173:613–6.
18. Eccles R. Physiology of nasal secretion. Eur J Respir Dis. 1983;62:115–9.
19. Jackson G, Dowling H, Spiesman I, Boand A. Transmission of the common cold to volunteers under controlled conditions. 1 the common cold as a clinical entity. Arch Intern Med. 1958;101:267–78.
20. Widdicombe J. Microvascular anatomy of the nose. Allergy. 1997;52:7–11.
21. Eccles R. Anatomy and physiology of the nose and control of nasal airflow. In: Adkinson N, Bochner B, Yunginger J, Holgate S, Busse W, Simons F, editors. Middleton's allergy, principles and practice. 6th ed. Philadelphia, PA: Mosby; 2003. p. 775–87.
22. Gwaltney JM, Phillips CD, Miller RD, Riker DK. Computed tomographic study of the common cold. N Engl J Med. 1994;330:25–30.
23. Falck B, Svanholm H, Aust R, Backlund L. The relationship between body posture and pressure in occluded maxillary sinus of man. Rhinology. 1989;27:161–7.
24. Whittet HB. Infraorbital nerve dehiscence: the anatomic cause of maxillary sinus "vacuum headache"? Otolaryngol Head Neck Surg. 1992;107:21–8.

25. Kubba H, Robson AK, Bearn MA. Epiphora: the role of rhinitis. Am J Rhinol. 1998;12:273–4.
26. Annamalai S, Kumar NA, Madkour MB, Sivakumar S, Kubba H. An association between acquired epiphora and the signs and symptoms of chronic rhinosinusitis: a prospective case-control study. Am J Rhinol. 2003;17:111–4.
27. Maini R, Mac Ewen CJ, Young JD. The natural history of epiphora in childhood. Eye. 1998;12:669–71.
28. Kilbourne E. Influenza in man. In: Influenza. New York: Plenum Medical Book Company; 1987. p. 157–218.
29. Eccles R, Loose I, Jawad M, Nyman L. Effects of acetylsalicylic acid on sore throat pain and other pain symptoms associated with acute upper respiratory tract infection. Pain Med. 2003;4:118–24.
30. Baracos V, Rodemann HP, Dinarello CA, Goldberg AL. Stimulation of muscle protein degradation and prostaglandin E2 release by leukocytic pyrogen (interleukin-1). A mechanism for the increased degradation of muscle proteins during fever. N Engl J Med. 1983;308:553–8.
31. Smith MB, Feldman W. Over-the-counter cold medications. A critical review of clinical trials between 1950 and 1991. JAMA. 1993;269:2258–63.
32. Atan Şahin ÖN, Gülen F. The approach to common cold in children. J Pediatr Res. 2015;2(1):1–6.
33. Arroll B, Kenealy T. Antibiotics for the common cold and acute purulant rhinitis. Cochrane Database Syst Rev. 2005;3:cd001107.
34. Sperber SJ, Sorrentino JV, Riker DK, Hayden FG. Evaluation of an alpha agonist alone and in combination with a non-steroidal anti-inflammatory agent in the treatment of experimental rhinovirus colds. Bull NY Acad Med. 1989;65:145–60.
35. Oliver SD, Rees TP, Daniel RJE. The pharmacokinetics and clinical activity of a soluble combination of ibuprofen and pseudoephedrine. Eur J Clin Res. 1996;8:269–80.
36. Bronstein AC, Spyker DA, Cantilena LR Jr, Green JL, Rumack BH, Giffin SL. 2009 annual report of the American Association of Poison Control Centers' National Poison Data System (NPDS): 27th annual report. Clin Toxicol. 2010;48:979–1178.
37. Hutton N, Wilson MH, Mellits ED, Baumgardner R, Wissow LS, Bonuccelli C, Holtzman NA, DeAngelis C. Effectiveness of an antihistamine-decongestant combination for young children with the common cold: a randomised, controlled clinical trial. J Pediatr. 1991;118:125–30.
38. Clemens CJ, Taylor JA, Almquist JR, Quinn HC, Mehta A, Naylor GS. Is an antihistamine-decongestant combination effective in temporarily relieving symptoms of the common cold in preschool children? J Pediatr. 1997;130:463–6.
39. Isbister GK, Prior F, Kilham HA. Restricting cough and cold medicines ic children. J Paediatr Child Health. 2012;48:91–8.
40. Morales-Carpi C, Torres-Chazarra C, Lurbe E, Torro I, Morales Olivas FJ. Cold medication containing oral phenylephrine as a cause of hypertension in children. Eur J Pediatr. 2008;167:947–8.
41. Kotler DP. Cachexia. Ann Intern Med. 2000;133:622–34.

Rhinitis in Children

Nagehan Küçükcan, Naif Yaseen Albar, and Cemal Cingi

37.1 Introduction

Rhinitis is a frequently occurring condition in which the mucosal lining of the nose becomes irritated and inflamed. The cardinal symptom is a blocked nose, although patients may often be more troubled by other symptoms, such as rhinorrhoea, frequent sternutation or nasal pruritus. The usual reasons for the nose to become inflamed are a viral infection or an atopic reaction to aeroallergens. Exposure to irritant substances may produce a similar symptomatic response, but there may be no evidence of mucosal inflammation. Rhinitis secondary to a viral infection has a maximum duration of 10 days and occurs within a coryzal illness. In cases of rhinitis that have a brief duration (between 7 and 10 days), it may be difficult to ascribe an aetiology, particularly in the absence of markers of infection such as pyrexia or malaise. On the other hand, where rhinitis is chronic, it is essential to distinguish between the various possible aetiologies, which include an infection, allergy, rhinitis of non-allergic and non-infectious types and persistent rhinosinusitis [1].

Nasal pruritus and eye symptoms are particularly frequent in allergic rhinitis, whilst the other symptoms of rhinitis, such as a blocked nose, nasal discharge or sternutation do not occur more frequently in any particular type of rhinitis. The symptoms of rhinitis, regardless of aetiology, may often flare up if the patient is

N. Küçükcan (✉)
Section of Otorhinolaryngology, Adana Çukurova State Hospital, Çukurova, Adana, Turkey

N. Y. Albar
Department of Otorhinolaryngology, Head and Neck Surgery, College of Medicine, King Abdulaziz University, Rabigh, Saudi Arabia

C. Cingi
Department of Otorhinolaryngology, Faculty of Medicine, Eskişehir Osmangazi University, Eskişehir, Turkey

© The Author(s), under exclusive license to Springer Nature Switzerland AG 2022
C. Cingi et al. (eds.), *Pediatric ENT Infections*,
https://doi.org/10.1007/978-3-030-80691-0_37

exposed to irritant substances or experiences significant changes in air temperature and moisture content. Indeed, these triggers may be more of an issue than coming into contact with allergenic substances. When this kind of non-allergenic exposure causes symptoms, it is generally termed non-specific nasal hyperreactivity. Allergic rhinitis occurs when an allergen, to which the patient has previously undergone sensitisation, triggers a specific IgE-mediated inflammatory response. Sensitisation to aeroallergens typically occurs in individuals with a genetic predisposition (shown by a positive family history) and to particular known triggers, notably pollen, house dust mite faeces, moulds or animal dander. This pattern helps in diagnosing individuals presenting during a particular season, or whose symptoms are exacerbated in particular environments, where a specific trigger is likely to be found [1].

37.2   Principal Causes of Rhinitis

The key conditions which may produce rhinitis are as follows [2]:

1. **Allergic rhinitis**
   - seasonal
   - year-round
2. **Non-allergic rhinitis**
   - Vasomotor
   - Gustatory
   - Non-allergic rhinitis with eosinophilia syndrome
3. **Mixed rhinitis**
4. **Mechanical ventilation-associated rhinitis**
5. **Occupational rhinitis**
6. **Rhinitis medicamentosa**
   - Intranasal decongestant sprays
   - Cocaine snorted via the nose
7. **Rhinitis occurring as a side effect of particular medications**
   - Oral contraceptives
   - Medications used to treat erectile dysfunction
   - Certain drugs used to control hypertension
   - Aspirin and other NSAIDs (this condition occurs more often in individuals suffering from asthma and/or chronic rhinosinusitis with intranasal polyp formation)
   - Certain antidepressant medications
   - Certain benzodiazepines
8. **Pregnancy**
9. **Atrophic rhinitis**
10. **Systemic diseases**
    - Hypothyroidism
    - Granulomatosis with polyangiitis (Wegener's)
    - Midline granuloma

- Sarcoidosis
- Cystic fibrosis
- Immotile cilia syndromes

37.3 Symptoms of Rhinitis

The symptoms of rhinitis consist of the following [2]:

- Sternutation
- Nasal discharge (via the nostrils or the nasopharynx)
- Feeling stuffy, blocked nose
- Nasal pruritus

Rhinosinusitis refers to a disease process that involves the nasal interior as well as the paranasal sinuses. It may also be referred to as simply sinusitis. There is a degree of symptomatic overlap with rhinitis, although rhinosinusitis also involves symptoms that point towards the involvement of the sinuses. A typical presentation features a blocked nose, drainage (which may be of pus) from the nasal cavity into the nasopharynx, pressure or pain over the face, cephalgia and, occasionally, hyposmia [2].

37.4 Specific Disorders Producing Rhinitis

37.4.1 Allergic Rhinitis

In cases of allergic rhinitis, there is nasal mucosal, ocular, eustachian tube, middle ear, sinusal and pharyngeal inflammation. Nasal inflammation is a central feature, but the involvement of the adjacent structures varies from case to case. Although the inflammatory reaction affecting the mucosa involves release of multiple different immunomodulatory molecules, these pathways all start with the binding of IgE to an antigen of external origin [3, 4].

Allergic disorders, in which an individual develops a hypersensitivity to a particular protein of external origin via the production of specific IgE (sIgE) to that allergen, are in part genetically determined. If an individual with a genetic susceptibility to develop allergy is exposed to particular extrinsic proteins, they will undergo sensitisation and sIgE will begin to be produced. The mast cells, present within the lining mucosae of the nose, bear sIgE located on the outer plasma membrane. If an aeroallergen is subsequently inhaled, sIgE may attach to it, triggering a cascade of immunomodulator release, both immediately and after a delay [4–6].

Histamine, tryptase, chymase, kinins, and heparin are some of the immunomodulators secreted in the immediate phase [5, 6]. Mast cells then rapidly switch on production of further immunomodulators, such as the leukotrienes and prostaglandin D2 [7–9]. The symptoms associated with AR, such as nasal discharge, blocked nose, sternutation, pruritus, erythema, excess lacrimation, ear fullness and postnasal discharge, arise due to the actions of the immune signalling molecules. The mucus-producing glands begin to produce excess mucus following stimulation. The permeability of nasal blood vessels increases, such that there is extravasation of plasma. The vessels dilate, resulting in the nose becoming congested and a sense of pressure. Sternutation and pruritus arise from stimulation of the sensory nerve endings. Since the timescale for all these events is no longer than a few minutes, this response phase is termed "immediate" or "early" [3].

37.4.1.1 Epidemiology

Allergic rhinitis affects some 3% to 19% of the American population annually, which amounts to between 30 and 60 million cases. Allergic rhinitis (AR) has its onset prior to the age of 20 years 80% of the time [10]. Cases of AR have been moderately increasing recently [11]. At present, the frequency of AR in adulthood is between 10 and 30%, whilst in childhood it is 40% of individuals [10]. According to the European Community Respiratory Health Survey, AR affects between 10% and 41% of adults [12]. The cumulative prevalence in males and females living in Scandinavia is 15% and 14%, respectively [3, 13].

Male children are more likely to be affected by AR than girls, but in adulthood the distribution between males and females is equal [3].

AR frequently has its onset in children, adolescents and young adults, although it may begin at any point in life. The mean age for a first episode is between the age of 8 and 11 years. In four out of five cases, AR starts before the twentieth birthday [14]. Estimates place the frequency of AR as a maximum of 4 in 10 children, with a decreasing frequency as age increases [15, 16].

37.4.1.2 Physical Findings

The general findings at physical examination of patients with long-term AR include the presence of "allergic shiners" (discoloured infraorbital skin, which is bluish or greyish) and a transverse skin crease on the nose. This latter arises because nasal pruritus drives the patient to keep rubbing the nose and push its tip upwards, an action known as the "allergic salute" [1].

Otoscopy of the anterior portion of the nasal lining may reveal normal-appearing mucosa, but may also offer diagnostic clues. The classical appearance of the mucosal lining in cases of AR is swollen and pallid. This pallor is not seen if rhinitis is of non-allergic type. If rhinosinusitis secondary to a viral infection occurs, the mucosa is beefy red, as also occurs in cases of rhinitis medicamentosa [1].

AR can be divided into three types: "intermittent", where symptoms only arise when the patient encounters a specific trigger (such as a cat), "seasonal" when the symptomatic presentation only occurs at a specific point in the year and "persistent/perennial" when symptoms are present throughout the year [17, 18]. Around 70% of cases of AR that is seasonal in type also feature allergic conjunctival inflammation. This conjunctivitis produces pruritus, erythema and tearing [1].

37.4.1.3 Diagnostic Tests

Cutaneous Prick Testing

This test works on the principle that a small amount of allergen, obtained in the form of an extract and placed under the skin by pricking the skin with a pointed lancet, provokes a wheal-and-flare cutaneous reaction, indicative of an immediate phase allergic response. There is some variety in precisely how the test is carried out, and it may be described as "scratch", "prick" or "puncture" allergy testing.

The IgE located on the mast cell membrane binds antigenic proteins in the extract. The mast cells then degranulate, releasing histamine and triggering the immediate phase of the allergenic response. This reaction typically occurs within 15–20 minutes of exposure to the extract. Degranulation of histamine produces the wheal-and-flare reaction. The wheal, which forms the central portion of the skin lesion, is a result of oedema, whilst the flare reflects vasodilation of the surrounding skin. Pruritus also results from the action of histamine. There is a broad correlation between the magnitude of the reaction and the extent of sensitisation to the allergen [3].

Total Serum IgE

Total serum IgE measurement indicates the sum of all types of IgE within the circulation, but does not indicate what the IgE will react against. Although a raised serum IgE level is more common in individuals with AR than in healthy individuals, a raised value lacks both sensitivity and specificity in detecting AR. Up to half of those suffering from AR do not have a raised IgE when measured and a fifth of healthy individuals may show a raised serum IgE. Accordingly, use of serum total IgE in the diagnosis of AR is not routine. However, in conjunction with other factors, this test may sometimes be useful [3].

Total Circulating Eosinophils

A raised value for circulating eosinophils, like a raised circulating IgE titre, is consistent with the presence of AR, but again lacks the sensitivity and specificity to be of much value diagnostically, except on particular occasions when used in conjunction with other tests [3].

Nasal Provocation (Allergen Challenge) Testing

The nasal provocation test is basically confined to research settings, seldom being employed for the clinical assessment of potential AR. The patient inhales the suspected aeroallergen or it is placed within his or her nasal cavity. Following this exposure, any symptoms produced can be noted, including nasal discharge. The degree to which the nose becomes congested may also be measured objectively. There are some experts who view the nasal provocation test as the diagnostic gold standard in AR [3, 19].

37.4.1.4   Treatment

Pharmacotherapy
The majority of patients with AR gain benefit from medication. In many cases of intermittent AR, prescription of an antihistamine by mouth and topical decongestant suffices for symptomatic control. If AR is more persistent, topical corticosteroid treatment may be more suitable [20]. Topical intranasal corticosteroids may be employed as an alternative to a regular course of antihistamine and decongestant, or may be used in conjunction. Generally speaking, the choice of a second-generation antihistamine is to be encouraged, as they are less sedating and have a more favourable side effect profile than the first-generation agents, which were formerly used. A number of other medications offer potential benefit, too, notably eye drops containing an antihistamine, intranasal sprays containing antihistamines, topical nasal cromolyn, topical anticholinergics by spray and brief duration systemic steroids. The last option should be reserved for a flare up with a high degree of severity [3].

Immunotherapy
Immunotherapy is an option to contemplate mainly where AR is very severe, other forms of treatment have failed, there is comorbidity or complications occur. It is common to offer immunotherapy alongside conventional pharmacological treatments and eradication of exposure to environmental allergenic triggers. Immunotherapy may be in subcutaneous (SCIT) or sublingual (SLIT) form [3, 21].

37.4.2 Non-allergic Rhinitis

Non-allergic rhinitis (NAR) is an umbrella term for several separate conditions that each produce an inflammatory response in the nose [22, 23]. It is important to differentiate between cases of AR and NAR, since only in the former does IgE play a major role. NAR may be diagnosed on clinical grounds alone or following cutaneous prick testing or radio-allergo-sorbent tests (RAST) [24].

AR and NAR do not differ in the chronicity or severity of the symptoms they may cause. NAR may also strongly resemble AR in terms of the pattern of symptoms, i.e. nasal discharge, sternutation, itching and nasal blockage, although this depends on the underlying cause. Symptoms vary in their time course, from brief duration to virtually always present. The inflammatory processes of both AR and NAR may trigger rhinosinusitis in an individual who is at risk, since they may prevent effective drainage from the sinuses [24].

There are 7 conditions which together make up NAR, namely rhinitis due to infection, vasomotor rhinitis, occupational rhinitis, hormone-related rhinitis, medication-related rhinitis, gustatory rhinitis and non-allergic rhinitis with eosinophilia syndrome (NARES). The correct diagnosis can be established and thus suitable treatment initiated by taking a comprehensive patient history and performing physical examination [24].

37.4.2.1 Rhinitis Due to Infection

Rhinitis of infectious type typically occurs due to an infection affecting the upper respiratory tract. Generally, the pathogen is a virus, with the majority of cases secondary to rhinovirus, coronavirus, adenovirus, parainfluenza virus, respiratory syncytial virus, or enterovirus. A viral episode of this sort typically has spontaneous resolution within a week to ten days. Rhinitis secondary to an infection has a characteristic appearance, ranging from clear to mucopurulent. It is rarely watery. Symptoms of pain or pressure over the face, hyposmia or anosmia and postnasal drip occur, as does coughing. If the pain is chronic and accompanied by swelling, with pus-filled rhinorrhoea and pyrexia, a bacterial infection may have supervened [24].

37.4.2.2 Vasomotor Rhinitis

It is thought that the cause for vasomotor rhinitis is disequilibrium of autonomic nervous control of the blood vessels supplying the nasal interior. This leads to overactivity by the parasympathetic division, such that blood vessels in the nose dilate and oedema accumulates. The patient may complain of nasal discharge, sternutation and a blocked nose. These symptoms may be worsened by exposure to cold inhaled air, powerful smells, stress, or breathing in irritating substances. It has been noted that there is a greater prevalence of anxiety and depression in female patients with vasomotor rhinitis than in healthy female controls [24, 25].

37.4.2.3 Occupational Rhinitis

In cases of occupational rhinitis, symptoms are confined to when the patient is in the place of work. The trigger for this condition is generally an airborne irritant substance that the patient breathes in, such as a metal salt, animal dander, latex rubber, chemicals or wood swarf. It is common for occupational rhinitis to be co-morbid with occupational asthma. Diagnosis of this condition can be made on clinical grounds (history) or following testing (nasal provocation or cutaneous prick testing). Ideally, treatment would consist of avoiding the trigger, but since avoidance is frequently not feasible, it may be necessary to start an intranasal steroid spray and an antihistamine of the second generation [24].

37.4.2.4 Hormone-Related Rhinitis

Rhinitis may become symptomatic at times when there is a degree of endocrine disturbance. The oestrogens exert their effects upon the autonomic nervous system through a variety of different actions, such as making the central parasympathetic centres more active, increasing the levels of acetylcholine and enhancing the action of acetylcholine transferase. If oestrogen levels are raised, the sympathetic system becomes less active due to stimulation of α2-adrenoceptors, which provide negative feedback to the system. Furthermore, oestrogen acts to raise the amount of hyaluronic acid present in the nasal mucosal lining. The endocrine causes for rhinitis which occur with the highest frequency are pregnancy, menstruation, puberty, provision of oestrogen-containing medications and thyroid underactivity, which may or may not have already been diagnosed. Treatment of hormone-related rhinitis aims to control the symptoms and to address any underlying endocrine disorder [24].

37.4.2.5   Medication-Related Rhinitis

There are a number of prescribed and illicit drugs which may provoke rhinitis, such as angiotensin-converting enzyme inhibitors, reserpine, guanethidine, phentolamine, methyldopa, beta-blockers, chlorpromazine, gabapentin, penicillamine, aspirin, non-steroidal anti-inflammatory agents, cocaine consumed by snorting, oestrogen supplements and oral contraceptive drugs [24].

37.4.2.6   Gustatory Rhinitis

This condition occurs when the patient consumes food, especially when it is hot or spicy. Rhinitis comes on an hour or two after eating and is apparent as a large volume of watery nasal discharge. The pathogenetic mechanism is stimulation of the tenth cranial nerve, resulting in dilation of nasal blood vessels [24].

37.4.2.7   Non-allergic Rhinitis with Eosinophilia Syndrome (NARES)

This condition may be the underlying cause in up to 20% of cases of rhinitis. It may also be referred to as eosinophilic rhinitis or perennial intrinsic rhinitis. One theory proposes that NARES is a precursor condition to the Samter triad, which consists of asthma, polyp formation within the nose and sensitivity to aspirin. NARES may also arise due to defective biochemical pathways related to the prostaglandins. Around 1 in 5 nasal smears performed on the general population contains eosinophilia, but not all such smears correspond to actual rhinitis. Nevertheless, eosinophilia is a cardinal feature of NARES, where it is observed in between 10 and 20% of nasal smears undertaken. The typical symptomatic presentation of NARES is a blocked nose, sternutation, nasal discharge, an itching nose and reduced ability to smell [24].

37.4.2.8   Treatment

Therapy for rhinitis should be chosen according to which disorder is responsible. Treatment is easier if the clinician is able to decide on whether a particular case represents AR or NAR first [24]. There are several classes of agents to consider, namely:

Anticholinergics

If a patient presents with nasal discharge alone, ipratropium is the first choice of treatment. However, it is not suitable as monotherapy if other symptoms, such as sternutation, pruritus or a blocked nose are present, as it does not benefit these symptoms. Thus, additional medication will be needed.

Intranasal Steroids

Currently, there is evidence to suggest that these agents work by inducing relaxation of smooth muscle cells, dampening down the degree of responsiveness of the airways and lowering the level of pro-inflammatory messengers, and reducing their effects. Nasal corticosteroids are especially valuable in treating nasal discharge, sternutation, itching and a blocked nose. These agents have value in treating cases of NARES, since they appear to prevent the recruitment of eosinophils and halt the pro-inflammatory cascade.

Antihistamines

These agents offer benefit in reducing the symptoms of nasal discharge, itching and sternutation. Since their action mainly occurs through prevention of histaminergic transmission, they are of greatest benefit in AR. In conditions where histamine does not play a key role, they are not helpful. Blockade of the histamine H1 receptor, which is both competitive and reversible, is common to all antihistamines. However, the second-generation agents, which entered the market later, also block the release of other pro-inflammatory signal molecules secreted by mast cells and basophils.

Sympathomimetic Agents

This class of agents are all based on the imidazoline molecule. They are agonists at the $\alpha2$-adrenoceptor, which causes constriction of blood vessels. When applied topically, they can bring down nasal swelling and reduce congestion.

Prescribing for Children

None of the causes of rhinitis other than AR is common in the paediatric population, but why this should be so is not known. Indeed, the precise incidence is also unclear. Only 2% at most of paediatric cases with eosinophilic infiltration of the nasal cavity are due to NARES. The newer (second generation) antihistamines by mouth help provide symptomatic relief. Whenever feasible, children should not be offered antihistamines of the first generation, as these may produce paradoxical disinhibition. Children with a nasal discharge, sternutation, itching and nasal blockage may benefit from intranasal steroids. Whilst studies with long-term follow-up have not found actual instances of delayed growth resulting from nasal steroids, the FDA still advises clinicians to check growth in children prescribed these agents. Some disorders affecting the sinuses and nose in children are related to laryngopharyngeal reflux. Thus, treatment may need to be for this condition [24–27].

References

1. Kalogjera L. Rhinitis in adults. Acta Med Croatica. 2011;65(2):181–7.
2. Peden D. An overview of rhinitis. In: Corren J, Feldweg AM (Eds.). UpToDate. Last updated: Dec 15, 2016. http://0210818vd.y.https.www.uptodate.com.proxy.kirikkale-elibrary.com/contents/an-overview-of-rhinitis?source=search_result&search=An%20overview%20of%20rhinitis&selectedTitle=1~150. Accessed 4 Sept 2017.
3. Sheikh J. Allergic Rhinitis. In: Kaliner MA (Ed.). Medscape. Updated: Apr 10, 2017. http://emedicine.medscape.com/article/134825-overview#a5. Accessed 4 Sept 2017.
4. Skoner DP. Allergic rhinitis: definition, epidemiology, pathophysiology, detection, and diagnosis. J Allergy Clin Immunol. 2001;108(1 Suppl):S2–8.
5. Walls AF, He S, Buckley MG, McEuen AR. Roles of the mast cell and basophil in asthma. Clin Exp Allergy. 2001;1:68.
6. Haberal I, Corey JP. The role of leukotrienes in nasal allergy. Otolaryngol Head Neck Surg. 2003;129(3):274–9.
7. Iwasaki M, Saito K, Takemura M, Sekikawa K, Fujii H, Yamada Y. TNF-alpha contributes to the development of allergic rhinitis in mice. J Allergy Clin Immunol. 2003;112(1):134–40.

8. Cates EC, Gajewska BU, Goncharova S, Alvarez D, Fattouh R, Coyle AJ. Effect of GM-CSF on immune, inflammatory, and clinical responses to ragweed in a novel mouse model of mucosal sensitization. J Allergy Clin Immunol. 2003;111(5):1076–86.

9. Salib RJ, Kumar S, Wilson SJ, Howarth PH. Nasal mucosal immunoexpression of the mast cell chemoattractants TGF-beta, eotaxin, and stem cell factor and their receptors in allergic rhinitis. J Allergy Clin Immunol. 2004;114(4):799–806.

10. World Allergy Organization (WAO), Pawanker R, Canonica GW, Holgate ST, Lockey RF, Blaiss MS. White book on allergy: update 2013. Milwaukee, WI: World Allergy Organization. p. 2013.

11. Björkstén B, Clayton T, Ellwood P, Stewart A, Strachan D, ISAAC Phase III Study Group. Worldwide time trends for symptoms of rhinitis and conjunctivitis: Phase III of the international study of asthma and allergies in childhood. Pediatr Allergy Immunol. 2008;19(2):110–24.

12. Heinrich J, Richter K, Frye C, Meyer I, Wölke G, Wjst M, et al. European Community respiratory health survey in adults (ECRHS). Pneumologie. 2002 May;56(5):297–303.

13. Nihlen U, Greiff L, Montnemery P, Lofdahl CG, Johannisson A, Persson C. Incidence and remission of self-reported allergic rhinitis symptoms in adults. Allergy. 2006 Nov.;61(11):1299–304.

14. Dykewicz MS, Fineman S, Skoner DP, Nicklas R, Lee R, Blessing-Moore J. Diagnosis and management of rhinitis: Complete guidelines of the joint task force on practice parameters in allergy, asthma and immunology. Ann Allergy Asthma Immunol. 1998;81(5 Pt 2):478–518.

15. U.S. Department of Health and Human Services. Agency for Healthcare Research and Quality. Management of Alllergic and Nonallergic rhinitis. May 2002. AHQR publication 02:E023, Boston, MA. Summary, Evidence Report/Technology Assessment: No 54. http://www.ahrq.gov/clinic/epcsums/rhinsum.htm. Last accessed August 3, 2007.

16. Settipane RA. Demographics and epidemiology of allergic and nonallergic rhinitis. Allergy Asthma Proc. 2001;22(4):185–9.

17. Bousquet J, Van Cauwenberge P, Khaltaev N, et al. Allergic rhinitis and its impact on asthma. J Allergy Clin Immunol. 2001;108:S147.

18. Brozek JL, Bousquet J, Baena-Cagnani CE, et al. Allergic rhinitis and its impact on asthma (ARIA) guidelines: 2010 revision. J Allergy Clin Immunol. 2010;126:466.

19. Gendo K, Larson EB. Evidence-based diagnostic strategies for evaluating suspected allergic rhinitis. Ann Intern Med. 2004;140(4):278–89.

20. Seidman MD, Gurgel RK, Lin SY, Schwartz SR, Baroody FM, et al. Clinical practice guideline: Allergic rhinitis. Otolaryngol Head Neck Surg. 2015;152(1 Suppl):S1–43.

21. Bozek A, Ignasiak B, Filipowska B, Jarzab J. House dust mite sublingual immunotherapy: a double-blind, placebo-controlled study in elderly patients with allergic rhinitis. Clin Exp Allergy. 2013;43(2):242–8.

22. Hellings PW, Klimek L, Cingi C, et al. Non-allergic rhinitis: position paper of the European academy of allergy and clinical immunology. Allergy. 2017;72(11):1657–65.

23. Settipane RA, Kaliner MA. Chapter 14: nonallergic rhinitis. Am J Rhinol Allergy. 2013;27(Suppl 1):S48–51.

24. Ramakrishnan VJ. Pharmacotherapy for Nonallergic Rhinitis. In: Meyers AD (Ed.). Medscape. Updated: Aug 16, 2017. http://emedicine.medscape.com/article/874171-overview#a2 (Accessed online at September 4, 2017).

25. Addolorato G, Ancona C, Capristo E, Graziosetto R, Di Rienzo L, Maurizi M, et al. State and trait anxiety in women affected by allergic and vasomotor rhinitis. J Psychosom Res. 1999;46(3):283–9.

26. Baek JH, Cho E, Kim MA, et al. Response to nonallergenic irritants in children with allergic and nonallergic rhinitis. Allergy Asthma Immunol Res. 2016;8(4):346–52.

27. Berger WE, Schonfeld JE. Nonallergic rhinitis in children. Curr Allergy Asthma Rep. 2007;7(2):112–6.

Acute Rhinosinusitis in Children

38

İsmail Aytaç, Cemal Cingi, and Andrew A. Winkler

38.1 Introduction

General practitioners and ENT specialists are called on to manage sinusitis in children. Despite sinusitis having been recognized as a disorder for hundreds of years, it is only recently that the condition has begun to be better understood in terms of scope, pathogenetic mechanism, appropriate diagnosis, therapy, and complications. Treating pediatric cases of acute sinusitis secondary to a coryzal illness with antibiotics for a brief period is associated with good outcomes. Nonetheless, chronic or recurrent cases of sinusitis present greater difficulties in management and lead to high levels of frustration. Management of chronic sinusitis depends on both eradicating the bacterial pathogens and treating underlying disorders that complicate the condition [1].

Therefore, the therapeutic strategy in pediatric chronic sinusitis is eradication of infection by antibiotic pharmacotherapy together with management of underlying conditions for a period of time adequate to permit symptoms to abate and the sinus to begin to function normally, including mucociliary clearance. This chapter will discuss medical treatment of sinusitis in children [1].

İ. Aytaç (✉)
Department of Otorhinolaryngology, Faculty of Medicine, Gaziantep University, Gaziantep, Turkey

C. Cingi
Department of Otorhinolaryngology, Faculty of Medicine, Eskişehir Osmangazi University, Eskişehir, Turkey

A. A. Winkler
Department of Otolaryngology, University of Colorado School of Medicine, Aurora, CO, USA

38.2 Pathophysiology

It is thought that the osteomeatal complex (OMC) plays a vital role in the development of sinusitis. The OMC is present at the time of birth, although is not fully developed at that point. The complex consists of the uncinate process, ethmoidal infundibulum, hiatus semilunaris, ethmoidal bulla, and frontal recess, and is located in the middle meatus. Blockage of the complex is hypothesized but has not been established as a cause of sinusitis in children. Sivasli et al. found that pneumatization of the middle and superior turbinates were the most common anatomic variation in children with chronic sinus disease, though they did not a correlation between sinusitis and these anatomic variations [2]. Others have found that alteration to the anterior ethmoids limits the ability of the complex to drain, which causes persistent maxillary sinusitis and, sometimes, frontal sinusitis [1].

When sinus mucosa becomes inflamed, there is impairment of the mucociliary drainage of the sinus to the ostia and onwards into the nasopharynx. Such inflammation is a frequent consequence of an upper airway viral infection or an allergic response within the nose. There are, furthermore, a number of further factors that may put patients at risk of chronic rhinosinusitis, in particular allergic rhinitis, abnormal anatomy, gastro-esophageal reflux disorder (GERD), immunodeficiencies, and ciliary dysfunction [1].

Santee et al. conducted a pediatric cohort study prospectively, which demonstrated an association between previous episodes of acute sinusitis and decreased levels of nasopharyngeal microbial flora belonging to particular taxa. The cohort consisted of healthy individuals aged between 49 and 84 months. The levels of *Faecalibacterium prausnitzii* and *Akkermansia* spp. were both below normal, whereas *Moraxella nonliquefaciens* organisms were more abundant than usual. This relative abundance of *M. nonliquefaciens* was also observed in those individuals who had an episode of acute sinusitis during the one-year study duration [3].

38.3 Causes

The etiology of rhinosinusitis may be conveniently classified by the pathogen responsible for disease and any comorbid conditions [1]:

- Bacteria responsible for acute or subacute sinusitis.
  - *Streptococcus pneumoniae*, 20–30% of cases.
  - Non-typeable *Haemophilus influenzae,* 15–20% of cases.
  - *Moraxella catarrhalis*, 15–20% of cases (lower frequency in adults).
  - *Streptococcus pyogenes* (beta-hemolytic), 5% of cases.
- Bacteria responsible for chronic sinusitis.
  - There are no single species that are characteristic.
  - It is common for multiple microbe species to be present.
  - The following pathogens are frequently isolated.
    Alpha-hemolytic Streptococcal species.

Staphylococcus aureus.

Coagulase-negative Staphylococci.

Non-typeable *H. influenzae* occurs with a higher frequency than in acute sinusitis.

Moraxella catarrhalis.

Bacterial anaerobes, such as *Peptostreptococci, Prevotella, Bacteroides,* and *Fusobacterium* spp.

Pseudomonas spp. occur with raised frequency if the patient has already been treated with multiple antibiotics. Their presence may indicate an underlying immunodeficiency.

- Sinusitis following upper respiratory tract infections of viral type (URTI).
    - URTI is the single biggest risk factor for the development of sinusitis.
    - Attending a day-care facility/nursery raises the risk of a URTI by 300%. The main route of transmission is by children touching each other's hands. Careful hand hygiene and smaller groups in nurseries are shown to help to reduce the spread of infection. It may be necessary to keep the pediatric patient away from a nursery for a period to break the cycle of repeated infections.
    - Even though the issue has been addressed in several research studies, no gold standard exists for the appropriate treatment of a URTI of viral origin. Results obtained to date with antiviral medications suggest potential benefit. Since there are numerous viral pathogens that may cause URTI, a sufficiently poly-valent vaccine to cover all cases represents a significant challenge.
- Allergic rhinitis (AR)-associated sinusitis.
    - Apart from a URTI of viral origin, AR is the risk factor for sinusitis with the highest frequency.
    - In children above the age of 9 years, a URTI of viral type is present between 10 and 15% of the time.
    - Eosinophilia leads to raised levels of major basic protein, resulting in mucosal toxicity that impairs mucociliary clearance.
    - The total IgE serological titer is raised in 60% of cases of refractory sinusitis, according to Shapiro et al [4] Cutaneous testing is also strongly positive.
    - If a patient is below the age of 4 years, less reliance can be placed on IgE tests.
    - Treatment should aim to reduce the degree of edema within the mucosa secondary to an allergic response as a way to prevent sinusitis repeatedly becoming symptomatic.
    - Any case exhibiting treatment resistance should prompt allergy tests, especially if the child's family members have clear signs of atopy or where there is evidence of another allergic disorder, such as eczema.
- Sinusitis associated with abnormal anatomy.
    - There are a number of ways in which anomalous anatomical configurations of the intranasal sidewall may lead to a propensity for developing sinusitis.

- Obstruction of the osteomeatal complex may be caused by concha bullosa, a condition in which the middle turbinate is aerated and enlarged.
- Maxillary sinusitis occurs more frequently if Haller cells are seen. These cells are below the orbit. Their presence makes the sinus ostium narrower than usual.
- Septal deviation around the middle turbinate may cause this structure to move laterally and obstruct the osteomeatal complex.
- An agger nasi prominence, hypoplasia of the maxillary sinus or enlargement of the ethmoidal bulla are also risk factors for sinusitis.
- Immunodeficiency.
  - The overall frequency of immunodeficiency is 0.5%.
  - By the time a child reaches the age of 7 years, antibody-mediated immune function is comparable with that of an adult. Chronic sinusitis becomes less common after this, as would be anticipated.
  - Up to one in three patients suffering from treatment-resistant rhinosinusitis are likely to be immunodeficient. This is particularly likely if the patient experiences early recurrence of bacterial infection after cessation of antimicrobial therapy.
  - The frequency of immunodeficiency in the general population exceeds that of cystic fibrosis or ciliary disorders. Common variable immune deficiency occurs with the highest frequency, followed by deficiencies of IgG and then deficiency of specific antibodies.
  - Immunodeficiency can result in symptoms of more marked severity.
  - Most often, immunodeficiencies present through repeated upper airway infections.
  - In any individual where pharmacotherapy fails to resolve symptoms in spite of aggressive treatment regimens, immunodeficiency must be included in the differential diagnosis.
  - The first investigations to undertake are total immunoglobulin titers, titers for IgG, IgE, IgM, and IgA, and assessment of response to anti-pneumococcal vaccination, tetanus toxoid, and anti-diphtherial vaccination.
- Asthma-associated sinusitis.
  - Patients with significant postnasal drainage of mucus may cause irritation of the distal airway, and this may make the symptoms of asthma worse.
  - Four out of five patients who have asthma have comorbid chronic rhinitis and it is known that infections of the upper airway can cause a deterioration of airway function in those patients with airway hyperreactivity.
  - Therapeutic interventions for chronic sinusitis may be beneficial in restoring normal lung function and lessening the reliance on bronchodilator medications.
  - Anfuso et al. [5] carried out a prospective, non-randomized study comparing children with chronic rhinosinusitis alone to those who also had comorbid asthma as well as ten control patients. There were 28 cases of chronic rhinosinusitis in the study, some of which had comorbid asthma. In the group with both disorders, there was more severe inflammation apparent in the mucosal

epithelium of the proximal airways. This finding supports the notion that successfully treatment of chronic asthma in children is enhanced by simultaneous treatment of rhinological disorders.

- Gastro-esophageal reflux disorder (GERD).
  - There is developing recognition of the role of GERD as a cause of asthmatic-type symptoms, persistent coughing, and dysphonia.
  - The apertures of the eustachian tubes or the sinus ostia may become inflamed as a result of the irritant action of refluxed gastric juices.
  - Up to 60% of cases of GERD may present with respiratory symptoms alone.
  - In pediatric patients, insufficient weight gain, chronic disease involving airway hyperreactivity or reflux during infancy are potent risk factors for GERD.
  - It has been suggested that pediatric patients suffering from chronic sinusitis resistant to pharmacotherapy be offered an empirical trial of treatment for GERD, though this has not been widely employed.
- Allergic fungal sinusitis.
  - The growth of a polyp or alterations within the mucosa secondary to allergic fungal sinusitis often affect only one side of the nose.
  - The allergic mucin produced in this condition by the nose and sinuses is said to possess a viscosity resembling that of peanut butter.
  - When examined under the microscope, there are numerous eosinophils and Charcot-Leyden crystals.
  - The fungal pathogens responsible for the majority of cases belong to the genus *Aspergillus*.
  - The condition may be treated operatively.
  - There is proven benefit from adjunctive immunotherapy. There is evidence from trials over a 3-year period that patients with allergic fungal sinusitis who underwent surgery and received immunotherapy had no further episodes of the disorder [6]. These trials did, however, suffer from certain limitations.
- Biofilms.
  - In one study, biofilms were present in 14 out of 18 specimens of mucosa taken during surgery on patients with chronic sinusitis but were also present in 2 out of 5 healthy controls [7].
  - Further research is required to delineate what part biofilms play in the disorder and the implications for treatment.

38.4 Signs and Symptoms of Acute Sinusitis

The most frequent presentation of acute sinusitis features a cough during the waking hours and nasal discharge. There are a number of further signs or symptoms seen in the condition, namely [1]:

- Nasal obstruction.
- A mild fever, that occurs infrequently.

- Middle ear infection is present in between 50 and 60% of cases.
- Irritability.
- Headache.

Some indicators of an infection of greater severity are [1]:

- Discharge of pus from the nose.
- High fever (a temperature exceeding 39 °C).
- Soft tissue swelling around the orbits.

38.5 Diagnosis

38.5.1 History

Infection may occur due to a number of conditions that result in the sinus becoming less well ventilated, including blockage of the sinus ostia, or a reduction in immune defense, either localized to the sinus or systemically. Unless these underlying conditions are treated, eradication of the infection becomes extremely challenging. When obtaining the history from the patient, certain signs and symptoms are indicative of specific types of sinusitis [1].

- Acute sinusitis.
  - This condition typically resolves symptomatically in less than 30 days.
  - If an upper airway infective episode has a duration exceeding 7–10 days, it is likely that acute sinusitis is also present.
  - Coughing during the waking hours and a nasal discharge are the most frequent features noted.
  - There are also a number of other ways the acute sinusitis may present, such as:
      Nasal obstruction.
      A mild fever that occurs infrequently.
      Middle ear infection in 50–60% of cases.
      Irritability.
      Headache.
  - Some indicators of an infection of greater severity are [1]:
      Purulent discharge from the nose.
      High fever (a temperature exceeding 39 °C).
      Soft tissue swelling around the orbits.
  - Provided there are no complications, 40% of cases recover without requiring any intervention.
- Recurrent acute sinusitis.

- – The clinical definition calls for bouts of acute sinusitis with a duration not exceeding 30 days, with intervening disease-free (symptom-free) periods with a duration of no less than 10 days.
- Subacute sinusitis.
  - – By definition, subacute sinusitis exists if the period for which signs and symptoms of acute sinusitis persist is between 30 and 90 days.
- Chronic sinusitis.
  - – In chronic sinusitis, signs or symptoms are present, but not prominent, for a period exceeding 90 days and these signs or symptoms fail to improve.
  - – In this condition, bouts of illness may occur on at least six separate occasions annually.
  - – In some cases, the presentation may involve flare-ups or acute attacks with no intervening symptom-free intervals.
  - – Coughing at night is more common than in the other forms of sinusitis.

38.5.2 Physical Examination

Any patient with suspected sinusitis requires a detailed examination of the head and neck. The examination should include otoscopic examination of the middle meatus, anterior rhinoscopy, and nasal endoscopy for inspection of the adenoids [8].

- Anterior rhinoscopy [1].
  - – Anterior rhinoscopy may be difficult in children.
  - – Inspect the middle turbinate and meatus, looking for pus or discharge from the sinus.
  - – It is often beneficial to employ a pharmacological agent such as oxymetazoline to promote vasoconstriction.
  - – If polyps are noted, the patient should be assessed for underlying cystic fibrosis.
- Nasal endoscopy [1].
  - – Nasal endoscopy allows for optimal visualization of the middle meatus and offers the most reliable way to visualize the sinus outflow tracts outside of the operating room (Fig. 38.1).
  - – Younger pediatric patients may tolerate the procedure less well than older children.
- Transillumination of the sinuses rarely provides useful diagnostic information.

Min et al. noted in their study [9] of 195 children that chronic sinusitis presents differently before and during adolescence. The researchers noted that coughing, nasal obstruction, and septal deviation were more common during adolescence, whereas prior to adolescence, difficulty sleeping and enlarged tonsils were a more frequent presentation. Furthermore, prior to adolescence, CT imaging scores were higher and the total serological IgE titer was more elevated.

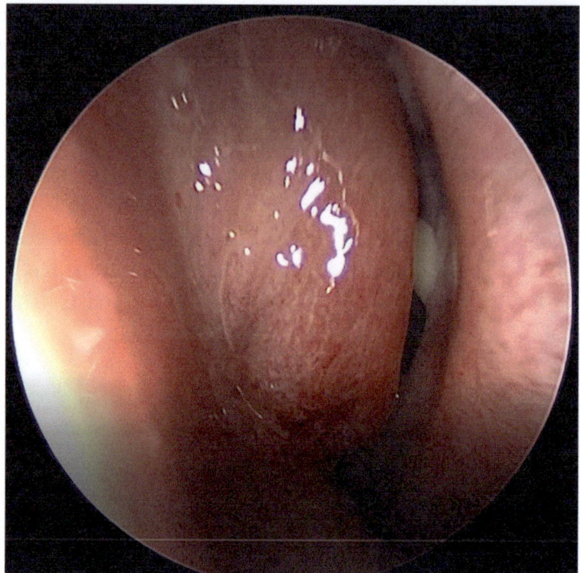

Fig. 38.1 Visualization of the middle turbinate and meatus with endoscopic imaging

38.6 Treatment

38.6.1 Antibiotics

Antibiotic treatment is appropriate in several circumstances, namely [1]:

- Prolonged acute sinusitis.
- Acute sinusitis of marked severity.
- Acute sinusitis in patients with systemic toxicity.
- Complicated acute sinusitis.

Antibiotic resistance is an increasingly pressing issue and should be administered judiciously when physical examination and history is consistent with acute sinusitis. Treatment duration should be between 10 or 14 days, or for seven days after symptoms have ceased [1]. The American Academy of Pediatrics issued sinusitis treatment guidelines in 2001, which have now been updated by Wald and colleagues [10]. The guidelines cover how to diagnose and treat acute bacterial sinusitis in a child or adolescent. They now include the category of "worsening course", referring to cases which initially begin to recover but then develop rhinorrhea de novo or more severely than before, coughing during the waking hours or fever. Additionally, it is now suggested that in cases where the symptoms of sinusitis (rhinorrhea with or without coughing during waking hours) persist longer than 10 days and do not improve, antibiotics may be started at once, or watchful waiting be undertaken for 3 more days. Finally, the evidence suggests that pediatric cases of acute sinusitis where no complications are suspected do not warrant radiological investigation. In terms of antibiotic choice, the drug of choice remains amoxicillin or amoxicillin-clavulanic acid [10].

Mahalingam et al. studied 98 cases of periorbital cellulitis in the setting of URTI/sinusitis. They concluded that combination therapy of ceftriaxone with metronidazole (cef/met) initiated at the beginning of hospitalization offered superior outcomes to monotherapy with amoxicillin-clavulanate acid or ceftriaxone. The cohort consisted of 26 adults and 72 children. On average, patients in whom the combined cef/met regimen was employed remained in hospital for 3.8 days, whereas monotherapy resulted in admissions lasting 4.5 or 5.8 days, depending on the agent employed [11].

38.6.1.1 Irrigation

Nasal saline irrigation is a safe and effective in treating sinusitis, whether acute or chronic. Irrigating the nasal cavity speeds up drainage by the mucociliary mechanism and promotes vasoconstriction. There is also the immediate effect of washing away pooled secretions, lowering bacterial load, and cleansing the nasal lining of allergens or irritating chemicals [12, 13].

Steroids.

Intranasal topical corticosteroids are vital to the treatment of comorbid allergic rhinitis. Nine out of ten patients with this condition reported feeling less stuffy and that their other symptoms had improved. The majority of topical intranasal steroids exhibit minimal systemic absorption, although side effects, such as pituitary under-activity and glaucoma, are known to occur in adults. In children, there have been cases of severe infection by varicella virus. There is a lack of pediatric safety data for most intranasal preparations. Thus, use should be weighed against potential harms [1].

38.6.1.2 Decongestants and Antihistamines

Nasal decongestant medications have varying levels of efficacy. Topical agents potentially offer relief to patients. It is advisable to discontinue the use of decongestants after the first 4 or 5 days, since injury to the mucosa can occur.

Mucolytics likewise offer varying levels of efficacy. They have not been shown yet to be effective in trials utilizing controls. The use of histamine blockers offers greatest benefit in patients suffering from allergic disorders [1].

38.6.1.3 Immunotherapy

This treatment offers efficacy in cases where a specific allergen has been identified and the condition has failed to respond to more conventional pharmacotherapy [1].

38.6.1.4 Optimization of Associated Medical Conditions

Allergic rhinitis.

To manage allergy the following strategies may be recommended: advise the patient to avoiding exposure to their allergen triggers, including environmental adaptations, use of topical intranasal corticosteroids, and second-generation histamine blockers. Immunotherapy is also a possibility [13].

Gastro-esophageal reflux (GERD).

In treating GERD, consultation with a pediatric or gastroenterology colleague is recommended. Conservative treatment consists of raising the head of the bed, avoiding eating just before sleep and adding a thickening agent to meals. Pharmacotherapeutic options consist of H2 blockers, prokinetic drugs, and proton pump inhibitors [1].

Immune deficiency.

In cases of immune deficiency, the involvement of an immunology specialist and, potentially, an infectious diseases physician is required. Pharmacotherapy often needs to be at the highest possible doses. Consideration should be given to injecting gamma-globulin intravenously, although the high financial costs involved and the numerous complications that may occur must also be considered [1].

Asthma.

Where possible, any factors that worsen asthma should be avoided. Pharmacotherapy includes bronchodilators and corticosteroids by inhalation [1].

Cystic fibrosis.

Measures thought to be of benefit include repeated nasal saline irrigation, intranasal corticosteroids, and irrigation with antibiotic solutions with action against *Pseudomonas*. There are no prospective studies to prove the benefit of antibiotic lavage.

Immotile cilia syndromes.

Medical therapy is the mainstay of treatment for genetic immotile cilia syndromes with surgery reserved for those with polyposis, progressive symptoms or exacerbation of sinusitis or lung disease. Consensus statements on immotile cilia syndrome nasal treatments are mainly anecdotal, but most agree that hypertonic 7% nasal saline irrigations and anticholinergics improve symptoms. Routine prophylactic antibiotics are generally not recommended but antibiotics should be used to treat acute sinusitis or if respiratory function is compromised [14].

Chronic sinusitis.

In cases of chronic rhinosinusitis, antibiotic treatment should be given for a minimum of four weeks and the agent chosen should be a second-line agent with a broad spectrum of activity and resistance to beta-lactamase deactivation. Where there is no clear improvement in the first seven days, a different antibiotic may be selected. Cultures obtained after a week may be valuable in revealing susceptibility patterns. In addition to antibiotic treatment, the other pharmacotherapeutic interventions may offer benefit, in particular intranasal corticosteroids. Optimization of comorbid conditions is another key to successful treatment of chronic sinusitis [1].

Acute rhinosinusitis complications.

Acute bacterial rhinosinusitis (ABRS) complications should be diagnosed when the patient develops signs of orbital and/or central nervous system (intracranial) involvement [10]. Periorbital and intraorbital infections are common complications of acute sinusitis and often occur secondary to acute ethmoidal sinusitis in healthy young children (Fig. 38.2a–b) [15]. Conventional radiographs can be used for imaging in acute sinusitis (Fig. 38.3), but it is recommended that children with potential orbital or intracranial complications of ABRS undergo contrast-enhanced computed

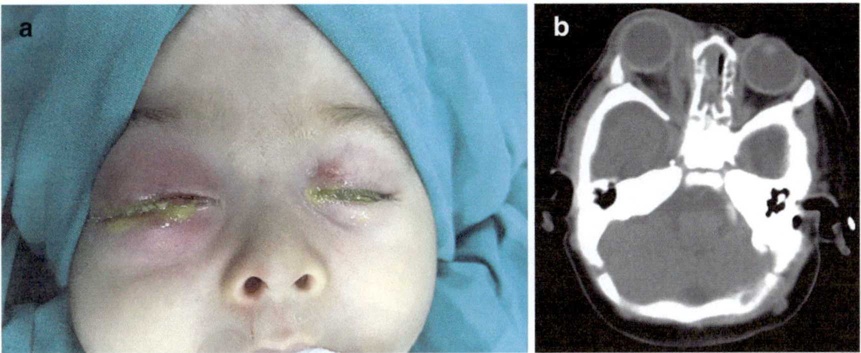

Fig. 38.2 (**a**, **b**) Inspection and tomography image of a 2-year-old pediatric patient who developed right periorbital cellulitis after ABRS

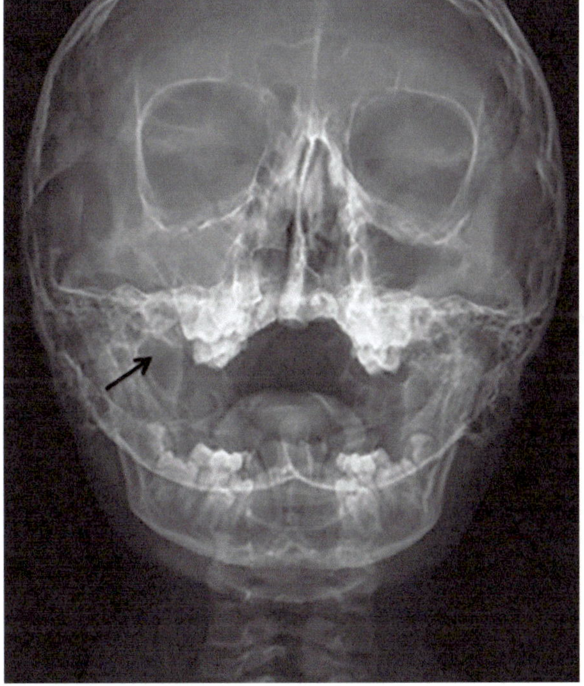

Fig. 38.3 Acute sinusitis image on conventional radiography

tomography (CT) imaging of the orbits, sinuses, and brain (Fig. 38.4). Magnetic resonance imaging (MRI) is an alternative [16]. Intracranial complications include meningitis, epidural or subdural abscess, brain abscess, and venous thrombosis. Rarely, complicated acute sinusitis can cause permanent blindness, neurological sequelae, or death if not treated promptly and appropriately [10].

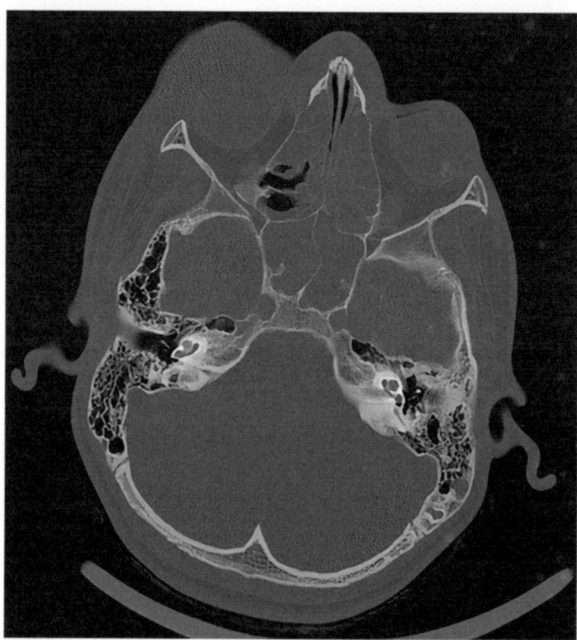

Fig. 38.4 Computed tomography image of a 16-year-old child who developed right periorbital abscess after ABRS

References

1. Ramadan HH. Medical Treatment of Pediatric Sinusitis. In: Meyers AD (Ed). Medscape. Updated: May 12, 2020. https://emedicine.medscape.com/article/873149-overview (Accessed online at October 15, 2020).
2. Sivasli E, Sirikci A, Bayazyt YA, et al. Anatomic variations of the paranasal sinus area in pediatric patients with chronic sinusitis. Surg Radiol Anat. 2003;24(6):400–5.
3. Santee CA, Nagalingam NA, Faruqi AA, et al. Nasopharyngeal microbiota composition of children is related to the frequency of upper respiratory infection and acute sinusitis. Microbiome. 2016;4(1):34.
4. Shapiro GG, Virant FS, Furukawa CT, et al. Immunologic defects in patients with refractory sinusitis. Pediatrics. 1991;87(3):311–6.
5. Anfuso A, Ramadan H, Terrell A, et al. Sinus and adenoid inflammation in children with chronic rhinosinusitis and asthma. Ann Allergy Asthma Immunol. 2015;114(2):103–10.
6. Mabry L, Marple BF, Folker RJ, Mabry CS. Immunotherapy for allergic fungal sinusitis: three years' experience. Otolaryngol Head Neck Surg. 1998;119(6):648–51.
7. Sanderson AR, Leid JG, Hunsaker D. Bacterial biofilms on the sinus mucosa of human subjects with chronic rhinosinusitis. Laryngoscope. 2006;116(7):1121–6.
8. Shin KS, Cho SH, Kim KR, et al. The role of adenoids in pediatric rhinosinusitis. Int J Pediatr Otorhinolaryngol. 2008;72(11):1643–50.
9. Min HJ, Chung HJ, Seong SY, et al. Differential characteristics of pediatric sinusitis who underwent endoscopic sinus surgery: children vs. adolescents. Clin Otolaryngol. 2016;41(5):579–84.

10. Wald ER, Applegate KE, Bordley C, et al. Clinical practice guideline for the diagnosis and management of acute bacterial sinusitis in children aged 1 to 18 years. Pediatrics. 2013;132(1):e262–80.
11. Mahalingam S, Hone R, Lloyd G, et al. The management of periorbital cellulitis secondary to sinonasal infection: a multicenter prospective study in the United Kingdom. Int Forum Allergy Rhinol. 2020;10(6):726–37.
12. Jeffe JS, Bhushan B, Schroeder JW Jr. Nasal saline irrigation in children: a study of compliance and tolerance. Int J Pediatr Otorhinolaryngol. 2012;76(3):409–13.
13. Wei JL, Sykes KJ, Johnson P, He J, Mayo MS. Safety and efficacy of once-daily nasal irrigation for the treatment of pediatric chronic rhinosinusitis. Laryngoscope. 2011;121(9):1989–2000.
14. Wise SK, Lin SY, Toskala E, et al. International consensus statement on allergy and rhinology: allergic rhinitis. Int Forum Allergy Rhinol. 2018;8(2):108–352.
15. Mener DJ, Lin SY, Ishman SL, Boss EF. Treatment and outcomes of chronic rhinosinusitis in children with primary ciliary dyskinesia: where is the evidence? A qualitative systematic review. Int Forum Allergy Rhinol. 2013;12:986–91.
16. Wald E, Kaplan S, Friedman E, Wood R. Acute bacterial rhinosinusitis in children: Clinical features and diagnosis. UpToDate. 2016; Update Jun 6, 2012. [online] [consulted on Nov 12, 2012]. https://www.uptodate.com/contents/acute-bacterial-rhinosinusitis-in-children-clinical-features-and-diagnosis#H13. (Accessed online at January 30, 2021)

Hale Aslan, Eda Çabuk Horoz, and Michael B. Soyka

Acute and chronic rhinosinusitis are common pediatric ailments. A recent study has identified that approximately 2% of ambulatory visits (<20 years of age) per year are due to chronic rhinosinusitis [1, 2]. Despite the lack of comprehensive prospective investigations, the European Rhinologic Society recently published guidelines in how to diagnose and treat pediatric CRS (pCRS) (EPOS2020) [3] Even if they are not life threatening, the child is deeply affected by his/her school performance and his/her sleep patterns thus affecting quality of life relevantly [2]. Our aim here is to reveal the innovations that exist in medical and surgical treatment while sharing basic information about pediatric chronic rhinosinusitis in the context of current literature and recent studies.

39.1 Introduction

The precise diagnosis of pediatric chronic rhinosinusitis in children is difficult because viral upper respiratory tract infections, adenoid hypertrophy, adenoiditis, etc. coincide in similar symptomatology and they may be clinically indistinguishable [3]. Due to the difficulty of defining the diseases correctly and the lack of proper studies, the epidemiological numbers differ significantly and tend to overestimate pCRS occurrence. In studies performing follow-up visits pCRS prevalence was estimated to be between 0.3 and 0.8 [4]. Since recent studies have shown significant improvements in terms of diagnostic and treatment modalities, many scientific communities have set out their approach guidelines accordingly [5, 6]. A major field of

H. Aslan (✉) · E. Ç. Horoz
Department of Otorhinolaryngology, Faculty of Medicine, Katip Çelebi University, İzmir, Turkey

M. B. Soyka
Department of Otorhinolaryngology, Head and Neck Surgery, University and University Hospital Zurich, Zurich, Switzerland

© The Author(s), under exclusive license to Springer Nature Switzerland AG 2022   451
C. Cingi et al. (eds.), *Pediatric ENT Infections*,
https://doi.org/10.1007/978-3-030-80691-0_39

information deficiency is the role of chronic rhinosinusitis in gastroesophageal reflux (GERD). Some studies have shown that treatment of GERD provides significant improvement in sinusitis symptoms [7]. However, its relevance remains unclear. Surgical treatment (adenotomy, less frequently followed by FESS) is often indicated in children, in the case of maximum medical treatment unresponsiveness [3]. In fact, although there are no radical changes in the medical and surgical treatment of chronic rhinosinusitis, adenotomy performed before endoscopic sinus surgery has been shown to improve eradication of biofilms [1]. However, the definition of optimal medical treatment in pediatric patients, as well as surgical intervention indications and the limits of surgery are less clear compared to adults [3].

39.2 Definition and Classification

Rhinosinusitis refers to the inflammation of the nose and one or more paranasal sinus(es). One must bear in mind that in children this might be clinically indistinguishable from adenoid obstruction or adenoiditis. In the European Position Paper on Rhinosinusitis and Nasal Polyps, a definition and treatment algorithm was defined based on the evidence that was updated and published in 2020 (Figs. 39.1 and 39.2):

The definition of pCRS according to EPOS 2020 is symptoms lasting >12 weeks.

- Presence of two or more symptoms with at least one of which being nasal obstruction or nasal discharge (anterior/posterior nasal discharge) with:

+/− Facial pain or pressure.

+/− Cough.

Fig. 39.1 Care pathways for pediatric CRS (EPOS 2020)

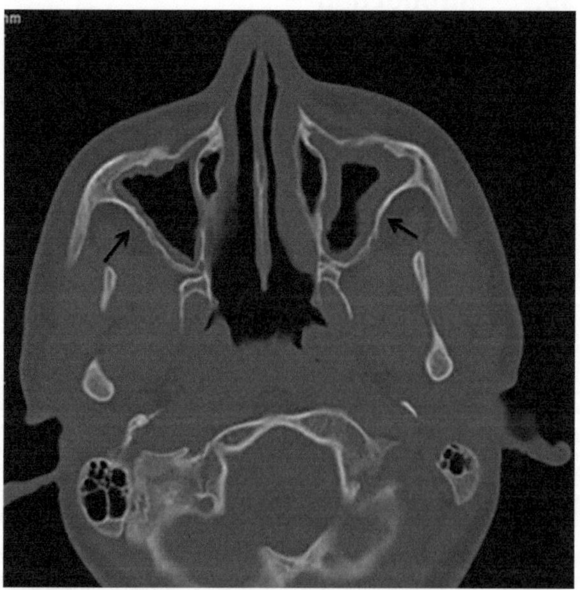

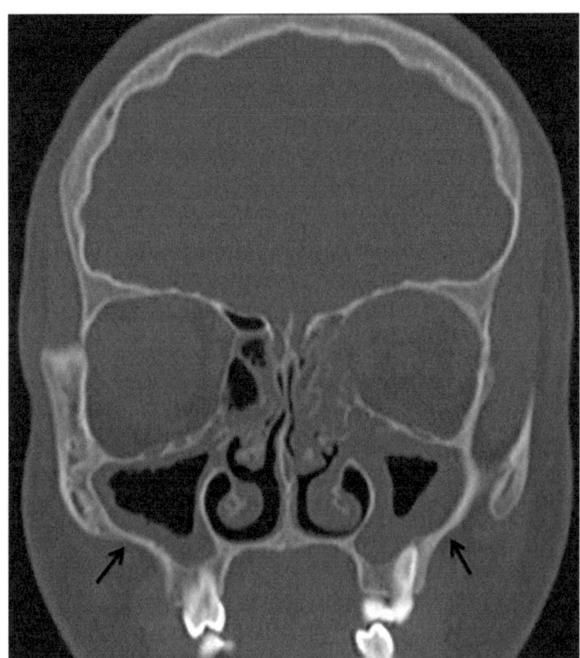

Fig. 39.2 Radiologic image of Woakes syndrome

And either.
-Endoscopic findings of.
- polyps.
-mucopurulent discharge and/or edema in the middle meatus.
Or
-CT changes in the osteomeatal complex and/or sinuses.

Classification

In contrast to adult CRS endotyping of pCRS and the distinction between type II and non-type II (i.e., Type I or Type III) inflammation is currently not recommended due to heterogeneity of endotypes. Therefore, the phenotypic distinction still is applied. Secondary pCRS, due to cystic fibrosis, primary ciliary dyskinesia or immunodeficiency needs to be classified accordingly.

Chronic Rhinosinusitis with Nasal Polyps (CRS with NP)

İn addition to the symptoms described above; chronic rhinosinusitis with nasal polyps is defined by the presence of bilateral nasal polyps in the middle/superior meatus and/or nasal cavity found by endoscopy.

Chronic Rhinosinusitis Without Nasal Polyps (CRS Without NP)

İn addition to the symptoms described above; chronic rhinosinusitis without nasal polyps is defined as the absence of polyps even after decongestion.

39.3 Pathophysiology and Microbiology

The exact pathogenesis of primary pCRS stays unclear and is most likely heterogenous [8]. Among the known conditions related to sinuses, recurrent viral upper respiratory tract infections, allergic and non-allergic rhinitis, ciliary dyskinesia, cystic fibrosis, immunodeficiency, reflux, and anatomical abnormalities may contribute or directly cause pCRS. Environmental and personal factors contribute to the development of pCRS and recurrent infections or exacerbations.

Adenoid hypertrophy and adenoiditis is not only difficult to be discerned from primary pCRS it is also most likely to contribute to its pathogenesis. There is increasing evidence that crypts in adenoid tissue may act as a reservoir for bacteria including biofilm formation. These biofilms can prevent effective treatment by inhibiting the penetration of antibiotics [9].

Similarly, to otitis prone children, patients exposed to passive smoking are prone to acute rhinosinusitis episodes. The situation is less clear in the pCRS group as evidence is missing. However, children exposed to smoke have a worse outcome after surgery and present with more severe symptoms [10–12].

Immunodeficiency plays a role in recurrent and chronic rhinosinusitis. This is particularly true in the immature immune systems of pediatric patients. Impaired humoral immunity and hypo-responsiveness to vaccination was found in a large proportion of pCRS patients, more often than in adults [8].

While allergic disposition by itself may turn the child prone to infection Costa Carcalho et al. provided evidence that primary or secondary immunodeficiency seem no to be the primary source of the disease in children with recurrent or chronic rhinosinusitis with respiratory allergies. Children with pCRS tend to have more often asthma and allergic rhinitis as comorbidities. In those patients with severe immunodeficiency secondary to chemotherapy Park et al. [13] showed that chronic sinusitis and invasive fungal sinusitis occurs more frequently. Therefore evaluation for humoral immunodeficiency seems extraordinarily important in patients with refractory pCRS.

Secondary rhinosinusitis is not only observed in immunocompromised children but obviously also in patients suffering from cystic fibrosis and primary ciliary dyskinesia. Cystic fibrosis (CF) is a common genetic disorder affecting the CFTR gene causing retention of thick secretions in the respiratory system and secondary damage to these organs. It is often accompanied by the colonization of P. aeruginosa and/or S. aureus. Almost all patients suffer from CRS, often presenting with nasal polyps. Therefore, pediatric patients presenting with CRS (especially with nasal polyps) should be screened for this disorder, despite negative newborn screening results. Heterozygous carriers of a CFTR mutation seem to be more prone to developing CRS. Primary ciliary dyskinesia (PCD) on the other hand is much less common and most often patients present with pulmonary problems and recurrent middle ear difficulties, i.e., otitis with effusion and acute infections. Nasal symptoms are not uncommon and CRS with the formation of polyps may be one of the findings leading to diagnosis. Beware that a full Kartagener's syndrome does not need to be present in all PCD patients (approx. 50%). Patients with nasal polyps that develop early in life may present with a condition referred to as the (pseudo-) Woakes syndrome. Although originally described as a necrotizing ethmoiditis it presents often in childhood leading to a widening of the nasal pyramid and an appearance of a hypertelorism. (Fig. 39.2).

Anatomic variations are other factors putatively associated with chronic rhinosinusitis. When the relationship between pneumatized middle concha, concha bullosa, and chronic and recurrent rhinosinusitis in children is investigated, Haruna et al. [14] discovered this anatomic variation in 4.6% of 95 patients, just as they have seen in it in older children with medial concha pneumatization. Opacification of the osteomeatal complex was also not found more frequently in patients with middle concha pneumatization. The authors could not establish a causal relationship between these anatomic variations and chronic recurrent rhinosinusitis. This study is actually a confirmation of other studies in the literature [15]. Likewise, there was no causal relationship between anatomical variations such as infraorbital cell or septal deviation. Therefore, there is no evidence for anatomic variations to cause pCRS.

There are few new studies showing the relationship between gastroesophageal reflux disease (GERD) and rhinosinusitis presenting controversial results. In a Brazilian pediatric study, sinusitis was detected in 10% of those with GERD, even though the group of patients who participated in the study was small. The relationship between rhinosinusitis and gastroesophageal reflux seems stronger in the pediatric population and most likely present in some patients. Clear and large studies are missing and therefore the link between the two disorders still needs to be investigated [16].

Finally, an interesting study by Pena et al. [17] revealed the results of glandular cell and mucin secretion in the infected and non-infected mucosa. Neither goblet cell hyperplasia nor increased MUC5AC gene expression was found to play a role in the thickened mucosa of children with chronic rhinosinusitis. MUC5B seems to be the predominant glandular mucin in the pCRS population [18].

39.4 Diagnostic Methods

The diagnosis of pCRS should follow clear definitions as mentioned above.

It is based on history and clinical findings primarily. The detailed medical and family history of the patient should be completed by a thorough physical examination [1]. Although not being a sufficient diagnostic method alone, pediatric patients with chronic nasal symptoms should be assessed by anterior rhinoscopy to judge on the state of the mucosa (i.e.) swelling or purulent discharge in the area of the inferior and middle turbinate. The second step should include rigid or flexible nasal endoscopy of the middle meatus and nasopharynx. Oral cavity examination can reveal purulent drainage, cobblestone appearance of the posterior pharynx wall or tonsillar hypertrophy and allows for posterior rhinoscopy [19]. The presence of nasal polyps in children is an unexpected finding, but the appearance should raise suspicion for CF, PCD, or allergic fungal rhinosinusitis [20].

After the anamnesis and the physical examination, appropriate diagnostic tests should be considered according to the accompanying symptoms in the patients. Both allergic rhinitis and rhinosinusitis can be associated with cough and wheezing [21]. Next to adenoid hypertrophy and adenoiditis, allergic as well as non-allergic rhinitis should be considered as differential diagnosis in suspected pCRS patients. In those where history is pointing towards allergies, thorough testing by skin prick in older children and/or serologic IgE measurements is mandatory. Parents and patients reporting nighttime cough, wheezing, or shortness of breath should undergo lung function testing, FeNO measurement, and specialist assessment after screening. Differential diagnosis includes postnasal drip as well as GERD and should be assessed accordingly.

Pediatric patients rarely report spontaneously about decreased or absent sense of smell despite being an important characteristic of pCRS. Careful history needs to be taken to specifically ask about this symptom and its occurrence. Patients in whom a sense of smell was never present could suffer from primary anosmia such as found in syndromic cases (Kallmann). Psychophysical testing for the sense of smell is available even for young patients.

In case of suspicion for secondary pCRS appropriate testing and specialist consultations are mandatory. Involvement of other organs like recurrent otitis or pneumonia may be suggestive. Screening for CF using a sweat test and potentially performing genetic testing need to be considered. Similarly, PCD is tested by (low) nasal NO measurement, high frequency video assessment of ciliary movement, using nasal brushing, mucociliary clearance test and possibly electron microscopy or genetic testing. Specialized pulmonological assessment obviously is a prerequisite. Immunodeficiencies, especially targeting the humoral system, need to be ruled out in case of recurrent acute or therapy resistant CRS. Furthermore, atypical microorganisms can point toward secondary origin [15]. CRS. Immunoglobulin levels including subclass analyses as well as vaccination antibodies and titer-increases after vaccination can help to screen these patients.

Middle meatal aspiration swabs can help identifying sinonasal colonization or infection. However, sinus aspirate culture is currently the only valid diagnostic method for diagnosing rhinosinusitis in patients who do not respond to conventional medical care, as it may be useful to guide further treatment [22]. In children, the data on the benefit of this approach are limited. Due to the fact that it is an invasive examination requiring general anesthesia it is rarely performed. In selected cases like immunocompromised children with suspected fungal rhinosinusitis it may be considered but needs to be weighed out against directly performing FESS with maxillary irrigation [23].

Plain film radiographs in the imaging of the sinuses and adenoids are absolutely in the aera of endoscopy, CT and MR scanning. Sinus Waters, Caldwell-Luc graphs show only pathologic findings in less than half of the patients. Loss of airflow, blurred appearance, fluid level, and opacification suggest sinusitis, but acute bacterial sinusitis, viral sinusitis, and allergic inflammation cannot be distinguished. Because of the high rates of false-positive and -negative results, they are not reliable tests [24].

Computed sinus tomography should be requested in the absence of appropriate medical treatment response, in the presence of unilateral symptoms or signs, in patients with persistent or recurrent disease, in the presence of sinusitis-related complications, in the presence of mechanical obstruction of the sinus and ahead if a surgery is planned. Otherwise, it should not be requested as a primary diagnostic tool [25]. Doses of CT radiation in children are considerably high. Hojreh et al. [26] suggests that if specific reconstruction algorithms and low dose protocols are used, a lower doses of CT images could be attained in children. These protocols are not yet in widespread use, but should be adopted. Cone beam (DVT) CT could present another innovative approach with lower doses of radiation if no contrast agent is needed. Magnetic resonance imaging (MR) may be considered in suspected intracranial spread of an infection, in situations such as brain abscess or epidural empyema as well as tumor suspicion [27].

39.5   Treatment

The treatment of CRS in children is divided into two: medical and surgical. The initial treatment of CRS should be medical except in cases of obvious anatomic obstruction. On the other hand, adenotomy may be one of the most important steps in diagnosing and treating true pCRS. More aggressive treatment approaches may be needed in cases with cystic fibrosis or mucociliary dyskinesias. In addition, the philosophy of protecting natural drainage routes may not apply to these patients. Gravity based drainage may be more effective [28].

39.6   Medical Treatment

Medical treatment of suspected pCRS usually starts with saline nasal sprays and rinsing. Saline seems to be beneficial in children with CRS according to a Cochrane review [29]. Literature, however, does not give us the answer about the amount, composition, and tonicity of the optimal solution. So far it is also unclear if additional drugs mixed with the saline rinses are of any benefit, antibiotic solutions seem not to be associated with a relevant additional improvement.

Treatment with nasal steroid sprays should be considered due to the good safety profile and good experience in the adult population and pediatric allergic rhinitis. There are no clinical randomized trials to support this in pCRS, but it is useful in suppressing disease-associated inflammation. Treatment of CRS can also significantly reduce asthma exacerbations in patients, particularly if they are accompanied by concurrent allergic rhinitis and asthma [30]. When the literature is reviewed, a modest benefit from using topical steroids has been shown. Currently, mometasone and fluticasone are the preferred choices for topical steroids in children due to their low systemic availability, local country-specific recommendations and age limits should be followed. There seems to be no long-term effect on growth nor the pituitary axis [31].

One study supports the use of systemic steroids in pCRS as an adjunct to antibiotic treatment [31, 32]. This, however, is limited by the concern of systemic side effects. The combination of antibiotics and nasal steroidal sprays is supported in a relatively new outcome-oriented clinical practice guide. However, these guidelines do not provide definitive information about the duration of antibiotic treatment [32]. Short-term antibiotic treatment in CRS has been shown to be inadequate to alleviate symptoms [33]. Despite the lack of data on long-term outcomes, the recommended treatment duration is usually between 3 and 6 weeks [34].

In fact, the ideal choice of antibiotics should be based on culture sensitivity. Fluoroquinolones may be considered in patients with cystic fibrosis due to the high incidence of Pseudomonas aeruginosa in these patients. Resistance to antibiotics in some countries is worrisome. The review of the current literature leads the EPOS 2020 group to state that there is insufficient evidence to include antibiotic treatment into routine patients with pCRS.

The role of anti-reflux treatment in pediatric chronic rhinosinusitis is controversial. Bothwell et al. [25] reported that 25 of the 28 children who were followed up with 2-year anti-reflux treatment avoided sinus surgery. Phipps found that approximately 60% of pediatric CRS patients who did not receive medical treatment had gastroesophageal reflux (GER), and 80% of them reported a decrease in sinonasal symptoms after anti-reflux treatment [35]. Conversely, a meta-analysis by Weaver found a weak (degree C) correlation between reflux and chronic rhinosinusitis. However, the evidence is low and most studies lack an adequate control group. This precludes any firm recommendation for routine anti-reflux treatment [26].

The role of a fungal infection in CRS is a controversial issue at the moment. Some advocate fungal etiology in CRS and use of topical amphotericin B as a treatment option, but there are only a few studies showing any benefit, as there is little theoretical data supporting this [36]. Although randomized placebo-controlled double-blind trial showed decreased tomographic and endoscopic mucosal thickness, there was no significant difference in patient symptoms. There is no study of the efficacy of nasal irrigation with amphotericin B in the pediatric population. Future tests of this hypothesis may include oral antifungal drugs, which could be more appropriate in the pediatric population. Until then, antifungal use in pediatric CRS cannot be widely recommended [37].

39.7 Surgical Treatment

As in adults, the indications for surgery should be provided step by step in children who fail to respond to maximal medical care. Some authors believe that the diagnoses of pCRS cannot be made before adenotomy has been performed. Therefore this type of simple and relatively safe procedure seems one of the first steps in its treatment. When choosing endoscopic sinus surgery as a treatment option, conservative approaches including anterior ethmoidectomy is often preferred. However, it is difficult to evaluate the results of sinus surgery in the pediatric population due to diversity of criteria used to measure success [31].

In patients with suspected invasive fungal sinusitis, rapid biopsy and staining is recommended. If invasion is present, the diseased tissue should be surgically excised and reversal of the immunodeficiency should be attained as soon as possible along with aggressive antifungal treatment.

39.7.1 Adenotomy/Adenoidectomy (AT)

In a study conducted by the participation of 175 participants of the American Pediatric Otorhinolaryngology Society, 55% of the participants used adenoidectomy as a routine assisting procedure and 81% of them applied it prior to endoscopic sinus surgery (ESS) [3]. Vandenberg and Heatley reported that 79% of 43 patients with chronic rhinosinusitis showed subjective improvement after adenoidectomy, and only 3 of them required FESS [38]. On the other hand, Ramadan reported less success of adenoidectomy compared to the ESS in chronic rhinosinusitis treatment. As a result of this study adenoidectomy has been identified as a primary treatment approach rather than an assisting measure of treatment in chronic rhinosinusitis [39].

There is growing evidence that removal of adenoid tissue removes biofilms buried in the crypts and on the adenoid tissue surface, and thus may be a source of recurrent infections [9]. Zuliani et al. have shown how mechanical debridement of nasopharyngeal biofilms (adenoidectomy) may explain improved clinical symptoms of sinusitis with surgery [30]. Many studies have shown that adenoidectomy in pediatric CRS is an effective and reliable method. Although not all symptoms are always treated that way due to the heterogeneity of etiologies, AT is a safe and relatively fast procedure that should be considered early in the diagnosis and treatment of pCRS (Table 39.1).

Table 39.1 Evidence supporting therapy of CRS in children (EPOS 2020)

Treatment	Level	Recommendation Score	Acceptability
Nasal saline wash	Ia	A	Yes
Gastroesophageal reflux treatment	III	C	No
Topical corticosteroid	IV	D	Yes
Long-term oral antibiotic	No data	D	Not clear
<4 weeks short-term antibiotic	Ib(−)[#]	A(−)*	No
Intravenous antibiotics	III(−)[##]	C(−)**	No

Ib(−)[#]: Negative resulted Ibstudy.
A(−)*:Suggestion level A for not using.
III(−)[##]: Negative resulted level III study.
C(−)**:Suggestion level C for not using.

39.7.2 Adenoidectomy and Antral Lavage

Some researchers have tried simultaneous adenoidectomy and antral lavage in patients under general anesthesia. This allowed both clearance of secretions in the sinuses and culturing for the identification of postoperative antibiotic therapy. Symptom relief rates were close to 80% and the success rate was higher when compared with sole AT [31].

39.7.3 Functional Endoscopic Sinus Surgery

In the surgical treatment of CRS, functional endoscopic sinus surgery (FESS) is the next step after failure of AT. In addition, FESS may be the first surgical option in patients whose adenoids are not large, and whose mucociliary clearance is impaired such as in primary ciliary dyskinesia [40]. The adoption of FESS in children is not so widespread, due to unjustified concerns of impaired mid face development. Bothwell et al. have not detected any difference in facial development when comparing FESS patients to those who did not have FESS over a follow-up period of 10 years [41].

Unlike in the early days of sinus surgeries, FESS aims at expanding the natural ostia and preserving the physiological drainage pathways [42]. Looking at FESS surgery literature in children, maxillary antrostomy and anterior ethmoidectomy are suggested at the beginning. This treatment is adequate in most cases. The clinical outcome is excellent, the symptom improvement interval ranges from 80% to 100% [43]. Paranasal sinus tomography (CT) should be performed prior to surgery to account for disease extension accompanying anatomic variation [28].

Postoperative care is important in pediatric FESS patients, and patients need to receive "maximal medical treatment" for several weeks after surgery. Irrigation with saline seems ideal, but it is difficult to perform it in the pediatric population [44]. After endoscopic sinus surgery, the recovery of the edematous mucosa lasts for 8 weeks while at the antral mucosa with nasal polyp healing progresses to a slower recovery period over 4 months [45]. Although second-look endoscopy was previously recommended to increase the chances of success, this paradigm has been abandoned, as it does not alter clinical results and requires additional anesthesia to the patient [46].

As a result, both adenoidectomy and FESS are effective treatments separately. However, clinicians should properly inform the child and his family about not to expect an absolute cure for the disease, even if there is improvement in the symptoms. Although FESS has a higher success rate than adenoidectomy, a step-by-step approach to surgical treatment is recommended. Adenoidectomy is a low-risk procedure that can be practiced by almost all otolaryngologists and has shown to provide significant benefits to children with CRS. FESS in the pediatric population is technically more demanding and the surgery should be performed only by those who are trained for FESS in children and rhinologists with adequate experience in pediatric CRS. A recent retrospective review of image guidance used in the pediatric FESS has shown that this technique may be useful for complex cases with involvement of the frontal sinus, sphenoid sinus, orbit, or skull base [47].

In the pediatric population, allergic fungal rhinosinusitis may manifest itself with nasal symptoms, atopy, headache, and ocular symptoms. FESS should be recommended as a first line treatment for patients suspected of allergic fungal sinusitis because allergic mucin is thick and not easily cleared from the sinuses. These patients have a high recurrence rate and after surgery they should be treated with maximal medical treatment including sinus irrigation and nasal steroids. In addition, immunotherapy could be considered in patients with fungal sensitization [48].

39.8 Conclusion

To choose the right treatment for the right patient a thorough patient's history needs to be obtained including the assessment of accompanying disorders like allergies. Treatment of pCRS starts with the exclusion of relevant differential diagnosis and is followed by medical treatment that usually includes saline rinses and topical corticosteroids. Adenotomy is often the first step when surgical therapy is chosen. FESS should only be performed by well-trained pediatric rhinosurgeons in the therapy of refractory and severe cases.

References

1. Gilani S, Shin JJ. The burden and visit prevalence of pediatric chronic rhinosinusitis. Otolaryngol Head Neck Surg. 2017 Dec;157(6):1048–52. https://doi.org/10.1177/0194599817721177.
2. Sami AS, Scadding GK. Rhinosinusitis in secondary school children-part 2: main project analysis of MSNOT-20 young persons questionnaire (MSYPQ). Rhinology. 2014;52:225–30.
3. Fokkens WJ, Lund VJ, Hopkins C, Hellings PW, Kern R, et al. European Position Paper on Rhinosinusitis and Nasal Polyps 2020. Rhinology. 2020;58(Suppl S29):1–464. https://doi.org/10.4193/Rhin20.600.
4. Westman M, Stjarne P, Bergstrom A, et al. Chronic rhinosinusitis is rare but bothersome in adolescents from a Swedish population-based cohort. J Allergy Clin Immunol. 2015;136:512–4.
5. American Academy of Pediatrics. Clinical practice guideline: management of sinusitis. Pediatrics. 2001;108:798–808.
6. Esposito S, Marseglia GL, Novelli A, et al. La rinusinusite in eta` pediatrica. Consensus Conference. Societa` Italiana di Infettivologia Pediatrica, Firenze, Giornale Italiano di Infettivologia. Pediatrica. 2006;3(Suppl. 1):3–29.
7. Slavin RG, Spector SL, Bernstein IL, et al. The diagnosis and management of sinusitis: a practice parameter update. J Allergy Clin Immunol. 2005;116(Suppl. 6):S13–47.
8. Steele RW. Chronic sinusitis in children. Clin Pediatr. 2005;44:465–71.
9. Coticchia J, Zuliani G, Coleman C, et al. Biofilm surface area in the pediatric nasopharynx: chronic rhinosinusitis vs obstructive sleep apnea. Arch Otolaryngol Head Neck Surg. 2007;133:110–4.
10. Ramadan HH. Surgical management of chronic sinusitis in children. Laryngoscope. 2004;114:2103–9.
11. Siedek V, Stelter K, Betz CS, Berghaus A, Leunig. Functional endoscopic sinus surgery--a retrospective analysis of 115 children and adolescents with chronic rhinosinusitis. Int J Pediatr Otorhinolaryngol. 2009;73:741–5.

12. Younis RT, Lazar RH. Criteria for success in pediatric functional Endonasal sinus Surg. Laryngoscope. 1996;106:869–73.
13. Costa Carvalho BT, Nagao AT, Arslanian C, et al. Immunological evaluation of allergic respiratory children with recurrent sinusitis. Pediatr Allergy Immunol. 2005;16:534–8.
14. Haruna S, Sawada K, Nakajima T, Moriyama H. Relationship between pediatric sinusitis and middle turbinate pneumatization–ethmoidal sinus pyocele thought to be caused by middle turbinate pneumatization. Int J Pediatr Otorhinolaryngol. 2005;69:375–9.
15. Jones NS. Acute and chronic sinusitis in children. Curr Opin Pulm Med. 2000;6:221–5.
16. Monteiro VR, Sdepanian VL, Weckx L, et al. Twenty-four-hour esophageal pH monitoring in children and adolescents with chronic and/or recurrent rhinosinusitis. Braz J Med Biol Res. 2005;38:215–20.
17. Pena MT, Aujla PK, Patel KM, et al. Immunohistochemical analyses of MUC5AC mucin expression in sinus mucosa of children with sinusitis and controls. Ann Otol Rhinol Laryngol. 2005;114:958–65.
18. Rose MC, Voynow JA. Respiratory tract mucin genes and mucin glycoproteins in health and disease. Physiol Rev. 2006;86:245–78.
19. Gwaltney JM. Acute community-acquired sinusitis. Clin Infect Dis. 1996;23:1209–23.
20. Hsin CH, Tsao CH, Su MC, Chou MC, Liu CM. Comparison of maxillary sinus puncture with endoscopic middle meatal culture in pediatric rhinosinusitis. Am J Rhinol. 2008;22:280–4.
21. Brent K. Transillumination and radiography in diagnosing sinusitis. Emerg Med News. 2003;25(1):13–4.
22. American Academy of Pediatrics Subcommittee on Management of Sinusitis and Committee on Quality Improvement. Clinical practice guideline: management of sinusitis. Pediatrics. 2001;108:798–808.
23. Ioannidis JP, Lau J. Technical report: evidence for the diagnosis and treatment of acute uncomplicated sinusitis in children: a systematic overview. Pediatrics. 2001;108(3):E57.
24. Herrmann BW, Forsen JW. Simultaneous intracranial and orbital complications of acute rhinosinusitis in children. Int J Pediatr Otorhinolaryngol. 2004;68:619–25.
25. Bothwell MR, Parsons DS, Talbot A, et al. Outcome of reflux therapy on pediatric chronic sinusitis. Otolaryngol Head Neck Surg. 1999;121:255–62.
26. Weaver EM. Association between gastroesophageal reflux and sinusitis, otitis media, and laryngeal malignancy: a systematic review of the evidence. Am J Med. 2003;115(Suppl 3A):81S–9S.
27. Georgalas C, Thomas K, Owens C, et al. Medical treatment for rhinosinusitis associated with adenoidal hypertrophy in children: an evaluation of clinical response and changes on magnetic resonance imaging. Ann Otol Rhinol Laryngol. 2005;114:638–44.
28. Huang WH, Fang SY. High prevalence of antibiotic resistance in isolates from the middle meatus of children and adults with acute rhinosinusitis. Am J Rhinol. 2004;18(6):387–91.
29. Harvey R, Hannan SA, Badia L, Scadding G. Nasal saline irrigations for the symptoms of chronic rhinosinusitis. Cochrane Database Syst Rev. 2007;3:CD006394.
30. Zuliani G, Carron M, Gurrola J, et al. Identification of adenoid biofilms in chronic rhinosinusitis. Int J Pediatr Otorhinolaryngol. 2006;70:1613–7.
31. Ramadan HH, Cost JL. Outcome of adenoidectomy versus adenoidectomy with maxillary sinus wash for chronic rhinosinusitis in children. Laryngoscope. 2008;118:871–3.
32. Keech DR, Ramadan H, Mathers P. Analysis of aerobic bacterial strains found in chronic rhinosinusitis using the polymerase chain reaction. Otolaryngol Head Neck Surg. 2000;123(4):363–7.
33. Park CS, Park YS, Park YJ, et al. The inhibitory effects of macrolide antibiotics on bone remodeling in chronic rhinosinusitis. Otolaryngol Head Neck Surg. 2007;137(2):274–9.
34. Bhattacharyya N. Antimicrobial therapy in chronic rhinosinusitis. Curr Allergy Asthma Rep. 2009;9(3):221–6.
35. Phipps CD, Wood WE, Gibson WS, et al. Gastroesophageal reflux contributing to chronic sinus disease in children. Arch Otolaryngol Head Neck Surg. 2000;126:831–6.
36. Ebbens FA, Scadding GK, Badia L, et al. Amphotericin B nasal lavages: not a solution for patients with chronic rhinosinusitis. J Allergy Clin Immunol. 2006;118:1149–56.

37. Lund VJ, Neijens HJ, Clement PA, et al. The treatment of chronic sinusitis: a controversial issue. Int J Pediatr Otorhinolaryngol. 1995;32(Suppl):21–35.
38. Vandenberg SJ, Heatley DG. Efficacy of adenoidectomy in relieving symptoms of chronic sinusitis in children. Arch Otolaryngol Head Neck Surg. 1997;123:675–8.
39. Ramadan HH. Adenoidectomy vs. endoscopic sinus surgery for the treatment of pediatric sinusitis. Arch Otolaryngol Head Neck Surg. 1999;125:1208–11.
40. Kaliner MA, Osguthorpe JD, Fireman P, et al. Sinusitis: bench to bedside – current findings, future directions. Otolaryngol Head Neck Surg. 1997;116:301–7.
41. Bothwell MR, Piccirillo JF, Lusk RP, et al. Long-term outcome of facial growth after functional endoscopic sinus surgery. Otolaryngol Head Neck Surg. 2002;126:628–34.
42. Hebert RL, Bent JP. Meta-analysis of outcomes of pediatric functional endoscopic sinus surgery. Laryngoscope. 1998;108:796–9.
43. Sobol SE, Samadi DS, Kazahaya K, et al. Trends in the management of chronic sinusitis: a survey of the American Society of Pediatric Otolaryngology. Laryngoscope. 2005;115:78–80.
44. Younis RT, Lazar RH. Criteria for success in pediatric functional endoscopic sinus surgery. Laryngoscope. 1996;106:869–73.
45. Huang HM, Lee HP, Liu CM, Lin KN. Normalization of maxillary sinus mucosa after functional endoscopic sinus surgery in pediatric chronic sinusitis. Int J Pediatr Otorhinolaryngol. 2005;69:1219–23.
46. Younis RT. The pros and cons of second-look sinonasal endoscopy after endoscopic sinus surgery in children. Arch Otolaryngol Head Neck Surg. 2005;131:267–9.
47. Rosenfeld RM. Pilot study of outcomes in pediatric rhinosinusitis. Arch Otolaryngol Head Neck Surg. 1995;121:729–36.
48. Parikh SR, Cuellar H, Sadoughi B, et al. Indications for image-guidance in pediatric sinonasal surgery. Int J Pediatr Otorhinolaryngol. 2009;73:351–6.

Abdullah Kınar, Cemal Cingi, and Nicolas Busaba

40.1 Introduction

Bacterial rhinosinusitis can lead to periorbital and intracranial complications when not adequately treated. In fact, it is not uncommon for the disease to present with signs and symptoms of associated complications, such as when infection spreads to the orbit or within the cranial cavity. The precise incidence of such complications has not been ascertained, although the rate in cases that require hospitalisation due to rhinosinusitis is around 5%, according to several publications [1–3].

The following signs and symptoms raise clinical suspicion of intracranial involvement [1, 4, 5]:

- Oedema surrounding the orbit or within the orbit, together with persistent cephalgia that is associated with vomiting.
- Vomiting and cephalgia of sufficient severity to cause hospitalisation, especially if the patient is an older child.
- Vomiting which fails to resolve within 24 hours.
- Obtunded level of consciousness.
- Localising neurological signs.
- Indicators of irritated meninges, such as nuchal rigidity.

A. Kınar (✉)
Section of Otorhinolaryngology, Afyonkarahisar State Hospital, Afyonkarahisar, Turkey

C. Cingi
Department of Otorhinolaryngology, Faculty of Medicine, Eskişehir Osmangazi University, Eskişehir, Turkey

N. Busaba
Department of Otolaryngology, Head and Neck Surgery, Harvard Medical School, Harvard University, Boston, MA, USA

C. Cingi et al. (eds.), *Pediatric ENT Infections*,
https://doi.org/10.1007/978-3-030-80691-0_40

The following are specific features of the presentation of rhinosinusitis complicated by involvement of the orbit or the cranial cavity [1, 6–10]:

- Periorbital (preseptal) cellulitis: The eyelids become oedematous and erythematous, as does the area around the orbit. However, the eyes maintain their full range of movement and are not proptotic. The condition is typically mild and responds to medical therapy.
- Orbital cellulitis: There is oedema around the orbit, eyelid erythema, pain with eye movement, chemotic/oedematous conjunctivae, proptosis, diplopia, acute loss of visual acuity, and ophthalmoplegia (eyes cannot move over their full range).
- Orbital subperiosteal abscess: There is peri-orbit oedema, eyelid is erythema, pain with eye movement, chemotic/oedematous conjunctivae, proptosis, ophthalmoplegia, diplopia, and at times acute loss of visual acuity [2, 11, 12]. Differentiating between a subperiosteal abscess and straightforward orbital cellulitis can be clinically challenging. Subperiosteal abscess is more likely if the orbit is noticeably displaced. However, the correct diagnosis is established via imaging or at the time of surgical exploration.
- Septic cavernous sinus thrombosis: This condition commonly presents with bilateral proptosis, ophthalmoplegia, periorbital swelling, cephalgia, and an altered mental status.
- Meningitis: This is characterised by pyrexia, neck stiffness/nuchal rigidity, and an altered mental status.
- Osteomyelitis of the frontal bone in conjunction with a subperiosteal abscess (Pott puffy tumour): In this condition, there is oedema affecting the frontal region and scalp, which is tender to palpation, which is frequently associated with cephalgia, photophobia, pyrexia, vomiting, and lethargy [13].
- Epidural abscess: Patients present with localising neurological signs, cephalgia, weariness, and nausea and vomiting. Fundoscopy reveals papilledema.
- Subdural abscess: In this condition, there is pyrexia, a grave headache, signs of irritated meninges, worsening neurological signs, fits and evidence of raised intracranial pressure, such as emesis and papilledema [14].
- Cerebral abscess: Patients present with cephalgia, nuchal rigidity, altered mental status, emesis, localising neurological signs, convulsions, involvement of oculomotor and abducens cranial nerves, and papilledema.

40.2 Preseptal Cellulitis

Preseptal cellulitis is common in the setting of acute rhinosinusitis. The blephara and soft tissues surrounding the orbit are affected, becoming acutely swollen and erythematous. The condition may be provoked by bacterial, viral, fungal, or helminthic pathogens. Direct extension of bacterial sinusitis, infection of nasolacrimal system, or an infection of surrounding soft tissue can be the culprits. In addition, injury to the blephara may also cause the condition [15].

Postseptal cellulitis (i.e. affecting the orbit itself) is generally a more serious condition than preseptal cellulitis. The presentation of both may exhibit marked similarities at the beginning. The key difference lies in the fact that preseptal infection does not extend beyond the soft tissues lying in front of the septum of the orbit [15].

Preseptal cellulitis may, however, progress into postseptal cellulitis. Abscesses may develop in the subperiosteum and the orbit itself. Once the orbit is involved, there is the possibility of thrombosis occurring within the cavernous sinus, or involvement of the meninges [15].

40.2.1 Orbital Septum

Classification of periorbital inflammation depends on where it occurs and how severe it is. A key anatomical structure that defines the region affected is the orbital septum, a slender membranous structure with its origin in the periosteum of the bony orbital wall. It has its insertion anteriorly on the tarsi. This structure forms a division between the more superficial portion of the eyelid and the orbit lying at greater depth, forming an obstacle to the spread of pathogens from the blephara into the eyeball itself [15].

40.2.2 Aetiology

Preseptal cellulitis may be caused by pathogens being directly deposited within the tissues or by extension from a nearby infected area. Orbital cellulitis and preseptal cellulitis often occur following an infection affecting the upper airway (upper respiratory tract infection; URTI), particularly the paranasal sinuses. Two large cases series identified URTI as a preceding event in almost two out of three instances where cellulitis occurred. Fifty percent of the time such individuals had sinusitis [15].

The pathogens occurring with the highest frequency are *Staphylococcus aureus*, *Staphylococcus epidermidis*, Streptococci, and anaerobic bacteria. These are the same agents responsible for bacterial infections of the upper airways and the outer blepharon. Typically, it is difficult to grow specific pathogens from blood or skin culture [15].

Studies of pathogens cultured from venous sampling in 1985, before the Hib (*H. influenzae* type b) polysaccharide vaccine entered into use, reveal that *H. influenzae* used to be the most prevalent organism identified [15–18]. According to one study predating the adoption of Hib vaccination, the presence of infection in the upper airways led to a 42% chance of positive blood culture. In cases where there was blepharal injury or infection of the eye originating externally, there was a 44% likelihood of a positive culture from aspirates drawn from below the skin [15].

40.2.3 Risk Factors

The following blepharal conditions all represent risk factors for preseptal cellulitis, where they are antecedent [15]:

- Stye
- Chalazion
- Insect bite [19]
- Traumatic injury [19, 20]
- Iatrogenic injury following a recent operation in the vicinity of the blephara [20]
- Iatrogenic, secondary to oral surgery
- Nasolacrimal system infections

An infection of the upper airway, particularly sinusitis [8], may occur at the same time as preseptal cellulitis or precede it slightly. Numerous systemic disorders are known to occur co-morbidly with preseptal cellulitis, such as:

- Varicella
- Asthma
- Sinonasal polyposis
- Neutropenia

40.2.4 Clinical Presentation

There may be mild to moderate pyrexia. Despite its being stated that leukocytosis and pyrexia are more common in postseptal cellulitis than preseptal cellulitis, the general consensus is that these two features are insufficient to permit distinguishing pre- from postseptal cellulitis. The following features may also be present:

- Pain
- Conjunctival inflammation
- Epiphora
- Blurring of vision

Preseptal cellulitis may produce erythematous swelling around the orbit, which, on occasion is sufficient to prevent patients from raising their eyelids on command [15].

40.2.5 Physical Examination

Since blepharitis may be a presentation of either pre- or postseptal cellulitis, the eye needs to be examined fully to make an accurate diagnosis. Clinicians should actively seek indications of a systemic disorder, particularly in paediatric cases.

Careful inspection of the blephara and adjoining structures is required to identify areas of trauma. Lymphadenopathy in the cervical, submandibular, and preauricular nodes should be assessed. Tender lymphadenopathy of a single preauricular node indicates possible conjunctival infection by an adenovirus. Conjunctival infection may be evident. Observe how the conjunctivae are draining [15].

All cases of blepharitis call for assessment of visual acuity and testing of pupillary reactivity. The signs that indicate preseptal infection has progressed to postseptal infection include restricted eye movement, visual impairment, and impairment to afferent pupillary responses. Afferent pupillary response deficit indicates compression of the second cranial nerve (optic nerve) and requires surgical exploration and drainage without delay [15].

40.2.6 Staging [21]

The degree to which the orbit is involved can be characterised by CT imaging [22]. The modified Chandler staging system is in use to delineate the levels of cellulitis, namely:

- Stage I - Preseptal cellulitis
- Stage II - Inflammation with an oedematous orbit
- Stage III - Abscess in the subperiosteum
- Stage IV - Abscess within the orbit
- Stage V - Cavernous sinus thrombosis

40.2.7 Treatment

There are a number of agents suitable for pharmacotherapy of preseptal cellulitis, namely [15]:

- Co-amoxiclav or ceftriaxone via intramuscular injection are suitable for treating specific non-hospitalised individuals.
- Cephalosporins belonging to the second generation or third generation are potentially useful for pharmacotherapy when culture results are unknown due to their broad-spectrum antibacterial efficacy.
- Synthetic penicillin which is penicillinase-resistant, such as nafcillin or oxacillin, may be used when *S. aureus* is suspected as the pathogen.

Cases that respond to intravascular treatment within 48 to 72 hours can be switched to oral pharmacotherapy and monitored for 24 hours to observe response.

A palpebral abscess may need to be drained operatively; [23] however this is not generally required if preseptal cellulitis is without complications. An infected nasolacrimal duct or dacryocystitis might also require surgical drainage if it develops acutely and begins pointing [15].

40.3 Orbital Cellulitis

The principal types of infection affecting the orbit itself and the adjoining structures are pre- and postseptal cellulitis. Orbital cellulitis refers to postseptal infection occurring within the orbital soft tissues. Preseptal cellulitis affects the palpebral soft tissues and the area surrounding the orbit but does not extend beyond the orbital septum. On occasion, distinguishing between pre- and postseptal cellulitis can be challenging [24].

There are number of aetiologies for postseptal cellulitis. This condition has an association with grave consequences. Up to 11% of individuals with postseptal cellulitis may lose their vision. Prompt diagnosis and early appropriate treatment are key to successful outcome [24].

40.3.1 Anatomy

The orbital septum is formed by a fascial plane which stretches from the periosteal layer around the margin of the orbit as far as the tendinous tissue of the levator muscle on the superior blepharon and the lower margin of the tarsus within the inferior blepharon [24].

40.3.2 Aetiology

Postseptal cellulitis may arise through the following pathogenic mechanisms [25]:

- Spread of an infection from the paranasal sinuses or other locations surrounding the orbit, e.g. the face, the eyeball, or the lacrimal canal.
- Direct introduction of a pathogen into the orbit due to trauma or a surgical procedure.
- Bacteria may enter the orbit via bacteraemia.

Postseptal cellulitis frequently occurs secondary to infected paranasal sinuses, as well as resulting from movement of pathogens out of the eyeball, the blephara, structures adjoining the eyes, or in the vicinity of the eye. Postseptal cellulitis can be secondary to an infected nasolacrimal, deep bone infection in the periorbital osseous structures, facial vein phlebitis, or odontogenic [24].

The single most frequent condition resulting in postseptal cellulitis, whatever the age of the patient, is ethmoid sinusitis which can be the cause in more than 90% of patients. The common pathogens are aerobic bacteria that do not sporulate. Sinusitis causes paranasal sinus mucosal oedema, which leads to obstruction of sinus ostia. The normal bacterial flora found within the sinus and upper airways overgrows and penetrates the swollen mucosal lining. Pus is then formed. Since there develops a relatively anaerobic environment within the sinus, pathogenic multiplication is favoured [24].

40.3.3 Traumatic Causes

Pathogens may be inoculated in a direct fashion into the orbital cavity following trauma (such as a fracture affecting the orbit) or be iatrogenic (i.e. after surgery). Any trauma that compromises the integrity of the orbital septum carries the risk of preseptal cellulitis. Inflamed tissue in the orbit appears between 48 and 72 hours after pathogenic inoculation [19]. If a foreign body remains within the wound, it may be a number of months before signs of inflammation appear [24].

A number of operations, notably orbital decompression, dacryocystorhinostomy, procedures on the blephara [26], strabismus correction, retinal surgery, and operations within the eye itself, are noted as events potentially precipitating postseptal cellulitis. Postsurgical endophthalmitis may spread to involve the soft tissues around the eyeball [24].

40.3.4 Bacterial Causes

The bacterial pathogens most frequently associated with postseptal cellulitis are Streptococci, *S. aureus* and *H. influenzae* type b. Other pathogens belonging to the genera *Pseudomonas, Klebsiella, Eikenella or Enterococcus are rare. In cases that occur in individuals who are older than 16 years, multi-microbial infection, both aerobes and anaerobes, become more common.*

40.3.5 Fungal Causes

The key fungal pathogens producing postseptal cellulitis belong to the genera *Mucor* or *Aspergillus*. These pathogens can invade the orbit. The risk of death is considerable where postseptal cellulitis secondary to a fungal pathogen occurs in the context of immunosuppression [24].

Mucormycetic invasive fungal sinusitis and orbital infection (zygomycosis, mucormycosis or phycomycosis) occurs in many countries [25–27], whereas the frequency of aspergillosis is highest where the climate is warm and with high humidity. Invasive fungal infection can lead to acute vasculitis producing thrombosis that develops over one day to one week [24]. Aspergillosis, on the other hand, can at times present as an indolent or chronic infection in contrast may be slowly developing and persistent, with a timescale of months or years [24].

40.3.6 Prognosis

Postseptal cellulitis may cause complications which affect the orbit or the cranial cavity. Between 7 and 9% of cases go on to from an abscess in the subperiosteum or the orbit, and irreversible visual damage may be caused by injury to the cornea following exposure or neurotrophic keratitis. The structures within the eye may be destroyed, and there may be the development of glaucoma or optic neuritis. The central retinal artery can become occluded. Patients may become blind following raised intraocular pressure or if a pathogen invades the second cranial nerve via the sphenoid sinus or orbital fissures. If infection spreads to the cranial nerves supplying the soft tissue surrounding the extra-ocular muscles or the muscles themselves, restriction of eye movement can develop [24].

40.3.7 Physical Examination

Proptosis of an eye or weakness of the extrinsic eye muscles are the key features to look for in postseptal cellulitis. Postseptal cellulitis may develop with frightening rapidity and cause complete physical exhaustion in a patient [24].

In addition to the features above, other possible signs are [24]:

- Loss of vision, defective colour vision, and Marcus Gunn pupil.
- Raised intraocular tension.
- Pain with eye movement.
- Chemotic conjunctivae.
- The orbit is painful and tender, even at onset.
- The blephara may take on a dark erythematous hue, the conjunctivae may be chemotic and bloodshot. Retropulsion of the eyeball may be difficult.
- Pus-filled rhinorrhoea may occur.

At the beginning, visual abnormalities may not be present. In paediatric cases with severe illness and where there is a high degree of oedema, assessment of visual ability may be challenging [24].

Additionally, the following features may be present [24]:

- Pyrexia
- Cephalgia
- Blepharal swelling
- Nasal discharge
- Worsening sense of being unwell

If there are numerous abscesses in the orbit or there is an abscess within the lacrimal gland, there is a possibility of methicillin-resistant *S. aureus* (MRSA).

40.3.8 Treatment

Any case of postseptal cellulitis calls for in-patient therapy without delay, and the patient should not be discharged while still pyrexial and a definite improvement in clinical condition has not been noted. In the past, if an abscess occurred subperiosteally or within the orbit, the lesion would be drained surgically in addition to pharmacotherapy with antibiotics [24].

An orbital compartment syndrome, when diagnosed, is an emergency indication for canthotomy and cantholysis. Individuals in whom the cornea becomes exposed will need to be provided with artificial lubrication for the cornea [24].

Where a case fails to respond to suitable antibiotic therapy in the first one to two days, operative drainage may be needed. This also applies when there is total opacification of the ipsilateral sinus(es) on imaging (such as CT or MRI), an abscess is present within the orbit, or an abscess of considerable size is present within the subperiosteum, even more so in adults. Once sited, drains must remain in situ over a number of days. Repeated procedures to drain the abscess may be called for. Where a fungal organism is responsible, the orbit needs to be debrided and in advanced cases exenteration of the orbit and sinus can be necessary [24].

40.4 Intracranial Complications

Postseptal cellulitis may cause complications which affect the orbit or the cranial cavity. Between 7 and 9% of cases go on to from an abscess in the subperiosteum or the orbit, and irreversible visual damage may be caused by injury to the cornea following exposure or neurotrophic keratitis. The structures within the eye may be destroyed, and there may be the development of glaucoma or optic neuritis. The central artery within the retina may become occluded. Patients may become blind following raised pressure within the orbit or if a pathogen invades the second cranial nerve via the sphenoid sinus.

If infection spreads to the nerves supplying the eye muscles or the muscles themselves, the eyes may develop restriction on their movement [24].

40.4.1 Cavernous Sinus Thrombosis

It may be challenging to differentiate between uncomplicated postseptal cellulitis and cavernous sinus thrombosis. This latter may result from paranasal sinusitis if the infected region (usually the middle third of the face, i.e. the orbit, mouth or paranasal sinuses) extends to involve the cavernous sinus. Moreover, cavernous sinus thrombosis and superior ophthalmic vein thrombosis may also themselves be the consequence of postseptal cellulitis [28].

In cases of cavernous sinus thrombosis that lack preseptal cellulitis, there is weakness of the external eye muscles but the eyes are at most slightly proptotic. The globe can be retropulsed normally. The ophthalmic and maxillary branches of the fifth cranial nerve have lessened sensation, the veins of the retina show dilatation, the orbit is congested and there may be other neurological signs, such as altered sensory perception. MRI with magnetic resonance venography (MRV) offers potential diagnostic benefit in cases of cavernous sinus thrombosis [24]. Treatment entails drainage of the infected sinus(es) or periorbital soft tissue in addition to prolonged intravenous antibiotics. Neurology and neurosurgery consultations should be obtained. These patients require hospitalisation, frequently in an intensive care setting.

References

1. Wald ER. Acute bacterial rhinosinusitis in children: clinical features and diagnosis. In: Kaplan SL, Wood RA, Isaacson GC, Torchia MM (Eds). UpToDate Last updated: May 13, 2019.
2. Brook I. Microbiology and antimicrobial treatment of orbital and intracranial complications of sinusitis in children and their management. Int J Pediatr Otorhinolaryngol. 2009;73:1183.
3. Clayman GL, Adams GL, Paugh DR, Koopmann CF Jr. Intracranial complications of paranasal sinusitis: a combined institutional review. Laryngoscope. 1991;101:234.
4. Goytia VK, Giannoni CM, Edwards MS. Intraorbital and intracranial extension of sinusitis: comparative morbidity. J Pediatr. 2011;158:486.
5. Hicks CW, Weber JG, Reid JR, Moodley M. Identifying and managing intracranial complications of sinusitis in children: a retrospective series. Pediatr Infect Dis J. 2011;30:222.
6. Sable NS, Hengerer A, Powell KR. Acute frontal sinusitis with intracranial complications. Pediatr Infect Dis. 1984;3:58.
7. Wassermann D. Acute paranasal sinusitis and cavernous sinus thrombosis. Arch Otolaryngol. 1967;86:205.
8. Whitaker CW. Intracranial complications of ear, nose, and throat infections. Laryngoscope. 1971;81:1375.
9. Germiller JA, Monin DL, Sparano AM, Tom LW. Intracranial complications of sinusitis in children and adolescents and their outcomes. Arch Otolaryngol Head Neck Surg. 2006;132:969.
10. Bair-Merritt MH, Shah SS, Zaoutis TE, et al. Suppurative intracranial complications of sinusitis in previously healthy children. Pediatr Infect Dis J. 2005;24:384.
11. Sultész M, Csákányi Z, Majoros T, et al. Acute bacterial rhinosinusitis and its complications in our pediatric otolaryngological department between 1997 and 2006. Int J Pediatr Otorhinolaryngol. 2009;73:1507.
12. Soon VT. Pediatric subperiosteal orbital abscess secondary to acute sinusitis: a 5-year review. Am J Otolaryngol. 2011;32:62.
13. Bambakidis NC, Cohen AR. Intracranial complications of frontal sinusitis in children: Pott's puffy tumor revisited. Pediatr Neurosurg. 2001;35:82.
14. Sàez-Llorens X, Guevara JN. Parameningeal infections. In: Cherry JD, Harrison G, Kaplan SL, et al., editors. Feigin and Cherry's textbook of pediatric infectious diseases. 8th ed. Philadelphia: Elsevier; 2018. p. 336.
15. Adams WG, Deaver KA, Cochi SL, Plikaytis BD, Zell ER, Broome CV, et al. Decline of childhood Haemophilus influenzae type b (Hib) disease in the Hib vaccine era. JAMA. 1993;269(2):221–6.
16. Ambati BK, Ambati J, Azar N, Stratton L, Schmidt EV. Periorbital and orbital cellulitis before and after the advent of Haemophilus influenzae type B vaccination. Ophthalmology. 2000;107(8):1450–3.
17. Barone SR, Aiuto LT. Periorbital and orbital cellulitis in the Haemophilus influenzae vaccine era. J Pediatr Ophthalmol Strabismus. 1997;34(5):293–6.
18. Donahue SP, Schwartz G. Preseptal and orbital cellulitis in childhood. A changing microbiologic spectrum. Ophthalmology. 1998;105(10):1902–5.
19. Babar TF, Zaman M, Khan MN, Khan MD. Risk factors of preseptal and orbital cellulitis. J Coll Physicians Surg Pak. 2009;19(1):39–42.
20. Chaudhry IA, Shamsi FA, Elzaridi E, Al-Rashed W, Al-Amri A, Arat YO. Inpatient preseptal cellulitis: experience from a tertiary eye care centre. Br J Ophthalmol. 2008;92(10):1337–41.
21. Eustis HS, Armstrong DC, Buncic JR, Morin JD. Staging of orbital cellulitis in children: computerized tomography characteristics and treatment guidelines. J Pediatr Ophthalmol Strabismus. 1986;23(5):246–51.
22. Ho CF, Huang YC, Wang CJ, Chiu CH, Lin TY. Clinical analysis of computed tomography-staged orbital cellulitis in children. J Microbiol Immunol Infect. 2007;40(6):518–26.
23. Anari S, Karagama YG, Fulton B, et al. Neonatal disseminated methicillin-resistant Staphylococcus aureus presenting as orbital cellulitis. J Laryngol Otol. 2005 Jan.;119(1):64–7.

24. Bergin DJ, Wright JE. Orbital cellulitis. Br J Ophthalmol. 1986 Mar.;70(3):174–8.
25. Boden JH, Ainbinder DJ. Methicillin-resistant ascending facial and orbital cellulitis in an operation Iraqi freedom troop population. Ophthal Plast Reconstr Surg. 2007;23(5):397–9.
26. Bullock JD, Fleishman JA. Orbital cellulitis following dental extraction. Trans Am Ophthalmol Soc. 1984;82:111–33.
27. Blomquist PH. Methicillin-resistant Staphylococcus aureus infections of the eye and orbit (an American ophthalmological society thesis). Trans Am Ophthalmol Soc. 2006;104:322–45.
28. van der Poel NA, de Witt KD, van den Berg R, de Win MM, Mourits MP. Impact of superior ophthalmic vein thrombosis: a case series and literature review. Orbit. 2018:1–7.

Nasal and Paranasal Sinus Infections in Children with Cystic Fibrosis

41

Ali Seyed Resuli, Cemal Cingi, and Glenis Scadding

41.1 Introduction

Cystic fibrosis (CF) is a chronic disease that involves multiple body systems and features repeated infective episodes affecting the bronchi, resulting in steadily worsening obstructive lung pathology and failure of the pancreas, which leads to malabsorption from the gut.

In the majority of cases of CF disorders of the sinuses and nose develop, resulting in referral to ENT specialists. It appears probable that the frequency and pathogenetic mechanism for other disorders affecting the head and neck, e.g. middle ear infections or pathology of the adenoids and tonsils, are little different in patients with CF from those without the condition [1, 2]. Interestingly, though, it seems that CF patients are less prone to otitis media than other people, although why this is so remains a mystery [3]. The focus of this chapter is disorders of the sinuses and nose in patients with CF [4].

CF is a genetic disorder with an autosomal recessive mode of inheritance. It involves mutated CF alleles on chromosome seven. The gene involved produces the CF transmembrane regulator (CFTR) protein, which transports chloride ions across the cellular outer membrane [5]. If this protein has defective function, chloride

A. S. Resuli (✉)
Department of Otorhinolaryngology, Faculty of Medicine, İstanbul Yeni Yüzyıl University, İstanbul, Turkey

C. Cingi
Department of Otorhinolaryngology, Faculty of Medicine, Eskişehir Osmangazi University, Eskişehir, Turkey

G. Scadding
University College London, Royal National Throat, Nose, and Ear Hospital (Honorary Consultant Physician in Allergy and Rhinology), London, UK

© The Author(s), under exclusive license to Springer Nature Switzerland AG 2022
C. Cingi et al. (eds.), *Pediatric ENT Infections*,
https://doi.org/10.1007/978-3-030-80691-0_41

regulation by the mucosal epithelium of the airways and exocrine glands is abnormal, and a viscous layer of mucus pools in these regions [6].

The clinical presentation of CF is dominated by infections in the lower portion of the respiratory tree, as well as pancreatic failure. However, virtually all sufferers from this disorder also experience chronic rhinosinusitis, since mucus pooling also occurs in the sinuses and nose [7–10]. Such disease within the sinuses can produce a high level of morbidity in itself, in addition to a postulated negative effect on any lung pathology, and for this reason, ENT specialists are frequently called upon to assess and treat individuals suffering from CF [6].

41.2 Sinonasal Manifestations in Cystic Fibrosis

Rhinosinusitis refers to inflammation of the nasal lining, occurring in conjunction with inflammation of at least a single sinus. The pathogenesis involves multiple elements, notably dysfunctional mucociliary clearance, infection, atopy, swelling of the mucosa and, on occasion, atypical anatomical conformation of the nasal interior or the sinuses surrounding the nose [6, 10]. As estimated by looking at symptomatic occurrence, abnormal findings on physical examination and imaging, almost 100% of CF patients experience rhinosinusitis [8–10]. It is probable that sinus disorders are so common in individuals with CF because of the abnormal consistency of sinonasal mucus, which prevents effective drainage by the mucociliary mechanism. When the ostia become obstructed, the cilia are damaged, with the result that an inflammatory oedematous process is set in motion. This process is also driven by the presence of pathogenic bacteria, notably Pseudomonas, *Staphylococcus aureus* and non-typeable *Haemophilus influenzae*, which colonise the sinuses. These are respiratory pathogens of both upper and lower tract [11]. It has also been proposed by researchers that mutation of the CFTR allele may itself be an independent risk factor for sinonasal disorders, since even non-CF patients with chronic rhinosinusitis are more likely to possess a single mutated allele [12, 13].

The presenting complaints occurring with highest frequency in cases of sinusitis in patients with CF are stuffiness and pus-filled rhinorrhoea. Other symptoms that are frequent are cephalgia, oral breathing and abnormalities of olfaction. There is some variation in the usual findings from physical examination, but the constant features are pus-filled discharge and altered sinonasal lining, causing the nose to be blocked. In paediatric CF cases, anterior rhinoscopy or nasal endoscopy may identify polyps in as many as 86% of individuals. The exact figures reported by researchers differ, depending on the population studied and the composition of any groups compared [14–20]. There may be hypertrophy of the turbinates as well as hyperplastic lymphoid tissue in the back of the throat.

41.3 Clinical Evaluation

The history plays a key role in deciding how to manage CF patients with sinonasal disease, hence a meticulously detailed history focusing on symptoms affecting the nose and sinuses is required [4].

Features that need to be asked about within the history are as follows [21]:

- Blocked nose
- Deteriorating rhinorrhoea
- Pain over the face
- Deterioration in coughing
- Pyrexia

Between 90% and 100% of CF patients have imaging results indicating a sinus disorder [22–24], but polyp formation in the nose is less predictable, affecting between 6 and 67% of cases [2]. The frequency of nasal polyp formation increases with rising age. At the age of 6 years, 19% of cases have polyps that can be identified at endoscopy. By the age of 18 years, this figure has risen to 45% [25]. There is a higher frequency of polyps noted for patients who are homozygous for the delta f508 mutated allele [26].

A mere 10% of individuals with CF actually experience symptoms of sinusitis, such as pain, rhinorrhoea, pyrexia, or postnasal drainage [22]. Accordingly, the majority of cases where imaging shows sinusitis are asymptomatic. There are two ways to explain this situation: either the patient truly has no symptoms despite active pathology; or individuals may have mentally adjusted to such a situation and no longer perceive it as being abnormal [27].

In deciding to treat sinusitis, more emphasis is placed on the patient's reported symptoms than on the results of imaging investigations.

When taking a history, doctors should also enquire about lung-related symptoms. Not only is there a strong correlation between bacterial bronchitis and chronic sinusitis, but sinusitis also affects the degree of responsivity of the bronchial airways and the longevity of diseased periods. Also organisms are found in the sinuses before colonising the lungs (please find this reference). A declining ability to tolerate exercise is frequently associated with flare-ups of acute sinusitis or deterioration in chronic sinusitis [28, 29].

41.4 Physical Assessment

In the majority of cases, those referred to ENT specialists have already been diagnosed with CF and the aim of referral is to assess the need for surgical interventions on the sinus. Patients need to be examined physically in a detailed and comprehensive way so that the nasal cavity and sinuses can be assessed and any other factors predisposing to sinusitis may be identified.

When inspecting the face, the clinician may note broadening of the bridge of the nose, arising from chronic nasal polyp formation. Occasionally, a polyp may even be visible, emerging from the nostrils. Anterior rhinoscopic examination may reveal oedema of the turbinates, pus-filled rhinorrhoea and polyps within the nose. Endoscopic evaluation may allow visualisation of polyps that are blocking the airway or the sinus ostium within the middle meatus. Pus may be seen discharging. It is not unusual to note the uncinate process projecting sufficiently to block part of the airway within the nose.

Assessment of the nasopharynx is similarly required. In a young patient, the adenoids may have hypertrophied and may be contributing to obstructed airflow within the nose. Just as with any other patient, CF sufferers need to have adenoidal hypertrophy treated prior to undertaking surgery on the sinuses [4].

## 41.5	Diagnosis

Sometimes CF may be diagnosed by an ENT specialist who notes the presence of multiple polyps in the nose of a paediatric patient with no other apparent health issues. On occasion, an individual with CF adapts to the condition to such an extent that they fail to present clinically at an early stage. Segal reports a frequency for CF of 1 in 16 children with nasal polyposis, but otherwise seemingly healthy [30]. The genetic abnormalities leading to CF vary, leading to a variety of severity in this disorder (pl find a reference).

CF children may be well grown and healthy looking therefore it is advisable to carry out the sweat chloride test on all paediatric cases presenting with polyp formation in the nose, to avoid missing a case of CF.

It is unusual, but possible, for paediatric cases of nasal polyposis to be seen in children who do not have CF. In such instances, the probable aetiology is allergic rhinitis of high severity, inflammatory responses linked to the Samter triad (asthma, intolerance of salicylates and polyp formation within the nose), Kartagener syndrome (organ reversal and non-motile cilia) or immune conditions of some other type. Diagnosis in such cases depends on thorough history-taking and physical examination, as well as the sweat test and a biopsy to examine the ciliary morphology, according to the presentation.

According to the research undertaken by Thamboo et al., the Sinonasal Outcome Test (SNOT-22), which consists of 22 questions, is suitable for screening paediatric CF cases for seemingly asymptomatic polyp formation within the nose. This research enrolled 37 children. If the SNOT-22 score was greater than 11, polyps could be accurately predicted 68.1% of the time, their absence predicted correctly 66.7% of the time, and the positive likelihood ratio was 1.82 [31].

### 41.5.1	CT Imaging

The degree of symptomatic discomfort and the severity as rated by CT imaging are only weakly correlated [32]. The symptomatic presentation is what guides how this condition is diagnosed and treated. The indications for undertaking CT imaging are to ascertain how extensive the condition is and to plan any surgical procedures. Axial and coronal sections are suitable, and no contrast agent is needed. CT should be employed sparingly in a growing child because of potential harm from being exposed to a source of radiation. The resulting imagery has often been put in the most appropriate format to assist with operative interventions (see following text). Accordingly, if the clinician ordering CT suspects that operative intervention may be called for, liaison with an ENT specialist is recommended first.

The radiological findings consistent with chronic sinusitis are an opacified lumen, movement of the lateral wall of the nasal cavity medially in the area of the middle meatus, and the uncinate process appears decalcified. These appearances are seen in above 90% of patients with CF [33]. At endoscopy, the medially displaced lateral wall of the nose is evident, as seen radiologically, but until recently this phenomenon had not been quantified. However, Herovchon et al. [34] have now quantified the degree of displacement in research using CT imaging that measured the angles created by the uncinate process.

In some 12% of patients, the lateral wall of the nose protrudes medially, whilst the maxillary sinus contains thick mucus. These findings most resemble a mucocoele, which requires surgical intervention [21, 27].

The maxillary and ethmoid sinuses are frequently hypoplastic and contain little air in individuals with chronic sinusitis. Likewise, the frontal sinuses are underdeveloped [35]. It is frequent to note the absence of a hollow space in the frontal sinus in a CF patient who has reached adolescence [4].

41.5.2 Nitric Oxide

By filtering, warming, and humidifying inhaled air, the nasal cavity and turbinates play critical physiological roles. Nitric oxide (NO), a reactive oxygen species that spreads to the bronchi and lungs to cause bronchodilatory and vasodilatory effects, is continually released by paranasal sinuses and is part of the innate immune system, being toxic to bacteria and viruses. Nasal NO levels tend to be very low in CF, probably secondary to sinus obstruction (37). This, along with reduced mucociliary clearance may allow infection to occur. Replacement of NO is being tested currently. Low nasal NO levels may also alert the astute ENT surgeon to the possible diagnosis and can provide a marker of the effectiveness of sinus surgery (38).

41.6   Treatment

41.6.1 Nasal Douching

Nasal douching with saline may be helpful in removing allergens, pollutants and infective agents. In rhinosinusitis cases, especially in patients with cystic fibrosis, nasal douching helps clear infected secretions and may improve nasal patency **(39).** Seawater may be superior to saline (40).

41.6.2 Antimicrobial Pharmacotherapy

The bacteria responsible for nasal and sinus infections are different in cases of CF from those typically seen, hence antibiotic pharmacotherapy also differs. Whereas Pseudomonas occurs in virtually all cases with CF, this is not the case in non-CF patients.

Treatment of patients with CF using antibiotics typically aims to control pathogenic microbes that are found along the whole length of the respiratory tract. Antimicrobial pharmacotherapy may be informed by cultured material from the middle meatus or from sputum. The organisms which are most often isolated are *Pseudomonas aeruginosa* and *Staphylococcus aureus* [36]. Usually, antibiotic agents by mouth are prescribed prophylactically to individuals with CF for prevention of respiratory infections (upper or lower) or for management of already existing infections [37]. Although the employment of antibiotics by inhalation, notably tobramycin, colistin or aztreonam is commonplace, since these agents may lessen bacterial colonisation and thus offer improvements in pulmonary function, whether this treatment has any actual benefit in upper respiratory infections is unclear [38–40]. One problem here is the known ototoxicity of aminoglycosides, such as tobramycin. These agents produce sensorineural deafness and injury to the labyrinth, following prolonged use [41]. This situation alone should prompt the involvement of ENT specialists in management of CF. It is known that chronic rhinosinusitis can be effectively treated with antibiotics given by mouth in non-CF cases [42], hence there may be a reason to try the same in CF cases, too. One study found that the dimensions of polyps within the nose in CF patients were reduced following prolonged systemic pharmacotherapy using macrolide antibiotics [43].

41.6.3 Corticosteroids

The usual benefit from intranasal corticosteroids lies in their reducing swelling of the nasal lining and enhancing mucociliary drainage. This applies both acutely and for lengthier periods. Using oral corticosteroid treatment for a brief period may offer benefit in acute infective episodes. Furthermore, they potentially lessen blood loss during surgical procedures to remove nasal polyps if given before the procedure begins. Steroid treatment is commonplace in managing lung-related symptoms suffered by CF patients. It may help in reducing nasal and sinus symptoms, too, but there is a regrettable lack of evidence to reveal exactly how steroid therapy administered orally affects the symptoms of sinus disease in patients with CF. The Cochrane Collaboration have released a review summarising the evidence from a number of trials in which steroids were administered by mouth to CF sufferers. There were definite benefits in reducing the rate lung disease progressed, making admission to hospital for respiratory problems less common and giving a higher life quality. There was a lack of direct evidence on symptoms of disease in the nose and sinuses [44]. However, since it is recognised that steroids by mouth do offer benefits in non-CF patients suffering from chronic sinusitis, it is not unreasonable to propose employing steroids for the treatment of sinusitis in CF cases, too [45, 46].

41.6.4 Other Therapies

Decongestant agents are less guaranteed to be beneficial. Antihistamine treatment not only lacks benefit but may even be harmful, since the secretions become even more viscid. In cases of CF, mucolytic agents typically offer no benefit. One exception to this principle is the employment of recombinant human deoxyribonuclease in infections of the lung and bronchi, where benefit has been shown. It reduces the viscoelasticity of sputum and improves breathing of (CF) patients [4].

41.6.5 Surgery

The evidence-base to support objective recommendations for when surgical interventions are appropriate in CF unfortunately does not yet exist. However, there are certain situations when it is reasonable to think about operative interventions, namely [4]:

- If the nose is significantly obstructed by intranasal polyp formation or the lateral wall of the nasal interior bulges medially, even despite aggressive pharmacotherapy, surgery may be appropriate.
- When it is noted at endoscopy or on CT imaging that the lateral wall of the nasal interior has shifted towards the midline, surgery may be warranted. This applies even if the patient has no symptoms of a blocked nose, since this phenomenon is highly likely to be due to a developing mucocele.
- Worsening of lung disease that seems to be linked to a deterioration in sinusitis, deterioration of lung function or decreased exercise tolerance, in spite of optimal pharmacotherapy, may be an indication for surgery.
- If no other cause than sinonasal disease can be ascribed to pain over the face or cephalgia, and this pain is reducing life quality.
- If the patient is dissatisfied with what has been achieved through optimal pharmacotherapy and remains troubled by nasal and sinus symptoms [27].

The situations in which operative interventions are contraindicated are as follows [4]:

- Obstructive lung disease of high severity, since general anaesthetics may be associated with intolerable risks.
- Deficiency of vitamin K and coagulation disorders of other causes. Patients with CF have inadequate activity by the pancreas and suffer from disorders of the liver and bile secretion. Thus, they may not absorb adequate vitamin K,

leading to a tendency to prolonged bleeding [47]. If the clotting profile performed prior to surgery indicates a lengthened prothrombin time (PT), the operation should not be undertaken until the PT has been brought back into the normal range.

- Hypoplasia of the sinus cavities may be considered relatively contraindicative for surgery. In CF patients, the maxillary, ethmoid and frontal sinuses may develop later than normal and contain less air than expected. It is common for hypoplasia affecting the sinuses to be noted on CT imaging. Given the additional risks that sinus hypoplasia imposes on surgical interventions, the imaging results need to be minutely checked and the operating surgeon should already have experience of this situation.

As with all patients presenting for sinus surgery, the approach in the past to CF cases was to employ simple polypectomy, open ethmoidectomy or the Caldwell-Luc method. Historically, polypectomy in CF cases has been associated with a decrease in symptoms at first but a greater than 80% risk that the lesions will recur [48–50]. More radical procedures, notably ethmoidectomy or Caldwell-Luc, offer a lower risk of recurrence of 45 to 60% in the two to eight years after the operation [46, 51]. As surgical interventions on the sinuses have developed in sophistication over the last few years, there has been increasing optimism that surgery can achieve higher success rates in CF cases, whilst becoming less invasive in nature. The safety and efficacy of surgery to the sinuses carried out endoscopically (ESS) has been demonstrated in numerous studies involving individuals suffering from CF [15, 52–57]. The benefits of ESS have been manifested as a decrease in nasal and sinus symptoms and a higher life quality in some studies [40, 57, 58], and as a lower risk of requiring redo operations than with conventional operations in others [59]. However, more radical types of operation on the sinuses may produce less benefit if the patient has CF. Georgalas et al. have recently published the results from a study of Draf type III (i.e. a modified Lothrop procedure done endoscopically) to drain the frontal sinus [60]. They examined long term outcomes, noting that, in their group of 122 cases, those patients who had CF were most at risk of the ostial entrance to the frontal sinus re-stenosing after surgery.

A procedure that possesses demonstrably equivalent efficacy to ESS in the treatment of chronic rhinosinusitis in patients without other disease is balloon catheter sinuplasty (BCS). This technique dates from 2006 [61]. Since its introduction, the technique has been specifically assessed in children with chronic rhinosinusitis to evaluate how efficacious and safe it is. Recently, results from research examining various cohorts suggest the technique is both safe and efficacious [62–65], whilst also benefitting from not requiring the excision of tissue, and preserving the integrity of the mucosae. It appears that BCS is especially suited for treating children with chronic rhinosinusitis, including those with CF. So far, studies focusing on the technique have not addressed CF cases in particular, but results from the use on other children are promising in terms of adding an extra option to the treatments clinicians have at their disposal to treat rhinosinusitis in paediatric CF cases.

41.6.6 Gene Therapy

This is a process in which a new, correct version of the CFTR gene is inserted into cells. Mutant copies of the CFTR gene remain, but the correct copy allows cells to make normal CFTR proteins. It is outwith the scope of this chapter, but more details can be found at https://www.cff.org/Research/Research-Into-the-Disease/Restore-CFTR-Function/Gene-Therapy-for-Cystic-Fibrosis

References

1. Cipolli M, Canciani M, Cavazzani M, et al. Ear disease is not a common complication in cystic fibrosis. Eur J Pediatr. 1993;152(3):265–6.
2. Halvorson DJ. Cystic fibrosis: an update for the otolaryngologist. Otolaryngol Head Neck Surg. 1999;120(4):502–6.
3. Haddad J Jr, Gonzalez C, Kurland G, et al. Ear disease in children with cystic fibrosis. Arch Otolaryngol Head Neck Surg. 1994;120(5):491–3.
4. Murray N. Sinonasal Manifestations of Cystic Fibrosis. In: Meyers AD (Ed). Medscape. Updated: May 23, 2019. https://emedicine.medscape.com/article/862538-overview (Accessed online at October 16, 2020).
5. Riordan JR, Rommens JM, Kerem BS, et al. Identification of the cystic fibrosis gene: cloning and characterization of complementary DNA. Science. 1989;245(4922):1066–73.
6. Oomen KP, April MM. Sinonasal manifestations in cystic fibrosis. Int J Otolaryngol. 2012;2012:789572. https://doi.org/10.1155/2012/789572.
7. Shatz A. Management of recurrent sinus disease in children with cystic fibrosis: a combined approach. Otolaryngology. 2006;135(2):248–52.
8. Tandon R, Derkay C. Contemporary management of rhinosinusitis and cystic fibrosis. Curr Opin Otolaryngol Head Neck Surg. 2003;11(1):41–4.
9. Cepero R, Smith RJH, Catlin FI, Bressler KL, Furuta GT, Shandera KC. Cystic fibrosis—an otolaryngologic perspective. Otolaryngology. 1987;97(4):356–60.
10. Kerrebijn JDF, Poublon RML, Overbeek SE. Nasal and paranasal disease in adult cystic fibrosis patients. Eur Respir J. 1992;5(10):1239–42.
11. Godoy JM, Godoy AN, Ribalta G, Largo I. Bacterial pattern in chronic sinusitis and cystic fibrosis. Otolaryngology. 2011;145:673–6.
12. Raman V, Clary R, Siegrist KL, Zehnbauer B, Chatila TA. Increased prevalence of mutations in the cystic fibrosis transmembrane conductance regulator in children with chronic rhinosinusitis. Pediatrics. 2002;109(1):E13.
13. Wang X, Moylan B, Leopold DA, et al. Mutation in the gene responsible for cystic fibrosis and predisposition to chronic rhinosinusitis in the general population. J Am Med Assoc. 2000;284(14):1814–9.
14. Cuyler JP, Monaghan AJ. Cystic fibrosis and sinusitis. J Otolaryngol. 1989;18(4):173–5.
15. Triglia JM, Nicollas R. Nasal and sinus polyposis in children. Laryngoscope. 1997;107(7):963–6.
16. Slieker MG, Schilder AGM, Uiterwaal CSPM, Van der Ent CK. Children with cystic fibrosis: who should visit the otorhinolaryngologist? Arch Otolaryngol. 2002;128(11):1245–8.
17. Ryan MW. Diseases associated with chronic rhinosinusitis: what is the significance? Curr Opin Otolaryngol Head Neck Surg. 2003;11:41–4.
18. Yung MW, Gould J, Upton GJG. Nasal polyposis in children with cystic fibrosis: a long-term follow-up study. Ann Otol Rhinol Laryngol. 2002;111(12):1081–6.
19. Smith TL, Mendolia-Loffredo S, Loehrl TA, Sparapani R, Laud PW, Nattinger AB. Predictive factors and outcomes in endoscopic sinus surgery for chronic rhinosinusitis. Laryngoscope. 2005;115(12):2199–205.

20. Sakano E, Ribeiro AF, Barth L, Neto AC, Ribeiro JD. Nasal and paranasal sinus endoscopy, computed tomography and microbiology of upper airways and the correlations with genotype and severity of cystic fibrosis. Int J Pediatr Otorhinolaryngol. 2007;71(1):41–50.
21. Brihaye P, Clement PA, Dab I, Desprechin B. Pathological changes of the lateral nasal wall in patients with cystic fibrosis (mucoviscidosis). Int J Pediatr Otorhinolaryngol. 1994;28(2–3):141–7.
22. Cepero R, Smith RJ, Catlin FI, et al. Cystic fibrosis--an otolaryngologic perspective. Otolaryngol Head Neck Surg. 1987;97(4):356–60.
23. Neely JG, Harrison GM, Jerger JF, et al. The otolaryngologic aspects of cystic fibrosis. Trans Am Acad Ophthalmol Otolaryngol. 1972;76(2):313–24.
24. Shwachman H, Kulcycki LL, Mueller HL. Nasal polyposis in patients with cystic fibrosis. Pediatrics. 1962;30:389–401.
25. Schraven SP, Wehrmann M, Wagner W, Blumenstock G, Koitschev A. Prevalence and histopathology of chronic polypoid sinusitis in pediatric patients with cystic fibrosis. J Cyst Fibros. 2011;10(3):181–6.
26. Babinski D, Trawinska-Bartnicka M. Rhinosinusitis in cystic fibrosis: not a simple story. Intl J Ped Otorhinol. 2008;72:619–24.
27. Nishioka GJ, Cook PR. Paranasal sinus disease in patients with cystic fibrosis. Otolaryngol Clin N Am. 1996;29(1):193–205.
28. Ramsey B, Richardson MA. Impact of sinusitis in cystic fibrosis. J Allergy Clin Immunol. 1992;90(3 Pt 2):547–52.
29. Nishioka GJ, Barbero GJ, Konig P, et al. Symptom outcome after functional endoscopic sinus surgery in patients with cystic fibrosis: a prospective study. Otolaryngol Head Neck Surg. 1995;113(4):440–5.
30. Segal N, Gluk O, Puterman M. Nasal polyps in the pediatric population. B-ENT. 2012;8(4):265–7.
31. Thamboo A, Santos RC, Naidoo L, Rahmanian R, Chilvers MA, Chadha NK. Use of the SNOT-22 and UPSIT to appropriately select pediatric patients with cystic fibrosis who should be referred to an otolaryngologist: cross-sectional study. JAMA Otolaryngol Head Neck Surg. 2014;140(10):934–9.
32. Sakano E, Ribeiro AF, Barth L, Neto AC, Ribeiro JD. Nasal and paranasal endoscopy computed tomography and microbiology of upper airways and the correlations with genotype and severity of cystic fibrosis. Intl J Ped Otorhinol. 2007;71:41–50.
33. April MM, Zinreich SJ, Baroody FM, Naclerio RM. Coronal CT scan abnormalities in children with chronic sinusitis. Laryngoscope. 1993;103(9):985–90.
34. Hervochon R, Teissier N, Blondeau JR, et al. Computed tomography description of the Uncinate process angulation in patients with cystic fibrosis and comparison with primary ciliary dyskinesia, nasal polyposis, and controls. Ear Nose Throat J. 2019;98(2):89–93.
35. Ledesma-Medina J, Osman MZ, Girdany BR. Abnormal paranasal sinuses in patients with cystic fibrosis of the pancreas. Radiological findings. Pediatr Radiol. 1980;9(2):61–4.
36. Desrosiers MY, Salas-Prato M. Treatment of chronic rhinosinusitis refractory to other treatments with topical antibiotic therapy delivered by means of a large-particle nebulizer: results of a controlled trial. Otolaryngol Head Neck Surg. 2001;125(3):265–9.
37. Anderson P. Emerging therapies in cystic fibrosis. Ther Adv Respir Dis. 2010;4(3):177–85.
38. Moss RB, King VV. Management of sinusitis in cystic fibrosis by endoscopic surgery and serial antimicrobial lavage. Reduction in recurrence requiring surgery. Arch Otolaryngol Head Neck Surg. 1995;121(5):566–72.
39. Franche GLDS, Abreu E, Silva F, Saleh CDS. Bacteriology of the middle meatus aspirate in patients with cystic fibrosis. Braz J Otorhinolaryngol. 2007;73(4):494–9.
40. Shapiro ED, Milmoe GJ, Wald ER. Bacteriology of the maxillary sinuses in patients with cystic fibrosis. J Infect Dis. 1982;146(5):589–93.
41. Hansen CR, Pressler T, Koch C, Høiby N. Long-term azitromycin treatment of cystic fibrosis patients with chronic *Pseudomonas aeruginosa* infection; an observational cohort study. J Cyst Fibros. 2005;4(1):35–40.

42. Pai VB, Nahata MC. Efficacy and safety of aerosolized tobramycin in cystic fibrosis. Pediatr Pulmonol. 2001;32(4):314–27.
43. Westerman EM, Le Brun PPH, Touw DJ, Frijlink HW, Heijerman HGM. Effect of nebulized colistin sulphate and colistin sulphomethate on lung function in patients with cystic fibrosis: a pilot study. J Cyst Fibros. 2004;3(1):23–8.
44. McCoy KS, Quittner AL, Oermann CM, Gibson RL, Retsch-Bogart GZ, Montgomery AB. Inhaled aztreonam lysine for chronic airway *Pseudomonas aeruginosa* in cystic fibrosis. Am J Respir Crit Care Med. 2008;178(9):921–8.
45. Tan KHV, Mulheran M, Knox AJ, Smyth AR. Aminoglycoside prescribing and surveillance in cystic fibrosis. Am J Respir Crit Care Med. 2003;167(6):819–23.
46. Cheng K, Ashby D, Smyth R. Oral steroids for cystic fibrosis. Cochrane Database Syst Rev. 2000;2:CD000407.
47. Rashid M, Durie P, Andrew M, et al. Prevalence of vitamin K deficiency in cystic fibrosis. Am J Clin Nutr. 1999;70(3):378–82.
48. Shwachman H, Kulzycki LL, Mueller HL, Flake CG. Nasal polyposis in patients with cystic fibrosis. Pediatrics. 1962;30:389–401.
49. Jaffe BF, Strome M, Khaw KT, Shwachman H. Nasal polypectomy and sinus surgery for cystic fibrosis a 10 year review. Otolaryngol Clin N Am. 1977;10(1):81–90.
50. Crockett DM, McGill TJ, Healy GB, Friedman EM, Salkeld LJ. Nasal and paranasal sinus surgery in children with cystic fibrosis. Ann Otol Rhinol Laryngol. 1987;96(4):367–72.
51. Vaidyanathan S, Barnes M, Williamson P, Hopkinson P, Donnan PT, Lipworth B. Treatment of chronic rhinosinusitis with nasal polyposis with oral steroids followed by topical steroids: a randomized trial. Ann Intern Med. 2011;154(5):293–302.
52. Keck T, Rozsasi A. Medium-term symptom outcomes after paranasal sinus surgery in children and young adults with cystic fibrosis. Laryngoscope. 2007;117(3):475–9.
53. Albritton FD, Kingdom TT. Endoscopic sinus surgery in patients with cystic fibrosis: an analysis of complications. Am J Rhinol. 2000;14(6):379–85.
54. Schulte DL, Kasperbauer JL. Safety of paranasal sinus surgery in patients with cystic fibrosis. Laryngoscope. 1998;108(12):1813–5.
55. Cuyler JP. Follow-up of endoscopic sinus surgery on children with cystic fibrosis. Arch Otolaryngol. 1992;118(5):505–6.
56. Nishioka GJ, Barbero GJ, Konig P, Parsons DS, Cook PR, Davis WE. Symptom outcome after functional endoscopic sinus surgery in patients with cystic fibrosis: a prospective study. Otolaryngology. 1995;113(4):440–5.
57. Jones JW, Parsons DS, Cuyler JP. The results of functional endoscopic sinus (FES) surgery on the symptoms of patients with cystic fibrosis. Int J Pediatr Otorhinolaryngol. 1993;28(1):25–32.
58. Khalid AN, Mace J, Smith TL. Outcomes of sinus surgery in adults with cystic fibrosis. Otolaryngology. 2009;141(3):358–63.
59. Moss RB, King VV. Management of sinusitis in cystic fibrosis by endoscopic surgery and serial antimicrobial lavage: reduction in recurrence requiring surgery. Arch Otolaryngol. 1995;121(5):566–72.
60. Georgalas C, Hansen F, Videler WMJ, Fokkens WJ. Long term results of Draf type III, (modified endoscopic Lothrop) frontal sinus drainage procedure in 122 patients: a single Centre experience. Rhinology. 2011;49:195–201.
61. Stewart AE, Vaughan WC. Balloon sinuplasty versus surgical management of chronic rhinosinusitis. Curr Allergy Asthma Rep. 2010;10(3):181–7.
62. Ramadan HH. Safety and feasibility of balloon sinuplasty for treatment of chronic rhinosinusitis in children. Ann Otol Rhinol Laryngol. 2009;118(3):161–5.
63. Ramadan HH, McLaughlin K, Josephson G, Rimell F, Bent J, Parikh SR. Balloon catheter sinuplasty in young children. Am J Rhinol Allergy. 2010;24(1):e54–6.
64. Ramadan HH, Terrell AM. Balloon catheter sinuplasty and adenoidectomy in children with chronic rhinosinusitis. Ann Otol Rhinol Laryngol. 2010;119(9):578–82.
65. Sedaghat AR, Cunningham MJ. Does balloon catheter sinuplasty have a role in the surgical management of pediatric sinus disease? Laryngoscope. 2011;121:2053–4.

Oral Candidiasis in Infants and Children

42

Ümran Öner, Fatih Öner, Cemal Cingi, and Torello M. Lotti

42.1 Introduction

The initial description of oral candidiasis (thrush) is owed to Francois Valleix, a French paediatrician, who noted infection by *Candida albicans* within the mouth in 1838. Generally, oral candidiasis afflicts only particular categories of patient: neonates and babies under 1 year of age, those prescribed antibiotics or taking corticosteroids, those with multiple endocrine abnormalities or immunodeficient individuals. Oral candidiasis is a possible initial presentation of human immunodeficiency virus (HIV) and is an ominous sign when seen at a late stage of HIV infection. The risk of oral candidiasis is higher in paediatric patients taking corticosteroids by inhalation [1]. (Figs. 42.1, 42.2, 42.3).

Thrush may produce both white- and red-coloured oral lesions, which may occur acutely or chronically [2]. There are four distinct ways in which the condition can present [3]:

Ü. Öner (✉)
Section of Dermatology, Erzurum Regional Training and Research Hospital, University of Health Sciences, Erzurum, Turkey

F. Öner
Section of Otorhinolaryngology, Erzurum Regional Training and Research Hospital, University of Health Sciences, Erzurum, Turkey

C. Cingi
Department of Otorhinolaryngology, Faculty of Medicine, Eskişehir Osmangazi University, Eskişehir, Turkey

T. M. Lotti
Department of Dermatology and Venereology, University of Studies Guglielmo Marconi, Rome, Italy

C. Cingi et al. (eds.), *Pediatric ENT Infections*,
https://doi.org/10.1007/978-3-030-80691-0_42

489

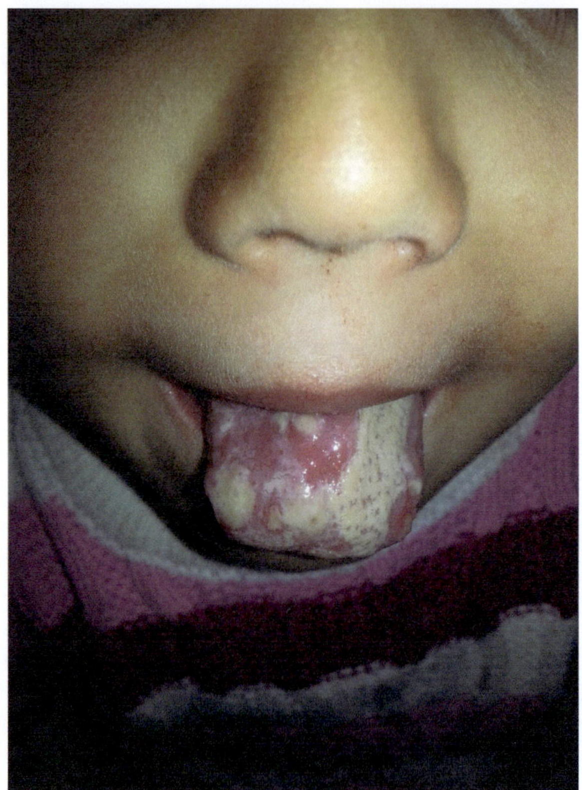

Fig. 42.1 Oral candidiasis in a children. "Courtesy of Ümran Öner"

- Acute pseudomembranous candidiasis is the most typical presentation. There are numerous white patches on the lingual, buccal and palatal surfaces.
- Chronic hyperplastic candidiasis: thickened white plaques occur on the inner cheek lining and the corners of the mouth.
- Acute atrophic (erythematous) candidiasis: There are red palatal plaques.
- Chronic atrophic candidiasis (denture stomatitis). This condition arises due to a dental prosthesis that is the wrong size or shape. It produces red plaques.

42.2　Pathophysiology

C. albicans appears as both a mould and yeast. Nearly half of the general population carry this organism within the oral cavity without symptoms. Oral T-lymphocytes and the presence of interleukin-17 usually ensure that Candidal numbers do not become excessive [4]. However, if a degree of immunodeficiency develops in an individual, the fungus may overgrow and become pathogenic.

C. albicans infections occur when there is disturbance of the normal oral flora, as occurs with dental prostheses, dry mouth, antibiotics, corticosteroid application to the nasopharynx or oral malignant neoplasia. Systemic immunodeficiency

Fig. 42.2 Oral candidiasis in a children. "Courtesy of Ümran Öner"

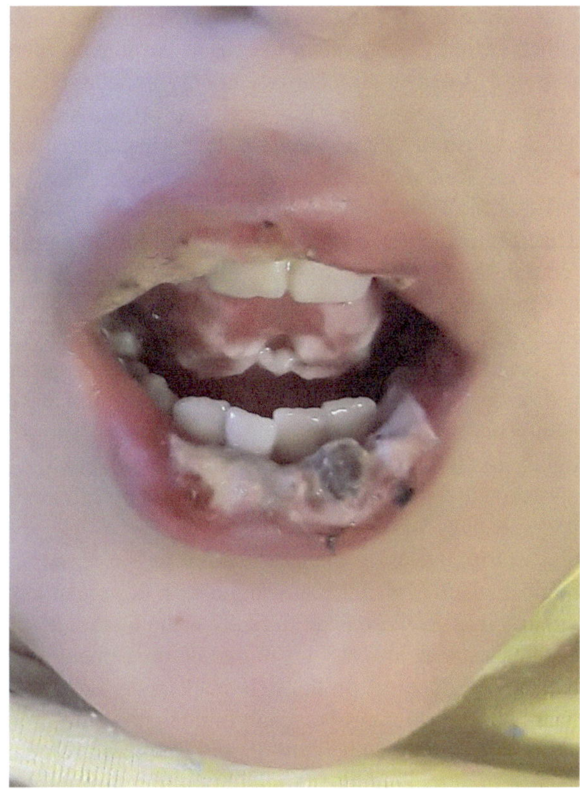

Fig. 42.3 Oral candidiasis in a children. "Courtesy of Ümran Öner"

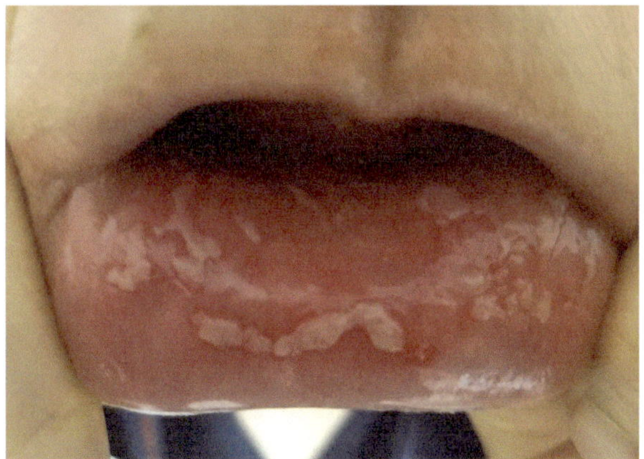

conditions also account for many cases, as occurs with immunosuppressant treatment, HIV infection and diabetes mellitus [5, 6].

The majority of cases of oral thrush are secondary to *C. albicans*, whilst individuals with severely depressed immune systems may sometimes develop candidiasis secondary to *C. tropicalis* or *C. stellatoidea*.

A key virulence factor of *Candida* species is secretion of aspartyl proteinases, which permit the organism to breach the mucosa and stimulate an inflammatory response. Aspartyl proteinases can only be secreted outside the candidal cell if the organism possesses the VPS4 (vacuolar protein-sorting associated protein-4) gene. This gene is thus a vital virulence factor in candidal infections [7].

It has been shown that candidal organisms may produce a subpopulation that exhibits high persistence, especially in cases where a dental prosthesis is in use. This subpopulation is generally not susceptible to antimicrobial agents and furthermore is able to manufacture a biofilm that resists eradication [8].

Oral candidiasis secondary to *C. albicans* occurs if the patient becomes relatively immunodeficient or the healthy oral microflora undergoes an alteration. Proliferation of yeast residing on the linings of the mouth causes the epithelium to desquamate cells and this causes a build-up of bacteria, keratin and dead cells. This accumulated matter becomes organised into a pseudomembranous structure, which then sticks tightly to the mucosal surface. The pseudomembrane is rarely very extensive, but occasionally there may be associated swelling and ulcer formation, with the mucosa underneath becoming necrotic [1].

Parturition, during which the baby passes through the mother's vagina, is the point at which neonatal colonisation with *C. albicans* occurs. Accordingly, oral candidiasis in a newborn is more likely if the mother is infected vaginally with yeasts. The fungus may also be transmitted by breastfeeding, if there is colonisation of the breast, by touching or through inadequate sterilisation of feeding bottle teats. Kissing the child may also result in transmission [1].

In both adulthood and childhood, asymptomatic carriage of *C. albicans* within the gut is a frequent occurrence. This may then be the source for the perineum to become seeded with *C. albicans*. Indeed, a nappy rash associated with *Candida* is common alongside oral candidiasis [1].

42.2.1 Chronic Mucocutaneous Candidiasis (CMC)

CMC is an umbrella term for a number of unusual syndromes where a candidal infection of mucous and cutaneous membranes exhibits treatment resistance to topically applied antifungal agents. CMC has an association with immunodeficiency, especially where this involves T-lymphocytic, dendritic cell or T-helper 17 abnormalities. It has been identified that immune defences against candida are weakened if particular molecular signals function abnormally. Some examples of immunodeficiency leading to CMC are excessive levels of interleukin-6, decreased synthesis of interleukin-23 and a lack of interleukin-17 [3].

42.3 Risk Factors

The risk for candidiasis is raised by multiple patient factors, but especially through immune deficiency, which may result from diabetes mellitus, antibiotic usage, immunosuppressant treatment, systemic corticosteroids or HIV, amongst other causes [3]:

- Compromised immune function: patients suffering from a variety of disorders are more likely to carry *Candida*, such as patients who are HIV positive, have diabetes, are using corticosteroids systemically, are taking steroids by inhalation/nebulisation, are immunosuppressed or who have a malignant neoplasm.
- Reduced saliva production results in higher numbers of *Candida* carried asymptomatically. Hyposalivation may be a side effect of medication, especially antipsychotics, Sjögren syndrome and treatment for cancer (radio- or chemotherapy).
- Inadequate mouth hygiene. Candidal organisms rise in number whilst patients sleep, but eating and cleaning the teeth lowers levels.
- Dental prostheses. Taking out and putting back dentures is associated with higher levels of *Candida* within saliva. This is likely to be due to the persistence of *C. albicans* in plaque formed on the prosthesis.
- Missing dentition results in there being a greater degree of skin overlapping the labial commissures, which is a risk factor for the development of angular cheilitis.
- Tobacco consumption causes a rise of between 30 and 70% in carriage of *Candida.*
- Antibiotic administration also raises the rate of carriage.
- If certain vitamins are deficient, thrush becomes more likely. One example is a low level of cobalamin. Iron-deficient patients are also at risk.

42.4 Aetiology

It is important not to forget the possibility of underlying immunodeficiency, e.g. secondary to HIV, if candidiasis recurs or in a child approaching his/her first birthday. Where candidiasis is chronic, the diagnosis may be CMC.

Administration of antibiotics systemically has the potential to disturb the healthy microbiota, allowing *Candida* to predominate.

Corticosteroid medications (by mouth or inhalation) have an association with oral candidiasis [1].

42.5 Differential Diagnosis

- Aphthous Ulcers
- Blastomycosis
- Histiocytosis
- Haemophagocytic lymphohistiocytosis

The following particularly apply in children:

- Candidiasis
- Cytomegalovirus infection
- Diphtheria

- Echoviral infection
- Enterovirus
- Oesophagitis
- Herpes simplex virus
- HIV infection
- Pharyngitis
- *Treponema pallidum* [1].

42.6 Diagnosis

42.6.1 History

Generally, the case comes to light when white flecks in the mouth are observed by the child's parent.

If candidiasis is severe, it may interfere with feeding.

Sometimes, the history may reveal that the child has been taking antibiotics or receiving corticosteroid treatment, which then reveals the likely trigger [1].

One study considered that candidiasis was reported less frequently than would be expected secondary to antibiotics with a known propensity to provoke the condition, such as amoxicillin or co-amoxiclav. The researchers felt there was a need for doctors prescribing antibiotics to have a greater awareness of the potential complications of use, as well as the advantages [9, 10].

If the infant is prone to diarrhoea, is not growing as expected, has enlargement of the liver and spleen, or has recurrent infective episodes, immunodeficiency should be suspected [11].

In addition, the mother should be asked about:

- Vaginal thrush, which may have put the infant at risk during birth.
- HIV-positive mothers may have transmitted the virus to their infant.

42.6.2 Physical Examination

At an early stage, there are minute flecks which evolve into larger plaques over time. The lesion adheres tightly to the mucosa and may only be detached with difficulty using an examination spatula, exposing a basal area of inflammation, which may feel tender and bleed.

Oral candidiasis can occur in conjunction with a fungal nappy rash. If an infant presents with a nappy rash, the clinician should also examine carefully the oral cavity [12].

42.6.2.1 Differentiation Between Oral Candidiasis and Tongue Coating

It is essential to examine patients who present with oral candidiasis meticulously, particularly in cases where the condition keeps occurring or if the child is older. The growth should be measured and note taken where any rash occurs. Check the lymph nodes and examine the spleen and liver for enlargement. Evaluate other possible areas that may be infected, as may occur in CMC [13–15].

42.6.2.2 Acute Pseudomembranous Candidiasis (Thrush)

Thrush presents as white plaques covering the lining of the buccal cavity, the lingual surface or elsewhere on the body. The initial flecks become plaques that join together and look like curdled milk. When the lesion is scraped off, underneath the basal area appears raw, reddened and sometimes haemorrhagic [3].

42.6.2.3 Chronic Hyperplastic Candidiasis

In chronic hyperplastic candidiasis, the lesions take the form of thickened, white-coloured plaques adhering to the cheek lining or the lingual surface. They feel hard and rough on examination. Whilst the plaques formed in thrush can be removed, albeit with difficulty, in this condition they are very firmly attached and do not detach [2].

The condition may produce nodules, which may have a homogeneous appearance or be speckled, and are not detachable. This speckled type of leukoplakia makes up between 3 and 50% of the plaques seen [16].

42.6.2.4 Acute Atrophic (Erythematous) Candidiasis

The dorsal aspect of the tongue, the lining of the cheek and the palate are all potentially affected in this condition. The lesions are areas of erythema. When present on the lingual dorsum, they appear as the loss of lingual papillae. The corners of the mouth may be inflamed. If patients are being administered antibiotics, there may be tender erythema of the oral cavity, in particular affecting the tongue [3].

42.6.2.5 Chronic Atrophic Candidiasis (Denture Stomatitis)

In this condition, the area covered by the denture when in the mouth becomes reddened and swollen. Patients may complain of pain or a burning sensation. It is unusual for the area underneath the lower denture to be affected. Angular cheilitis may also be seen [3].

There are three distinct patterns for stomatitis related to dentures, namely [3]:

- The inflamed area is confined to one point or there are tiny areas of hyperaemia.
- The entire area where the denture fits has an erythematous mucosa.
- In granular (inflammatory papillary hyperplastic) atrophic candidiasis, the area affected is the central bony palate and the alveolar ridge. The mucosal lining may have become hyperplastic.

42.6.2.6   Angular Stomatitis (perlèche, Angular Cheilitis)

Perleche is one of the forms that erythematous candidiasis may assume. The angles of the mouth are where the lesions occur. Patients complain of feeling sore, they have redness and fissures may be seen. The condition is linked to both fungal and bacterial pathogens (i.e. *Candida* spp. and mainly *Staphylococcus aureus*) [3].

There are a number of conditions besides mucosal candidiasis in which angular cheilitis may be seen, in particular deficiency states of cobalamin or iron, Down syndrome, orofacial granulomatosis and Crohn disease. It is also seen in HIV-positive patients or diabetic individuals [3].

42.6.2.7   Median Rhomboid Glossitis (Glossal Central
Papillary Atrophy)

This condition is a further subtype of erythematous candidiasis. It features an erythematous area of atrophy seen on the dorsal aspect of the tongue, towards the rear of the mouth. This condition is most often encountered in patients consuming tobacco or who are HIV positive [3].

42.6.3 Tests

If the clinician considers oral candidiasis the most likely explanation, the most straightforward way to verify the suspicion is by using a spatula to detach the lesion. An area of potentially haemorrhagic inflammation should be seen underlying the lesion.

Although fungal culture of a plaque is feasible, it is seldom actually necessary. Gram staining reveals yeast that are positive to the stain, large and ovoid in appearance.

Tooyama et al. have evaluated various potential tests to use for laboratory-based confirmation of a clinical diagnosis of oral candidiasis [17]. The researchers concluded that the most appropriate method was concentrated rinse sampling.

Typically, the first step in laboratory investigation of potential candidiasis is cytological. The lesion is scraped and a smear prepared. The smear can be treated with 10% potassium hydroxide solution followed by heating gently. This process destroys the human cells and reveals the fungus. Candidal species have the appearance of budding yeasts and are pseudohyphal. If the condition keeps recurring or resists treatment, mycological culture may be of value in giving a definitive diagnosis and indicating antimicrobial susceptibility. This information is of particular value where the lesion keeps returning, previous therapy has failed or the host is immunosuppressed [18].

It is possible to test for an antibody-linked immune response using an agglutinin, complement-fixation, precipitin, immunofluorescence or enzyme-linked immuno-assay (ELISA) test for *Candida*. The healthy immune response to superficial candidal infections including within the mouth is mainly cellular. If candidal antigens provoke a delayed hypersensitivity response or if evaluation of cellular immune responses in the laboratory are positive, this reveals that a cellular immune response to *Candida* exists.

If a clinician suspects the patient is suffering from CMC, it is appropriate to investigate for underlying HIV infection, folate or B12 deficiency, iron level (ferritin), haemoglobin level and full blood count. In appropriate circumstances, thyroid hormones and adrenal function should be evaluated, given the association between endocrine disease and oral candidiasis and CMC [3].

42.6.4 Histological Appearances

Slides can be Gram stained and treated with KOH to reveal Gram-positive yeast and pseudohyphae [1].

42.7   Medical Treatment

Despite the opinion expressed by some clinicians that oral candidiasis is a self-limiting condition in a newborn child with no underlying disorder, the literature provides no evidence to confirm the validity of this view [19].

Candidiasis typically resolves more quickly if antifungal agents are administered [20]. Initial treatment for oral candidiasis involves fluconazole or nystatin as an oral suspension. There are several alternatives also available. It is unusual for treatment-resistant *Candida* to be encountered, but the agent must come into contact with the fungus to be effective, and thus the suspension must be swirled throughout the entire mouth. This issue does not occur in systemic agents. Fluconazole has a higher success rate in treatment than nystatin [21].

Paediatric patients need to be instructed to swirl the antifungal solution around the mouth before swallowing it, provided they are old enough to do so. Adults should do likewise. If patients do not follow this procedure, a posterior pharyngeal or oesophageal infection may prove difficult to eradicate. In a young child, the caregiver needs to daub a millilitre or two of the solutions on the buccal mucosa each time the child takes the medication. It is also feasible to paint the agent onto the plaques using a non-absorbent swab or applicator. Timing administration to occur between mealtimes permits the agent to stay on the oral surfaces for longer.

Patients should not swallow solutions of Gentian violet. If it is not possible to obtain this agent as a solution, an alternative form is as a medicated lozenge [1].

Since topically applied antifungal agents such as this have little systemic absorption, they are associated with very reduced entry into the circulation and thus few side effects and minimal contraindications. The only currently used antifungal which has reduced effectiveness against *C. albicans* is itraconazole. Where it is not feasible to swirl nystatin around, or if nystatin remains too little time in the oral cavity and thus therapy does not succeed, the second choice involves either gentian violet or fluconazole by mouth [1].

42.7.1 Pharmacotherapy

Pharmacotherapy for candidiasis consists of both topical preparations and systemic medication, although the former is the preferred first line treatment. Indications for systemic treatment include a marked degree of severity, candidiasis within the oesophagus or the failure of topical treatment. The *Clinical Practice Guideline for the Management of Candidiasis* from the Infectious Diseases Society of America (IDSA) [22] is a key reference, on the basis of which the following approach may be suggested:

For pharmacotherapy of the oropharynx [14]:

- Mild cases may be treated with Nystatin suspension q.d.s. over 7–14 days. Alternatively clotrimazole 10 mg medicated lozenges five times a day for 7–14 days.
- If the case is moderate or severe, fluconazole 100–200 mg o.d. over 7–14 days.
- If treatment resistance to fluconazole is observed, itraconazole solution 200 mg o.d. for 4 weeks or less.
- HIV-positive individuals must be offered antiretroviral treatment whenever possible.
- Dentures: antifungal treatment is needed together with disinfection of the prosthesis.
- Swirling Chlorhexidine around the moth is potentially beneficial in oral candidiasis. The same applies to certain essential oils [23].

Antifungal pharmacotherapy.
These agents produce their effects through interfering with nucleic acid turnover (RNA and DNA) or cause the fungus to undergo an increase in cytotoxic peroxide within the cell [1].

42.7.2 Nystatin (Mycostatin, Nilstat, Nystex)

This agent is effective for candidiasis of the mouth. It has only minimal tendency to be absorbed from unbroken skin, the gut or vaginally. The agent is produced by *Streptomyces noursei.* It both kills the fungus and prevents replication. These effects are observed in a number of yeasts as well as fungi resembling yeasts. The agent binds to sterols contained within the plasma membrane of the fungus and causes leakage of the cell contents into the extracellular space [1].

42.7.3 Amphotericin B Deoxycholate (Fungizone Oral Suspension)

This molecule is naturally synthesised by certain strains of *Streptomyces nodosus.* It may prevent replication or cause fungal death. This agent becomes bound to sterols, such as ergosterol, within the plasma membrane of the fungus and results in leakage of cellular contents, which kills the fungus [1].

42.7.4 Clotrimazole (Mycelex Troches)

This agent changes the properties of the fungal plasma membrane. It is especially beneficial if the patient is not immunodeficient. Where unavailable as a suspension (such as in the USA), medicated lozenges are available, but suffer from concerns about raised liver function test values and side effects within the gut [1].

42.7.5 Miconazole Oral (Daktar)

This agent interferes with the manufacture of ergosterol, thereby rendering the plasma membrane more permeable. The leakiness of the membrane results in the loss of essential cellular components and this kills the fungus.

42.7.6 Gentian Violet

Gentian violet has the advantages of both high efficacy in treatment-resistant infections and low cost. Unfortunately, it produces an intense stain on the mucosal surfaces and on any clothes that come into contact with it. This may be unacceptable to some patients [1].

42.7.7 Fluconazole (Diflucan)

Fluconazole is an azole-type antimicrobial that is readily absorbed from the gut. It damages the fungal plasma outer membrane and is excreted renally.

This agent prevents microbial reproduction. It is available by mouth and is non-naturally occurring. It is classified as a bistriazole. The mechanism of action is inhibition of candidal cytochrome P450 and alpha-demethylation of sterols at position C14. This results in the fungus being unable to produce ergosterol from lanosterol and hence it causes damage to the outer plasma membrane [1].

42.8 Complications

Although it seldom occurs, candidiasis that affects a major portion of the trachea and oesophagus may make swallowing impossible or create severe respiratory problems in a patient with no apparent risk factors.

There are reports of candidal infection of the bronchi and lungs.

Individuals who are markedly immunosuppressed are at risk of disseminated candidiasis.

Thrush frequently extends to cause inflammation of the oesophagus in cases of immunocompromise. According to one study, candidal oesophagitis is the most frequently observed opportunistic infection in individuals who have progressed on to the acquired immune deficiency syndrome (AIDS) [1].

References

1. Kumar M. Thrush. In: Steele RW (Ed). Medscape. Updated: Jan 17, 2019. https://emedicine. medscape.com/article/969147-overview (Accessed online at October 15, 2020).
2. Millsop JW, Fazel N. Oral candidiasis. Clin Dermatol. 2016 Jul-Aug.;34(4):487–94.
3. Gupta S. Mucosal candidiasis medication. In: James WD (Ed). Medscape. Updated: Mar 27, 2020. https://emedicine.medscape.com/article/1075227-medication#3 (Accessed online at October 15, 2020).
4. Conti HR, Peterson AC, Brane L, Huppler AR, Hernández-Santos N, Whibley N, et al. Oral-resident natural Th17 cells and γδ T cells control opportunistic Candida albicans infections. J Exp Med. 2014;211(10):2075–84.
5. Meighani G, Aghamohammadi A, Javanbakht H, Abolhassani H, Nikayin S, Jafari SM, et al. Oral and dental health status in patients with primary antibody deficiencies. Iran J Allergy Asthma Immunol. 2011;10(4):289–93.
6. Alnuaimi AD, Wiesenfeld D, O'Brien-Simpson NM, Reynolds EC, McCullough MJ. Oral Candida colonization in oral cancer patients and its relationship with traditional risk factors of oral cancer: a matched case-control study. Oral Oncol. 2015;51(2):139–45.
7. Rane HS, Hardison S, Botelho C, Bernardo SM, Wormley F Jr, Lee SA. Candida albicans VPS4 contributes differentially to epithelial and mucosal pathogenesis. Virulence. 2014;5(8):810–8.
8. Lafleur MD, Qi Q, Lewis K. Patients with long-term oral carriage harbor high-persister mutants of Candida albicans. Antimicrob Agents Chemother. 2010;54(1):39–44.
9. Gillies M, Ranakusuma A, Hoffmann T, Thorning S, McGuire T, Glasziou P, et al. Common harms from amoxicillin: a systematic review and meta-analysis of randomized placebo-controlled trials for any indication. CMAJ. 2015;187(1):E21–31.
10. Pullen LC. Amoxicillin Adverse Effects Underreported, Underrecognized. Medscape Medical News. Available at http://www.medscape.com/viewarticle/835143. November 19, 2014.; Accessed: June 16, 2015.
11. Pappas PG, Kauffman CA, Andes D, et al. Clinical practice guidelines for the management of candidiasis: 2009 update by the Infectious Diseases Society of America. Clin Infect Dis. 2009;48(5):503–35.
12. Hoppe JE. Treatment of oropharyngeal candidiasis and candidal diaper dermatitis in neonates and infants: review and reappraisal. Pediatr Infect Dis J. 1997;16(9):885–94.
13. Kalfa VC, Roberts RL, Stiehm ER. The syndrome of chronic mucocutaneous candidiasis with selective antibody deficiency. Ann Allergy Asthma Immunol. 2003;90(2):259 64.
14. Liu X, Hua H. Oral manifestation of chronic mucocutaneous candidiasis: seven case reports. J Oral Pathol Med. 2007;36(9):528–32.
15. Rowen JL. Mucocutaneous candidiasis. Semin Perinatol. 2003 Oct.;27(5):406–13.
16. Sitheeque MA, Samaranayake LP. Chronic hyperplastic candidosis/candidiasis (candidal leukoplakia). Crit Rev Oral Biol Med. 2003;14(4):253–67.
17. Tooyama H, Matsumoto T, Hayashi K, Kurashina K, Kurita H, Uchida M, et al. Candida concentrations determined following concentrated oral rinse culture reflect clinical oral signs. BMC Oral Health. 2015;15:150.
18. Lalla RV, Patton LL, Dongari-Bagtzoglou A. Oral candidiasis: pathogenesis, clinical presentation, diagnosis and treatment strategies. J Calif Dent Assoc. 2013;41(4):263–8.

19. Raucher HS. Should we be treating oral thrush? Pediatr Infect Dis J. 1998;17(3):267.
20. Lewis MAO, Williams DW. Diagnosis and management of oral candidosis. Br Dent J. 2017;223(9):675–81.
21. Lyu X, Zhao C, Yan ZM, Hua H. Efficacy of nystatin for the treatment of oral candidiasis: a systematic review and meta-analysis. Drug Des Devel Ther. 2016;10:1161–71.
22. Pappas PG, Kauffman CA, Andes DR, Clancy CJ, Marr KA, Ostrosky-Zeichner L, et al. Executive summary: clinical practice guideline for the Management of Candidiasis: 2016 update by the Infectious Diseases Society of America. Clin Infect Dis. 2016;62(4):409–17.
23. Karbach J, Ebenezer S, Warnke PH, Behrens E, Al-Nawas B. Antimicrobial effect of Australian antibacterial essential oils as alternative to common antiseptic solutions against clinically relevant oral pathogens. Clin Lab. 2015;61(1–2):61–8.

Parotitis in Children

43

Fatma Deniz Aygün, Haluk Çokuğraş, and Judith R. Campbell

43.1 Introduction

The parotid glands, bordered anteriorly by the masseter, posteriorly by the sternocleidomastoid, and superiorly by the zygomatic arch, are located side of the face bilaterally in the preauricular area, over the mandibular ramus [1]. The parotid gland's principal function is to secrete saliva, essential for mucosal lubrication, digestion of food, and immunity. The secretions prevent the ascension of bacteria into the gland, protect oral mucosa, gums and teeth. The parotid duct, also known as the Stensen duct, appears at the anterior border of the upper part of the parotid gland and allows saliva to drain from the parotid duct into the mouth.

The parotid gland is the most frequently inflamed salivary gland. Acute parotitis is characterized by sudden swelling, erythema, induration, and tenderness over the parotid gland [2]. Any process disrupting salivary flow through the parotid duct can lead to parotitis. Acute parotitis is classified as suppurative or nonsuppurative.

43.2 Suppurative Parotitis

Parotid gland infections are more common in immunocompromised, postoperative, elderly patients with an incidence of 0.01–0.02% of all hospital admissions [3]. Acute suppurative parotitis is rarely seen in children; most reported childhood cases are between 7 months and 14.6 years [4].

F. D. Aygün (✉) · H. Çokuğraş
Division of Pediatric Infectious Diseases, Department of Pediatrics, Cerrahpaşa Faculty of Medicine, İstanbul University-Cerrahpaşa, İstanbul, Turkey

J. R. Campbell
Section of Infectious Diseases, Department of Pediatrics, Baylor College of Medicine, and Infectious Disease Service, Texas Children's Hospital, Houston, TX, USA

Suppurative parotitis is commonly a polymicrobial infection caused by aerobic and anaerobic bacteria ascending from the oral cavity, but *Staphylococcus aureus* is the most frequent single pathogen [5]. However, other gram-positive organisms, including *Streptococcus pyogenes,* viridans group streptococci, and gram-negative organisms (*Escherichia coli, Klebsiella pneumoniae,* other Enterobacteriaceae, *Moraxella catarrhalis,* and *Eikenella corrodens)* are the other reported causative agents. Gram-negative organisms are more common among hospitalized patients. *Peptostreptococcus* spp., *Prevotella* spp., *Fusobacterium* spp., *Propionibacterium acnes, Actinomyces israelii, Eubacterium lentum, Bacteroides* spp., and *Porphyromonas assacharolytica* are anaerobic bacteria that also cause suppurative parotitis.

Invasion of *Mycobacterium tuberculosis* or *Mycobacterium avium intracellulare* via either spread from an adjacent focus or a lymphatic route can lead to granulomatous parotitis. *Francisella tularensis, Actinomyces,* and *Brucella* species are the other causes of granulomatous parotitis. *Bartonella henselae, Treponema pallidum,* and *Burkholderia pseudomalle* are rarely reported to cause parotitis. *Streptococcus pneumonia* and *Haemophilus influenzae* can lead to recurrent parotitis [4–8].

43.2.1 Suppurative Parotitis: Pathogenesis

Acute suppurative parotitis may develop due to the parotid gland's retrograde contamination by the oral cavity bacteria. Patients with poor oral hygiene, dental abscesses, or chronic tonsillitis are more susceptible to this suppurative condition [5]. The stasis of salivary flow due to dehydration, some medications like anticholinergics, antihistamines, antipsychotics drugs, neoplasms of the oral cavity, sialolithiasis, stenosis, anatomic anomalies, autoimmune processes, cystic fibrosis, and diabetes are other contributing conditions that can lead to acute parotitis [5, 8]. Tracheostomy and immunosuppression are the other risk factors. Hematogenous spread during bacteremia may also be the pathogenesis, especially in neonates. Prematurity, insufficient breastfeeding, excessive oral suctioning, nasogastric tube feeding, and dehydration due to environmental hot weather are the possible mechanisms of acute neonatal suppurative parotitis [9].

43.2.2 Suppurative Parotitis: Clinical Manifestations

Acute bacterial parotitis is characterized by the sudden onset of usually unilateral local pain, tenderness, and a firm, erythematous swelling of the preauricular and postauricular areas of the mandible (Figs. 43.1 and 43.2) [4, 5]. High fever, chills, trismus, and dysphagia may be present.

Fluctuation generally is not a prominent physical examination finding because of the dense parotid fascia over the gland. Involvement of the glandular parenchyma and stretching of the thick parotid capsule leads to severe pain. Facial nerve palsy can rarely accompany suppurative parotitis. Purulent discharge from the Stensen

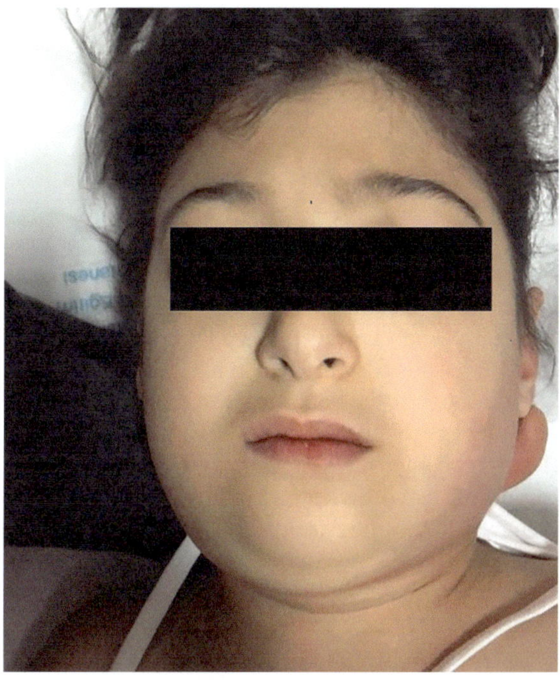

Fig. 43.1 Left cheek swelling and slight effacement of the corner of the mandible. Courtesy Emine Hafize Erdeniz

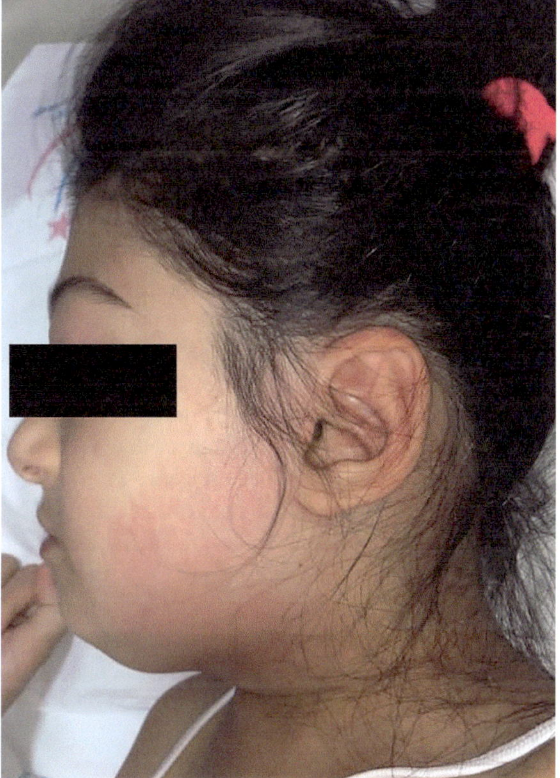

Fig. 43.2 Swelling and erythema of the parotid region that spreads to the cheek. Courtesy Emine Hafize Erdeniz

duct is the pathognomonic finding of suppurative parotitis [4, 5, 10]. In severe cases, the infection can extend to adjacent tissues such as the ear, face, or along fascial planes to the mediastinum.

43.2.3 Suppurative Parotitis: Diagnosis

The diagnosis is usually made upon the characteristic clinical findings. Trauma, lymphadenitis, neoplasia, intraglandular abscess, and parotid gland duct anomalies should be considered in the differential diagnosis. The laboratory findings are usually nonspecific; however, leukocytosis is commonly present, and elevated serum amylase level is present in up to half of them.

Ultrasound is the noninvasive and preferred imaging technique that reveals diffusely enlarged gland with edema, increased vascularity, and a coarse pattern. However, computed tomography (CT) is the most useful imaging method [5] because of its ability to differentiate soft tissue densities within the gland and is preferred if the ultrasound findings are not clear. Magnetic resonance imaging (MRI) can assess ductal abnormalities and parenchymal diseases of the parotid gland. X-ray sialography is contraindicated in the acute stage of infection due to rupture risk [3, 7]. Gram stain and the culture of the purulent drainage material from the Stensen duct can confirm the diagnosis and yield the causative organism.

43.2.4 Suppurative Parotitis: Treatment

Since suppurative parotitis is a potentially life-threatening clinical condition with the risk of invasion to deep fascial spaces of the head and neck, treatment is the appropriate selection of intravenous antibiotics to treat the causative organisms.

Antibiotics that target *S. aureus*, other gram-positive organisms, and anaerobes should be included in the treatment. A combination of penicillinase-resistant penicillins, first-generation cephalosporins, and clindamycin with an aminoglycoside is the treatment of choice, especially in immunocompetent patients [5]. Vancomycin or linezolid should be used for likely or culture-proven methicillin-resistant *S. aureus* (MRSA) infections [5, 7, 11]. Comorbid diseases like chronic renal insufficiency, diabetes mellitus, hemodialysis, and intravenous drug usage are the risk factors for MRSA infections. In cases of immunocompromised hosts, either piperacillin-tazobactam or meropenem plus vancomycin or linezolid will be the appropriate empiric therapy for Enterobacteriaceae, *Pseudomonas aeruginosa,* and *S. aureus* pending culture results. The spectrum of the antibiotic treatment should be narrowed once microbiologic results are available. Surgical drainage may be warranted if there is no clinical improvement after 48 hours of treatment with empiric intravenous antibiotics. A period of 10–14 days of therapy is often adequate depending on the severity of the infection and the host's immune status. Good oral hygiene, locally applied heat, adequate hydration, and avoidance of anticholinergic medications are also often helpful.

43.2.5 Suppurative Parotitis: Complications

Complications of untreated suppurative parotitis include massive swelling of the neck causing respiratory obstruction, osteomyelitis of facial bones, and septicemia [5]. Trigeminal neuritis, facial nerve paralysis, septic jugular thrombophlebitis (Lemierre disease), salivary fistula, and mediastinitis are the other rare complications of acute suppurative parotitis [7, 8].

43.3   Nonsuppurative Parotitis

Autoimmune diseases, metabolic conditions, like diabetes mellitus or gout, benign and malignant tumors, sialolithiasis, alcoholism, uremia, sarcoidosis, and viral pathogens are the nonsuppurative causes of parotitis.

43.3.1 Juvenile Recurrent Parotitis

Juvenile recurrent parotitis (JRP) is a rare, generally unilateral, nonsuppurative, and non-obstructive parotid inflammation characterized by repeated episodes of pain, swelling that may accompany fever and malaise. In childhood, JRP was historically the second most common inflammation of the parotid gland after mumps. In regions with high immunization rates, JRP may be more common. Genetic inheritance, allergy, retrograde infection, and autoimmunity are the suggested causative factors. The onset of the disease is between 3 and 6 years of age with a male predilection. At least 2 episodes of recurrent unilateral or bilateral swelling during the last 6 months in children age < 16 years are the suggested diagnosis criteria of JRP. Juvenile recurrent parotitis is a self-limiting disease and usually resolves after puberty, but it is necessary to exclude Sjogren's syndrome, lymphoma, and human immunodeficiency virus (HIV) infection [12, 13].

Treatment is composed of a conservative and symptomatic approach during relapses, aiming to prevent gland parenchyma damage and relieve symptoms. Analgesics, massage, warm application on the parotid gland, chewing gum, and sialogogic agents can be considered. Corticosteroids and antibiotics are among various regimes, but the most suitable treatment for JRP remains unknown. Sialendoscopy with or without ductal corticosteroid infusion is a treatment choice recommended in the current literature [12–14].

43.3.2 Chronic Recurrent Parotitis

Chronic recurrent parotitis (CRP) is another form of nonsuppurative parotitis characterized by unilateral or bilateral, intermittent or persistent, and painful swelling of the involved gland. The etiology of CRP is multifactorial, and the main problem is obstructive salivary drainage or decreased salivary production. The retrograde infections causing the stasis of saliva, allergic, genetic, hereditary factors, and immune deficiency are suggested etiologic factors that facilitate chronic parotitis [15]. Chronic recurrent parotitis and JRP can be considered similar clinical conditions, but CRP is most common in middle-aged females. Cases of CRP can lead to progressive gland destruction that affects life quality, but JRP usually resolves after puberty.

Reducing recurrence frequency can be achieved with judicious use of antibiotics, analgesics, and mouth rinses. Bilateral sialendoscopy and lavage with intraductal hydrocortisone, ductal ligation, ductoplasty, tympanic neurectomy can be the treatment of choices, but only total parotidectomy contentious can completely resolve the symptoms [15, 16].

43.3.3 Nonsuppurative Parotitis: Miscellaneous Causes

Liver cirrhosis, vitamin B12 deficiency, metabolic disorders, autoimmune diseases such as Sjögren's syndrome, and sarcoidosis can lead to parotitis [5]. Acute parotitis was reported to develop after noninvasive ventilation. Positive airway pressure transmitted to the oral cavity during noninvasive ventilation causes retrograde airflow and can obstruct the parotid duct [17]. Kawasaki disease might be considered an uncommon cause of nonsuppurative parotitis and might be considered in children with parotitis unresponsive to antibiotics and prolonged fever [18].

43.4 Mumps and Other Viral Causes of Acute Parotitis

Mumps virus is the classic and primary virus to cause parotitis, but cytomegalovirus, Epstein-Barr virus (EBV), herpes simplex virus (HSV), influenza A virus, parainfluenza viruses, adenovirus, coxsackievirus, echoviruses, and human herpesvirus six are other viral agents associated with parotitis [5]. Chronic parotitis is frequently reported in HIV infection in children that have not received antiretroviral therapy. This condition s more common in children than adults.

Mumps, also called epidemic parotitis, is a contagious infectious disease characterized by unilateral or bilateral swelling of the parotid or other salivary glands. Mumps was first described in the fifth century BC by Hippocrates. In 1935, Johnson and Goodpasture demonstrated the disease experimentally using a bacteria-free, filter-sterilized preparation of macerated monkey parotid tissue [19, 20]. Mumps is caused by the mumps virus belonging to the Paramyxoviridae family having a negative-sense, single-stranded ribonucleic acid (RNA) genome.

43.4.1 Mumps: Epidemiology

Mumps occurs worldwide, and it is endemic among the unvaccinated community. Humans are the only natural host for the mumps virus, but it is reported in laboratory experiments that hamsters, chicken embryos, and non-human primates can be infected by the virus [20]. The mumps virus can spread through contact with contaminated surfaces, airborne droplets, or fomites. Mumps may affect people of any gender and age, with the highest incidence among children between 5 and 9 years of age. The disease is usually asymptomatic in about one-third of the infected children, but it can cause more severe complications among adults, especially in males. Although sporadic outbreaks can occur at any time of year, it is common in late winter and early spring [21–23].

43.4.2 Mumps: Clinical Manifestations

The incubation period is between 14 and 24 days (range 12–25 days). The mumps virus is transmissible via saliva droplets in the air from 3 days before to 4 days after the onset of parotitis. The patients are typically infectious from 3 days before until 9 days after onset of symptoms [23, 24]. After entering the upper respiratory mucosa, the virus spreads to regional lymph nodes, resulting in viremia during the early acute phase. The viremia typically occurs in the salivary glands, but the virus can settle in the pancreas, kidney, liver, gonads, thyroid gland, inner ear, and nervous system. Symptoms typically begin with a few days as chills, myalgia, headache, and a slight temperature rise may occur 24 h before the onset of parotid swelling. Around 20% of all cases may have very mild illness or no symptoms. Mumps can present as a lower respiratory tract infection, especially in young children [23, 24].

The hallmark of mumps is generally bilateral parotid gland swelling. Parotitis usually develops 2–3 weeks after exposure and lasts for 2–3 days, but it may persist for a week or more. On physical examination, parotid swelling may obscure the mandible's angle and lift the earlobe up and out. The submandibular and sublingual glands may also be swollen. The orifice of the Stensen duct is erythematous and enlarged [5, 23, 24]. Serum and urine amylase levels may be elevated due to tissue damage and inflammation in the parotid gland. Leukopenia with a relative lymphocytosis can be demonstrated [24].

43.4.3 Mumps: Complications

The settling of the mumps virus in various organs in the early phase of viremia can lead to complications that may occur in the absence of parotitis. The complications can develop even in fully immunized individuals.

43.4.3.1 Orchitis and Epididymitis

Unilateral orchitis is the most common extra-salivary gland manifestation of mumps that can develop in approximately 10–20% of infections in post-pubertal men. Symptoms are typically seen in the first 8 days of the parotid swelling but occasionally may precede it or even manifest itself present without the parotid swelling [23].

It results in swelling, severe pain, and tenderness at the affected site. Epididymitis almost always accompanies orchitis. In about 60–80% of cases, orchitis is unilateral, and 10–40% of patients are bilateral. Both germ cells and Leydig cells are involved, associated with reduced levels of testosterone production. Orchitis can be associated with oligospermia and hypofertility, but sterility is rare even in bilateral cases [25].

43.4.3.2 Oophoritis

Mastitis and oophoritis, manifesting as pelvic pain, fever, and vomiting, occur in 5–10% of mumps cases in post-pubertal women. Oophoritis has been associated with premature menopause and infertility, but such cases are sporadic [26].

43.4.3.3 Mumps: Neurologic Complications

Mumps virus is highly neurotropic, and aseptic meningitis is the most common neurologic complication. Pleocytosis of the cerebrospinal fluid (CSF) is present in half of the cases, but clinical meningitis occurs in 1–10% of patients and encephalitis in <0.5% [23]. Mumps can lead to aseptic meningitis or encephalitis, which begins 3–14 days after the onset of parotitis, often after fever and parotitis have subsided. However, the central nervous system (CNS) signs can be present concurrently with parotitis, and as many as 50% of patients with mumps meningitis lack a clear history of parotid gland involvement.

Neurologic symptoms consist of headache, back pain, vomiting, stiff neck, or drowsiness. Seizures, coma, and focal deficits can accompany severe cases. The cerebrospinal fluid examination may consist of a normal protein content, normal or mildly depressed glucose content, and modest lymphocytic pleocytosis, usually between 50 and 300 white blood cell (WBC)/mm^3 [23, 27]. Most of the patients recover completely with no permanent deficits. Hydrocephalus has been rarely reported [27].

43.4.3.4 Mumps: Sensorineural Hearing Loss

Sensorineural hearing loss has been reported in approximately 4% of mumps cases. Hearing loss is typically unilateral, but bilateral cases are also reported. Degeneration of the organ of Corti and the stria vascularis has been demonstrated in histopathological examination in patients developing mumps deafness. Mumps virus was also isolated from the inner ear after sudden deafness, and post-labyrinthine disorder is reported with mumps deafness. The hearing loss is usually transient but can be permanent [28–31]. There is no specific antiviral therapy for mumps, so vaccination against mumps is essential to prevent mumps-associated hearing loss [23].

43.4.3.5 Mumps: Pancreatitis

Pancreatitis diagnosed as severe epigastric pain and tenderness can occur during mumps in approximately 4% of cases. The clinical course is mostly benign; although there are conflicting reports on the association between mumps pancreatitis and diabetes mellitus, most cases resolve with conservative management [32].

43.4.3.6 Mumps: Cardiac Involvement

While this is rarely symptomatic, interstitial lymphocytic myocarditis and pericarditis have been reported during mumps, leading to endocardial fibroelastosis. Electrocardiographic abnormalities, including ST-segment depression, can be observed in 15% of patients [33].

43.4.3.7 Mumps: Other Complications

Arthropathy, autoimmune hemolytic anemia, thyroiditis, thrombocytopenia, hepatitis, retinitis, and interstitial nephritis are the other rare complications of mumps. The women who acquire mumps during the first trimester of pregnancy can suffer from spontaneous abortion, but the mumps virus does not appear to cause congenital malformations [24, 34].

43.4.4 Mumps: Diagnosis

The clinical features and the physical examination findings are usually enough to diagnose mumps. The laboratory confirmation may be necessary in atypical cases or during a possible mumps outbreak. Detection of mumps virus is done via culture or serologic tests. The enzyme immunoassay test (EIA) is the most commonly used in detecting mumps immunoglobulin (Ig) M and IgG antibodies. The IgM antibody can be detected in the first days of infection and remains positive for up to 4 weeks, rarely for months [23, 24, 34]. A fourfold rise in serum mumps IgG antibody titer between acute and convalescent phases is diagnostic but is not useful for establishing a mumps infection diagnosis in previously vaccinated individuals. An IgG antibody cross-reactivity between the mumps and parainfluenza viruses can occur in serologic testing. Detection of mumps virus in body fluids by reverse-transcriptase polymerase chain reaction (RT-PCR) can be performed. RT-PCR results may be falsely negative in vaccinated individuals due to the virus's lower quantities [34].

43.4.5 Mumps: Treatment

There is no specific antiviral treatment for mumps. Supportive and symptomatic treatment with an antipyretic and analgesic agent such as acetaminophen. Orchitis can be managed with bed rest, cold packs. Pancreatitis can be managed with analgesic agents and intravenous fluids [23, 34].

43.4.6 Mumps: Prevention

Mumps is a vaccine-preventable disease. The two doses of live attenuated measles, mumps, and rubella vaccine (MMR) must be administered to subcutaneously all children at 12 months of age and between 4 and 6 years or at the beginning of primary school [23]. MMR vaccine is very safe and effective. Measles, mumps, rubella, and varicella combination vaccine (MMRV) is another live attenuated vaccine licensed for use in children 12 months through 12 years of age. However, MMRV was associated with an approximately twofold increased risk of febrile seizures compared with separate injections of MMR and varicella vaccines. MMR and varicella vaccines can be administered at the same visit, but at different sites, for children 12 through 48 months of age [35, 36].

In a mumps outbreak setting, individuals incompletely immunized against mumps should receive two doses of MMR separated by at least 28 days. In cases of a mumps outbreak, intense exposure setting, high attack rate may necessitate the third dose of MMR vaccine. Following the exposure, immunoglobulin is not effective as post-exposure prophylaxis [37].

References

1. Kochhar A, Larian B, Azizzadeh B. Facial nerve and parotid gland anatomy. Otolaryngol Clin N Am. 2016;49:273–84.
2. Greenberg JS, Breiner MJ. Anatomy, head and neck, auriculotemporal nerve. Treasure Island (FL): StatPearls Publishing; 2020.
3. Fattahi TT, Lyu PE, Van Sickels JE. Management of acute suppurative parotitis. J Oral Maxillofac Surg. 2002;60:446–8.
4. Stoesser N, Pocock J, Moore CE, et al. Pediatric suppurative parotitis in Cambodia between 2007 and 2011. Pediatr Infect Dis J. 2012;31:865–8.
5. Campbell JR. Parotitis. In: Cherry JD, Harrison GJ, Kaplan SL, Steinbach WJ, Hotez PJ, editors. Feigin and Cherry's textbook of pediatric infectious diseases. 8th ed. Philadelphia, PA: Elsevier; 2019. p. 134–6.
6. Brook I. The bacteriology of salivary gland infections. Oral Maxillofac Surg Clin North Am. 2009;21:269–74.
7. Al-Dajani N, Wootton SH. Cervical lymphadenitis, suppurative parotitis, thyroiditis, and infected cysts. Infect Dis Clin North Am. 2007;21:523–41.
8. Patel P, Scott S, Cunningham S. Challenging case of parotitis. J Am Osteopath Assoc. 2017;117:137–40.
9. Avcu G, Belet N, Karli A, Sensoy G. Acute suppurative parotitis in a 33-day-old patient. J Trop Pediatr. 2015;61:218–21.
10. Hernandez S, Busso C, Walvekar RR. Parotitis and sialendoscopy of the parotid gland. Otolaryngol Clin N Am. 2016;49:381–93.
11. Brook I. Acute bacterial suppurative parotitis: microbiology and management. J Craniofac Surg. 2003;14:37–40.
12. Nahlieli O, Shacham R, Shlesinger M, et al. Juvenile recurrent parotitis: a new method of diagnosis and treatment. Pediatrics. 2004;114:9–12.
13. Garavello W, Redaelli M, Galluzzi F, Pignataro L. Juvenile recurrent parotitis: a systematic review of treatment studies. Int J Pediatr Otorhinolaryngol. 2018;112:151–7.
14. Roby BB, Mattingly J, Jensen EL, et al. Treatment of juvenile recurrent parotitis of childhood: an analysis of effectiveness. JAMA Otolaryngol Head Neck Surg. 2015;141:126–9.
15. Nahlieli O, Bar T, Shacham R, Eliav E, Hecht-Nakar L. Management of chronic recurrent parotitis: current therapy. J Oral Maxillofac Surg. 2004;62:1150–5.
16. Mahalakshmi S, Kandula S, Shilpa P, et al. Chronic recurrent non-specific parotitis: a case report and review. Ethiop J Health Sci. 2017;27:95–100.
17. Alaya S, Mofredj A, Tassaioust K, et al. Acute parotitis as a complication of non-invasive ventilation. J Intensive Care Med. 2016;31:561–3.

18. Li Y, Yang Q, Yu X, Qiao H. A case of Kawasaki disease presenting with parotitis: a case report and literature review. Medicine (Baltimore). 2019;98:e15817.
19. Johnson CD, Goodpasture EW. The etiology of mumps. Am J Hyg. 1935;21:46–57.
20. Rubin S, Eckhaus M, Rennick LJ, et al. Molecular biology, pathogenesis and pathology of mumps virus. J Pathol. 2015;235:242–52.
21. Barrabeig I, Costa J, Rovira A, et al. Viral etiology of mumps-like illnesses in suspected mumps cases reported in Catalonia. Spain Hum Vaccin Immunother. 2015;11:282–7.
22. Gupta RK, Best J, MacMahon E. Mumps and the UK epidemic 2005. BMJ. 2005;330:1132–5.
23. American Academy of Pediatrics. Mumps. In: Kimberlin DW, Brady MT, Jackson MA, Long SS, editors. Red Book: 2018 Report of the committee on infectious diseases. 31st ed. Itasca, IL: American Academy of Pediatrics; 2018. p. 567–73.
24. Hviid A, Rubin S, Muhlemann K. Mumps. Lancet. 2008;371:932–44.
25. Choi HI, Yang DM, Kim HC, et al. Testicular atrophy after mumps orchitis: ultrasonographic findings. Ultrasonography. 2020;39:266–71.
26. Shahabi P, Asadzadeh S, Bannazadeh Baghi H, et al. Pregnancy after mumps: a case report. J Med Case Rep. 2019;13:379.
27. Bale JF Jr. Measles, mumps, rubella and human parvovirus B19 infections and neurologic disease. Hand Clin Neurol. 2014:1345–53.
28. Hashimoto H, Fujioka M, Kinumaki H. An office-based prospective study of deafness in mumps. Pediatr Infect Dis J. 2009:28173–5.
29. Morita S, Fujiwara K, Fukuda A, et al. The clinical features and prognosis of mumps-associated hearing loss: a retrospective, multi-institutional investigation in Japan. Acta Otolaryngol. 2017;137:44–7.
30. Kawashima Y, Ihara K, Nakamura M, et al. Epidemiological study of mumps deafness in Japan. Auris Nasus Larynx. 2005;32:125–8.
31. Noda T, Kakazu Y, Komune S. Cochlear implants for mumps deafness: two paediatric cases. J Laryngol Otol. 2015;129:38–41.
32. Rawla P, Bandaru SS, Vellipuram AR. Review of infectious etiology of acute pancreatitis. Gastroenterology Res. 2017;10:153–8.
33. Kahlfuss S, Flieger RR, Mankertz A, et al. Pericardial tamponade in an adult suffering from acute mumps infection. Case Rep Med. 2016;2016:7980936.
34. Clemmons N, Hickman C, Lee A, Marin M, Patel M. Mumps. In: Sandra W. Roush SW, Baldy LM, Hall MAK (eds). Centers for Disease Control and Prevention Manual for the Surveillance of Vaccine-Preventable Diseases, https://www.cdc.gov/vaccines/pubs/surv-manual/chpt09-mumps.html (accessed: Nov 1, 2020).
35. McLean HQ, Fiebelkorn AP, Temte JL, et al. Prevention of measles, rubella, congenital rubella syndrome, and mumps, 2013: summary recommendations of the advisory committee on immunization practices (ACIP). MMWR. 2013;62:1.
36. MacDonald SE, Dover DC, Simmonds KA, Svenson LW. Risk of febrile seizures after first dose of measles-mumps-rubella-varicella vaccine: a population-based cohort study. CMAJ. 2014;186:824.
37. Ogbuanu IU, Kutty PK, Hudson JM, et al. Impact of a third dose of measles-mumps-rubella vaccine on a mumps outbreak. Pediatrics. 2012;130:e1567–74.

Acute Tonsillopharyngitis in Children

44

Necdet Demir, Nuray Bayar Muluk, and Dennis Chua

44.1 Introduction

Tonsillopharyngitis can be defined as a condition in which the pharynx and/or palatine tonsils become acutely infected and is accompanied by sore throat, difficulty swallowing, pyrexia and lymphadenopathy in the cervical region. It can be diagnosed clinically, diagnosis being confirmed microbiologically or via the rapid antigen test [1].

Inflammation solely affecting the tonsils of the pharynx is tonsillitis, but, as the adenoids and lingual tonsils are frequently also involved, pharyngitis may be an equally appropriate term to use. For our purposes we can equate pharyngotonsillitis with adeno-tonsillitis, noting that lingual tonsillitis has a meaning restricted to inflammation occurring in the lymphoid tissue situated at the lingual base [2].

The pharynx may be inflamed or irritated by various pathogens: viruses, such as the Adenoviridae, Enteroviridae and Epstein-Barr virus [EBV] occur in juveniles and are treated routinely on a conservative basis; pathogenic bacteria such as GABHS necessitate antibacterial chemotherapy. However, in all cases in which children are affected, regardless of aetiology, care must be taken to prevent dehydration or other common clinical sequelae [3].

N. Demir (✉)
Section of Otorhinolaryngology, VM Medical Park Pendik Hospital, Pendik, İstanbul, Turkey

N. Bayar Muluk
Department of Otorhinolaryngology, Faculty of Medicine, Kırıkkale University, Kırıkkale, Turkey

D. Chua
Section of Otorhinolaryngology, and Ear, Nose, and Throat Surgeons Medical Centre, Mount Elizabeth Hospital, Singapore, Singapore

C. Cingi et al. (eds.), *Pediatric ENT Infections*,
https://doi.org/10.1007/978-3-030-80691-0_44

44.2 Aetiology

Tonsillitis and its sequelae are caused by both host and parasite factors; thus overcrowding and malnutrition are implicated as are the following pathogens, which account for the majority of cases: Herpes simplex, EBV, Cytomegalovirus, other members of the Herpesviridae, the Adenoviridae and the Measles virus [2].

Tonsillopharyngitis is generally secondary to viral infection: commonly, a coryza-causing virus, e.g. rhinovirus, adenovirus, influenza virus, respiratory syncytial virus; more rarely, EBV (Epstein-Barr virus, the infectious agent in mononucleosis) or HIV (human immunodeficiency virus).

Bacteria cause less than one in three cases of tonsillopharyngitis; however, in these cases, the usual pathogens responsible are Group A Streptococci and typically this so-called "strep throat" afflicts children aged between 5 and 15 years old, being less often seen in children younger than 3, or older adults. If untreated, the illness may be complicated by tonsillar abscess and cellulitis, rheumatic fever or glomerulonephritis. On occasion, gonococcal infection or diphtheria may present as tonsillopharyngitis [4].

Of the between 15% and 30% of cases attributable to bacterial causes, anaerobes are a key cause, but the majority of infections are with the GABHS organism, Streptococcus pyogenes. This organism has the ability to bind to adhesin molecules found in the epithelium of the tonsil and, indeed, antibody coating of the pathogen may be a key step in the development of tonsillitis secondary to bacterial infection [2].

Acute pharyngitis on rare occasions may be due to Mycoplasma pneumoniae, Corynebacterium diphtheriae or Chlamydia pneumoniae and the sexually transmitted pathogen Neisseria gonorrhoea is also a possible cause. Whilst the UK and Nordic countries consider Arcanobacterium haemolyticum a significant cause of acute pharyngitis, the USA does not count the organism as a significant pharyngitic pathogen. A. haemolyticum is associated with a dermatological eruption resembling Scarlatina [2].

Tonsillopharyngitis in a pyrexial patient experiencing a sudden sore throat and whose tonsils are exuding pus, with neck glands painful to the touch, usually resolves on its own within a 2–5-day period and is most likely due to Streptococcus pyogenes. This organism is also referred to as Group A Streptococcus (GAS). Sore throats of longer duration are rarely due to GAS [5].

44.3 Epidemiology

The peak occurrence of the condition is in the paediatric age range, with the caveat that it is rare in those younger than 2 years of age. Aetiology is age-related, cases in those aged 5–15 typically being Streptococcal in origin, whilst in younger children a virus is suspected. Peritonsillar abscess (PTA) has a predilection for adolescents, but may occur at a younger age [2].

Pharyngitis is frequent in upper respiratory tract infection. The carrier rate in children is 2.5–10.9%. 15.9% of school age children on average were carriers of GAS according to one study [6, 7].

44.4   Symptoms

Acute tonsillitis in children presents with sore throat, pyrexia, halitosis, dysphagia, odynophagia and cervical lymphadenopathy. The obstructed airway may lead to mouth breathing, snoring or sleep-disordered breathing such as momentarily ceasing to breathe whilst asleep or sleep apnoea. Patients are commonly debilitated and lethargic. Whilst adequate symptomatic resolution is frequent within 3–4 days, even well-treated cases may last up to a fortnight.

A patient with seven episodes of tonsillitis in 1 year, 5 for 2 years running, or 3 in each year for a 3-year period, all of which have been proven microbiologically as streptococcal should be diagnosed with recurrent streptococcal tonsillitis. In such cases, chronic sore throat, foetid breath, longstanding cervical lymphadenopathy and tonsillitis may be seen. Carriers can easily infect children [2].

A child suffering from tonsillopharyngitis will exhibit pyrexia, sore throat, halitosis, dysphagia, odynophagia and cervical lymph glands which are painful to touch.

44.5   Diagnosis

44.5.1   Examination

Acute tonsillitis is apparent when a pyrexial patient has swollen and erythematous tonsils, possibly with exuded pus. If petechiae are visible on the palate, Streptococcus pyogenes (a Group A β-haemolytic organism) or EBV may be responsible, the former usually occurring in the age range 5–15 years.

Lymph nodes painful on palpation and a stiff neck are seen in acute tonsillitis. Mucous membranes and skin turgor should be assessed to determine fluid status. In adolescents and younger children, EBV-associated infectious mononucleosis needs to be excluded; especially if acute tonsillitis is present alongside lymphadenopathy in the neck, axilla and/or groin, an enlarged spleen, lethargy and malaise and slight elevation in temperature. EBV tonsillitis may produce a greyish membrane over inflamed tonsils, removal of which does not result in bleeding. The palate may have an eroded mucosa with bruising of the hard palate [2].

44.5.2 Investigations

The Gold Standard for diagnosing GABHS infection is by throat swab and culture. Antibiotics are the most effective (90–95%) in this group and can definitely be employed. Given the problems associated with bacterial resistance, swab and culture of throat organisms in cases of tonsillitis may be considered essential. It is ineffective to rely solely on clinical observation and on whether exudates are seen, erythema and lymphadenopathy observed and pyrexia recorded to distinguish between tonsillitis secondary to a virus or secondary to GABHS [2]. Thus, microbiological culture, despite a potential delay of up to 2 days, remains the best way to diagnose accurately. Whilst sensitivity and specificity for GABHS are both generally high using the throat culture method, it is worth bearing in mind that the protocol followed in obtaining the swab and the culture medium employed does have some effect on the final result.

Where appropriate, Monospot, Full blood count and electrolyte should be performed [2].

There are also Rapid Antigen Detection Tests (RADT) to which the majority of clinical settings have access and which is helpful when treatment needs to begin without delay. In combination with throat culture, RADT achieves high reliability. RADT alone is 70–90% as sensitive and 95–100% as specific as throat culture [3].

Thus, a form of RADT and culture is standard in most settings, even more so in the Developed World. Where testing has needed to be performed serially, RADT then culture for the RADT test negatives has shown highest efficacy and has the potential to reduce unwarranted antimicrobial therapy through restricting antibiotic prescribing to cases confirmed by either initial screen or subsequent culture [8].

Serum immunoglobulin titres (antistreptolysin-O, antideoxyribonuclease-B (anti-DNAse-B)) may be used to demonstrate antecedent infection in cases of acute rheumatic fever, glomerulonephritis and the other sequelae of Group A streptococcal pharyngitis [2].

Virology. In cases of suspected EBV, a full blood count can support the diagnosis by detecting atypical leucocytes as can a Monospot or other heterophile antibody detection method. A subclinical hepatitic picture is also seen in EBV with mildly elevated transaminases [3].

Nonetheless, monospot testing may produce false negatives in patients aged under 6 years as well as in the initial symptomatic 7-day period. Monospot has a 90% true positive rate in adolescents whose diagnosis is eventually proven serologically [3].

In a viral epidemic, such as H1N1 influenza, where sore throat features as a presenting complaint, it is at the clinician's discretion whether to investigate a possible streptococcal aetiology at the initial time of presentation or subsequently after symptoms have continued for some time [3].

Imaging studies in the form of X-rays are of no diagnostic merit in acute tonsillitis except where there has been a progression to deeper seated infection behind the oropharyngeal fascia. In the latter case, lateral plain film or contrast-enhanced CT are indicated [2].

44.6 Treatment

44.6.1 Medical Treatment

Patients with acute tonsillitis require little beyond ensuring adequate hydration and absorbing sufficient calories alongside adequate analgesia and antipyretic. If the patient cannot eat and drink enough, antibiotic therapy, fluids and analgesia will need to be provided intravenously. Patients with good oral intake do not need hospitalization and indeed IV fluids may be provided outside hospital if a suitably qualified attendant is available. Steroidal therapy supplied via an IV line may be indicated to reduce severe throat oedema [2].

To prevent the possibility of too readily diagnosing bacterial cause and thus over-prescribing antimicrobial therapy, a clinical scoring method should precede sending swabs for culture or using RADT. Treatment aims to alleviate symptoms, shorten the time for which a patient remains contagious, and obviate suppuration locally or systemic involvement. In an ideal world, prescribing antimicrobials would only happen following laboratory confirmation. Where RADT is unfeasible or results in a probable false negative, culture remains the diagnosis test par excellence and if the clinician has confidence in the eventual diagnosis, antimicrobial therapy can be undertaken. The first line is usually Penicillin with Amoxicillin an acceptable alternative. Co-amoxiclav should not be used empirically. Nor are the Macrolides to be used first line except where a Penicillin reaction may occur and to treat carriers of GABHS [9].

Antibiotic treatment versus GABHS causing acute pharyngitis aims to [5]:

Alleviate the harshness of symptoms and shorten their length. Likewise in cases complicated by suppuration, reduce the likelihood of other, non-suppuration-related conditions such as acute rheumatic fever.

The best evidence for a role of antibiotics in achieving this is found in acute rheumatic fever, whereas glomerulonephritis and PANDAS (paediatric autoimmune neuropsychiatric disorder associated with group A streptococci syndrome) have less conclusive evidence [10]. PANDAS is covered elsewhere but the evidence for antibiotics having a preventive effect is inconclusive [5].

Diminution of Transmissivity to Others in Proximity Via a Reduction in Infective Potential

A patient with symptoms of pharyngitis due to a documented GABHS infection, whether detected by RADT or culture, warrants treatment with antibiotics [11]. Infection with Group C or G Streptococci can also be treated with antibiotics to alleviate symptoms. Which antibiotic to employ in these situations will be discussed below, but, given that acute rheumatic fever is not a consequence of Group C or G streptococci, 5 rather than 10 days' prescription is adequate [12–14].

Streptococcal infection (or the less seldom encountered Corynebacterium diphtheriae and Neisseria gonorrhoeae) is a clear indication for antibiotic prescription. Other bacterial agents responsible for pharyngitis are not effectively treated by antimicrobials and entails unjustified financial burdens, side-effects and contributes to microbial resistance [5].

44.6.1.1 Timing of Therapy

Antibiotics may be started empirically where a case of pharyngitis presents with clinical and epidemiological features strongly suggestive of GABHS, but does not yet have positive laboratory testing. Where such confirmation from the laboratory is not forthcoming, stopping the antibiotic is best [5].

A latent period of 48–96 h is normal in GABHS pharyngitis. Systemic symptoms, including fever, abate normally within 3 or 4 days regardless of antibiotic use. [15] Research has shown that Penicillin produces symptomatic improvement up to 48 h earlier if administered in the first 2 days, compared with placebo. [16–20].

Some patients with negative RADT will have swabs that culture the pathogen. Even if these patients are improving clinically, they still need antimicrobial treatment to diminish the chance of passing on the infection [5].

On area of controversy concerns whether treating too early may in fact suppress the patient's immunoglobulin response and act to promote recurrent pharyngitis. A study of cases of GABHS pharyngitis comparing those receiving treatment at first consultation versus a second group in which treatment did not begin within the first 48 hours, concluded that the first group had eightfold more recurrent infection. [17].

44.6.1.2 Antibiotics for Group A Streptococcus

The treatment armamentarium in GABHS pharyngitis includes Penicillin and derivatives (such as Ampicillin and Amoxicillin), the Cephalosporins, Macrolides and Clindamycin. [21]. It does not include Sulphonamides, Fluoroquinolones or Tetracyclines since organisms are either resistant or are simply not eradicated in the pharynx by these drugs. Penicillin which has been administered intramuscularly is currently the sole agent proven in controlled trials to obviate the first signs of rheumatic fever [22, 23].

44.6.2 Surgery

Tonsillectomy should be offered where: the patient has had pharyngitis of streptococcal origin, for which microbiological documentation exists, more than six times in 1 year; more than five times per year for 2 years in succession: three episodes of either infectious tonsillitis or adenitis for three consecutive years even with adequate drug treatment; chronic (recurrent) tonsillitis in a carrier of Streptococcus, where antibiotics not deactivated by the β-lactamase enzyme have failed to eradicate carriage [2].

Children with the following may also be offered tonsillectomy: several allergies or sensitivities to antimicrobials; PFAPA (periodic fever, aphthous stomatitis, pharyngitis and adenitis); previous peritonsillar abscess [24].

Only seldomly is acute lingual tonsillitis a reason for surgery, but if this otherwise rare condition occurs many times or is severe, tonsillitis may be offered. If the tonsils have hypertrophied due to mononucleosis and continue to impinge symptomatically on the airway after the illness resolves, they may need to be removed surgically [2].

44.6.2.1 Tonsillectomy Indications

The following are sufficient in themselves to indicate a tonsillectomy [25]:

Tonsillomegaly leading to upper airway partial occlusion, great difficulty swallowing, disordered sleep or cardiopulmonary involvement.

Medical treatment followed by surgical drainage of the peritonsillar abscess (provided this was not when the disease was acute) which failed.

Febrile convulsions secondary to tonsillitis.

Histopathologically mandated.

Whilst in the following cases, tonsillectomy may be needed: [25].

Infectious tonsillitis occurring more than three times in 12 months even when otherwise adequately treated medically.

Ongoing dysgeusia or halitosis secondary to chronic tonsillar infection which fails to respond medically.

Streptococcal carriage not eradicable by antimicrobials unaffected by beta-lactamase.

Hypertrophic tonsil on one side which is likely to be cancerous.

The following methods may be employed for tonsillar dissection and excision [26–29]:

Cold steel methods (such as curette or scissors).

Monopolar cautery.

Bipolar cautery (microscopically assisted or not).

COBLATION (radiofrequency ablation, can reduce tonsillar bulk).

Titanium-bladed Scalpel of harmonic type.

Microdebrider-assisted intracapsular tonsillectomy or use of other powered instrumentation.

Haemostasis may be achieved intraoperationally by the following: [25].

Sponge pressure lasting minutes.

Administration of bismuth subgallate.

Tie use.

Cautery employing suction.

Bipolar cautery.

References

1. Sasaki CT. Tonsillopharyngitis. MSD Manual. https://www.msdmanuals.com/professional/ear,-nose,-and-throat-disorders/oral-and-pharyngeal-disorders/tonsillopharyngitis (Accessed online at August 11, 2020).
2. Shah UK. Tonsillitis and peritonsillar abscess. In: Meyers AD (Ed.). Medscape. Updated: Jan 19, 2017. http://emedicine.medscape.com/article/871977-overview (Accessed August 11, 2020).

3. Simon HK. Pediatric pharyngitis. In: Steele RW (Ed.). Medscape. Updated: Apr 26, 2016. http://emedicine.medscape.com/article/967384-overview#a4 (Accessed online at August 11, 2020).

4. Sasaki CT. Tonsillopharyngitis (Tonsillitis; Pharyngitis). Merck Manual Consumer version. http://www.merckmanuals.com/home/ear,-nose,-and-throat-disorders/mouth-and-throat-disorders/tonsillopharyngitis#v8369892 (Accessed online at August 11, 2020).

5. Pichichero ME. Treatment and prevention of streptococcal tonsillopharyngitis. In: Sexton DJ, Edwards MS, Bond S (Eds.). UpToDate. https://www.uptodate.com/contents/treatment-and-prevention-of-streptococcal-tonsillopharyngitis (Accessed online at August 11, 2020).

6. Pichichero ME, Casey JR. Defining and dealing with carriers of group a streptococci. Contemp Pediatr. 2003;1:46.

7. Wald ER. Commentary: antibiotic treatment of pharyngitis. Pediatr Rev. 2001;22(8):255–6.

8. Ayanruoh S, Waseem M, Quee F, Humphrey A, Reynolds T. Impact of rapid streptococcal test on antibiotic use in a pediatric emergency department. Pediatr Emerg Care. 2009;25(11):748–50.

9. Piñeiro Pérez R, Hijano Bandera F, Alvez González F, Fernández Landaluce A, Silva Rico JC, Pérez Cánovas C, Calvo Rey C, Cilleruelo Ortega MJ. Consensus document on the diagnosis and treatment of acute tonsillopharyngitis. An Pediatr. 2011;75(5):342. https://doi.org/10.1016/j.anpedi.2011.07.015.

10. Potter EV, Svartman M, Mohammed I, Cox R, Poon-King T, Earle DP. Tropical acute rheumatic fever and associated streptococcal infections compared with concurrent acute glomerulonephritis. J Pediatr. 1978;92(2):325.

11. Harris AM, Hicks LA, Qaseem A. High value care task force of the American College of Physicians and for the Centers for Disease Control and Prevention. Appropriate antibiotic use for acute respiratory tract infection in adults: advice for high-value care from the American College of Physicians and the Centers for Disease Control and Prevention. Ann Intern Med. 2016;164(6):425–34.

12. Gerber MA, Baltimore RS, Eaton CB, et al. Prevention of rheumatic fever and diagnosis and treatment of acute Streptococcal pharyngitis: a scientific statement from the American Heart Association Rheumatic Fever, Endocarditis, and Kawasaki Disease Committee of the Council on Cardiovascular Disease in the Young, the Interdisciplinary Council on Functional Genomics and Translational Biology, and the Interdisciplinary Council on Quality of Care and Outcomes Research: endorsed by the American Academy of Pediatrics. Circulation. 2009;119(11):1541–51.

13. Meier FA, Centor RM, Graham L Jr, Dalton HP. Clinical and microbiological evidence for endemic pharyngitis among adults due to group C streptococci. Arch Intern Med. 1990;150(4):825–9.

14. Turner JC, Hayden FG, Lobo MC, et al. Epidemiologic evidence for Lancefield group C beta-hemolytic streptococci as a cause of exudative pharyngitis in college students. J Clin Microbiol. 1997;35(1):1–4.

15. Brink WR, Rammelkamp CH Jr, Denny FW, Wannamaker LW. Effect in penicillin and aureomycin on the natural course of streptococcal tonsillitis and pharyngitis. Am J Med. 1951;10(3):300–8.

16. Randolph MF, Gerber MA, DeMeo KK, Wright L. Effect of antibiotic therapy on the clinical course of streptococcal pharyngitis. J Pediatr. 1985;106(6):870–5.

17. Pichichero ME, Disney FA, Talpey WB, et al. Adverse and beneficial effects of immediate treatment of group a beta-hemolytic streptococcal pharyngitis with penicillin. Pediatr Infect Dis J. 1987;6(7):635–43.

18. Krober MS, Bass JW, Michels GN. Streptococcal pharyngitis. Placebo-controlled double-blind evaluation of clinical response to penicillin therapy. JAMA. 1985;253(9):1271–4.

19. Del Mar CB, Glasziou PP, Spinks AB. Antibiotics for sore throat. Cochrane Database Syst Rev. 2000;3:CD000023.

20. Gilbert GG, Pruitt BE. School health education in the United States. Hygie. 1984;3(4):10–5.

21. Betriu C, Sanchez A, Gomez M, et al. Antibiotic susceptibility of group a streptococci: a 6-year follow-up study. Antimicrob Agents Chemother. 1993;37:1717.

22. Denny FW, Wannamaker LW, Brink WR, et al. Prevention of rheumatic fever; treatment of the preceding streptococcic infection. J Am Med Assoc. 1950;143:151.
23. Wannamaker LW, Rammelkamp CH Jr, Denny FW, et al. Prophylaxis of acute rheumatic fever by treatment of the preceding streptococcal infection with various amounts of depot penicillin. Am J Med. 1951;10:673.
24. Baugh RF, Archer SM, Mitchell RB, Rosenfeld RM, Amin R, Burns JJ, et al. Clinical practice guideline: tonsillectomy in children. Otolaryngol Head Neck Surg. 2011;144(1 Suppl):S1–30.
25. Drake AF. Tonsillectomy. In: Meyers AD (Ed.). Medscape. Updated: Oct 23, 2015 http://reference.medscape.com/article/872119-overview#a10 (Accessed online at August 11, 2020).
26. Carr MM, Muecke CJ, Sohmer B, Nasser JG, Finley GA. Comparison of postoperative pain: tonsillectomy by blunt dissection or electrocautery dissection. J Otolaryngol. 2001;30(1):10–4.
27. Pizzuto MP, Brodsky L, Duffy L, Gendler J, Nauenberg E. A comparison of microbipolar cautery dissection to hot knife and cold knife cautery tonsillectomy. Int J Pediatr Otorhinolaryngol. 2000;52(3):239–46.
28. Lee KC, Bent JP 3rd, Dolitsky JN, Hinchcliffe AM, Mansfield EL, White AK. Surgical advances in tonsillectomy: report of a roundtable discussion. Ear Nose Throat J. 2004;83(8 Suppl 3):4–13.
29. Nelson LM. Radiofrequency treatment for obstructive tonsillar hypertrophy. Arch Otolaryngol Head Neck Surg. 2000;126(6):736–40.

Chronic Tonsillopharyngitis

45

Mehmet Emrah Ceylan, İbrahim Çukurova, and Eugenio De Corso

45.1 Introduction

Tonsillitis, whether chronic or recurrent, leads to repeated episodes of tonsillar inflammation, which have a negative effect on the life quality of patients. Repeated episodes of tonsillitis and pharyngitis affect many children, to the extent that they appear a part of their everyday life. Whilst antibiotics are effective in reducing symptoms in the short term, it is frequent for tonsillitis to reappear. The reason for this recurrence is that a number of pathogenic bacteria are able to form a biofilm within the moisture-rich and warm tonsillar crevices which protects the pathogen and allows it to reinfect the host [1].

Chronic tonsillitis is resistant to eradication and may cause the formation of tonsilloliths. If tonsillitis occurs at least twice within a period of 1 year, it may be classified as recurrent. Tonsillitis, whether chronic or recurrent, leads to repeated inflammation involving the tonsils and is associated with a major impairment to the patient's quality of life [2, 3]. Although tonsillitis is extremely common in children, cases rarely occur in a child before the second birthday. The peak age range for Streptococcal tonsillitis is between the ages of 5 and 15 years. Tonsillitis due to viruses generally occurs in children who are younger than this [4]. Numerous researchers have found that, on average, the carriage rate of group A Streptococci in children of school age is 15.9% [5, 6].

M. E. Ceylan (✉)
Section of Otorhinolaryngology, Davraz Yaşam Hospital, Davraz, Isparta, Turkey

İ. Çukurova
Section of Otorhinolaryngology, Tepecik Training and Research Hospital, İzmir University of Health Sciences, İzmir, Turkey

E. De Corso
Department Head and Neck Surgery, Institute of Otorhinolaryngology, Catholic University of Sacred Heart, Rome, Italy

© The Author(s), under exclusive license to Springer Nature Switzerland AG 2022
C. Cingi et al. (eds.), *Pediatric ENT Infections*,
https://doi.org/10.1007/978-3-030-80691-0_45

45.2 Epidemiology

The frequency of tonsillitis is very high in a large number of children and, indeed, is often regarded as an integral part of childhood. It has been shown in one study that tonsillectomy is indicated in approximately 3 in 10 cases of peritonsillar abscess [6], whilst the frequency of paediatric recurrent tonsillitis was 11.7% in Norway and 12.1% in Turkey [7]. It is common in such cases that antibiotic treatment does cause an abatement of symptoms, but recurrence of symptoms then follows [8]. Pathogenic bacteria are able to form a biofilm within the moisture-rich and warm tonsillar crevices, which protects the pathogen and allows it to reinfect the host, as has been discovered by researchers from the Washington University School of Medicine [9]. One group of researchers used a novel microscopy technique to visualise biopsies from cases of chronic tonsillitis, with 70.8% of the slides revealing a biofilm when this method was used [10]. A different study noted that the epithelial covering of the tonsils and adenoids of patients awaiting adenotonsillectomy for an indication of chronic tonsillitis or adenoiditis was frequently coated with a biofilm [11]. Similar biofilm formation has also been noted in a number of other diseases of the ear, nose and throat, namely chronic rhinosinusitis and chronic otitis media [12, 13].

45.3 Pathophysiology

The majority of patients with chronic tonsillitis are infected with a variety of bacteria simultaneously, in particular Streptococci (α-haemolytic and β-haemolytic), *Staphylococcus aureus*, *Haemophilus influenzae* and *Bacteroides* spp. A study which examined the bacterial flora on the surface and core of the tonsils in 30 paediatric patients who underwent tonsillectomy found that whether a child received antibiotic treatment 6 months earlier or not made no difference to bacterial prevalence at the time surgery was performed [14]. It is thought that the dimensions of the tonsil have a bearing on chronic bacterial tonsillitis. The tonsillar dimensions influence the prevalence of aerobic bacteria and the abundance of T cells and B cells. Where there is tonsillar or adenoidal hypertrophy, the bacterial pathogen with the highest frequency is *H. influenzae*. The results of microbiological analysis of tonsillectomy specimens for resistance to penicillin or to synthesis of beta-lactamases indicate that there is no difference between cases where the tonsillectomy indication was pharyngitis due to recurrent group A β-haemolytic Streptococci and where the indication was hypertrophied tonsillar tissue [15].

Localised immunological responses play a key role in the pathogenesis of chronic tonsillitis. Tonsillitis causes an alteration in where dendritic cells and antigen-presenting cells are concentrated. Dendritic cells migrate away from the outer epithelial layers towards the crypts and regions outside the follicles. It may be possible to distinguish between recurrent episodes of tonsillitis and chronic tonsillitis on the basis of different patterns of immune signals. One study utilised these patterns to draw the conclusion that recurrent tonsillitis was more common in childhood, whilst in adulthood candidates for surgery generally suffered from chronic tonsillitis [16].

45.4   Biofilms

Biofilms consist of a system of different microbial organisms joined together within a watery matrix made up of extracellular polymeric substances (ESPs). Biofilms are responsible for a variety of infective conditions characterised by persistence, such as plaque formation on teeth, infections in cystic fibrosis, and infections of the urinary tract, the deep bone and the ear [9, 17, 18]. Biofilms are of ancient origin and arose as a way for microbes to survive and flourish in challenging situations by co-operating in the production and maintenance of a balanced community [19, 20].

The biofilm that develops results from strong evolutionary selective pressure brought about by harsh conditions, including exposure to chemicals or antibiotics [21, 22]. The microbes within the biofilm are able to profit in three ways from forming a film: first, the film offers escape from the damaging environment within the host; second, the film allows bacteria to survive in a location where there is abundant nutrition; and third, microbes derive advantages from co-operation that are otherwise unavailable [23]. Biofilms have now been noted to occur as a key virulence factor in numerous infective disorders in humans. They are a factor in infections by bacteria in at least 65–80% of cases [17, 24–27]. Biofilms present a severe problem for human health given their role in increasing resistance to antibiotics and their propensity to form when an indwelling medical device is present [28]. There are four key steps in how a biofilm is created: (1) bacteria must be able to adhere to a surface, (2) colonies begin to form, (3) the biofilm reaches maturity and (4) bacteria can break off from the film and be disseminated to other parts of the host [29].

When bacteria break away from the biofilm, they are carried along by a body fluid, but are also capable of movement by themselves. After they seed in a locality, they begin the process of biofilm formation once again [19, 30].

45.5   Recurrent and Chronic Tonsillitis

Chronic tonsillitis is a major health condition, whether it occurs in a child or adult [31, 32]. There is disagreement as to precisely what qualifies recurrent tonsillitis as severe, but the following all contribute to a high degree of severity: at least five episodes of confirmed tonsillitis annually; symptoms that persist beyond a year; and an adverse impact on the patient, preventing normal activities [33, 34]. According to one study, the risk of developing recurrent tonsillitis at some point in life for the general population is 11.7% (95% CI, 11.0–12.3%) and females are significantly more at risk than males [7]. The usual treatment for recurrent tonsillitis is operative, but antibiotic pharmacotherapy is employed for cases where tonsillectomy criteria are not satisfied or the patient has a contraindication to surgery [35, 36].

Tonsillectomy is an operation which has been carried out on children for more than a century. It may also be coupled with removal of the adenoids. However, despite this long history, the clinical benefit derived remains the subject of debate. Even 70 years ago, in the early 1950, the BMJ opined: "it is better to delay a decision than to hurry it, and above all to avoid operating on tonsils which have been recently inflamed" [37]. According to one study, there was still a 60% chance of pharyngitis in the 12 months following tonsillectomy [38]. Another study cautioned about complications that may endanger life from this type of surgery. Research following up a cohort of individuals who underwent tonsillectomy 20 years postoperatively noted that the risk of chronic, immunologically related disorders was higher in the operated individuals than in controls, with a mean relative risk of 9.41 (95% confidence interval between 1.13 and 78.14) [39]. Against this, a different study conducted in adult patients established an association between tonsillectomy and better health outcomes and life quality over the long term, as well as cost-effectiveness [40].

45.6 Physical Examination

When physically examining the patient, a key initial consideration is to establish if the airway or the ability to swallow are compromised. To enable inspection of the throat, ask the patient to open his or her mouth but not stick the tongue out. A tongue blade may be used to carefully depress the tongue in the middle. The same instrument may be used to retain the tongue whilst examining the mouth lining, teeth and saliva ducts. Examination of the nasopharynx is possible using a flexible endoscope in particular patients, especially if there is a marked degree of spasm of the jaw muscles [41].

45.7 Treatment

N-Acetyl-cysteine (NAC) possesses antioxidant properties and can inhibit bacterial growth and biofilm formation [42] by interfering with the production of ESPs [43] and disrupting already formed biofilms [44]. It has been discovered that NAC inhibits the ability of *S. pneumoniae* or *H. influenzae* to attach to the epithelium of the oropharynx, at least in vitro [43]. Chronic infection results in elevation of prostaglandins. NAC is effective in depressing prostaglandin levels whilst also breaking up biofilms [45–48]. Non-steroidal anti-inflammatory agents (NSAIDs) also inhibit biofilm development and can prevent fungal infections entirely [49].

45.7.1 Tonsillectomy

The indications for tonsillectomy are as follows [41]:

- Pharyngitis confirmed by culture as due to Streptococci occurs at least seven times in 1 year.
- Or pharyngitis of streptococcal origin occurs five times yearly consecutively over 2 years.

- Or tonsillitis with or without adenoiditid occurs at least three times each year over a period of three consecutive years, even though appropriately managed medically.
- Tonsillitis is chronic or recurrent and occurs in association with carriage of streptococci. The organisms have not been eradicated by antibiotic agents that can resist beta-lactamase degradation.

References

1. Abu Bakar M, McKimm J, Haque SZ, Majumder MAA, Haque M. Chronic tonsillitis and biofilms: a brief overview of treatment modalities. J Inflamm Res. 2018;11:329–37. https://doi.org/10.2147/JIR.S162486.
2. American Academy of Otolaryngology Tonsillitis. 2018. [Accessed January 6, 2018]. http://www.entnet.org/content/tonsillitis.
3. Hayes K. Chronic and recurrent tonsillitis: what to know. 2017. [Accessed January 6, 2018]. Available from: https://www.verywell.com/chronic-and-recurrent-tonsillitis-1191984.
4. Shah UK. Tonsillitis and peritonsillar abscess. Drugs & diseases. Otolaryngology and Facial Plastic Surgery Medscape; [Accessed January 6, 2018]. Available from: https://emedicine.medscape.com/article/871977-overview#a6.
5. Pichichero ME, Casey JR. Defining and dealing with carriers of group a streptococci. Contemp Pediatr. 2003;20(1):46–53.
6. Wald ER. Commentary: antibiotic treatment of pharyngitis. Pediatr Rev. 2001;22(8):255–6.
7. Kvestad E, Kvaerner KJ, Roysamb E, Tambs K, Harris JR, Magnus P. Heritability of recurrent tonsillitis. Arch Otolaryngol Head Neck Surg. 2005;131(5):383–7.
8. Ward D. Bacterial biofilms may be source of recurrent tonsillitis Medicine & Health. Washington University in St. Louis; 2018. [Accessed January 6, 2018]. Available from: https://source.wustl.edu/2003/09/bacterial-biofilms-maybe-source-of-recurrent-tonsillitis/.
9. Chole RA, Faddis BT. Anatomical evidence of microbial biofilms in tonsillar tissues: a possible mechanism to explain chronicity. Arch Otolaryngol Head Neck Surg. 2003;129(6):634–6.
10. Kania RE, Lamers GE, Vonk MJ, et al. Demonstration of bacterial cells and glycocalyx in biofilms on human tonsils. Arch Otolaryngol Head Neck Surg. 2007;133(2):115–21.
11. Al-Mazrou KA, Al-Khattaf AS. Adherent biofilms in adenotonsillar diseases in children. Arch Otolaryngol Head Neck Surg. 2008;134(1):20–3.
12. Saylam G, Tatar EC, Tatar I, Özdek A, Korkmaz H. Association of adenoid surface biofilm formation and chronic otitis media with effusion. Arch Otolaryngol Head Neck Surg. 2010;136(6):550–5.
13. Sanderson AR, Leid JG, Hunsaker D. Bacterial biofilms on the sinus mucosa of human subjects with chronic rhinosinusitis. Laryngoscope. 2006;116(7):1121–6.
14. Woolford TJ, Hanif J, Washband S, Hari CK, Ganguli LA. The effect of previous antibiotic therapy on the bacteriology of the tonsils in children. Int J Clin Pract. 1999;53(2):96–8.
15. Shah UK. Which bacteria are involved in the pathophysiology of chronic tonsillitis? In: Meyers AD (Ed). Medscape. Updated: Apr 06, 2020. https://www.medscape.com/answers/871977-53769/which-bacteria-are-involved-in-the-pathophysiology-of-chronic-tonsillitis (Accessed online at October 15, 2020).
16. Bussi M, Carlevato MT, Panizzut B, Omede P, Cortesina G. Are recurrent and chronic tonsillitis different entities? An immunological study with specific markers of inflammatory stages. Acta Otolaryngol Suppl. 1996;523:112–4.
17. Costerton JW, Stewart PS, Greenberg EP. Bacterial biofilms: a common cause of persistent infections. Science. 1999;284(5418):1318–22.

18. Donlan RM, Costerton JW. Biofilms: survival mechanisms of clinically relevant microorganisms. Clin Microbiol Rev. 2002;15(2):167–93.
19. Hall-Stoodley L, Costerton JW, Stoodley P. Bacterial biofilms: from the environment to infectious disease. Nat Rev Microbiol. 2004;2(2):95–108.
20. Mai-Prochnow A, Lucas-Elio P, Egan S, et al. Hydrogen peroxide linked to lysine oxidase activity facilitates biofilm differentiation and dispersal in several gram-negative bacteria. J Bacteriol. 2008;190(15):5493–501.
21. Tilahun A, Haddis S, Teshale A, Hadush T. Review on biofilm and microbial adhesion. Int J Microbiol Res. 2016;7(3):63–73.
22. Brown MRW, Gilbert P. Microbiological quality assurance: a guide towards relevance and reproducibility of Inocula. Boca Raton, NY: CRC Press; 1995.
23. Jefferson KK. What drives bacteria to produce a biofilm? FEMS Microbiol Lett. 2004;236(2):163–73.
24. Chambers JR, Sauer K. The MerR-like regulator BrlR impairs *Pseudomonas aeruginosa* biofilm tolerance to colistin by repressing PhoPQ. J Bacteriol. 2013;195(20):4678–88.
25. Joo HS, Otto M. Molecular basis of in-vivo biofilm formation by bacterial pathogens. Chem Biol. 2012;19(12):1503–13.
26. Lebeaux D, Chauhan A, Rendueles O, Beloin C. From in vitro to in vivo models of bacterial biofilm-related infections. Pathogens. 2013;2(2):288–356.
27. Costerton JW. Introduction to biofilm. Int J Antimicrob Agents. 1999;11(3–4):217–21.
28. Donlan RM. Biofilm formation: a clinically relevant microbiological process. Clin Infect Dis. 2001;33(8):1387–92.
29. Landini P, Antoniani D, Burgess JG, Nijland R. Molecular mechanisms of compounds affecting bacterial biofilm formation and dispersal. Appl Microbiol Biotechnol. 2010;86(3):813–23.
30. Hall-Stoodley L, Stoodley P. Biofilm formation and dispersal and the transmission of human pathogens. Trends Microbiol. 2005;13(1):7–10.
31. Wagner S, Jung H, Nau F, Schmitt H. Relevance of infectious diseases in a pediatric practice. Klin Padiatr. 1993;205(1):14–7.
32. Potera C. Forging a link between biofilms and disease. Science. 1999;283(5409):1837–9.
33. Management of sore throat and indications for tonsillectomy. Edinburgh: Scottish Intercollegiate Guidelines Network, Royal College of Physicians; [Accessed January 11, 2018]. (National Clinical Guideline No. 34). Available from: http://www.sdl.academic.chula.ac.th/Sore%20Throat/Sign.pdf.
34. McKerrow WS. Recurrent tonsillitis. Am Fam Physician. 2002;66(9):1735–6.
35. El Hennawi DED, Geneid A, Zaher S, Ahmed MR. Management of recurrent tonsillitis in children. Am J Otolaryngol. 2017;38(4):371–4.
36. Georgalas CC, Tolley NS, Narula A. Tonsillitis. BMJ Clin Evid. 2009;2009:0503.
37. Gale AH. Refresher course for general practitioners: pros and cons of tonsillectomy. Br Med J. 1951;1(4698):133–5.
38. Burton MJ, Glasziou PP, Chong LY, Venekamp RP. Tonsillectomy or adenotonsillectomy versus non-surgical treatment for chronic/recurrent acute tonsillitis. Cochrane Database Syst Rev. 2014;19(11):CD00.
39. Johansson E, Hultcrantz E. Tonsillectomy—clinical consequences twenty years after surgery? Int J Pediatr Otorhinolaryngol. 2003;67(9):981–8.
40. Senska G, Atay H, Pütter C, Dost P. Long-term results from tonsillectomy in adults. Dtsch Arztebl Int. 2015;112(50):849–55.
41. Shah UK. Tonsillitis and Peritonsillar Abscess Treatment & Management. In: Meyers AD (Ed). Medscape. Updated: Apr 06, 2020. https://emedicine.medscape.com/article/871977-overview (Accessed online at October 15, 2020).
42. Schwandt LQ, Van Weissenbruch R, Stokroos I, Van Der Mei HC, Busscher HJ, Albers FW. Prevention of biofilm formation by dairy products and N-acetylcysteine on voice prostheses in an artificial throat. Acta Otolaryngol. 2004;124(6):726–31.

43. Riise GC, Qvarfordt I, Larsson S, Eliasson V, Andersson BA. Inhibitory effect of N-acetylcysteine on adherence of *Streptococcus pneumoniae* and *Haemophilus influenzae* to human oropharyngeal epithelial cells in vitro. Respiration. 2000;67:552–8.
44. Hansen EN, Zmistowski B, Parvizi J. Periprosthetic joint infection: what is on the horizon? Int J Artif Organs. 2012;35(10):935–50.
45. Ricciotti E, Fitz Gerald GA. Prostaglandins and inflammation. Arterioscler Thromb Vasc Biol. 2011;31(5):986–1000.
46. Kiecolt-Glaser JK. Stress, food, and inflammation: psychoneuro-immunology and nutrition at the cutting edge. Psychosom Med. 2010;72(4):365–9.
47. Hsieh CC, Hsieh SC, Chiu JH, Wu YL. Protective effects of N-acetylcysteine and a prostaglandin E1 analog, alprostadil, against hepatic ischemia: reperfusion injury in rats. J Tradit Complement Med. 2014;4(1):64–71.
48. Blasi F, Page C, Rossolini GM, et al. The effect of N-acetylcysteine on biofilms: implications for the treatment of respiratory tract infections. Respir Med. 2016;117:190–7.
49. Witkin SS, Jeremias J, Ledger WJ. A localized vaginal allergic response in women with recurrent vaginitis. J Allergy Clin Immunol. 1988;81(2):412–6.

Peritonsillar Abscess in Children

46

Murat Songu, Ahmet Erdem Kilavuz, and Felicia Manole

46.1 Introduction

Peritonsillar abscess (PTA) is a suppurative infection that leads to a collection of purulent material between the capsule of the palatine tonsil and pharyngeal muscles and is the most common abscess of the head and neck region. It is usually unilateral but can rarely be bilateral. Peritonsillar abscess (also known as quinsy) is the commonest of all deep neck infections.

The incidence of PTA in children is 14 cases per 100,000 population. Approximately 25–30% of patients with a peritonsillar abscess is in the pediatric age group [1]. Although it is rare compared to pre-antibiotic era, an evidence-based review has shown that in recent years the incidence of PTA has increased by 18%. It is suggested that this could be a result of the current trends of fewer tonsillectomy operations performed and reduced antibiotic prescribing in primary care [2].

It is the most common complication of acute tonsillitis. Most infections occur in the superior tonsillar pole, but occurrence in the middle and inferior tonsillar areas is also possible. In some occasions, it may have multiple loculations within the peritonsillar space [3].

The development of the abscess is gradual, usually starts with peritonsillar cellulitis, following acute tonsillitis. PTA occurs after the failure of medical treatment,

M. Songu (✉)
Section of Otorhinolaryngology, Medicana International İzmir Hospital, İzmir, Turkey

A. E. Kilavuz
Department of Otorhinolaryngology, Faculty of Medicine, Acıbadem Mehmet Ali Aydınlar University, İstanbul, Turkey

F. Manole
Department of Otorhinolaryngology, Faculty of Medicine and Pharmacy, University of Oradea, Oradea, Bihor, Romania

© The Author(s), under exclusive license to Springer Nature Switzerland AG 2022   533
C. Cingi et al. (eds.), *Pediatric ENT Infections*,
https://doi.org/10.1007/978-3-030-80691-0_46

or lack thereof, at these stages. An alternative theory suggests that a PTA is formed in a group of salivary glands in the supratonsillar fossa, known as Weber glands [4].

Although Group A beta-hemolytic streptococci can be recovered in a significant portion of the abscesses, mixed anaerobic and aerobic bacteria are the main pathogen of PTA [5]. The frequency of methicillin-resistant Staphylococcus aureus (MRSA) is growing to be greater in PTA bacterial cultures recently, which is probably due to increasing prevalence of antibiotic resistance [6].

46.2   Clinical Presentation

Patients complain of fever, sore throat, odynophagia, and trismus. The examination may be difficult because of the limited opening of the mouth. Patients with PTA manifest a muffled voice; drooling, unilateral swelling, and erythema of the superior tonsillar pole; edema and deviation of the uvula to the opposite side; and bulging of the posterolateral part of the soft palate. Snoring and other obstructive sleep apnea symptoms may occur due to narrowing of the upper airway. This could lead to a potential respiratory distress. There may also be a localized ear pain on the affected side. Lymphatic drainage of the PTA is to the ipsilateral jugulodigastric nodes, so there may be a unilateral cervical lymphadenopathy [7] (Figs. 46.1 and 46.2).

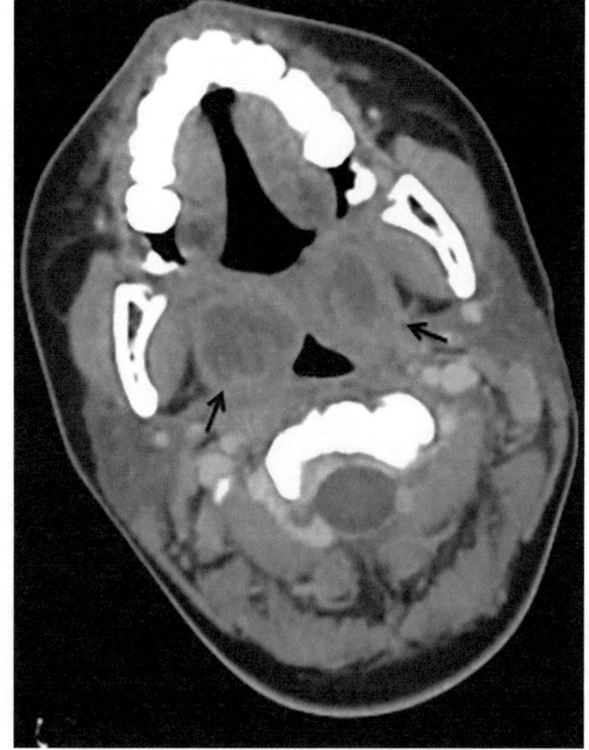

Fig. 46.1 Bilateral peritonsillar abscesses in an 11-year-old girl with fever, odynophagia, and severe sore throat. Contrast-enhanced axial neck CT images demonstrate rim enhancing fluid collections (arrows) in bilateral peritonsillar region. After immediate surgical incision and drainage, Streptococcus pyogenes as the most commonly cultured pathogen was identified (Courtesy of Esin Kurtulus Ozturk MD)

Fig. 46.2 Bilateral peritonsillar abscesses in an 11-year-old girl with fever, odynophagia, and severe sore throat. Coronal neck CT images demonstrate rim enhancing fluid collections (arrows) in bilateral peritonsillar region. After immediate surgical incision and drainage, Streptococcus pyogenes as the most commonly cultured pathogen was identified (Courtesy of Esin Kurtulus Ozturk MD)

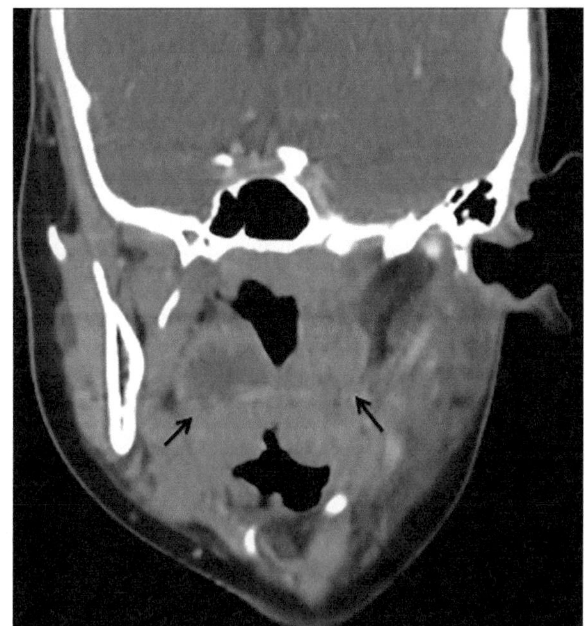

46.3 Diagnosis

The diagnosis of a peritonsillar space infection is usually made clinically, but it may be difficult to differentiate between cellulitis and an early abscess because the pathogenesis is similar and patients present with similar symptoms [8]. No method to differentiate between the two is ideal; however, observing the patient's response to intravenous antibiotics up to 48 h, attempting a needle aspiration or using a radiological modality such as computerized tomography (CT) or ultrasonography (US) could be beneficial. In CT, PTA appears as a low-attenuation mass with a ring-enhancing wall. Whereas peritonsillar cellulitis manifests loss of the fat planes, lack of ring enhancement and soft tissue swelling and edema [9]. Intraoral US is more accurate than the transcutaneous approach. However, this may be difficult to perform in children with limited mouth opening. PTA appears as an echo-free cavity with an irregular border, whereas peritonsillar cellulitis is seen as a homogeneous or striated area with no distinct fluid collection [10].

Laboratory tests provide secondary benefits when if the clinician is certain of the diagnosis. However, a complete blood count (CBC) may show a leukocytosis with neutrophil predominance. Whereas in infectious mononucleosis, a lymphocyte predominance with atypical lymphocytosis is expected. Serum electrolyte levels may assist if the patient's oral intake is impaired. Both aerobic and anaerobic cultures from aspirated purulent may be studied for antibiotic sensitivity. That being said, some experts believe this is unnecessary because almost all patients respond following drainage and antibiotic therapy, regardless of culture results. Culture may be sterile if the patient is currently taking antibiotics [11].

46.4 Treatment and Complications

46.4.1 Medical Treatment

Medical treatment should provide hydration, analgesia, and antibiotherapy. Evaluating the degree of upper airway obstruction is vital. An anxious, ill-appearing child with drooling and posturing must be approached cautiously. Airway obstruction may require immediate airway management, such as intubation or tracheotomy. Hospitalization may be needed especially in young children or patients with the impaired oral intake. However, older children may be managed as an outpatient, with oral medication after drainage [12].

Paracetamol and/or ibuprofen could be considered for pain and fever management. Evidence for the use of corticosteroids in PTA is limited; however, the use of corticosteroids is not uncommon. Several studies have explored the use of corticosteroid therapy in other inflammatory conditions of the pharynx; however, the relevance of these studies to PTA is not clear [1].

Antibiotic treatment should cover group A Streptococcus, S. aureus, and oral flora anaerobes. For inpatient management, penicillin and metronidazole appear to be a sensible choice [13]. Due to increasing penicillin resistance, intravenous ampicillin plus sulbactam could be considered as a logical choice [14]. A combination of intravenous ceftriaxone and clindamycin or a carbapenem (i.e., imipenem, meropenem) is used for severe or complicated cases [15]. A beta-lactam antibiotic such as amoxicillin plus clavulanate could be used as a drug of choice in outpatient management [16]. Some authors suggest that intramuscular clindamycin is an excellent choice and can be safely prescribed on an outpatient basis following needle aspiration, thereby reducing both antibiotic and hospital costs [17].

46.4.2 Surgical Treatment

The aim of surgical treatment is to drain purulent material from peritonsillar space. The surgical options are needle aspiration, incision and drainage, and tonsillectomy. Needle aspiration could be performed either as the definitive drainage procedure or to confirm the presence of pus before performing incision and drainage. The procedure can be done using topical anesthesia. In 90% of cases, the point of entry should be a superior-medial aspect of the tonsil. Some authorities recommend 3-point aspiration, with the first site being superior and medial and the other two sites progressively 0.5–1 cm more inferior and lateral [18]. Complications include respiratory distress, aspiration, and hemorrhage. The success rate of needle aspiration is more than 90%. Similar success rates were found in studies that compared needle aspiration to incision and drainage [19]. If symptoms do not resolve with needle aspiration, the patient may either undergo a second needle aspiration or one of the other drainage procedures. Performing needle aspiration is not recommended for uncooperative child, very young child, the anticipation of airway management problems, and bleeding diathesis [2].

Incision and drainage provides wider drainage; however, it is more painful than needle aspiration. Some studies suggest incision and drainage may resolve pain faster than aspiration [20]. Contraindications to incision and drainage are an uncertain diagnosis, uncooperative child, very young child, and potential of airway management problems.

Tonsillectomy is usually performed if abscess fails to resolve with other drainage techniques. It is preferred and defined as the definitive therapy, by some authorities. When performed in the acute stages of a PTA, tonsillectomy procedure is also called as quinsy tonsillectomy, abscess tonsillectomy, or tonsillectomy à chaud. Quinsy tonsillectomy has a clear role in intolerant children and in patients with persistent peritonsillar abscess who could benefit in overall reduced recovery time [2]. There is still controversy regarding the rate of postoperative bleeding after abscess tonsillectomy; however, evidence suggests that quinsy tonsillectomy as a procedure carries no greater risk of post-tonsillectomy hemorrhage than a routine tonsillectomy [21].

Interval tonsillectomy is performed several weeks after the resolution of PTA. This procedure could be suggested to those patients with a previous history of recurrent pharyngitis or previous episodes of peritonsillar abscess. Interval tonsillectomy may provide a more difficult dissection than quinsy tonsillectomy and result in an overall longer recovery time. However, interval tonsillectomy allows a more planned operation without the patient being acutely unwell [2, 22].

46.4.3 Complications

PTA may lead to fatal complications. Many historians believe that a PTA may have been the source of US President George Washington's asphyxiation [23]. Possible complications include airway compromise, aspiration of abscess contents following incision or spontaneous drainage, aspiration pneumonia, parapharyngeal abscess, septic thrombophlebitis involving the internal jugular vein (Lemierre syndrome) or internal carotid artery leading pseudoaneurysm or rupture of the carotid artery, sepsis, mediastinitis, necrotizing fasciitis and various complications of group A streptococcus infection [24].

References

1. Millar KR, Johnson DW, Drummond D, Kellner JD. Suspected peritonsillar abscess in children. Pediatr Emerg Care. 2007;23:431–8.
2. Powell J, Wilson JA. An evidence-based review of peritonsillar abscess. Clin Otolaryngol. 2012;37:136–45.
3. Hromadkova P. Peritonsillar abscess in children. Bratislavskelekarskelisty. 2006;107:272.
4. Klug TE, Rusan M, Fuursted K, Ovesen T. Peritonsillar abscess: complication of acute tonsillitis or Weber's glands infection? Otolaryngol Head Neck Surg. 2016;155:199–207.
5. Brook I, Frazier EH, Thompson DH. Aerobic and anaerobic microbiology of peritonsillar abscess. Laryngoscope. 1991;101:289–92.
6. Brook I. Role of methicillin resistant Staphylococcus aureus in head and neck infections. J Laryngol Otol. 2009;123:1301–7.

7. Tom LWC, Jacobs IN. Diseases of the oral cavity, oropharynx, and nasopharynx. In: Ballenger's otorhinolaryngology, head and neck surgery. 16th ed. Hamilton: BC Decker Inc.; 2003. p. 1039–40.

8. Brodsky L, Sobie SR, Korwin D, Stanievich JF. A clinical prospective study of peritonsillar abscess in children. Laryngoscope. 1988;98:780–3.

9. Maroldi R, Farina D, Ravanelli M, Lombardi D, Nicolai P. Emergency imaging assessment of deep neck space infections. In: Seminars in Ultrasound, CT and MRI. New York: Elsevier; 2012. p. 432–42.

10. Scott PMJ, Loftus WK, Kew J, Ahuja A, Yue V, Van Hasselt CA. Diagnosis of peritonsillar infections: a prospective study of ultrasound, computerized tomography and clinical diagnosis. J Laryngol Otol. 1999;113:229–32.

11. Schraff S, McGinn JD, Derkay CS. Peritonsillar abscess in children: a 10-year review of diagnosis and management. Int J Pediatr Otorhinolaryngol. 2001;57:213–8.

12. Souza DLS, Cabrera D, et al. Comparison of medical versus surgical management of peritonsillar abscess: a retrospective observational study. Laryngoscope. 2016;126:1529–34.

13. Prior A, Montgomery P, Mitchelmore I, Tabaqchali S. The microbiology and antibiotic treatment of peritonsillar abscesses. Clin Otolaryngol. 1995;20:219–23.

14. Plum AW, Mortelliti AJ, Walsh RE. Microbial flora and antibiotic resistance in peritonsillar abscesses in upstate New York. Ann Otol Rhinol Laryngol. 2015;124:875–80.

15. Côrte FC, Firmino-Machado J, Moura CP, Spratley J, Santos M. Acute pediatric neck infections: outcomes in a seven-year series. Int J Pediatr Otorhinolaryngol. 2017;99:128–34.

16. Lamkin RH, Portt J. An outpatient medical treatment protocol for peritonsillar abscess. Ear Nose Throat J. 2006;85:658.

17. Ozbek C, Aygenc E, Unsal E, Ozdem C. Peritonsillar abscess: a comparison of outpatient IM clindamycin and inpatient IV ampicillin/sulbactam following needle aspiration. Ear Nose Throat J. 2005;84:366.

18. Savolainen S, Jousimies-Somer HR, Mäkitie AA, Ylikoski JS. Peritonsillar abscess: clinical and microbiologic aspects and treatment regimens. Arch Otolaryngol Head Neck Surg. 1993;119:521–4.

19. Weinberg E, Brodsky L, Stanievich J, Volk M. Needle aspiration of peritonsillar abscess in children. Arch Otolaryngol Head Neck Surg. 1993;119:169–72.

20. Qureshi H, Ference E, Novis S, Pritchett CV, Smith SS, Schroeder JW. Trends in the management of pediatric peritonsillar abscess infections in the US, 2000–2009. Int J Pediatr Otorhinolaryngol. 2015;79:527–31.

21. Lehnerdt G, Senska K, Jahnke K, Fischer M. Post-tonsillectomy haemorrhage: a retrospective comparison of abscess-and elective tonsillectomy. Acta Otolaryngol. 2005;125:1312–7.

22. Simon LM, Matijasec JW-D, Perry AP, Kakade A, Walvekar RR, Kluka EA. Pediatric peritonsillar abscess: quinsy ie versus interval tonsillectomy. Int J Pediatr Otorhinolaryngol. 2013;77:1355–8.

23. Scheidemandel HHE. Did George Washington die of quinsy? Arch Otolaryngol. 1976;102:519–21.

24. Bulgurcu S, Arslan IB, Demirhan E, Kozcu SH, Cukurova I. Neck abscess: 79 cases. Northern Clin Istanbul. 2015;2:222.

Retropharyngeal and Parapharyngeal Abscesses in Children

47

Aylin Eryılmaz, Sema Başak, and Andrey Lopatin

47.1 Introduction

Lymphadenitis, cellulitis, or abscess located in the deep neck spaces are defined as deep neck infection. The majority of deep neck infections in the pediatric age group are seen in the first 6 years [1]. Early childhood shows a significant clustering, especially for retropharyngeal abscesses. The reason for such clustering is the presence of lymph nodes in the retropharyngeal space, which are active in the first years of life, and regress as the child grows.

Deep neck spaces are divided by the fascia and areolar tissue networks surrounding the neck structures. Infections involving retropharyngeal and parapharyngeal spaces are not common in both children and adults, but their early diagnosis and initiation of appropriate treatment are vital as they can lead to life-threatening complications such as sepsis, meningitis, and mediastinitis. In this section, retropharyngeal and parapharyngeal abscesses in the pediatric age group are discussed.

47.1.1 Retropharyngeal Space

The retropharyngeal space extends from the skull base to the second thoracic vertebra. The buccopharyngeal fascia, a part of the middle layer of the deep cervical

A. Eryılmaz (✉) · S. Başak
Department of Otorhinolaryngology, Faculty of Medicine, Aydın Adnan Menderes University, Aydın, Turkey

A. Lopatin
Policlinic №1, Medical Department, Business Administration of the President of Russian Federation, Moscow, Russia

C. Cingi et al. (eds.), *Pediatric ENT Infections*,
https://doi.org/10.1007/978-3-030-80691-0_47

fascia, forms the anterior wall, and the alar fascia forms the posterior wall. The space is laterally adjacent to the carotid sheath. Because of the close relationship between the medial superior constrictor muscle and the prevertebral fascia in the midline, the retropharyngeal space is divided into the right and left. Therefore, the inflammation is usually unilateral, except in extraordinary circumstances. The retropharyngeal space contains connective tissue and a lymph node chain. Pharynx, nasopharynx, adenoid, middle ear, paranasal sinuses, nasal cavity, and the lymphatic vessels of the surrounding muscles drain into these lymph nodes. The retropharyngeal space neighbors the carotid sheath, superior mediastinum, and parapharyngeal space.

47.1.2 Parapharyngeal Space

The parapharyngeal space looks like an inverted pyramid extending from the midskull base to the hyoid bone. This space is confined by the pterygomandibular raphe anteriorly, the prevertebral fascia posteriorly, the superior constrictor muscle medially, and the parotid gland deep lobe and medial pterygoid muscle laterally. It is divided by the styloid protrusion into two parts called the prestyloid/poststyloid. The anterior prestyloid part contains the internal maxillary artery, auriculotemporal, lingual, and inferior alveolar nerves, pterygoid muscles, the parotid gland deep lobe, fat tissue, and the lymph nodes. The poststyloid part includes the carotid artery, internal jugular vein, cervical sympathetic chain, IX, X, XI, and XII cranial nerves. The parapharyngeal region is bordering the peritonsillar, submandibular, retropharyngeal, and parotid spaces.

47.2 Etiology

Deep neck phlegmon and abscesses in children occur mostly because of upper respiratory tract infections [2]. In adults, odontogenic infections are the most common source of deep neck space inflammation. Intraoral lacerations, neck or pharyngeal trauma, and foreign body swallowing are the other etiological factors [3]. Especially in children, sharp foreign bodies penetrate the hypopharynx or esophagus walls and infect adjacent areas, such as the retropharyngeal space. Oral/oropharyngeal surgical applications and endoscopic interventions may cause iatrogenic retropharyngeal or parapharyngeal infections. Circumstances of delivery, neonatal intensive care unit staying, and head and neck trauma are predisposing factors also [2]. It has been reported that congenital neck cysts and other anomalies may be a significant risk factor, especially in recurrent deep neck infections [4]. During history taking, all possible etiological factors should be questioned thoroughly, and this information should be considered in the differential diagnosis.

47.2.1 Microbiology

Deep neck abscesses are mostly polymicrobial infections (anaerobic and aerobic). *Streptococcus viridans, Streptococcus pyogenes, Staphylococcus epidermis,* and *Staphylococcus aureus* are the most common aerobic microorganisms, whereas the most common anaerobic microorganisms are *Bacteroides, Fusobacterium,* and *Peptostreptococcus.* Causative pathogens may differ in adults and children [5]. It has been reported that age-dependent differences in causative pathogens can also be seen in the pediatric group. Coticcha et al. detected *S. aureus* in 79% cases of deep neck infections in children under 1 year. In the same study, *Group A Streptococcus* was more common in this age group [2]. Another study revealed *Community-Acquired Methicillin-Resistant S. aureus* (CAMRSA) in 61% of pediatric deep neck abscesses [6, 7].

47.3   History and Examination Findings

Evaluating only the clinical presentation does not allow for making a precise diagnosis in retropharyngeal and parapharyngeal infections. A detailed examination of the teeth and a complete ENT examination should be done. While evaluating the oral cavity and oropharynx, the soft palate, uvula, palatine tonsils, and the posterior pharyngeal wall should be examined meticulously. Swelling or displacement of the walls of oral and pharyngeal cavities are the typical clinical signs. Retropharyngeal and parapharyngeal infections may show some differences in terms of symptoms and examination findings. The type of inflammation (lymphadenitis, cellulitis, or abscess) influences individual clinical presentations. The most common initial symptom is fever [3, 8, 9]. It should be kept in mind that complaints such as sore throat, restriction in neck movements, neck tissue swelling, trismus, torticollis, dysphagia, drooling, hoarse voice, and respiratory distress are not always associated with infections of the deep neck region.

47.3.1 Retropharyngeal Infection

Infections of the retropharyngeal region present themselves with typical symptoms, such as dysphagia, drooling, neck pain, neck swelling, restricted neck movements, restlessness, respiratory distress, and fever. The neck is tilted towards the sick side and cannot be flexed. Unilateral bulging of the posterior pharynx wall can be seen when pharyngoscopy is performed. If the infection presents with local lymphadenitis, the swelling is limited to a particular area. In case of cellulitis or abscess formation, the swelling can be observed along the entire length of the pharynx walls [5]. The infection can spread to the posterior mediastinum, leading to fatal complications.

47.3.2 Parapharyngeal Infection

Infection of the parapharyngeal spaces involving the neck fascia may spread to other deep neck regions. Alternatively, inflammation may propagate to this region from the neighboring areas. The infections of the prestyloid and poststyloid spaces present with different symptoms. For infection involving the prestyloid part, trismus, and swelling of the submandibular region, especially in the angulus mandible area, unilateral displacement of the pharyngeal wall is typical. In contrast, poststyloid infections manifest with more uncertain symptoms; therefore correct diagnosis is usually doubtful. If the pharyngeal wall is not displaced and pterygoid muscles are not involved, trismus may not be present. The most critical finding suggesting the diagnosis of parapharyngeal abscess is restricted neck motions [8]. There is a high risk of fatal neurovascular complications such as internal jugular vein thrombosis, carotid artery erosion, or pseudoaneurysm in this particular group of patients. Ipsilateral Horner's syndrome and/or IX, X, XI, XII cranial nerve palsy often complicate poststyloid region infections. Sichel et al. stated that poststyloid infections are more common in children while prestyloid in adults [10]. The age difference occurs depending on the etiology of the infections. Acute cervical lymphadenitis usually precedes parapharyngeal abscess formation in children, while the abscess results from spreading infection from adjacent deep neck spaces in adults [10].

47.4　Laboratory Tests

Laboratory tests give information about the presence of acute infection. Therefore, complete blood count, sedimentation rate, C-reactive protein (CRP) test, serum glucose, electrolytes, and coagulation studies should be performed. Leukocytosis (WBC >12,000) in the complete blood count is the most common laboratory finding [3]. Culture of purulent material obtained by aspiration and blood cultures help to prescribe an appropriate treatment. In immunocompromised or clinically suspicious patients, anaerobic cultures, fungal cultures, and cultures for atypical pathogens such as mycobacteria should be considered [5].

47.5　Imaging Techniques

As with all infections involving deep neck spaces, imaging is of utmost importance in diagnosing and treating retropharyngeal and parapharyngeal infections. Imaging methods should be chosen according to patients' complaints, clinical presentations, and complications.

47.5.1 Conventional X-Rays

Using lateral neck radiographs in the management of deep neck infections is controversial. Plain X-rays are cheap and easy-to-perform examinations, especially in

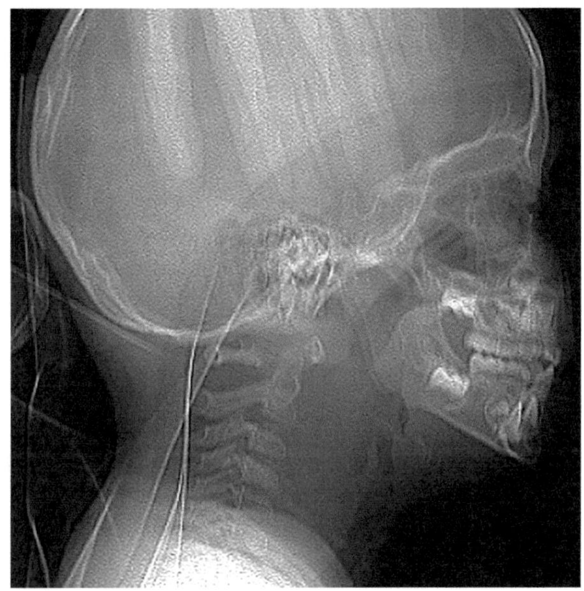

Fig. 47.1 Lateral radiography in a child with retropharyngeal abscess

children. Lateral neck radiographs in a child with uncomplicated retropharyngeal abscess avoid unnecessary computed tomography (CT) associated radiation exposure [8]. However, Nagy et al. reported that lateral neck radiographs have 83% sensitivity, while contrast-enhanced (CT) sensitivity is 100% [11]. Soft tissue thickness of over 5 mm at the second cervical vertebra level and 14 mm at the sixth cervical vertebra level on lateral neck radiographs in children are considered pathological. Besides, air-fluid level, "thumbprint sign," and thickening of arytenoids can be seen. It should be kept in mind that lateral radiographs may lead to diagnostic confusions because of crying, swallowing, breathing, and abnormal position at the time of the procedure. Plain X-rays do not help in diagnosis of the deep neck infections other than those in the retropharyngeal space. If the dental origin is suspected, panoramic view radiography should be performed. Chest examination should be done if complaints such as dyspnea, tachycardia, and/or cough are present (Fig. 47.1).

47.5.2 Computed Tomography

CT provides excellent visualization of the head and neck bone and soft tissue structures. CT imaging enhanced with contrast media significantly improves visualization. Therefore, CT is the standard radiological technique in diagnosing deep neck infections (Fig. 47.2). CT scans precisely detect the location and the borders of inflamed tissues allowing for the correct surgery planning. The size of inflamed area on CT greater than 2.0 cm^2 directly correlates with the presence of pus that can be drained during surgery in 89% of the patients [3]. CT can evaluate neighboring neurovascular structures and exclude other pathological conditions requiring surgical intervention.

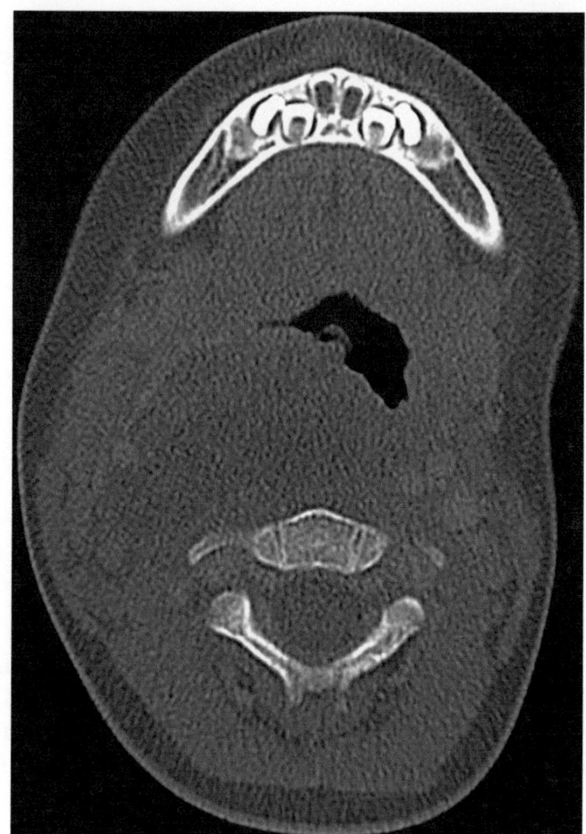

Fig. 47.2 Computed tomography in a child with retropharyngeal abscess

47.5.3 Ultrasonography

Ultrasonography (USG) is a noninvasive, cheap, and rapid procedure with no radiation exposure, it needs no sedation, and needle aspiration can be performed under USG control when necessary. Sethia et al. considered USG as the first option in evaluating head and neck infections in children [12]. They reported that USG reduces the use of CT with the same diagnostic accuracy. This is essential for children who are more susceptible to radiation's adverse effects than adults. Head and neck CT, especially in the pediatric age group, carries a high risk of complications; it holds the third order regarding the risk of developing thyroid microcarcinomas [13]. USG has been shown to be an equally sensitive and more specific diagnostic tool than CT for diagnosing lateral neck abscesses in children [14]. However, the use of USG is limited in profound parapharyngeal and retropharyngeal spaces infections with excessive neck edema.

47.5.4 Magnetic Resonance Imaging

The advantages of magnetic resonance imaging (MRI) are the lower radiation exposure and better soft tissue imaging when compared to CT. However, MRI may require general anesthesia, especially in young children; therefore, it is a second-line option to diagnose potential complications, not for routine use [5].

47.6   Treatment

47.6.1 Medical Treatment

Empirical antibiotic treatment must cover the entire spectrum of the potential pathogens. It must reach a sufficient concentration in the infected area, cause minimal toxicity and maximum efficacy, avoiding antibiotic resistance development [15].

Empirical treatment must cover the *Streptococci group A, S. aureus*, and respiratory anaerobes. Initial treatment can be upgraded accordingly as soon as the results of culture and the recovered pathogen sensitivity get ready. Amoxicillin/clavulanic acid or clindamycin are the first-line therapy. Ampicillin-sulbactam may not be effective against methicillin-resistant S. aureus (MRSA). Vancomycin can be the second-line option for patients who do not respond to initial treatment. Parenteral therapy should be carried out until the patient's body temperature comes to the normal level and the symptoms resolve completely; then, an oral antibiotic can be prescribed for up to 14 days. A systematic review reported that 52% of pediatric patients could be successfully managed with medical treatment only [16].

In pediatric deep neck infections, systemic corticosteroid therapy significantly reduces the need for surgery. Surgical drainage was necessary for 36% of the patients in the dexamethasone group and 53% in the non-dexamethasone group ($p = 0.043$). The hospital stay was shorter in the dexamethasone group. However, it has been stated that larger case series are required for statistically significant conclusions [17]. Antibiotic and corticosteroid therapy have been routinely used in the other case series [15]. Medical treatment response has to be monitored within the first 24–48 h of treatment. In case of no response, a control CT is required.

47.6.2 Surgical Treatment: Indications, Predictive Factors, Preoperative Assessment, and Methods

If medical therapy fails and especially when an abscess or/and upper airway obstruction develop, parapharyngeal and retropharyngeal infections require surgical treatment [18]. Retropharyngeal space may be surgically drained through an intraoral approach if a typical bulging of the posterior pharyngeal wall is present and patient has no dyspnea. A transoral incision on the posterior pharyngeal wall should be done with the patients in head-down position so as to avoid pus aspiration. If the infection is more complicated and spreads to the neighboring areas and critical vascular structures, an approach along the anterior border of sternocleidomastoid muscle must be used.

An intraoral approach to the lateral pharyngeal space is usually confined by the opening and drainage of a peritonsillar abscess. The external approach along the inferior margin of the mandible facilitates more adequate drainage of this particular area.

A prospective study enrolled 12 children with parapharyngeal infections. Initial surgical drainage and intravenous (IV) antibiotic treatment were performed in five cases where inflammation was not limited to the parapharyngeal space. The other seven children were followed up with IV antibiotic (amoxicillin-clavulanic acid) only. The assessment performed 2 days later revealed clinical improvement in five of these seven children, and they continued antimicrobial treatment. No improvement was observed in the remaining two cases. The authors believe that surgery is indicated only in those cases where control CT scans show increase of infection severity. If this does not occur, IV antibiotic therapy has to be continued. The mean duration of hospital stay in this study was 11 [9–14] days. Five patients recovered within the first 48 h. It is worthy of note that in this series inflammation was found to be limited to the posterior parapharyngeal area in all patients, showing that most infections of this location were caused by lymphadenitis [18, 19].

In the other study 54 children with parapharyngeal and retropharyngeal abscesses confirmed by CT received antibiotic treatment and surgical drainage or an antibiotic only [20]. Younger patients required surgery more frequently. Among 27 children with the abscess size on CT smaller than 25 mm, treatment with antibiotic monotherapy was conducted in 13, and antibiotic + surgical drainage in 14. Comparison of treatment results and duration of hospital stay showed no significant difference between the two treatment options. In the group of 27 children with an abscess size greater than 25 mm treated with antibiotic only, 23 children needed surgical drainage. The fever persisted longer in the group requiring surgical drainage comparing to the antibiotic group [20]. Another study concluded that if the infection was limited by the area of necrotic lymph nodes rather than fascial planes, the mediastinal spread in children was less than in adults; therefore children more often could be followed up closely with antibiotic treatment for a while [21].

In a retrospective study, 32 children with parapharyngeal and retropharyngeal abscesses were prescribed IV ampicillin-sulbactam or clindamycin. Patients not responding to medical treatment were found to have larger abscesses than those who had responded (5.38 cm^2 vs. 1.53cm^2). When surgery was required, the intraoral approach was found to be safe and sufficient if the infection did not spread behind the medial part of parapharyngeal and retropharyngeal spaces [22].

In the other study, the need for surgical drainage was investigated in 93 children with deep neck infections. The age, leukocyte value, and CRP value were not predictive, whereas the predictive cutoff value for radiologically measured abscess size was 2.5 cm [23]. Surgical drainage appeared to be necessary in cases of the airway obstruction, immunosuppressed and unresponsive to antibiotic treatment patients, and those who developed complications [15].

A multicenter study analyzed a series of 153 children with deep neck abscesses. The study has shown that an abscess size over 3 cm, high leukocyte value, and the need for hospital referral were found to be a predictive value. Indications for surgical intervention included the presence of peripheral rim involvement on CT, a CRP value >41.25 mg/L, a sedimentation rate >56 mm/h, and a neutrophil/lymphocyte ratio >8.02 [24]. The patients undergoing surgery were usually younger than 4 years; they had airway obstruction symptoms, complications, abscess size over 2.2 cm, did not improve clinically after 48 hours of IV antibiotics, or required hospitalization in an intensive care unit [5].

Surgical drainage of the infection in the medial parapharyngeal space extending towards the skull base utilizes tonsillectomy, the lymph nodes and abscess cavity exposure by means of the tonsillar fossa muscles dissection under microscopic control to prevent carotid injury [25].

A study investigating the timing of surgical drainage in adults and children has shown that abscess-related morbidity and mortality increased 2.38-fold when the drainage was performed after 3 days in adults. In contrast, morbidity and mortality rates did not changed when the drainage was postponed in children. Multivariate regression analysis revealed that statistically significant postoperative mortality and morbidity-related factors in children were female gender, congenital malformations, preoperative sepsis, and septic shock. Delayed surgical drainage had prolonged the time spent in the hospital [26].

47.7 Complications

Complications such as airway obstruction, sepsis, aspiration due to abscess rupture, internal jugular vein thrombosis, carotid artery erosion, and mediastinitis occur quite often in patients with deep neck infections [27–29]. Airway obstruction is the most common among these complications. Therefore, endoscopic examination of the patients' upper airways, especially intubated, is very important (Fig. 47.3). If not prevented, abscess rupture may develop, and the patient may die because of aspiration.

When 45 cases with pediatric deep neck abscesses were examined, compression or partial stenosis of the internal carotid arteries was detected, especially in those with lateral parapharyngeal and retropharyngeal abscesses. This can be explained by an inflammatory or autoimmune process in the artery wall. The authors stressed that even in the absence of threatening clinical presentations, potentially fatal complications (thrombosis, sepsis, pseudoaneurysm, perforation) must be kept in mind [30]. A pediatric patient with carotid artery occlusion due to retropharyngeal abscess needs antibiotic therapy and anticoagulants [31]. Angiography and coil embolization can be indicated in retropharyngeal and parapharyngeal abscesses, causing a pseudoaneurysm of the internal carotid artery and ischemic stroke which can be fatal [32]. Observation from a pediatric hospital has shown that 15 out of 130

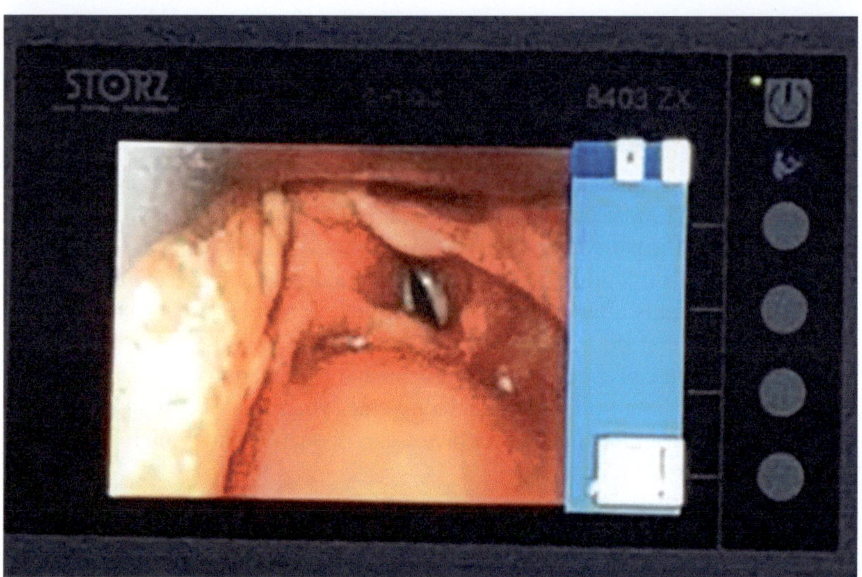

Fig. 47.3 Retropharyngeal abscess, airway obstruction; intubation using a video camera

patients with retropharyngeal abscess developed complications with airway obstruction, and multiple abscesses being the most common among them [33]. Seven of these patients needed follow-up in the intensive care unit, five required bronchoscopy, and seven patients have been intubated for 5 ± 3 days after surgical draining. Another study dealing with deep neck infections in kids under 5 years of age also revealed airway obstruction as the most common complication in 8.2% ($n = 42$) cases [34].

A retropharyngeal abscess complicated by IX, X, and XII cranial nerve palsy probably caused by compression of the carotid area has been described [35]. This observation points out the necessity of careful cranial nerve examination in patients with deep neck infections.

A retrospective study has shown that 9.4% of pediatric patients with retropharyngeal/parapharyngeal abscesses developed complications ($n = 13$), and mediastinitis was the most common one ($n = 9$). That is why a control CT is necessary when clinical presentations do not regress within 48 h. The scanning area must cover the upper mediastinum to check whether it is intact or not. The higher rate of complications was associated with younger age and the abscess location. In this study, S. aureus was the most common bacterial pathogen in complicated cases, and MRSA strains were recovered in four cases [36].

MRSA infection is closely related with the risk of mediastinitis development in pediatric patients with retropharyngeal abscess [37]. Most of these patients require intensive care, revision surgeries, and multiple courses of IV antibiotic therapy. Transthoracic surgery may be required in these children as well. Upon discharge, the physician must instruct parents to control their child's condition carefully, paying particular attention to such complaints as dyspnea, neck pain, sore throat, neck swelling, and fever. Control outpatient examination in the clinic within several days after discharge is obligatory.

References

1. Adil E, Tarshish Y, Robertson D, et al. The public health impact of pediatric deep neck space infections. Otolaryngol Head Neck Surg. 2015;153(6):1036–41.
2. Coticchia JM, Getnick GS, Yun RD, et al. Age-, site-, and time-specific differences in pediatric deep neck abscesses. Arch Otolaryngol Head Neck Surg. 2004;130(2):201–7.
3. Page NC, Bauer EM, Lieu JE. Clinical features and treatment of retropharyngeal abscess in children. Otolaryngol Head Neck Surg. 2008;138(3):300–6.
4. Nour YA, Hassan MH, Gaafar A, et al. Deep neck infections of congenital causes. Otolaryngol Head Neck Surg. 2011;144:365–71.
5. Lawrence R, Bateman N. Controversies in the management of deep neck space infection in children: an evidence-based review. Clin Otolaryngol. 2017;42(1):156–63.
6. Naidu SI, Donepudi SK, Stocks RM, et al. Methicillin-resistant Staphylococcus aureus as a pathogen in deep neck abscesses: a pediatric case series. Int J Pediatr Otorhinolaryngol. 2005;69:1367–71.
7. Fleisch AF, Nolan S, Gerber J, et al. Methicillin-resistant Staphylococcus aureus as a cause of extensive retropharyngeal abscess in two infants. Pediatr Infect Dis J. 2007;26:1161–3.
8. Grisaru-Soen G, Komisar O, Aizenstein O, et al. Retropharyngeal and parapharyngeal abscess in children--epidemiology, clinical features and treatment. Int J Pediatr Otorhinolaryngol. 2010;74(9):1016–20.
9. Sudhanthar S, Garg A, Gold J, et al. Parapharyngeal abscess: a difficult diagnosis in younger children. Clinical Case Rep. 2019;7(6):1218–21.
10. Sichel J, Attal P, Hocwald E, et al. Redefining parapharyngeal space infections. Ann Otol Rhinol Laryngol. 2006;115(2):117–23.
11. Nagy M, Backstrom J. Comparison of the sensitivity of lateral neck radiographs and computed tomography scanning in pediatric deep-neck infections. Laryngoscope. 1999;109(5):775–9.
12. Sethia R, Mahida JB, Subbarayan RA, et al. Evaluation of an imaging protocol using ultrasound as the primary diagnostic modality in pediatric patients with superficial soft tissue infections of the face and neck. Int J Pediatr Otorhinolaryngol. 2017;96:89–93.
13. Zhang Y, Chen Y, Huang H, et al. Diagnostic radiography exposure increases the risk for thyroid microcarcinoma: a population-based case-control study. Eur J Cancer Prev. 2015;24(5):439–46.
14. Collins B, Stoner JA, Digoy GP. Benefits of ultrasound vs. computed tomography in the diagnosis of pediatric lateral neck abscesses. Int J Pediatr Otorhinolaryngol. 2014;78(3):423–6.
15. Sousa Menezes A, Ribeiro DC, Guimarães JR, et al. Management of pediatric peritonsillar and deep neck infections- cross- sectional retrospective analysis. World J Otorhinolaryngol Head Neck Surg. 2019;5(4):207–14.
16. Carbone PN, Capra GG, Brigger MT. Antibiotic therapy for pediatric deep neck abscesses: a systematic review. Int J Pediatr Otorhinolaryngol. 2012;76(11):1647–53.
17. Tansey JB, Hamblin J, Mamidala M, et al. Dexamethasone use in the treatment of pediatric deep neck space infections. Ann Otol Rhinol Laryngol. 2020;129(4):376–9.
18. Sichel JY, Dano I, Hocwald E, et al. Nonsurgical management of parapharyngeal space infections: a prospective study. Laryngoscope. 2002;112(5):906–10.
19. Sichel JY, Gomori JM, Saah D, et al. Parapharyngeal abscess in children: the role of CT for diagnosis and treatment. Int J Pediatr Otorhinolaryngol. 1996;35(3):213–22.
20. Wong DK, Brown C, Mills N, et al. To drain or not to drain - management of pediatric deep neck abscesses: a case-control study. Int J Pediatr Otorhinolaryngol. 2012;76(12):1810–3.

21. Kirse DJ, Roberson DW. Surgical management of retropharyngeal space infections in children. Laryngoscope. 2001;111(8):1413–22.
22. Johnston D, Schmidt R, Barth P. Parapharyngeal and retropharyngeal infections in children: argument for a trial of medical therapy and intraoral drainage for medical treatment failures. Int J Pediatr Otorhinolaryngol. 2009;73(5):761–5.
23. Wilkie MD, De S, Krishnan M. Defining the role of surgical drainage in paediatric deep neck space infections. Clin Otolaryngol. 2019;44(3):366–71.
24. Donà D, Gastaldi A, Campagna M, et al. Deep neck abscesses in children: an Italian retrospective study. Pediatr Emerg Care. 2020;2020:24. https://doi.org/10.1097/PEC.0000000000002037.
25. Okumura Y, Hidaka H, Noguchi N, et al. Intraoral drainage under surgical microscopy with tonsillectomy for parapharyngeal abscesses. J Laryngol Otol. 2015;129(6):595–7.
26. Cramer JD, Purkey MR, Smith SS, et al. The impact of delayed surgical drainage of deep neck abscesses in adult and pediatric populations. Laryngoscope. 2016;126(8):1753–60.
27. Goldenberg D, Golz A, Joachims HZ. Retropharyngeal abscess: a clinical review. J Laryngol Otol. 1997;111(6):546–50.
28. Goldenberg NA, Knapp-Clevenger R, Hays T, et al. Lemierre's and Lemierre's-like syndromes in children: survival and thromboembolic outcomes. Pediatrics. 2005;116(4):e543–8.
29. Waggie Z, Hatherill M, Millar A, et al. Retropharyngeal abscess complicated by carotid artery rupture. Pediatr Crit Care Med. 2002;3(3):303–4.
30. Derinkuyu BE, Boyunağa Ö, Polat M, et al. Association between deep neck space abscesses and internal carotid artery narrowing in pediatric patients. Turk J Med Sci. 2017;47(6):1842–7.
31. Elliott M, Yong S, Beckenham T. Carotid artery occlusion in association with a retropharyngeal abscess. Int J Pediatr Otorhinolaryngol. 2006;70(2):359–63.
32. Ruff MW, Nasr DM, Klaas JP, et al. Internal carotid artery Pseudoaneurysm and ischemic stroke secondary to retropharyngeal and parapharyngeal abscess. J Child Neurol. 2017;32(2):230–6.
33. Elsherif AM, Park AH, Alder SC, et al. Indicators of a more complicated clinical course for pediatric patients with retropharyngeal abscess. Int J Pediatr Otorhinolaryngol. 2010;74(2):198–201.
34. Jain A, Singh I, Meher R, et al. Deep neck space abscesses in children below 5 years of age and their complications. Int J Pediatr Otorhinolaryngol. 2018;109:40–3.
35. Ohara T, Okamoto T, Naganuma H, et al. A pediatric case of retropharyngeal abscess causing multiple instances of cranial nerve palsy. Nihon Jibiinkoka Gakkai Kaiho. 2015;118(5):657–61.
36. Baldassari CM, Howell R, Amorn M, et al. Complications in pediatric deep neck space abscesses. Otolaryngol Head Neck Surg. 2011;144(4):592–5.
37. Wright CT, Stocks RM, Armstrong DL, et al. Pediatric mediastinitis as a complication of methicillin-resistant Staphylococcus aureus retropharyngeal abscess. Arch Otolaryngol Head Neck Surg. 2008;134(4):408–13.

Uvulitis in Children

48

İsmail Zafer Ecevit and Olcay Y. Jones

48.1 Introduction

The term uvula comes from "uva," the Latin word for grape. The palatine uvula or uvula is located at the back edge of the soft palate as a projecting soft tissue in the midline of the oropharynx. It is composed of muscle fibers surrounded by connective tissue with blood vessels, lymph nodes, and the abundance of palatine glands. It is covered by an epithelial layer in continuum with the oral mucosa. Although it is often overlooked during the physical exam, the uvula is a highly sophisticated accessory tissue: mechanically, it is involved in speech and swallowing as a part of the soft palate; it also produces large quantities of saliva as a part of the digestive process in the oral cavity [1]. Isolated uvulitis described as enlarged uvula due to inflammation that can be secondary to bacterial infection, allergy, chemical exposures, and trauma is quite uncommon [2, 3]. It often manifests with an acute onset that can be life-threatening due to the risk of airway obstruction.

48.2 Epidemiology

The incidence of uvulitis is not known but the isolated inflammation of the uvula is rare. Infectious uvulitis is more common among children compared to adults and often associated with streptococcal pharyngitis and tonsillitis [2]. This is likely to be

İ. Z. Ecevit (✉)
Division of Pediatric Infectious Diseases, Department of Pediatrics, Faculty of Medicine, Başkent University, Ankara, Turkey

O. Y. Jones
School of Medicine and Health Sciences, George Washington University, Washington, DC, USA

C. Cingi et al. (eds.), *Pediatric ENT Infections*,
https://doi.org/10.1007/978-3-030-80691-0_48

from the anatomical proximity of the uvula with the Waldeyer's tonsillar ring. The diagnosis of *Streptococcus pyogenes* uvulitis is often overlooked as it usually does not pose serious concerns for the airway patency or require hospital admissions. This appears to be a common pattern for uvulitis as shown in the largest case series in the literature that involves 15 patients [4]. Among those with acute uvulitis from various causes, only one required hospital stay due to the associated peritonsillar abscess. Another case report emphasizes the potential for co-presence of uvulitis and epiglottitis, and the importance of full evaluation of these patients [5, 6]. Relatively limited involvement of uvula during common pharyngitis has been of interest; the role of innate immunity and the particular importance of macrophages and gamma delta T cells have been suggested [7].

48.3 Etiology

Causes of the uvulitis may be infectious or noninfectious (Table 48.1). Bacterial infections and trauma following the use of instruments in the airway are the most common etiologies. Bacterial uvulitis is usually associated with other upper respiratory tract infections such as epiglottitis and tonsillopharyngitis [2, 8].

The most common bacterial cause is *S. pyogenes* (group A streptococcus) and streptococcal uvulitis usually occurs associated with pharyngitis [2, 9]. *Haemophilus influenzae* type b (Hib), the second most common bacteria, may cause isolated uvulitis or

Table 48.1 Etiology of infectious and noninfectious uvulitis

Infectious causes
Streptococcus pyogenes (group A streptococcus)
Haemophilus influenzae type b
Streptococcus pneumoniae
Fusobacterium nucleatum
Beta-lactamase producing *Prevotella intermedia*
Candida albicans
Mycobacterium leprae
Noninfectious causes
Kawasaki disease
Cannabis inhalation
Marijuana use
Cocaine
Sauna hazard
Lisinopril
Mephedrone
Traumatic adenoidectomy
Endotracheal, oral, nasal tubes
Suction catheter
Upper gastrointestinal endoscopy Ecobalium elaterium
Angioedema (Quincke's edema)

uvulitis with epiglottitis or bacteremia especially in children not immunized with Hib vaccine [8, 10–14]. Brook [15] described two children with uvulitis due to anaerobic bacteria; the first had *Fusobacterium nucleatum* isolated from blood and Hib from the uvular surface. The second patient had beta-lactamase-producing *Prevotella intermedia* in blood culture. In another report, an adult patient with uvulitis and epiglottitis grew *Streptococcus pneumoniae* from her blood culture [13]. *Mycobacterium lepra* (leprosy) infection [16] can present with uvular involvement ranging from enanthemas and ulcers to intense fibrosis with partial loss or destruction of the uvula in about 10% of patients. *Candida albicans* uvulitis has been reported among immunocompetent toddlers [17]. Uvular involvement can be associated with viral infections such as enteroviruses, adenovirus, herpes simplex virus, varicella-zoster virus, and Epstein-Barr virus. However, isolated uvulitis has not been reported due to viral infections. The role of viruses on uvular involvement has not been fully studied.

Trauma is the most common cause of noninfectious causes of uvulitis. Traumatic uvulitis has been described after endotracheal, orogastric, or nasal tubes, endoscopy, oropharyngeal suctioning after traumatic adenoidectomy, and laryngeal mask airway use [18–25]. Uvular edema and inflammation may follow cannabis, marijuana, or cocaine inhalation due to thermal irritation or allergic reaction [26–29]. Mephedrone induced uvulitis after nasal inhalation has been reported [30].

Angioedema of the uvula, also known as Quincke's disease, caused by angiotensin-converting enzyme inhibitors (ACE-I) is reported [31, 32]. Isolated uvular edema has been described in a patient taking lisinopril, an antihypertensive ACE-I drug. Hereditary angioneurotic edema (Quincke's edema) results from congenital and acquired C1 inhibitor deficiency (C1INH) or dysfunctional C1INH protein can be present by uvular edema [32, 33]. Life-threatening uvular angioedema has been reported after intranasal application of *Ecbalium elaterium* (the wild or squirting cucumber) juice as a homeopathic remedy for sinusitis [34].

Uvulitis associated with Kawasaki disease has been described in two children [35]. Although mucocutaneous findings of lips and tongue are included in the diagnostic criteria, the changes in uvula are often overlooked among children with Kawasaki disease.

48.4 Pathogenesis

Infectious uvulitis is acute cellulitis with distinguished features of inflammation and edema. Infection occurs by direct invasion of microorganisms after oropharyngeal colonization. Uvular edema may be associated with swelling of the tonsils and hypopharynx [10].

Traumatic procedures may cause uvulitis related to compression injury and ischemia or irritation [21, 23, 36]. Histological examination has revealed abscesses and ulcers on the uvular mucosa after endotracheal tube placement in an adult patient [37].

Mephedrone, a sympathetic stimulant of the amphetamine family, seems to be a type-1 hypersensitivity reaction [30, 38]. Crack cocaine and marijuana burns at high temperature and inhalation cause thermal injury to mucous membranes.

48.5 Clinical Manifestations

Bacterial uvulitis is characterized by enlarged edematous or bullous-appearing and erythematous uvula. The uvula enlarges several times to normal size. The most common symptoms of infectious uvulitis are fever, difficulty swallowing, odynophagia, sore throat, and respiratory distress [2, 4]. The patients are usually leaning forward and may suffer from drooling, spitting, odynophagia, muffled voice or hoarseness, and gagging sensation. Uvulitis may cause cough, stridor, and foreign body sensation to the throat and rarely may lead to complete upper respiratory tract obstruction. The most common associated symptom of group A streptococcal uvulitis is pharyngitis [8, 9]. In this case, the uvula is bright red. *H. influenzae* type b uvulitis usually has been reported in children who did not vaccinate against Hib and coexist with epiglottitis [8, 9, 14]. Uvulitis and epiglottitis may have similar symptoms. In the case of uvulitis with concurrent epiglottitis, upper airway obstruction usually is seen and diagnosis of epiglottitis can be missed [9]. Bacterial uvulitis may be associated with peritonsillar abscess and epiglottitis [4, 6].

A swollen uvula caused by angioedema (Quincke's edema) is usually present with pale and edematous uvula without erythema [39–41]. It is not painful. Most patients are young and otherwise healthy. The patient usually suffers from dysphagia, muffled voice, gagging, and occasional sign of respiratory distress due to upper airway obstruction. Due to allergy, rash and swelling of the lips may be present but rare [42]. Edematous and enlarged uvula can obscure the posterior pharynx [22].

Uvula may be ecchymotic in traumatic patients. Uvulitis with cannabis inhalation can be present with upper airway obstruction [26]. In patients with uvulitis of unknown etiology, the main symptoms are sore throat and dysphagia [4].

48.6 Diagnosis

The diagnosis of uvulitis is easy with a red and swollen uvula [3, 43]. It may be covered with exudate. Fever usually indicates possible infectious uvulitis. History of drug use or exposure to new medicine or food should be asked.

Clinical presentations of uvulitis sometimes similar to epiglottitis with sitting upright position stooped forward and drooling saliva from the open month. While a patient is in a sitting upright position, the uvula would fall backward causing partial obstruction of the oropharynx. Due to severe airway obstruction and respiratory distress in patients with epiglottitis, all patients with uvulitis should be investigated for concurrent epiglottitis [6, 10, 12]. A detailed history and physical examination can give clues for the etiology of uvulitis. Uvulitis with concurrent epiglottitis caused by Hib is suspected in a toxic-appearing child with high fever and respiratory distress especially, the child is between 3 months and 5-year-old age and did not have a history of Hib vaccination. If the patient has associated epiglottitis, a tongue depressor should be avoided for physical examination. A lateral neck X-ray is necessary to rule out epiglottitis.

For patients with upper airway obstruction, flexible fiberoptic laryngoscopy may be needed to visualize the degree of involvement of the supraglottic structures. Computed tomography (CT) or magnetic resonance imaging (MRI) with contrast should be obtained in doubt of peritonsillar or retropharyngeal abscess and/or cellulitis.

Both blood and surface culture of uvula and pharynx for aerobic and anaerobic bacteria are necessary to determine the etiology before antimicrobial therapy.

In patients with compression uvulitis due to oropharyngeal and nasopharyngeal tubes, endotracheal intubation, or endoscopy, appearing of the distal uvula may be erythematous, ecchymotic, or whitish-gray [20, 23, 24]. Traumatic uvulitis should be suspected in a child with uvular edema after extubation [24].

Detecting tetrahydrocannabinol in urine and blood samples may be useful if marijuana use is suspected. Specialized tests including serum levels of total and specific IgE and C1 esterase inhibitor (C1 INH) to rule out allergic reactions or angioedema may be necessary with allergy and immunology consultation [44].

48.7 Differential Diagnosis

Infectious and noninfectious diseases should be thought of in the differential diagnosis of uvulitis. All cases with uvulitis should be carefully evaluated for possible etiologies. Angioedema, hereditary angioneurotic edema, epiglottitis, peritonsillar abscess, retropharyngeal abscess, gingivostomatitis, severe pharyngitis, oro/nasopharyngeal instrumentation, and illicit drug use should be differentiated from infectious uvulitis.

In patients with cellulitis and fever, the infectious etiology of uvulitis needs to be ruled out. Epiglottitis should always be considered as an associated infection with uvulitis especially in patients with fever and respiratory difficulty. But sometimes the patient may not have respiratory distress [6]. Epiglottitis associated with uvulitis can be diagnosed with the presence of a thumb sign on lateral neck X-ray.

For patients with a severe sore throat, difficulty of swallowing, respiratory distress after surgery, endotracheal tube placement, or laryngeal mask airway, uvulitis should be considered.

History of exposure to new drugs or foods may suggest allergic uvular edema. Hereditary angioneurotic edema is the most common cause of recurrent uvula edema and patients usually have a history of similar episodes in the family. Hereditary angioneurotic edema episodes are frequently associated with abdominal pain.

48.8 Treatment

Patients with uvulitis must be carefully managed. Patients with respiratory distress should be hospitalized. To prevent airway obstruction, keeping the patient in proper positioning with an upright position and stooped forward is recommended.

Treatment of uvulitis is based on the etiology. If the bacterial infection seems likely, antibiotic therapy effective for group A streptococcus, *S. pneumoniae*, and

Hib should be given immediately to prevent life-threatening complications such as bacteremia. The decision for parenteral or oral therapy depends on clinical findings, age, and immunization status of the patient. Ceftriaxone and cefotaxime have good coverage for these pathogens, especially penicillin non-sensitive *S. pneumoniae*, beta-lactamase-producing *H. influenzae*, and group A streptococcus (Table 48.2). If the patient has an allergy to beta-lactam antibiotics such as penicillin or cephalosporins and infection is caused by penicillin-resistant *S. pneumoniae*, levofloxacin is the appropriate choice unless there is no effective option for antimicrobial therapy.

Clinically stable patients without respiratory distress can be treated with empiric oral antibiotic regimens. The patients with confirmed streptococcal infection associated with pharyngitis can be treated with oral penicillin V. Amoxicillin-clavulanate, cefuroxime axetil, and cefdinir are other alternatives for penicillin-susceptible *S. pneumonia* infection. Antibiotic treatment can be modified if the organism is identified and susceptibilities are determined. A 7–10 day course of treatment usually will be enough; initial parenteral antibiotic therapy can be switched to oral therapy if the patient is afebrile and clinically stable [3].

The experience of treatment of *Candida* uvulitis is not enough to recommend specific antifungal treatment. One reported candidal uvulitis in a child was treated with topical nystatin and another child improved without treatment [17].

Topical or nebulized epinephrine and steroids are beneficial for preventing severe upper airway obstruction in severe cases of uvular swelling with infectious or non-infectious uvulitis [20, 26, 30, 39, 45, 46]. Dexamethasone or its equivalent steroid is recommended but the optimal dose has not been established; dexamethasone up to 1 mg/kg every 6–12 h for 24–48 h have been reported [47]. In comparison, a single dose of oral dexamethasone (0.6 mg/kg, maximum 10 mg) can provide significant improvement of pain and inflammation as shown in children with severe or exudative acute pharyngitis from group A beta-hemolytic streptococcus [48]. Careful follow-up and hospital admission will be needed particularly if high dose steroids are indicated. Analgesics, topical or nebulized lidocaine should be used for severe pain [20, 23, 26]. If the patient has severe edema leading to airway obstruction, an otolaryngologist should be consulted. Needle decompression, uvulectomy or intubation, and tracheostomy (cricothyrotomy) may be necessary [22, 31, 42, 49].

Table 48.2 Recommended antibiotics and dosages for bacterial uvulitis

Antibiotic	Dose for children
Amoxicillin-clavulanate	45 mg/kg/day po, q12h
Ceftriaxone	50–100 mg/kg/day IV, qd or q12h
Cefotaxime	150–200 mg/kg/day IV, q8h
Cefuroxime	30 mg/kg/day po, q12h
Cefdinir	14 mg/kg/day po, q12h
Penicillin V	25–50 mg/kg/day, q12h
Levofloxacin	6 months to 5 years old: 20 mg/kg/day IV, q12d ≥5 years old: 10 mg/kg/day IV, qd

If there is strong evidence of allergic reaction, prompt treatment with parenteral or topical epinephrine, diphenhydramine and steroids are essential to preserving the patency of upper airways [39]. Angioedema will require an understanding of the underlying mechanism and assuring absence of iatrogenic agents; histamine-mediated angioedema is treated with antihistamines, steroids, and epinephrine; on the other hand, bradykinin-mediated angioedema will require targeted treatment to downregulate kinin pathway [50].

References

1. Finkelstein Y, Meshorer A, Talmi YP, Zohar Y, Brenner J, Gal R. The riddle of the uvula. Otolaryngol Head Neck Surg. 1992;107:444–50.
2. Kotloff KL, Wald ER. Uvulitis in children. Pediatr Infect Dis. 1983;2:392–3.
3. Wald ER. Uvulitis. In: Cherry JD, Harrison GJ, Kaplan SL, Steinbach WJ, Hotez PJ, editors. Feigin and Cherry's textbook of pediatric infectious diseases. 8th ed. Philadelphia: Elsevier; 2019. p. 116–7.
4. McNamara R. Clinical characteristics of acute uvulitis. Am J Emerg Med. 1994;12:51–2.
5. De Pieri C, Valentini E, Pusiol A, Passone E, Gamalero L, Cogo PE. Infective uvulitis in a child. Pediatr Emerg Care. 2020;36(8):384–8. https://doi.org/10.1097/PEC.2258.
6. Shomali W, Holman K. Concurrent uvulitis and epiglottitis. Cleve Clin J Med. 2016;88:712–4.
7. Olofsson K, Hellström S, Hammarström ML. Human uvula: characterization of resident leukocytes and local cytokine production. Ann Otol Rhinol Laryngol. 2000;109:488–96.
8. Li KI, Kiernan S, Wald ER, Reilly JS. Isolated uvulitis due to *Haemophilus influenzae* type b. Pediatrics. 1984;74:1054–7.
9. Aquino V. Terndrup TE uvulitis in three children: etiology and respiratory distress. Pediatr Emerg Care. 1992;8:206–8.
10. Jerrard DA, Olshaker J. Simultaneous uvulitis and epiglottitis without fever or leukocytosis. Am J Emerg Med. 1996;14:551–2.
11. Lathadevi HT, Karadi RN, Thobbi RV, Guggarigoudar SP, Kulkarni NH. Isolated uvulitis: an uncommon but not a rare clinical entity. Indian J Otolaryngol Head Neck Surg. 2005;57:139–40.
12. McNamara R, Koobatian T. Simultaneous uvulitis and epiglottitis in adults. Am J Emerg Med. 1997;15:161–3.
13. Westerman EL, Hutton JP. Acute uvulitis associated with epiglottitis. Arch Otolaryngol Head Neck Surg. 1986;112:448–9.
14. Wynder SG, Lampe RM, Shoemaker ME. Uvulitis and *Hemophilus influenzae* bacteremia. Pediatr Emerg Care. 1986;2:23–5.
15. Brook I. Uvulitis caused by anaerobic bacteria. Pediatr Emerg Care. 1997;13:221.
16. Costa A, Nery J, Olivera M, Cuzzi T, Silva M. Oral lesions in leprosy. Indian J Dermatol Venereol Leprol. 2003;69:381–5.
17. Krober MS, Weir MR. Acute uvulitis apparently caused by *Candida albicans*. Pediatr Infect Dis J. 1991;10:73.
18. Arigliani M, Dolcemascolo V, Passone E, Vergine M, Cogo P. Uvular trauma after laryngeal mask airway use. J Pediatr. 2016;176:217.
19. Casati A, Caldi M, Colnaghi E, Torri G. A rare post-anesthesia complication causing upper airway obstruction. Acta Anaesthesiol Scand. 1997;41:1221–2.
20. Gilmore T, Mirin M. Traumatic uvulitis from a suction catheter. J Emerg Med. 2012;43:479–80.
21. Harris MA, Kumar M. A rare complication of endotracheal intubation. Lancet. 1997;350:1820–1.
22. Partridge RA, McNamara RM. Traumatic uvulitis. Ann Emerg Med. 1992;21:1407.
23. Peghini P, Saicedo J, Al-Kawas F. Traumatic uvulitis. A rare complication of upper GI endoscopy. Gastrointest Endosc. 2001;53:818–20.

24. Ziahosseini K, Ali S, Simo R, Malhotra. Uvulitis following general anesthesia. BMJ Case Rep. 2014;2014:2014205038. https://doi.org/10.1136/bcr-2014-205038.
25. Tabboush ZS. Airway obstruction from uvular edema after traumatic adenoidectomy. Anesth Analg. 2000;91:494.
26. Boyce SH, Quigley MA. Uvulitis and partial upper airway obstruction following cannabis inhalation. Emerg Med. 2002;14:106–8.
27. Guarisco JL, Cheney ML, LeJeune FE Jr, Reed HT. Isolated uvulitis secondary to marijuana use. Laryngoscope. 1998;98:1309–12.
28. Macfarlane R, Hart J, Henry JA. A man with massive uvula. Lancet. 2002;359:492.
29. Mallat A, Robertson J, Brock-Utne JG. Preoperative marijuana inhalation-an airway concern. Can J Anaesth. 1996;43:691–3.
30. Murphy A, Haughey R. Mephedrone-induced uvulitis. Anesthesia. 2014;69:189–90.
31. Kuo DC, Barish RA. Isolated uvular angioedema associated with ACE inhibitor use. J Emerg Med. 1995;13:327–30.
32. Wong AYS, Wong TW, Lau CC. A case of angioedema involving the tongue and uvula. J Emerg Med. 2000;7:162–5.
33. Bork K, Gül D, Hardt J, Drwald G. Hereditary angioedema with normal C1 inhibitor: clinical symptoms and course. Am J Med. 2007;120:987–92.
34. Satar S, Gökel Y, Toprak N, Sebe A. Life-threatening uvular angioedema caused by *Ecobalium elaerium*. Eur J Emerg Med. 2001;8:337–9.
35. Kazi A, Gauthier M, Lebel MH, Farrel CA, Lacroix J. Uvulitis and supraglottitis: early manifestations of Kawasaki disease. J Pediatr. 1992;120:564–7.
36. Diaz JH. Is uvular edema a complication of endotracheal intubation? Anesth Analg. 1993;76:1139–41.
37. Cheng LHH, Halfpenny D. Treatment of an enlarged uvula. Br J Oral Maxillofac Surg. 2008;46:490–1.
38. Kinsey CM, Howell M. A 27-year-old woman with a swollen uvula, chest pain, and elevated creatinine phosphokinase levels. Chest. 2008;133:809–11.
39. Claes P, Devue K, Beckers R, Delooz HH, Corne LC. Sudden drooling and supine gagging: an important emergency? Eur J Emerg Med. 2005;5:255–6.
40. Deutsch ES, Zazal GH. Quincke's edema, revisited. Arch Otolaryngol Head Neck Surg. 1991;117:100–2.
41. Evans TC, Roberge RJ. Quincke's disease of the uvula. Am J Emerg Med. 1987;5:211–6.
42. Roberts JR. Acute angioedema of the uvula. Emerg Med News. 2001;23:7–12.
43. Woods CR. Clinical features and treatment of uvulitis in children and adolescents. In Kaplan SL, Torchia MM (ed). Uptodate,com; last updated 2009, https://somepomed.org/articulos/contents/mobipreview.htm?16/23/16752?source=see_link&anchor=H10. Accessed 14 Dec 2020.
44. Wagenaar-Bos IG, Drouet C. Aygoren-Pursun E, et al functional C1-inhibitor diagnostics in hereditary angioedema: assay evaluation and recommendations. J Immunol Methods. 2008;338:14–20.
45. Neustein SM. Acute uvular edema after regional anesthesia. J Clin Anesth. 2007;19:365–6.
46. Roberge RJ, Sullivan T. Topical epinephrine therapy of acute uvulitis. Am J Emerg Med. 1997;15:331–2.
47. Hawkins DB, Crockett DM, Shum TK. Corticosteroids in airway management. Otolaryngol Head Neck Surg. 1983;91:593–6.
48. Schams SC, Goldman RD. Steroids as adjuvant treatment of sore throat in acute bacterial pharyngitis. Can Fam Physician. 2012;58:52–4.
49. Hawke M, Kwok P. Acute inflammatory edema of the uvula (uvulitis) as a cause of respiratory distress: a case report. J Otolaryngol. 1987;16:188–90.
50. Bernstein JA, Cremonesi P, Hoffmann TK, Hollingsworth J. Angioedema in the emergency department: a practical guide to differential diagnosis and management. Int J Emerg Med. 2017;10(1):15. https://doi.org/10.1186/s12245-017-0141-z.

Epiglottitis (Supraglottitis)

49

Mehmet Özgür Pınarbaşlı, Erkan Özüdoğru,
and Klara Van Gool

49.1 Introduction

Epiglottitis (supraglottitis) is the bacterial infection of the epiglottis and peripheral laryngeal structures. It was first described in 1878 as the case report named "angina epiglottidea anterior" [1]. It threatens life by causing obstruction in upper respiratory tract due to edema secondary to infection. Although the incidence of epiglottitis decreased due to vaccination, it is still seen in the pediatric and adult age groups. These patients usually present to pediatric clinics; however, otolaryngologists should also diagnose the disease and apply necessary treatments.

49.2 Epidemiology

Epiglottitis can be seen in all age groups but it is most common among children between the ages of 2 and 8 [2, 3]. Its incidence in children is three times higher than that of adults [4, 5]. It has been reported in newborns and cases under 1 year of age [6]. It can be seen in all seasons but its incidence increases in winter months. There's no information about the sex-specific incidence of epiglottitis in the literature.

M. Ö. Pınarbaşlı (✉) · E. Özüdoğru
Department of Otorhinolaryngology, Faculty of Medicine, Eskişehir Osmangazi University, Eskişehir, Turkey

K. Van Gool
Department of Otorhinolaryngology, Head and Neck Surgery, University Hospital Antwerpen, Antwerpen, Belgium

49.3 Etiology

In acute epiglottitis, etiology can be divided into infective and noninfective causes. Infective causes are mostly bacterial and are most common among children. The most common cause of this disease is *Haemophilus influenzae type b (Hib)* [7, 8]. However, the incidence of *Hib* in the etiology has decreased considerably due to recent *Hib* vaccination programs [9, 10]. *Hib* was replaced by A group beta-hemolytic streptococcus, *streptococcus pneumoniae,* and *Staphylococcus aureus* [2, 11]. Particularly in children with immunodeficiency, rarely klebsiella, pseudomonas, candida, and viruses are also detected [1, 12, 13]. Noninfective causes include traumas on the upper respiratory tract, trauma from foreign bodies (injury by fishbone), and thermal burns [11, 14].

49.4 Clinical Course

Epiglottitis is an acute presentation that shows a rapid onset in a period of 2–6 h [15]. Patients usually present to pediatric emergency departments of hospitals with symptoms of high fever, sore throat, irritability, excessive drooling of saliva in the mouth, respiratory distress, and difficulty in swallowing. Children are restless and intoxicated. In patients, due to the progression of supraglottic edema, airway obstruction results in dyspnea and stridor symptoms. Children usually prefer to sit upright and extend their heads. In this sitting position, called the "tripod position," the supraglottic airway is maximally open [1, 9, 16].

Additionally, due to supraglottic edema and swollen epiglottis, children cannot swallow their saliva and drool. The drooling, dysphonia, dysphagia, and dyspnea presentation seen more often in the case of pediatric epiglottitis is defined as a 4D finding [17]. Other common signs include a cough, hoarseness, and muffled voice [1, 18].

Infections such as acute otitis media, pneumonia, and meningitis can often occur in children with epiglottitis infection [16].

49.5 Diagnosis

Diagnosis is usually made with the clinic. A red-pink swollen epiglottis observed during the physical examination is sufficient for diagnosis [2]. However, if the respiratory distress of the patient is severe, examination with a tongue depressor, nasopharyngolaryngoscopy, or bronchoscopy should not be performed. These examinations should be performed under operating room conditions after appropriate conditions are provided. Diagnostic methods such as blood draw, radiological examinations which increase anxiety in children, should be delayed until airway safety is achieved.

A lateral neck radiography can be performed to support the diagnosis. This radiography should be performed on children who do not have too much respiratory distress in the company of an anesthesiologist or otolaryngologist [18]. In the radiography, the image referred to as "thumb sign" caused by edema and thickening in the epiglottis and arytenoids is identified [19]. The thumb sign is more common in pediatric cases than in adult cases. Although the thumb sign is said to be pathognomic in children diagnosed with epiglottitis, it has been reported that this finding may not be detected in approximately 20% of the patients in one study and approximately 50% of the patients in another study [7, 20, 21]. Also, anteroposterior chest X-ray may also be performed to rule out croup and the presence of a foreign body [22].

In patients, leukocyte count increases and neutrophil dominance is observed. Left shift is observed in peripheral smear. Blood cultures may be taken to detect the factor. It is also stated in the literature that direct swab from epiglottis can be taken by direct laryngoscopy from children intubated due to respiratory distress [4].

49.6 Differential Diagnosis

In particular, the differential diagnosis should be done with croup, foreign body aspiration, peritonsillar abscess, and parapharyngeal abscess. The absence of fever, good general condition, and sudden onset of respiratory distress should suggest noninfectious conditions such as spasmodic croup, foreign body aspiration, and angioneurotic edema [16]. Anteroposterior chest radiography may be used to rule out foreign body presence. In addition, the subglottic stenosis seen in the same radiography (pencil tip view) should bring croup to mind [16]. Hoarseness and barking cough, which are the typical characteristics of croup, are not seen in acute epiglottitis. Drooling and talking with a muffled voice should suggest acute epiglottitis, retropharyngeal abscess, or peritonsillar abscess. In oral examination, swelling around the tonsils, deviation of the uvula to the opposite side, and the presence of trismus should bring peritonsillar abscess into mind [19]. In lateral cervical radiography, an air-fluid level seen in the prevertebral and retropharyngeal region should suggest a retropharyngeal abscess and a neck tomography should be performed [19].

49.7 Complications

Especially in children without *Hib* vaccination, hematogenous spread of the infectious agent may result in infections such as pneumonia, acute otitis media, pericarditis, and meningitis [2]. Hypoxic damage to the central nervous system and other organs may occur, especially in cases of complete obstruction of the respiratory tract. Post-obstructive pulmonary edema and hypoxia have also been encountered in cases of sudden resolution of the obstruction [2].

49.8 Treatment

There are two important points in the treatment of acute epiglottitis. The first is to provide airway safety. The other is empirical antibiotic therapy after airway safety is provided. Children with suspected acute epiglottitis should be taken to operating room conditions without delay. The necessary conditions for intubation and tracheotomy should be provided in the presence of an anesthesiologist and an otolaryngologist in the operating room. Intubation tubes in appropriate sizes, video laryngoscope, flexible nasopharyngolaryngoscope, rigid bronchoscope, and tracheotomy set should be kept available. Children with severe respiratory distress should be given orotracheal intubation. Children without severe respiratory distress may be followed up in intensive care settings. In some studies, elective intubation was recommended because it would prevent the complications of emergency intubation [19, 23]. During intubation, it is recommended that a tube that is one size smaller than the age-appropriate intubation tube of the child is used [1, 2]. In situations where it is not possible to do intubation, airway safety must be provided by opening emergency tracheotomy.

After ensuring airway safety, epiglottis and other supraglottic structures are assessed by direct laryngoscopy or flexible nasopharyngolaryngoscopy. If the abscess is observed in the epiglottis or vallecula region, incision and drainage should be performed. Blood culture and swab cultures may be obtained. Patients should be started on empirical iv antibiotic therapy and taken to the intensive care unit until the culture results are reported.

Empirical antibiotic therapy should be effective against infectious agents such as *Hib*, beta-hemolytic streptococcus, and *Streptococcus pneumoniae*. For this purpose, the most commonly used antibiotics are Ceftriaxone (100 mg/kg/day/iv), cefotaxime (200 mg/kg/day/iv), and sulbactam ampicillin (100 mg/kg/day/iv) [1, 2, 7, 9, 19]. In the literature, it is said that it is not necessary to use anti-anaerobic agents such as metronidazole because anaerobic microorganisms are not found in culture results [7]. However, if the presence of an abscess is detected in the examination, we think that it is appropriate to add antibiotics effective against anaerobes to treatment after drainage. Vancomycin should be initiated in patients with methicillin-resistant *Staphylococcus aureus* (MRSA) [19].

Antibiotic therapy should be continued for at least 10 days after extubation. Intubated patients should be followed up in the intubated state in intensive care unit for 24–72 h on average [1, 7, 16, 18]. Extubation should be decided according to the status of abatement of edema and infection in the supraglottic structures after daily endoscopic examinations.

The use of steroids in acute epiglottitis treatment is controversial. Although the patients have been reported to be extubated in a shorter time upon abatement of infection and edema in supraglottic structures after steroid use and spend a shorter time in intensive care and have shorter hospitalization times, there are also published articles reporting that these times were unchanged [7, 10, 24]. We believe that using a single daily dose of 1 mg/kg of prednisolone or dexamethasone for 3–4 days in children is effective in resolving edema in supraglottic structures.

In conclusion, acute epiglottitis is a life-threatening serious infection that causes acute respiratory distress following rapid progression in children. When acute epiglottitis is suspected, children should be examined under operating room conditions, started on necessary treatments and followed in intensive care units. These examinations and follow-ups should be done in conjunction with a pediatrician, an anesthesiologist, and an otolaryngologist.

References

1. Stroud RH, Friedman NR. An update on inflammatory disorders of the pediatric airway: epiglottitis, croup, and tracheitis. Am J Otolaryngol. 2001;22(4):268–75.
2. Tezer H. Severe respiratory tract infections in pediatric cases. ANKEM Derg. 2014;28:125–33.
3. Mathoera RB, Wever PC, Van Dorsten FRC, Balter SGT, De Jager CPC. Epiglottitis in the adult patient. Neth J Med. 2008;66:373–7.
4. Oz F. Larenks Ödemi. Solunum. 2003;6(5):257–64.
5. Wurtele P. Acute epiglottis in children and adults: a large-scale incidence study (review). Otolaryngol Head Neck Surg. 1990;103:902.
6. Rosenfeld RM, Fletcher MA, Marban SL. Acute epiglottis in a newborn infant. Pediatr Infect Dis J. 1992;11:594–5.
7. Glynn F, Fenton JE. Diagnosis and management of supraglottitis (epiglottitis). Curr Infect Dis Rep. 2008;10:200–4.
8. Shah RK, Robertson DW, Jones DT. Epiglottitis in the Hemophilus influenza type b vaccine era: changing trends. Laryngoscope. 2004;114:557–60.
9. Koturoglu G, Kurugol Z. Croup syndromes and acute epiglottitis. Turkiye Klinikleri J Pediatr Sci. 2011;7(4):93–7.
10. Guldfred LA, Lyhne D, Becker BC. Acute epiglottitis: epidemiology, clinical presentation, management and outcome. J Laryngol Otol. 2008;122(8):818–23.
11. Roosevelt GE. Acute inflammatory upper airway obstruction (croup, epiglottitis, laryngitis, and bacterial tracheitis). In: Kliegman RM, Stanton BF, St. Geme JM, Schor NF, Behrman RE, editors. Nelson textbook of pediatrics. 19th ed. Philadelphia: Elsevier; 2011. p. 1445–50.
12. Beil EP, Sole DP. A rare case of Candida epiglottitis in an immunocompetent child. Pediatr Emerg Care. 2017;35:26–7. https://doi.org/10.1097/PEC.0000000000001082.
13. Slijepcevic A, Strigenz D, Wiet G, Elmaraghy CA. EBV epiglottitis: primary supraglottic viral infection in a pediatric immunocompetent host. Int J Pediatr Otorhinolaryngol. 2015;79(10):1782–4.
14. Kulick R, Selbest SM, Baker MD. Thermal epiglottitis after swallowing hot beverages. Pediatrics. 1988;81:441.
15. Yener M, Yılmaz YZ. Larenks Enfeksiyonları. Klinik Gelişim. 2012;25:23–8.
16. Blackstock P, Adderhey RJ, Steward DJ. Epiglottitis in young infants. Anesthesiology. 1987;67(1):97–100.
17. Hughes AL, Karter N, Swanson DS. Laryngeal infections. In: Valdez TA, Vallejo JG, editors. Infectious diseases in pediatric otolaryngology. New York: Springer; 2016. p. 151–63.
18. Üçsel R. Üst Solunum Yolu Obstruksiyonları. Pediatr Dent. 2007;57:119–28.
19. Mandal A, Kabra SK, Lodha R. Upper airway obstruction in children. Indian J Pediatr. 2015;82(8):737–44.
20. Loos GD. Pharyngitis, croup and epiglottitis. Prim Care. 1990;17(2):335–45.
21. Madhotra D, Fenton JE, Makura ZG, et al. Airway intervention in adult supraglottitis. Ir J Med Sci. 2004;173:197–9.
22. Abdallah C. Acute epiglottitis: trends, diagnosis and management. Saudi J Anaesth. 2012;6(3):279–81.
23. Hammer J. Acquired upper airway obstruction. Paediatr Respir Rev. 2004;5:25–33.
24. Katori H, Tsukuda M. Acute epiglottitis: analysis of factors associated with airway intervention. J Laryngol Otol. 2005;119:967–72.

Laryngitis, Laryngotracheitis (Croup), and Bacterial Tracheitis in Children

50

Belgin Gülhan, Hasan Tezer, and Ulugbek S. Khasanov

50.1 Introduction

The widely used term, croup, is derived from the word *"kropan,"* meaning cry aloud [1]. In old times until 1900 years, most croup-like diseases were identified as diphtheria. In the year 1883, differentiation anticipated Klebs' discovery of *Corynebacterium diphtheriae.* In 1948, Rabe [2] made a classification of infectious croup as the bacterial or nonbacterial origin and found that mostly was viral in origin.

If the patient has prolonged expiration with wheezing, then the tracheobronchial airway is affected up to the subglottic area. In this case, terms laryngotracheitis and laryngotracheobronchitis are preferred. These terms are used instead of croup in some areas of the world [1]. For the most common type of croup, laryngotracheitis can be also used. In severe laryngotracheitis patients, the term laryngotracheobronchitis can be also chosen. Laryngotracheobronchitis is an extensive form of laryngotracheitis and it is associated with bacterial superinfection [3].

In this chapter, infectious causes of croup as laryngitis, laryngotracheitis, and bacterial tracheitis are highlighted. Acute epiglottitis which is also a cause of croup syndrome is not discussed in this chapter.

B. Gülhan (✉)
Section of Pediatric Infectious Diseases, Ankara City Training and Research Hospital, University of Health Sciences, Ankara, Turkey

H. Tezer
Division of Pediatric Infectious Diseases, Department of Pediatrics, Faculty of Medicine, Gazi University, Ankara, Turkey

U. S. Khasanov
Department of Otorhinolaryngology and Stomatology, Tashkent Medical Academy, Tashkent, Uzbekistan

50.2 Laryngitis

Laryngitis is a common manifestation of infection with many respiratory viruses in children, adolescents, and adults. In closed population groups (school or military camps), outbreaks of laryngitis are caused most frequently by adenovirus types 4 and 7, and community outbreaks most often are seen in association with influenza viruses. Adenovirus and *Streptococcus pyogenes* (group A beta-hemolytic streptococcus) infections can cause laryngitis [3].

Usually, the disease starts with an upper respiratory tract infection (URTI). At the time of infection, cough, sore throat, and hoarseness are observed in laryngitis [3]. The specific clinical manifestation is hoarseness. Other symptoms depend on the causative infectious agent. Adenoviruses and influenza viruses cause the most severe instances of laryngitis. With these viruses, fever usually occurs, and sore throat, headache, muscle aches and pains, and prostration are common symptoms. In contrast, patients with laryngitis resulting from rhinovirus, parainfluenza virüs (PIV), or respiratory syncytial virüs (RSV) infections have minimal or no fever and few systemic complaints. The patients often present with nasal findings like coryza and nasal stiffness. Occasionally, in some patients, a secondary bacterial infection of the upper respiratory tract can also be observed. These patients have persistent hoarseness [1].

Patients with laryngitis should rest their voice and increase fluid intake. The clinicians should order throat culture if *S. pyogenes* infection is suspected. If the throat culture is positive, penicillin or a suitable antimicrobial agent should be given. In children and adolescents with prolong, hoarseness sinusitis should be considered. If laryngeal symptoms persist, the laryngoscopic examination should be performed to exclude tumors, foreign bodies, and other chronic diseases [1]. For the relief of symptoms of laryngitis, humidified air is not efficacious [4, 5].

50.3 Laryngotracheitis (Croup)

The "croup" is often used to identify different respiratory diseases characterized by cough, inspiratory stridor, and hoarseness. These symptoms and signs result from an obstruction in the laryngeal region. Primarily, croup is a *laryngotracheitis*. It covers diseases in a wide spectrum from laryngitis to laryngotracheobronchitis and laryngotracheobroncho-pneumonitis. The etiology of croup syndromes is diverse. The consideration of noninfectious possibilities in the differential diagnosis is very crucial (Table 50.1) [3].

50.3.1 Epidemiology

In general, croup usually is observed in children 6 months to 3 years of age. Its annual incidence is highest in the second year of life at approximately 5% [6–8]. It is rare over the age of 6. On the other hand, croup can be also observed in small

Table 50.1 Clinical considerations and differential diagnosis in croup syndromes (Adopted from Ref. [1])

Infectious	Mechanical	Allergic
Acute epiglottitis Laryngitis Laryngeal diphtheria Laryngotracheitis Laryngotracheobronchitis Laryngotracheobronchopneumonitis Bacterial tracheitis Spasmodic croup	Foreign body Secondary to trauma resulting from intubation Extrinsic or intrinsic mass	Acute angioneurotic edema

infants at the age of 3 months and in adolescents. Boys are more likely to develop the disease than girls with a male-to-female ratio of approximately 1.4:1 [7–10].

In a study, a family history of croup was found the most significant risk factor for croup and recurrent croup. In the multivariable analysis, the odds ratio (OR) for the parents having a history of croup was 3.2 for recurrent croup [11]. In this study, parental smoking was not found to be an increased risk factor for the croup. However, smoking is a risk factor for other respiratory infections [11, 12].

Croup cases are mostly seen in the autumn and early winter period. Between 1998 and 2010, hospitalization due to PIV-related croup in the USA was calculated as 8481 per year (0.4 per 1000 children) and the annual cost was 58 million dollars [13]. Most patients have mild and transient symptoms. Less than 1% of patients require hospitalization. However, croup is a major reason for hospital admissions (3.2–5.1% of emergency room admissions) under the age of 2 [10, 14]. In a 6-year study evaluating the period between 1999 and 2005, the rate of patients admitted to the emergency department due to croup was 5.6%. Among those discharged home, 4.4% had a repeat ED visit within 48 h [10].

In most children, the disease is transmitted by close person-to-person contact with large droplets or by airborne transmission [1].

50.3.2 Etiology

Viruses are responsible for the most acute infection episodes of the upper airway tract. However, bacterial tracheitis and epiglottitis are caused mostly by bacteria (Table 50.2) [3]. The most common etiological agent is human PIV type 1 (PIV-1) [15–17]. Human PIV type 2 (PIV-2) sometimes causes croup outbreaks. Human PIV type 3 (PIV-3) seldomly causes croup and causes more severe clinical conditions than PIV-1 and PIV-2. HPIV-1 and HPV-2 are responsible for most of the croup cases, while PIV-3 is responsible for a minority of cases. Human PIV type 4 (PIV-4) appears as a lower respiratory tract infection rather than croup [18, 19].

Enterovirus (especially coxsackie types A9, B4, and B5, and echovirus types 4, 11, and 21), rhinovirus, RSV, influenza virus, and human bocavirus are other

Table 50.2 Etiologic agents of laryngotracheitis (Adopted from Ref. [1, 7])

Virus
Human parainfluenza virus type 1 (most common)
Human parainfluenza virus type 2
Human parainfluenza virus type 3 (more severe croup than type 1 and 2)
Rhinovirus
Enterovirus (coxsackievirus types A9, B4, and B5, and echovirus types 4, 11, and 21)
Respiratory syncytial virüs (RSV)
Influenza viruses (A and B)
Bocavirus
Human metapneumovirus
Coronavirus (including HCoV-NL63 and SARS-CoV-2)
Measles virus
Adenovirus
Herpes simplex viruses (HSVs)
Bacteria
Mycoplasma pneumonia
Corynebacterium diphtheria

etiological agents [17]. In literature, a sound relationship has been identified between human metapneumovirus and coronavirus (HCoV NL63) infections and croup in pediatric age [20–22]. But some studies showed that human metapneumovirus mostly causes lower respiratory tract infection [23]. Coronaviruses were known to cause croup, and also recently, three pediatric patients with croup-associated severe acute respiratory syndrome *coronavirus* 2 (*SARS-CoV-2*) infection were reported [24].

Sometimes the cause of croup can be bacteria such as *Mycoplasma pneumoni*a. The most common secondary bacterial agents are *Staphylococcus aureus, S. pyogenes, and Streptococcus pneumonia* [7].

50.3.3 Clinical Features and Diagnosis

The prodromal phase of croup lasts 12–48 h. It is associated with pharyngitis, rhinorrhea, fever (low-grade), and with or without cough. After these symptoms, the gradual development of barking cough, hoarseness, and inspiratory stridor is observed. Fever may or may not accompany these symptoms. Symptoms may exacerbate at nighttime, with excitement and crying. Mild croup lasts for 3–7 days. However, severe croup can last up to 2 weeks [25].

The diagnosis of croup is mostly based on the history and physical examination findings. Radiological or laboratory findings are not necessary for diagnosis. Radiological findings can be used in the differentiation of other diseases in the differential diagnosis [1]. To provide surveillance studies, diagnosis and treatment of influenza and isolation in cases requiring hospitalization, nasopharyngeal or oropharyngeal multiplex polymerase chain reaction (PCR) respiratory viruses panel

Table 50.3 Westley croup score (Adopted from Ref. [29])

Clinical situation	Assessment of score
Level of consciousness	Normal, including sleep = 0, disoriented = 5
Cyanosis	None = 0, with agitation = 4, at rest = 5
Stridor	None = 0, with agitation = 1, at rest = 2
Air entry	Normal = 0, decreased = 1, markedly decreased = 2
Retractions	None = 0 mild = 1 moderate = 2 severe = 3

The severity of score: ≤ 2 indicates mild, 3–7 moderate, 8–11 severe, ≥ 12 respiratory failure.

Table 50.4 Assessment of the severity of croup (Modified from Ref. [29])

Mild
• Barking cough
• Stridor
• Retractions (suprasternal and/or intercostal): Mild
Moderate
• Barking cough
• Stridor which can be observed at rest
• Retractions (suprasternal and/or intercostal) which can be visible at rest
• Agitation
Severe
• Barking cough
• Inspiratory stridor (occasionally expiratory)
• Retractions (suprasternal and/or intercostal) which are marked or severe
• Distress or agitation: significant
• Lethargy (possible)

can be used where many agents can be detected from a sample [26, 27]. Also, viral culture and/or rapid diagnostic tests that detect viral antigens are performed on secretions from the nasopharynx or throat. It is not necessary in most cases to detect the etiologic agent causing croup.

Clinically, the severity of the disease is determined by the following signs: the presence or absence of stridor at rest, degree of chest wall retractions, air entry, presence or absence of pallor or cyanosis, and mental status. These findings have created the score to evaluate the response to corticosteroid and nebulized epinephrine therapy, namely the *Westley Croup Score* (WCS) (Table 50.3) [28].

Although there are no universally accepted standards for assessing disease severity, some tools can be useful in estimating the severity of croup (Table 50.4).

50.3.4 Differential Diagnosis

In the differential diagnosis of croup, bacterial tracheitis is the most important disease. It also carries a high risk of airway obstruction. Similarly, foreign material blockage and angioneurotic edema are other causes of obstruction in the upper airway. In these diseases, symptoms are usually observed abruptly; the patient is afebrile and other clues of the infection are absent. Laryngotracheobronchitis and laryngotracheobronchopneumonia patients have signs of lower airway tract infection like pneumonia. These help the clinician in the differential diagnosis of these diseases from spasmodic croup and laryngotracheitis. In unvaccinated patients with possible exposure, laryngeal diphtheria should be also kept in mind.

Deep neck infections such as retropharyngeal or peritonsillar abscess may have findings mimicking the airway obstruction. Extrinsic compressing of the airway (vascular ring) and intraluminal obstruction from masses (laryngeal web, laryngeal papilloma, subglottic hemangioma) are the other possible causes of upper airway obstruction. Patients with these diseases usually have chronic repeated complaints [1, 3, 29].

50.3.5 Complications

The child should be observed for the following complications: hypoxemia and cardiorespiratory failure, pulmonary edema, pneumothorax and pneumomediastinum, mechanical problems caused by tracheotomies and nasotracheal tubes, and secondary bacterial infections. Children with a history of croup have an increased prevalence of bronchial reactivity [1].

50.3.6 Treatment

The main treatment tools of croup in children are the management of hypoxia and stabilization of the airway. The treatment of children diagnosed with acute spasmodic and infectious croup is also possible at home [3].

In children with croup, the consensus is that patients should be made as relaxed as possible. The treatment that is applied should not scare or disturb the child because excitement causes an increase in symptoms [30]. In children with respiratory distress, oxygen should be administered. The humidified air is not an effective treatment option for croup [30–33].

50.3.6.1   Nebulized Epinephrine

Nebulized epinephrine is an agreed therapy in moderate and severe cases. Epinephrine diminishes laryngeal mucosal edema. It constricts capillary arterioles. Nebulized racemic epinephrine (0.05 mL/kg per dose (maximum of 0.5 mL) of a 2.25 percent solution diluted to 3 mL total volume with normal saline) or L-epinephrine (0.5 ml/kg/dose, max. Dose 5 mL of 1:1000 dilution) can be also used. The activity period of racemic epinephrine is less than 2 h. L-epinephrine and racemic epinephrine are equally effective [34]. Patients should be observed for 2–3 h.

If the croup symptoms do not reappear, no rest stridor is present and pulse oximetry, color, and level of consciousness are normal and the patients have received steroids, then the patients can be discharged. Nebulized epinephrine should be used attentively in tachycardic patients, and in patients with Fallot tetralogy and ventricular outlet obstruction due to possible cardiovascular signs like tachycardia and hypertension may be observed [3, 35, 36].

50.3.6.2 Corticosteroids

Corticosteroids diminish edema in laryngeal mucosa edema. Corticosteroid use in croup is investigated extensively. Corticosteroids improve croup scores, decrease the need for epinephrine, shorten the duration of stay in the emergency department, and reduce unplanned admissions to hospitals [37–40]. In meta-analyses of randomized trials, patients treated with corticosteroids have distinctive recovery [41–43]. In another meta-analysis of 10 trials (1679 children), glucocorticoids reduced the rate of return visits and hospital admission or readmission compared with placebo [38]. The classical dosage of *dexamethasone* is thought to be 0.6 mg/kg intramuscular or peroral. Instead, other doses like 0.30 and 0.15 mg/kg have been also suggested [37, 41]. Low-dose dexamethasone (0.15 mg/kg) may also have similar effects to higher doses. In a noninferiority study of comparison between dexamethasone 0.6 mg/kg with a dose of 0.15 mg/kg and prednisolone 1 mg/kg, there was no difference in treatment in terms of doses and steroid type [42].

Prednisolone of doses at 1 mg/kg per oral (single dose) is an alternative treatment to oral dexamethasone [44]. However, the risk of recurrence of croup symptoms is increased with the use of a single dose of prednisolone compared to the use of dexamethasone [38, 42].

Nebulized budesonide (2 mg/4 ml of water) and intramuscular dexamethasone have an identical clinical impact; oral and intramuscular dexamethasone have similar effects on disease. Nebulized budesonide can be used as an alternative agent in patients who cannot take dexamethasone orally and cannot be treated with intravenous or intramuscular [29].

Beclomethasone, betamethasone, and *fluticasone* were also studied in some trials but not routinely used in clinical settings [45–47]. Steroids are contraindicated in patients with varicella or tuberculosis (unless the patient is under appropriate antituberculosis treatment) [3]. Steroids may increase the risk of complications of varicella after exposure to the varicella virus. The other complications are disseminated disease or bacterial superinfection [48].

50.3.6.3 Other Treatment Modalities

In croup, there is no indication of antibiotics. In small pediatric patients with the age of less than 4 years, cough and cold medications should not be given [3]. Cold weather also may improve symptoms in mild croup, but there is no study on this subject.

Administration of heliox, helium, and oxygen as a mixture is useful in croup. Heliox may decrease the work of breathing in children with severe croup by reducing turbulent airflow. However, there is no satisfying evidence in the literature for recommending it in severe croup cases. There is limited data to recommend it as general use in children with severe croup [49–51]. If a child has progressive stridor, respiratory distress, severe resting stridor, hypoxia, depressed mental status, cyanosis, need for reliable observation, or decreased oral intake, hospitalization is essential [3]. Antitussives, decongestants, and sedatives generally do not play a role in the management of croup.

According to the severity of the disease, the treatment modalities of croup are shown in Table 50.5 [29].

50.4　Bacterial Tracheitis

As a definition, bacterial tracheitis is the infection of the trachea. Although rare, it is a potentially life-threatening disease [3]. In bacterial tracheitis, there is an invasion of bacterial infection to the tracheal soft tissues. However, bacterial tracheitis

Table 50.5　Treatment of croup (Adopted from Ref. [1, 14, 29])

	Mild	Moderate	Severe
	Barky cough, hoarseness; no stridor, no or minimal chest wall retractions at rest	Stridor and chest wall retractions at rest; no agitation	Stridor, sternal contractions at rest, accompanied by agitation or fatigue
Therapy			
Decongestants, cough suppressants, antibiotics	Not recommended	Not recommended	Not recommended
Humidification	Not proven beneficial	No effect	No effect
Corticosteroids	Dexamethasone (0.6 mg/kg, one dose PO)	Dexamethasone (0.6 mg/kg, one dose PO or IM)	Dexamethasone (0.6 mg/kg, one dose PO or IM)
Nebulized epinephrine	Not recommended	Nebulized racemic epinephrine (0.25–0.5 mL of 2.25% racemic epinephrine in 3 mL of normal saline, can be used every 20 min or L-epinephrine (5 of 1:1000 solution)	Nebulized racemic epinephrine (0.25–0.5 mL of 2.25% racemic epinephrine in 3 mL of normal saline, can be used every 20 min or L-epinephrine (5 mL of 1:1000 solution)
Disposition	Discharge home	Discharge to home if no stridor and no retractions at rest. If no improvement in 4 h, consider hospitalization	Observe for 2 h *Good response*: no recurrence, no stridor, no retractions at rest. Discharge to home possible *Poor response*: stridor, retractions at rest after two epinephrine doses. Hospitalize

IM intramuscular; *PO* per oral.

occurs more commonly than generally noticed. The situation constantly leads to increased respiratory effort. This may cause total airway obstruction and/or respiratory arrest [51].

50.4.1 Epidemiology

Tracheitis is a significant reason for reversible airway obstruction in children. Bacterial tracheitis is also named pseudomembranous or bacterial croup. It is a potentially lethal condition that mainly affects pediatric patients [52]. Tracheitis is responsible for 5–14% of the cases with upper-airway obstruction who require intensive care [53, 54]. In a study evaluating the years between 1993 and 2007, the estimated incidence of bacterial tracheitis was determined as 0.1 per 100,000 people [55]. The mean age of diagnosis is between 5 and 7 years and slightly have seen predominancy in males [3]. Bacterial tracheitis is usually seen in the first 6 years of life. In a study in which 300 cases were compiled, the age range was calculated as 10–78 months [56]. Also in this study, it was observed that the number of males was higher (male-to-female ratio of 1.3:1).

Bacterial tracheitis may follow a primary viral infection. Most cases of bacterial tracheitis are seen following a viral upper respiratory tract infection in previously healthy children [57]. Bacterial tracheitis complications developed in 21 (0.3%) of 6769 patients under the age of 18 who were hospitalized due to influenza infection between 2003 and 2010 in the United States (US) [58].

The most common cause of bacterial tracheitis in all case series was methicillin-sensitive *S. aureus* (MSSA) [57, 58]. Other commonly isolated bacteria include *S. pneumoniae, S. pyogenes*), alpha-hemolytic streptococci, and *Moraxella catarrhalis* which is more common among younger children [1, 59].

50.4.2 Clinical Manifestation

The affected child has symptoms of acute airway obstruction. The most common symptoms are stridor, tachypnea, fever, cough, a husky voice, or increased secretions from the nose and mouth. In the first 2–7 days, symptoms of the disease are mild or moderate. Later the clinical situation usually worsens acutely. In terms of clinical signs, the patient can lie straight and does not salivate. Dysphagia is not expected. Bacterial tracheitis should be kept in mind if the child is febrile with a toxic appearance and if the symptoms do not get better with nebulized epinephrine. On visualization, there is inflammation in the subglottic area, edema of the tracheal mucosa, and voluminous purulent endotracheal secretions in the airways. There is mild inflammation in epiglottis which is unremarkable, different from findings in bacterial epiglottitis [1, 3, 51, 57]. Other uncommon but reported symptoms and signs include neck pain, orthopnea, choking, dysphagia, dysphonia, and syncope [57].

50.4.3 Diagnosis

History, clinical suspicion, and complete physical examination are essential for the tracheitis diagnosis. For differential diagnosis of tracheitis from pneumonia, chest radiography is usually used. Direct laryngoscopy and bronchoscopy can help to the conclusive diagnosis of tracheitis. This procedure should be made by a pediatric otolaryngologist preferably in the operative room [57]. The presence of purulent tracheal secretion, pseudomembranes, and tracheal inflammation with normal-appearing epiglottis and larynx are clues for the diagnosis. In 38–100% of the cases, endotracheal intubation is needed. Later, bacterial cultures (aerobic and anaerobic) and viral cultures (if indicated) should be obtained in the procedure [1, 58].

50.4.4 Treatment

The mainstay of the treatment is airway management, the stabilization of the airway. Many patients require endotracheal intubation. If there are signs of severe airway obstruction (e.g., hypoxia, marked retractions, depressed level of consciousness) airway control precedes diagnostic evaluation.

Antimicrobial treatment should be initiated in a child with the course suggestive of bacterial tracheitis. Empiric treatment should comprise antistaphylococcal agents. Current empiric treatment includes vancomycin initially 45–60 mg/kg per day intravenously divided every 6–8 h, dose and frequency are individualized based on serum concentration or clindamycin 40 mg/kg per day in three divided doses, and a third-generation cephalosporin (e.g., cefotaxime 150 mg/kg per day every 6–8 h intravenously or ceftriaxone 50–100 mg/kg mg/kg per day divided every 12–24 h, usual maximum daily dose: 2000 mg per day (higher maximum daily doses as high as 4000 mg per day for human immunodeficiency virus [HIV]-(exposed or -positive) patients [59]. If MSSA is isolated, treatment should be changed to oxacillin 150 mg/kg per day every 6 h intravenously or another antistaphylococcal penicillin [1, 3] such as ampicillin-sulbactam or a first-generation cephalosporin.

If direct laryngoscopy is suggestive of bacterial tracheitis, an artificial airway should be strongly considered. Supplemental oxygen is usually essential. Children with tracheitis are more prone to airway obstruction. In this case, appropriate antimicrobials and aggressive supportive care help extubation within 3–4 days. If the patient is an immune-compromised host, antivirals, antifungals, or immune modulators can be given. In immune-compromised patients, fungal tracheitis often has a poor prognosis [1, 3, 56, 60].

References

1. Tovar Padua LJ, Cherry JD. Croup (laryngitis, laryngotracheitis, spasmodic croup, laryngotracheobronchitis, bacterial tracheitis, and laryngotracheobranchopneumonitis) and epiglottitis (supraglottis). In: Cherry JD, Harrison GJ, Kaplan SL, Steinbach WJ, Hotez PJ, editors. Feigin

and Cherry's textbook of pediatric infectious diseases. 8th ed. Philadelphia: Elsevier; 2019. p. 175–90.

2. Rabe EF. Infectious croup; etiology. Pediatrics. 1948;2(3):255–65.

3. Rodrigues KK, Roosevelt GE. Acute inflammatory upper airway obstruction (croup, epiglottitis, laryngitis, and bacterial tracheitis). In: Kliegman RM, editor. Nelson textbook of pediatrics. 21st ed. Philadelphia: Elsevier; 2020. p. 2202–6.

4. Neto GM, Kentab O, Klassen TP, et al. A randomized controlled trial of mist in the acute treatment of moderate croup. Acad Emerg Med. 2002;9:873–9.

5. Scolnik D, Coates AL, Stephens D, et al. Controlled delivery of high vs low humidity vs mist therapy for croup in emergency departments: a randomized controlled trial. JAMA. 2006;295:1274–80.

6. Denny FW, Murphy TF, Clyde WA, et al. Croup: an 11-year study in pediatric practice. Pediatrics. 1983;71:871–96.

7. Cherry JD. Clinical practice. Croup N Engl J Med. 2008;358:384–91.

8. Bjornson CL, Johnson DW. Croup. Lancet. 2008;371(9609):329–39.

9. Segal AO, Crighton EJ, Moineddin R, et al. Croup hospitalizations in Ontario: a 14-year time-series analysis. Pediatrics. 2005;116:51–5.

10. Rosychuk RJ, Klassen TP, Metes D, et al. Croup presentations to emergency departments in Alberta, Canada: a large population-based study. Pediatr Pulmonol. 2010;45:83–91.

11. Pruikkonen H, Dunder T, Renko M, et al. Risk factors for croup in children with recurrent respiratory infections: a case-control study. Paediatr Perinat Epidemiol. 2009;23:153–9.

12. Salzman MB, Filler HF, Schechter CB. Passive smoking and croup. Arch Otolaryngol Head Neck Surg. 1987;113:866–8.

13. Abedi GR, Prill MM, Langley GE, et al. Estimates of parainfluenza virus-associated hospitalizations and cost among children aged less than 5 years in the United States, 1998-2010. J Pediatric Infect Dis Soc. 2016;5:7–13.

14. Ortiz-Alvarez O. Acute management of croup in the emergency department. Paediatr Child Health. 2017;22:166–73.

15. Peltola V, Heikkinen T, Ruuskanen O. Clinical courses of croup caused by influenza and parainfluenza viruses. Pediatr Infect Dis J. 2002;21:76–8.

16. Counihan ME, Shay DK, Holman RC, et al. Human parainfluenza virus-associated hospitalizations among children less than five years of age in the United States. Pediatr Infect Dis J. 2001;20:646–53.

17. Rihkanen H, Rönkkö E, Nieminen T, et al. Respiratory viruses in laryngeal croup of young children. J Pediatr. 2008;152:661–5.

18. Frost HM, Robinson CC, Dominguez SR. Epidemiology and clinical presentation of parainfluenza type 4 in children: a 3-year comparative study to parainfluenza types 1-3. J Infect Dis. 2014;209:695–702.

19. Xiao NG, Duan ZJ, Xie ZP, et al. Human parainfluenza virus types 1-4 in hospitalized children with acute lower respiratory infections in China. J Med Virol. 2016;88:2085–91.

20. Kuypers J, Martin ET, Heugel J, et al. Clinical disease in children associated with newly described coronavirus subtypes. Pediatrics. 2007;119:e70–6.

21. Sung JY, Lee HJ, Eun BW, et al. Role of human coronavirus NL63 in hospitalized children with croup. Pediatr Infect Dis J. 2010;29:822–6.

22. Van der Hoek L, Sure K, Ihorst G, et al. Croup is associated with the novel coronavirus NL63. PLoS Med. 2005;2:e240.

23. Døllner H, Risnes K, Radtke A, Nordbø SA. Outbreak of human metapneumovirus infection in Norwegian children. Pediatr Infect Dis J. 2004;23:436–40.

24. Venn AMR, Schmidt JM, Mullan PC. A case series of pediatric croup with COVID-19. Am J Emerg Med. 2020;43:287. https://doi.org/10.1016/j.ajem.2020.09.034.

25. Johnson D, Williamson J. Croup: duration of symptoms and impact on family functioning. Pediatr Res. 2001;49:83A.

26. McCulloh RJ, Andrea S, Reinert S, Chapin K. Potential utility of multiplex amplification respiratory viral panel testing in the management of acute respiratory infection in children: a retrospective analysis. J Pediatric Infect Dis Soc. 2014;3:146–53.
27. Couturier MR, Barney T, Alger G, et al. Evaluation of the FilmArray® respiratory panel for clinical use in a large children's hospital. J Clin Lab Anal. 2013;27:148–54.
28. Westley CR, Cotton EK, Brooks JG. Nebulized racemic epinephrine by IPPB for the treatment of croup: a double-blind study. Am J Dis Child. 1978;132:484–7.
29. Toward Optimized Practice (TOP) Working Group for Croup. Clinical practice guideline for diagnosis and management of croup, 2008 (revised 2015). https://actt.albertadoctors.org/CPGs/Lists/CPGDocumentList/croup-guideline.pdf. Accessed 21 Nov 2020.
30. Kaditis AG, Wald ER. Viral croup: current diagnosis and treatment. Pediatr Infect Dis J. 1998;17:827–34.
31. Brook I. Aerobic and anaerobic microbiology of bacterial tracheitis in children. Clin Infect Dis. 1995;20:222–3.
32. Geelhoed G. Croup Pediatr Pulmonol. 1997;23:370–4.
33. Klassen T. Croup: a current perspective. Pediatr Clin North Am. 1999;46:1167–78.
34. Waisman Y, Klein BL, Boenning DA, et al. Prospective randomized double-blind study comparing L-epinephrine and racemic epinephrine aerosols in the treatment of laryngotracheitis (croup). Pediatrics. 1992;89:302–6.
35. Bjornson C, Russell K, Vandermeer B, et al. Nebulized epinephrine for croup in children. Cochrane Database Syst Rev. 2013:CD006619.
36. Lee JH, Jung JY, Lee HJ, et al. Efficacy of low-dose nebulized epinephrine as a treatment for croup: a randomized, placebo-controlled, double-blind trial. Am J Emerg Med. 2019;37:2171.
37. Kairys SW, Olmstead EM, O'Connor GT. Steroid treatment of laryngotracheitis: a meta-analysis of the evidence from randomized trials. Pediatrics. 1989;83:683–93.
38. Gates A, Gates M, Vandermeer B, et al. Glucocorticoids for croup in children. Cochrane Database Syst Rev. 2018;8:CD001955.
39. Tibballs J, Shann FA, Landau LI. Placebo-controlled trial of prednisolone in children intubated for croup. Lancet. 1992;340:745–8.
40. Bjornson CL, Klassen TP, Williamson J, et al. A randomized trial of a single dose of oral dexamethasone for mild croup. N Engl J Med. 2004;351:1306–13.
41. Johnson DW, Jacobson S, Edney PC, et al. A comparison of nebulized budesonide, intramuscular dexamethasone, and placebo for moderately severe croup. N Engl J Med. 1998;339:498–503.
42. Ausejo M, Saenz A, Pham B, et al. The effectiveness of glucocorticoids in treating croup: a meta-analysis. BMJ. 1999;319:595–600.
43. Russell K, Wiebe N, Saenz A, et al. Glucocorticoids for croup. Cochrane Database Syst Rev. 2011;1:CD001955.
44. Garbutt JM, Conlon B, Sterkel R, et al. The comparative effectiveness of prednisolone and dexamethasone for children with croup: a community-based randomized trial. Clin Pediatr (Phila). 2013;52:1014–21.
45. Eboriadou M, Chryssanthopoulou D, Stamoulis P, et al. The effectiveness of local corticosteroids therapy in the management of mild to moderate viral croup. Minerva Pediatr. 2010;62:23.
46. Amir L, Hubermann H, Halevi A, et al. Oral betamethasone versus intramuscular dexamethasone for the treatment of mild to moderate viral croup: a prospective, randomized trial. Pediatr Emerg Care. 2006;22:541–4.
47. Roorda RJ, Walhof CM. Effects of inhaled fluticasone propionate administered with metered-dose inhaler and spacer in mild to moderate croup: a negative preliminary report. Pediatr Pulmonol. 1998;25:114–7.
48. Dowell S, Bresee J. Severe varicella associated with steroid use. Pediatrics. 1993;92:223–8.
49. Moraa I, Sturman N, McGuire TM, et al. Heliox for croup in children. Cochrane Database Syst Rev. 2018;10(10):CD006822.
50. DiCecco R, Rega P. The application of heliox in the management of croup by an air ambulance service. Air Med J. 2004;23:33–5.

51. Walner DL. The utility of radiographs in the evaluation of pediatric upper airway obstruction. Ann Otol Rhinol Laryngol. 1999;108:378–83.
52. Jones R, Santos JI, Overall JC. Bacterial tracheitis. JAMA. 1979;242:721–6.
53. Chan PW, Goh A, Lum L. Severe upper airway obstruction in the tropics requiring intensive care. Pediatr Int. 2001;43:53–7.
54. Chiu TF, Huang LM, Chen JC, et al. Croup syndrome in children: five-year experience. Acta Paediatr Taiwan. 1999;40:258–61.
55. Tebruegge M, Pantazidou A, Yau C, et al. Bacterial tracheitis - tremendously rare, but truly important: a systematic review. J Pediatr Infect Dis. 2009;4:199–209.
56. Tebruegge M, Pantazidou A, Thorburn K, et al. Bacterial tracheitis: a multi-centre perspective. Scand J Infect Dis. 2009;41:548–57.
57. Stroud RH, Friedman NR. An update on inflammatory disorders of the pediatric airway: epiglottitis, croup, and tracheitis. Am J Otolaryngol. 2001;22:268–75.
58. Huang YL, Peng CC, Chiu NC, et al. Bacterial tracheitis in pediatrics: 12-year experience at a medical center in Taiwan. Pediatr Int. 2009;51:110–3.
59. American Academy of Pediatrics. Systemic antimicrobials with dosage forms and usual dosages. In: Bradley JS JS, Nelson JD, Barnett ED, et al., editors. Nelson's pediatric antimicrobial therapy. 26th ed. Itasca: American Academy of Pediatrics; 2020.
60. Salamone FN, Bobbitt DB, Myer CM, et al. Bacterial tracheitis reexamined: is there a less severe manifestation? Otolaryngol Head Neck Surg. 2004;131:871–6.

HPV-Related Recurrent Respiratory Papillomatosis in Childhood

51

Hakan Çelikhisar, Zafer Kurugöl, and Khassan M. Diab

51.1 Introduction

Recurrent respiratory papillomatosis (RRP) commonly exacts a heavy toll on children and their relatives, resulting from the morbidity of the condition itself, the necessary therapeutic interventions and the psychological burden it imposes. It occurs with a relatively low frequency, but the viruses responsible (human papillomaviruses 6 and 11) are widely prevalent. Recurrent respiratory papillomatosis creates considerable morbidity in the form of dysphonia, blockage to the airway, and the need for operative intervention to occur repeatedly. Although papillomas can develop anywhere along the length of the upper airway, the most commonly affected region is the vocal cord. Hence, the usual first indication of the condition is a voice problem. The process of phonation relies on unimpeded vibration of the cords as the pressure below the glottis exceeds that above. However, papilloma growth alters the resonating character of the cords and produces an abnormal mucosal wave. Surprisingly, even though the voice is one of the most distinctive individual traits possessed by human beings, alterations in the way a small child speaks may pass unnoticed. Nonetheless, the unimpeded development of papillomas can threaten the

H. Çelikhisar (✉)
Section of Pulmonology, İzmir Metropolitan Multicipality Eşrefpaşa Hospital, İzmir, Turkey

Z. Kurugöl
Division of Pediatric Infectious Diseases, Department of Pediatrics, Faculty of Medicine, Ege University, İzmir, Turkey

K. M. Diab
Federal State Budgetary Institution, Scientific and Clinical Center of Otorhinolaryngology of the Medico-Biological Agency, and Ministry of Health, Pirogov Russian National Research Medical University, Moscow, Russia

© The Author(s), under exclusive license to Springer Nature Switzerland AG 2022
C. Cingi et al. (eds.), *Pediatric ENT Infections*,
https://doi.org/10.1007/978-3-030-80691-0_51

patency of the airway and produce both dyspnoea and stridor. Treatment aims above all else to lessen these symptoms, by excising the papilloma. Even where a radical surgical approach is adopted, however, the papilloma will usually regrow [1–3].

Over the last 10 years, human papillomaviruses (HPVs) have been the focus of intensive research. This virus family is extremely varied, but all share a tropism for keratinocytes within the epidermis or the mucosa [1, 2]. Human papillomavirus gains entry into the cells at the base of the epithelium. A variety of infectious conditions affecting the skin or mucosae result from HPV invasion. There are a number of modes of transmission, including sexual activity, close physical contact with infected people or clothing, and vertical transmission from a pregnant woman with HPV to her child. The resulting infection may be symptomatic or asymptomatic [1–4]. Cutaneous and genital condylomata, recurrent respiratory papillomatosis (RRP), low-grade and high-grade squamous intraepithelial lesions (SILs) and cervical carcinoma are all conditions resulting from HPV infection. At present, cervical carcinoma is the second most common malignancy in women worldwide [5].

It has recently been found that HPV is present within the mouth in between 6 and 10% of children and adolescents, whilst the frequency of HPV in normal adults is 5–8%. A key condition resulting from cutaneous or oral mucosal infection by HPV-2 or 4 (usually) is verruca vulgaris. Within the mouth, this lesion typically occurs on keratinised portions of the mucosa, such as the labial, gingival and palatal surfaces. Verruca vulgaris is most frequent in children, but may occur in adults, too. The lesion is highly contagious. Another lesion, focal hyperplasia of the epithelium (eponymously referred to as Heck's disease) results from infection by HPV-13 and 32. It is usually seen in paediatric patients, but the incidence is also rising in patients with HIV. The lesions, which are multiple, sessile and nodular, are found on the labial or lingual mucosa. This condition frequently resolves spontaneously and is highly unlikely to recur once it resolves [2].

Guidelines for managing HPV have recently been issued in the form of Proceedings from the 4th Workshop on Paediatric Virology held in September 2018 in the Greek capital, Athens [6].

51.2 Microbiology

The HPVs are diminutive, capsid viruses that lack an envelope. Their genome consists of 8000 base pairs, with eight genes, two of which are the structural proteins, L1 and 2, that encapsulate the genome. It has been possible to genetically engineer cell cultures to express the L1 protein. This protein undergoes self-assembly even when other viral proteins are not present, forming a virus-like particle (VLP), which has been used as the target for vaccines against the HPVs. L1 is the key pathogenicity factor, a smaller role being played by L2. The mechanism the virus uses to replicate is tied to the process through which epithelium differentiates. The virus can infect the basal cell layer of the epithelium since there are minute gaps in the integrity of the epithelium. There are heparan sulphate proteoglycans which facilitate attachment of the virions to the stem cells of the base layer. As the layers migrate upwards and differentiate, the virus expresses different genes, eventually expressing L1, L2 and E4 as the cell reaches the top level. These genes are needed for the virus to enclose its genome prior to release. When the virally infected cell is desquamated after a brief period, the HPV virions are scattered, ready to infect further basal cells [6, 7].

51.3 Background

There has been intensive research into HPVs in both young and older children, covering cutaneous and genital condylomata, RRP in boys and girls below and above the age of 1 year and the occurrence of cervical squamous intraepithelial lesions in girls during adolescence [5, 8]. The beginning of this research push was in 1978, with the publication of the first study investigating paediatric cases of HPV, authored by Pfister and zur Hausen [9]. Studies have been undertaken all across the globe to understand HPV in children, taking advantage of advances in molecular methods, notably PCR (polymerase chain reaction). This area of study has achieved prominence alongside the development and clinical deployment of vaccines targeting HPV. This chapter reviews the history of efforts to understand HPV in children, which have led up to our current knowledge of HPV in this age group [6, 9].

51.4 HPV Infection of the Larynx in Neonates and Children

In children, infection with HPV may result in cutaneous or anogenital condylomata as well as papilloma growth in the larynx or mouth. Papillomas in the larynx secondary to HPV infection generally appear during infancy, with a pronounced tendency to recur. The condition has usually been referred to as juvenile onset recurrent respiratory papillomatosis (JO-RRP) [10]. The usual viral subtypes isolated in this condition are HPV-6 and HPV-11 [10]. It is thought that HPV is transmitted to the infant vertically, from an infected mother [11]. The typical accompanying clinical presentation is of increasing dysphonia, stridor and potentially a grave blockage of the airway. The condition is mostly diagnosed following a laryngoscopic examination, where characteristic lesions are seen. In some cases, a histopathological diagnosis may be needed. Juvenile onset recurrent respiratory papillomatosis rarely causes death and treatment usually produces a good initial outcome. Nonetheless, the condition may progress with different degrees of severity and frequently it reduces the patient's life quality [10].

There are a variety of therapeutic techniques, which generally all have the goal of keeping the airway unobstructed whilst causing minimal injury to the larynx itself. The usual tried-and-tested approach is to operate on the papillomas, excising them with a microdebrider, ablating them with lasers or employing both techniques together [12]. Unfortunately, the nature of the disorder is such that recurrence swiftly occurs and there is no alternative but to keep excising the papillomas surgically. Repeated operations render complications more probable, including laryngeal injury. In the light of this issue, pharmacotherapeutic strategies have been advocated, especially when used in conjunction with surgery. Three of the agents used in this way are cidofovir [13], interferon [14] and indole-3-cardinol [15]. Interferon has the disadvantage of a large number of adverse effects, which constrains its usage. It is not fully understood precisely how cidofovir exerts its clinical effect, but there are indications that papilloma formation recurs less swiftly if this agent is used adjunctively with surgery [13]. The precise place of cidofovir in treatment of RRP has yet to be fully determined; hence this agent should only be used with caution and after fully informing the child and his/her guardian of the potential for untoward consequences [12, 14]. The research literature has proposed a number of other approaches, too, including laser angiolysis, cis-retinoic acid treatment, bevacizumab [15, 16] and celecoxib [17]. Vaccinating already infected individuals is also possible [18]. Bevacizumab inhibits the action of vascular endothelial growth factor and appears to improve outcomes when combined with surgical treatment [12, 16]. The cyclooxygenase-2 enzyme is overexpressed in papillomas, and thus a potential target for therapy against HPV. Celecoxib appears capable of inhibition of the cyclooxygenase-2 enzyme, but there is no clear evidence so far to show that this action retards the development of papillomas nor in preventing their regrowth [10, 15]. Some researchers have claimed that vaccination against HPV not only prevents infection occurring with the virus in the first place and thus growth of papillomas, but may even reduce the degree of papilloma regrowth and potentially actually make the lesions remit [18]. It is anticipated that the frequency of laryngeal papillomas will fall in newborns and older children as the uptake of vaccination increases.

51.5 Effective Methods by Which the Uptake of HPV Vaccination in Adolescents Can Be Increased

Despite a global rise in the number of adolescents vaccinated against HPV, take-up of vaccination is still less than for other vaccines [19–21]. A number of reasons for this low uptake have been put forward, linked to social and demographic factors [22–25]. The most frequently cited reasons for low uptake are being unaware of the risks posed by being infected with HPV and anxiety about how safe vaccination actually is [22, 24, 25]. Parents' documented objections are that the vaccine is insufficiently effective or that they consider their child to be at low risk of HPV. There are also concerns that prevention is inconsistent. Recent reports cite concern about the financial cost of vaccination as a reason to decline vaccination [22, 26]. There is evidence that parents and adolescents themselves commonly feel a need to be better informed about the consequences of HPV and how to protect themselves, prior to consenting to vaccination [27]. The key factors influencing their decision are the advice offered by clinicians, opinions gleaned from the Internet, the school environment and mass media. These factors are of consistent importance. Judgements made by healthcare professionals about a female patient's suitability for vaccination also potentially prevent vaccination, regardless of what the patient herself may wish.

If the aim is to increase the level of individuals vaccinated against HPV, recognition of the opposing socio-cultural factors needs to be taken [19]. To promote trust in the vaccine, vaccination information needs to be easily understood, easy to find and may need to be modified to make it more culturally appropriate. Basing vaccine programmes within schools has been shown to increase the uptake of the HPV vaccine [27, 28]. Objection to the cost is avoidable by providing the vaccine free at the point of care via systems offering universal healthcare coverage. It must be admitted, though, that there remains a need for a detailed evaluation of the vaccination programmes currently in place and research to identify suitable innovation that will lead to higher numbers of adolescents accepting vaccination (Table 51.1).

Table 51.1 Principal findings from the "4th Workshop on Paediatric Virology" on HPV infections and how to prevent them in children [6]

HPV vaccination	The latest figures show that the strategy of making up for missed opportunities to vaccinate Swedish young women has succeeded and is now having a significant effect on reducing the frequency of HPV. There is a need for further research to assess the state of the policies and vaccination programmes currently in place and to look into new ways to increase the appeal of HPV vaccines and their uptake in adolescents
HPV and neonatal prematurity	If it can be clearly and validly shown that HPV infection is associated with premature birth, this information may be useful in marketing the vaccine to young women. If it turns out that there is no genuine association with prematurity, this will be an important finding for doctors and pregnant women, who will no longer need to fear such an outcome. This issue of possible causality can be settled by a prospective type of cohort study in which there are higher numbers enrolled
HPV-related JO-RRP	At present, management of JO-RRP involves considerable difficulty and causes significant frustration. It calls for repeated intervention to preserve the voice and keep the airway open. Thus, research that can precisely inform the correct therapeutic approach is a vital necessity if clinicians are to improve the life quality of paediatric patients with this condition. Management needs to be put on a firm foundation of evidence. For this to occur, the data currently available need to be meticulously evaluated and the different management approaches compared for their strengths and weaknesses. Since JO-RPP is the result of HPV being transmitted from mother to child, as vaccine uptake improves, it is to be hoped that the condition will begin to decline in frequency
HPV-related conjunctival papilloma	A sessile limbal conjunctival papilloma calls for watchful waiting or excision close to its borders. If such a papilloma shows features indicating dysplasia or malignant transformation, it will need to be surgically removed and cryotherapy employed adjunctively
HPV-related HNSCC as a vaccination target	The vaccines currently licensed to prevent HPV are effective against HPV infections of the anus or genitalia. At the current time, however, the efficacy of these agents on HPV infections of the oral cavity and their ability to prevent HNSCC secondary to HPV has yet to be definitively established in a trial

HPV human papilloma viruses, *JO-RRP* juvenile onset recurrent respiratory papillomatosis, *HNSCC* head and neck squamous cell carcinoma [6].

51.6 Treatment

Sadly, at present, there is no curative treatment available. The first step in therapy is operative, with the goal of preventing dysphonia and keeping the airway patent, whilst endeavouring to avoid any complications resulting from surgical removal. Whilst there are a number of pharmacotherapeutic interventions that may be employed adjunctively, surgery to remove papillomas remains the key management option.

51.6.1 Surgical

Treatment through surgery presents risks to both the patient and the surgeon. In particular, treatments that may release viable viral fragments may endanger surgical staff and appropriate prophylactic measures are therefore recommended.

Over the last decade, the surgical instrument used most frequently to excise papillomas formed on the larynx or trachea is the electric microdebrider with a laryngeal blade attachment. A study comparing a carbon dioxide laser with a microdebrider as the instrument employed in excision of RRP noted that the latter entailed a shorter operation and period under anaesthesia, as well as not causing thermal trauma around the lesion, as occurred with the laser [29]. The American Society of Paediatric Otolaryngology conducted a survey in 2004 of surgeons' preferences in treating RRP, revealing a clear preference for microdebridement rather than CO_2 laser ablation [30]. It should be acknowledged, nonetheless, that no RCT has yet pitted carbon dioxide laser ablation against microdebridement for papilloma removal within the larynx. A 2009 study by Holler et al. compared prospectively 11 paediatric cases of RRP, managed either by microdebridement or carbon dioxide laser ablation [31]. The outcome measure was improvement in dysphonia, assessed using an objective acoustic measure. The microdebrider had demonstrable superiority.

A number of other types of laser have now entered into surgical use for RRP, two of which are a 585 nm pulsed dye laser and a 532 nm pulsed potassium-titanyl-phosphate laser. Both these lasers are angiolytic. There is absorption of the laser energy by haemoglobin molecules; thus the vessels within papillomas are selectively ablated. With these newer tools, an older child or adult can be treated in the clinic. Hartnick et al. performed a longitudinal study with a prospective methodology that enrolled 23 children. They discovered that the longer wavelength laser is more suitable for radical operative excision when the papilloma is located at the anterior commissure, since it produces a lower level of trauma to the surrounding epithelium [32].

Although a tracheotomy may be performed from time to time as a life-preserving treatment in a child with severe RRP that completely blocks the airway, surgeons mostly prefer to avoid this intervention as it results in chronic inflammation. This inflammation may then lead to extensive of the HPV infection to the distal portions of the airway. Where a tracheotomy is unavoidable, it is recommended that the cannula be removed at the earliest opportunity, once it is safe to manage RRP using an endoscopic approach.

51.6.2 Adjuvant Treatments

There are multiple agents which have found employment adjunctively in cases of RRP. The criterion for employing such an agent that is most commonly applied is where the child requires surgical intervention on more than four occasions annually, where the papilloma recurs in a very short period and threatens the patency of the airway and where papilloma formation occurs lower down the respiratory tract at several locations. Gallagher and Derkay [33] wrote a detailed review of the many pharmacotherapeutic agents that have been trialled as adjuvant therapy in RRP, such as aciclovir, ribavirin, indole-3-carbinol, cyclooxygenase-2 inhibitors, retinoids, and zinc. The agents that have been most widespread and generated the most research interest are interferon and cidofovir.

There have been two RCTs which examined the role of interferon [34, 35]. In each case, interferon offered benefit when used with severe RRP. This benefit continued whilst interferon was being administered, but not afterwards.

There are two methods used to reduce the size of papillomas: excision using the endoscope or microlaryngoscopic ablation. Debridement should be restricted as far as practicable to the papilloma itself, sparing any adjoining epithelium. If the surrounding tissues are damaged, there may be scar formation or stenotic narrowing, causing irreversible dysphonia with or without risking the patency of the airway. Histopathological tissue diagnosis is essential at first presentation. Thereafter, biopsy is helpful to check for dysplastic change or progression towards malignancy.

Over time there has been an improvement in the techniques used to reduce the mass of papillomatous tissue. At first, surgery was undertaken with microlaryngeal tools, including forceps used to obtain cup biopsies. One danger in this approach is inadvertent avulsive injury to adjacent, undiseased epithelium, resulting in scarring. To allow for a higher level of accuracy, ENT specialists then began employing lasers for ablation. Lasers may be fired in direct line of sight or via fibre optics in the case of carbon dioxide lasers. Laser surgery runs the risk of starting a fire within the airway or trauma to other structures. There are also lengths of viral DNA present in the smoke created by the laser. One study performed on calves with bovine papillomavirus noted that exposure to the smoke plume produced serious side effects, in particular pyrexia, symptoms consistent with influenza-like illness, convulsions, a reduction in weight gain and leucopenia.

Cidofovir has been introduced in many settings as a treatment for RRP. It is generally injected directly into the papilloma, but may also be administered systemically via intravenous injection. Cidofovir is an analogue of the cytosine nucleotide. This agent then inhibits the action of DNA polymerase. When used in cytomegalovirus infection, cidofovir targets the viral DNA polymerase. However, since HPV does not produce its own DNA polymerase, a different mechanism applies. Whatever the precise mode of action, there have been numerous case series, involving small numbers of cases, where cidofovir seems to offer benefit. Up to now, a single RCT featuring double-blinding and placebo control has been conducted to assess the role of cidofovir in RRP. This trial, by McMurray et al. [36], noted benefit that was statistically significant in the group receiving the active agent. One outcome measure used was the Derkay score for disease severity. It is important to note, nonetheless, that benefit was also noted in the placebo group. The study suffered from a significant limitation in the dose tested. Since cidofovir exhibits toxicity at higher doses, the regulator permitted a maximum dose of 0.3 mg/mL to be injected into the papilloma. This dosage was significantly lower than the usual off-label prescriptions then in use. At a somewhat later time, regulatory approval was granted for a much higher dose of 5 mg/mL. Cidofovir also has a potentially carcinogenic effect and thus the RRP Task Force suggested in 2005 that the agent only be considered where other treatment modalities had repeatedly failed [37, 38]. However, more recently, research using histopathological examination of papilloma tissue from cases of RRP has not found that dysplasia progresses, and the authors concluded that further research was needed [39].

A number of case reports conclude that RRP is less prone to recur when gastro-oesophageal reflux disease (GORD) is well controlled. McKenna and Brodsky [40] reported on a limited number of paediatric patients suffering from RRP in 2005. Where RRP had exhibited treatment resistance to earlier attempts at control, managing GORD well gave improved control of RRP. More research is needed to fully understand the implications of this finding, but at present it seems beneficial to start children on GORD treatment if they have aggressive RRP.

There are multiple adjuvant agents where there is anecdotal evidence for efficacy and a biological rationale for their use. The evidence base for the majority of such agents is relatively weak, since studies have enrolled few patients, the natural history of RRP lesions varies considerably and there are no RCTs so far.

At present the most promising approach to preventing RRP appears to be to vaccinate individuals against HPV. Currently, 3 prophylactic HPV vaccines are licensed in many countries of the world: bivalent vaccine protecting against genotypes 16/18, quadrivalent vaccine protecting against genotypes 6/11/16/18, and nonavalent vaccine protecting against genotypes 6/11/16/18/31/33/45/52/58 [39, 41].

51.7 Future Perspectives

There has been a noticeable increase in research into the effects of HPV in paediatric patients since HPV vaccines are licensed for use in the United States [42, 43]. This research had as its rationale the resolution of lingering concerns about how effective vaccination actually is and how safe [44, 45]. This research focuses on the ideal age at which vaccination should be offered (compared to current recommendations) and addresses the question of whether males as well as females should undergo vaccination for HPV [46]. There has been research which looked at the epidemiological variants affecting whether adolescents agree to be vaccinated and what techniques are most effective at raising the numbers receiving the vaccine. Since the programmes to vaccinate against HPV have now been underway for some time, it is expected that a deeper understanding of how HPV is transmitted to infants will emerge, along with a deeper appreciation of the natural history of infections in the paediatric age range. There remains a need for studies to elucidate in precise detail these issues. HPV remains an area with plentiful research potential and clinicians will be faced with the need to treat HPV-associated lesions for a considerable time to come.

References

1. Mammas IN, Sourvinos G, Spandidos DA. The paediatric story of human papillomavirus (review). Oncol Lett. 2014;8(2):502–6. https://doi.org/10.3892/ol.2014.2226.
2. Scasso F, Ferrari G, DE Vincentiis GC, Arosio A, Bottero S, Carretti M, Ciardo A, Cocuzza S, Colombo A, Conti B, Cordone A, DE Ciccio M, Delehaye E, Della Vecchia L, DE Macina I, Dentone C, DI Mauro P, Dorati R, Fazio R, Ferrari A, Ferrea G, Giannantonio S, Genta I, Giuliani M, Lucidi D, Maiolino L, Marini G, Marsella P, Meucci D, Modena T, Montemurri B, Odone A, Palma S, Panatta ML, Piemonte M, Pisani P, Pisani S, Prioglio L, Scorpecci A, Scotto DI Santillo L, Serra A, Signorelli C, Sitzia E, Tropiano ML, Trozzi M, Tucci FM, Vezzosi L, Viaggi B. Emerging and re-emerging infectious disease in otorhinolaryngology. Acta Otorhinolaryngol Ital. 2018;38:S1–S106. https://doi.org/10.14639/0392-100X-suppl.1-38-2018.
3. Stavinoha R, Buchinsky FJ. Recurrent respiratory papillomatosis. In: Licameli GL, Tunkel DE, editors. Pediatric otorhinolaryngology: diagnosis and treatment. Thieme Medical and Scientific Publishers; 2013. p. 109–13.
4. Mammas IN, Sourvinos G, Spandidos DA. Human papilloma virus (HPV) infection in children and adolescents. Eur J Pediatr. 2009;168:267–73.
5. Zur Hausen H. Papillomaviruses in the causation of human cancers - a brief historical account. Virology. 2009;384:260–5.
6. Mammas IN, Dalianis T, Doukas SG, Zaravinos A, Achtsidis V, Thiagarajan P, Theodoridou M, Spandidos DA. Paediatric virology and human papillomaviruses: an update. Exp Ther Med. 2019;17(6):4337–43. https://doi.org/10.3892/etm.2019.7516.
7. Mammas IN, Greenough A, Theodoridou M, et al. Paediatric virology and its interaction between basic science and clinical practice (review). Int J Mol Med. 2018;41(3):1165–76. https://doi.org/10.3892/ijmm.2018.3364.
8. Syrjänen S. Current concepts on human papillomavirus infections in children. APMIS. 2010;118:494–509.
9. Pfister H, Zur Hausen H. Seroepidemiological studies of human papilloma virus (HPV-1) infections. Int J Cancer. 1978;21:161–5.
10. Donne AJ, Clarke R. Recurrent respiratory papillomatosis: an uncommon but potentially devastating effect of human papillomavirus in children. Int J STD AIDS. 2010;21:381–5. https://doi.org/10.1258/ijsa.2010.010073.
11. Silverberg MJ, Thorsen P, Lindeberg H, Grant LA, Shah KV. Condyloma in pregnancy is strongly predictive of juvenile-onset recurrent respiratory papillomatosis. Obstet Gynecol. 2003;101:645–52. https://doi.org/10.1016/S0029-7844(02)03081-8.
12. Ivancic R, Iqbal H, de Silva B, Pan Q, Matrka L. Current and future management of recurrent respiratory papillomatosis. Laryngoscope Investig Otolaryngol. 2018;3:22–34. https://doi.org/10.1002/lio2.132.
13. Derkay CS, Volsky PG, Rosen CA, Pransky SM, McMurray JS, Chadha NK, Froehlich P. Current use of intralesional cidofovir for recurrent respiratory papillomatosis. Laryngoscope. 2013;123:705–12. https://doi.org/10.1002/lary.23673.

14. Gerein V, Rastorguev E, Gerein J, Jecker P, Pfister H. Use of interferon-alpha in recurrent respiratory papillomatosis: 20-year follow-up. Ann Otol Rhinol Laryngol. 2005;114:463–71. https://doi.org/10.1177/000348940511400608.

15. Rosen CA, Bryson PC. Indole-3-carbinol for recurrent respiratory papillomatosis: long-term results. J Voice. 2004;18:248–53. https://doi.org/10.1016/j.jvoice.2003.05.005.

16. Sidell DR, Nassar M, Cotton RT, Zeitels SM, de Alarcon A. High-dose sublesional bevacizumab (avastin) for pediatric recurrent respiratory papillomatosis. Ann Otol Rhinol Laryngol. 2014;123:214–21. https://doi.org/10.1177/0003489414522977.

17. Limsukon A, Susanto I, Soo Hoo GW, Dubinett SM, Batra RK. Regression of recurrent respiratory papillomatosis with celecoxib and erlotinib combination therapy. Chest. 2009;136:924–6. https://doi.org/10.1378/chest.08-2639.

18. Young DL, Moore MM, Halstead LA. The use of the quadrivalent human papillomavirus vaccine (gardasil) as adjuvant therapy in the treatment of recurrent respiratory papilloma. J Voice. 2015;29:223–9. https://doi.org/10.1016/j.jvoice.2014.08.003.

19. Mammas IN, Theodoridou M, Sourvinos G, Spandidos DA. Exploring effective interventions to increase adolescents' vaccination against human papillomavirus (HPV). Int J Mol Med. 2018;42:S17.

20. Mammas IN, Spandidos DA. Paediatric virology as a new educational initiative: an interview with Nobelist professor of virology Harald zur Hausen. Exp Ther Med. 2017;14:3329–31. https://doi.org/10.3892/etm.2017.5008.

21. Zur Hausen H, Mammas IN, Spandidos DA. HPV vaccination in boys: determining the clinical relevance of this strategy. Exp Ther Med. 2017;14:3327–8. https://doi.org/10.3892/etm.2017.5005.

22. Mammas IN, Theodoridou M, Koutsaftiki C, Bertsias G, Sourvinos G, Spandidos DA. Vaccination against human papillomavirus in relation to financial crisis: the 'evaluation and education of Greek female adolescents on human papillomaviruses' prevention strategies' ELEFTHERIA study. J Pediatr Adolesc Gynecol. 2016;29:362–6. https://doi.org/10.1016/j.jpag.2015.12.007.

23. Einstein MH, Schiller JT, Viscidi RP, Strickler HD, Coursaget P, Tan T, Halsey N, Jenkins D. Clinician's guide to human papillomavirus immunology: knowns and unknowns. Lancet Infect Dis. 2009;9:347–56. https://doi.org/10.1016/S1473-3099(09)70108-2.

24. Fisher H, Trotter CL, Audrey S, MacDonald-Wallis K, Hickman M. Inequalities in the uptake of human papillomavirus vaccination: a systematic review and meta-analysis. Int J Epidemiol. 2013;42:896–908. https://doi.org/10.1093/ije/dyt049.

25. Kessels SJ, Marshall HS, Watson M, Braunack-Mayer AJ, Reuzel R, Tooher RL. Factors associated with HPV vaccine uptake in teenage girls: a systematic review. Vaccine. 2012;30:3546–56. https://doi.org/10.1016/j.vaccine.2012.03.063.

26. Mammas IN, Theodoridou M. Financial crisis and childhood immunization: when parents disagree. Acta Paediatr. 2013;102:e145–6. https://doi.org/10.1111/j.1651-2227.2012.02773.x.

27. Gottvall M, Stenhammar C, Grandahl M. Parents' views of including young boys in the Swedish national school-based HPV vaccination programme: a qualitative study. BMJ Open. 2017;7:e014255. https://doi.org/10.1136/bmjopen-2016-014255.

28. Batista Ferrer H, Trotter CL, Hickman M, Audrey S. Barriers and facilitators to uptake of the school-based HPV vaccination programme in an ethnically diverse group of young women. J Public Health (Oxf). 2016;38:569–77. https://doi.org/10.1093/pubmed/fdv073.

29. Patel N, Rowe M, Tunkel D. Treatment of recurrent respiratory papillomatosis in children with the microdebrider. Ann Otol Rhinol Laryngol. 2003;112(1):7–10.

30. Schraff S, Derkay CS, Burke B, Lawson L. American Society of Pediatric Otolaryngology members' experience with recurrent respiratory papillomatosis and the use of adjuvant therapy. Arch Otolaryngol Head Neck Surg. 2004;130(9):1039–42.

31. Holler T, Allegro J, Chadha NK, et al. Voice outcomes following repeated surgical resection of laryngeal papillomata in children. Otolaryngol Head Neck Surg. 2009;141(4):522–6.

32. Hartnick CJ, Boseley ME, Franco RA Jr, Cunningham MJ, Pransky S. Efficacy of treating children with anterior commissure and true vocal fold respiratory papilloma with the 585-nm pulsed-dye laser. Arch Otolaryngol Head Neck Surg. 2007;133(2):127–30.
33. Gallagher TQ, Dcrkay CS. Pharmacotherapy of recurrent respiratory papillomatosis: an expert opinion. Expert Opin Pharmacother. 2009;10(4):645–55.
34. Leventhal BG, Kashima HK, Weck PW, et al. Randomized surgical adjuvant trial of interferon alfa-n1 in recurrent papillomatosis. Arch Otolaryngol Head Neck Surg. 1988;114(10):1163–9.
35. Healy GB, Gelber RD, Trowbridge AL, Grundfast KM, Ruben RJ, Price KN. Treatment of recurrent respiratory papillomatosis with human leukocyte interferon. Results of a multicenter randomized clinical trial. N Engl J Med. 1988;319(7):401–7.
36. McMurray JS, Connor N, Ford CN. Cidofovir efficacy in recurrent respiratory papillomatosis: a randomized, double-blind, placebo- controlled study. Ann Otol Rhinol Laryngol. 2008;117(7):477–83.
37. Donne AJ, Hampson L, He XT, et al. Potential risk factors associated with the use of cidofovir to treat benign human papillomavirus- related disease. Antivir Ther. 2009;14(7):939–52.
38. Derkay C. Multi-disciplinary task force on recurrent respiratory Papillomas. Cidofovir for recurrent respiratory papillomatosis (RRP): a re-assessment of risks. Int J Pediatr Otorhinolaryngol. 2005;69(11):1465–7.
39. Gupta HT, Robinson RA, Murray RC, Karnell LH, Smith RJ, Hoffman HT. Degrees of dysplasia and the use of cidofovir in patients with recurrent respiratory papillomatosis. Laryngoscope. 2010;120(4):698–702.
40. McKenna M, Brodsky L. Extraesophageal acid reflux and recurrent respiratory papilloma in children. Int J Pediatr Otorhinolaryngol. 2005;69(5):597–605.
41. Bishai D, Kashima H, Shah K. The cost of juvenile-onset recurrent respiratory papillomatosis. Arch Otolaryngol Head Neck Surg. 2000;126(8):935–9. Erratum in: Arch Otolaryngol Head Neck Surg 2009;135(2):208
42. FUTURE II Study Group. Quadrivalent vaccine against human papillomavirus to prevent high-grade cervical lesions. N Engl J Med. 2007;356:1915–27.
43. Paavonen J, Naud P, Salmerón J, et al. Efficacy of human papillomavirus (HPV)-16/18 AS04-adjuvanted vaccine against cervical infection and precancer caused by oncogenic HPV types (PATRICIA): final analysis of a double-blind, randomised study in young women. Lancet. 2009;374:301–14.
44. Rafle AE. Challenges of implementing human papillomavirus (HPV) vaccination policy. BMJ. 2007;335:375–7.
45. Mammas I, Maher F, Theodoridou M, Spandidos DA. Human papilloma virus (HPV) vaccination in childhood: challenges and perspectives. Hippokratia. 2011;15:299–303.
46. Mammas IN, Spandidos DA. Vaccination against human papillomavirus in childhood: the next rubella analogue? J BUON. 2012;17:389–90.

Odontogenic İnfections in Children

Mustafa Altıntaş, Koray Gençay, and Mario Milkov

52.1   Introduction

Odontogenic infections are the infection of the alveolus, jaws, or face that originates from a tooth or from its supporting structures. They are very frequent in children so they are important for pediatricians, otorhinolaryngologists, and pediatric dentists.

The most common causes of odontogenic infections are dental caries, deep fillings or failed root canal treatment, pericoronitis, and periodontal disease. The infection starts locally around a tooth and may remain localized to the region where it started, or may spread into adjacent or distant areas. The course of the infection depends on the virulence of the bacteria, host resistance factors, and the regional anatomy. Dentoalveolar region infection, submental space infection, submandibular space infection, sublingual space infection, retropharyngeal space infection, buccal space infection, masticator space infection, and canine space infection are the clinical presentations of odontogenic infections. The first and most important element in treating dental infections is the elimination of the primary source of the infection with antibiotics as adjunctive therapy [1–3].

M. Altıntaş (✉)
Section of Otorhinolaryngology, Antalya Training and Research Hospital, University of Health Sciences, Antalya, Turkey

K. Gençay
Department of Pedodontics, Faculty of Dentistry, İstanbul University, İstanbul, Turkey
e-mail: koray@istanbul.edu.tr

M. Milkov
Department of Otorhinolaryngology, Faculty of Medicine, Varna University, Varna, Bulgaria

C. Cingi et al. (eds.), *Pediatric ENT Infections*,
https://doi.org/10.1007/978-3-030-80691-0_52

52.2 Clinical Manifestations of Odontogenic Infections in Children

The clinical presentation of an odontogenic infection is highly variable depending on the source of the infection whether the infection is localized or if it has become disseminated. Like all infections, the clinical signs and symptoms are pain/tenderness, redness, and swelling. Patients with superficial dental infections present with localized pain, cellulitis, and sensitivity to tooth percussion and temperature. However, patients with deep infections or abscesses that spread along the fascial planes may present with swelling, fever, and sometimes difficulty swallowing, opening the mouth, or breathing. In single space infection cases the most commonly involved fascial space is the buccal space (60%) followed by canine space (13%).

52.3 Clinical Presentation of Odontogenic Infections Varies by Location

- Dentoalveolar infections are usually present by swelling of the alveolar ridge with periodontal, periapical, and subperiosteal abscess.
- Submental space infections mostly exist as firm midline swelling beneath the chin (Fig. 52.1). Submandibular space infections manifest as swelling of the submandibular triangle through the neck. Mandibular incisors may the cause of infection [1–3].
- Mandibular molar infections cause submandibular space infection. Trismus is typical.
- The swelling of the mouth floor with the possible elevation of the tongue and dysphagia is the sign of sublingual space infection.

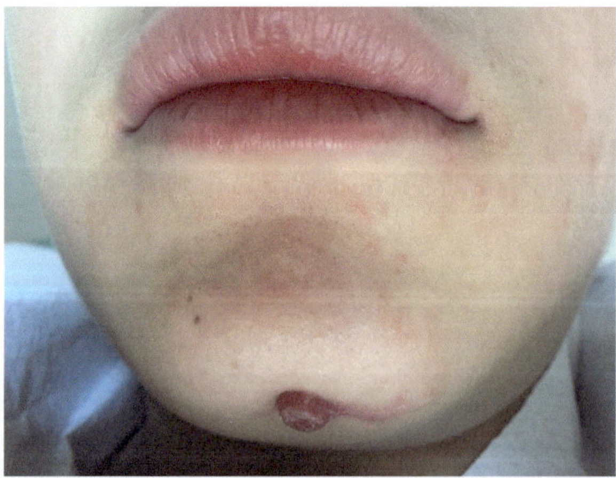

Fig. 52.1 Extraoral sinus tract due to dentoalveolar infection (Courtesy of Mutlu E and Gencay K)

- Infections of the molars seldom cause retropharyngeal space infections. Stiff neck, sore throat, dysphagia, and raspy voice are the significant symptoms.
- The retropharyngeal space infection has a high potential to spread to the mediastinum.
- Premolar or molar tooth infections may cause buccal space infection and swelling of the cheek.
- Masticator space infection usually goes with swelling on either side of the mandibular ramus and is caused by the mandibular third molar infection. Trismus is present.
- Canine space infection presents by the swelling of the anterior cheek with loss of the nasolabial fold and possible extension to the infraorbital region [2–4].

52.4 Microbiology and Treatment Principles

Orofacial odontogenic infections are mixed aerobic–anaerobic infections, and the bacteriology often excogitates the existence of commensal oral flora [4]. The pathogenesis of odontogenic infection is polymicrobial, consisting of various facultative anaerobes, such as the streptococci viridans group and the Streptococcus anginosus group, and strict anaerobes, especially anaerobic cocci, Prevotella and Fusobacterium species [3–5].

Amoxicillin possesses antimicrobial activity against major pathogens in orofacial odontogenic infections, but β-lactamase production has restricted the effectiveness of amoxicillin against the resistant strains of Staphylococcus aureus, Bacteroides, Prevotella, and Porphyromonas. For the management of orofacial infections, the use of amoxicillin/clavulanate and clindamycin is recommended because of stability against β-lactamases [4, 5].

Microorganisms that show low susceptibility to one or more of the standard antibiotic therapy regimes have a significantly higher chance of causing serious health problems, a tendency of spreading and are more likely to require an inpatient management with admission of IV antibiotics. Penicillin continues to be a highly effective antibiotic to be used against viridans streptococci, group C Streptococci, and prevotella, whereas clindamycin could not be shown to be effective as an empirical drug of choice for a high number of odontogenic infections [6].

52.5 Management of Odontogenic Infections in Children

There is a paucity of data regarding medical and surgical management of odontogenic infections among pediatric patients [7], with almost no clear-cut guidelines and little literature on how localized infections should be managed. So the applied management of odontogenic infections in children is similar to that of adults [7]. Guidelines seem to be in consensus that in localized dentoalveolar infection/abscess, it is most important to remove the source of infection either by incision and drainage, extraction, or pulpal opening of the teeth [7–9]. Systemic antibiotic therapy is only required when patient is immunocompromised or there are signs of a systemic spread [9–12]. In cases of spreading infection such as odontogenic facial cellulitis or where signs of systemic involvement are present, prompt attention should be given because severe complications can occur rapidly especially in children [10]. Hospital admission and intravenous antibiotic therapy is necessarily followed by immediate surgical intervention as this contributes to a more rapid cure [13]. In-patient management often requires a multidisciplinary approach whereby there is a confluence of dental and medical management with pediatric infection and ENT collaboration.

Although immediate intervention of some sort is recommended by dentists, the statement is not clear on the prescription of antibiotics, the need for an intracanal medicament and whether infections drained through the pulp should be left open for drainage or not [9]. Numerous studies have reported the inadvertent use of antibiotics to contain odontogenic infections in children with no immediate intervention, leaving the tooth to be treated days later [14, 15]. Older protocols which are still followed suggest removal of the source supplemented with an antibiotic course [16]. Defensive prescription to stay away from lawsuits and behavioral problems in children that impede active intervention encourage the above practice. More recently, emphasis on responsible use of antibiotics due to the global rise in drug-resistant bacterial strains has been highlighted [17]. Comparatively, there are clearer guidelines for spreading odontogenic infections and more studies reported [7, 13, 17]. Further studies regarding the management of odontogenic infections, both spreading and localized, in pediatric patients should be performed.

52.6 Special Conditions

52.6.1 Ludwig's Angina

It is a diffuse cellulitis in the submandibular, sublingual, and submental spaces, characterized by its propensity to spread rapidly to the surrounding tissues. Early recognition and treatment for Ludwig's angina are of paramount importance due to the myriad of complications that can occur in association with Ludwig's angina. Known complications of Ludwig's angina include carotid arterial rupture or sheath abscess, thrombophlebitis of the internal jugular vein, mediastinitis, empyema, pericardial effusion, osteomyelitis of the mandible, subphrenic abscess, aspiration pneumonia, and pleural effusion. Many Ludwig's angina cases were reported that evolved from a chronic odontogenic infection. They usually present with perioral swelling with the involvement of bilateral submandibular and sublingual areas, accompanied by excruciating pain, chills, fever, and vomiting. They may be treated with clindamycin and cefoxitin for infection and vigorously hydrated. The potentially lethal clinical condition should be well understood. Early recognition and aggressive treatment will help to prevent complications from Ludwig's angina (Fig. 52.2) [19].

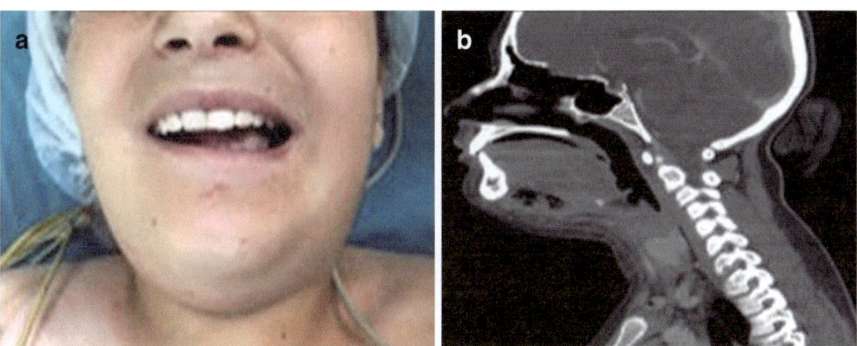

Fig. 52.2 (**a**) Ludwig angina, seen with swelling and hyperemia in the submental region. (**b**) 12-year-old patient sagittal contrast-enhanced CT image that shows air densities in the mouth floor [18]

52.6.2 The Periapical Infection

It is the most common form of odontogenic infection and is caused by invasion of the root canal system of the tooth by microorganisms (Fig. 52.3). This acute apical infection entails a concomitant infection of the root canal and the periradicular tissues, because the latter is an extension of the former. Once the microorganisms enter the periapical tissues via the apical foramen, they induce an inflammatory process that can lead to the formation of an abscess. In most cases the infection is localized intraorally, but in some instances it may spread into distal areas and result in severe complications, such as sinusitis, airway obstruction, cavernous sinus thrombosis, brain abscess, or even death [20].

52.6.3 Pericoronitis

It is another common cause of odontogenic infection. The primary cause is the accumulation of bacteria and food debris that gets trapped in the space between the overlapping gum of a partially exposed (erupted) mandibular third molar and the crown of the tooth (Fig. 52.4). Most cases are chronic and consist of a mild persistent inflammation of the mandibular third molar area. Pericoronitis can, however, become a serious infection associated with fever, swelling, and an abscess that has the ability to spread if left untreated. On occasions the symptoms can become severe because of the rapid spread of infection, requiring that the patient be hospitalized for intravenous antibiotics and possibly extraction of tooth in an operating room under general anesthesia. Because of the close proximity to the pharynx, airway obstruction becomes a strong possibility [22].

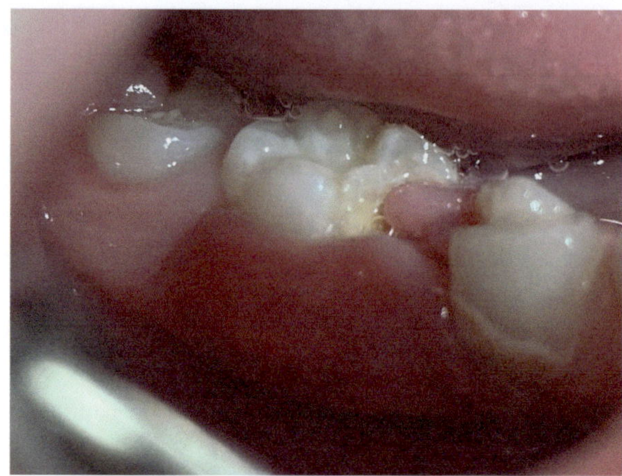

Fig. 52.3 Periapical abscess in a second primary tooth (Courtesy of Mutlu E and Gencay K)

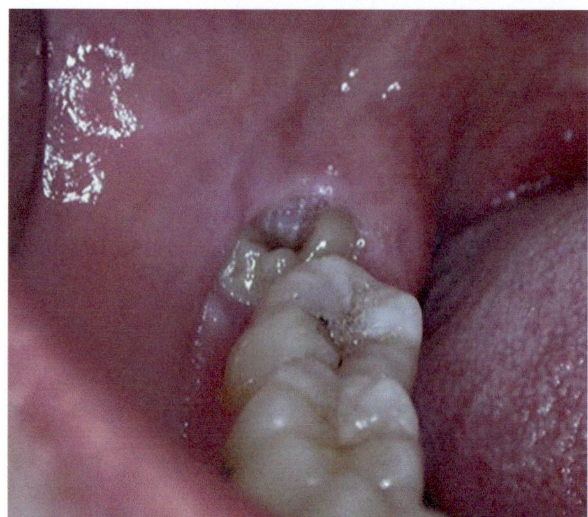

Fig. 52.4 Pericoronitis due to eruption of third molar [21]

52.6.4 Dental Abscess

Acute dental abscess is a frequent and sometimes underestimated disease of the oral cavity. The acute dental abscess usually occurs secondary to caries, trauma, or failed endodontic treatment. After the intact pulp chamber is opened, colonization of the root canals takes place with a variable set of anaerobic bacteria, which colonize the walls of the necrotic root canals forming a specialized mixed anaerobic biofilm. Asymptomatic necrosis is common. However, abscess formation occurs when these bacteria and their toxic products breach into the periapical tissues through the apical foramen and induce acute inflammation and pus formation (Fig. 52.5). The main

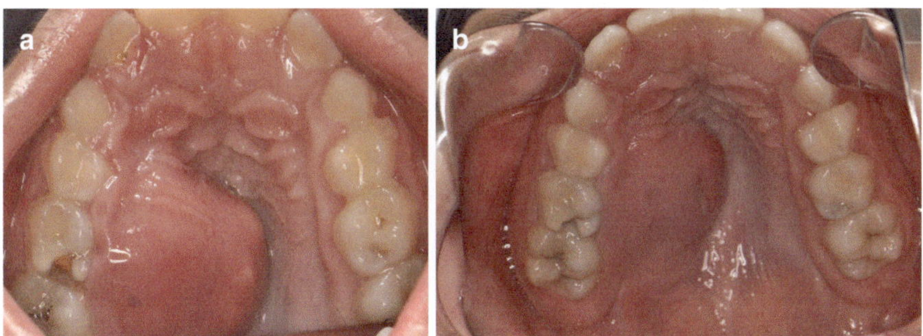

Fig. 52.5 A case of 9-year-old patient. Massive swelling in the palatal area (**a**). Surgical incision is made (**b**). (Courtesy of Mutlu E, Kasmoglu Y and Gencay K)

signs and symptoms of the acute dental abscess which are often referred to as a periapical abscess or infection are pain, swelling, erythema, and suppuration usually localized to the affected tooth, even if the abscess can eventually spread causing a severe odontogenic infection which is characterized by local and systemic involvement culminating in sepsis syndrome.

The vast majority of dental abscesses respond to antibiotic treatment; however, in some patients surgical management of the infection may be indicated [2, 23].

52.6.5 Facial Cellulitis

Cellulitis of odontogenic origin is an acute, deep, and diffuse inflammation of the subcutaneous tissue that spreads through the spaces between the tissue cells to several anatomic regions, tissue spaces, and throughout the aponeurotic plane because of the infection of one or several teeth or due to dental or supportive tissue-associated pathologies (Fig. 52.6) [24].

It has various clinical presentations, from a harmless, isolated process to a progressive, diffuse clinical condition that may cause complications. If cellulitis is detected at an early stage, it usually has a soft and smooth consistency with inflammatory signs, its edges are poorly defined, and, sometimes, the underlying epidermis is not raised up. In the advanced stage, the area is indurated [25, 26]. The intraoral examination includes assessing the level of mouth opening, which may be restricted by the presence of pain and trismus. The clinical characteristics include cleft effacement and tooth mobility or extrusion.

The general symptoms of head and neck infections vary. Sepsis presents with apathy, weakness, discomfort, fever spikes, sweating, thready pulse, leukocytosis, and, sometimes, marked secondary anemia. Muscle spasm or immobilization of adjacent muscles causes trismus, torticollis, and stiffness. Neural involvement causes pain in the affected sensory nerve and motor nerve paralysis. Dysphagia,

Fig. 52.6 Facial cellulitis originated by odontogenic infection. (Courtesy of Mutlu E and Gencay K)

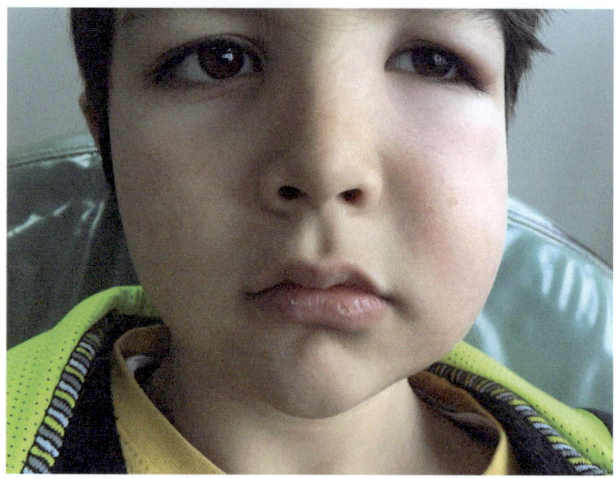

dysphonia, and aphonia may also occur, depending on the site of infection [24, 25]. The treatment of facial cellulitis of odontogenic origin in children depends on the patient's general status and the course of the clinical condition. The main objective is to control and eliminate the causative agent, which, in some cases, requires the specialized care of a pediatrician and hospital management [24–26].

52.7 Complications of Odontogenic Infections

The two most severe intracranial complications of orofacial infections are cavernous sinus thrombosis and brain abscess (Fig. 52.7). Odontogenic infections may involve the cavernous sinus through an anterior and posterior pathway, that is to say as a retrograde septic thrombophlebitis from the infraorbital space to the inferior ophthalmic vein through the inferior orbital fissure into the cavernous sinus, or via the pterygoid venous plexus to the inferior petrosal sinus into the cavernous sinus [27].

The patient with cavernous sinus thrombosis may present with fever, headache, nausea, vomiting, supraorbital paresthesia, proptosis, photophobia ophthalmoplegia, chemosis, and ocular pain. Drainage of the infraorbital or infratemporal spaces and treatment of the responsible tooth are mandatory. High-dose intravenous antibiotics able to cross the blood brain barrier are indicated. The role for anticoagulation and steroids in these patients is not clear.

Very few brain abscesses can be ascribed to dental origin. Bacteria can reach the brain as direct propagation or via the bloodstream. Brain abscesses present with fever, headache, and focal neurological deficits. Computed tomography scan and magnetic resonance imaging are pathognomonic. The microbiological pattern of the brain abscess reflects the original infective site [28].

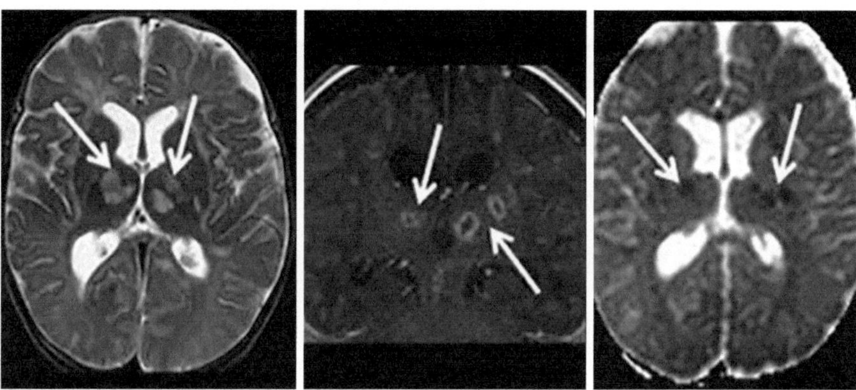

Fig. 52.7 MR imaging shows a 13-day-old child patient affected by brain abscesses from beta-hemolytic streptococcus infection [30]

Intravenous adequate antibiotic therapy is mandatory. Surgical options include aspiration or excision. Adequate monitoring must take place in neurological intensive care unit. Repeated aspiration may be necessary, but it may avoid residual neurological deficits associated with excision. Mortality rates is 20% [28, 29].

52.8 Conclusions

An early and adequate diagnosis of facial infections of odontogenic origin by the primary care pediatrician, an appropriate antibiotic use, and dental treatment are key for the rapid resolution of this condition. Essentially, patients with rapidly progressing facial cellulitis of odontogenic origin, trismus, general status compromise, or oral antibiotic therapy failure should be referred for hospitalization. A timely diagnosis and hospital management may prevent severe complications.

It is imperative to have a pediatric dentist available at the hospital due to the high prevalence of this type of conditions and the complications that may develop if not managed adequately.

Further studies on this topic are required and it is necessary to insist on oral hygiene and periodic dental exams, which are essential to prevent and treat dental cavities and periodontal disease and avoid their progression.

References

1. Bertossi D, Barone A, Iurlaro A, Marconcini S, De Santis D, Finotti M, Procacci P. Odontogenic orofacial infections. J Craniofac Surg. 2017;28(1):197–202.
2. Ogle OE. Odontogenic infections. Dent Clin N Am. 2017;61(2):235–52. https://doi.org/10.1016/j.cden.2016.11.004.

3. Lim SW, Lee WS, Mani SA, Kadir K. Management of odontogenic infection in paediatric patients: a retrospective clinical study. Eur Arch Paediatr Dent. 2020;21(1):145–54. https://doi.org/10.1007/s40368-019-00466-0.

4. Shakya N, Sharma D, Newaskar V, Agrawal D, Shrivastava S, Yadav R. Epidemiology, microbiology and antibiotic sensitivity of odontogenic space infections in Central India. J Maxillofac Oral Surg. 2018;17(3):324–31. https://doi.org/10.1007/s12663-017-1014-y.

5. Santosh AN, Viresh AN, Sharmada BK. Microbiology and antibiotic sensitivity of odontogenic space infection. Int J Med Dent Sci. 2014;3(1):303–13.

6. Heim N, Faron A, Wiedemeyer V, Reich R, Martini M. Microbiology and antibiotic sensitivity of head and neck space infections of odontogenic origin. Differences in inpatient and outpatient management. J Craniomaxillofac Surg. 2017;45(10):1731–5. https://doi.org/10.1016/j.jcms.2017.07.013.

7. Rush DE, Abdel-Haq N, Zhu JF, et al. Clindamycin versus Unasyn in the treatment of facial cellulitis of odontogenic origin in children. Clin Pediatr (Phila). 2007;46:154–9.

8. AAPD Clinical Affairs Committee American Academy of Pediatric Dentistry. Guideline on management considerations for pediatric oral surgery and oral pathology. Pediatr Dent. 2015;37:85–94.

9. AAPD Clinical Affairs Committee American Academy of Pediatric Dentistry. Guideline on use of antibiotic therapy for pediatric den- tal patients. Pediatr Dent. 2016;38:325–7.

10. Flynn TR. What are the antibiotics of choice for odontogenic infections, and how long should the treatment course last? Oral Maxillofac Surg Clin N Am. 2011;23:519.

11. Robertson DP, Keys W, Rautemaa-Richardson R, et al. Management of severe acute dental infections. BMJ. 2015;350:h1300.

12. Segura-Egea JJ, Gould K, Sen BH, et al. European Society of Endodon-tology position statement: the use of antibiotics in endodontics. Int Endod J. 2018;51:20–5.

13. Thikkurissy S, Rawlins JT, Kumar A, et al. Rapid treatment reduces hospitalization for pediatric patients with odontogenic-based cellulitis. Am J Emerg Med. 2010;28:668–72.

14. Al-Malik M, Al-Sarheed M. Pattern of management of oro-facial infection in children: a retrospective. Saudi J Biol Sci. 2017;24:1375–9.

15. Cherry WR, Lee JY, Shugars DA, et al. Antibiotic use for treating dental infections in children a survey of dentists' prescribing practices. J Am Dent Assoc. 2012;143:31–8.

16. Fouad AF, Rivera EM, Walton RE. Penicillin as a supplement in resolving the localized acute apical abscess. Oral Surg Oral Med Oral Pathol Oral Radiol Endod. 1996;81:590–5.

17. Gibson MP, Levin L. Editorial: antibiotics in dentistry: be responsible! Quintessence Int. 2018;49:7–8.

18. Bükülmez A, Bucak A, Balıkoğlu P, et al. A rare case in children: Ludwig Angina. Kocatepe Tıp Dergisi. 2020, 21(3):281–4.

19. Pak S, Cha D, Meyer C, Dee C, Fershko A. Ludwig's Angina. Cureus. 2017;9(8):e1588. https://doi.org/10.7759/cureus.1588.

20. Harjunmaa U, Doyle R, Järnstedt J, Kamiza S, Jorgensen JM, Stewart CP, Shaw L, Hallamaa L, Ashorn U, Klein N, Dewey KG, Maleta K, Ashorn P. Periapical infection may affect birth outcomes via systemic inflammation. Oral Dis. 2018;24(5):847–55. https://doi.org/10.1111/odi.12817.

21. Moloney J, Stassen LF. Pericoronitis: treatment and a clinical dilemma. J Ir Dent Assoc. 2009;55(4):190–2.

22. Nuwwareh S. Managing a patient with pericoronitis. J Can Dent Assoc. 2013;79:169.

23. Robertson D, Smith AJ. The microbiology of the acute dental abscess. J Med Microbiol. 2009;58(Pt 2):155–62. https://doi.org/10.1099/jmm.0.003517-0.

24. Grandas Ramírez AL, Velásquez CS. Prevalencia de celulitis odontogénica en pacientes de 0 a 18 años que asistieron a la Fundación HOMI-Hospital de la Misericordia de Bogotá entre Febrero de 2009 a Febrero de 2011. Acta Odontol Col. 2012;2(1):71–85.

25. Kara A, Ozsurekci Y, Tekcicek M, et al. Length of hospital stay an management of facial cellulitis of odontogenic origin in children. Pediatr Dent. 2014;36(1):e18–22.

26. Batista Sánchez T, Martínez Chacón M, Rojas Escobar R, et al. Celulitis facial odontógena en pacientes del Hospital Lenin de Holguín. CCM. 2017;21(2):34–6.
27. Ogundiya DA, Keith DA, Mirowski J. Cavernous sinus thrombosis and blindness as complications of an odontogenic infection: report of a case and review of literature. J Oral Maxillofac Surg. 1989;47:1317–21.
28. Corson MA, Postlethwaite KP, Seymour RA. Are dental infections a cause of brain abscess? Case report and review of the literature. Oral Dis. 2001;7:61–5.
29. Pedrazzoli M, Colletti G, Ferrari M, et al. Mesenchymal phosphaturic neoplasm in the maxillary sinus: a case report. Int J Oral Maxillofac Surg. 2010;39:1027–32.
30. Mameli C, Genoni T, Madia C, et al. Brain abscess in pediatric age: a review. Childs Nerv Syst. 2019;35:1–12. https://doi.org/10.1007/s00381-019-04182-4.

Neck Infections in Children

53

Emine Ünal Evren, Hakan Evren, and Charles M. Myer III

53.1 Introduction

Although it is rare for a pus-forming lesion to develop in the neck in a child, when it does, the situation may become grave and ensuring patency of the airway may become an emergency situation. Infection can track along the spaces in the neck and spread into adjacent structures, e.g. the mediastinum and the vertebral spine. Since the neck is a series of complicated anatomical structures and symptoms in paediatric cases may be less obvious, accurate diagnosis and treatment depends on the alertness of clinicians to the danger. Paediatric cases may begin with, for example, upper respiratory symptoms, eating or drinking less, cervical discomfort, cervical lymphadenopathy or trismus. These symptoms may quickly worsen to the point where the airway gets blocked, a thrombosis forms in the jugular vein, there is inflammation of the mediastinum or sepsis develops. The key steps in the clinical management of cervical infections are administration of the correct antibiotic, surgical drainage and circumventing complications [1]. Cervical infections encompasses pus-forming cervical adenitis, abscess formation (peritonsillar, retropharyngeal or parapharyngeal), pus-forming thyroiditis, infection of an embryological remnant (cervical cyst), in addition to complications of operative

E. Ü. Evren (✉) · H. Evren
Department of Infectious Diseases and Microbiology, University of Kyrenia,
School of Medicine, Kyrenia, Turkish Republic on Northern Cyprus (TRNC), Cyprus

C. M. Myer III
Department of Otolaryngology, Head and Neck Surgery, College of Medicine,
and Cincinnati Children's Hospital and Medical Center, University of Cincinnati,
Cincinnati, OH, USA

C. Cingi et al. (eds.), *Pediatric ENT Infections*,
https://doi.org/10.1007/978-3-030-80691-0_53

procedures, radiation exposure, injury, and human or animal bites. How these manifest clinically and how they should be treated form the material for this chapter.

53.2　Suppurative Cervical Adenitis in Children

Suppurative cervical adenitis is a condition in which there is enlargement, inflammation and tenderness of the cervical lymph nodes secondary to infection by a range of pathogens. There are lymph nodes situated along the entire length of the lymphatic system, with greater density at key points, such as in the cervical region. Cervical lymphadenitis is a common occurrence in the paediatric population due to the frequency of infective episodes affecting the oropharynx.

53.2.1　Acute Viral Lymphadenitis

Paediatric cervical adenitis is generally the result of infection with viruses [2]. Adenopathy following a viral infection usually occurs following an infective episode of the upper respiratory tract (URTI). It is mostly bilateral, affects several nodes and enlargement is mild and not accompanied by redness of the skin or heat. This type of adenopathy does not often produce pus and typically leads to recovery within a brief period. The most frequently implicated viral pathogens in cervical lymphadenopathy are rhinovirus, parainfluenza and influenza viruses, respiratory syncytial virus, adenovirus, reovirus and coronavirus. Cytomegalovirus and Epstein-Barr Virus are also frequently isolated [3]. Acute cervical adenitis secondary to virus infections is often in association with pyrexia and symptoms of an URTI. Exanthems, conjunctivitis and enlarged spleen and liver may also occur with certain pathogens. Cases of pharyngitis and tonsillitis cause lymphadenitis in the anterior and posterior neck lymph glands. In 90% of cases of kerato-conjunctivitis due to adenovirus, lymphadenitis is preauricular [4]. If lymphadenitis precedes an URTI of viral aetiology, there is no necessity for additional tests to confirm the diagnosis, nor does the condition require separate treatment.

53.2.2　Acute Bacterial Lymphadenitis

If a single lymph node on one side of the neck suddenly enlarges and becomes painful to touch in a child under school age, it is often a result of infection by a bacterium. The lymph nodes most commonly affected in this way are the submandibular, upper cervical, submental, occipital or lower cervical. The majority (between 40 and 80%) of cases of one-sided adenitis in children aged 1–4 years are due to *Staphylococcus aureus* or *Streptococcus pyogenes* [5]. An older child who is suffering from periodontal disease or tooth decay may be susceptible to infection by anaerobes, such as Bacteroides, Peptococcus, Propionibacterium, Fusobacterium or Peptostreptococcus spp. [6]. Rather less commonly, one of the following pathogens may be identified: *Francisella tularensis, Pasteurella multocida, Yersinia pestis,* or *Haemophilus influenzae* type B [4]. The usual case presentation is of pyrexia, throat ache and coughing, or otalgia. When examined physically, there may be evidence of pharyngitis, tonsillitis, acute otitis media or impetigo. Infection with *P. multocida* occurs in the context of being bitten by an animal, whilst Yersinia cases occur when fleas bite the head or neck, most often in the west of the USA. The most likely pathogens should be considered when prescribing first-line antimicrobial agents. Agents which are not deactivated by beta-lactamase generally provide cover for Staphylococci or Streptococci. It may be necessary to admit severely affected children to hospital for careful monitoring. Older children with periodontal disease need to be covered for anaerobes, which are susceptible to penicillin V or clindamycin. Currently, the majority of Staphylococcal cultures obtained from cases of cervical adenitis remain sensitive to methicillin. Unfortunately, research also indicates an increasing degree of methicillin resistance amongst strains of *S. aureus* carried asymptomatically in the nasopharynx in children [7, 8]. Cases where there is no response to a suitable initial empirical trial of antibiotic may need to receive cover for methicillin-resistant *S. aureus* (MRSA). A typical course of antibiotics lasts 10 days and goes on a minimum of 5 days after the acute phase of the illness has passed. In the majority of patients, symptoms should alleviate following 2–3 days' suitable therapy. 25% of cases have a fluctuant mass which can often be managed with antimicrobial therapy and aspirating the mass with a needle. Any such aspirate needs to be sent to the laboratory for Gram and acid-alcohol fast staining, culture (both aerobically and anaerobically) and mycobacterial culture. In children with immunocompromise, the potassium hydroxide test is required, as is mycological culture.

53.2.3 Mycobacterial Lymphadenitis

Persistent cervical lymphadenitis may also result from infection by *Mycobacterium tuberculosis* or atypical mycobacteria. In either case, the presentation is more or less identical. Cervical nodes quickly become enlarged, but do not exceed 3 cm in diameter, whilst the skin which overlies the nodes turns pink or lilac-red and resembles parchment. The nodes exhibit fluctuance and a sinus tract may naturally develop, so that the lesion drains spontaneously. It is rare for constitutional symptoms to occur [4]. Purified protein derivative (PPD) testing of the skin can develop positivity in atypical mycobacterial infection, but this is less florid a reaction (the indurated area does not exceed 15 mm in diameter) than occurs where *M. tuberculosis* is present [9]. Lymphadenitis due to *M. tuberculosis* calls for 12–18 months' worth of multiple antibiotics with activity against the pathogen. Nodes begin to regress in under 3 months. Since atypical mycobacteria are rarely sensitive to antituberculous agents, operative removal of the affected nodes is the best option. If suppurative occurs, multiple drainage procedures may be necessary.

53.2.4 Cat Scratch Disease

Cat scratch disease is characterised by lymphadenitis in the area draining skin where a typical papular lesion appears. It is due to *Bartonella henselae*. The regional adenopathy appears after the papular lesion has developed, but this papule may already have disappeared when lymphadenopathy is observed. The most frequent regional nodes involved are axillary or cervical (50% and 28%, respectively). A textbook case will feature a single, enlarged lymph node that is painful to touch and exceeds 4 cm in diameter. Mild pyrexia, malaise and myalgia may feature. In between 30 and 50% of patients, pus may be formed. Serology provides diagnostic confirmation. Whilst the lesion generally resolves without intervention and minus complications, patients may recover more swiftly when Azithromycin is administered [10]. Rifampin, gentamicin, ciprofloxacin, trimethoprim and sulfamethoxazole, and clarithromycin are the agents which may be needed in cases that develop complications.

53.2.5 Other Infections

In paediatric cases, adenitis is not generally linked to Nocardia spp., but where this occurs, it is usually due to immunocompromise. Nocardia inhabit soil and rotting plant matter. Infection occurs by inhaling the organisms or by a break in the skin. A pustule develops. To isolate the organism, the pustule contents are cultured. Sulfonamides are the first-line treatment.

Where Actinomyces, a commensal in the mouth, invades locally, cervicofacial actinomycosis can develop. This is seen as a brawny area of induration, followed by the nodes becoming involved. Diagnosis is by histopathology. The characteristic appearances are of sulphur granules. Intravenous antibiotic pharmacotherapy is needed at first, after which oral antibiotics are administered for a period from 3 months to a year. Penicillin is first line.

Toxoplasma infections may also be revealed by the presence of cervical lymphadenopathy. Generally it is a serological diagnosis and specific treatment is not needed, unless symptoms reach a high level of severity, when pyrimethamine, sulfadiazine, and leucovorin are administered in combination over approximately 4–6 weeks.

Histoplasmosis, blastomycosis, and coccidiomycosis are infections with fungi. These pathogens are saprophytic and live in the soil. They inhabit particular areas of the USA. The presentation is as a lung infection, following which adenitis may develop. Cases can be diagnosed by serology or cutaneous testing. The majority of patients with such infections recover without any intervention, but cases where symptoms reach a severe level are treated with long-term administration of antifungal agents [11].

53.3 Peritonsillar Cellulitis and Abscess

Infection that occurs in between the palatine tonsillar capsule and the muscles of the pharynx results in inflammation, i.e. peritonsillar cellulitis. When pus gathers in this area, it is known as quinsy or PTA (peritonsillar abscess). The usual progression is from inflammation of the tonsil or pharynx itself (i.e. pharyngitis or tonsillitis) to a localised cellulitis (i.e. phlegmon), before abscess formation occurs [12].

Amongst deep cervical infections in children and adolescents, the type with the highest frequency is PTA, which is present in over half such occurrences [13]. It is more common in adolescence, but is possible even at younger ages [14]. It has been shown in a population-based study that doctors had proposed a diagnosis of potential PTA in 14 children out of every 100,000 population [15].

PTA frequently involves multiple pathogens. The most commonly isolated organisms are *Streptococcus pyogenes*, *Streptococcus anginosus*, *Staphylococcus aureus*, and anaerobic bacteria affecting the respiratory system, such as Fusobacteria, Prevotella and Veillonella spp. [16].

PTA presents clinically as a severe throat ache (typically on one side), pyrexia and vocal muffling, the "hot potato" voice. Sialorrhoea may occur. Up to two out of three cases of PTA cases suffer from trismus, since the lesion irritates the internal pterygoid muscle and causes reflex spasm. This feature helps in distinguishing between quinsy and tonsillitis or pharyngitis [17]. It is frequent for cervical oedema and pain to occur and there may be otalgia present on the side of the lesion [18]. The child may take less by mouth due to pain, tiredness and feeling irritable.

Physical examination in a paediatric case of quinsy reveals oedema and fluctuance of the tonsil, whilst the uvula is shifted towards the unaffected side [19]. Whilst it is possible to observe tonsillar enlargement with exudate and reddening of the throat in a child suffering from peritonsillar cellulitis, it is rare to find the uvula shifted over, or trismus [17]. Quinsy and cellulitis may both cause lymph node enlargement in the cervical and submandibular regions. PTA seldom occurs on both sides simultaneously, but if it does, the upper airway may become blocked and the patient snores [20].

Quinsy is generally a clinical diagnosis that does not depend on laboratory investigations or radiology, provided the uvula is shifted medially together with the tonsil. Where clinical doubt exists, intraoral or submandibular ultrasonographic studies may confirm an abscess is present before it is aspirated. On occasion, a PTA may be diagnosed on a CT scan that has been obtained to evaluate a suspected pharyngeal or cervical infection. Laboratory investigations may, however, assist in grading the severity and need for intervention. Suitable investigations include full blood count and microbiological testing (including culture for *S. pyogenes* plus Gram stain of the aspirated fluid) [19]. Imaging studies are required on occasion where it is unclear whether the lesion represents PTA or another deep cervical infection or epiglottitis.

A differential diagnosis of cases of PTA needs to consider alternative explanations for a painful throat, blockage of the upper airway and oedema within the pharynx. Some key diagnoses to exclude are epiglottitis, retropharyngeal abscess, an abscess within the parapharyngeal recess and severe inflammation of the pharynx and tonsils.

Antibiotics and support are sufficient to treat peritonsillar cellulitis, but PTA may require being drained surgically [21]. In paediatric cases without complicating features (i.e. no airway obstruction or bacteraemia) and where the abscess is small, antibiotic therapy may also suffice [22].

Empirical treatment of PTA is guided by the need to target Group A Streptococci, *S. aureus* and anaerobic bacteria found in the respiratory tract. If the lesion is drained and the fluid cultured, a more appropriate antibiotic may later be identified. PTA often involves more than one pathogen, however, and not all such pathogens may show up on laboratory culture [23]. Depending on local prevalence of MRSA, methicillin resistance may need to be considered. Ampicillin with sulbactam or clindamycin administered parenterally are suitable for empirical therapy. This empirical therapy can be supplemented with vancomycin or linezolid if there is no response or MRSA is thought to be present [19]. The intravenous antibiotics should go on until there is no fever and the patient is better clinically. Oral treatment should then be commenced, so that the total course of treatment is 2 weeks [24]. Suitable agents for administration by mouth are co-Amoxiclav or Clindamycin or Linezolid.

Surgical drainage of PTA performed in the course of a tonsillectomy, plus administration of antibiotics and appropriate support measures, is sufficient for the lesion to resolve in 9 out of 10 cases [21]. Whether steroid administration is of value in treating PTA is not yet clear from the evidence so far [25].

Cases that do not respond fall into the following categories: the clinical situation has been complicated; atypical pathogens are involved; there is an underlying complicating condition (such as a congenital cyst or open tract) [23]. Management may involve further imaging studies or revision surgery, possibly with the addition of further antibiotics to broaden coverage.

Although PTA seldom leads to complications, when they occur, there is a risk of death occurring. Pathogens may track into the deeper cervical structures and enter the circulation. The following may develop: blockage of the airway, septicaemia, thrombus formation in the internal jugular vein, inflammation of the mediastinum and necrotising fasciitis [22].

53.4 Paediatric Retropharyngeal Infections

The retropharyngeal space covers the area between the skull base and the posterior mediastinum. Within this space there are two groups of lymph glands which are noticeable in young children, but regress prior to the onset of puberty [26]. These lymphatics provide drainage to the nasopharynx, posterior paranasal sinuses and the middle ear. Approximately 50% of cases of infection in the retropharynx are found to occur with URTI as a result of this connection [27]. Given that URTIs are most common when patients are aged between 2 and 4 years, it is unsurprising that this is also the most common age for cellulitis or an abscess of the retropharynx to occur [28].

Retropharyngeal abscesses frequently involve multiple pathogens. The most commonly isolated organisms are *Streptococcus pyogenes*, *S. aureus*, and anaerobic bacteria affecting the respiratory system [13].

Retropharyngeal abscesses have different features depending on the point at which they present. They may exhibit features of pharyngitis and inflammation or may present as blockage to the upper portion of the aerodigestive tract. The following symptoms may occur: dysphagia, sialorrhoea, taking less by mouth, a stiff neck, voice that sounds different from usual, breathing difficulty, pain in the chest or trismus [29, 30].

When the oropharynx is seen, there may be oedematous mucosa evident posteriorly, typically only on one side. If swelling is midline, one must consider tuberculous spondylitis or Pott's disease. The anterior cervical lymph nodes are often painful to touch. Palpation may reveal a mass if the pathogen has tracked laterally into the pharyngeal space. If a child's breathing is markedly compromised, they are usually assessed within the operating theatre.

Blood films from cases of retropharyngeal abscess generally exhibit leucocytosis with neutrophilia and stab cells. If the lesion is aspirated, the drained fluid should be sent for both aerobic and anaerobic culture [19]. Routine pharyngeal culture plus rapid diagnostic testing for Group A Streptococcal species is also required. In the absence of evident blockage to the airway and a retropharyngeal infection is not deemed likely, the first stage in investigation may be lateral cervical plain X-ray. If a retropharyngeal infection is strongly suspected, however, contrast-enhanced CT needs to be requested. Flexible nasopharyngoscopy may provide valuable information.

Important competing diagnoses to exclude are other causes of throat pain, blockage of the upper airway and a stiff neck, such as epiglottitis, croup, tracheitis secondary to bacterial infection, other deep neck space infections, uvulitis, angioedema or neoplasia [19].

Guidelines for treating a retropharyngeal abscess depend on the bacteria responsible and the evidence from observational research on treatment outcomes. In paediatric cases where the airway is greatly under threat, securing the airway is the top priority, followed by an operation to drain the lesion. Even where a patient's condition is stable, if CT indicates an abscess at least 2.5 cm in diameter (i.e. a mature abscess), drainage is the preferred option. How a retropharyngeal abscess that is not causing any blockage of the airway should best be dealt with remains controversial [31]. Certain practitioners advise that any abscess be drained without delay and antibiotic pharmacotherapy commenced, whilst other clinicians believe that a 1 to 2 day empirical trial of antibiotic therapy is warranted first, especially for smaller lesions [32, 33].

Empirical antimicrobial therapy needs to target the most likely pathogens responsible, i.e. *S. pyogenes*, *S. aureus* and anaerobic bacteria found within the respiratory tract. Parenteral ampicillin sulbactam or clindamycin is the usual first line, but these agents may not be effective if antibiotic-resistant organisms are involved, such as MRSA. In cases where first-line therapy fails, the addition of vancomycin or linezolid is generally the best way to cover Gram-positive cocci that may be resistant to other agents [34]. Where the airway is under threat or fatality may result from another cause, the abscess exceeds 2.5 cm in diameter or the lesion does not regress with pharmacotherapy, the abscess should be drained in theatre [35].

Retropharyngeal abscesses are seldom complicated, but where this happens, the following may occur: septicaemia, blockage of the airway, inflammation of the mediastinum, thrombus formation in the internal jugular vein, carotid artery rupture and aspiration pneumonia if the abscess bursts and its contents enter the airway [13].

53.5   Parapharyngeal Abscess

The parapharyngeal space (also known as the pharyngomaxillary space) has connections to all the other important fascial spaces in the neck. The superior pharyngeal constrictor muscle lies medial to the space, whilst laterally, the space borders on the pterygoid muscle. An infection that begins in the pharynx or affects the teeth may produce a parapharyngeal abscess, just as occurs with infections of the other key spaces deep within the neck [30, 36]. The most frequent pathogens responsible are *S. pyogenes*, *S. aureus* or anaerobic bacteria that inhabit the respiratory tree [37, 38]. On physical examination, limitation of cervical motion is seen, as are tender lymph nodes on one side of the neck and a pain in the neck. Other ways in which a parapharyngeal abscess presents are pyrexia, throat ache, oedema and painful swallowing [39]. CT imaging is confirmatory. However, since CT involves exposing a child to radiation, CT should not be performed in a young child unless the diagnosis is highly likely. The condition can be managed with parenteral antibiotics plus possible operative drainage of the abscess. First-line antibiotic therapy is ampicillin sulbactam and clindamycin [29, 30]. Where the condition is not recovering within 48 hours of commencing parenteral antibiotics, an operation to drain the abscess is needed [37]. It has been noted in the literature that the following occur as complications: thrombus formation in the internal jugular vein and neurological damage to the cranial nerves or cervical chain [40, 41].

53.6   Other Cervical Infections

Pus-producing thyroid inflammation, infected embryologic cysts, and infections following injury, bites, surgery or radiation exposure account for the other infections of the neck.

53.6.1 Suppurative Thyroiditis

The thyroid may become infected through a range of causes, including spread via the circulation and direct extension from a deep cervical infection. Suppurative thyroiditis is accompanied by pyrexia, pain, tenderness, redness, difficulty swallowing, difficulty speaking, a hoarse voice or an inflamed throat. *S. aureus*, *S. pyogenes* or *S. pneumoniae* are the leading causes. Appropriate antibiotic selection and draining the lesion at operation are the ways in which suppurative thyroiditis is treated. When present in the left thyroid lobe, one must consider a persistent fistula from piriform sinus.

53.6.2 Infected Embryological Remnant Cysts

Embryological anomalies, e.g. cystic hygroma, pharyngeal and bronchial cleft cysts or thyroglossal duct cysts, may become apparent when a cervical infection develops. Infection within these anomalies calls for broad-acting antimicrobials. Penicillin or an appropriate cephalosporin may be prescribed alongside clindamycin to destroy oral pathogens.

53.6.3 Infections Following Bites, Injury, Radiation Exposure or Operative Injury

It is fairly frequent for children to be bitten by animals or another human and such injuries may develop into infections, usually with bacteria from the mouth of the assailant. *Pasteurella multocida* is frequently the infective agent in animal bites. Bite-related infections, whether the child was bitten by an animal or another human, are best treated initially with penicillin, co-amoxiclav or moxifloxacin.

Infectious complications are possible after maxillofacial injury, radiation exposure or surgery to the neck. These conditions need to be carefully watched for. The typical pathogens responsible are *S. aureus* and *Pseudomonas aeruginosa*. Antibiotics selection should be guided by culture result and susceptibility testing [42].

References

1. Côrte FC, Firmino-Machado J, Moura CP, Spratley J, Santos M. Acute pediatric neck infections: outcomes in a seven-year series. Int J Pediatr Otorhinolaryngol. 2017;99:128–34.
2. Peters TR, Edwards KM. Cervical lymphadenopathy and adenitis. Pediatr Rev. 2000;21(12):399.
3. Leung AK, Robson WLM. Childhood cervical lymphadenopathy. J Pediatr Health Care. 2004;18(1):3–7.
4. Chesney P. Cervical lymphadenitis and neck infections. Principles and practice of pediatric infectious diseases. 2nd ed. London: Churchill Livingstone; 2003. p. 165–76.
5. Kelly CS, Kelly RE Jr. Lymphadenopathy in children. Pediatr Clin North Am. 1998;45(4):875–88.
6. Bodenstein L, Altman R. Cervical lymphadenitis in infants and children. Semin Pediatr Surg. 1994;3:134–41.
7. Anwar M, Jaffery G, Rehman KB, Tayyib M, Bokhari S. Staphylococcus aureus and MRSA nasal carriage in general population. J College Phys Surg--Pakistan: JCPSP. 2004;14(11):661–4.
8. Creech CB, Kernodle DS, Alsentzer A, Wilson C, Edwards KM. Increasing rates of nasal carriage of methicillin-resistant Staphylococcus aureus in healthy children. Pediatr Infect Dis J. 2005;24(7):617–21.
9. Spyridis P, Maltezou HC, Hantzakos A, Scondras C, Kafetzis D. Mycobacterial cervical lymphadenitis in children: clinical and laboratory factors of importance for differential diagnosis. Scand J Infect Dis. 2001;33(5):362–6.
10. Bass JW, Freitas BC, Freitas AD, Sisler CL, Chan DS, Vincent JM, Person DA, Claybaugh JR, Wittler RR, Weisse ME. Prospective randomized double blind placebo-controlled evaluation of azithromycin for treatment of cat-scratch disease. Pediatr Infect Dis J. 1998;17(6):446–52.
11. Gosche JR, Vick L. Acute, subacute, and chronic cervical lymphadenitis in children. Semin Pediatr Surg. 2006;2:99–106.
12. Goldstein N. Hammerschlag, MR. Peritonsillar, retropharyngeal, and parapharyngeal abscesses. In: Feigin RD, Cherry JD, Demmler GJ, Kaplan SL, editors. Textbook of pediatric infectious diseases. 5th ed. Philidelphia: Saunders; 2004. p. 178.
13. Ungkanont K, Yellon RF, Weissman JL, Casselbrant ML, GonzÁAlez-Valdepeña H, Bluestone CD. Head and neck space infections in infants and children. Otolaryngol Head Neck Surg. 1995;112(3):375–82.

14. Friedman NR, Mitchell RB, Pereira KD, Younis RT, Lazar RH. Peritonsillar abscess in early childhood: presentation and management. Archiv Otolaryngol–Head Neck Surg. 1997;123(6):630–2.
15. Millar KR, Johnson DW, Drummond D, Kellner JD. Suspected peritonsillar abscess in children. Pediatr Emerg Care. 2007;23(7):431–8.
16. Klug TE. Peritonsillar abscess: clinical aspects of microbiology, risk factors, and the association with parapharyngeal abscess. Clin Infect Dis. 2009;49:1467–2.
17. Szuhay G, Tewfik TL. Peritonsillar abscess or cellulitis? A clinical comparative paediatric study. J Otolaryngol-Head Neck Surg. 1998;27(4):206.
18. Galioto NJ. Peritonsillar abscess. Steroids. 2008;8(13):14.
19. Tebruegge M, Curtis N. Infections related to the upper and middle airways. In: principles and practice of pediatric infectious diseases. Amsterdam: Elsevier; 2012. p. 205–13.
20. Simons JP, Branstetter BF IV, Mandell DL. Bilateral peritonsillar abscesses: case report and literature review. Am J Otolaryngol. 2006;27(6):443–5.
21. Herzon FS, Martin AD. Medical and surgical treatment of peritonsillar, retropharyngeal, and parapharyngeal abscesses. Curr Infect Dis Rep. 2006;8(3):196.
22. Yellon R. Head and neck space infections. Pediatric otolaryngol. 2003;2:1681–701.
23. Beahm E, Elden L. In: Burg FD, Ingelfinger JR, Polin RA, Gerson AA, editors. Bacterial infections of the neck. Current pediatric therapy. 18th ed. Philadelphia: Saunders; 2006. p. 1117.
24. Apostolopoulos NJ, Nikolopoulos TP, Bairamis TN. Peritonsillar abscess in children. Is incision and drainage an effective management? Int J Pediatr Otorhinolaryngol. 1995;31(2–3):129–35.
25. Chau JK, Seikaly HR, Harris JR, Villa-Roel C, Brick C, Rowe BH. Corticosteroids in peritonsillar abscess treatment: a blinded placebo-controlled clinical trial. Laryngoscope. 2014;124(1):97–103.
26. McClay JE, Murray AD, Booth T. Intravenous antibiotic therapy for deep neck abscesses defined by computed tomography. Archiv Otolaryngol–Head Neck Surg. 2003;129(11):1207–12.
27. Philpott C, Selvadurai D, Banerjee A. Paediatric retropharyngeal abscess. J Laryngol Otol. 2004;118(12):919–26.
28. Dawes LC, Bova R, Carter P. Retropharyngeal abscess in children. ANZ J Surg. 2002;72(6):417–20.
29. Page NC, Bauer EM, Lieu JE. Clinical features and treatment of retropharyngeal abscess in children. Otolaryngol Head Neck Surg. 2008;138(3):300–6.
30. Craig FW, Schunk JE. Retropharyngeal abscess in children: clinical presentation, utility of imaging, and current management. Pediatrics. 2003;111(6):1394–8.
31. Saluja S, Brietzke SE, Egan KK, Klavon S, Robson CD, Waltzman ML, Roberson DW. A prospective study of 113 deep neck infections managed using a clinical practice guideline. Laryngoscope. 2013;123(12):3211–8.
32. Vural C, Gungor A, Comerci S. Accuracy of computerized tomography in deep neck infections in the pediatric population. Am J Otolaryngol. 2003;24(3):143–8.
33. Kirse DJ, Roberson DW. Surgical management of retropharyngeal space infections in children. Laryngoscope. 2001;111(8):1413–22.
34. Pesola A, Sihvonen R, Lindholm L, Patari-Sampo A Clindamycin resistant emm 33 Streptococcus pyogenes emerged among invasive infections in Helsinki metropolitan area, Finland, 2012 to 2013. Eurosurveillance; 2015
35. Wilkie MD, De S, Krishnan M. Defining the role of surgical drainage in paediatric deep neck space infections. Clin Otolaryngol. 2019;44(3):366–71.
36. Oh J-H, Kim Y, Kim C-H. Parapharyngeal abscess: comprehensive management protocol. Orl. 2007;69(1):37–42.
37. Dudas R, Sterwint J. Retropharyngeal abscess. Pediatr Rev. 2006;27(6):e45–6.
38. Chang L, Chi H, Chiu N-C, Huang F-Y, Lee K-S. Deep neck infections in different age groups of children. J Microbiol Immunol Infect. 2010;43(1):46–52.
39. Grisaru-Soen G, Komisar O, Aizenstein O, Soudack M, Schwartz D, Paret G. Retropharyngeal and parapharyngeal abscess in children—epidemiology, clinical features and treatment. Int J Pediatr Otorhinolaryngol. 2010;74(9):1016–20.

40. Sudhanthar S, Garg A, Gold J, Napolova O. Parapharyngeal abscess: a difficult diagnosis in younger children. Clin Case Rep. 2019;7(6):1218–21.
41. Huang C-M, Huang F-L, Chien Y-L, Chen P-Y. Deep neck infections in children. J Microbiol Immunol Infect. 2017;50(5):627–33.
42. Bennett JE, Dolin R, Blaser MJ. Mandell, Douglas, and Bennett's principles and practice of infectious diseases. Amsterdam: Elsevier; 2014.

Infections of Congenital Neck Masses

54

Fatih Yücedağ, Nuray Bayar Muluk,
and Gabriela Kopacheva-Barsova

54.1 Introduction

Congenital masses of the head and neck already exist by the time the child is born, but they may pass unrecognised up to the point when they later cause a problem [1]. A child with a noticeable neck mass may present perinatally or in a paediatric general clinic. Taking a detailed history and noting the features of the lesion leads to a targeted list of potential diagnoses, at which point the case may be referred to an appropriate specialist with expertise in managing head and neck masses. These lesions develop through anomalous embryological development processes and may be of cystic, solid or vascular type. Typically they present when infection develops. Such lesions may be neoplasms; however, this is rarely the case. Indeed, lesions of the head and neck represent a mere 5% of all cancers encountered in childhood [2].

Paediatric masses in the head and neck region in young children are of many different types. The many individual kinds may be classified into congenital, inflammatory or neoplastic in type [3]. Performing a meticulous examination of the head and neck and ordering appropriate investigations form the basis of diagnosis. There are specific patterns to the presentation, which are a result of the embryological development and anatomical configuration of this part of the body. Clinicians need to understand these subjects well to appreciate the varying natural historical features of particular masses [1–4].

F. Yücedağ (✉)
Section of Otorhinolaryngology, Karaman State Hospital, Karaman, Turkey

N. Bayar Muluk
Department of Otorhinolaryngology, Faculty of Medicine, Kırıkkale University, Kırıkkale, Turkey

G. Kopacheva-Barsova
Department of Otorhinolaryngology, Faculty of Medicine, Cyril and Methodius University of Skopje, Skopje, Republic of North Macedonia

© The Author(s), under exclusive license to Springer Nature Switzerland AG 2022
C. Cingi et al. (eds.), *Pediatric ENT Infections*,
https://doi.org/10.1007/978-3-030-80691-0_54

The lesions that occur with the highest frequency are all cystic in nature—dermoid, branchial or from the thyroglossal duct. Typically, surgical excision of these lesions is required to prevent them becoming infected. Failure to remove the lesions results in recurrent infections and significant risk for the affected individual.

Cysts of the thyroglossal duct characteristically present as a swollen area in the midline slightly inferior to the chin. Operative excision is recommended to stop the development of infection and fistulation.

Cysts of the branchial cleft similarly occur in the midline. They are highly prone to infection and thus excision is strongly recommended.

Dermoid cysts typically occur facially, on the neck or in the scalp area. They sometimes enlarge and are prone to infection. Excision is required.

54.2   Cysts of the Thyroglossal Duct

These lesions occur with the highest frequency of any midline paediatric lesion occurring congenitally. The commonest way for them to present is with a cystic mass located near to the hyoid bone in the midline. The lesion is not painful. The majority of such lesions come to clinical attention before the age of 5 years. In a straightforward thyroglossal cyst, the lesions are observed to move upwards during deglutition or when the patient sticks his/her tongue out. This is due to the lesion being attached to the hyoid bone and the foramen caecum. In early embryonic development, the thyroid develops as an out-pouching of the tongue in the region where the anterior and posterior muscular groups abut each other. The thyroid begins its descent as the embryo increases in length, moving close to the future hyoid bone. The median portion of the thyroidal primordium lengthens, and the thyroglossal duct is formed as the gland moves caudally. Before week 5 of embryological development, the thyroglossal duct has usually been obliterated, but a trace persists as the future foramen caecum. If the thyroglossal duct does not undergo obliteration prior to formation of the hyoid bone, the thyroglossal duct becomes a sinus that may enlarge to become a thyroglossal cyst [5, 6].

54.2.1 Management by Surgery

Unless the thyroglossal cyst creates complications, its removal is generally straightforward. ENT surgeons remove the lesion via a transverse incision. The head of the child needs to be somewhat raised and the neck put in extension. The surgeon needs to dissect carefully around the lesion to find its full extent. The thyroglossal cyst needs to be removed together with the central portion of the hyoid, to which it is attached. The lesions need to be removed as an entire specimen; otherwise there is a high risk it will regrow. To assist with removing the cyst in its entirety, the surgeon may depress the basal tongue by placing a finger in the patient's oral cavity. Suturing of the tract at its proximal border completes the resection procedure [7].

54.3   Branchial Cleft Cysts

Around 1 in 3 neck masses present since birth are branchial cleft cysts lined by epithelium. These cysts are not malignant and may be noticed at any point in life. Most arise from the second branchial cleft. They present as a mass which is not painful to touch and exhibits fluctuance. The usual location is just in front of the sternocleidomastoid muscle.

Branchial cleft cysts may become noticeable following an infective episode affecting the upper respiratory tract in which the cyst initially enlarges and then shrinks again [7, 8]. This lesion develops when remnants of the cervical sinus are trapped and unable to form an opening either internally or externally. They thus form a cystic lesion lined by epithelium. It has been suggested that the lesions actually originate from cells which normally give rise to Waldeyer's ring. In fact, it is fairly uncommon to find a lesion that is composed purely of branchial cleft cells, with most lesions composed of two different populations of cells [9, 10].

The type of mass that is most frequently seen with a lateral distribution are cysts of the branchial cleft. In between 2 and 3% of cases, they are found on both sides. There is an increased risk in patients with a positive family history, but otherwise they are not more common in males than females, or in particular ethnic groups. They occur in children more often than in adults [11].

Branchial cleft structures normally undergo complete involution in utero, but when this does not occur, cell rests may from a cyst, when there is no opening towards the gut or externally, or a fistula where such an opening does exist. The vast majority (9 out of 10) of branchial cleft cysts have a lining composed of stratified squamous epithelium [9, 10].

54.3.1 Specific Features of Cysts from Each Level

54.3.1.1   First Branchial Cleft Cyst

Between 5 and 25% of branchial cleft cysts are from the first cleft. These lesions are of two kinds: Work's type 1 and 2. The former occurs as a cyst in the pre-auricular region. These patients have a second external auditory meatal structure consisting of cells exclusively derived from the ectoderm. The vestibulocochlear nerve is medial to the course of the cystic tract, which runs alongside the external ear canal before terminating in the middle portion of the middle ear. Type 2 lesions, by contrast, are found in three locations: at the mandibular angle, in the pre-auricular or submandibular regions. This type is more common than Work's type 1. It consists of cells of mesodermal as well as ectodermal origin. In 57% of cases, the vestibulocochlear nerve is medial to the lesion, but in 30% the nerve is lateral. The cystic tract terminates in the external auditory meatus or in the vicinity of the meatus [11].

54.3.1.2   Second Branchial Cleft Cyst

These lesions are the ones occurring with highest frequency, being thought to account for approaching 95% of cases where a branchial cleft cyst is present. The cystic tract is bounded on one side by the internal and on the other by the external carotid artery. The vestibulocochlear nerve lies superficial to the cyst, whereas the hypoglossal and glossopharyngeal nerves lie deep to the lesion. Where the cyst possesses a sinus, its opening is found in the tonsillar fossa. Structures which are derived embryologically from the second branchial arch, e.g. the handle of the malleus, the crus longum of the incus and the crura and head of the stapes, are above the cyst, whereas those with an origin from the third branchial arch, e.g. the major cornu of the hyoid bone, are below the cyst [11].

54.3.1.3 Third Branchial Cleft Cyst

The most frequent location for a third branchial cleft cyst to occur is antero-inferiorly within the neck, on the left-hand side. Their presentation may be in the form of an abscess, a cervical mass or as inflammation of the thyroid. The vagus and hypoglossal nerves and the common carotid artery lie deep to the lesion, whereas the glossopharyngeal nerve is more superficial. If the lesion has a sinus tract, it pierces the thyrohyoid membrane at a higher level than the superior laryngeal nerve, terminating within the superior piriform sinus [11].

54.3.1.4 Fourth Branchial Cleft Cyst

Fourth branchial cleft cysts occur infrequently. The usual presentation is of a mass located infero-anteriorly on the neck, underneath the platysma muscle and in front of the sternocleidomastoid. It follows a complex course: initially, it winds around the hypoglossal nerve before passing behind the common carotid artery and the thyroid gland. It runs alongside the recurrent branch of the vagus nerve. It pierces the cricothyroid membrane at a lower level than the superior laryngeal nerve. At this point on its course, it lies superficial to the recurrent laryngeal nerve. The tract then terminates at the apical aspect of the piriform sinus [11].

54.3.2 Evaluation and Treatment

A number of imaging techniques are available to assess a potential branchial cleft cyst, including ultrasonography, computed tomographic scans (CT) and magnetic resonance imaging (MRI). Ultrasonography is an appropriate investigation in the case of cystic lesions of considerable size. On CT, these lesions appear as cystic, with a clearly circumscribed border and enhanced by contrast. CT offers valuable information about the relationship of the lesion to surrounding structures, both those lying deeper and those more superficial, and this is of value in identifying the subtype. There may be an enhanced appearance to the wall of the lesion if MRI is undertaken using gadolinium contrast agent. MRI offers particular advantage in assessment of type 2 cysts arising from the first branchial cleft due to better visualisation of the parotid gland and the nervous tissues found in the vicinity of the lesion [11, 12].

Therapy for branchial cleft cysts relies on operative removal of the whole lesion. In cases where the presence of a cyst become obvious due to infection, removal needs to wait until the infection has completely resolved. It is better if possible not to cut into and attempt to drain the lesion before undertaking removal, as it may complicate procedures to ensure the entire lesion is excised. Removal of a portion of the thyroid is potentially necessary to adequately treat cysts of the third and fourth branchial cleft. If the cyst opens into the piriform sinus and this is observable by direct laryngoscopy, finding the exact location of the lesion will be more straightforward. In the opinion of some experts, cauterisation of the fistulous opening of a third or fourth branchial cyst offers efficacy in treatment [11, 12].

54.4 Dermoid Cyst

Dermoid cysts are non-malignant lesions that occur due to anomalous embryological development of the cutaneous tissues, resulting in ectodermally derived cells being trapped in anomalous locations [13, 14]. The lesion consists of cysts with a lining of stratified, squamous epithelium. Within the wall there are fully developed organs usually found in skin. The interior of the cyst is occupied by keratin and hair. Although dermoid cysts are classified as congenital lesions, they may not be diagnosed for some time after the patient is born. However, there is a 40% chance the lesion will be recognised at the time of birth, whilst the remaining 60% of cases are usually discovered before children reach their fifth birthday. Most lesions of this type appear before the age of 1 year and enlarge only gradually. The most frequent locations (84% of cases) for cysts of this kind are the head and neck [15, 16].

54.4.1 Aetiology and Epidemiology

Very little is known about the exact reasons why dermoid cysts form. Histopathologically, the lesions are classified as genuine hamartomas. Entrapment of cutaneous-forming embryonic cells during development is the main event in their pathogenesis. A study by Prior et al. [15, 16] identified no particular risk factors for their occurrence. Patient sex, histological characteristics and age were not correlated.

Dermoid cysts make up a considerable proportion of masses in children discovered on the skull, or scalp in particular, estimated at between 15.4 and 58.5%. They are typically congenital and present before the age of 6 years around 70% of the time [14–18]. Their occurrence has, however, been noted in adult patients, too [15, 16]. Pollard et al. noted that the lesion had a slight female predilection, but this finding has not been repeated in studies since then [16]. The majority of published cases refer to Caucasian patients, although the lesion has no discernible ethnic or racial bias.

54.4.2 Pathophysiology

Dermoid cysts are caused by anomalous development of skin organs in utero. Ectodermally derived cells that are destined normally for the outer surface of the body become entrapped in deeper layers when the skin fuses during development. Their characteristic locations are in the line of the cranial sutures or the anterior fontanelle, which relates to the way they become entrapped [14, 16]. Most patients present with dermoid cysts in the head and neck area. However, the lesion can potentially occur in any location on the body. Within those cases that do present on the head and neck, the lesion's favoured location is frontally, occipitally or supra-orbitally. The commonest place to see a dermoid cyst is the lateral third of the eyebrow.

54.4.3 Evaluation and Treatment

Dermoid cysts are capable of expanding as they mature, and this growth may be into the skull or the spinal column [14, 16]. Accordingly, imaging studies are required prior to taking a biopsy specimen or removing the lesion, particularly where the cyst lies on the midline or in the scalp region [15]. Aspirating the contents of the cyst or obtaining a tissue biopsy risks introducing an infection which could result in osteomyelitis, meningeal or cerebral involvement [15, 16]. Dermoid cysts in the region of the nose are the midline congenital malformation to affect the nose with the highest rate of occurrence. Research indicates there is a risk of between 10 and 45% that such a lesion extends into the cranial cavity. MRI is the most suitable imaging modality to discover whether the lesion extends into the cranial cavity or the spine. It is also reported that dermoid cysts occurring on the forehead or at the pterion are more likely to erode into the bone. If it is suspected that the tumour is eroding the osseous tissues, CT is more suitable to evaluate the extent of destruction of bone. Sometimes high-resolution ultrasound scanning may be useful in visualising a part of the tumour that lies at depth [16].

Ultrasonography of dermoid cysts reveals an evenly textured, hypoechoic lesion that is clearly differentiated from surrounding tissues [15]. Fistulography may be used selectively if it is suspected the lesion impinges on a deep tract. Dacryocystographic study may also occasionally be needed. In any case, if a dermoid cyst is thought to extend into the spine or cranial cavity, a neurosurgical opinion is highly advisable [13, 16].

Dermoid cysts have a characteristic tendency to enlarge gradually and are capable of resulting in destruction of osseous tissues, expanding into the interior of the skull or the spine [13, 17]. This expansion and invasion is a risk factor for meningitis or a cerebral abscess. If a dermoid cyst is not large, surgery to excise it may not be urgently required, since such lesions may not change for many years and can sometimes begin to shrink. In the majority of cases, nonetheless, it is advisable to ensure removal by a surgeon experienced in taking out the lesion without disruption to its boundaries, since the possibility of expansion remains high [13, 16].

Operating without delay may also permit a less traumatic surgical intervention and the cutaneous incision may be less extensive, allowing for a superior cosmetic result. Operative removal also permits the entire lesion to be examined histopathologically, since there is a small possibility that a malignancy may mimic a dermoid cyst by presenting as a single mass on the head or neck in a paediatric patient. In the majority of cases, the lesion may be directly approached and removed by carefully dissecting around the borders of the mass. Should the cyst be inadvertently punctured whilst being excised, any remaining elements require removal with a curette and the site needs to be irrigated extensively [13, 18].

Where the wall of the cyst is adherent to other essential structures, it may be necessary to leave part of the lesion in place [15], albeit in the knowledge that the lesion may well recur [15]. This is one reason to elect for excision at the earliest opportunity, since there is an association between removing a cyst intact and a low rate of recurrence. One new surgical option, for dermoid cysts that are small, is removal with the endoscope. However, where a dermoid cyst has extended into the cranial cavity, the only option may be craniotomy [15–20].

54.5 Macrocystic Lymphatic Malformations

Macrocystic malformations of lymphatic tissue, which used to be known as "cystic hygromas," have a frequency of 1 in 2000 live births. The majority are found within the head and neck. Such lesions may even be noted within the first trimester of pregnancy, as ultrasonographic techniques have developed. It is usually recommended that total operative removal is needed for a cure, but sclerotherapy has been recommended in certain cases where the lesion has no complications and is not impinging upon the airway in any way. There are some case reports and small case series in the literature which indicate the possibility of different approaches, such as pharmacotherapy with sildenafil, propranolol or sirolimus. It has even been reported that the lesions may spontaneously regress, but this appears to be an uncommon occurrence. It is not unusual for a macrocystic malformation to become infected, in which case antibiotic pharmacotherapy is frequently efficacious, after which the lesion may be removed at a convenient time or subjected to sclerotherapy [21–24].

References

1. Dremmen MHG, Tekes A, Mueller S, et al. Lumps and bumps of the neck in children–neuro-imaging of congenital and acquired lesions. J Neuroimaging. 2016;26:562–80.
2. Goins MR, Beasley MS. Pediatric neck masses. Oral Maxillofac Surg Clin North Am. 2012;24:457–68.
3. Dickson PV, Davidoff AM. Malignant neoplasms of the head and neck. Semin Pediatr Surg. 2006;15(2):92–8.
4. Bodenstein L, Altman RP. Cervical lymphadenitis in infants and children. Semin Pediatr Surg. 1994;3(3):134–41.
5. Garcia E, Osterbauer B, Parham D, Koempel J. The incidence of microscopic thyroglossal duct tissue superior to the hyoid bone. Laryngoscope. 2019;129(5):1215–7.
6. Unsal O, Soytas P, Hascicek SO, Coskun BU. Clinical approach to pediatric neck masses: retrospective analysis of 98 cases. North Clin Istanb. 2017;4(3):225–32.
7. Ross J, Manteghi A, Rethy K, Ding J, Chennupati SK. Thyroglossal duct cyst surgery: a ten-year single institution experience. Int J Pediatr Otorhinolaryngol. 2017;101:132–6.

 8. Koch EM, Fazel A, Hoffmann M. Cystic masses of the lateral neck - proposition of an algorithm for increased treatment efficiency. J Craniomaxillofac Surg. 2018;46(9):1664–8.
 9. Coste AH, Lofgren DH, Shermetaro C. Branchial cleft cyst. Treasure Island: StatPearls Publishing; 2020.
10. Lee DH, Yoon TM, Lee JK, Lim SC. Clinical study of second branchial cleft anomalies. J Craniofac Surg. 2018;29(6):e557–60.
11. Allen SB, Goldman J. Branchial cleft cysts. Treasure Island: StatPearls Publishing; 2020.
12. Teo NW, Ibrahim SI, Tan KK. Distribution of branchial anomalies in a paediatric Asian population. Singapore Med J. 2015;56(4):203–7.
13. Shahjahan Shareef S, Ettefagh L. Dermoid cyst. Treasure Island: StatPearls Publishing; 2020.
14. Julapalli MR, Cohen BA, Hollier LH, Metry DW. Congenital, ill-defined, yellowish plaque: the nasal dermoid. Pediatr Dermatol. 2006;23(6):556–9.
15. Nakajima K, Korekawa A, Nakano H, Sawamura D. Subcutaneous dermoid cysts on the eyebrow and neck. Pediatr Dermatol. 2019;36(6):999–1001.
16. Orozco-Covarrubias L, Lara-Carpio R, Saez-De-Ocariz M, Duran-McKinster C, Palacios-Lopez C, Ruiz-Maldonado R. Dermoid cysts: a report of 75 pediatric patients. Pediatr Dermatol. 2013;30(6):706–11.
17. Prior A, Anania P, Pacetti M, Secci F, Ravegnani M, Pavanello M, Piatelli G, Cama A, Consales A. Dermoid and epidermoid cysts of scalp: case series of 234 consecutive patients. World Neurosurg. 2018;120:119–24.
18. McAvoy JM, Zuckerbraun L. Dermoid cysts of the head and neck in children. Arch Otolaryngol. 1976;102(9):529–31.
19. Sorenson EP, Powel JE, Rozzelle CJ, Tubbs RS, Loukas M. Scalp dermoids: a review of their anatomy, diagnosis, and treatment. Childs Nerv Syst. 2013;29(3):375–80.
20. Reissis D, Pfaff MJ, Patel A, Steinbacher DM. Craniofacial dermoid cysts: histological analysis and inter-site comparison. Yale J Biol Med. 2014;87(3):349–57.
21. Forrester MB, Merz RD. Descriptive epidemiology of cystic hygroma: Hawaii, 1986 to 1999. South Med J. 2004;97:631–6.
22. Ninh TN, Ninh TX. Cystic hygroma in children: a report of 126 cases. J Pediatr Surg. 1974;9:191e5.
23. Chen M, Lee CP, Lin SM, Lam YH, Tang RYK, Tse HY, et al. Cystic hygromadetected in thefirst trimester scan in Hong Kong. J Matern Fetal Neonatal Med. 2014;27:342e5. https://doi.org/10.3109/14767058.2013.818122.
24. Gilony D, Schwartz M, Shpitzer T, Feinmesser R, Kornreich L, Raveh E. Treatment of lymphatic malformations: a more conservative approach. J Pediatr Surg. 2012;47:1837e42. https://doi.org/10.1016/j.jpedsurg.2012.06.005.

Pediatric Ear, Nose, and Throat Field Infectious Disease Emergencies

55

Muhammed Evvah Karakılıç, Mustafa Çanakçı, and Emmanuel P. Prokopakis

55.1 Introduction

ENT infections are the most common cause of admittance to pediatric emergency services. Families who are susceptible to children's illnesses apply to the emergency department for almost all ear, nose, and throat infections that are important or not. These diseases usually progress with high fever, and for families, high fever in their children is a reason for panic and emergency unit admission.

Most of the oral and throat infections in the pediatric age group are viral. While adenoviruses, coronaviruses, enteroviruses, rhinoviruses, herpes simplex, influenza, Ebstein Barr, and influenza constitute the majority of viral infections, cytomegalovirus, human immunodeficiency virus, parainfluenza family are seen less frequently. Although measles is rare, it is a critical infection that should not be forgotten.

Group A beta-hemolytic streptococci (GABHS) are the most common among bacterial agents, while Hemophilus influenza type B, and staph. Aureus is seen more rarely [1, 2]. Early-onset of GABHS diagnosis and treatment in emergency services or primary care areas is vital for managing complications.

M. E. Karakılıç (✉) · M. Çanakçı
Department of Emergency Medicine, Faculty of Medicine, Eskişehir Osmangazi University, Eskişehir, Turkey
e-mail: mcanakci@ogu.edu.tr

E. P. Prokopakis
Department of Otorhinolaryngology, School of Medicine, University of Crete, Heraklion, Crete, Greece

55.2 Acute Pharyngitis

55.2.1 Definition and Etiology

Acute pharyngitis is a clinical condition that is very common in childhood, can be applied in all seasons, and should be considered because of possible complications and essential diseases in the differential diagnosis. It is essential to differentiate superficial and deep infections in all age groups. Especially in patients with a toxic appearance, drooling, stridor changes, phonation changes, trismus, and torticollis cause red flags in patients presenting with a sore throat [2].

General symptoms are sore throat, fever, odynophagia, headache, abdominal pain, vomiting, cough, coryza, diarrhea, arthralgia, myalgia, and lethargy. However, it is widely known that most infections are self-limiting and regress within days [2, 3].

Due to the Covid-19 pandemic, children with a sore throat should be questioned in terms of possible cases [4]. In order to prevent the spread of the disease, appropriate isolation methods should be provided. Although the most important causes of fever in the pediatric age group are pharyngitis and otitis media, patients should be swabbed if deemed necessary.

It is known that the most common causes of acute pharyngitis are viral [5]. Adenoviruses, coronaviruses, enteroviruses, rhinoviruses, herpes simplex, influenza, Epstein Barr, and influenza are frequent pathogens causing pharyngitis [2, 3]. GABHS, group C and G streptococci, and mycoplasma pneumonia are common bacteria in pharyngitis [3].

55.3 Viral Pharyngitis

55.3.1 Definition and Etiology

As mentioned above, there are many different infection source microorganisms. Almost all of these microorganisms cause patients to consult a doctor with similar complaints. In infants, the clinic is mostly uneasy, fever, general indulgence, not sucking, while sore throat, anorexia, fever, and odynophagia are observed in the play age and school age. Apart from these common infections, clinically significant EBV, CMV, and HIV should be evaluated.

Classical fever, pharyngitis, and anterior cervical lymphadenopathy in children also in EBV infections [6]. It progresses asymptomatically in most children [7]. Especially in children under 4 years of age, the heterophile antibody test may be falsely negative in diagnosis. Therefore, IgM and IgG tests and EBV DNA evaluation can be performed in case of clinical suspicion [2, 7, 8]. Since exudative pharyngitis may be seen, pruritic maculopapular eruptions may be characteristic after prescribed penicillin antibiotics [2, 3].

CMV infections also come with symptoms similar to EBV. Negative monospot test used to detect heterophile antibodies in diagnosis and contact with a person infected with CMV may be guiding. Besides, lymphadenopathy is less common than EBV, and splenomegaly is not an expected finding. It can be diagnosed with IgM and IgG. If these two viral infections are suspected, the CMV immunoglobulin level would be a more appropriate approach for both viruses [2].

"Acute retroviral syndrome" that develops after HIV infection comes with symptoms similar to EBV at a rate of 50–70%. Unlike EBV and CMV, there are no exudative lesions, and there is no significant tonsillar hypertrophy, its onset is sudden, the presence of mucocutaneous ulcers, and high-risk social history should suggest HIV, especially in adolescents [2].

55.3.2 Treatment

Symptomatic treatment is sufficient for local manifestations of all viral infections. Antiviral treatments are not indicated in children without other systemic findings [2, 8, 9].

Although there are studies on acyclovir in EBV infections, it is still stated that it is not required for most patients. Besides, corticosteroid therapy is not routinely recommended. Patient-specific evaluation should be made, and profit-loss rates should be carefully evaluated [10, 11]. It will be necessary for EBV infections to monitor liver functions due to complications and rest in splenic rupture [6, 8].

55.3.3 Helpful Measures

The use of hot and cold drinks can provide relief. Herbal teas with honey or lemon can be consumed, but honey is not recommended to be used in children under 12 months due to the risk of botulism [8, 12]. Ice absorption and cold dessert eating can be provided. Randomized controlled studies on chlorhexidine and benzydamine have also shown that these two agents help relieve symptoms [9, 13]. Sucking hard candies may be preferred to lozenges in children over five years old. It may be recommended to gargle with warm water over the age of 6. Also, chewing gum is not recommended due to the sorbitol's possibility of the chewing gum worsening the symptoms [8].

55.3.4 Analgesia

Oral intake is reduced in most children due to pain. Therefore, 10–15 mL/kg acetaminophen (max. 1 g or 4 g/day) every 4–6 h or 10 mg/kg every 6 h (2.4 g daily at max 600 mg) are recommended. It has been stated that ibuprofen is more effective in the sore throat because its anti-inflammatory effect is more pronounced [14]. However, it has been validated with meta-analyses that both agents are effectively relieving sore throat [15]. It should be kept in mind that the use of nonsteroidal anti-inflammatory drugs (NSAIDs) in children with severe dehydration will cause acute kidney injury [16]. Complications should be evaluated if there is no improvement or worsening in the patients' symptoms within 3 days [17].

Although studies have shown that a single dose of low-dose steroid use effectively reduces sore throat, its safety is controversial due to the lack of many studies in children. Also, adverse effects, recurrence and relapse rates, lack of statistically significant difference between placebo at times of return to school limit its use [18].

55.3.5 Complications

Self-limiting many viral disease factors observe recovery without causing complications. Especially for EBV, splenomegaly, hepatitis, and malignancies that may develop as latent should not be forgotten. Also, Lemierre's syndrome that develops after EBV is a severe thrombotic condition that can be life-threatening [2].

55.4   Bacterial Pharyngitis

55.4.1 Definition and Etiology

The most common cause of acute bacterial pharyngitis is Group A Beta-Hemolytic Streptococci (GABHS). It is seen in 15–30% of all pharyngitis [19]. In a meta-analysis performed in patients under 18 years of age, GABHS was detected in 37% (32%–43%–95% CI) of patients presenting with sore throat and in 24% (21%–26%–95% CI) of children under 5 years of age [20]. It is more common in winter and early spring [2, 8].

It is common in children under 3 years of age to present with nasal congestion, subfebrile fever (<38.3 C), and painful cervical lymphadenopathy. Fever, headache, nausea and vomiting, abdominal pain, decreased oral intake, and sore throat is common symptoms in 3 and above. Typically, it has a sudden onset. Poorness and sub-dermal fever may be observed under 1 year of age [21]. Painful anterior cervical lymphadenopathy and exudative lesions are significant findings on physical examination.

Group C and G streptococcus families are less common than GABHS. In another study, GABHS was detected in 22.8% of all throat cultures, while non-GABHS bacteria were detected in 3%. The most frequent ones were C and G types. Lymphadenopathy was found to be less, cough and rhinorrhea were more common in those infected with Group C and G streptococci [22]. It is also thought that this group is detected as a carrier in patients with viral pharyngitis.

Neisseria gonorrhea is rare and difficult to diagnose. The complaints are similar to other bacterial infections. It is mostly detected in sexually active adolescents. There may be an association of proctitis, vaginitis, and urethritis. If spawned in the prepubertal age group, care should be taken about abuse [2].

Although Corynebacterium diphtheriae is observed very rarely in developed countries after vaccination, it is one of the critical microorganisms that we may encounter in the future due to the increase in vaccine antibodies in recent years. Due to localized necrosis caused by diphtheria exotoxins, respiratory mucosa may be affected, and cardiac and neurological complications may be observed. There is a GABS-like exudative appearance, but these exudates are in the form of pseudo-membranes and can be removed [2].

Fusobacterium necoplanum causes thrombophlebitis of the jugular vein. It usually occurs in adolescents and young adults. Fever above 39°, respiratory symptoms, unilateral neck swelling, and pain are common findings [2, 3].

55.4.2 Diagnosis

The gold standard method for all infections is throat culture. The sensitivity of rapid antigen tests developed for GABHS is between 80 and 90%. Even if the test is negative, a throat culture is recommended when GABS is suspected [21]. Since the antigen test has a high specificity, culture is unnecessary if it is positive. A standard classification system for antigen testing is Centor criteria. According to Centor criteria, the presence of exudative lesions, painful anterior cervical lymph-adenopathy, fever (>38.3), and the absence of cough are evaluated [23, 24]. There are controversial results in studies conducted in the pediatric age group according to the modified center criteria, but it is stated that the priority will be rapid testing and culture [25].

For Neisseria gonorrhea, throat culture and nucleic acid amplification methods can be used. Loeffler medium is used in the diagnosis of diphtheria [2].

55.4.3 Treatment

Antibiotherapy is especially important for GABHS to avoid complications. Since GABHSs are sensitive to penicillin, it is recommended to give penicillin treatment with a narrow spectrum. Although there are different regimens, the most frequently used are two doses of penicillin for 10 days or one dose of benzathine penicillin plus a single oral penicillin dose. Information on drugs is given in Table 55.1.

In the treatment of Neisseria, a single dose of 250 mg im ceftriaxone or oral azithromycin can be used [26]. Penicillins and first-generation cephalosporins are also used in Fusobacterium infections. Penicillin g (300,000 U every 12 h for <10 kg, can be used every 12 h for>10 kg) is continued until oral administration. After oral intake, penicillin V 250 mg QID is completed for 14 days [27]. After 14 days, culture is recommended again, as 21% of patients are still culture-positive [27]. In addition to antibiotherapy, 20,000–40,000 U antitoxin in pharyngeal-laryngeal disease, 40,000–60,000 U antitoxin in nasopharyngeal disease, and 80,000–120,000 U antitoxin in disease lasting more than 3 days and diffuse neck swelling are recommended [28].

Table 55.1 Antibiotic regimens used in GABHS treatment [8]

Drug	Dosing
Penicillin V	• if ≤27 kg: 250 mg two to three times daily for 10 days • if >27 kg: 500 mg two to three times daily for 10 days
Amoxicillin	• 50 mg/kg per day orally (maximum 1000 mg per day) for 10 days • may be administered once daily or in two or three equally divided doses
Penicillin G benzathine	• if ≤27 kg: Penicillin G benzathine (Bicillin L-A) 600,000 units IM • if >27 kg: Penicillin G benzathine (Bicillin L-A) 1.2 million units IM
Cephalexin	• 40 mg/kg/day divided twice daily for 10 days (maximum 500 mg/dose)
Cefuroxime	• 10 mg/kg/dose orally twice daily for 10 days (maximum 250 mg/dose)
Cefdinir	• 7 mg/kg/dose orally every 12 h for 5 to 10 days or 14 mg/kg/dose every 24 h for 10 days (maximum 600 mg/day)
Azithromycin	• 12 mg/kg (maximum 500 mg/dose) on day 1 followed by 6 mg/kg/dose (maximum 250 mg/dose) once daily on days 2 through 5
Clarithromycin	• 7.5 mg/kg/dose (maximum 250 mg per dose) orally twice daily for 10 days
Clindamycin	• 7 mg/kg/dose (maximum 300 mg per dose) orally three times daily for 10 days

55.4.4 Complications

GABHS has non-suppurative and suppurative complications. Non-suppurative complications; acute rheumatoid fever (ARF), poststreptotoxic glomerulonephritis (PSGN), and pediatric autoimmune neuropsychiatric disorders associated with streptococci (PANDAS). Suppurative complications are necrotizing fasciitis, peritonsillar abscess/cellulitis, otitis media, and sinusitis [28].

55.5   Uvulitis

55.5.1 Definition and Etiology

In isolation, inflammation of the uvula can be both infectious and non-infectious. The most common bacterial agent associated with pharyngitis is GABHS. In patients who are not immunized, the most common cause is Hemophilus influenza type B and accompanies epiglottitis. Other causes are Fusobacterium nucleatum, Prevotella intermedia, and C. Albicans [29].

The most common complaints are sore throat and snagging sensation. If there is difficulty in swallowing and accompanying complications, there may be respiratory distress [2, 29].

55.5.2 Diagnosis

It is placed clinically. Antigen testing can be done for GABHS. Culture should be performed if the diagnosis of H. influenza is suspected [2]. Since uvula edema may be due to non-infectious reasons, a detailed history should be taken. In particular, hyperemia and pain suggest infectious causes in the foreground [29].

55.5.3 Treatment

Treatment for the detected microorganism should be done. However, it should be kept in mind that the uvula may become inflamed due to angioedema. In this case, in terms of airway safety, steroid therapy, antihistamines, and if anaphylaxis is in question, adrenaline should be used in treatment [2].

55.6   Epiglottitis

55.6.1 Definition and Etiology

Acute inflammatory edema of the epiglottis is called epiglottitis. It leads to rapidly progressing and life-threatening airway obstruction [2, 30]. Thanks to Hemophilus influenza vaccination, it occurs in 5 people out of 100,000 children a year. In developed countries, this rate is 0.6–0.8 per 100,000 [31]. Streptococci, staphylococci, pseudomonas, Serratia spp. are the main microorganisms that can cause epiglottitis. Candida albicans may be the cause of epiglottitis in immunosuppressed patients [32].

Sudden onset of fever, stridor, drooling, and hot potato sound are seen, and cough is not a common finding. 80% of the patients come with shortness of breath and stridor, 79% with voice change, 57% with fever, and 50% with a sore throat [29]. Children appear to be severely toxic and use their hands to support the back, bringing the head into hyperextension to maintain airway patency; This position is called the tripod position [2, 30].

55.6.2 Diagnosis

The diagnosis is often made clinically. In older children, epiglottis can be visualized directly, but it should be kept in mind that these maneuvers may worsen airway obstruction. Although imaging methods are unnecessary in the classical presentation, lateral neck radiography can be performed in cases whose clinical picture is not fully established, but the suspicion continues. In this graph, the thumb sign of the epiglottis is significant [33].

55.6.3 Treatment

Since airway obstruction may develop rapidly, patients need aggressive airway management. In cases of angioedema and anaphylaxis, antihistamines, steroids, and adrenaline should be given. Information should be given to the pediatric

Table 55.2 Treatment regimens that can be used for epiglottitis [29]

Drug	Dosage
Ceftriaxone Or	50–100 mg/kg daily 1 or 2 doses max 2 g
Cefotaxime and	150–200 mg/kg 4 doses max 10 g (QID)
Vancomycin	40–60 mg/kg 3–4 doses max 2 g
Clindamycin	30–40 mg/kg 3 doses max 2.7 g
Oxacillin	150–200 mg/kg 4 doz max 12 g (QID)

otorhinolaryngologist in the early period. One should be prepared for the need for a surgical airway [2, 29].

The child should be evaluated by sitting in a comfortable position. If not agitated, oxygen can be given to the nasal passage, and nebulized adrenaline can be given to reduce airway edema [34]. Awake nasotracheal intubation can be tried in patients with spontaneous breathing. The use of supraglottic airway devices is contraindicated. If endotracheal intubation fails, the surgical airway should be provided without delay [29].

Since the blamed strains are Hemophilus spp., Streptococcus, Staphylococcus aureus, wide spectrum cephalosporin and vancomycin should be started, and treatment should be treated last at least 7–10 days (Table 55.2).

The steroid for mucosal edema is controversial. It should be preferred in selected patients [31, 34]. All patients should be followed up in the intensive care unit [29, 31].

55.7 Peritonsillar Abscess

55.7.1 Definition and Etiology

Peritonsillar abscess (PTA) is the most common deep neck infection in children and adolescents and accounts for at least 50 percent of cases [35, 36]. It is most common in adolescents and young adults but can also occur in younger children [37]. Although the number of patients with a pre-diagnosis of the peritonsillar abscess with clinical suspicion increases up to 40 per 100,000, the number of patients diagnosed with abscess by aspiration is 3 in 100,000 [38]. The dominant bacterial species are Streptococcus pyogenes (group A streptococcus [GABHS]), Streptococcus anginosus, Staphylococcus aureus (including methicillin-resistant S. aureus [MRSA]) and respiratory anaerobes (including Fusobacteria, Prevotella, and Veillonella species).

Typically, severe sore throat, fever, hot potato voice, and drooling are seen. Trismus is observed in 65% of the cases. Trismus is important in differentiating from other superficial infections [35, 39].

55.7.2 Diagnosis

Trismus presence makes examination difficult. In examining this patient group, surgical airway materials should be kept ready, and aggressive and repetitive examinations should be avoided. Pushing the uvula and severe swelling in the tonsils suggest peritonsillar abscess in the foreground. There is no specific laboratory and imaging method for diagnosis. However, contrast-enhanced neck computed tomography can be used to differentiate it from retropharyngeal abscess [2, 40].

55.7.3 Treatment

Especially young children require inpatient treatment. Uncomplicated patients can tolerate aspiration and can tolerate oral procedure can be treated on an outpatient basis with close follow-up [41, 42]. If this patient group is suspected, a rapid consultation with an ENT specialist is required [2, 40].

Empirical treatment should include group A streptococci, Staphylococcus aureus, and respiratory anaerobes. Empirical treatment can be changed as needed based on culture results or clinical response to treatment if drainage is performed [43].

If drainage is not done, methicillin-resistant S. aureus (MRSA) treatment should be arranged depending on the prevalence of MRSA in the community and whether the patient is colonized with MRSA [2, 40].

Amoxicillin-clavulanate (45 mg/kg per dose every 12 h in children [maximum single dose 875 mg) or clindamycin in a patient responding to parenteral clindamycin (10 mg/kg every 8 h in children [maximum single dose 600 mg); Linezolid (<12 age: 30 mg/kg per day in three doses; age 12 years: 20 mg/kg regimens per day in two doses can be used in children [44].

Surgical incision, drainage, and tonsillectomy are the most important methods to be chosen for patients who do not respond to 24-h medical treatment. Medical follow-up was found to be more successful in patients younger than 6 years old [45]. In studies comparing needle aspiration with other surgical methods, it was found that patients tolerated aspiration better, although there were similar success rates [46, 47].

Although corticosteroids were observed to be better in reducing pain, they did not benefit other conditions [48, 49].

Symptoms should subside within 24 h in assessing response to treatment. Patients who do not have symptomatic relief or worsen after 24 h should be reassessed immediately [40, 49].

55.7.4 Complications

Early diagnosis and proper management of peritonsillar infection is critical. Although peritonsillar abscess (PTA) complications occur rarely, they cause significant morbidity and mortality. Airway obstruction, aspiration pneumonia, Lemierre's syndrome, mediastinitis, and necrotizing fasciitis can be seen [40].

55.8 Retropharyngeal Abscess

55.8.1 Definition and Etiology

The area where the upper border of the skull base, the lower border of the 2nd vertebra, the anterior border of the posterior pharyngeal wall and the posterior border of the prevertebral fossa is called the retropharyngeal region [50]. It is an essential area in terms of lymphatic spread since bilateral lymph nodes are in this region. Although the lymph nodes are obliterated after the age of 4, it is still necessary to be careful in terms of lymphatic drainage. Lymphatic drainage and direct spread speak in abscesses formed in this area [2, 50].

It is usually seen after URTI and pharyngitis. Fever is often present but is not seen in approximately 10% of patients [51, 52]. As with peritonsillar abscess, severe sore throat, fever, hot potato voice, drooling, keeping the head in the sniffing position. Sliding in the posterior oropharynx and pushing in the uvula are important findings [2, 50].

55.8.2 Diagnosis

Imaging methods can be used after clinical suspicion. Initial imaging includes soft tissue lateral neck radiography. To limit false-positive results, the radiograph should be taken during inspiration with the neck extended. The retropharyngeal space in C2 is diagnostic of twice the diameter of the vertebral body or greater than half the width of the C4 vertebral body. Gas can also be seen in this area. Contrast-enhanced CT may show necrotic nodes, inflammatory phlegmon, or fluid collection in the abscess. CT is useful for diagnosing and defining the extent of infection and surgical planning [50, 51].

55.8.3 Treatment

Ensuring airway safety of patients should be a priority. If there is suspicion in patients who will undergo CT for imaging, intubation should be performed, and mortality that may occur during imaging is prevented. IV/IO should be opened, fluid therapy should be started, and antibiotherapy should be given. The most common are Staphylococcus aureus, Streptococcus viridans, and oral anaerobes. While localized abscesses and cellulitis show complete recovery with antibiotics, surgery is required in all other cases. Surgical drainage is required in the presence of airway obstruction, abscess larger than 2.5 cm^2, and ongoing symptoms despite IV antibiotherapy [53, 54].

Empirically, ampicillin-sulbactam (15 mL/ kg QID) or clindamycin (50 mg/kg) can be started at a dose. The treatment regimen can be changed according to the aspiration result [50].

55.8.4 Complications

Early diagnosis and proper management of retropharyngeal infection is critical. Although peritonsillar abscess (PTA) complications occur rarely, they cause significant morbidity and mortality. Airway obstruction, aspiration pneumonia, Lemierre's syndrome, mediastinitis, and necrotizing fasciitis can be seen [50].

55.9 Ear Infections

Although ear pain is a common complaint in the pediatric age group, it is seriously important due to complications caused by infectious conditions. Ear functions must work properly, especially for learning to be learned. For this reason, both the prevention and treatment of infective conditions and the prevention of complications are required.

55.9.1 Acute Otitis Media

Acute otitis media (AOM) is common in the pediatric age group. It is an infection of the middle ear cavity characterized by the symptoms and signs of middle ear inflammation accompanying moderate to severe bulging in the tympanic membrane or ear discharge.

AOM is most common in the 6–24 month interval [55] and is slightly more common in boys than in girls [56, 57]. With the inclusion of conjugated pneumococcal vaccine in the national vaccination program in many countries, the incidence of AOM has decreased significantly [58–60]. The most important risk factor for AOM is age [61]. This condition is associated with immature anatomy, weak immunity, and genetic predisposition. In addition to age, season (most often autumn, winter), underlying diseases, family history, going to daycare, exposure to tobacco smoke, and pacifier use can be counted among other risk factors. Breastfeeding is protective [62–66].

A viral upper respiratory tract infection (URTI) often plays a role in initiating AOM [67]. Eustachian dysfunction causes poor ventilation and negative middle ear pressure, as well as accumulation of secretions produced by the middle ear mucosa. Microbial growth in middle ear secretions progresses to suppurative infection. Middle ear effusion can last for weeks to months following treatment of middle ear infection [65, 68, 69].

Among the bacterial agents, the most common are S. pneumoniae, untyped H. influenzae, and Moraxella catarrhalis [57, 70, 71]. Among the viral pathogens,

RSV, influenza virus, and human metapneumovirus most frequently cause AOM [72–74]. In young infants (<2 months), the most common bacterial causes of AOM are the same as in older children; Dual infection of Streptococcus pneumoniae and Haemophilus influenzae has been detected in children with resistant AOM and/or recurrent otitis media [75]. Rarely, Mycobacteria tuberculosis, Corynebacterium diphtheriae, Clostridium tetani, and parasitic and fungal agents can also cause AOM [76, 77].

Symptoms can be confused with classic URI symptoms [78–80]. A most common symptoms are ear pain, swelling, discharge, hearing loss, and fever in children [80]. Ear pain is the most common complaint and is the most predictive complaint about AOM [78, 79]. However, ear pain is less frequent in children younger than 2 years compared to other age groups [81].

AOM may also manifest itself with nonspecific symptoms such as fever, restlessness, sleep disturbance, sucking/feeding disorder, vomiting, and diarrhea in young children, especially infants [79, 80].

55.9.2 Diagnosis

Otoscopic examination is indispensable for the diagnosis of AOM [81]. Before the examination, if there is an obstructive serum in the external auditory canal, it should be removed [82, 83]. With otoscopic examination, each quadrant of the tympanic membrane should be systematically evaluated in position, movement, transparency, color, and other findings [83].

55.9.3 Tympanic Membrane Findings

The presence of fluid in the middle ear, bulging tympanic membrane, decreased or no membrane movement when assessed by pneumatic otoscope; the appearance of opaque, yellow, or white-colored membranes are the classic otoscopic examination findings of AOM [84]. However, not all of them are always visible.

1. Bulging tympanic membrane:
   Bulging tympanic membrane is the most important and distinctive feature of AOM from otitis media with effusion (EOM) [85–87]. Bulging tympanic membrane is indicative of both acute inflammation and middle ear effusion (MEE). Children with MEE without acute inflammation findings have EOM [81].

   Bulging first manifests itself in the posterosuperior region where the eardrum is the softest.

   When the tympanic membrane swells, the stalk of the malleus becomes indistinct [88]. When there is less amount of infected middle ear fluid, the tympanic membrane may appear thick/plump rather than bulging.

   It has been observed that the predictive value of the tympanic membrane in terms of AOM varies between 83 and 99%. In another study, when looking at the relationship between examination findings and diagnosis of AOM, 92% of children with AOM had bulging tympanic membrane, while no bulging tympanic membrane was observed in children with or without effusion in otitis media with effusion [86].

2. Acute perforation with purulent otorrhea:
   Acute perforation of the membrane with purulent otorrhea without otitis externa makes the diagnosis of AOM [89].
3. Retraction of the membrane:
   Retraction or absence of movement in the tympanic membrane during the examination with airtight pneumatic otoscopy is an indication of MEE [83].
4. Turbid or opaque tympanic membrane:
   When there is fluid in the middle ear cavity, all or part of the tympanic membrane (air-fluid level) may appear cloudy or opaque. However, this is not a finding that distinguishes AOM from EOM. The opacification of the tympanic membrane without bulging is usually a finding suggestive of EOM [20, 86].
5. The tympanic membrane's color:
   The white or pale yellow appearance of the tympanic membrane is a finding indicating infected pus fluid in the common ear cavity and suggesting AOM. Middle ear fluid that is not infected as in OME usually appears gray or blue [81].

A red or hemorrhagic tympanic membrane may indicate acute inflammation but is a nonspecific finding. Erythema in the tympanic membrane can be caused by vasodilation due to traumatization of the canal, URI, crying, or high fever [90].

In the diagnosis of AOM, erythema in the membrane is less critical than the membrane's position and mobility [85, 86]. A study in which otoscopic findings were evaluated, AOM was diagnosed in only 15 percent of people with erythematous tympanic membrane without bulging or impaired movement [86].

55.9.4 Other Findings

- Bulla: It can be seen in the inflamed tympanic membrane during AOM.
- Bubbles or air-liquid levels: suggest EOM more than AOM [86]. Air-liquid levels give fluctuation by pneumatic otoscopy.
- Myringosclerosis (asymptomatic whitish plaques of calcium and phosphate crystals in the tympanic membrane): Chronic otitis media may be caused by perforation, a myringotomy (with or without tympanostomy tube insertion), or trauma. Myringosclerosis moves with the tympanic membrane during pneumatic otoscopy [81].
- Perforation of the tympanic membrane: It may be caused by increased middle ear pressure leading to central ischemia and necrosis [81].
- AOM cause atrophic areas: atrophic areas have increased mobility.
- Retraction pockets: AOM can be seen as a sequela and predisposing to cholesteatoma development [81].

- Cholesteatoma: Desquamation is a benign proliferation of the stratified squamous epithelium. It may appear as a cyst, oily white debris, or mass in the tympanic membrane [81].

The first thing to consider in the differential diagnosis of AOM is EOM. It is crucial to diagnose AOM correctly and differentiate it from EOM to prevent unnecessary antibiotic use and the proliferation of resistant organisms [91, 92].

Otitis media with effusion (EOM) is an uninfected effusion in the middle ear with reduced mobility of the tympanic membrane and an opaque or cloudy appearance. However, these findings can be seen in both AOM and EOM. EOM usually occurs before or after AOM develops. Although AOM and EOM are on an alternating spectrum, other otoscopic findings may be helpful [83].

55.9.5 Treatment

Systemic and local signs and symptoms of AOM usually resolve within 48–72 h [65, 93]. In children treated with analgesia and observation, symptoms and signs improve more slowly than those given appropriate antibiotic treatment [93].

Pain is a common feature of AOM and can be severe [94]. Analgesic treatment is recommended in children with AOM, whether they are treated with antibiotics or not [89]. Oral ibuprofen or acetaminophen is recommended for pain control in children with AOM [95, 96].

Topical procaine or lidocaine preparations (if available) are an alternative to oral analgesics for children 2 years old, but should not be used in children with tympanic membrane perforation [96].

It found that antihistamines and decongestants' efficacy in the treatment of AOM did not prevent surgery or other complications in AOM [97]. In addition, treatment with antihistamines may prolong the duration of middle ear effusion [67]. In children with AOM and known or suspected nasal allergies, an oral decongestant or antihistamine can provide symptomatic relief in nasal congestion [96].

Although antibacterial treatment is important in the treatment of AOM, 48–72 h of observation is the second option that can be chosen. It would be appropriate to select these situations, especially according to the patient's clinical condition and age [96].

Antibiotic treatment should be started immediately, especially in children under 2 years of age. Antibiotic treatment should also be initiated immediately in patients over 2 years of age who have immunosuppressed status, have toxic appearance, have persistent otalgia for more than 48 h, and have a fever of 39 degrees and above, and bilateral AOM [89, 96].

Observation may be preferred in patients over 2 years of age with good general condition and mild symptoms, and it would be logical to make a joint decision with the parent.

Recurrence has decreased with the use of antibiotics in AOM. Small-scale side effects such as nausea are observed, and it is stated that there is no difference with placebo in terms of meningitis [93].

American Academy of Pediatrics (AAP) guidelines (2013) for children aged 6 months to 2 years with unilateral AOM and mild symptoms (i.e., mild ear pain for <48 h and temperature <102.2 °F [39 °C]) advises observation by parents and care provider [89]. However, given the high rate of treatment failure among children with unilateral non-severe AOM, initially managed by observation and analgesia [98], it would be appropriate to treat such children with antimicrobial therapy. Amoxicillin is the agent of choice in patients who have not recently received beta-lactam treatment, and who do not have purulent conjunctivitis, and who do not have a history of recurrent AOM. Amoxicillin dosage is 90 mg/kg per day and divided into two doses (a maximum of 3 g/day is recommended).

Children younger than 2 years old can be treated for 10 days, and children ≥2 years old for 5–7 days [89, 96].

Beta-lactam resistance should be considered, and a beta-lactamase antibiotic should be added in patients who have recently received beta-lactam therapy or have purulent conjunctivitis or a history of recurrent AOM that does not respond to amoxicillin. Amoxicillin-clavulanate is recommended [86, 88].

The dose was 90 mg/kg amoxicillin per day and 6.4 mg/kg clavulanate per day divided into two doses (we recommend a maximum daily dose of the amoxicillin component 3 g). 16-year-old adolescents who can take large tablets can use 1–2 g of amoxicillin and 62.5 to 125 mg of clavulanate-release amoxicillin-clavulanate every 12 h [89].

Children under 2 years of age require 10 days of treatment, and children ≥2 years of age 5 to 7 days of treatment.

Cephalosporins can be used in patients with mild sensitivity to a penicillin [96]. Cefdinir 14 mg/kg per day orally in one or two doses (maximum 600 mg/day) for 10 days, Cefpodoxime 10 mg/kg per day orally in two doses (maximum 400 mg/day) for 10 days, Cefuroxime suspension 30 mg/kg per day orally divided in two doses (maximum 1 g / day) for 10 days, Cefuroxime tablets 250 mg orally every 12 h for 10 days, Ceftriaxone 50 mg/kg intramuscularly once per day (maximum 1 g/day) for one to three doses.

Macrolides or clindamycin should be used in patients with severe reactions to penicillin. Azithromycin 10 mg/kg per day orally (maximum 500 mg/day) as a single dose on day 1 and 5 mg/kg per day (maximum 250 mg/day) for days 2 through 5. Clarithromycin 15 mg/kg per day orally divided into two doses (maximum 1 g/day). The optimal dose for clindamycin therapy for AOM is uncertain; we suggest 20–30 mg/kg per day orally divided into three doses (maximum 1.8 g/day) [96, 99].

In a prospective study, tympanocentesis, in which middle ear fluid was drained entirely in combination with antimicrobial therapy, was associated with treatment failure, susceptibility to otitis, and a reduced risk of tympanostomy tube placement [92]. Even if the otitis media is not drained, tympanocentesis allows the fluid drainage, reducing the middle ear's pressure and pain [96].

55.10 Nasal Infections

Acute rhinosinusitis occurs as a result of an infection of one or more paranasal sinuses. It is mostly referred to as viral rhinosinusitis because it is associated with viral pathogens that cause the common cold [100, 101].

Fever usually does not occur in viral rhinosinusitis. Even if it does, it regresses within 48 h. Nasal discharge and cough begin to regress in 72 h. The headache is usually not severe and resolves within a few days by limiting itself. In bacterial rhinosinusitis, a fever above 39 degrees is seen for more than 3 days. If there is no change in nasal discharge and cough, severe headaches with poor general conditions indicate the disease's severity. Without treatment, symptoms persist for more than 10 days [102].

Acute sinusitis is defined as the inflammation episodes of the paranasal sinuses where the symptoms improve in less than 30 days, Subacute sinusitis symptoms improve within 30 to 90 days, and chronic sinusitis is defined as the inflammation episodes of the paranasal sinuses with persistent symptoms (cough, rhinorrhea, nasal congestion) that last longer than 90 days. It is usually associated with underlying non-infectious conditions such as allergic or host factors [103, 104].

55.11 Acute Bacterial Rhinosinusitis (ABRS)

Acute bacterial rhinosinusitis (ABRS) is a common problem in children. ABRS develops in about 6–9% of viral upper respiratory tract infections in children [105, 106].

The clinical signs of ABRS are similar to those of viral upper respiratory tract infection [107]. Help distinguish between clinical course, duration and severity of symptoms, viral URIs, and ABRS [91, 106].

Cough is present in most illnesses and becomes more pronounced as the disease progresses [106]. Anterior or postnasal discharge, obstruction, and/or nasal obstruction are also seen. Similar to cough, nasal complaints are observed in approximately 75% of the patients. Mild erythema and edema of the nasal conchae can be seen with mucopurulent anterior nasal discharge. Drainage from the posterior ethmoids may lead to the accumulation of purulent material in the posterior pharynx [102].

Fever is observed, but it is often not one of the main complaints. A fever of 39 °C (102.2 °F) for at least three consecutive days is an indication that ABRS will be severe. Fever that occurs in uncomplicated viral URTI usually occurs early in the disease and regresses within 3 days [101].

Nonspecific symptoms such as headache, facial pain, sinus tenderness, and sore throat can also be seen in varying degrees, although less frequently in young children [108, 109].

55.11.1 Diagnosis

The diagnosis of uncomplicated acute bacterial rhinosinusitis (ABRS) in children is usually made clinically.

- Symptoms and signs consistent with sinus inflammation (daytime cough and/or nasal symptoms)
- Clinical course suggestive of bacterial rather than viral infection
- If symptoms are present without improvement for >10 and <30 days, or
- Severe symptoms (poor appearance, fever $\geq$39 ° C (102.2 °F) and purulent, runny nose for $\geq$3 days) or
- Worsening symptoms (increase in respiratory symptoms, new onset of severe headache or fever, or recurrence of fever after initial recovery) [110–112]

55.12 Complicated ABRS

Imaging methods are used in cases where orbital and intracranial complications of ABRS are suspected [106, 112]. CT is the first method of choice since sedation is not often required, and it shows the sinus anatomy better [110].

Microbiological evaluation is not usually necessary for children with uncomplicated ABRS. If it looks toxic or has orbital or intracranial complications, it is recommended to not respond to immunocompromised and antimicrobial therapy [100].

Although there are different systems in determining the disease's degree, it is estimated that the disease will have a severe prognosis at 8 points and above, according to a frequently used system (Table 55.3).

Table 55.3 Complicated sinusitis scoring system [113]

Symptom	Puan
Abnormal nasal or postnasal discharge	
Minimal	1
Severe	2
Nasal congestion	1
Cough	2
Malodorous breath	1
Facial tenderness	3
Erythematous nasal mucosa	1
Fever	
<38.5 °C	1
$\geq$38.5 °C	2
Headache (retro-orbital)/irritability	
Severe	3
Mild	1

55.12.1 Treatment

There is no need for hospitalization of the patients without any complications. Inpatient treatment will be appropriate in patients who need sinus aspiration and who have immunization status. Empirical treatment should cover S. pneumoniae, H. influenzae, and M. catarrhalis. It should include its treatment. Penicillin and beta-lactamase antibiotics will be sufficient in most patients. The drugs to be used are given in Table 55.4 [110, 114, 115].

55.12.2 Complications

Children with untreated bacterial rhinosinusitis are at risk of severe complications. Complications may arise from the orbital or intracranial spread [116].

Findings suggestive of intracranial expansion are as follows [102, 117, 118]:
- Coexistence of periorbital/orbital edema with persistent headache and vomiting
- Vomiting for more than 24 h
- Change in consciousness

Table 55.4 Outpatient and inpatient regimens in the treatment of sinusitis

Outpatient treatment	
Amoxicillin-clavulanate	45 mg/kg$^\Delta$ per day orally divided in 2 doses (maximum 1.75 g/day
Amoxicillin	90 mg/kg per day orally divided into 2 doses (maximum 4 g/day)
Cefpodoxime	10 mg/kg per day orally divided into 2 doses (maximum 400 mg/day)
Cefdinir	14 mg/kg per day orally divided in 1 or 2 doses (maximum 600 mg/day)
Levofloxacin	10–20 mg/kg per day orally divided into 1 or 2 doses (maximum 500 mg/day)
Ceftriaxone	50 mg/kg per day IV or IM once (maximum 1 g/day), followed 24 h later by appropriate oral therapy
Inpatient treatment	
Ampicillin sulbactam	200–400 mg/kg per day IV divided every 6 h (QID) (maximum 8 g ampicillin component/day), or
Ceftriaxone	100 mg/kg per day IV divided every 12 h (BID) (maximum 2 g/day)
Levofloxacin	10–20 mg/kg per day IV divided every 12 or 24 h (maximum 500 mg/day)
Second step	
Addition of vancomycin	(60 mg/kg per day IV) divided every 6 h (QID) (maximum 4 g/day) and possibly,
Metronidazole	(30 mg/kg per day IV) divided every 6 h (QID) (maximum 4 g/day)

- Focal neurological deficits
- Meningeal irritation signs (e.g., neck stiffness)

Clinical signs specific to orbital and intracranial complications of rhinosinusitis are as follows [119, 120]:
- Perceptual (periorbital) cellulitis
- Orbital cellulitis
- Orbital subperiosteal abscess
- Septic cavernous sinus thrombosis
- Meningitis
- Epidural abscess
- Subdural abscess
- Brain abscess
- Headache
- Neck stiffness
- Mental status changes
- Vomiting
- Focal neurological deficits
- Seizures
- Third and sixth cranial nerve paralysis
- Papilledema

References

1. Shapiro DJ, Lindgren CE, Neuman MI, Fine AM. Viral features and testing for streptococcal pharyngitis. Pediatrics. 2017;139:5.
2. Caglar D, Kwun R. Mouth and throat disorders in infants and children. In: Tintinalli J, editor. Tintinalli's emergency medicine a comprehensive study guide. 9th ed. New York: McGraw-Hill Education; 2020.
3. Evaluation of sore throat in children—UpToDate [Internet]. [cited 24 Dec 2020]; https://www.uptodate.com/contents/evaluation-of-sore-throat-in-children?search=pharyngitis&source=search_result&selectedTitle=3~150&usage_type=default&display_rank=3.
4. Kenmoe S, Kengne-Nde C, Ebogo-Belobo JT, Mbaga DS, Fatawou Modiyinji A, Njouom R. Systematic review and meta-analysis of the prevalence of common respiratory viruses in children < 2 years with bronchiolitis in the pre-COVID-19 pandemic era. PLoS One. 2020;15(11):e0242302.
5. Herath VCK, Carapetis J. Sore throat: is it such a big deal anymore? J Infect. 2015;71(Suppl 1):S101–5.
6. Epstein-Barr Virus (EBV) infectious mononucleosis (mono): background, pathophysiology, epidemiology; 2020 [cited 24 Dec 2020]. https://emedicine.medscape.com/article/222040-overview
7. Horwitz CA, Henle W, Henle G, Goldfarb M, Kubic P, Gehrz RC, et al. Clinical and laboratory evaluation of infants and children with Epstein-Barr virus-induced infectious mononucleosis: report of 32 patients (aged 10-48 months). Blood. 1981;57(5):933–8.
8. Acute pharyngitis in children and adolescents: symptomatic treatment—UpToDate [Internet]. [cited 24 Dec 2020]. https://www.uptodate.com/contents/acute-pharyngitis-in-children-and-adolescents-symptomatic-treatment?search=Acute%20pharyngitis%20in%20children%20

and%20adolescents:%20Symptomatic%20treatment&source=search_result&selectedTitle= 1~150&usage_type=default&display_rank=1.

9. Cingi C, Songu M, Ural A, Yildirim M, Erdogmus N, Bal C. Effects of chlorhexidine/ benzydamine mouth spray on pain and quality of life in acute viral pharyngitis: a prospective, randomized, double-blind, placebo-controlled, multicenter study. Ear Nose Throat J. 2010;89(11):546–9.

10. Tynell E, Aurelius E, Brandell A, Julander I, Wood M, Yao QY, et al. Acyclovir and prednisolone treatment of acute infectious mononucleosis: a multicenter, double-blind, placebo-controlled study. J Infect Dis. 1996;174(2):324–31.

11. van der Horst C, Joncas J, Ahronheim G, Gustafson N, Stein G, Gurwith M, et al. Lack of effect of peroral acyclovir for the treatment of acute infectious mononucleosis. J Infect Dis. 1991;164(4):788–92.

12. Bisno AL. Acute pharyngitis. Massachusetts Medical Society; 2009 [cited 24 Dec 2020]. https://www.nejm.org/doi/10.1056/NEJM200101183440308

13. Cingi C, Songu M, Ural A, Erdogmus N, Yildirim M, Cakli H, et al. Effect of chlorhexidine gluconate and benzydamine hydrochloride mouth spray on clinical signs and quality of life of patients with streptococcal tonsillopharyngitis: multicentre, prospective, randomised, double-blinded, placebo-controlled study. J Laryngol Otol. 2011;125(6):620–5.

14. Pierce CA, Voss B. Efficacy and safety of ibuprofen and acetaminophen in children and adults: a meta-analysis and qualitative review. Ann Pharmacother. 2010;44(3):489–506.

15. Marseglia GL, Alessio M, Da Dalt L, Giuliano M, Ravelli A, Marchisio P. Acute pain management in children: a survey of Italian pediatricians. Ital J Pediatr. 2019;45(1):156.

16. Moghal NE, Hegde S, Eastham KM. Ibuprofen and acute renal failure in a toddler. Arch Dis Child. 2004;89(3):276–7.

17. Weglowski J, Caglar D, Sharieff G, Whiteman P. An evidence-based approach to the evaluation and treatment of pharyngitis in children. Pediatr Emerg Med Pract. 2011;8(12):1–25.

18. de Cassan S, Thompson MJ, Perera R, Glasziou PP, Del Mar CB, Heneghan CJ, et al. Corticosteroids as standalone or add-on treatment for sore throat. Cochrane Database Syst Rev. 2020;5:CD008268.

19. Kronman MP, Zhou C, Mangione-Smith R. Bacterial prevalence and antimicrobial prescribing trends for acute respiratory tract infections. Pediatrics. 2014;134(4):e956–65.

20. Shaikh N, Leonard E, Martin JM. Prevalence of streptococcal pharyngitis and streptococcal carriage in children: a meta-analysis. Pediatrics. 2010;126(3):e557–64.

21. Shulman ST, Bisno AL, Clegg HW, Gerber MA, Kaplan EL, Lee G, et al. Clinical practice guideline for the diagnosis and management of group a streptococcal pharyngitis: 2012 update by the Infectious Diseases Society of America. Clin Infect Dis Off Publ Infect Dis Soc Am. 2012;55(10):1279–82.

22. Frost HM, Fritsche TR, Hall MC. Beta-hemolytic nongroup A streptococcal pharyngitis in children. J Pediatr. 2019;206:268–73.

23. Centor RM, Witherspoon JM, Dalton HP, Brody CE, Link K. The diagnosis of strep throat in adults in the emergency room. Med Decis Mak Int J Soc Med Decis Mak. 1981;1(3):239–46.

24. Harris AM, Hicks LA, Qaseem A. High value care task force of the American College of Physicians and for the Centers for Disease Control and Prevention. Appropriate antibiotic use for acute respiratory tract infection in adults: advice for high-value care from the American College of Physicians and the Centers for Disease Control and Prevention. Ann Intern Med. 2016;164(6):425–34.

25. Vasudevan J, Mannu A, Ganavi G. McIsaac modification of Centor score in diagnosis of streptococcal pharyngitis and antibiotic sensitivity pattern of Beta-hemolytic streptococci in Chennai, India. Indian Pediatr. 2019;56(1):49–52.

26. Bissessor M, Whiley DM, Fairley CK, Bradshaw CS, Lee DM, Snow AS, et al. Persistence of Neisseria gonorrhoeae DNA following treatment for pharyngeal and rectal gonorrhea is influenced by antibiotic susceptibility and reinfection. Clin Infect Dis Off Publ Infect Dis Soc Am. 2015;60(4):557–63.

27. Kneen R, Pham NG, Solomon T, Tran TM, Nguyen TT, Tran BL, et al. Penicillin vs. erythromycin in the treatment of diphtheria. Clin Infect Dis Off Publ Infect Dis Soc Am. 1998;27(4):845–50.
28. Treatment and prevention of streptococcal pharyngitis - UpToDate [Internet]. [cited 24 Dec 2020]. https://www.uptodate.com/contents/treatment-and-prevention-of-streptococcal-pharyngitis?search=Treatment%20and%20prevention%20of%20streptococcal%20pharyngitis&source=search_result&selectedTitle=1~150&usage_type=default&display_rank=1.
29. Epiglottitis (supraglottitis): Clinical features and diagnosis - UpToDate [Internet]. [cited 24 Dec 2020]. https://www.uptodate.com/contents/epiglottitis-supraglottitis-clinical-features-and-diagnosis?search=uvulitis&source=search_result&selectedTitle=1~3&usage_type=default&display_rank=1.
30. Abdallah C. Acute epiglottitis: trends, diagnosis and management. Saudi J Anaesth. 2012;6(3):279–81.
31. Cherry JD. Epiglottitis (supraglottitis). In: Feigin RD, editor. Textbook of pediatric infectious diseases. 6th ed. Philadelphia: Saunders; 2009.
32. Chen C, Natarajan M, Bianchi D, Aue G, Powers JH. Acute epiglottitis in the immunocompromised host: case report and review of the literature. Open Forum Infect Dis. 2018;5:3.
33. Matsuura H, Fukumura T. Thumb and vallecula signs in acute infectious epiglottitis. CMAJ Can Med Assoc J J Assoc Medicale Can. 2017;189(41):E1289.
34. Sobol SE, Zapata S. Epiglottitis and croup. Otolaryngol Clin North Am. 2008;41(3):551–66.
35. Ungkanont K, Yellon RF, Weissman JL, Casselbrant ML, González-Valdepeña H, Bluestone CD. Head and neck space infections in infants and children. Otolaryngol--Head Neck Surg Off J Am Acad Otolaryngol-Head Neck Surg. 1995;112(3):375–82.
36. Schraff S, McGinn JD, Derkay CS. Peritonsillar abscess in children: a 10-year review of diagnosis and management. Int J Pediatr Otorhinolaryngol. 2001;57(3):213–8.
37. Friedman NR, Mitchell RB, Pereira KD, Younis RT, Lazar RH. Peritonsillar abscess in early childhood. Presentation and management. Arch Otolaryngol Head Neck Surg. 1997;123(6):630–2.
38. Millar KR, Johnson DW, Drummond D, Kellner JD. Suspected peritonsillar abscess in children. Pediatr Emerg Care. 2007;23(7):431–8.
39. Szuhay G, Tewfik TL. Peritonsillar abscess or cellulitis? A clinical comparative paediatric study. J Otolaryngol. 1998;27(4):206–12.
40. Peritonsillar cellulitis and abscess - UpToDate [Internet]. [cited 24 Dec 2020]. https://www.uptodate.com/contents/peritonsillar-cellulitis-and-abscess?search=Peritonsillar%20cellulitis%20and%20abscess&source=search_result&selectedTitle=1~18&usage_type=default&display_rank=1.
41. Goldstein NA. Peritonsillar, retropharyngeal, and parapharyngeal abscesses. In: Feigin RD, editor. Textbook of pediatric infection diseases. 6th ed. Philadelphia: Saunders; 2009.
42. Yellon RF. Head and neck space infections. In: Bluestone CD, editor. Pediatric otolaryngology. 4th ed. Philadelphia: Saunders; 2003.
43. Beahm ED. Bacterial infections of the neck. In: Burg FD, editor. Current pediatric therapy. 18th ed. Philadelphia: Saunders; 2006.
44. Apostolopoulos NJ, Nikolopoulos TP, Bairamis TN. Peritonsillar abscess in children. Is incision and drainage an effective management? Int J Pediatr Otorhinolaryngol. 1995 Mar;31(2–3):129–35.
45. Blotter JW, Yin L, Glynn M, Wiet GJ. Otolaryngology consultation for peritonsillar abscess in the pediatric population. Laryngoscope. 2000;110(10 Pt 1):1698–701.
46. Johnson RF, Stewart MG, Wright CC. An evidence-based review of the treatment of peritonsillar abscess. Otolaryngol--Head Neck Surg Off J Am Acad Otolaryngol-Head Neck Surg. 2003;128(3):332–43.
47. Powell J, Wilson JA. An evidence-based review of peritonsillar abscess. Clin Otolaryngol Off J ENT-UK Off J Neth Soc Oto-Rhino-Laryngol Cervico-Facial Surg. 2012;37(2):136–45.

48. Ozbek C, Aygenc E, Tuna EU, Selcuk A, Ozdem C. Use of steroids in the treatment of peritonsillar abscess. J Laryngol Otol. 2004;118(6):439–42.

49. Chau JKM, Seikaly HR, Harris JR, Villa-Roel C, Brick C, Rowe BH. Corticosteroids in peritonsillar abscess treatment: a blinded placebo-controlled clinical trial. Laryngoscope. 2014;124(1):97–103.

50. Retropharyngeal infections in children - UpToDate [Internet]. [cited 24 Dec 2020]. https://www.uptodate.com/contents/retropharyngeal-infections-in-children?search=retropharyngeal%20abscess&source=search_result&selectedTitle=1~40&usage_type=default&display_rank=1.

51. Georget E, Gauthier A, Brugel L, Verlhac S, Remus N, Epaud R, et al. Acute cervical lymphadenitis and infections of the retropharyngeal and parapharyngeal spaces in children. BMC Ear Nose Throat Disord. 2014;14:8.

52. Nazir KA, Fozia PA, Ul Islam M, Shakil A, Patigaroo SA. Paediatric acute retropharyngeal abscesses: an experience. Afr J Paediatr Surg AJPS. 2013;10(4):327–35.

53. Page NC, Bauer EM, Lieu JEC. Clinical features and treatment of retropharyngeal abscess in children. Otolaryngol--Head Neck Surg Off J Am Acad Otolaryngol-Head Neck Surg. 2008;138(3):300–6.

54. Wilkie MD, De S, Krishnan M. Defining the role of surgical drainage in paediatric deep neck space infections. Clin Otolaryngol Off J ENT-UK Off J Neth Soc Oto-Rhino-Laryngol Cervico-Facial Surg. 2019;44(3):366–71.

55. Todberg T, Koch A, Andersson M, Olsen SF, Lous J, Homøe P. Incidence of otitis Media in a Contemporary Danish National Birth Cohort. PLoS One. 2014;9(12):e111732.

56. Van Dyke MK, Pirçon J-Y, Cohen R, Madhi SA, Rosenblüt A, Macias Parra M, et al. Etiology of acute otitis media in children less than 5 years of age. Pediatr Infect Dis J. 2017;36(3):274–81.

57. Kaur R, Morris M, Pichichero ME. Epidemiology of acute otitis media in the postpneumococcal conjugate vaccine era. Pediatrics. 2017;140:3.

58. Pichichero M, Kaur R, Scott DA, Gruber WC, Trammel J, Almudevar A, et al. Effectiveness of 13-valent pneumococcal conjugate vaccination for protection against acute otitis media caused by Streptococcus pneumoniae in healthy young children: a prospective observational study. Lancet Child Adolesc Health. 2018;2(8):561–8.

59. Kawai K, Adil EA, Barrett D, Manganella J, Kenna MA. Ambulatory visits for otitis media before and after the introduction of pneumococcal conjugate vaccination. J Pediatr. 2018;201:122–7.

60. Wiese AD, Huang X, Yu C, Mitchel EF, Kyaw MH, Griffin MR, et al. Changes in otitis media episodes and pressure equalization tube insertions among young children following introduction of the 13-valent pneumococcal conjugate vaccine: a birth cohort-based study. Clin Infect Dis Off Publ Infect Dis Soc Am. 2019;69(12):2162–9.

61. Acute otitis media in children: Epidemiology, microbiology, and complications - UpToDate [Internet]. [cited 24 Dec 2020]. https://www.uptodate.com/contents/acute-otitis-media-in-children-epidemiology-microbiology-and-complications?search=acute%20otitis%20media%20children&source=search_result&selectedTitle=3~150&usage_type=default&display_rank=3.

62. Pagano AS, Wang E, Yuan D, Fischer D, Bluestone C, Marquez S, et al. Cranial indicators identified for peak incidence of otitis media. Anat Rec Hoboken NJ. 2017;300(10):1721–40.

63. Rovers MM, Numans ME, Langenbach E, Grobbee DE, Verheij TJ, Schilder AG. Is pacifier use a risk factor for acute otitis media? A dynamic cohort study. Fam Pract. 2008;25(4):233–6.

64. Leach AJ, Wigger C, Andrews R, Chatfield M, Smith-Vaughan H, Morris PS. Otitis media in children vaccinated during consecutive 7-valent or 10-valent pneumococcal conjugate vaccination schedules. BMC Pediatr. 2014;14(1):200.

65. Rovers MM, Schilder AGM, Zielhuis GA, Rosenfeld RM. Otitis media. Lancet Lond Engl. 2004;363(9407):465–73.

66. Bowatte G, Tham R, Allen KJ, Tan DJ, Lau M, Dai X, et al. Breastfeeding and childhood acute otitis media: a systematic review and meta-analysis. Acta Paediatr Oslo Nor. 2015;104(467):85–95.

67. Chonmaitree T, Trujillo R, Jennings K, Alvarez-Fernandez P, Patel JA, Loeffelholz MJ, et al. Acute otitis media and other complications of viral respiratory infection. Pediatrics. 2016;137:4.
68. Winther B, Alper CM, Mandel EM, Doyle WJ, Hendley JO. Temporal relationships between colds, upper respiratory viruses detected by polymerase chain reaction, and otitis media in young children followed through a typical cold season. Pediatrics. 2007;119(6):1069–75.
69. Alper CM, Winther B, Mandel EM, Hendley JO, Doyle WJ. Rate of concurrent otitis media in upper respiratory tract infections with specific viruses. Arch Otolaryngol Head Neck Surg. 2009;135(1):17–21.
70. Coker TR, Chan LS, Newberry SJ, Limbos MA, Suttorp MJ, Shekelle PG, et al. Diagnosis, microbial epidemiology, and antibiotic treatment of acute otitis media in children: a systematic review. JAMA. 2010;304(19):2161–9.
71. Casey JR, Adlowitz DG, Pichichero ME. New patterns in the otopathogens causing acute otitis media six to eight years after introduction of pneumococcal conjugate vaccine. Pediatr Infect Dis J. 2010;29(4):304–9.
72. Ruohola A, Meurman O, Nikkari S, Skottman T, Salmi A, Waris M, et al. Microbiology of acute otitis media in children with tympanostomy tubes: prevalences of bacteria and viruses. Clin Infect Dis Off Publ Infect Dis Soc Am. 2006;43(11):1417–22.
73. Heikkinen T, Thint M, Chonmaitree T. Prevalence of various respiratory viruses in the middle ear during acute otitis media. N Engl J Med. 1999;340(4):260–4.
74. Stockmann C, Ampofo K, Hersh AL, Carleton ST, Korgenski K, Sheng X, et al. Seasonality of acute otitis media and the role of respiratory viral activity in children. Pediatr Infect Dis J. 2013;32(4):314–9.
75. Dagan R, Leibovitz E, Greenberg D, Bakaletz L, Givon-Lavi N. Mixed pneumococcal-nontypeable Haemophilus influenzae otitis media is a distinct clinical entity with unique epidemiologic characteristics and pneumococcal serotype distribution. J Infect Dis. 2013;208(7):1152–60.
76. Berman S. Otitis media in developing countries. Pediatrics. 1995;96(1 Pt 1):126–31.
77. Ding Y, Geng Q, Tao Y, Lin Y, Wang Y, Black S, et al. Etiology and epidemiology of children with acute otitis media and spontaneous otorrhea in Suzhou. China Pediatr Infect Dis J. 2015;34(5):e102–6.
78. Niemela M, Uhari M, Jounio-Ervasti K, Luotonen J, Alho OP, Vierimaa E. Lack of specific symptomatology in children with acute otitis media. Pediatr Infect Dis J. 1994;13(9):765–8.
79. Kontiokari T, Koivunen P, Niemelä M, Pokka T, Uhari M. Symptoms of acute otitis media. Pediatr Infect Dis J. 1998;17(8):676–9.
80. Laine MK, Tähtinen PA, Ruuskanen O, Huovinen P, Ruohola A. Symptoms or symptom-based scores cannot predict acute otitis media at otitis-prone age. Pediatrics. 2010;125(5):e1154–61.
81. Acute otitis media in children: clinical manifestations and diagnosis - UpToDate [Internet]. [cited 24 Dec 2020]. https://www.uptodate.com/contents/acute-otitis-media-in-children-clinical-manifestations-and-diagnosis?search=Acute%20otitis%20media%20in%20children:%20Clinical%20manifestations%20and%20diagnosis&source=search_result&selectedTitle=1~150&usage_type=default&display_rank=1.
82. Barriga F, Schwartz RH, Hayden GF. Adequate illumination for otoscopy. Variations due to power source, bulb, and head and speculum design. Am J Dis Child. 1986;140(12):1237–40.
83. Jones WS, Kaleida PH. How helpful is pneumatic otoscopy in improving diagnostic accuracy? Pediatrics. 2003;112(3 Pt 1):510–3.
84. Shaikh N, Hoberman A, Kaleida PH, Rockette HE, Kurs-Lasky M, Hoover H, et al. Otoscopic signs of otitis media. Pediatr Infect Dis J. 2011;30(10):822–6.
85. Rothman R, Owens T, Simel DL. Does this child have acute otitis media? JAMA. 2003;290(12):1633–40.
86. Shaikh N, Hoberman A, Rockette HE, Kurs-Lasky M. Development of an algorithm for the diagnosis of otitis media. Acad Pediatr. 2012;12(3):214–8.
87. Tähtinen PA, Laine MK, Ruohola A. Prognostic factors for treatment failure in acute otitis media. Pediatrics. 2017;140:3.

88. Pelton SI. Otoscopy for the diagnosis of otitis media. Pediatr Infect Dis J. 1998;17(6):540–3.
89. Lieberthal AS, Carroll AE, Chonmaitree T, Ganiats TG, Hoberman A, Jackson MA, et al. The diagnosis and management of acute otitis media. Pediatrics. 2013;131(3):e964–99.
90. Isaacson G. Acute otitis media and the crying child. Pediatr Infect Dis J. 2016;35(12):e399–400.
91. Wald ER. To treat or not to treat. Pediatrics. 2005;115(4):1087–9.
92. Pichichero ME. Acute otitis media: part I. improving diagnostic accuracy. Am Fam Physician. 2000;61(7):2051–6.
93. Venekamp RP, Sanders SL, Glasziou PP, Del Mar CB, Rovers MM. Antibiotics for acute otitis media in children. Cochrane Database Syst Rev. 2015;6:CD000219.
94. Rovers MM, Glasziou P, Appelman CL, Burke P, McCormick DP, Damoiseaux RA, et al. Antibiotics for acute otitis media: a meta-analysis with individual patient data. Lancet Lond Engl. 2006;368(9545):1429–35.
95. Sjoukes A, Venekamp RP, van de Pol AC, Hay AD, Little P, Schilder AG, et al. Paracetamol (acetaminophen) or non-steroidal anti-inflammatory drugs, alone or combined, for pain relief in acute otitis media in children. Cochrane Database Syst Rev. 2016;12:CD011534.
96. Acute otitis media in children: Treatment - UpToDate [Internet]. [cited 24 Dec 2020]. https://www.uptodate.com/contents/acute-otitis-media-in-children-treatment?search=Acute%20otitis%20media%20in%20children:%20Treatment&source=search_result&selectedTitle=1~150&usage_type=default&display_rank=1.
97. Coleman C, Moore M. Decongestants and antihistamines for acute otitis media in children. Cochrane Database Syst Rev. 2008;3:CD001727.
98. Hoberman A, Ruohola A, Shaikh N, Tähtinen PA, Paradise JL. Acute otitis media in children younger than 2 years. JAMA Pediatr. 2013;167(12):1171–2.
99. Kozyrskyj A, Klassen TP, Moffatt M, Harvey K. Short-course antibiotics for acute otitis media. Cochrane Database Syst Rev. 2010;9:CD001095.
100. Cohen JS, Agrawal D. Nose and sinus disorders in infants and children. In: Tintinalli J, editor. Tintinalli's emergency medicine a comprehensive study guide. 9th ed. New York: McGraw-Hill Education; 2020.
101. Acute bacterial rhinosinusitis in children: clinical features and diagnosis - UpToDate [Internet]. [cited 24 Dec 2020]. https://www.uptodate.com/contents/acute-bacterial-rhinosinusitis-in-children-clinical-features-and-diagnosis?search=Acute%20bacterial%20rhinosinusitis%20in%20children:%20Clinical%20features%20and%20diagnosis&source=search_result&selectedTitle=1~66&usage_type=default&display_rank=1.
102. Acute bacterial rhinosinusitis in children: Microbiology and management - UpToDate [Internet]. [cited 24 Dec 2020]. https://www.uptodate.com/contents/acute-bacterial-rhinosinusitis-in-children-microbiology-and-management?search=Acute%20bacterial%20rhinosinusitis%20in%20children:%20Microbiology%20and%20management&source=search_result&selectedTitle=1~66&usage_type=default&display_rank=1.
103. Shapiro GG, Virant FS, Furukawa CT, Pierson WE, Bierman CW. Immunologic defects in patients with refractory sinusitis. Pediatrics. 1991;87(3):311–6.
104. Peters AT, Spector S, Hsu J, Hamilos DL, Baroody FM, Chandra RK, et al. Diagnosis and management of rhinosinusitis: a practice parameter update. Ann Allergy Asthma Immunol Off Publ Am Coll Allergy Asthma Immunol. 2014;113(4):347–85.
105. Carson JL, Collier AM, Hu SS. Acquired ciliary defects in nasal epithelium of children with acute viral upper respiratory infections. N Engl J Med. 1985;312(8):463–8.
106. DeMuri GP, Gern JE, Moyer SC, Lindstrom MJ, Lynch SV, Wald ER. Clinical features, virus identification, and sinusitis as a complication of upper respiratory tract illness in children ages 4–7 years. J Pediatr. 2016;171:133–9.
107. Lusk RP, Stankiewicz JA. Pediatric rhinosinusitis. Otolaryngol Neck Surg. 1997;117(3_suppl):S53–7.
108. Williams JW Jr, Simel DL. Does this patient have sinusitis?: diagnosing acute sinusitis by history and physical examination. JAMA. 1993;270(10):1242–6.
109. Kogutt MS, Swischuk LE. Diagnosis of sinusitis in infants and children. Pediatrics. 1973;52(1):121–4.

110. Chow AW, Benninger MS, Brook I, Brozek JL, Goldstein EJC, Hicks LA, et al. IDSA clinical practice guideline for acute bacterial rhinosinusitis in children and adults. Clin Infect Dis. 2012;54(8):e72–112.
111. Meltzer EO, Hamilos DL, Hadley JA, Lanza DC, Marple BF, Nicklas RA, et al. Rhinosinusitis: developing guidance for clinical trials. J Allergy Clin Immunol. 2006;118(5 Suppl):S17–61.
112. Wald ER, Applegate KE, Bordley C, Darrow DH, Glode MP, Marcy SM, et al. Clinical practice guideline for the diagnosis and management of acute bacterial sinusitis in children aged 1 to 18 years. Pediatrics. 2013;132(1):e262–80.
113. Wald ER, Nash D, Eickhoff J. Effectiveness of amoxicillin/clavulanate potassium in the treatment of acute bacterial sinusitis in children. Pediatrics. 2009;124(1):9–15.
114. Rosenfeld RM, Piccirillo JF, Chandrasekhar SS, Brook I, Ashok Kumar K, Kramper M, et al. Clinical practice guideline (update): adult sinusitis. Otolaryngol--Head Neck Surg Off J Am Acad Otolaryngol-Head Neck Surg. 2015;152(2 Suppl):S1–39.
115. Jackson MA, Schutze GE. Diseases C on I. The use of systemic and topical fluoroquinolones. Pediatrics. 2016;138:5.
116. Brook I. Microbiology and antimicrobial treatment of orbital and intracranial complications of sinusitis in children and their management. Int J Pediatr Otorhinolaryngol. 2009;73(9):1183–6.
117. Goytia VK, Giannoni CM, Edwards MS. Intraorbital and intracranial extension of sinusitis: comparative morbidity. J Pediatr. 2011;158(3):486–91.
118. Hicks CW, Weber JG, Reid JR, Moodley M. Identifying and managing intracranial complications of sinusitis in children: a retrospective series. Pediatr Infect Dis J. 2011;30(3):222–6.
119. Matos RJP, Júlio S, Marques P, Santos M. Intracranial complications of acute rhinosinusitis in pediatric age: the role of endoscopic sinus surgery. Acta Otorrinolaringológica Gallega. 2020;0:13.
120. Bair-Merritt MH, Shah SS, Zaoutis TE, Bell LM, Feudtner C. Suppurative intracranial complications of sinusitis in previously healthy children. Pediatr Infect Dis J. 2005;24(4):384–6.

Oropharyngeal Manifestations of Common Viral Exanthems and Systemic Infectious Diseases in Children

56

Nazan Dalgıç, Emin Sami Arısoy, and Gail J. Demmler-Harrison

56.1 Introduction

The oral cavity is an anatomical region that plays a critical role in many physiological processes such as digestion, respiration, and speech. It is constrained anteriorly by the lips, laterally by the cheeks, superiorly by the hard and soft palate, and posteriorly bordered by the circumvallate papillae and the junction of the hard and soft palate.

The oral cavity is sterile right before birth but gets colonized shortly after that. However, studies have identified the presence of the human microbiome before birth [1]. There is a substantial microbiota inside the mouth living in symbiosis with the host. The oral microbiome reflects the collection of genomes from a diverse microbiota that includes bacteria, fungi, and viruses within the mouth [1].

Several infectious diseases manifest oropharyngeal symptoms and signs in previously healthy children and may be diagnosed by identifying their characteristics. Numerous bacterial, viral, and fungal infections can affect the oral cavity directly or secondarily due to systemic disease [2, 3]. Therefore, the diagnostic approach necessitates examining the oral cavity and pharynx in detail and

N. Dalgıç (✉)
Section of Pediatric Infectious Diseases, İstanbul Şişli Etfal Training and Research Hospital, İstanbul, Turkey
e-mail: nazandalgic@ttmail.com

E. S. Arısoy
Division of Pediatric Infectious Diseases, Department of Pediatrics, Faculty of Medicine, Kocaeli University, Kocaeli, Turkey

G. J. Demmler-Harrison
Section of Infectious Diseases, Department of Pediatrics, Baylor College of Medicine, and Infectious Disease Service, Texas Children's Hospital, Houston, TX, USA

© The Author(s), under exclusive license to Springer Nature Switzerland AG 2022 651
C. Cingi et al. (eds.), *Pediatric ENT Infections*,
https://doi.org/10.1007/978-3-030-80691-0_56

throughout the body. Color of the oropharyngeal mucosa, presence of lesions on the mucosal surfaces and palate, evaluation of the tongue, gingivae, and teeth should be scrutinized.

The severity of symptoms and signs is partly linked to the age at which the child is infected. However, children with immune deficiency, such as human immunodeficiency virus (HIV) infection and leukemia, have an increased risk for recurrent infections in the oral cavity [2].

Physicians should know about oropharyngeal manifestations of infectious diseases for an accurate diagnosis and early treatment, preventing complications and sequelae. The oral and pharyngeal signs of some selected systemic infectious diseases in children are highlighted in this chapter.

56.2 Measles

Measles is an acute, exanthematous, and highly contagious systemic infectious disease. The measles virus is included in the Paramyxoviridae family as a member of the genus *Morbillivirus*. The respiratory route spreads measles, and the initial infection point is the respiratory epithelium. The virus progresses to the regional lymph nodes, reaching the reticuloendothelial system by causing viremia. After the measles virus infects leukocytes, it enters the thymus, spleen, lymph nodes, liver, skin, and lungs with secondary viremia.

The incubation period is 10–14 days. The early symptoms are a gradually increasing fever accompanied by conjunctivitis, rhinitis, and cough. This severe influenza-like upper respiratory disease evolves to an exanthematous stage with a characteristic red spotty rash starting on the face and neck, covering most of the body [4].

The distinctive oral lesions of measles termed "Koplik spots" appear early in the infection as the prodromal manifestation and typically occurs 1 to 3 days before skin rash development. Koplik spots occur in 95% of patients with measles, develop characteristically on the buccal or labial mucosa, but sometimes the hard or soft palate. Koplik spots appear as 1–3 mm blue-white or grayish blotches surrounded by a bright red border, elevates on an erythematous base, then increase the number and coalesce into small patches. Koplik spots almost always disappear by the time the cutaneous rash appears.

Measles is diagnosed utilizing clinical, epidemiological, and laboratory features. The infection can be detected by a positive serologic test result for measles immunoglobulin (Ig) M antibody, a significant increase in measles IgG antibody concentration in paired acute and convalescent serum specimens, isolation of measles virus, or identification of measles RNA from clinical samples, such as blood, urine, throat, or nasopharyngeal secretions. The differential diagnosis of measles mainly includes erythema infectiosum (fifth disease), scarlet fever, rubella, viral hemorrhagic fevers, and drug eruptions. No specific antiviral therapy is available [5].

56.3 Rubella

Rubella, also known as German measles, is a systemic infectious disease primarily affecting the skin and lymph nodes. Rubella virus is an enveloped, positive-stranded RNA virus classified as a *Rubivirus* in the Togaviridae family. The virus spreads through nasopharyngeal secretions from infected individuals via droplets of mucus and saliva and replicates in the nasopharyngeal tissues and lymph nodes. Viremia lasts 5–7 days. The patients spread the virus 7 days before to 14 days after the onset of rash. The incubation period is 12–23 days.

Rubella is characterized by absent or minimal prodromal symptoms, an exanthem of 3-day duration, and generalized poly-micro-lymphadenopathy, mainly on retro-auricular and sub-occipital areas. In the prodromal period, low-grade fever, weakness, swelling of the lymph nodes, and upper respiratory tract infection symptoms may be observed [5]. The characteristics rash of rubella appears first on the face and behind the ears as small light red patches and then spread gradually throughout the body, increasing the diameter over time become a maculopapular eruption. The rash generally disappears in less than 24 h [5, 6]. Runny rose, mild conjunctivitis, mild pharyngitis, headache, arthralgia, and myalgia may also appear as other symptoms and signs in rubella. In approximately half of the cases, the disease is asymptomatic [5].

In 1898, Forchheimer described pinhead-sized, rose-red colored macular lesions on the soft palate and uvula developed at approximately the rash time and disappeared less than 24 h. At present, this enanthem is not seen as described previously in children with rubella by Forchheimer; however, small, petechial lesions known as Forchheimer's sign occasionally may be seen on the soft palate and uvula [6].

Rubella infection is commonly diagnosed by detecting rubella-specific IgM antibodies that can be seen as early as 4 days after rash onset. The infection can also be diagnosed by a fourfold rise in rubella IgG antibody concentrations between acute and convalescent sera. There is no specific treatment for rubella. Antipyretics and analgesics can be used as needed to relieve symptoms [7].

56.4 Mumps

Mumps virus, also known as the epidemic agent of parotitis, is an RNA virus in the Paramyxoviridae family. The virus is spread by contact with infectious respiratory tract secretions and saliva and causes an acute generalized infection, mainly in the ages of 5–15 years [8]. The incubation period usually is 16–18 days, but clinical onset may start from 12 to 25 days after exposure [5].

In one-third of patients with mumps infection, subclinical or mild respiratory tract symptoms and signs occur. In others, prodromal symptoms such as fever, loss of appetite, malaise, and headache are common. Usually, within the subsequent 2 days, unilateral or bilateral earache and parotid tenderness develop in most cases [8, 9].

Swelling of the unilateral or bilateral parotid gland occurs during the following 2–3 days. The orifice of the Stensen duct generally is seen as erythematous and swollen, and secretions from the duct are clear [9, 10].

When the affected parotid gland grows to maximum, fever, pain, and tenderness start to regress, the gland returns to its average size within a week. Due to the frequent involvement of the submandibular and sublingual glands, gonads, pancreas, nervous system, and other organs, mumps can be widespread or systemic. The infection spontaneously resolves within 1–2 weeks leading to lifelong protection. Other viral, bacterial, or autoimmune causes of parotitis such as Sjögren's disease are included in the differential diagnosis of mumps in children. Treatment is supportive for mumps infection; specific antiviral therapy is not available [5, 8, 10].

56.5 Roseola Infantum

Roseola infantum, also known as the sixth disease or exanthema subitum, is a generally benign acute febrile exanthematous illness of young children. Roseola is caused by infection mainly with human herpesvirus (HHV)-6, or occasionally with HHV-7 acquired at a young age. The infection is generally transmitted by asymptomatic shedding of virus in secretions of close contacts. The average incubation period is 9–10 days [5, 11].

Roseola infantum has a characteristic clinical course of high fever of 3- to 4-day duration, and then the appearance of an erythematous macular or maculopapular rash. The illness usually occurs with the apparent abrupt onset of fever. It is characterized by a light pink, non-itchy, morbilliform rash that appears on the trunk with a sudden decline of high fever after 3–4 days. The rash can last 1–3 days, but it can disappear quickly [11–13].

During the febrile period, most children appear to be alert, happy, and playful. With high fever, children rarely seem irritable or sick, suggesting a more severe illness. A febrile seizure is a frequent complication. Enlargement of the retro-auricular, sub-occipital, and cervical lymph nodes is sometimes also noted [12].

Examination of the oral cavity most commonly reveals mild inflammation of the pharynx and tonsils. Small exudative follicular lesions are occasionally observed on the tonsils. In some cases, small ulcerative lesions on the tonsillar pillars, uvula, and soft palate are seen. The soft palate lesions generally consist of only erythematous macules and maculopapules, presumably because of the hyperplasia of lymphoid follicles in the submucosa [14]. Mild maculopapular enanthems on the soft palate and uvula are also named Nagayama spots [15].

The clinical course is sufficiently specific and different to assure an accurate diagnosis of roseola with the absence or minimal clinical or laboratory findings during the febrile phase. Mostly, roseola is clinically diagnosed based on its characteristics: fever for 3–4 days, followed by a sudden rash development while fever declines in a young child [5, 11, 15].

Diagnosis can also be made by serology or virus detection by molecular techniques such as polymerase chain reaction (PCR) test in body fluids and tissues.

Roseola infantum is a mostly benign and self-limited illness, and recovery is almost always complete without significant sequelae. Therefore the management of roseola is composed of fever control with antipyretics and supportive treatment such as adequate fluid intake [12, 15].

56.6   Herpes Simplex Virus (HSV) Infections

Herpes simplex virus (HSV), included in the Herpesviridae family, is categorized into HSV-1 and HSV-2 subtypes based on biological and serologic differences. HSV is a leading pathogenic virus causing mucocutaneous illnesses in the oral cavity and genitalia [16]. A significant association is known between HSV-1 and oropharyngeal infection, meningoencephalitis, and dermatitis above the waistline. On the other side, HSV-2 is mainly associated with genital and anal infections. Nevertheless, HSV-1 and HSV-2 can cause primary and recurrent infections in the oropharyngeal and genital regions due to the different sexual practices [17, 18].

Herpes simplex virus replication occurs at the portal of entry on mucosae, leading to sensory nerve endings infection. Then, HSV transports to regional neural ganglions to establish latency. Primary HSV infections are usually presented with prodromal and systemic symptoms such as fever, malaise, headache, nausea, vomiting, and lymphadenopathy [17, 18]. Primary HSV-1 infections generally occur at younger ages and often cause painful mucocutaneous lesions; however, the infection sometimes can be asymptomatic. Oral HSV-1 infection is frequently accompanied by acute generalized marginal gingivitis and vesicles and ulcerations on the oral mucosa, following prodromal symptoms [18, 19]. Adolescents may present with herpetic tonsillitis. Neonatal HSV 1 or HSV 2 skin, eye mouth disease may also present with an ulcerative lesion on the palate, tongue, or oral mucosa.

The leading agent of oral herpes and gingivostomatitis is HSV-1. The disease primarily develops in children and adolescents not been exposed to the virus previously. The incubation period is 2–14 days, with an average of 4 days. Primary herpetic gingivostomatitis mostly starts with local and systemic findings. Fever, malaise, and headache are together with swollen and tender cervical lymph nodes, and the illness resembles the prodromal phase of influenza infection. Within one to a few days, lesions appear as intraepithelial vesicles on the oral mucosa, gingivae, hard palate, and vermillion border of the lips. Then the vesicles burst rapidly to form shallow erosions and ulcers on the erythematous base [3, 18]. A grayish pseudomembrane then covers the erosions and ulcers, which may coalesce spontaneously or be infected secondary to bacteria. The gingiva is characteristically red, swollen, and tender, and the mouth is highly painful; most patients do not want to eat. Ulcers are very contagious and heal in 3–5 days by crusting [16]. Primary herpetic gingivostomatitis heals entirely in about 14 days. Then the virus becomes latent in a sensory ganglion, often trigeminal ganglion.

Several factors such as fever, emotional and physical stress, and systemic illness may trigger the reactivation of HSV-1 [18]. Secondary to activating this type of factors or suppressing or compromising the immune system, the virus transports to peripheral nerves, and recurrence of herpes occurs. The frequency and severity of herpetic lesion recurrences are variable. Recurrent HSV-1 labialis, called "cold sores" or "fever blisters," emerges as single or grouped vesicles in the perioral region, usually on the vermilion border of the lips [17]. Recurrent lesions frequently occur with itching and burning sensation on more keratinized lips, adjacent gingiva, and palate. Recurrent herpes lesions can be seen anywhere in the immune-suppressed patient, including non-keratinizing oral mucosa areas.

Primary HSV gingivostomatitis is usually diagnosed clinically, and its current treatment is primarily supportive of antipyretics and analgesics. Topical anesthetics can be useful to relieve pain. In immune-competent patients, topical antiviral agents (acyclovir, penciclovir, docosanol) have only limited activity for therapy of herpes labialis and are not recommended. Oral acyclovir may be used in immune-competent children with herpetic gingivostomatitis presented within 72 to 96 h of disease onset if they cannot drink or have significant pain [17, 18]. Limited data also support a small therapeutic benefit of oral acyclovir for primary and recurrent HSV and herpetic gingivostomatitis in immunocompetent hosts.

Neonatal HSV-1 and HSV-2 infections with skin, eye, mouth (SEM) manifestations may also present with oral lesions, especially on the palate. Neonatal SEM HSV disease is considered a medical emergency should be thoroughly evaluated immediately for other infection sites and treated with intravenous acyclovir.

56.7 Varicella (Chickenpox)

Varicella is the primary infection of the varicella-zoster virus (VZV), a Herpesvidae family member. As predominantly a childhood disease, it is a highly contagious but mostly mild and self-limiting acute infectious disease. Varicella arises commonly in young children, although older individuals can be affected. Most cases are presented between 1 and 10 years of age. Varicella generally occurs in late winter and early spring but can occur throughout the year [20]. The viral transmission is occurred primarily by respiratory secretions, mainly saliva droplets, sneezing, and coughing from a person infected or direct contact with the vesicular skin rash fluid. Contagion starts from 2 days before the appearance of vesicles and goes to the crusting phase of the skin rash. The incubation period is usually 14–16 days but can be between 10 and 21 days [21].

Varicella is characterized by a pruritic exanthem that progresses through erythema, papule, vesicle, and crusting stages. The rash is commonly accompanied by fever and mild to moderate systemic symptoms and signs. The first lesions generally appear on the head and neck, but new ones quickly develop on the trunk, extremities, oral, conjunctival, respiratory, and genital mucous membranes [5]. The rash is more common on the trunk and head than on the limbs. In immune-competent patients, symptoms and signs are usually mild to moderate, but a severe case can have severe constitutional symptoms and more than a thousand skin lesions [20].

Oral lesions often involve the buccal mucosa, palate, and lips [21]. The presence and number of oral cavity enanthemas are related to the severity of the infection.

Oral manifestations are relatively common and may precede skin lesions. The places involved most frequently in the oral cavity are the palate and edge of the lips' vermilion, followed by the buccal mucosa [22]. The oral cavity enanthemas begin as 3–4 mm opaque-white vesicles, which ruptures and forms 1–3 mm ulcers. Oral lesions are manifested in approximately one to third of mild varicella cases, and sometimes a few oral ulcers appear and heal in 1–3 days. However, in severe cases, oral lesions may be several and persist for 5–10 days [5, 22]. Gingival lesions sometimes resemble those seen in primary HSV infections, but varicella's oral lesions tend to be relatively painless [20].

The varicella diagnosis is primarily clinical, with the appearance of characteristic itchy vesicles crusting in a few days. Serological confirmation is seldomly needed. After the primary infection, the VZV remains latent in the dorsal root ganglions, and endogenous reactivation of the virus later results in herpes zoster (shingles).

Serious complications such as pneumonia, secondary bacterial infections, central nervous system involvement, and even death are sometimes seen [20].

Treatment for varicella and herpes zoster in children is mainly symptomatic with antipyretics for fever, and antihistamines for pruritus, except in older cases >12 years old for whom antiviral therapy indicated because the complication rate is usually higher. Acyclovir, valacyclovir, and famciclovir are the antiviral drugs available for VZV infections' specific treatment [21].

Varicella can be prevented by vaccination. The vaccination is about 80–85% effective in the prevention of varicella and highly (>95%) effective in the prevention of severe disease [20].

56.8   Epstein-Barr Virus (EBV) Infection

Epstein-Barr virus (EBV) is included in the Herpesviridae family, a significant pathogenic virus infecting the cells in the oropharyngeal cavity, and B cells as the target and reservoir. The viral transmission in children happens following contact with saliva and oral secretions of the infected individuals on fingers, toys, or other objects. Adults generally become infected through intimate contact such as kissing; thus, the EBV infection is nick-named as "kissing disease." The virus replicates within epithelial cells of the oropharynx and remains in the host for life. The incubation period of EBV infection is around 8 weeks [23].

EBV infections are usually seen in early childhood but commonly asymptomatic in infants and children. However, adolescents and young adults are at a greater risk for symptomatic disease, and the infection generally results in infectious mononucleosis (IM). In symptomatic individuals, fever, pharyngitis, and lymphadenopathies are the classical triad of EBV infection, and upper respiratory tract symptoms, hepatosplenomegaly, and oral signs are the other main manifestations [23–25].

After entering the body, EBV passes to B lymphocytes and bloodstream by multiplying in mucous and salivary gland cells. Shortly after the onset of the disease, fever and sore throat usually are the leading manifestations. Then, tonsillopharyngitis, lymphadenopathies, and hepatosplenomegaly may develop [23, 24].

Significant lymphadenopathy is seen in more than 90% of cases and characteristically appears as enlarged symmetrically and tender nodes. In EBV infection, the most involved lymph nodes are in the anterior and posterior cervical chains. The pharynx and tonsils are inflamed, but there is no exudate over the tonsils at the beginning. As the disease progresses, the white exudates become apparent on the swollen, hyperplastic tonsils. Then, exudate patches evolve to become thick opaque white membrane plaques, while the uvula is red and edematous [23, 25]. The exudates remain for 7–10 days or even longer and cover both tonsils completely; however, the patient is in good general condition. As the membrane matures, crypt exudates' color often turns yellowish while whiteness mainly retains [22].

In some cases, the inflammatory edema causes the patients to have difficulty swallowing and breathing due to excessive respiratory congestion, facing death danger. The lingual tonsils, located on the tongue's base and extend from the circumvallate papillae to the epiglottis, can also become hyperplastic and compromise the airway. Because of tonsillar hyperplasia, pharyngeal edema, epiglottal swelling, and arytenoid hypertrophy, deaths due to respiratory difficulties have been reported [22–24].

Sharply demarcated, symmetrically distributed, numerous petechiae are also seen at the hard and soft palate junction in about 25% of patients with EBV infection, but these small clusters of hemorrhages are not pathognomic. The petechiae generally disappear within 24–48 h. In patients with EBV infection, parotid lymphoid tissue's enlargement with or without facial nerve palsy is rarely reported. Oral lesions other than lymphoid enlargement also may be encountered. Necrotizing ulcerative gingivitis (NUG) is relatively common compared to NUG-like pericoronitis and necrotizing ulcerative mucositis [22, 26].

Complications rarely occur but most commonly arise in children. Hepatitis, myocarditis, autoimmune hemolytic anemia, aplastic anemia, thrombocytopenia, splenic rupture, encephalitis, seizures, and hemophagocytic lymphohistiocytosis can occur as complications of EBV infections.

In addition to IM, EBV is also associated with lymphoproliferative disorders, oral hairy leukoplakia, various types of lymphoid and epithelial malignancies, including lymphomas (most notably African Burkitt lymphoma), smooth muscle tumors, and nasopharyngeal, gastric, hepatocellular, salivary lymphoepithelial, and oral squamous cell carcinomas [22–24].

The management of EBV infection is primarily supportive. The oral-pharyngeal lesions do not necessitate treatment and resolve spontaneously [23]. Antiviral medication and corticosteroids may be needed in some patients.

56.9 Non-poliovirus Enteroviral Infections

Enteroviruses (EVs), members of the Picornaviridae family, are subclassified as polioviruses and non-polio EVs. Polioviruses largely have been eradicated by vaccination; however, the non-polio EVs continue to cause disease worldwide.

Non-polio EVs contain over 100 different serotypes, previously subclassified as echoviruses, group A and B coxsackieviruses, and enumerated EVs. According to the current classification system, non-polio EVs are grouped into four species as EV A through D, based on genetic similarity, however, some serotype names are retained [22, 27]. Enteroviruses are spread by respiratory and fecal-oral routes, and prenatally from mother to infant, in the peripartum period, and possibly via breast-feeding [22].

Hand-foot-and-mouth disease (HFMD), herpangina, and acute lymphonodular pharyngitis are closely related and not entirely separated three clinical patterns manifested lesions in the oral cavity caused by non-polio EVs [22]. The severity of the illness varies by strain in all three clinical conditions. Most strains cause a self-limiting disease; however, some strains can produce illness with significant complications and even deaths. Both HFMD and herpangina may be encountered in epidemics with the same strain. In addition, acute lymphonodular pharyngitis is generally regarded as a variant of herpangina.

Hand-foot-and-mouth disease is a commonly encountered exanthematous illness in children and adults. It presents a clinical picture characterized by an oral vesicular eruption and a macular, maculopapular, and papulovesicular rash in various parts of the body, mainly in the hands and feet, but it can also involve the buttocks and genitalia. In most HFMD cases, coxsackievirus A16 is the etiologic agent. Nevertheless, the disease is also caused by coxsackievirus A5, A7, A9, A10, B2, and B5, EV71, and echovirus 11. Enterovirus 71 has caused HFMD outbreaks accompanied by neurologic involvement in the Asia-Pacific region [27–29].

Hand-foot-and-mouth disease is highly contagious, and the etiologic virus is transmitted through infected saliva. After 3–5 days of the incubation period, oral lesions appear within 1–2 days [28]. Erythematous macules appear initially on the tongue, gingiva, buccal mucosa, and palate, rapidly evolving into 2–3 mm vesicles on an erythematous base. The labial mucosa, buccal mucosa, and tongue are the most common sites. The vesicles are rarely seen because they rapidly erode and become ulcerated, surrounded by an erythematous halo, and heal typically in 1 week. The ulcers are painful, they may interfere with eating, and their total number ranges from 1 to 30 and averages 5 to 10. Each lesion typically measures 2–7 mm in diameter but may be >1 cm. In approximately half of the patients, the tongue is involved, may be edematous and tender, in addition to the ulcers [22, 29]. In HFMD, anterior regions of the mouth are more frequently involved, and the oral lesions are more numerous.

Skin manifestations consist of a mixture of groped 5–10 papules and vesicles located on the toes, heels, and dorsal and lateral of the hand and foot generally appear after oral lesions. Vesicles erode and evolve rapidly into ulcers with an erythematous halo around them [22].

Herpangina is a benign clinical condition manifested with fever and a painful popular, vesicular, and ulcerative oral enanthem. It can be distinguished from HFMD and primary herpetic gingivostomatitis clinically. Several non-polio EV serotypes, most commonly coxsackievirus A serotypes, are responsible. Herpangina usually is caused by coxsackievirus A1 to A6, A8, A10, or A22. However, it also may be caused by coxsackievirus A7, A9, A16, and B2 to B6, echovirus 9, 16, or 17, or enterovirus 71. The clinical presentation is characterized by an acute onset of fever, sore throat, and dysphagia, but anorexia, headache, vomiting, diarrhea, rhinorrhea, cough, and myalgia may rarely be accompanied. Nevertheless, most cases are subclinical or mild [22, 27, 30].

The oral lesions typically are in small numbers (commonly 2–6), appear as red punctate macules, turn into erythematous papules to evolve into fragile vesicles within hours or days in the posterior pharynx, mainly on the soft palate, uvula, or tonsillar pillars, and then rapidly ulcerate. The ulcerations average 2–4 mm in diameter and usually take 7–10 days to heal. However, the systemic manifestations resolve within a few days [22, 28, 29].

Acute lymphonodular pharyngitis, a less encountered clinical entity caused by coxsackievirus A10, is characterized by fever, sore throat, and mild headache, which may last 4–14 days. The pharyngeal lesions look like the lesions in herpangina but remain in the form of papules without evolving into vesicles and ulcers. Yellow to dark-pink nodules appear on the soft palate or tonsillar pillars in low numbers (one to five), representing hyperplastic lymphoid aggregates, and disappear within 10 days without vesiculation or ulceration [22].

The diagnosis of HFMD and herpangina is generally based on clinical manifestations. However, reverse transcriptase (RT)-PCR assay and culture help confirm the clinical diagnosis [27]. Since the non-polio EV infections are generally self-limited, treatment is symptomatic, such as antipyretics used for fever and analgesics for painful oral lesions.

56.10 Human Papillomavirus (HPV) Infections

Over 200 HPVs are categorized by genotype, grouped into cutaneous and mucosal types [31]. Most HPV infections are asymptomatic, and 90% resolve spontaneously. Nevertheless, the persistency of HPV infection can cause benign epithelial proliferation (warts) of the mucous membranes and skin, cancers of the head and neck, and lower anogenital tract. The cutaneous HPV types cause various kinds of benign skin warts. Certain mucosal HPV types with low risk are associated with warts or papillomas of mucous membranes, including the oral, nasal, upper respiratory tract, conjunctival, and anogenital areas [32]. Other mucosal HPV types with high risk are associated with precancers and cancers, including oropharyngeal, cervical, and anogenital cancers.

Oral HPV infections are linked to sexual behavior, but evidence supports mouth-to-mouth transmission. In addition, in infants, most HPV infections are acquired from the mother during the intrauterine period, during delivery, or later via saliva [33]. The role of the mother is central in infecting her offspring. The oral cavity may be the first site that HPV enters into the body. Some oral HPV infections may be persistent, which is mandatory for the associated malignant transformation. However, the malignant evolution of HPV-related lesions requires additional cofactors.

Squamous papilloma, condyloma acuminatum, verruca vulgaris, and focal epithelial hyperplasia (Heck's disease) are the HPV-related oral cavity lesions [31]. Oral papillomas and condylomas can develop at any age, caused by the most prevalent HPV types with low-risk HPV-6 and HPV-11 as in the genital tract [33]. Heck's disease, not seen in the genital tract, is a specific benign neoplastic condition in oral mucosa caused by HPV-13 and HPV-32, characterized by multiple white to pinkish papules with slightly pale, smooth, or roughened surface placed diffusely in the oral cavity.

Cancers of the cervix, vagina, vulva, penis, anus, and oropharynx (back of the throat, base of the tongue, and tonsils) are attributed as HPV-related invasive cancers. Cervical and oropharyngeal cancers are the most common HPV-attributable cancers among women and men, respectively [32].

Recurrent respiratory papillomatosis (RRP) is a rare but potentially life-threatening benign, often multi-focal tumor of the respiratory tract with laryngeal predilection. It is characterized by multiple recurring warty excrescences (papillomas) on the mucosal surface in the larynx or other areas of the upper respiratory tract [33–35]. Recurrent respiratory papillomatosis is named juvenile-onset RRP when it develops before 18 years of age; onset in adults also occurs. Juvenile RRP is attributed to transmission of HPV-6 or HPV-11 from a mother to infant during delivery and is diagnosed most commonly between 2 and 5 years of age [33]. The typical manifestations of RRP are voice change (e.g., hoarseness), stridor, or abnormal cry. Recurrent respiratory papillomatosis can result in respiratory tract obstruction in small children, and repeated surgeries are often needed. The diagnosis of RRP may be challenging unless it is not considered. For any child presenting with a voice disturbance with or without stridor, the possibility of RRP should be kept in mind [34, 35].

56.11 Human Immunodeficiency Virus (HIV) Infection

After the onset of the human immunodeficiency virus (HIV) and acquired immune deficiency syndrome (AIDS) pandemic, several oral manifestations accompanied by HIV infection have been gradually recognized. Importantly, none of these findings are specific to HIV infection and AIDS, which can also be detected in immune-compromised patients and even in normal individuals for other reasons. However, clinical presentations in patients with HIV infection are often more severe and atypical.

The 1993 consensus classification of EC-Clearinghouse and World Health Organisation (WHO) Collaborating Centre on oral manifestations related to HIV infection in adults is universally used [36]. This classification divides the oral presentations of HIV disease into three groups as strongly associated, less commonly associated, and seen in HIV infection [22, 36]. Seven oral lesions are known to be strongly associated with HIV: oral candidiasis, oral hairy leukoplakia, Kaposi's sarcoma, linear gingival erythema, necrotizing ulcerative gingivitis, necrotizing ulcerative periodontitis, and non-Hodgkin lymphoma [22, 36]. These manifestations involve more than half of adults with HIV infection and about 80% of those diagnosed with AIDS. Similar data have also been found in children, with a very high incidence of oral lesions [22, 36, 37].

Oral candidiasis, HSV infections, linear gingival erythema, parotid salivary gland enlargement, and recurrent aphthous ulcerations are the most common oral lesions in children with HIV disease [38, 39]. HIV-related gingivitis, periodontitis, and oral neoplastic lesions such as oral hairy leukoplakia, Kaposi sarcoma, and non-Hodgkin lymphoma are much less common in children than in adults [38]. Children with HIV infection are more susceptible to bacterial infections, mainly with encapsulated bacteria such as *Streptococcus pneumoniae*, in contrast to adults. An oral infection focus can become a source for septicemia in HIV-infected children, creating a life-threatening problem. Thus, appropriate oral health necessitates being routinely maintained in children with HIV infection [38, 40]. Regularly chlorhexidine gluconate 0.12% mouth rinse usage helps minimize candidiasis, gingivitis, and the oral cavity's superinfections [38].

HIV-related oral manifestations are critical diagnostic and prognostic indicators [22]. And there are significant reverse correlations between viral load and CD4 + T cell count, and oral lesions [22, 38, 39]. In this context, with the launch of highly active antiretroviral therapy (HAART), the prevalence of HIV-related oral lesions has shown a significant decrease in children [37, 39]. Because of the oral lesions, HIV-infected children are disturbed during teeth brushing and swallowing, thus avoiding their oral health-related care. Intervening and treating oral lesions in HIV-infected children provide them to reach a better quality of life [3, 37].

56.12 Conclusion

Several systemic pediatric infectious diseases can cause symptoms and signs in the oral cavity. In pediatric patients, a detailed ear, nose, and throat examination should always be an integral part of systemic physical examination; it may render specific findings for diseases' diagnosis.

References

1. Xiao J, Fiscella KA, Gill SR. Oral microbioma: possible harbinger for children's health. Int J Oral Sci. 2020;12(1):12.
2. Chi AC, Neville BW, Krayer JW, Gonsalves WC. Oral manifestations of systemic disease. Am Fam Physician. 2010;82:1381–8.
3. Li X, Kolltveit KM, Tronstad L, Olsen I. Systemic diseases caused by oral infection. Clin Microbiol Rev. 2000;13:547–58.
4. Sallberg M. Oral viral infections of children. Periodontology. 2000;49:87–95.
5. Chaves RF, Rodrigues CRT, Brum SC, Barbosa CCN, De Oliveira NG. Oral manifestations of systemic diseases infectious in children. J Surg Clin Dent. 2014;2:29–35.
6. Cherry JD, Baker A. Rubella virus. In: Cherry JD, Harrison GJ, Kaplan SL, Steinbach WJ, Hotez PJ, editors. Feigin and Cherry's textbook of pediatric infectious diseases. 8th ed. Philadelphia: Elsevier; 2019. p. 1601–22.

7. Glick M, Siegel MA. Viral and fungal infections of the oral cavity in immunocompetent patients. Infect Dis Clin North Am. 1999;13:817–31.
8. Hviid A, Rubin S, Muhlemann K. Mumps. Lancet. 2008;371:932–44.
9. American Academy of Pediatrics. Mumps. In: Kimberlin DW, Brady MT, Jackson MA, Long SS, editors. Red book: 2018 report of the committee on infectious diseases. 31st ed. Itasca: American Academy of Pediatrics; 2018. p. 567–73.
10. Campbell JR. Parotitis. In: Cherry JD, Harrison GJ, Kaplan SL, Steinbach WJ, Hotez PJ, editors. Feigin and Cherry's textbook of pediatric infectious diseases. 8th ed. Philadelphia: Elsevier; 2019. p. 134–6.
11. Stone RC, Micali GA, Schwartz RA. Roseola infantum and its causal human herpesviruses. Int J Dermatol. 2014;53:397–403.
12. Wright JM, Taylor PP, Allen EP, et al. A review of the oral manifestations of infections in pediatric patients. Pediatr Infect Dis. 1984;3:80–8.
13. Syrjanen S. Viral infections in oral mucosa. Scand J Dent Res. 1992;100:17–31.
14. Cherry JD. Roseola infantum (exanthem subitum). In: Cherry JD, Harrison GJ, Kaplan SL, Steinbach WJ, Hotez PJ, editors. Feigin and cherry's textbook of pediatric infectious diseases. 8th ed. Philadelphia: Elsevier; 2019. p. 559–61.
15. Caserta MT. Human herpesviruses 6 and 7 (roseola, exanthem subitum). In: Long SS, Prober CG, Fischer M, editors. Principles and practice of pediatric infectious diseases. 5th ed. Philadelphia: Elsevier; 2018. p. 1081–8.
16. Fatahzadeh M, Schwartz RA. Human herpes simplex virüs infections: epidemiology, pathogenesis, symptomatology, diagnosis, and management. J Am Acad Dermatol. 2007;57:737–63.
17. American Academy of Pediatrics. Herpes simplex. In: Kimberlin DW, Brady MT, Jackson MA, Long SS, editors. Red book: 2018 report of the committee on infectious diseases. 31st ed. Itasca: American Academy of Pediatrics; 2018. p. 437–49.
18. Balasubramaniam R, Kuperstein AS, Stoopler ET. Update on oral herpes virus infections. Dent Clin N Am. 2014;58:265–80.
19. Crimi S, Fiorillo L, Bianchi A, et al. Herpes virus, oral clinical signs and QoL: systematic review of recent data. Viruses. 2019;11(5):463.
20. Heininger U, Seward JF. Varicella. Lancet. 2006;368:1365–76.
21. Gould D. Varicella zoster virus: chickenpox and shingles. Nurs Stand. 2014;28:52–8.
22. Neville BW, Damm DD, Allen CM, Chi AC. Viral infections. In: Oral and maxillofacial pathology. 4th ed. St. Louis: Elsevier; 2016. p. 224–6.
23. Luzuriaga K, Sullivan JL. Infectious mononucleosis. N Engl J Med. 2010;362:1993–2000.
24. Clarkson E, Mashkoor F, Abdulateef S. Oral viral infections: diagnosis and management. Dent Clin N Am. 2017;61:351–63.
25. Santosh ABR, Muddana K. Viral infections of oral cavity. J Family Med Prim Care. 2020;9:36–42.
26. Kikuchi K, Inouea H, Miyazaki Y, Idea F, Kojima M, Kusama K. Epstein - Barr virus (EBV)-associated epithelial and non-epithelial lesions of the oral cavity. Jpn Dent Sci Rev. 2017;53:95–109.
27. American Academy of Pediatrics. Enterovirus (nonpoliovirus). In: Baker CJ, editor. Red Book® atlas of pediatric infectious diseases. 4th ed. Elk Grove: American Academy of Pediatrics; 2020. p. 189–93.
28. Repass G, Palmer WC, Stancampiano FF. Hand, foot, and mouth disease: identifying and managing an acute viral syndrome. Cleve Clin J Med. 2014;81:537–43.
29. Nervi SJ. Hand-foot-and-mouth disease (HFMD). In: Bronze MS (ed). Medscape.com, updated: 2018, https://emedicine.medscape.com/article/218402 Accessed 29 Dec 2020.
30. Romero JR. Hand, foot, and mouth disease and herpangina. In: Edwards MS, Drutz JE, Torchia MM (ed). Uptodate.com, updated 2020, https://www.uptodate.com/contents/hand-foot-and-mouth-disease-and-herpangina Accessed 30 Dec 2020.
31. Betz SJ. HPV-related papillary lesions of the oral mucosa: a review. Head Neck Pathol. 2019;13:80–90.

32. American Academy of Pediatrics. Human papillomaviruses. In: Baker CJ, editor. Red book atlas of pediatric infectious diseases. 4th ed. Elk Grove: American Academy of Pediatrics; 2020. p. 460–4.
33. Syrjänen S. Oral manifestations of human papillomavirus infections. Eur J Oral Sci. 2018;126(Suppl. 1):49–66.
34. Zacharisen MC, Conley SF. Recurrent respiratory papillomatosis in children: masquerader of common respiratory diseases. Pediatrics. 2006;118:1925–31.
35. Tasca RA, Clarke RW. Recurrent respiratory papillomatosis. Arch Dis Child. 2006;91:689–91.
36. Classification and diagnostic criteria for oral lesions in HIV infection. EC-clearinghouse on oral problems related to HIV infection and WHO collaborating centre on oral manifestations of the immunodeficiency virus. J Oral Pathol Med. 1993;22:289–91.
37. Lauritano D, Moreo G, Oberti L, et al. Oral manifestations in HIV-positive children: a systematic review. Pathogens. 2020;9:88–103.
38. Simos C, Gonzales BE. Infections of the oral cavity. In: Cherry JD, Harrison GJ, Kaplan SL, Steinbach WJ, Hotez PJ, editors. Feigin and Cherry's textbook of pediatric infectious diseases. 8th ed. Philadelphia: Elsevier; 2019. p. 96–108.
39. Araújo JF, Oliveira AEF, Carvalho HLCC, Roma FRVO, Lopes FF. Most common oral manifestations in pediatric patients HIV positive and the effect of highly active antiretroviral therapy. Cien Saude Colet. 2018;23:115–22.
40. Leggott PJ. Oral manifestations of HIV infection in children. Oral Surg Oral Med Oral Pathol. 1992;73:187–92.

Periodic Fever, Aphthous Stomatitis, Pharyngitis, and Cervical Adenitis Syndrome (PFAPA Syndrome)

Ercan Kaya, Melek Kezban Gürbüz, and Jeffrey C. Bedrosian

57.1 Introduction

PFAPA syndrome is a repetitive disease with no clear etiology, characterized by a sudden onset of high fever, aphthous stomatitis, pharyngitis, and cervical lymphadenopathy episodes. This disease is more frequently seen in males under the age of 5 and regresses in adolescence.

It was described for the first time by Marshall et al. in 1987. A few years later, this disease (periodic fever, aphthous stomatitis, pharyngitis, cervical adenitis) began to be referred to as the acronym, PFAPA syndrome [1–3]. The disease is typically classified within the group of periodic fever syndromes. In addition to PFAPA, this group includes diseases such as FMF (familial Mediterranean fever), tumor necrosis factor receptor-associated periodic syndrome (TRAPS), and cryopyrin-associated autoinflammatory syndrome (CAPS).

In their daily practice, pediatricians and ENT specialists often encounter fever and pharyngitis in pediatric patients. Although these symptoms are usually associated with infections, when the fever recurs regularly, parents begin to seriously worry about their children. Therefore, PFAPA syndrome should be considered in the differential diagnosis in patients presenting with periodic fever. While detailed physical examination and evaluation are very important in patients presenting with periodic fever and pharyngitis, laboratory tests are not particularly useful in the diagnosis of PFAPA syndrome. However, laboratory tests are important in distinguishing other diseases that cause periodic fever. The diagnosis is mostly based on

E. Kaya (✉) · M. K. Gürbüz
Department of Otorhinolaryngology, Faculty of Medicine, Eskişehir Osmangazi University, Eskişehir, Turkey

J. C. Bedrosian
St. Luke's Medical Center, Rhinology and Skull Base Surgery, Bethlehem Otolaryngology Office of Specialty Physician Associates, Bethlehem, PA, USA

© The Author(s), under exclusive license to Springer Nature Switzerland AG 2022
C. Cingi et al. (eds.), *Pediatric ENT Infections*,
https://doi.org/10.1007/978-3-030-80691-0_57

good knowledge of the syndrome and past medical history as well as examination findings [1–3].

57.2 Epidemiology

The frequency of PFAPA syndrome is unclear, though the frequency of the diagnosis has increased since description of the syndrome. This is thought to be due to the fact that PFAPA is prioritized in the differential diagnosis by clinicians, especially in the presence of recurrent fever and other symptoms. Its incidence is estimated to be approximately 2/10,000 [4]. Førsvoll et al.'s prospective study on evaluation of the prevalence of PFAPA syndrome in Norwegian children found an incidence of 2.3/10,000; however, more detailed epidemiological studies have not been conducted yet worldwide [5]. Although there is no ethnic predisposition among patients with PFAPA syndrome, it has been reported in studies that it is more common in males [6].

57.3 Etiopathogenesis

Although infection and autoimmune mechanisms have been considered in its pathophysiology, there is no proven pathophysiological mechanism so far and no clear link to an autoimmune or infectious etiology [2]. Although infectious causes are considered primarily due to the appearance of tonsillitis during attacks, throat cultures taken during attacks are generally detected as normal throat flora [2, 7]. No common infectious agent identified during attacks has been reported in the literature, though there are rare case reports of microorganisms found [8]. In addition, the long duration of the disease without progression, self-limitation and significant response to corticosteroid therapy in this syndrome reduces the possibility of infectious pathology [9].

In the past, PFAPA syndrome was thought to occur due to abnormal cytokine responses in the presence of infection [2, 9]. Stojanov et al.'s first study on PFAPA reported increased IL-6 and IFN-gamma serum concentrations, significantly increased IL-1beta, TNF-alpha, and IL-12p70 levels, and lower levels of anti-inflammatory IL-4, intracellular IL-4 and IL-10 or serum IL-10 levels compared to the control group during febrile PFAPA attacks. Continuous pro-inflammatory cytokine activation and decreased anti-inflammatory response and increased pro-inflammatory mediators during attack periods suggest a disorder of the immune response in PFAPA syndrome [9]. Chronic febrile attacks in autoinflammatory diseases (FMF, Cyclic Neutropenia, HyperIGD syndrome, TRAPS), other than PFAPA syndrome, which is accompanied by recurrent fever attacks, have been ascribed to a defect that regulates the inflammatory response in the immune system [10]. In their second study on PFAPA, Stojanov et al. found that complementary (C1QB, C2, SERPING1), IL- [1–]associated (IL-1β, IL-1RN, CASP1, IL18RAP) and IFN-induced (AIM2, IP-10/CXCL10) genes are significantly overexpressed during

PFAPA attacks [11]. IL-1β and IL-18 are pro-inflammatory cytokines that play a key role in the innate immune response, defense against pathogens and inflammation. The initiation of the effects of both IL-1β and IL-18 is via inflammasome, which are cytoplasmic protein complexes that may be associated with the pathogenesis of autoinflammatory diseases [12]. In a Japanese study conducted in patients with PFAPA syndrome, IL-1β, IL-1ra, IL-6, and sTNFR1 increased only during the attack period, while serum TNF-α and IL-18 levels were found to be high in both attack and non-attack periods [13]. Similar results were obtained in studies investigating cytokine levels in serum, and a study conducted by Patricia M et al. found similar rates in both groups when tonsillectomy specimens of patients with PFAPA syndrome and tonsillar hypertrophy were compared in terms of levels of IL-1β, TNF-α, TGF-β, IL-17, and IFN-γ [6]. In summary, immune system dysregulation triggered by a possible external factor is seen as the main factor in the etiopathogenesis of PFAPA syndrome [12].

57.4 Clinical Signs

In PFAPA syndrome, attacks that start before the age of 5 typically recur in 4–6-week intervals throughout the year [1, 14]. For the diagnosis of PFAPA, at least one of the symptoms of aphthous stomatitis, pharyngitis, and adenitis cardinal should appear in the presentation in addition to periodic fever attacks [1]. Frequently, patients will be diagnosed with concurrent acute tonsillitis (Figs. 57.1, 57.2). Symptoms such as nausea, weakness, headache, vomiting, abdominal pain, diarrhea, arthralgia, cough, myalgia, runny nose, and rash may also be seen [11, 15, 16]. These complaints resolve automatically within 4–5 days [1].

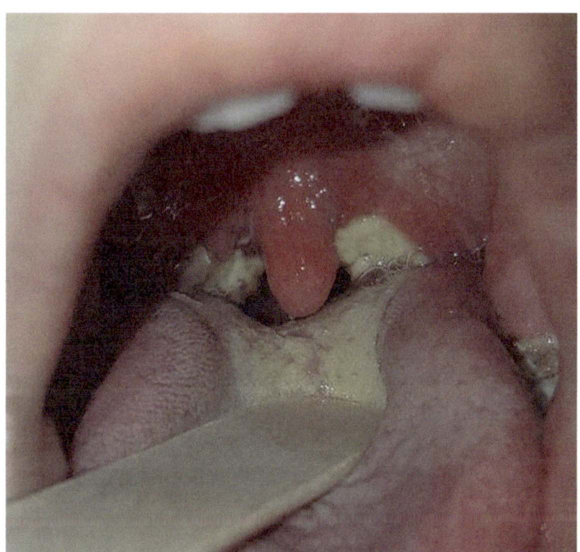

Fig. 57.1 Tonsillitis-like appearance in the patient with PFAPA syndrome

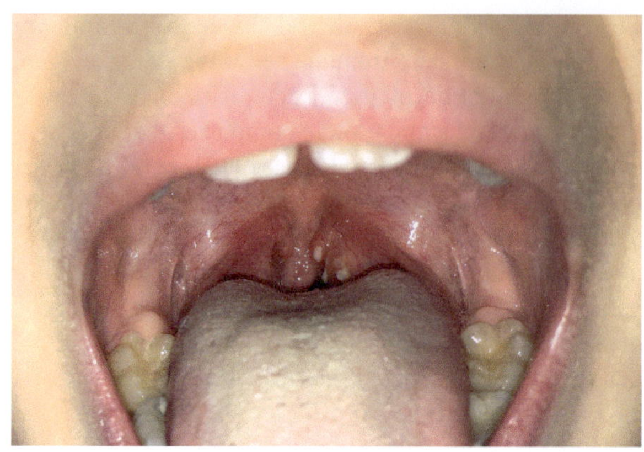

Fig. 57.2 Tonsillitis-like appearance in the patient with PFAPA syndrome

57.5 Diagnostic Criteria

- -Fever recurring in regular intervals as from less than 5 years of age.
- -It's accompanied by at least one of the following without any symptoms of URTI.
- -Aphthous stomatitis, Cervical lymphadenitis, Pharyngitis.
- -Patient being asymptomatic between attacks.
- -Normal growth and development.
- -Cyclic neutropenia should have been ruled out in the differential diagnosis.

Additionally, significant improvement in fever attacks with the administration of a single dose of oral steroid is also recommended as a diagnostic criterion [7].

57.6 Diagnosis

There is no laboratory test specific to the syndrome. During attacks, leukocytosis, thrombocytosis, and a markedly elevated acute phase response are observed. Acute phase response returns to normal levels after fever resolves. Biochemical tests and autoimmunity indicators are normal in patients. All cultures taken from children with PFAPA remain sterile.

Although no specific laboratory test can be identified for PFAPA syndrome, studies are underway. There are studies evaluating procalcitonin (PCT) and C-reactive protein (CRP) levels to differentiate PFAPA attacks from acute bacterial and viral infections or to help diagnose the syndrome [15, 17]. Tekin M et al. examined Mean Platelet Volume (MPV) values in the attack and non-attack periods of patients with PFAPA syndrome, compared them with those of the control group, and found lower MPV values [18]. Yamazaki T. et al. measured CD64, which is a member of the family of receptors that define neutrophils and monocytes, and found significantly increased CD64 levels during the attack, in contrast to CD64 levels similar to those of the control group before the attack [19]. In conclusion, although there is no test that ensures definitive diagnosis of PFAPA, PFAPA syndrome is diagnosed in the light of the diagnostic criteria supported by laboratory findings.

57.7 Differential Diagnosis

Fever secondary to infection is frequently observed in pre-school children. However, fever in PFAPA syndrome is of periodic character and can be observed not only in this syndrome but also in other various syndromes. Therefore, in the approach to periodic fever complaint, conditions such as PFAPA syndrome, mevalonate kinase deficiency (Hyper IgD syndrome), familial Mediterranean fever (FMF), cyclic neutropenia, tumor necrosis factor receptor-associated periodic syndrome (TRAPS), Cryopyrinopathies (CAPS), and familial cold autoinflammatory syndrome should also be kept in mind. Conventionally, although the diseases mentioned above are known as diseases that cause periodic fever syndrome, they have been defined and examined as immune-induced autoinflammatory diseases for the past 20 years. In this group, recurrent fever attacks are accompanied by various systemic complaints and increased acute phase reactants that cannot be explained by infection [20, 21].

Fever episodes are quite regular in cyclic neutropenia; however, they are not as high and resistant as in PFAPA syndrome. Moreover, aphthous ulcers in cyclic neutropenia are deeper, more painful, and long lasting than in PFAPA syndrome. Cyclic neutropenia may be easily differentiated from PFAPA by the accompanying neutropenia.

Familial Mediterranean fever (FMF) is the alternative diagnosis with the highest prevalence. Unlike PFAPA syndrome, which occurs with regular cycles, familial Mediterranean fever (FMF) is not a periodic disease and is characterized by random attacks. While abdominal pain is common in PFAPA, it is not as severe as in FMF. Although aphthous lesions are seen in both, pharyngitis and cervical lymphadenopathy are nonexistent in FMF. Arthritis, pleuritis, and erysipelas-like erythema are seen only in FMF. In addition, FMF does not respond to individual doses of glucocorticoids [20].

In mevalonate kinase deficiency (Hyper IgD syndrome), there is autoinflammation not accompanied by T cellular response. It can mimic PFAPA significantly in terms of symptoms. Arthritis, arthralgia, nausea, diarrhea, vomiting and hepatosplenomegaly, which are not seen in PFAPA Syndrome, can be frequently seen in mevalonate kinase deficiency. In laboratory tests, the IgD level is typically >100 U/ml. However, young children might have normal IgD levels. Disease response to corticosteroids is minimal. The most valuable diagnostic method is to demonstrate increased mevalonic acid level in urine between attacks [20, 22].

Among hereditary periodic fever syndromes, TRAPS is the most frequently mentioned disease after FMF. TRAPS involves acute attacks characterized by fever, pain, and inflammatory findings, like other autoinflammatory syndromes. Though ranging from 5 days to several weeks, the duration of attacks is approximately 1–2 weeks. During an attack, fever, musculosed lethal symptoms, skin manifestations, eye symptoms and abdominal findings can be seen. Body temperature is generally above 38 °C, which persists in almost all patients during the attack. Severe myalgia is the major clinical manifestation of TRAPS, observed in almost all patients, distinguishing TRAPS from PFAPA.

Also, familial cold auto-inflammatory syndromes, cold urticaria, Muckle-Wells syndrome, neonatal onset multisystem autoinflammatory disease (NOMID), and chronic infantile neurological cutaneous and articular syndrome (CINCA) can rarely cause recurrent fever under the heading of cryopirinopathies.

57.8 Adults PFAPA

PFAPA syndrome was initially considered a disease specific to the pediatric population. It usually starts before the age of 5 and resolves spontaneously in adolescence. In addition to this classical knowledge, some studies which conducted long-term follow-up of patients diagnosed with PFAPA syndrome in childhood reported that the disease continued for a long time in a small percentage of patients [23, 24]. Since the first adult patient with this disease was reported in 2008, many cases of PFAPA syndrome from not only the pediatric age group, but also from the adult age group, have been reported [14, 16, 25–28]. Therefore, the age range of this syndrome has expanded today. Cantarini L et al.'s study defined the following to facilitate the diagnosis of PFAPA syndrome in adult patients: erythematous pharyngitis and/or cervical lymphadenitis accompanied by repetitive fever attacks, increased inflammatory markers, and absence of complaints in the absence of attacks [29].

Rigante D et al. compared 85 children and 30 adult patients with PFAPA syndrome and reported longer periods of fever attacks in adult patients, compared to shorter episodes in pediatric patients. Also, joint symptoms, myalgia, headache, fatigue, ocular findings, and rashes were more common in adults [30].

Treatment of adult patients is similar to the treatment of pediatric patients. During febrile attacks, pediatric patients do not usually respond to fever-reducing medications, whereas they respond within hours to kg/1 mg of corticosteroid therapy. Rigante D et al. reported that they also achieved successful results with NSAIDs and low-dose corticosteroids (25 mg) in adult patients [30]. Alternative therapies are also being investigated, including studies reporting that anakinra and canakinumab, which are among the group of IL-1 inhibitors, are effective when there is no response to corticosteroid treatment in adult patients [31, 32].

57.9 Treatment

Due to the lack of clearly defined pathophysiology of PFAPA syndrome, there is currently no disease-specific treatment. The goal of treatment is to control symptoms during fever attacks. In most of the cases, complaints remit over time or disappear spontaneously. However, in the pediatric patient group (especially under the age of 5), fever attacks generally affect not only children but also their parents. Antipyretic and nonsteroidal anti-inflammatory agents used during febrile attacks generally do not show much efficacy, although corticosteroids may effectively resolve febrile attacks within hours. The dose of corticosteroids is generally similar in many treatment protocols: a single dose in the range of 0.5–2 mg/kg is used [33]. Often a single dose of 1 mg/kg prednisone is used, though beta-methasone (0.1–0.2 mg/kg) can also be used [33, 34]. Although a single dose of corticosteroid is administered during a febrile episode, the same dose may be repeated 2 days later if the febrile period continues [33]. Reported values for the rate of resolving a febrile attack of a single dose corticosteroid were 63%, 84%, and 90% [35, 36].

Colchicine, which is often used in the treatment of FMF (familial Mediterranean fever), is an alternative treatment of PFAPA syndrome, as there are similarities between FMF and PFAPA syndrome in terms of clinical and laboratory findings. Several studies demonstrated that colchicine significantly reduces the frequency of febrile episodes compared to corticosteroids [37, 38]. It is estimated that PEFAPA patients with heterozygous MEFV mutations can respond better to this medication. Colchicine can be considered as a second-line treatment in patients with PFAPA syndrome, where the frequency of febrile attacks cannot be controlled with corticosteroids [33].

Cimetidine, which is an immune modulating H2 antagonist, was first proposed by Feder in 1992 in the prophylactic treatment of PFAPA syndrome [39]. However, subsequent studies demonstrating low treatment efficacy have made it a less preferred alternative therapy [3, 36].

Since patients with inflammatory diseases are likely to have low vitamin D levels, the relationship between PFAPA syndrome and vitamin D level has been investigated. Patients with PFAPA syndrome were found to have significantly decreased levels of vitamin D compared to controls [40]. Stagi S. et al. found that the frequency of febrile attacks decreased significantly with vitamin D supplementation during febrile attacks [41].

IL-1 blockers such as anakinra, rilonacept and canakinumab have also started to be used in treatment due to the increased IL-1β effect in pathogenesis [11, 42]. StojanovS et al.'s first study demonstrated inflammasome-mediated activation and increased IL-1β during febrile attacks of patients with PFAPA syndrome and reported positive clinical responses with the use of anakinra, an IL-1 receptor antagonist [9]. These medications are mostly preferred in the treatment of patients with resistant PFAPA syndrome [43]. Due to the problems in the immune pathways in the pathogenesis of PFAPA syndrome, Buongiorno A et al. considered using Pidotimod, an immunomodulating medication, in therapy and reported significant response to treatment [44]. However, these studies are limited studies conducted in a small number of patients. Nevertheless, innovative searches for the treatment of PFAPA syndrome continue to be more directed towards pathogenesis.

Tonsillectomy has been an alternative treatment option, as well. However, its mechanism of action is not fully understood. In many patients with PFAPA syndrome, inflammation is thought to start from tonsils, prompting irregular systemic responses to that inflammation. Therefore, tonsillectomy acts to remove the tissue that initiates the inflammatory response. Indeed, while there has been a range of publications discussing the effectiveness of tonsillectomy, it is commonly accepted that patients with PFAPA benefit from tonsillectomy, promoting subsequent disease remission [20].

57.10 Prognosis

Although there's a limited number of studies on the prognosis and long-term follow-up of patients with PFAPA syndrome in the literature, it has been reported that the disease usually resolves spontaneously within an average of 6.3 years. The disease may persist for years in small groups of patients, though the frequency of attacks and the severity of symptoms during attacks decrease significantly with age.

References

1. Marshall GS, Edwards KM, Butler J, et al. Syndrome of periodicfever, pharyngitis, andaphthousstomatitis. J Pediatr. 1987;110:43–6.
2. Long SS. Syndrome of periodic fever, Aphthousstomatitis, pharyngitis, and adenitis (PFAPA)—what it isn't. What is it ? J Pediatr. 1999;135:1–5.
3. Thomas KT, Feder HM Jr, Lawton AR, et al. Periodicfeversyndrome in children. J Pediatr. 1999;135(1):15–21.
4. Jamilloux Y, Belot A, Magnotti F, et al. Geoepidemiology and immunologic features of autoinflammatory diseases: a comprehensive review. Clin Rev Allergy Immunol. 2017;54(3):454–79.
5. Førsvoll J, Kristoffersen EK, Øymar K. Incidence, clinicalcharacteristicsandoutcome in Norwegianchildrenwithperiodicfever, aphthousstomatitis, pharyngitisandcervicaladenitissyndrome; a population-basedstudy. Acta Paediatr. 2013;102(2):187–92.
6. Valenzuela PM, Araya A, Pérez CI, et al. Profile of inflammatory mediators in tonsils of patients with periodic fever, aphthous stomatitis, pharyngitis, and cervicaladenitis (PFAPA) syndrome. Clin Rheumatol. 2013;32(12):1743–9.
7. Padeh S, Brezniak N, Zemer D, et al. Periodicfever, aphthous stomatitis, pharyngitis, and adenopathy syndrome: clinical characteristics and outcome. J Pediatr. 1999;135(1):98–101.
8. Ryan ME, Ferrigno K, O'Boyle T, et al. Periodic fever and skin lesions caused by disseminated Mycobacterium chelonae infection in an immunocompetent child. Pediatr Infect Dis J. 1996;15(3):270–2.
9. Stojanov S, Hoffmann F, Kéry A, et al. Cytokine profile in PFAPA syndrome suggests continuous inflammation and reduced anti-inflammatory response. Eur Cytokine Netw. 2006;17(2):90–7.
10. Kolly L, Busso N, von Scheven-Gete A, et al. Periodic fever, aphthous stomatitis, pharyngitis, cervicaladenitis syndrome is linked to dysregulated monocyte IL-1β production. J Allergy ClinImmunol. 2013;131(6):1635–43.
11. Stojanov S, Lapidus S, Chitkara P, et al. Periodicfever, aphthous stomatitis, pharyngitis, and adenitis (PFAPA) is a disorder of innate immunity and Th1 activation responsive to IL-1 blockade. Proc Natl Acad Sci USA. 2011;108(17):7148–53.
12. Theodoropoulou K, Vanoni F, Hofer M. Periodic fever, aphthous stomatitis, pharyngitis, and cervical adenitis (PFAPA) syndrome: a review of the pathogenesis. Curr Rheumatol Rep. 2016;18(4):18.
13. Kubota K, Ohnishi H, Teramoto T, et al. Clinical and genetic characterization of Japanese sporadic cases of periodic fever, aphthous stomatitis, pharyngitis and adenitis syndrome from a single medical center in Japan. J Clin Immunol. 2014;34(5):584–93.
14. Cazzato M, Neri R, Possemato N, et al. A case of adult periodicfever, aphthous stomatitis, pharyngitis, and cervical adenitis (PFAPA) syndrome associated with endocapillary proliferative glomerulonephritis. Clin Rheumatol. 2013;1:S33–6.
15. Yazgan H, Keleş E, Yazgan Z, et al. C-reactive protein andprocalcitoninduringfebrilattacks in PFAPA syndrome. Int J Pediatr Otorhinolaryngol. 2012;76(8):1145–7.
16. Colotto M, Maranghi M, Durante C, et al. PFAPA syndrome in a young adult with a history of tonsillectomy. Intern Med. 2011;50(3):223–5.

17. Kraszewska-Głomba B, Szymańska-Toczek Z, Szenborn L. Procalcitonin and C-reactive protein-based decision tree model for distinguishing PFAPA flares from acute infections. Bosn J Basic Med Sci. 2016;16(2):157–61.
18. Tekin M, Toplu Y, Kahramaner Z, et al. The mean platelet volume levels in children with PFAPA syndrome. Int J Pediatr Otorhinolaryngol. 2014;78(5):850–3.
19. Yamazaki T, Hokibara S, Shigemura T, et al. Markedly elevated CD64 expressions on neutrophils and monocytes are useful for diagnosis of periodic fever, aphthous stomatitis, pharyngitis, and cervicaladenitis (PFAPA) syndrome during flares. Clin Rheumatol. 2014;33(5):677–83.
20. Harel L, Hashkes PJ, Lapidus S, et al. The first international conference on periodic fever, aphthous stomatitis, pharyngitis, adenitis syndrome. J Pediatr. 2018;193:265–74.
21. Hashkes PJ, Toker O. Autoinflammatory syndromes. Pediatr Clin North Am. 2012;59:447–70.
22. Kara A. Periyodik Ateş Sendromları. Turkiye Klinikleri J Pediatr Sci. 2011;7(4):140–5.
23. Wurster VM, Carlucci JG, Feder HM Jr, et al. Long-term follow-up of children with periodic fever, aphthous stomatitis, pharyngitis, and cervical adenitis syndrome. J Pediatr. 2011;159(6):958–64.
24. Onderka CE, Ridder GJ. Periodic fever, aphthous stomatitis, pharyngitis and cervical adenitis (PFAPA syndrome) Trea. Dtsch Med Wochenschr. 2012;137(10):471–5.
25. Padeh S, Stoffman N, Berkun Y. Periodic fever accompanied by aphthous stomatitis, pharyngitis and cervical adenitis syndrome (PFAPA syndrome) in adults. Isr Med Assoc J. 2008;10(5):358–60.
26. Cantarini L, Vitale A, Bartolomei B, et al. Diagnosis of PFAPA syndrome applied to a cohort of 17 adults with unexplained recurrent fevers. Clin Exp Rheumatol. 2012;30(2):269–71.
27. Kutsuna S, Ohmagari N, Tanizaki R, et al. The first case of adult-onset PFAPA syndrome in Japan. Mod Rheumatol. 2016;26(2):286–7.
28. Hernández-Rodríguez J, Ruíz-Ortiz E, Tomé A, et al. Clinical and genetic characterization of the autoinflammatory diseases diagnosed in an adult reference center. Autoimmun Rev. 2016;15(1):9–15.
29. Cantarini L, Vitale A, Sicignano LL, et al. Diagnostic criteria for adult-onset periodic fever, aphthous stomatitis, pharyngitis, and cervical adenitis (PFAPA) syndrome. Front Immunol. 2017;8:1018.
30. Rigante D, Vitale A, Natale MF, et al. A comprehensive comparison between pediatric and adult patients with periodic fever, aphthous stomatitis, pharyngitis, and cervical adenopathy (PFAPA) syndrome. Clin Rheumatol. 2017;36(2):463–8.
31. Lopalco G, Rigante D, Vitale A, et al. Canakinumab efficacy in refractory adult-onset PFAPA syndrome. Int J Rheum Dis. 2017;20(8):1050–1.
32. Cantarini L, Vitale A, Galeazzi M, et al. A case of resistant adult-onset periodic fever, aphthous stomatitis, pharyngitis and cervicaladenitis (PFAPA) syndrome responsive to anakinra. Clin Exp Rheumatol. 2012;30(4):593.
33. Vanoni F, Theodoropoulou K, Hofer M. PFAPA syndrome: a review on treatment and outcome. Pediatr Rheumatol Online J. 2016;14(1):38.
34. Rocco R. Periodic fever, aphthous stomatitis, pharyngitis and adenitis: PFAPA syndrome in Argentina. An Pediatr (Barc). 2011;74(3):161–7.
35. Ter Haar N, Lachmann H, Özen S, et al. Treatment of autoinflammatory diseases: results from the Eurofever Registry and a literature review. Ann Rheum Dis. 2013;72(5):678–85.
36. Wurster VM, Carlucci JG, Feder HM Jr, et al. Long-termfollow-up of children with periodic fever, aphthous stomatitis, pharyngitis, and cervical adenitis syndrome. J Pediatr. 2011;159(6):958–64.
37. ButbulAviel Y, Tatour S, GershoniBaruch R, et al. Colchicine as a therapeutic option in periodic fever, aphthous stomatitis, pharyngitis, cervical adenitis (PFAPA) syndrome. Semin Arthritis Rheum. 2016;45(4):471–4.
38. Tasher D, Stein M, Dalal I, et al. Colchicine prophylaxis for frequent periodic fever, aphthous stomatitis, pharyngitis and adenitis episodes. Acta Paediatr. 2008;97(8):1090–2.
39. Feder HM Jr. Cimetidine treatment for periodic fever associated with aphthous stomatitis, pharyngitis and cervical adenitis. Pediatr Infect Dis J. 1992;11(4):318–21.

40. Mahamid M, Agbaria K, Mahamid A, et al. Vitamin D linked to PFAPA syndrome. Int J Pediatr Otorhinolaryngol. 2013;77(3):362–4.
41. Stagi S, Bertini F, Rigante D, et al. Vitamin D levels and effects of vitamin D replacement in children with periodic fever, aphthous stomatitis, pharyngitis, and cervical adenitis (PFAPA) syndrome. Int J Pediatr Otorhinolaryngol. 2014 Jun;78(6):964–8.
42. Ali NS, Sartori-Valinotti JC, Bruce AJ. Periodicfever, aphthous stomatitis, pharyngitis, and adenitis (PFAPA) syndrome. Clin Dermatol. 2016;34(4):482–6.
43. Rigante D, Gentileschi S, Vitale A, et al. Evolving frontiers in the treatment of periodic fever, aphthous stomatitis, pharyngitis, cervical adenitis (PFAPA) syndrome. Isr Med Assoc J. 2017;19(7):444–7.
44. Buongiorno A, Pierossi N. Effectiveness of pidotimod in combination with bacterial lysates in the treatment of the PFAPA (periodicfever, aphthous stomatitis, pharyngitis, and cervicaladenitis) syndrome. Minerva Pediatr. 2015;67(3):219–26.

Preseptal Cellulitis and Other Facial Skin Infections in Children

58

Bilge Aldemir Kocabaş, Ergin Çiftçi, and Tobias Tenenbaum

58.1 Introduction

Facial infections in the pediatric age group are very common. Understanding these infections is important for improving patient outcomes and treating patients. Insect bites, traumatic injuries, viruses, and rarely bacteremia can be initiating causes. Comprehensive patient history and physical examination for diagnosis are important as in all diseases. Although preseptal cellulitis is localized in the periorbital and adjacent structures, other facial infections are not specific to the face. Other facial infections can be classified into two categories as purulent and nonpurulent. Impetigo, furuncles, and carbuncles are all defined in the purulent infection class. Cellulitis, erysipelas, and necrotizing fasciitis are each one, examples of nonpurulent infection. As bacterial infections, fungi and viruses such as enterovirus, herpes simplex virus (HSV), and varicella-zoster virus (VZV) can also be causative agents for facial infections. In all these circumstances, pathogenic microorganisms harm surrounding tissues and lead to an inflammatory reaction presented as erythema, warmth, and pain.

B. A. Kocabaş (✉)
Section of Pediatric Infectious Diseases, Antalya Training and Research Hospital, University of Health Sciences, Antalya, Turkey

E. Çiftçi
Division of Pediatric Infectious Diseases, Department of Pediatrics, Faculty of Medicine, Ankara University, Ankara, Turkey

T. Tenenbaum
Division of Pediatric Infectious Diseases, University Children's Hospital Mannheim, Heidelberg University, Mannheim, Germany

58.2   Preseptal (Periorbital) Cellulitis

Timely diagnosis and appropriate therapy are necessary to reduce the serious complications in orbital infections. The terms "periorbital cellulitis" or "preseptal cellulitis" are used as an infection in the eyelids that is restricted to anterior regions of orbital septum [1, 2]. The orbital septum is a thin stratum of fascia that extends vertically from the periosteum of the orbital margin to the tarsal plate within the eyelids. It supplies a barrier that reduces the spread of infectious agents into deeper orbital and retro-orbital structures. The eye's anatomy has a critical role in the spreading of infection from nearby tissues [1]. Veins draining the ethmoid and maxillary sinuses, orbit, skin of the eye, and periorbital tissues create a valveless anastomosis. The venous system of the orbit facilitates the spreading of infection to surrounding structures such as the cavernous sinus [3]. In a close anatomical connection, the frontal sinus composes the upper wall of the orbit, while the maxillary sinus composes the inferior wall. The frontal maxillary process, lacrimal bone, lamina papyracea of the ethmoid bone, and a part of the sphenoid bone are all composed of the medial wall of the orbit. Infection in the mucosa of paranasal sinuses can spread to the bone and intra-orbital contents. The septum is an effective barrier to prevent the extension of infection to the orbit [4–8].

While the incidence of preseptal cellulitis is higher than orbital cellulitis, both are more frequently seen in children than in adults [1]. Orbital cellulitis is more severe than preseptal cellulitis and it can cause serious complications such as loss of vision, meningitis, intracranial abscess, cavernous sinus thrombosis, and even death [2, 5]. Subperiosteal abscess, orbital abscess, orbital cellulitis, cavernous sinus thrombosis, pan ophthalmitis, and endophthalmitis are posterior infections of the orbital septum and can cause eye swelling.

Clinical manifestations are very suggestive for the diagnosis of preseptal cellulitis. The eyelid edema and hyperemia without proptosis are usually diagnostic for preseptal cellulitis. But sometimes, edema can make it difficult to evaluate eye movements and proptosis in some patients with intense eyelid swelling. Radiologic examinations are indicated in these cases [1, 5, 7].

In a patient with cellulitis on the eyelids and around, the clinical examination should be fulfilled carefully. If ocular movement and pupil functions are normal and no proptosis exists, preseptal cellulitis should be considered. Computed tomography (CT) and magnetic resonance imaging (MRI) demonstrate eyelids edema and inflammation of subcutaneous tissues anterior to the orbital septum; however, CT is commonly recommended to be restricted only in the cases with suspected orbital cellulitis. Posterior involvement of the orbital septum is suggestive of orbital cellulitis. Preseptal cellulitis can spread posteriorly to the septum if left untreated. Prompt initiated antibiotic therapy and monitoring for signs of sepsis can achieve to prevent complications and spread of infection [7–10].

Preseptal cellulitis is common in the pediatric age group and can be originated from bacteremia, sinusitis, trauma, or infected wound (e.g., pyoderma, hordeolum, conjunctivitis, dacryocystitis, insect bite) (Fig. 58.1) [1–3]. In the etiology of periorbital cellulitis, Haemophilus influenzae type b (Hib) was the most frequent

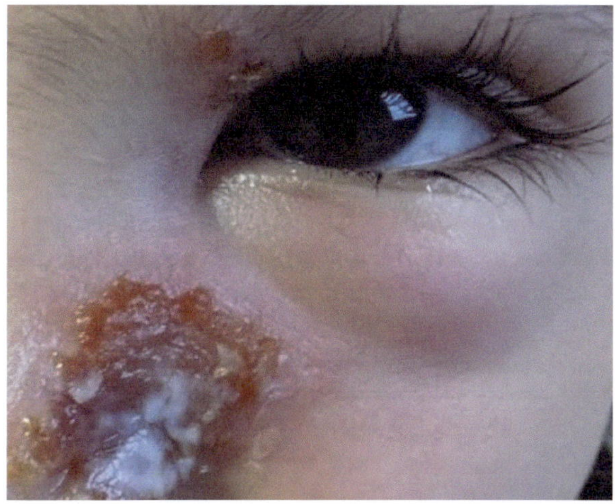

Fig. 58.1 Preseptal cellulitis secondary to bullous impetigo (Courtesy Bilge Aldemir Kocabaş, MD)

microorganism before developing the Hib vaccine. Currently, *Streptococcus pyogenes* (group A β-hemolytic streptococci [GABHS]), *Streptococcus pneumoniae,* and *Staphylococcus aureus* are the common etiologic agents [1, 3, 7].

Infectious sources of preseptal cellulitis can be classified into three categories: the first is localized infections belongs to the conjunctiva, eyelids, or contiguous structures (conjunctivitis, dacryocystitis, dacryoadenitis, chalazion, impetigo, traumatic bacterial cellulitis, etc.), the second is hematogenous dissemination the pathogens of the nasopharynx to the periorbital tissues, and the third one is acute sinusitis [1, 5, 10, 11].

Typical symptoms of preseptal cellulitis are unilateral ocular pain, erythema, and eyelid swelling. Chemosis (conjunctival swelling) may be seen in severe cases. Painful eye movements, restricted ocular motility, and proptosis are the findings of deeper orbital involvement and are absent in cases with preseptal cellulitis. These symptoms are concerned with soft tissue infection behind the orbital septum, called "orbital cellulitis" [1, 12–15].

Even though preseptal cellulitis is a more different clinical form from orbital cellulitis, these circumstances might often be confused or seen concomitantly. Clinical symptoms and physical examination findings are mostly helpful in the differential diagnosis. Occasionally, it is hard to distinguish preseptal cellulitis and early-stage orbital cellulitis according to physical examination findings. For the reason that the eyelid connective tissue structure is so weak, in case of infection, mild proptosis may not be noticed on account of significant edema around the eyes [2, 5, 8]. If the eye movements could not be evaluated due to severe eyelid edema, it is suggested that these patients should be given therapy as orbital cellulitis until differentiate the diagnosis. For ruling out the diagnosis of orbital cellulitis, CT should be performed. Radiological imaging methods take a crucial role in identifying the orbital infection size and complications and determining the most proper procedure in the treatment [1, 2, 9, 16]. Magnetic resonance imaging is beneficial for the diagnosis of abscesses but it is generally insufficient for bone tissue. Thus, CT is the method of radiology of choice preferred in the diagnose of orbital infections [13–16].

58.2.1 Post-traumatic Preseptal Cellulitis

Puncture wounds on the face or scalp are the most responsible etiologies for post-traumatic preseptal cellulitis [1, 3, 8]. It also may occur after blunt trauma without an obvious entry wound. Although *S. pyogenes* and *S. aureus* are the most frequent causative agents, sometimes it is seen with polymicrobial etiology especially after dirty wounds. Other bacterial causes include anaerobes such as *Bacteroides, Peptococcus*, and *Peptostreptococcus*. Infection by aerobic gram-negative bacilli is uncommon. *Pasteurella multocida* is a common organism in patients with post-traumatic preseptal cellulitis after cat and dog bites. Cellulitis frequency of secondary to methicillin-resistant S. aureus (MRSA) is increasing especially in endemic areas for MRSA [1–3, 10, 12].

Clinical symptoms and signs are predominantly determined by the interval and severity of the injury and the infecting agents. The involved area is erythematous, edematous, and tender [1–3]. The fluctuation of subcutaneous tissue may be seen if an abscess has developed. The swelling of the uninvolved contralateral eyelids may occur due to lymphedema. Vision is unaffected and ophthalmoplegia and proptosis are absent. Evaluation of the eye may be impossible as a result of severe eyelid edema in some patients. Neuroimaging is required in these cases to assess the globe and rule out orbital cellulitis. The ophthalmological examination is very important in patients with severe post-traumatic preseptal cellulitis because of the potential for globe injury [1, 3, 8, 16].

58.2.2 Nontraumatic Preseptal Cellulitis

Apart from the traumatic preseptal cellulitis, sinusitis is the main etiological factor for nontraumatic form in the majority of the cases (Fig. 58.2). The remaining predisposing factors are insect bites, conjunctival infections, or a dental abscess, which cause facial cellulitis [10–13].

Before the Hib vaccination program, this organism frequently was a cause of nontraumatic preseptal cellulitis in children [1]. *S. pneumoniae* is the most common cause of preseptal cellulitis in children, nowadays [6, 8, 12]. A variety of other bacterial agents may cause preseptal cellulitis, but they are seen less commonly. Other organisms, including *Trichophyton* spp., *Bacillus anthracis*, and *Mycobacterium tuberculosis* can be causative agents, rarely. Palpebral myiasis has also been reported as an etiological agent [8, 12, 17].

Adenovirus is another cause of preseptal cellulitis in children [1, 12, 18]. Unnecessary treatment with antibiotics generally is applied because it can mimic bacterial infection. The swelling of the lid may be prominent, but erythema usually is minimal. Preauricular lymphadenopathy often occurs in older children, and marked conjunctival hyperemia with or without chemosis and subconjunctival hemorrhage may be present. Photophobia also may be noticed in cases of concurrent punctate keratopathy. A history of recent contact with another infected person

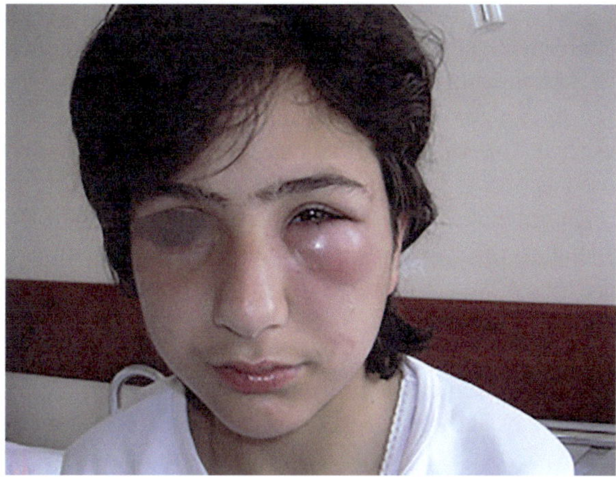

Fig. 58.2 Preseptal cellulitis secondary to sinusitis (Courtesy Ergin Çiftçi, MD)

frequently is noted. Care should be taken to prevent from spreading the infection to medical personnel, family members, and others [1, 3, 8].

Hospitalization is important for children with signs of systemic toxicity and younger than 1 year of age those with inadequate *H. influenzae* type b immunization. A sepsis workup should be initiated for children with signs of systemic toxicity and extremely young children. If orbital involvement is suspected and/or clinical diagnosis is unclear, the patient should be consulted with an ophthalmologist first, then a CT can be taken. Blood cultures in patients with preseptal cellulitis usually are negative. Also, it is difficult to obtain the microorganism in the infection site cultures. Even so, blood cultures in children under 2 years are more likely to be positive. The culture of conjunctival discharge is rarely having significant diagnostic benefits [1, 9, 12, 15].

58.2.3 Treatment of Preseptal Cellulitis

Preseptal cellulitis is common in the pediatric ages, and treatment with timely diagnosis and appropriate antimicrobial therapy does not result in any morbidity and mortality in almost all cases. Empirical antibacterial treatment with anti-staphylococcal and antistreptococcal antibiotics should be initiated, Also, mainly in severe and problematic cases, both aerobic and anaerobic coverage should be targeted.

Gram stain and culture of mucopurulent material will help identify the responsible agent. Radiological imaging modalities have a critical role to determine the spread of orbital infection and choose appropriate treatment methods. Oral antimicrobial therapy is sufficient in most cases. Outpatient treatment with oral antibiotics is reasonable for older, less acutely ill children. Antibiotic treatment should be continued for 7–10 days for preseptal cellulitis [8, 12, 14].

For oral antimicrobial treatment amoxicillin-clavulanic acid is the treatment of choice with a dose of 45 mg/kg per day divided into two doses, or 80–90 mg/kg per day when penicillin-resistant *Streptococcus pneumoniae* is a concern. Cefuroxime (20 mg/kg per day, divided into two doses), cefdinir (14 mg/kg per day, divided every 12 h), and cefpodoxime (10 mg/kg per day divided into two doses) can be used as other alternatives.

In general, more severe cases should always be treated intravenously first and switch to oral therapy after 3–5 days if the patient is afebrile for at least 24 h and otherwise have improved clinically. Intravenous treatment should be given for infants and those with signs of serious systemic infection. Ampicillin-sulbactam (150 to 200 mg/kg per day, divided into four doses) is preferred as the treatment of choice in parenteral therapy, but a cephalosporin such as cefuroxime (100–150 mg/ kg per day, in three doses) can also be used. In proven penicillin allergy, cefuroxime intravenously is an option, then is orally maintained or switch to cefpodoxime. If there is a suspicion of MRSA infection or hemodynamically instability, vancomycin can be added to therapy with doses of 40–60 mg/kg per day.

Tetanus prophylaxis can be administered according to the patient's immunization and trauma status. Surgical drainage of large abscesses may be required if a rapid response to antimicrobial therapy does not occur [1, 3, 13–16]. Intracranial expansion of infection should be suspected in patients with complaints of headache, and persistent fever despite intravenous antibiotics. When antibiotic treatment fails, other noninfectious causes should be explored. Some conditions such as lipoblastomatosis, Langerhans histiocytosis, and dermoid cysts can mimic preseptal cellulitis [19–21].

58.3 Other Facial Skin Infections

The epidermal skin layer provides the primary barrier to invasion by microorganisms and interface between the body and the environment. A dermal layer composed of collagen end elastic fibers gives skin its elasticity. Other cell elements, including mast cells, blood and lymph vessels, and cutaneous nerves may be involved in skin infections. The subcutaneous fat lamina is just underneath the dermis, contributes to thermal stability [22–25].

Colonization is defined as the presence of a microorganism on the skin without either clinical symptoms or signs of infection. Normal bacterial skin colonization is defined in two ways, resident and transient flora. Resident flora predominates and includes typical nonpathogens, such as *Propionibacterium acnes*, and *Staphylococcus epidermidis* in addition to other anaerobic diphtheroid and micrococci. Transient flora includes pathogenic organisms, such as streptococci, *S. aureus*, gram-negative enteric organisms, and *Candida albicans*. These pathogens usually are present in smaller amounts than the resident flora and can be removed by skin cleansing. Damaged skin, contact with animate and inanimate environmental sources, and exposure to antimicrobial agents or indwelling devices can modify the skin flora and predispose to infection by the resident or acquired transient flora. Predisposing factors to infection are preexisting skin disease, poor hygiene, minor trauma, and impaired host immunity [26–28].

Bacterial facial skin infections are classified according to the involved anatomical layer: (a) for the epidermis infection; impetigo, (b) infection of the superficial dermis; folliculitis, (c) for the deep dermis infection; furuncles, carbuncles, and (d) infection of subcutaneous tissues; erysipelas, cellulitis, fasciitis.

58.3.1 Impetigo

Impetigo or pyoderma is a superficial skin infection that affects solely the epidermis. It is seen especially in summer due to insect bites, burns, chickenpox, and cutaneous injuries which are facilitating factors for the entry of microorganisms. It is common in children, especially on exposed body regions such as the legs and face [22, 28, 29]. Although *S. aureus* and *S. pyogenes* are the two most responsible microorganisms in the impetigo etiology, *S. aureus* is responsible for plenty of them. Impetigo generally onsets like a red macula, then transforms to vesicles which have cloudy fluid. The vesicles rupture and leave a thick, yellow-colored, and wet crust that is surrounded by the erythema. There are multiple lesions of various ages on the affected skin. Generally, patients with impetigo have no constitutional symptoms but are often accompanied by an inflammatory reaction of regional lymph nodes.

At the beginning of infection, the differential diagnosis may necessitate being made with vesicular skin lesions such as in VZV and HSV infections. However, in these infections, vesiculae usually contain whitish fluid and not pus, and transformation of lesions into the pustular and crusted stage is typical in impetigo [26–29]. Although impetigo has a mild clinical course it is quite contagious, and the child should be isolated until an effective treatment has been given. Impetigo lesions first begin on the face and then generally affect other parts of the body by scratching and touching with the fingers [22–25].

Two clinical types of impetigo as nonbullous and bullous exist. The nonbullous form is more common and typically occurs on the face and extremities. Initially, vesicles or pustules occur on reddened skin. Then, the vesicles or pustules rupture, and the characteristic honey-colored (yellow-brown) crusts are left. Both forms of impetigo have no or minimal pain, are not accompanied by erythema of the surrounding skin, and structural symptoms are usually absent. Itching may occur, most cases have regional adenopathy, and about half of the patients have leukocytosis.

Impetigo is often diagnosed according to the clinical appearance Gram-positive cocci in chains or clusters are seen in Gram stain procedures or *S. aureus* or *S. pyogenes* are isolated in cultures. Swab cultures are diagnostic for causative agents in a patient who has not taken antibiotics previously. Spontan resolution is possible without treatment, and cure is recorded within 2 weeks without scarring. Recurrent or persistent impetigo may be a warning for an immunodeficiency as chronic granulomatous disease (CGD) or an indication for a chronic nasal *S. aureus* carriage [22, 28–30].

58.3.1.1 Nonbullous Impetigo

The most common form of impetigo is nonbullous impetigo. Though *S. aureus* is the most frequently etiological organism, *S. pyogenes* (GABHS) can be responsible in some cases with nonbullous impetigo. Staphylococci usually spread from the nose to the normal face skin and cause infection. In contrast, the skin becomes colonized with GABHS within 10 days before impetigo occurred [1–3, 26]. *S. pyogenes* is colonized to the skin and triggered impetigo lesions and then may spread to the other skin regions. Both staphylococci and *S. pyogenes* can compose nonbullous impetigo and cannot be distinguished clinically unless microorganism cultured from the lesion. While *S. aureus* can be isolated from impetigo lesions in all ages in childhood, *S. pyogenes* is generally isolated from older children. Impetigo related to *S. pyogenes* is unconventional under 2 years of age, except in endemic areas. The staphylococcal types in nonbullous impetigo etiology are variable. While group 2 phage is generally not responsible for the nonbullous impetigo, it is associated with staphylococcal toxic shock syndrome (STSS) and staphylococcal scalded skin syndrome (SSSS). Several serotypes of *S. pyogenes* termed "impetigo strains" are different from those that cause pharyngitis, cause nonbullous impetigo (Fig. 58.3) [26–28, 31].

58.3.1.2 Bullous Impetigo

Bullous impetigo which primarily affects infants and young children is a bacterial skin infection. Whereas both *S. pyogenes* and *S. aureus* can be responsible for the etiology of nonbullous impetigo, bullous impetigo is almost always attributed to *S. aureus*; the majority of are from phage group II strains of *S. aureus* that produce exfoliative toxin A are responsible for bullous impetigo. This toxin induces loss of cell adhesion on the surface of the epidermis. Flaccid and transparent bullae, which have yellow-colored fluid, develop commonly on the face skin (Fig. 58.4). Bullae are quite fragile and can easily rupture. After rupturing, they leave a thin

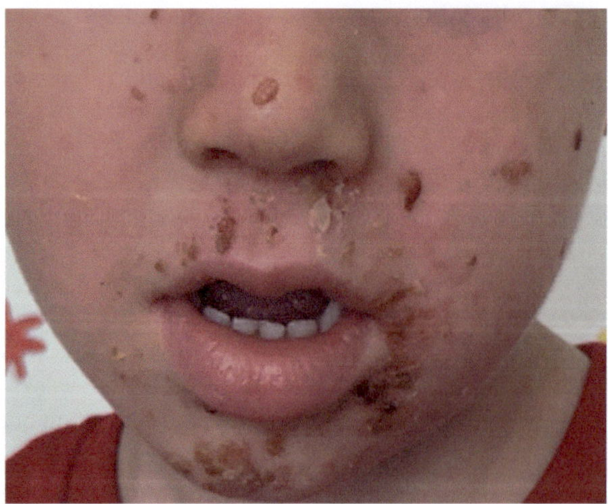

Fig. 58.3 Nonbullous impetigo caused by *Streptococcus pyogenes* (Courtesy Bilge Aldemir Kocabaş, MD)

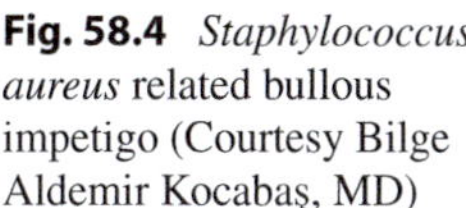

Fig. 58.4 *Staphylococcus aureus* related bullous impetigo (Courtesy Bilge Aldemir Kocabaş, MD)

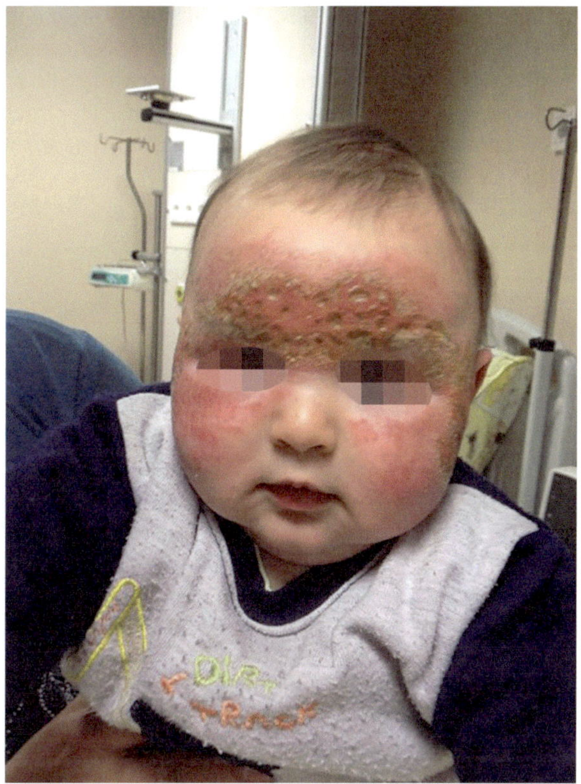

brown-colored crust. They have generally no surrounding erythema and regional adenopathy. Lesions of bullous impetigo develop on intact skin unlike those of non-bullous impetigo [22, 28, 29, 31].

Obtaining wound cultures from an intact blister or moist plaque should be done for detecting the etiological agent. If the patient appears ill, blood cultures should also be taken. Pathology of bullous impetigo is characterized by edema in the papillary dermis with a mixed inflammation of lymphocytes and neutrophils, and acantholytic cells in the subcorneal area of the epidermis. These findings as similar to those in pemphigus lesions. For that reason, if staphylococci cannot be cultured from the bullae, it may be difficult to differentiate diagnosis. Histopathological findings of nonbullous impetigo are the same as the bullous form but blister formation is slight [22–26].

Especially in the case of unresponsive to treatment, other differential diagnoses should be considered. In the differential diagnosis; bullous mastocytosis, epidermolysis bullosa, herpetic infections, and scalded skin syndrome, burns, contact dermatitis, erythema multiforme, bullous dermatosis, pemphigus, and bullous pemphigoid should be kept in mind [24–26].

Local antiseptics such as octenidine, antimicrobial soaps with povidone-iodine or chlorhexidine, and additional zinc ointments with or without bacitracin are sufficient for limited lesions. Topically used fusidic acid cream can be applied in cases with more extensive lesions. Oral antibiotics such as amoxicillin-clavulanic acid are infrequently required. Oral therapy of bullous and nonbullous impetigo is suggested in patients with numerous lesions. Mupirocin can be applied for MRSA nasal carriage, but then also body washings (e.g., with Octenidin) need to be included, too [22–30].

58.3.2 Folliculitis

Folliculitis is an infection of hair follicles and adjacent tissues (Fig. 58.5). A more serious form of folliculitis caused by *S. aureus* is "folliculitis barbae." It is a recurrent inflammatory form that involves deeper and multiple hair follicles in the face and neck. Erythematous follicular pustules and papules develop, especially on the face and scalp. The upper lip and chin are mostly involved parts of the face. Papules can join and form plaques, and heal with scarring. *S. aureus* carriage is a predisposing factor for the development of folliculitis. This form is scarcely seen in childhood except for the adolescent period. Systemic symptoms are generally not seen in the course of the disease. That is why only local antiseptic measures are enough for treatment. Systemic antibiotherapy and eradication of nasal MRSA carriage are needed for the treatment of intractable cases [22–31].

"Hot tub folliculitis," which is caused by *P. aeruginosa*, is characterized by pruritic follicular macules, papules, and pustules. The organism can be cultured from the pus. Papules and pustules may progress to nodules that completely erythematous to violaceous 8–48 h after the exposure. This condition is related to especially poorly chlorinated hot tubs/whirlpools/swimming pools, and contaminated water slides [22–28]. The lesions show density in covered and moist regions of the body (in the distribution of the wet bathing suit, etc.). Identification of the distribution of

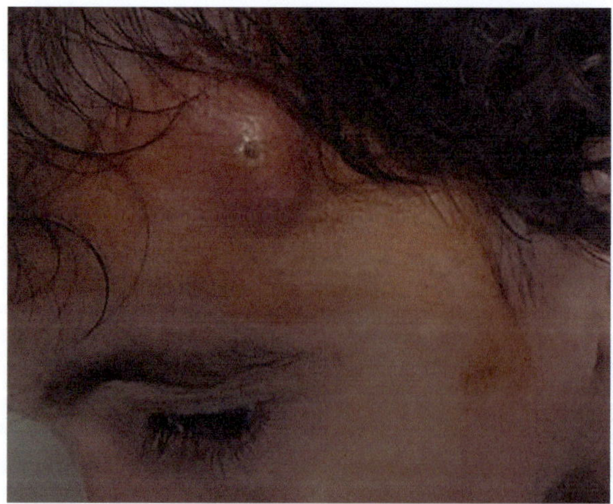

Fig. 58.5 Folliculitis and an abscess formation (Courtesy Bilge Aldemir Kocabaş, MD)

folliculitis may help to diagnosis. While folliculitis produced by *S. aureus* is limited to the scalp and/or face, Pseudomonas folliculitis generally occurs on exposed areas of skin to contaminated water. Fever, malaise, and lymphadenopathy can occur in some patients. The lesions usually regress spontaneously in 1–2 weeks and heal with hyperpigmentation. In cases with hot tub folliculitis that does not resolve spontaneously after several weeks and also cases with constitutional symptoms, systemic antibiotics effective to *P. aeruginosa* (such as ciprofloxacin 20 mg/kg/day, in adolescents) should be administered. As pseudomonas folliculitis can cause serious complications in immunocompromised children, they should be kept away from hot tubs [22–28].

58.3.3 Furuncles and Carbuncles

Furuncle (boil) is a painful and suppurative lesion of hair follicles. It is seen especially in the areas rich in hair follicles as the face, neck, axilla, and buttocks. The most common causative agent in carbuncles and furuncles is *S. aureus*. Conditions that abrade the dermis can facilitate microorganisms to invade the perifollicular skin (Fig. 58.6). If the lesion progress into the dermis and subcutaneous tissues, it can serve as a focus for cellulitis and skin abscess. Obesity, preexisting dermatitis, hyperhidrosis, anemia, malnutrition, diabetes, and other immunodeficiency states are predisposing factors for the development of furuncle. Community-acquired *S. aureus* infections can be spread by skin contact during sports activities and sharing personal hygiene equipment [22–32].

The lesion onsets as a red painful nodule and quickly forms into a hot, painful, raised from the surface, and indurated lesion within a diameter of 1–2 cm. It is characterized by a yellowish area in the center. When the lesion ruptures (either spontaneous or surgical), a yellowish, purulent, and creamy necrotic discharge drains from

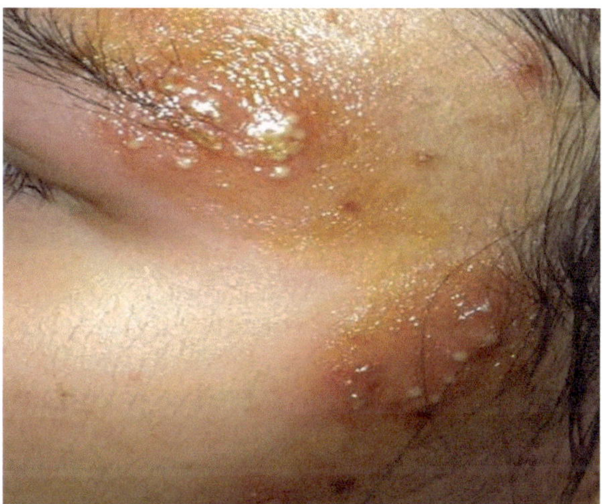

Fig. 58.6 *Staphylococcus aureus* related furuncle (Courtesy Bilge Aldemir Kocabaş, MD)

the lesion. Autoinoculation and secondary foci can frequently occur. As generally any systemic symptoms do not accompany the infection, local ointments are usually adequate. In recurrent episodes, nasal culture for *S. aureus* carriage and topical eradication treatment may be needed. When furuncles onset around the upper lip or nares, they could be severe by causing septic situations as cavernous sinus thrombophlebitis. As a consequence, furuncles in these sites recommended being treated with high dose systemic antibiotics intravenously including flucloxacillin (125–250 mg every 6 h), cefazolin (100–150 mg/kg/day divided into three or four doses), or (cefuroxime, 75 to 100 mg/kg/day divided into three doses) [22–28].

Carbuncle is a kind of skin infection but is deeper-seated different from the furuncles. Several hair follicles are affected and infection progresses into the deep locations of subcutaneous tissue with coalescence and spreading. Inflammatory reactions in surrounding connective tissue are accompanied by a group of follicles accompanied with multiple drainage points. Fever and leukocytosis secondary to inflammation and also bacteremia can be seen. Carbuncles are mostly localized at the basement of the neck. The lesions leave a firm, hypertrophic, and violet-colored scar while healing. Fever and malaise are usually existing. In cases with bacteremia, parenteral antibiotic therapy is required. Wearing loose-fitting clothes and regular bathing with antimicrobial soaps can be preventive for furuncle and carbuncle. Application of a hot and moist compress and an incision when indicated are recommended for drainage of lesions. In the treatment of large or numerous furuncles and carbuncles, it is recommended that given systemic antibiotics according to culture and sensitivity testing results. Incision or drainage is the suggested treatment choice for large furuncles, carbuncles, and abscesses [22–29, 32].

58.3.4 Erysipelas

Erysipelas is superficial cellulitis of the skin involving lymphatic vessels. It is characterized by a bright erythematous plaque with a distinct, elevated border. The affected area is demarcated with a sharp line from the unaffected skin [22–27, 32–34]. Erysipelas most often involves the face, although the trunk or lower extremity can be affected. The affected skin is tender and warm and may have a peau d'orange appearance (Fig. 58.7). Large, tender bullae might be seen in the erythematous zone. The patient usually is toxic and highly febrile. Cellulitis rapidly enlarges on the affected skin in a few hours with the demarcation line. Erysipelas is most commonly seen in young children and the elderly. GABHS is the most common ctiological organism for erysipelas [22, 32, 34].

Histopathologic findings include intense edema and vascular dilation of the dermis and uppermost subcutaneous tissue. Involvement of lymphatic channels and tissue spaces with polymorphonuclear leukocytes is a typical finding. Surgical wounds or disruption of skin barriers can be a source of entry; however, the initial lesion cannot be seen in some patients [22–27].

The diagnosis generally is recognized on clinical grounds, and group A β-hemolytic streptococcus traditionally has been isolated by aspiration of the

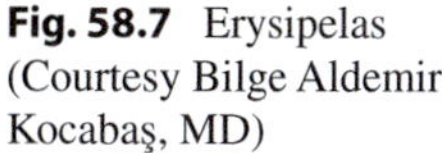

Fig. 58.7 Erysipelas (Courtesy Bilge Aldemir Kocabaş, MD)

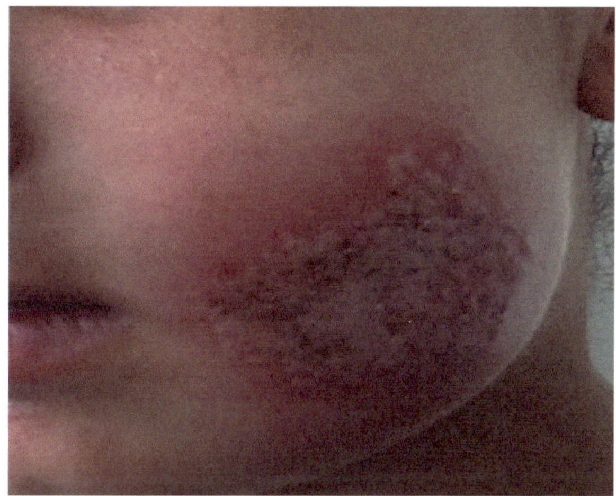

advancing margin of the lesion. A few case reports have identified other streptococci (including groups B, C, and G), *Moraxella* spp., *H. influenzae*, and *S. pneumoniae* as etiologic agents [22, 25, 33].

Erysipelas has a classic clinical appearance, and appropriate diagnosis and therapy result in a prompt clinical response in most cases. Appropriate empirical antibiotic treatment includes amoxicillin-clavulanic acid (45 mg/kg per day divided into two doses; dosing in severe infections or when penicillin-resistant *S. pneumoniae* is a concern is 80 to 90 mg/kg per day divided into two doses), cefpodoxime (10 mg/kg/day divided into two doses), cefdinir (14 mg/kg/day, divided every 12 h), cephalexin (25–50 mg/kg/day divided into 3–4 doses), and cefuroxime (30 mg/kg/day divided into two doses) [32, 33].

58.3.5 Facial Cellulitis

Facial cellulitis is an entity different from preseptal or orbital cellulitis and is divided into two forms as nonodontogenic and odontogenic. Trauma, skin, or sinus infections are included in the etiology of nonodontogenic facial cellulitis. But it sometimes can be idiopathic. Odontogenic facial cellulitis is originated from the dentition and its adjacent periodontal structure (Fig. 58.8). Correct and early diagnosis of the infection source prevents subsequent complications [22–28].

The diagnosis of cellulitis is made when the subcutaneous tissues and dermis are involved in a clinical process manifested as localized edema, erythema, warmth, and tenderness of the tissues. The leading edge of the involved site may be notable, but it is not raised and well-demarcated as in erysipelas. Infection usually is caused by *S. aureus* and GABHS; however, infection also is caused by *Streptococcus agalactiae* (group B streptococcus) especially in neonates, and *S. pneumoniae*. Frequently, patients have a history of antecedent trauma at the site of involvement. If possible, getting local cultures are recommended, but in practice, it rarely is

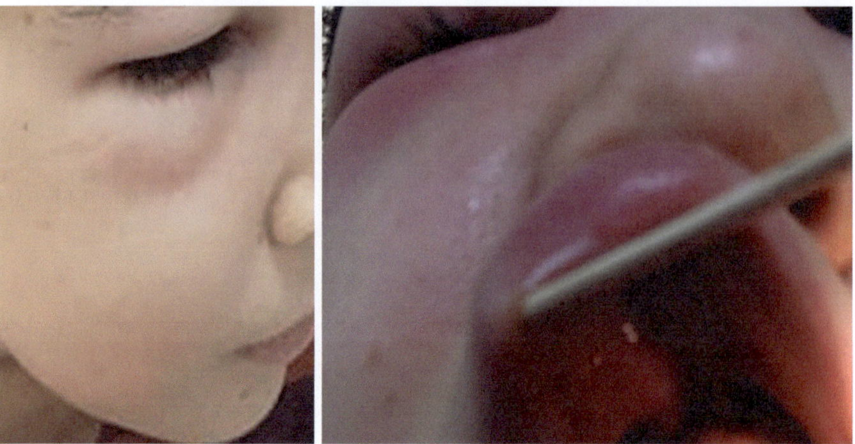

Fig. 58.8 Facial cellulitis due to a dental abscess (Courtesy Bilge Aldemir Kocabaş, MD)

performed. Blood cultures are valuable in patients with the disease caused by *S. pneumoniae, S. agalactiae,* and *H. influenzae* type b [22–28, 32–34].

Group B streptococcal cellulitis occurs in neonates and generally is seen as part of invasive, late-onset disease. Unilateral involvement of the face or submandibular sites occurs most commonly. When cellulitis occurs in an infant younger than 3 months old, group B streptococcal bacteremia should be suspected, even if other signs of systemic infection are absent [22–26, 32, 33].

H. influenzae type b cellulitis often involves the face of the infants. A violaceus hue of the cellulitic area, which some researchers thought to be pathognomonic, might be observed. This process nearly always was the result of hematogenous seeding by *H. influenzae* type b, and meningitis occurred in 15 to 20 percent of such patients [22–27].

Cellulitis can be treated with antibiotics effective against *S. aureus* and *S. pyogenes*. Deeper or necrotizing infections, poor adherence to therapy, severely immunocompromised conditions, or failing the outpatient treatment are the indications of hospitalization and parenterally antibiotherapy including cefazolin, 100–150 mg/kg/day divided into three or four doses; flucloxacillin, 125–250 mg every 6 h; or ceftriaxone, 50 mg/kg per dose once or twice per day intravenously [32–37].

58.3.6 Necrotizing Fasciitis

Necrotizing fasciitis is an infection that affects the subcutaneous tissues and fascia and resulted in necrosis. The rapidly progressive bacterial infection leads to a fulminant course and high mortality rate [22–25, 38, 39]. The infection quickly invades the subcutaneous tissue and also superficial muscle fascia and finally causes extensive necrosis. A good outcome is possible only with prompt and aggressive (both medical and surgical) treatment.

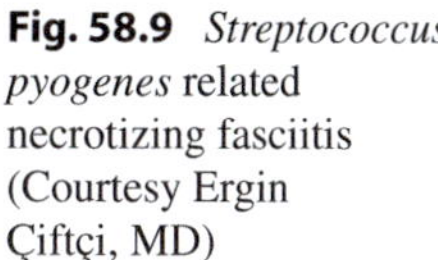

Fig. 58.9 *Streptococcus pyogenes* related necrotizing fasciitis (Courtesy Ergin Çiftçi, MD)

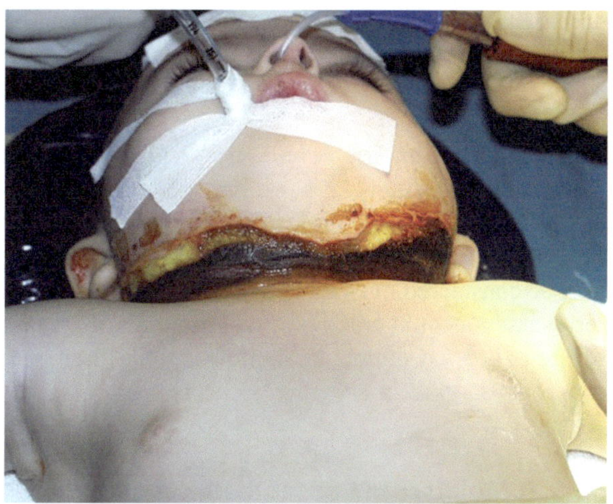

Necrotizing fasciitis seen in children commonly is caused by *S. pyogenes*. Skin trauma caused by varicella (Fig. 58.9), burns, or eczema facilitates infection. An association has been noted among varicella, ibuprofen use, and invasive *S. pyogenes* infection, but there is no sufficient evidence for confirming this connection. Congenital or acquired immunodeficiencies are risk factors for necrotizing fasciitis [22, 38, 39].

In the children with necrotizing fasciitis, a high degree of fever and irritability are indispensable clinical findings. Swelling of soft tissue usually is seen, but the erythema may be subtle. There is intense pain with palpation of the involved skin in the physical examination. Within the first 24–48 h after onset of the infection, bleb formation and a dusky appearance occur on the involved area due to thromboses and ischemia. Skin necrosis is seen in the later phase and is related to a poor prognosis. Identification of the signs of toxic shock syndrome is critical because mortality rates are high in patients with fasciitis. Although *S. pyogenes* is a unique pathogen in the etiology, most patients have a mixed infection with other aerobes (MRSA, groups B and C streptococci) and anaerobes (*Clostridium* spp.) [22, 30, 36–39].

As the findings are not specific in the early phase of necrotizing fasciitis, the diagnosis should not be made according to the appearance of the involved site. Radiographs are generally normal and not diagnostic. MRI is the preferred method for imaging soft tissue. MRI helps demonstrate the edema of the soft tissue infiltrating the fascial planes. If it is impossible to be performed MRI in a short time, surgical intervention should not be postponed. Laboratory findings of toxic shock syndrome should be well known and investigated in any pediatric patient with fasciitis. A microbiological diagnosis can be made by isolating bacteria from blood, or tissue culture [22, 36, 38].

Surgical debridement of necrotic tissue is the most important part of the management of necrotizing fasciitis, and an increased mortality rate is inevitable when debridement is delayed more than 24 h. Repeated examinations should be evaluated during the following 24–48 h for additional surgical debridements. Careful administration of fluids, pain control, management of multisystem organ failure, and administration of proper parenteral antimicrobial therapy should be initiated immediately.

Acceptable empiric antibiotic regimens include intravenous penicillin (50.000–100.000 units/kg per dose every 6 h) or ceftriaxone (75–100 mg/kg per day) plus clindamycin for its antitoxin and other effects against toxin-elaborating strains of streptococci and staphylococci. The use of intravenous immunoglobulin may be considered in cases of toxic shock syndrome-associated fasciitis. Elaborate serial assessment is crucial for determining the treatment response. Persistent and severe pain is an important sign of ongoing tissue necrosis and an indication for additional surgical intervention [35–39].

58.3.7 Molluscum Contagiosum

Molluscum contagiosum is a common viral skin infection of children and adolescents, and Poxviruses are responsible for the disease [22–27, 40]. It is mostly seen in patients under 5–10 years old, although it can be seen at any age. The transmission route of disease is close contact. Replication and hyperplasia occur after viral entry to the cell following close contact. Typical lesions are 1–5 mm, dome-shaped, skin-colored or pink papules with a distinctive central umbilication. In children, molluscum contagiosum is seen most frequently on the face and neck. Periocular lesions may lead to secondary keratoconjunctivitis or trachoma. Atypical lesions of molluscum contagiosum are seen more commonly in acquired or other immuno-compromised states. Lesions in immunocompromised patients often are large, situated more deeply in the epidermis, and may number in hundreds. Patients with atopic dermatitis may be predisposed to develop more severe molluscum contagiosum infection [40–42].

Although molluscum contagiosum often persists in immunocompromised patients, they generally resolve spontaneously from several months to 3–5 years in healthy children. Treatment can be considered in patients with intractable and diffuse infections. No definitive treatment choices are available for molluscum contagiosum. Most treatments, similar to those used for warts, are destructive. Destructive treatment can result in adverse effects such as irritation, pain, dyspigmentation, or scarring. These should be considered when making a treatment decision [22, 41, 42].

58.3.8 Herpes Simplex Virus Infections

Herpes simplex virus (HSV) infection is a self-limited, painful viral infection. It is characterized by grouped vesicles on an erythematous base and mostly recurrent dermatitis. Mucocutaneous involvement is common. Though HSV type 1 is usually associated with orofacial disease, HSV type 2 is more related to genital infection [25–27, 43, 44]. After the acquisition of the virus from mucosal surfaces and abraded skin, primary infection occurs and the virus moves to the adjacent dorsal ganglia. Infection persists for life in a latent form until reactivation by factors such as trauma, stress, illness, immunosuppression, or sunlight.

Primary infection usually occurs in childhood, and it is generally asymptomatic. In symptomatic cases, the disease is called "primary herpetic gingivostomatitis," characterized by fever, malaise, submandibular adenopathy with tenderness, and vesicles and erosions on the buccal mucosa, tongue, the palate, or lips (Fig. 58.10). Primary herpetic gingivostomatitis is caused by HSV type 1 (HSV-1) [22, 27, 43].

After primary infection, the virus remains in the trigeminal ganglion in a latent form. If the responsible factors for reactivation occur HSV causes the disease called "herpes labialis." Reactive infection of latent virus is generally asymptomatic. When symptomatic, it causes "herpes labialis" which manifests as single or grouped vesicles in the perioral region, usually on the vermilion border of the lips (called "cold sores" or "fever blisters"). Prodromal symptoms in the form of itching and burning appear 12–24 h before the emergence of the vesicles. In recurrent cases, identification of these prodromal symptoms can be useful for promptly starting anti-viral therapy [43–45].

Conjunctivitis and keratitis can be seen during both primary and recurrent HSV infection. Disseminated infection and encephalitis are the causes of mortality and occur especially in neonates or immunocompromised cases [22, 27, 43].

Testing for HSV to confirm the diagnosis in the skin or mucosal lesions is rarely needed but should be performed if lesions occur in atypical areas (i.e., not labial herpes). PCR is the diagnostic test of choice for HSV infections. Serologic tests have limited indications in confirming the diagnosis of acute HSV-1 infection because antibody titers are not correlated with the presence of lesions. Viral culture, direct fluorescent antibody (DFA), and Tzanck smear are rarely used tests in the present day.

Intravenous acyclovir (30 mg/kg/day divided into three doses) is suggested especially in immunocompromised patients with cutaneous HSV infection. If herpes

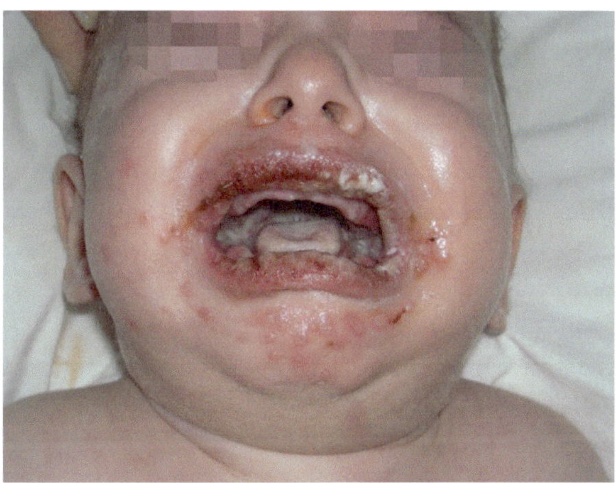

Fig. 58.10 Primary herpetic gingivostomatitis (Courtesy Bilge Aldemir Kocabaş, MD)

lesions in the face close to the eyes and/or nose, parenteral acyclovir therapy also should be preferred, even if there is no immunodeficiency status [43–45].

58.3.9 Varicella-Zoster Virus (VZV) Infections

Varicella-zoster virus (VZV) is one of the herpesviruses. VZV causes two clinical forms of the disease. Varicella (chickenpox) is the primary infection and causes latent infection. Herpes zoster (shingles) is the reactivated type of the disease and is characterized by localized skin lesions at the same dermatome. Varicella is characterized by pruritic, generalized, and vesicular rash typically consisting of 250 to 500 lesions in varying stages (papules, vesicles, crusting) (Fig. 58.11). After primary infection occurs, VZV spreads from mucosal and epidermal lesions to local sensory nerves. It remains latent in the dorsal ganglion cells of the sensory nerves. Reactivation of the latent infection (herpes zoster) can be seen more frequently in the elderly and immunosuppressive conditions, but also children.

Herpes zoster is a painful dermatomal dermatitis. Lesions begin with paresthesia and pain in a dermatome and develop into clusters of vesicles which are restricted in a unilaterally dermatomal region. Vesicles can be disseminated in immunocompromised patients. Some of the patients have malaise and fever. In more than half of the cases, virus activation can be seen in the thoracic dermatomes. The nasociliary nerve can be involved in the tip and side of the nose (cranial nerve V) are affected [22, 46–49]. Only symptomatic treatment is sufficient in the majority of the patients. However, postherpetic neuralgia (ongoing dysesthesias and pain after the lesions) is important morbidity, especially in adults. It is rarely seen in children and zoster is generally associated with mild symptoms in this age group. Sometimes, adolescents can suffer from neuralgia unlike young children [47–49]. When the patient scratches the lesions, bacterial superinfection with agents of skin flora including *S. pyogenes* and *S. aureus* can develop.

Herpes zoster is mostly diagnosed based on its characteristic typical presentation. Diagnostic testing (e.g., serologic methods, polymerase chain reaction to detect VZV DNA from skin lesions, direct fluorescent antibody staining of VZV-infected cells) might be used for patients with atypical presentations or to rule out infection with herpes simplex virus. Acyclovir is required in patients with disseminated and ophthalmic zoster (Fig. 58.12) [45–49].

58.3.10 Tinea Faciei

Tinea faciei otherwise known as facial ringworm is a variant of ringworm that generally affects the face regions such as the forehead, nose, around the eyes, chin, and cheeks (Fig. 58.13). The disease commonly spread through direct contact with infected animals, infected people, contaminated objects, or the soil. Dermatophyte infections of the face in children are characterized by erythematous, scaly plaques

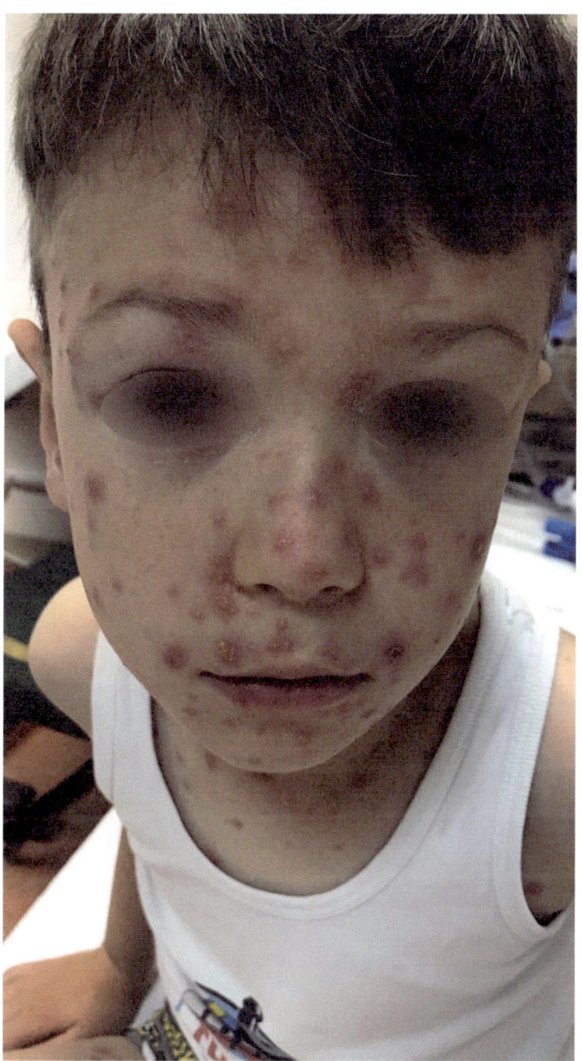

Fig. 58.11 Varicella vesicles (Courtesy Bilge Aldemir Kocabaş, MD)

that may be unilateral or occur in a "butterfly" distribution, mimicking cutaneous findings of systemic lupus erythematosus and other collagen vascular diseases. Differential diagnosis includes seborrheic, atopic, and contact dermatitis [19, 22, 27, 50].

Light microscopy examination with potassium hydroxide should show spores in infected skin scrapings from advancing margins of lesions. Fungal culture on Sabouraud dextrose agar provides a growth medium selective for dermatophytes and may aid in differentiating various species. Rarely, a biopsy may be required for a definitive diagnosis.

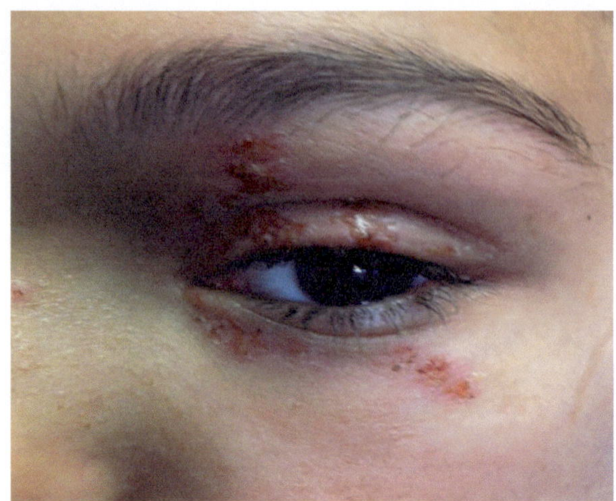

Fig. 58.12 Ophthalmic herpes zoster infection (Courtesy Bilge Aldemir Kocabaş, MD)

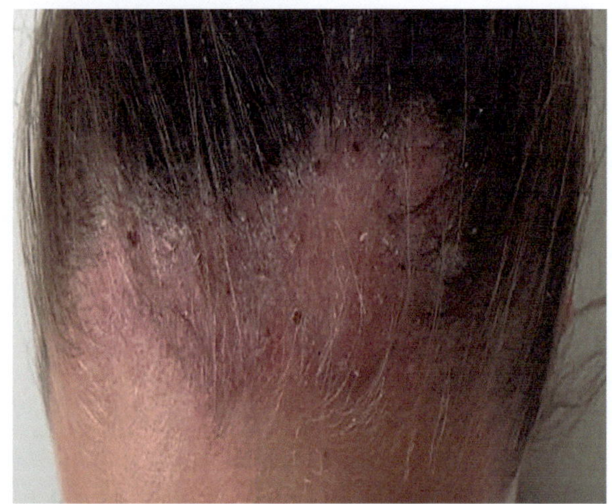

Fig. 58.13 Tinea faciei and capitis (Courtesy Bilge Aldemir Kocabaş, MD)

Localized lesions of tinea faciei, generally respond to a 2 to 4-week course of topical antifungal agents including terbinafine, butenafine, naftifine, azoles, ciclopirox, and tolnaftate. The severe or refractory disease may require oral antifungal medications including terbinafine tablets: 62.5 mg per day for 10–20 kg, 125 mg per day for 20–40 kg and 250 mg per day for above 40 kg, fluconazole 6 mg/kg once weekly, itraconazole 3–5 mg/kg per day, griseofulvin microsize 10 to 20 mg/kg per day or griseofulvin ultra-micro size 5 to 15 mg/kg per day [25, 27, 50].

58.3.11 Seborrheic Dermatitis

Seborrheic dermatitis is an infection characterized by desquamation and inflammation of areas rich from sebaceous glands such as the face, scalp, and upper trunk. Red lesions coated with white to yellowish and oily scales on the scalp, eyebrows, cheeks, nasolabial folds, and ears are typical [22, 27, 28, 51]. Complications such as secondary bacterial infection, lichenification, and otitis externa can be seen. This infection has usually a chronic course with exacerbations. Stress and conditions free from moisture are triggered factors for the relapses. There is a relationship between the disease and genetic factors. Also, studies indicate a significant role of Malassezia, lipophilic yeast, in seborrheic dermatitis. Impaired cell-mediated immunity is a risk factor for fungal survival on the skin [22, 27, 51].

In infants, seborrheic dermatitis has a self-limited course and generally resolves spontaneously in weeks to several months. The initial treatment may include simple skincare measures. In the more extensive or persistent cases, either a short course of low-potency topical corticosteroids once daily for 1 week or ketoconazole 2% cream or shampoo twice per week for 2 weeks can be used. Shampoos containing zinc pyrithione or selenium sulfide and other topical antimycotics are also effective and commonly used [22, 51].

58.3.12 Tuberculosis of the Skin

Immune deficiencies, malnutrition, and poor hygiene are predisposing factors for cutaneous tuberculosis. *Mycobacterium bovis*, *Mycobacterium tuberculosis*, and sometimes by bacillus Calmette-Guérin (BCG) vaccine can be responsible for the cutaneous disease [22–27]. In the conditions with the host immune system is weakened, mycobacteria multiply intracellularly within macrophages after entry of the mycobacterium to the skin. After that, progressive disease occurs.

If *M. bovis* or *M. tuberculosis* penetrates the skin or mucous membrane due to the trauma in an uninfected and nonimmune person primary cutaneous tuberculosis (tuberculous chancre) can occur [52, 53]. The disease is seen mostly on the lower extremities, face, and genitals. The initial lesion is seen after 3–4 weeks later from the break of the tissue and invasion with the organism. A reddish or brown papule progressively expands to get a shallow, hard, and demarcated ulcer. Sometimes satellite abscesses can be seen. Some lesions have a crust as in the impetigo, and others cluster and form verrucous at the margins. The primary lesion also can present as a painless ulcer on the palate, gingiva, or conjunctiva. Regional lymphadenopathy without pain may occur several weeks after the development of the primary lesion. Also, these can be accompanied by lymphadenitis, lymphangitis, and finally, perforation and ulceration of the skin surface called scrofuloderma. If the lesions are left untreated, they heal with scarring within a year. Also, they may reactivate, form lupus vulgaris, or, rarely, progress to the acute miliary form. Thus, anti-tuberculous therapy is indicated in these patients [22, 27, 52].

Lupus vulgaris is a chronic, rare, progressive form of cutaneous tuberculosis. It is seen in patients with a moderate to a high degree of tuberculin sensitivity due to the previous infection. It is more common in females than in males. This form of tuberculosis develops as a result of direct expansion from underlying joints or lymph nodes, through the hematogenous or lymphatic spread. Infrequently, it may be followed by inoculation of the BCG vaccine.

It frequently follows pulmonary tuberculosis or cervical adenitis. The majority of cases have lesions on the neck and head, frequently on the nose or cheek. Typically, the characteristic lesion is a plaque composed of nodules with apple jelly color when investigated by diascopy. Solitary or multiple lesions of variable size and form may develop. Ulceration and scarring are observed in the course of the disease. Spontaneous healing can be seen centrally. Lesions typically show recurrence within the area of atrophy.

The infection is chronic. Generally, the plaques persist and progress over many years. Deformities may be caused by vegetative masses and ulceration of the buccal, nasal, or conjunctival mucosa; the gingiva; the palate; or the oropharynx. Squamous cell carcinoma may develop after several years of lupus vulgaris. Small size lesions can be excised. Anti-tuberculous therapy (4-drug regimen include isoniazid, pyrazinamide, rifampin, and either ethambutol or streptomycin for at least two months following the complete resolution of skin lesions.) usually prevents further dissemination and induces involution [22, 52–55].

58.4 Conclusion

Various facial infections can be seen in the pediatric age group. The causes of these infections can range from insect bites and simple abrasions to serious traumatic injuries and the spread of infections from neighboring tissues. Facial infections can be caused by a variety of bacteria, fungi, and even viruses. Clinical findings vary from mild to severe depending on the affected anatomical region and the causative microorganism. Initial treatment should be selected taking into account the potential pathogens and the regional antimicrobial resistance pattern. Treatment should finally be guided according to antibiotic susceptibility results and clinical treatment response. With proper treatment, the prognosis is generally good.

References

1. Olitsky SE, Hug D, Plummer LS, et al. Orbital infections. In: Kliegman RM, Stanton BF, St Geme JW, Schor NF, editors. Nelson textbook of pediatrics. 21st ed. Philadelphia: Elsevier; 2020. p. 3391–3.
2. Baiu I, Melendez E. Periorbital and orbital cellulitis. JAMA. 2020;323:196.
3. Baht A. Ocular infections. In: Cherry JD, Harrison GJ, Kaplan SL, Steinbach WJ, Hotez PJ, editors. Feigin and Cherry's textbook of pediatric infectious diseases. 8th ed. Philadelphia: Elsevier; 2019. p. 578–97.
4. Sciarretta V, Dematte M, Fameti P, et al. Management of orbital cellulitis and subperiosteal orbital abscess in pediatric patients: a ten-year review. Int J Pediatr Otorhinolaryngol. 2017;96:72–6.
5. Aldemir-Kocabaş B, Karbuz A, Özdemir H, Çiftçi E, İnce E. Periorbital and orbital cellulitis: from presentation to outcome. J Pediatr Inf. 2014;8:148–52.
6. Williams KJ, Allen RC. Paediatric orbital and periorbital infections. Curr Opin Ophthalmol. 2019;30:349–55.

7. Gonzalez MO, Durairaj VD. Understanding pediatric bacterial preseptal and orbital cellulitis. Middle East Afr J Ophthalmol. 2010;17:134–7.

8. Wald ER. Periorbital and orbital infections. In: Long SS, Prober CG, Fischer M, editors. Principles and practice of pediatric infectious diseases. 5th ed. Philadelphia: Elsevier; 2018. p. 517–22.

9. Gupta S, Sharma S. Orbital cellulitis: defining a multidisciplinary approach as the need of the hour. Indian J Otolaryngol Head Neck Surg. 2019;71:464–9.

10. Mohd-Ilham I, Muhd-Syafi AB, Khairy-Shamel ST, Shatriah I. Clinical characteristics and outcomes of paediatric orbital cellulitis in Hospital Universiti Sains Malaysia: a five-year review. Singapore Med J. 2020;61:312–9.

11. Ekhlassi T, Becker N. Preseptal and orbital cellulitis. Dis Mon. 2017;63:30–2.

12. Seltz LB, Smith J, Durairaj VD, et al. Microbiology and antibiotic management of orbital cellulitis. Pediatrics. 2011;127:566–72.

13. Ryan JT, Preciado DA, Bauman N, et al. Management of pediatric orbital cellulitis in patients with radiographic findings of subperiosteal abscess. Otolaryngol Head Neck Surg. 2009;140:907–11.

14. Bedwell J, Bauman NM. Management of pediatric orbital cellulitis and abscess. Curr Opin Otolaryngol Head Neck Surg. 2011;19:467–73.

15. Cohen N, Erisson S, Anafy A, et al. Clinicians need to consider surgery when presented with some markers for severe paediatric orbital cellulitis. Acta Paediatr. 2020;109:1269–70.

16. Crosbie RA, Clement WA, Kubba H. Paediatric orbital cellulitis and the relationship to underlying sinonasal anatomy on computed tomography. J Laryngol Otol. 2017;131:714–8.

17. Missotten GS, Kalpoe JS, Bollemeijer JG, Schalij-Delfos NE. Myiasis of the upper eyelid. J AAPOS. 2008;12:516–7.

18. Kaufman HE. Adenovirus advances: new diagnostic and therapeutic options. Curr Opin Ophtalmol. 2011;22:290–3.

19. Kempster R, Ang GS, Galloway G, Beigi B. Langerhans cell histiocytosis mimicking preseptal cellulitis. J Pediatr Ophthalmol Strabismus. 2009;46:108–11.

20. Dutton JJ, Escaravage GK Jr, Fowler AM, Wright JD. Lipoblastomatosis: case report and review of the literature. Ophthal Plast Reconstr Surg. 2011;27:417–21.

21. Dizon M, Ozturk A, Redett RJ, Izbudak I. Neuroimaging findings in a child with dumbbell-shaped frontosphenoidal dermoid cyst presenting as preseptal cellulitis. Pediatr Radiol. 2009;39:850–3.

22. Diiorio DA, Humphrey SR. Cutaneous and fungal infections. In: Kliegman RM, Stanton BF, St Geme JW, Schor NF, editors. Nelson textbook of pediatrics. 21st ed. Philadelphia: Elsevier; 2020. p. 3549–68.

23. Pasternack MS, Swartz MN. Skin and soft tissue infections. In: Bennett JE, Dolin R, Blaser MJ, editors. Mandell, Douglas and Bennett's principles and practice of infectious diseases. 9th ed. Philadelphia: Elsevier; 2020. p. 1282–316.

24. Cherry JD. Skin infections. In: Cherry JD, Harrison GJ, Kaplan SL, Steinbach WJ, Hotez PJ, editors. Feigin and Cherry's textbook of pediatric infectious diseases. 8th ed. Philadelphia: Elsevier; 2019. p. 539–59.

25. Stevens DL, Bisno AL, Chambers HF, et al. Practice guidelines for the diagnosis and management of skin and soft tissue infections: 2014 update by the infectious diseases society of America. Clin Infect Dis. 2014;59:10–52.

26. Lawrence HS, Nopper AJ. Superficial bacterial skin infections and cellulitis. In: Long SS, Prober CG, Fischer M, editors. Principles and practice of pediatric infectious diseases. 5th ed. Philadelphia: Elsevier; 2018. p. 437–44.

27. Faergemann J, Dahlen G. Facial skin infections. Periodontology. 2009;49:194–209.

28. Sladden MJ, Johnston GA. Common skin infections in children. BMJ. 2004;329:95–9.

29. Dollani LC, Marathe KS. Impetigo/staphylococcal scalded skin disease. Pediatr Rev. 2020;41:210–2.

30. Kumar N, David MZ, Boyle-Vavra S, Sieth J, Daum RS. High Staphylococcus aureus colonization prevalence among patients with skin and soft tissue infections and controls in an urban emergency department. J Clin Microbiol. 2015;53:810–5.
31. Chang AY, Scheel A, Dewyer A, et al. Prevalence, clinical features and antibiotic susceptibility of group a streptococcal skin infections in school children in urban Western and northern Uganda. Pediatr Infect Dis J. 2019;38:1183–8.
32. Klotz C, Courjon J, Michelangeli C, Demonchy E, Ruimy R, Roger PM. Adherence to antibiotic guidelines for erysipelas or cellulitis is associated with a favorable outcome. Eur J Clin Microbiol Infect Dis. 2019;38:703–9.
33. Brindle R, Williams OM, Barton E, Featherstone P. Assessment of antibiotic treatment of cellulitis and erysipelas: a systematic review and meta-analysis. JAMA Dermatol. 2019;155:1033–40.
34. Allmon A, Deane K, Martin KL. Common skin rashes in children. Am Fam Physician. 2015;92:211–6.
35. Lane RD, Sandweiss DR, Corneli HM. Treatment of skin and soft tissue infections in a pediatric observation unit. Clin Pediatr (Phila). 2014;53:439–43.
36. Lin YT, Lu PW. Retrospective study of pediatric facial cellulitis of odontogenic origin. Pediatr Infect Dis J. 2006;25:339–42.
37. Schweinfurth JM. Demographics of pediatric head and neck infections in a tertiary care hospital. Laryngoscope. 2006;116:887–9.
38. Creech CB. Myositis, pyomyositis, and necrotizing fasciitis. In: Long SS, Prober CG, Fischer M, editors. Principles and practice of pediatric infectious diseases. 5th ed. Philadelphia: Elsevier; 2018. p. 473–9.
39. Zundel S, Lemaréchal A, Kaiser P, Szavay P. Diagnosis and treatment of pediatric necrotizing fasciitis: a systematic review of the literature. Eur J Pediatr Surg. 2017;27:127–37.
40. Alikhan A, Shwayder T. Molluscum contagiosum. In: Irvine AD, Hoeger PH, Yan AC, editors. Harper's textbook of pediatric dermatology. 3rd ed. Hong Kong: Wiley-Blackwell; 2011. p. 461–8.
41. Forbat E, Al-Niaimi F, Ali FR. Molluscum contagiosum: review and update on management. Pediatr Dermatol. 2017;34:504–15.
42. Van der Wouden JC, Van der Sande R, Kruithof EJ, Sollie A. Wa van Suijlekom-Smit L, Koning S Interventions for cutaneous molluscum contagiosum. Cochrane Database Syst Rev. 2017;17:CD004767.
43. Stanberry LR. Herpes simplex virus. In: Kliegman RM, Stanton BF, St Geme JW, Schor NF, editors. Nelson textbook of pediatrics. 21st ed. Philadelphia: Elsevier; 2020. p. 1701–8.
44. Caviness AC, Oelze LL, Saz UE, et al. Direct immunofluorescence assay compared to cell culture for the diagnosis of mucocutaneus herpes simplex virus infections in children. J Clin Virol. 2010;49:58–60.
45. Ahluwalia J, Han A, Kusari A, Eichenfield LF. Recurrent herpes labialis in the pediatric population: prevalence, therapeutic studies, and associated complications. Pediatr Dermatol. 2019;36:808–14.
46. Vrcek I, Choudhury E, Durairaj V. Herpes zoster ophthalmicus: a review for the internist. Am J Med. 2017;130:21–6.
47. Weinmann S, Naleway AL, Koppolu P, et al. Incidence of herpes zoster among children: 2003-2014. Pediatrics. 2019;144:e20182917.
48. Rosamilia LL. Herpes zoster presentation, management, and prevention: a modern case-based review. Am J Clin Dermatol. 2020;21:97–107.
49. LaRussa PS, Marin M, Gershon AA. Varicella-zoster virus. In: Kliegman RM, Stanton BF, St Geme JW, Schor NF, editors. Nelson textbook of pediatrics. 21st ed. Philadelphia: Elsevier; 2020. p. 1709–15.
50. Farag AGA, Hammam MA, Ibrahem RA, et al. Epidemiology of dermatophyte infections among school children in Menoufia governorate. Egypt Mycoses. 2018;61:321–5.
51. Borda LJ, Perper M, Keri JE. Treatment of seborrheic dermatitis: a comprehensive review. J Dermatolog Treat. 2019;30:158–69.

52. Singal A, Sonthalia S. Cutaneous tuberculosis in children: the Indian perspective. Indian J Dermatol Venereol Leprol. 2010;76:494–503.
53. Sethuraman G, Ramesh V. Cutaneous tuberculosis in children. Pediatr Dermatol. 2013;30:7–16.
54. Pace Spadaro E, XuerebDingli J, Doffinger R, Dinakantha K, Betts A, Pace D. BCG induced lupus vulgaris: an unexpected adverse event. Arch Dis Child. 2017;11:312–38.
55. Sellami K, Boudaya S, Chaabane H, et al. Twenty-nine cases of lupus vulgaris. Med Mal Infect. 2016;46:93–5.

Tuberculosis in the Ear, Nose, and Throat Field in Children

Emine Manolya Kara, Ayper Somer, and Hesham Negm

59.1 Introduction

Tuberculosis (TB) is among the most lethal communicable diseases around the globe [1]. The disease is caused by *Mycobacterium tuberculosis* (MTB) complex (MTBC) bacteria, including *M. tuberculosis, Mycobacterium africanum, Mycobacterium bovis, Mycobacterium canetti*, and *Mycobacterium microti* [2]. About one-quarter of the world's population is estimated to be infected with *M. tuberculosis*. According to the World Health Organization (WHO), TB accounted for ten million new cases and almost 1.2 million deaths in 2019 [3]. Tuberculosis often accompanies human immunodeficiency virus (HIV) infection in middle or low-income countries. Disease burden is pronounced in the advanced form of the disease with low CD4 cell count [3].

Although the most common form of TB is the pulmonary disease, extrapulmonary tuberculosis (EPTB) accounts for 15% of newly diagnosed cases. Of those; TB of the head and neck region constitute 10–35% [4]. Except for tuberculous lymphadenitis (TL), ear, mastoid, nose, oropharynx, larynx, and thyroid involvement is quite rare, representing <1% of all cases [4, 5].

E. M. Kara (✉) · A. Somer
Division of Pediatric Infectious Diseases, Department of Pediatrics, Faculty of Medicine, İstanbul University, İstanbul, Turkey

H. Negm
Department of Otorhinolaryngology, Faculty of Medicine, Cairo University, Cairo, Egypt

59.2 Tuberculous Lymphadenitis

Tuberculous lymphadenitis is the most frequent form of EPTB. Tuberculosis of the cervical lymph nodes is defined as scrofula. It can be observed in up to 60% of all TL cases [6]. Previously, TL was considered a disease of childhood; however, the peak age of the disease has shifted towards early adulthood in recent years [7]. While most of the historical scrofula cases were associated with the consumption of unpasteurized milk contaminated with *M. bovis*, the disease is caused mainly by *M. tuberculosis* transmission via aerosol or droplet particles in the current day [1]. Although rare, Bacille Calmette-Guérin (BCG) vaccination may cause lymphadenitis in the cervical region (Fig. 59.1) [8]. This is more pronounced in the presence of underlying immunodeficiency.

Tuberculous lymphadenitis may occur in the cervical, submandibular, and supraclavicular regions, often as a result of the spread from a pulmonary or abdominal focus within several weeks to 6–12 months after primary infection [2, 9]. The lymph node involvement usually starts with lymphoid hyperplasia and granuloma formation. Caseification necrosis develops over time. Lymphadenopathy (LAP) is typically unilateral, firm, discrete, and often fixed to the underlying tissue (Fig. 59.2) [9]. However, when liquefaction occurs, the node can fluctuate as named cold abscess (Fig. 59.3), become erythematous, drain spontaneously, and sinus formation may occur as named scrofuloderma (Figs. 59.4 and 59.5). The incidence of the bilateral disease is reported as 26% in some series [10]. Systemic signs and symptoms are usually absent. Low-grade fever may be encountered.

In TB endemic countries, any children with persistent (>4–6 weeks) cervical LAP unresponsive to standard antimicrobial therapy should raise the suspicion of TB [11, 12]. Tuberculin skin test (TST) and interferon-gamma release assays (IGRAs) show high sensitivity and specificity [1, 13]. IGRAs are superior to TST in BCG vaccinated children, countries with low TB burden, and in the presence of

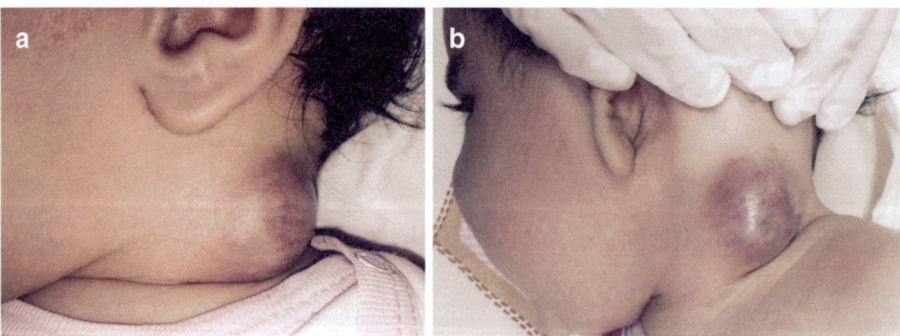

Fig. 59.1 (**a** and **b**) BCG lymphadenitis in a previously healthy 10-month old girl (Courtesy Emine Manolya Kara, MD)

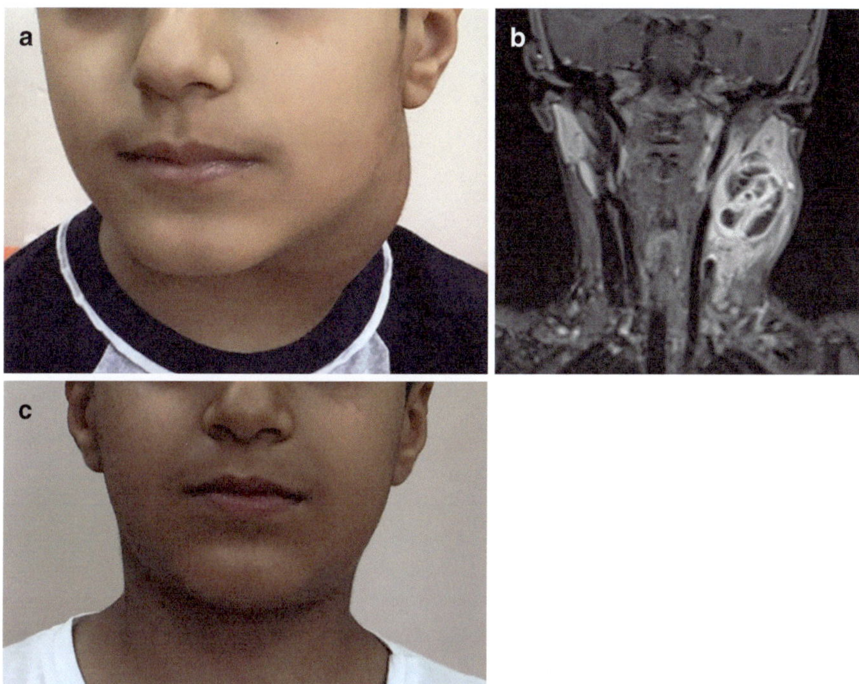

Fig. 59.2 (**a**) Cervical non-tender lymphadenopathy lasting for 3 weeks. (**b**) Magnetic resonance imaging of the neck shows abscess formation with contrast enhancement of relevant lymph node. Fine needle aspiration revealed a positive PCR test for *M. tuberculosis*. (**c**) Complete resolution of adenopathy was seen after 6 months of anti-tuberculosis therapy (Courtesy Nevin Hatipoğlu, MD)

Fig. 59.3 Tuberculous lymphadenitis, a cold abscess (Courtesy Nevin Hatipoğlu, MD)

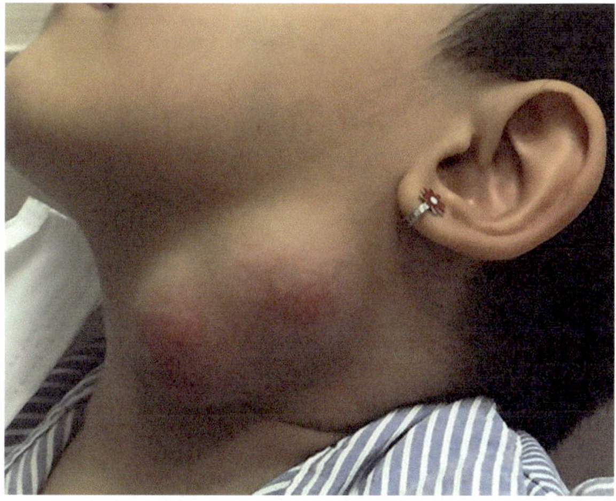

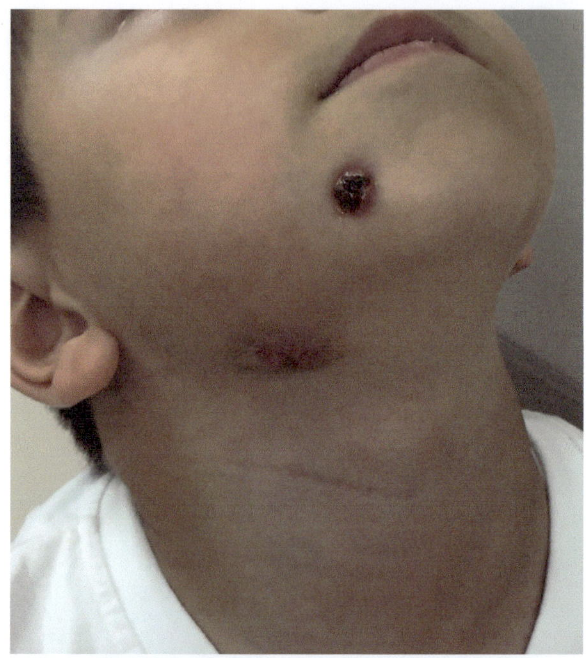

Fig. 59.4 Scrofuloderma, sinus tract formation, and spontaneous drainage (Courtesy Nevin Hatipoğlu, MD)

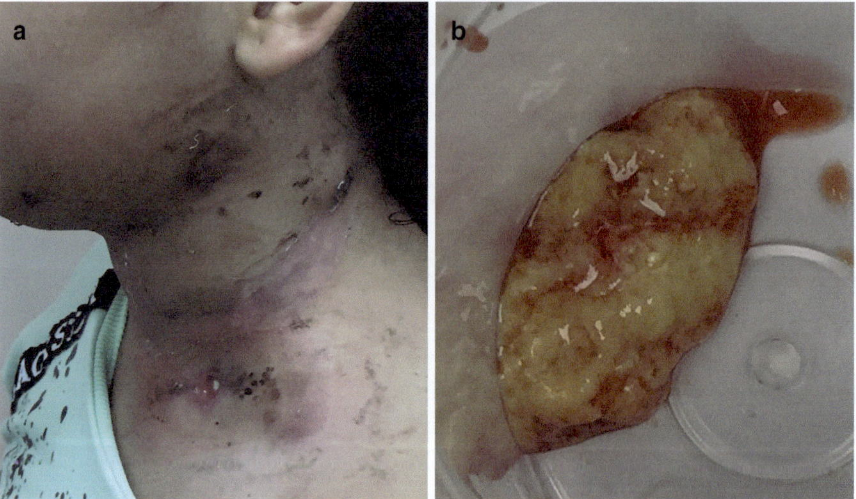

Fig. 59.5 (**a**) Submandibular and supraclavicular tuberculous lymphadenitis. (**b**) Caseous material drained from supraclavicular adenopathy with positive acid-fast bacilli on microscopy and PCR test for *M. tuberculosis* (Courtesy Nevin Hatipoğlu, MD)

NTM exposure [9]. However, neither negative results can rule out, nor positive values are sufficient to establish the diagnosis. Fine needle aspiration (FNA) from the cold abscess and/or excisional biopsy is required for further investigation. *Xpert MTB/RIF* assay as a new revolutionary—cartridge-based nucleic acid amplification—test simultaneously detecting MTBC and resistance to rifampin (R) in less than 2 h can also be performed in aspirate and biopsy materials [11, 13]. The culture of the lymph node material is the gold standard method for the diagnosis [1].

Concomitant TL and pulmonary tuberculous involvement incidence can be up to 20–40% in countries, where TB is endemic [11]. In non-endemic countries, this ratio is usually less than 10%. Even so, an initial chest radiograph which may reveal pleural thickening and calcifications should be performed to evaluate the presence of pulmonary TB.

Ultrasonography (US) is the first-line imaging method in LAP evaluation [14]. It has advantages over other examination modalities of being inexpensive, noninvasive, time-saving, and able to guide procedures such as FNA and core-needle biopsy. The key US features of TL include hypo echogenicity, strong internal echoes, thin echogenic layers, soft tissue changes, and displaced hilar vascularity [14].

It is emphasized that sono-elastography, which has been used in recent years, is more successful in distinguishing benign from malignant LAPs compared to other US modalities and may replace surgical node biopsy in the future [15]. Contrast-enhanced computed tomography (CT) and magnetic resonance imaging (MRI) are much more informative than the US in evaluating the anatomical location, characteristics, and surrounding tissue. Therefore, it is also indicated in the presence of lymphatic and vascular malformations, malignancies for detailed anatomic evaluation before surgery [11].

Several infectious diseases (e.g., pyogenic infections, cat scratch disease, toxoplasmosis, tularemia, brucellosis, fungal infections), non-infectious diseases (e.g., Kawasaki disease, sarcoidosis, Rosai-Dorfman disease, Kikuchi-Fujimoto disease [Kikuchi's histiocytic necrotizing lymphadenitis], Castleman disease), congenital malformations, malignancies, and Nontuberculous mycobacteria (NTM) lymphadenitis should be considered in the differential diagnosis of TL [2]. It cannot be easy to differentiate MTBC from NTM lymphadenitis since the examination findings are similar [1, 16]. Both can cause indolent, painless, slowly growing, firm LAP with or without fistula. Chest radiography may be normal in each form. However, TST induration size is often ≥15 mm in MTB lymphadenitis, whereas NTM infection usually causes a cross-reaction of 10 mm or less [1]. IGRAs may be useful in differentiating MTB from NTM lymphadenitis in children with rare exceptions (e.g., *Mycobacterium kansasii, Mycobacterium marinum, Mycobacterium szulgai, Mycobacterium flavescens*). Besides, TL can be observed in children at any age; however, most cases with NTM lymphadenitis are under the age of 5 [16]. Tuberculous lymphadenitis may resolve spontaneously if left untreated. However, in most cases, the integrity of the node capsule is broken, and the infection spreads to adjacent tissues resulting in sinus tract formation often the indication for surgery.

The treatment of solitary TL should include a three-drug regimen. After two months of induction therapy with isoniazid (H), 10–15 mg/kg/day, maximum 300 mg/day; R, 15–20 mg/kg/day, maximum 600 mg/day; and pyrazinamide (Z) 30–40 mg/kg/day, maximum 2 g/day, the therapy should be continued with HR for 4 months [12].

Common side effects of isoniazid include most commonly mild hepatic enzyme elevations, hepatitis, or hypersensitivity reactions. Altered pyridoxine metabolism can cause peripheral neuritis and convulsions, mainly in malnourished children. Pyridoxine supplementation is recommended in the presence of nutritional deficiency, symptomatic HIV infection, and pregnancy [12].

Rifampicin can cause an influenza-like reaction, orange discoloration of body fluids, vomiting, pruritus, hepatotoxicity, and thrombocytopenia, whereas pyrazinamide can yield gastrointestinal tract discomfort, hepatotoxicity, hyperuricemia, and arthralgia.

Tuberculous lymphadenitis usually responds well to anti-TB therapy. Regression of lymph nodes to average size may require months to years. Paradoxical enlargement of the lymph nodes can be observed after the initiation of anti-TB treatment in up to 20% of the patients [11]. This phenomenon has been attributed to an immune response to dying MTB. Most of these reactions occur between 3 weeks and 4 months of the therapy and pronounced in patients with HIV infection. Non-steroidal anti-inflammatory agents and corticosteroids can be used in selective cases [11].

On the other side, the treatment strategy for NTM-related lymphadenitis is the surgical excision of all affected lymph nodes. Clarithromycin and rifabutin with or without ethambutol (E) may be preferred in NTM lymphadenitis cases not suitable for surgery. When left untreated, spontaneous regression may occur in 9–12 months [16].

59.3 Tuberculosis of the Ear and Mastoids

M. tuberculosis infection of the middle ear and mastoid cells is called tuberculous otitis media (TOM). At present, it is infrequent, accounting for approximately 0.04% of all chronic suppurative otitis media (OM) cases [17]. TOM occurs in three ways: the aspiration of MTB through the eustachian tube, hematogenous dissemination from the primary focus, and direct implantation through a perforated tympanic membrane [18].

In middle and low-income countries, unpasteurized milk consumption infected with *M. bovis* is the primary cause of TOM. Nontuberculous Mycobacteria, mainly *M. abscessus* can be responsible for otitis media with or without mastoiditis in children with tympanostomy tubes [1, 2, 9]. Tuberculous mastoiditis often complicates undiagnosed and untreated TB of the middle ear [9]. Nevertheless, some experts state that TB mastoiditis mostly develops secondary to hematogenous spread. Pulmonary involvement may accompany up to 90% of TOM or TB mastoiditis cases [17]. Tuberculous otitis media should be considered in the presence of persistent ear discharge in patients with pulmonary TB.

Clinical findings such as membrane perforation, unresolved ear discharge, and hearing loss are often the same as in chronic OM. The disease may accompany facial paralysis and preauricular LAP [9, 19]. Mastoiditis frequently causes postauricular swelling and pain. The eardrum looks dull and thickened in the beginning, then seen often damaged with multiple perforations in the later stages [19].

A CT scan demonstrates soft tissue density swelling within the tympanic cavity without evidence of cholesteatoma. Middle ear structures may also be destructed. Ziehl-Neelsen stain from ear discharge may reveal MTB, though it is infrequent due to the low bacterial load in the pus [9]. The culture of the ear drainage sample may yield nonspecific bacterial growth.

Microbiologic tests mainly culture and polymerase chain reaction (PCR) test and histologic examination should be performed from tissue and pus material if surgery is done. Histological findings demonstrate classical TB microscopy with granuloma formation, caseous necrosis, multinucleated giant Langerhans cells. Miliary (superficial infection), granulomatous (bony involvement), and caseous type (sequestration and massive necrosis) of inflammation may be demonstrated [17, 20].

The most serious complication is the extension of the disease to the central nervous system. Perforation, hearing loss (sensorineural, conductive, or mixed type), and labyrinth fistula may be encountered in untreated patients [19]. Facial nerve palsy can occur in up to 20% of the cases [18].

Standard four-drug anti-TB therapy with HRZE in the first two months of the induction phase, followed by HR for a total of 6–9 months (depending on the presence of bone involvement) is recommended. Surgical intervention may be required for complications.

59.4 Laryngeal Tuberculosis

In the early twentieth century, laryngeal tuberculosis (LTB) was a common form of TB. However, in the present-day LTB accounts for only 1% of all cases [21]. It is even rarer in the pediatric age group.

Primary LTB occurs as a result of the direct invasion of MTBC mycobacteria into the larynx. Bronchogenic extension from pulmonary TB, lymphatic, or hematogenous dissemination may also lead to LTB. It has been stated in ancient sources that LTB is observed in the posterior pharynx as a result of exposure to infected sputum in patients who are bedridden for a long time [22]. The predominance of anterior laryngeal involvement in the literature supports the idea of spreading through blood and lymphatics. Smoking, diabetes, HIV infection, and other immune deficiency states are facilitating risk factors [22].

LTB mostly accompany pulmonary TB disease in children. The isolated LTB disease usually confused with laryngeal carcinoma, is sporadic especially in the elderly. The clinical manifestation of LTB showed variation in time because of the widespread use of antibiotics and corticosteroids. The most common symptoms are nonspecific like sore throat, hoarseness, croup-like cough, and dysphagia [23]. Stridor and severe dyspnea due to laryngeal obstruction may be encountered [21]. The constitutional symptoms as fatigue, weight loss, fever, night sweats, and hemoptysis are frequently observed [21]. Any laryngeal sign resistant to standard medical treatment lasting more than 2 weeks should raise the suspicion of LTB.

On laryngoscopy, edematous changes, hyperemia, leukoplakia, and ulceroglandular mass lesions can be seen. The lesions are usually on vocal cords but can also be observed on arytenoids, epiglottis, sub-glottic regions, and posterior commissure [24]. The patients may be misdiagnosed as acute epiglottitis or leukoplakia initially. The disease is usually confused with larynx cancer in the advanced form since shares similar clinical symptoms and findings [24]. They both can be presented with hoarseness, cough, stridor, dysphagia, and hemoptysis. Systemic symptoms such as night sweats, fever, and weight loss may be observed. Cervical LAP may accompany. Smoking is blamed for both LTB and larynx cancer. In a study evaluating LTB cases, most of the lesions were found to be ulceroglandular, mimicking malignancy. Sputum microscopy can yield MTB in up to 20% of patients with LTB [25]. Histologic examination demonstrates epithelioid granulomatous inflammation with caseification. Syphilis, fungal infections, amyloid accumulation, and granulomatosis with polyangiitis should be evaluated in the differential diagnosis in the presence of a granulomatous lesion. LTB has a favorable prognosis with standard anti-TB therapy (HRZE for 2 months, followed by HR for 4 months). Complete resolution occurs within 2–9 months.

59.5   Tuberculosis of the Nasopharynx and Paranasal Sinuses

Nasopharyngeal TB (NPTB) often accompanies the pulmonary disease. Primary NPTB is very rare even in regions with a high burden of TB [26]. Like TOM, pasteurization of cow's milk and effective anti-TB therapy decreased the incidence of NPTB dramatically. In the literature, several pathophysiological mechanisms have been mentioned like insemination of infected droplet material from inhaled air, secondary lymphatic, or hematogenous spread from primary focus or extension from adenoids. Primary NPTB occurs via direct contact of the MTB during nasal ventilation [27].

Symptoms and findings are nonspecific. Systemic symptoms as fever, malaise, night sweats, weight loss, and cough), local symptoms as epistaxis, runny nose, postnasal drip, and nasal obstruction), and otogenic complaints (hearing impairment, fullness sensation, otitis media) can be observed. Upper and middle jugular, retropharyngeal, and a posterior group of cervical lymph nodes may be involved. Nasal septal ulceration and perforation of septal cartilage can occur. Invasion of cavernous sinus or skull base and extension outside the nasopharynx has also been reported [28]. Lymph nodes are usually bilaterally affected.

Tuberculosis of the paranasal sinuses is even rarer. Most of the reported cases represent the involvement of maxillary sinuses [29]. Purulent nasal discharge, bleeding, deteriorated smell sensation, fronto-ethmoidal swelling and headache may be the presenting signs. Visual disturbances may further occur in severe cases with the invasion of the orbit [29].

Direct nasopharynx examination reveals mucosal irregularity, white patches, and ulcerative mass lesions. It may be hard to differentiate NPTB from cancer. CT and MRI can demonstrate polypoid mass and diffuse mucosal thickening, but insufficient for diagnosis [26]. A biopsy is often necessary. Differential diagnosis also includes granulomatous diseases like sarcoidosis, syphilis, leprosy, fungal infections, and autoimmune disorders like Churg-Strauss syndrome, polyarteritis nodosa, and Wegener granulomatosis.

Caseating granulomatous inflammation is the typical histopathologic finding. Mycobacterial culture from sputum or tissue samples yielding *Mycobacterium* spp. is the gold standard for diagnosis. The culture methods may also detect drug sensitivity. With the appropriate 6 months of anti-TB therapy (2 months of HRZE, followed by 4 months of HR) the disease carries a favorable prognosis.

59.6 Tuberculosis of the Oral Cavity

Almost 0.1–5% of all TB diseases occupy the oral cavity [30]. Infected sputum may inoculate directly to oral mucosa or disseminate from a distant focus via a hematogenous route. In recent years, the emergence of drug-resistant TB and acquired immune deficiency syndrome (AIDS) have drawn attention to TB in the oral cavity again [30]. Oral TB is found to account for up to 1.33% of HIV-associated opportunistic infections [31]. Similarly, TB cases associated with anti-tumor necrosis factor (anti-TNF) therapy has increasingly been reported [32].

Despite the oral cavity being the first contact point of inhaled droplets or aerosol, the incidence of TB is very low. This is mainly due to the protective role of saliva against bacillary invasion. Also, the presence of saprophytes, the thickness of protective epithelial covering, and resistance of muscles to bacterial invasion decrease the incidence of TB in the oral cavity [33]. Therefore, patients with oral tubercular lesions often have a history of persistent local trauma, poor oral hygiene, or inflammation. Any area with a damaged mucosal barrier may favor the colonization and infection of MTB.

A systematic review focusing on the TB of the oral cavity revealed that the tongue was the most commonly affected site, followed in the frequency by the mandible, gingivae, lips, buccal mucosa, soft and hard palate [30]. Gingival involvement is more common in children than in adults. The disease may either be caused by *M. bovis* infection via unpasteurized milk or more frequently secondary to contact with infected sputum contaminated with *M. tuberculosis*. Although pain, odynophagia, burning sensation, excessive salivation, halitosis, and intra-oral bleeding are frequent symptoms, patients may be asymptomatic initially. A previous study demonstrated that 0.62% of the tonsillectomy samples were positive for TB [34].

Tonsillar hypertrophy, oropharyngeal edema, ulcerative lesions with ill-defined margins, and necrotic base can be observed during examination. These lesions are unresponsive to antibiotics or corticosteroids. A biopsy is required to rule out systemic diseases such as syphilis, Wegener's granulomatosis, sarcoidosis, Behcet's disease, Crohn's disease, and oral cancer [30]. Oral tubercular lesions may also coexist with oral malignancy in 3% of cases in adults [35].

Histopathologic samples rarely stain positive for acid-fast bacilli. Typical granuloma formation consisting of epithelioid histiocytes and multinucleate giant cells may not be observed in patients with advanced HIV infection [36]. A standard four-drug 6-month treatment regimen of 2HRZE/4HR is recommended. Surgery may be required for complications.

59.7   Tuberculosis of the Salivary Glands

The salivary glands are generally protected from TB. There are several inhibitory factors like the clearing effect of salivary flow, proteolytic enzymes, and thiocyanate ions presenting antibacterial action. If primary salivary gland TB occurs, it is frequently unilateral parotid gland invasion. Submandibular salivary glands are most commonly involved in systemic TB [37]. Persistent oral trauma, poor oral hygiene, dental infection, Stensen duct obstruction, systemic illnesses like diabetes, immunosuppression, Sjogren's disease), and certain medications (e.g., antihistaminic and anticholinergic drugs) may predispose to infection [37].

The mycobacteria can reach the parotid gland via direct passage from the oral cavity, by blood vessels, or lymphatic channels. Approximately one-quarter of the patients have pulmonary disease [37]. The primary parotid TB can be presented as acute suppurative sialadenitis or maybe more chronic, which can be misdiagnosed as a tumor. It is more common in patients with immune deficiency states. Parotid abscesses and/or periauricular fistula may be encountered. Ultrasonography, which has a high sensitivity for superficial lobe involvement, is the initial study of choice [37]. Ultrasonography can also aid the FNA biopsy. CT or MRI may be preferred for detailed anatomical examination. Exploratory parotidectomy may be essential in indeterminate cases. An incisional biopsy is contraindicated due to the risk of cutaneous fistula formation.

Actinomycosis, pyogenic parotitis, HIV infection, mumps, sarcoidosis, Sjogren's syndrome, and malignancy should be evaluated in the differential diagnosis. The disease carries a good prognosis with standard 6-month anti-TB therapy (2HRZE/4HR).

59.8   Tuberculosis of the Thyroid Gland

Primary TB of the thyroid gland occurs at an estimated rate of 0.1% to 0.4% of TB cases [38]. Only rare case reports are available in the literature. As in salivary glands, the thyroid gland is relatively spared from TB. The firm thyroid capsule, high iodine levels, colloid which has a bactericidal action, and rich gland vascularization are thought to be the possible protective mechanisms [38]. The clinical presentation is usually subacute. The thyroid gland may be tender and swollen. Cystic mass lesions can be palpated. The patient is usually euthyroid, though thyrotoxicosis and hypothyroidism have also been reported [39].

Radiologic findings are nonspecific and often indistinguishable from malignancy. Histopathologic examination is required for diagnosis. Autoimmune disorders, granulomatous thyroiditis, infectious etiology, and malignancy should be evaluated in the differential diagnosis. A six-month standard regimen (2HRZE/4HR) as in the treatment of pulmonary TB remains the recommended regimen.

59.9 Conclusion

Primary tuberculosis of the ENT region is sporadic. The disease usually accompanies pulmonary TB. Since the clinical symptoms and signs are unremarkable, several differential diagnoses including malignancy should be considered. Standard anti-TB therapy is often successful, and the outcome is favorable.

References

1. Chiang SS, Starke JR. Mycobacterium tuberculosis. In: Long SS, Prober CG, Fischer M, editors. Principles and practice of pediatric infectious diseases. 5th ed. Philadelphia: Elsevier; 2018. p. 790–806.
2. Cruz AT, Starke JR. Tuberculosis. In: Cherry J, Harrison GJ, Kaplan SL, Steinbach WJ, Hotez PJ, editors. Feigin and Cherry's textbook of pediatric infectious diseases. 8th ed. Philadelphia: Elsevier; 2019. p. 957–88.
3. World Health Organization. Global tuberculosis report 2020. Geneva: World Health Organization; 2020. p. 1–208.
4. Qian X, Albers AE, Nguyen DTM, et al. Head and neck tuberculosis: literature review and meta-analysis. Tuberculosis. 2019;116:78–88.
5. Vaamonde P, Castro C, García-Soto N, Labella T, Lozano A. Tuberculous otitis media: a significant diagnostic challenge. Otolaryngol Head Neck Surg. 2004;130:759–66.
6. Geldmacher H, Taube C, Kroeger C, et al. Assessment of lymph node tuberculosis in northern Germany: a clinical review. Chest. 2002;121:1177–82.
7. Perlman DC, D'Amico R, Salomon N. Mycobacterial infections of the head and neck. Curr Infect Dis Rep. 2001;3:233–41.
8. Goraya JS, Virdi VS. Bacille Calmette-Guérin lymphadenitis. Postgrad Med J. 2002;78:327–9.
9. Schaaf HS, Garcia-Prats AJ. Diagnosis of the most common forms of extrathoracic tuberculosis in children. In: Starke JR, Donald PR, editors. Handbook of child and adolescent tuberculosis. New York: Oxford University Press; 2016. p. 177–99.
10. Agarwal AK, Sethi A, Sethi D, et al. Tubercular cervical adenitis: clinicopathologic analysis of 180 cases. J Otolaryngol Head Neck Surg. 2009;38:521–5.
11. Spelman D. Tuberculous lymphadenitis. In: Bernardo J, Baron EL (eds). Uptodate.com. 2020; https://www.uptodate.com/contents/tuberculous-lymphadenitis. Accessed 3 Dec 2020.
12. American Academy of Pediatrics. Tuberculosis. In: Kimberlin DW, Brady MT, Jackson MA, Long SS, editors. Red Book: 2018 report of the committee on infectious diseases. 31st ed. Itasca: American Academy of Pediatrics; 2018. p. 829–53.
13. Acharya B, Acharya A, Gautam S, et al. Advances in diagnosis of tuberculosis: an update into molecular diagnosis of *Mycobacterium tuberculosis*. Mol Biol Rep. 2020;47:4065–75.
14. Chou C, Yang TL, Wang CP. Ultrasonographic features of tuberculous cervical lymphadenitis. J Med Ultrasound. 2014;3:158–63.
15. Heřman J, Sedláčková Z, Fürst T, et al. The role of ultrasound and shear-wave elastography in evaluation of cervical lymph nodes. Biomed Res Int. 2019;2019:4318251.
16. Tebruegge M, Curtis N. Mycobacterium nontuberculosis species. In: Long SS, Prober CG, Fischer M, editors. Principles and practice of pediatric infectious diseases. 5th ed. Philadelphia: Elsevier; 2018. p. 806–12.
17. Aremu SK, Alabi BS. Tuberculous otitis media: a case presentation and review of the literature. BMJ Case Rep. 2010;2010:1–4.

18. Cho YS, Lee HS, Kim SW, et al. Tuberculous otitis media: a clinical and radiologic analysis of 52 patients. Laryngoscope. 2006;116:921–7.
19. Hand JM, Pankey GA. Tuberculous otomastoiditis. Microbiol Spectr. 2016;4:1–4.
20. Sebastian SK, Singhal A, Sharma A, Doloi P. Tuberculous otitis media - series of 10 cases. J Otolaryngol. 2020;15:95–8.
21. Swain SK, Behera IC, Sahu MC. Primary laryngeal tuberculosis: our experiences at a tertiary care teaching hospital in Eastern India. J Voice. 2019;33:812.
22. Bhat VK, Latha P, Upadhya D, Hegde J. Clinicopathological review of tubercular laryngitis in 32 cases of pulmonary Kochs. Am J Otolaryngol. 2009;30:327–30.
23. Agarwal R, Gupta L, Singh M, et al. Primary laryngeal tuberculosis: a series of 15 cases. Head Neck Pathol. 2019;13:339–43.
24. Suhail A, Ahmed MS, Sobani ZU, Ghaffar S. Laryngeal tuberculosis presenting as laryngeal carcinoma. J Pak Med Assoc. 2012;62:167–8.
25. Jindal SK, Jindal A, Agarwal R. Upper respiratory tract tuberculosis. Microbiol Spectr. 2016;4:6.
26. Darouassi Y, Aljalil A, Hanine A, et al. Nasopharyngeal tuberculosis: report of four cases and review of the literature. Pan Afr Med J. 2019;33:150.
27. Srirompotong S, Yimtae K, Jintakanon D. Nasopharyngeal tuberculosis: manifestations between 1991 and 2000. Otolaryngol Head Neck Surg. 2004;131:762–4.
28. Martínez A, Lede Á, Fernández JA. Primary rhinopharyngeal tuberculosis: an unusual location. Acta Otorrinolaringol. 2011;62:401–3.
29. Sanehi S, Dravid C, Chaudhary N, Venkatachalam VP. Tuberculosis of paranasal sinuses. Indian J Otolaryngol Head Neck Surg. 2008;60:85–7.
30. Kakisi OK, Kechagia AS, Kakisis IK, Rafailidis PI, Falagas ME. Tuberculosis of the oral cavity: a systematic review. Eur J Oral Sci. 2010;118:103–9.
31. Miziara ID. Tuberculosis affecting the oral cavity in Brazilian HIV-infected patients. Oral Surg Oral Med Oral Pathol Oral Radiol Endod. 2005;100:179–82.
32. Ferreira S, Vaz-Marques P. Tuberculous tonsillitis in a patient treated with an anti-TNF agent. Eur J Case Rep Intern Med. 2017;4(8):690.
33. Pekiner FN, Erseven G, Borahan MO, Gümrü B. Natural barrier in primary tuberculosis inoculation: oral mucous membrane. Int J Tuberc Lung Dis. 2006;10:1418.
34. Ricciardiello F, Martufi S, Cardone M, et al. Otorhinolaryngology-related tuberculosis. Acta Otorhinolaryngol Ital. 2006;26:38–42.
35. Krawiecka E, Szponar E. Tuberculosis of the oral cavity: an uncommon but still a live issue. Postepy Dermatol Alergol. 2015;32:302–6.
36. Jain P, Jain I. Oral manifestations of tuberculosis: step towards early diagnosis. J Clin Diagn Res. 2014;8:18–21.
37. Chaudhary P, Chaudhary B, Munjewar CK. Parotid tuberculosis. Indian J Tuberc. 2017;64:161–6.
38. Laitman BM, Samankan S, Hwang S, Chai RL. Primary thyroid tuberculosis: an uncommon presentation of a thyroid mass. Ear Nose Throat J. 2020;14:1–3.
39. Chaudhary A, Nayak B, Guleria S, et al. Tuberculosis of the thyroid presenting as multinodular goiter with hypothyroidism: a rare presentation. Indian J Pathol Microbiol. 2010;53:579–81.

Cervical Lymphadenitis due to Nontuberculous Mycobacterial Infection in Children

60

Selda Hançerli Törün, Ayper Somer, and Lyalikov Sergey Aleksandrovich

60.1 Introduction

Nontuberculous mycobacteria (NTM) are ubiquitous in soil, water, and man-made environments [1]. There have been more than 130 NTM species identified, only a few are responsible as an infectious agent. Lymphadenitis, skin and soft tissue infection, pulmonary disease, and disseminated disease are the leading NTM associated diseases. Disseminated infections almost always are associated with impaired cell-mediated immunity, as found in children with hematopoietic stem cell transplants, congenital immune defects, or advanced human immunodeficiency virus (HIV) infection [2]. Cervical lymphadenitis due to NTM will be reviewed in this chapter.

60.2 Microbiology and Epidemiology

Nontuberculous mycobacteria, also named atypical mycobacteria, are peculiar species that are not classified as *Mycobacterium tuberculosis* complex. They are ubiquitous organisms detected dispersedly in the environment, found in water, soil, milk, other food, domestic and wild animals, and depending on the geographic region the prevalence varies [1]. The healthcare-associated transmission via medical equipment has been reported.

S. H. Törün (✉) · A. Somer
Division of Pediatric Infectious Diseases, Department of Pediatrics, Faculty of Medicine, İstanbul University, İstanbul, Turkey

L. S. Aleksandrovich
Department of Pediatrics, Grodno State Medical University, Grodno, Belarus

The most common species isolated in children are *Mycobacterium avium* complex (MAC; includes *Mycobacterium intracellulare* and *M. avium*), *Mycobacterium abscessus, Mycobacterium fortuitum,* and *Mycobacterium marinum*. Several new species recently identified by nucleic acid amplification testing but yet cannot be grown by routine culture methods have been isolated in lymph nodes of children with cervical adenitis [2–4].

M. fortuitum, Mycobacterium chelonae, Mycobacterium smegmatis, and *M. abscessus* commonly are referred to as "rapidly growing" mycobacteria (RGM), because growth sufficient for identification can be achieved in the laboratory within 3 to 7 days, whereas MAC, *Mycobacterium szulgai,* and *M. marinum* usually proliferate in an adequate amount for identification in several weeks. RGM has been associated with infections vastly dispersed in the body such as a wound, bone, soft tissue, pulmonary, central venous catheter, and middle-ear infections. Other mycobacterial strains classified as non-pathogenic have caused infections in immunocompromised hosts, or foreign body infections (Table 60.1) [2, 3].

When the NTM disease first described *Mycobacterium scrofulaceum* was the predominant etiological species, but MAC is currently isolated in 70% to 90% of culture-positive NTM lymphadenitis. In Northern and Central Europe, NTM lymphadenitis is most frequently caused by *Mycobacterium malmoense*. Because of unusual growth requirements (optimal incubation temperature of 30 °C and iron supplementation), the prominence of *Mycobacterium haemophilum* as a cause of cervical lymphadenitis previously was underestimated, currently, the incidence of

Table 60.1 Classification of nontuberculous mycobacterial species causing human disease

Rapidly growing nontuberculous mycobacteria	Slowly growing nontuberculous mycobacteria
M. fortuitum complex	Photochromogens
M. fortuitum	*M. marinum*
M. porcinum	*M. kansasii*
M. peregrinum	Scotochromogens
M. chelonae	*M. scrofulaceum*
M. abscessus	*M. gordonae*
M. abscessus subspecies *bolletii*	Nonchromogens
M. abscessus subspecies *abscessus*	*M. avium* complex
M. abscessus subspecies *massiliense*	*M. avium*
M. mucogenicum	*M. chimaera*
M. smegmatis	*M. intracellulare*
	M. terrae complex
	M. simiae
	M. xenopi
	M. haemophilum
	M. malmoense
	M. szulgai
	M. asiaticum
	M. ulcerans

M. haemophilum in some series approaches to 25%. *Mycobacterium kansasii, M. chelonae, Mycobacterium simiae,* and *M. fortuitum* are other relatively rare causes of NTM-related lymphadenitis [2–4].

As for the varying species in tuberculosis low-burden countries, MAC and *M. scrofulaceum* are more prevalent in Australia and the United States (US). In the United Kingdom, Scandinavia, and Northern Europe, *M. malmoense* and *M. haemophilum* are the most common mycobacteria causing peripheral lymphadenitis [3, 4]. The increase in NTM-associated lymphadenitis in these low-burden countries where BCG vaccination was discontinued suggests that BCG may have a preventive effect in the development of NTM-related lymphadenitis [5].

60.3 Pathogenesis

The usual portal of entry for NTM species is believed to be any disturbance in the cutaneous or mucosal barrier as in the skin (e.g., cutaneous lesions caused by *M. marinum*), oropharyngeal mucosa (the presumed portal of entry for cervical lymphadenitis), gastrointestinal or respiratory tract for disseminated MAC, and respiratory tract (including tympanostomy tubes for otitis media), surgical sites (especially for central vascular catheter infection), and with penetrating trauma (needles and organic material most often associated with *M. abscessus* and *M. fortuitum*) [2–4].

The pathogenicity of NTM ranges from asymptomatic colonization to even visceral dissemination (lung, gut, bone, and skin) in the presence of impaired cell-mediated immunity. The most common presentation of NTM-related disease in immunocompetent children is chronic cervicofacial lymphadenitis and it is most frequently caused by MAC [2].

The risk of mycobacterial disease increases with immunosuppressive treatments used for several severe childhood conditions. In particular, children with leukemia receiving chemotherapy or bone marrow transplantation (BMT) have a higher risk of developing NTM infections. Solid-organ transplantation or BMT for other disorders are also identified as conditions with increased risk. NTM infections have also been reported in HIV-positive children. HIV infection strongly influences the pathogenesis of the mycobacterial disease as well known in tuberculosis by causing a progressive decline in CD4 T-cell immunity, resulting in a higher risk of clinical disease, with more frequent extrapulmonary involvement, atypical radiographic signs, and paucibacillary disease, potentially hindering timely diagnosis.

Several inherited diseases are also associated with the predisposition of NTM-related diseases. Some of the congenital lung disorders such as cystic fibrosis, primary ciliary dyskinesia, and pulmonary alveolar proteinosis lead to defects in the airway clearance. As NTM infections are increasingly reported in adults with cystic fibrosis, children are also vulnerable. Chronic granulomatous disease, T-cell related primary immunodeficiencies, and some other hereditary deficiencies are conferring a predisposition to mycobacterial diseases [2–4].

60.4 Clinical Features

Lymphadenitis is the most common manifestation of NTM infection in children younger than 12 years of age with a peak incidence of 1 to 5 years of age. In contrast, children older than 12 years of age with mycobacterial adenitis generally have *M. tuberculosis* complex infection [3].

The children with NTM lymphadenitis are typically healthy and present with a painless mass that reluctant to standard antibiotic therapy and without fever or other systemic signs of illness. NTM lymphadenitis generally presents as a unilateral, non-tender node, smaller than 4 cm in diameter, and slowly enlarges over several weeks [6]. The overlying skin gradually changes from pink to violaceous and thins to become parchment-like. Spontaneous drainage following fistula formation often occurs and may lead to significant disfiguration of the surrounding skin. It is usually encountered in the cervical and submandibular region, and more rarely parotid region (Fig. 60.1). The interval between symptom onset and diagnosis ranges from 4 to 12 weeks.

60.5 Radiographic Features

The most important tool in the diagnosis of NTM disease is radiologic evaluation. Ultrasonographic features of NTM lymphadenitis are decreased echogenicity; and in the advanced stages, intranodal liquefaction, matted nodes, and soft tissue edema

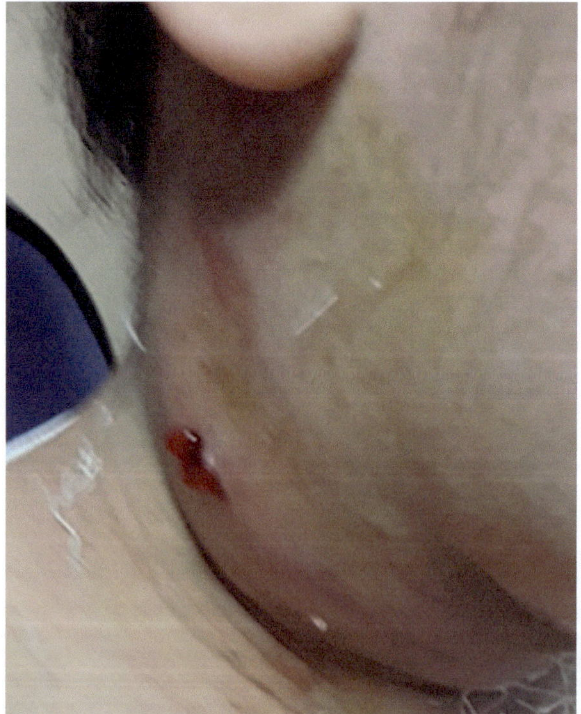

Fig. 60.1 Pustulated lymphadenitis due to NTM in anterior cervical region (Courtesy İstanbul University, Faculty of Medicine, Department of Pediatrics, Division of Pediatric Infectious Diseases)

[7]. Contrast-enhanced axial computerized tomography (CT) scans demonstrate asymmetric cervical lymphadenopathies and adjacent low-density, necrotic, ring-enhancing masses involving the subcutaneous fat and skin. Inflammatory stranding of the subcutaneous fat is typically minimal or absent, unlike conventional bacterial abscesses. Calcifications, cysts structure, and necrotic areas are frequently observed.

Magnetic resonance imaging (MRI) generally demonstrates low signal intensity lesions with ring enhancement. If the cervical mass is necrotic, there will be low and high signal intensity in the center of the mass in T1- and T2-weighted images, respectively [8].

60.6 Laboratory Features

Consultation with the laboratory should be done to ensure that culture specimens are handled correctly. For example, isolation of *M. haemophilum* requires the culture to be maintained at 30 °C and the addition of the heme-containing medium for isolation. Contamination of cultures or transient colonization occurs commonly because these organisms are dispersed widely in the environment.

Repeated isolation on culture media of a single species from any site, and an acid-fast bacilli smear-positive sample and are more likely to indicate disease than culture contamination or transient colonization. Isolation of NTM from sites that usually are sterile, such as blood, lymph node aspirates, middle ear or mastoid aspirates, or surgically excised tissue, is the most reliable diagnostic test.

Identification in culture may exclude differential diagnoses. Culture media may be solid (Löwenstein-Jensen) or liquid. Incubation usually takes 45–60 days. A liquid medium (Bactec MGIT 960) allows earlier diagnosis, with faster bacterial growth (1–2 weeks).

In patients with clinically suspected NTM lymphadenitis, it is also possible to identify mycobacterial DNA fragments molecularly by polymerase chain reaction (PCR). Although it is not a routine test, PCR is a confirmatory and sensitive technique for the diagnosis of NTM [3].

60.7 Diagnosis

The definitive diagnosis of NTM infection requires isolation of the organism. Patients with NTM infection may be tested positive with tuberculin skin test (TST), because the purified protein derivative (PPD) preparation, derived from *M. tuberculosis*, shares several antigens with NTM species. The TST has suboptimal sensitivity and it is unreliable in the differentiation of *M. tuberculosis* infection from infection with NTM and previous BCG vaccination. These TST reactions usually have less than 10 mm of induration but can measure more than 15 mm [3]. In a study of 174 children with cervicofacial lymphadenitis with no exposure to *M. tuberculosis* and had not received BCG vaccination, TST with >5 mm of induration at 48 h had a sensitivity, specificity, and positive and negative predictive value of 70%, 98%, 98%, and 64%, respectively, for NTM (confirmed by positive culture and/or polymerase chain reaction) [9].

Positive acid-fast smear with negative molecular testing would support the diagnosis of NTM infection. Moreover, several opportunistic infections may complicate the diagnosis. For example, NTM, BCG, and Nocardia are acid-fast and can cause positive sputum smears. The distinction can only be possible through culture or molecular techniques.

In an observational study of 29 children with culture-confirmed NTM lymphadenitis, 17 (59%) had induration ≥15 mm; the majority of these children had *M. avium* complex (MAC) or *M. haemophilum* lymphadenitis [10]. In children with suspected NTM lymphadenitis and TST ≥5 mm induration, interferon-gamma release assays may be helpful.

Immunodiagnostic tests such as the IFN-γ release assays (IGRAs) are more specific and are based on the T cell mediated IFN-γ release after stimulation with specific *M. tuberculosis* antigens. These tests are proved to have better specificity worldwide. IGRAs use 2 or 3 antigens to detect infection with *M. tuberculosis*. Although these antigens are not found on *M. avium-intracellulare* and most other NTM species, cross-reactions are possible with infection caused by *M. kansasii, M. marinum*, and *M. szulgai*. Hermansen's [11] study showed an overall low positivity rate (4%) in patients with NTM without RD1 (specific genomic area in MTB, called the region of difference), especially in children with MAC lymphadenitis (100% Quantiferon Gold In-Tube test [QFT] negative). Thus, in a child presenting with cervical lymphadenitis, a negative QFT may help distinguish NTM from tuberculosis lymphadenitis.

Histopathologic examination is one of the most important techniques for diagnosing NTM lymphadenitis. Caseating necrosis, Langerhans giant cells, granulomatous inflammation, and calcification can be seen. The presence of micro-abscesses, non-caseating granulomas, ill-defined granulomas, and a small number of giant cells are more prominent in non-tuberculous adenitis when compared with tuberculous adenitis [3]. When bacteriological studies fail to confirm an etiology, histopathological studies should be considered, especially in clinical presentations compatible with tuberculosis disease but also with other causes. Lymph nodes, pleura, pericardium, and lung are potentially useful biopsy specimens in the setting of suspected intrathoracic tuberculosis. Numerous granulomas in various stages of development, some with central caseous necrosis, are among the classical findings. However it should be kept in mind granulomatous inflammation is not specific for the diagnosis of tuberculosis, especially in regions where environmental NTM or fungi are common.

60.8 Differential Diagnosis

The differential diagnosis of NTM lymphadenitis includes other infectious causes of unilateral lymphadenitis (e.g., *Streptococcus pyogenes, Staphylococcus aureus, Bartonella henselae, M. tuberculosis*, viral infections, toxoplasmosis), benign cysts, and malignancy. It is important to differentiate tuberculous from NTM cervical lymphadenitis because their treatment protocols are different and culture is necessary for definitive diagnosis. Tuberculous lymphadenitis is more often associated with a strongly positive TST, abnormal chest radiograph, history of constitutional symptoms, and contact with a case of active tuberculosis. Nodes in acute bacterial lymphadenitis often are larger, evolve rapidly, and are more tender and erythematous; fever is prominent, and white cell count and C-reactive protein are typically elevated [3].

60.9 Management

Surgical excision of infected lymph nodes is considered to be the most effective treatment, and this approach has been recommended in many studies [11–15]. For patients with NTM or suspected NTM lymphadenitis and no evidence of pulmonary or disseminated disease, surgical excision without antimicrobial therapy as the initial intervention will be the most appropriate treatment if excision can be performed safely and surgical excision of NTM lymphadenitis is recommended by the American Thoracic Society, Infectious Diseases Society of America, and the American Academy of Pediatrics Committee on Infectious Diseases [2, 16]. Various surgical procedures are suggested: incision with drainage, curettage of fistulized zones, or complete resection of pathological adenopathies. The incision with drainage and curettage of fistulized zones was associated with a 55% relapse compared to only 5% with complete resection of lymph nodes and infected tissue. The relative risk of relapse after minimal surgery is almost 11 times greater than after complete resection.

Despite the current recommendations for complete resection of NTM cervicofacial lymphadenitis, we have had to treat extensive lesions whereby complete excision is not always possible or recommended. Many NTM species are relatively resistant in vitro to anti-tuberculosis drugs. If the diagnosis is uncertain and the surgical risks (e.g., facial nerve injury) preclude surgical excision, fine-needle aspiration may help establish the microbiologic diagnosis with minimal procedural risk. Chemotherapeutic treatment of MAC infection is less successful because of isoniazid, rifampin, and pyrazinamide resistance [5]. The approach to therapy should be directed by the following: (1) the species causing the infection; (2) the results of drug susceptibility testing; (3) the site(s) of infection; (4) the patient's immune status; and (5) the need to treat a patient presumptively for tuberculosis while awaiting culture reports that subsequently reveal NTM.

In a randomized trial comparing antimycobacterial therapy with clarithromycin and rifabutin with surgical excision, 66% of patients treated with antibiotics were cured, 32% developed draining fistula, and 78% had adverse effects related to medication or disease (e.g., headache, fever, fatigue, tooth discoloration, abdominal pain, vomiting) [17]. It is important to warn families about the possibility of developing a draining fistula before starting antimycobacterial therapy. When antimicrobial treatment for NTM lymphadenitis is undertaken, and *M. tuberculosis* is not a concern, empiric therapy is a macrolide (azithromycin or clarithromycin) in combination with ethambutol and/or rifampin (or rifabutin). Therapy with azithromycin or clarithromycin combined with rifampin or ethambutol may be beneficial for children in whom surgical excision is incomplete or for children with recurrent disease. The duration of therapy for NTM infection is a minimum of 3–6 months or longer due to the severity of the disease.

When antimicrobial therapy is undertaken in young (preschool-aged) children with suspected NTM lymphadenitis in whom *M. tuberculosis* remains a concern (e.g., pending culture results in children with risk factors for *M. tuberculosis*, TST with ≥15 mm of induration), the empiric antimicrobial regimen should include coverage for both NTM and *M. tuberculosis*.

The antibiotic regimen may need to be altered if a species other than MAC is isolated:

- *M. simiae*: Clarithromycin, rifabutin, clofazimine streptomycin, and moxifloxacin are sensitive in vitro tests [18].
- *M. fortuitum*: *M. fortuitum* is susceptible to macrolides, amikacin, carbapenems, fluoroquinolones, and trimethoprim-sulfamethoxazole [19, 20]. Because of inducible macrolide resistance, macrolide therapy alone is not recommended [21].

NTM lymphadenitis has been shown to recur at a rate of 7% within 5 years in one study [22]. Follow-up of patients is recommended.

60.10 Conclusion

NTM lymphadenitis incidence peaks in children under 5 years old of age. Although it varies according to epidemiological data, MAC and *M. scrofulaceum* were the predominant etiological agent. Surgery is considered in first-line treatment. Antimicrobial therapy is recommended to continue for 3–6 months in cases. Since there is a possibility of recurrence, it is recommended to follow these patients for 5 years.

References

1. Falkinham JO 3rd. Ecology of nontuberculous mycobacteria - where do human infections come from? Semin Respir Crit Care Med. 2013;34:95–102.
2. American Academy of Pediatrics. Nontuberculous mycobacteria. In: Kimberlin DW, Brady MT, Jackson MA, Long SS, editors. Red book: 2018 report of the committee on infectious diseases. 31st ed. Itasca: American Academy of Pediatrics; 2018. p. 853–61.
3. Linam WM, Jacobs RF. Other mycobacteria. In: Cherry JD, Harrison GJ, Kaplan SL, Steinbach WJ, Hotez PJ, editors. Feigin and Cherry's textbook of pediatric infectious diseases. 8th ed. Philadelphia: Elsevier; 2019. p. 988–95.
4. Tebruegge M, Curtis N. Mycobacterium nontuberculosis species. In: Long SS, Prober CG, Fischer M, editors. Principles and practice of pediatric infectious diseases. 5th ed. Philadelphia: Elsevier; 2018. p. 806–12.

5. Schaaf HS, Garcia-Prats AJ. Diagnosis of the most common forms of extrathoracic tuberculosis in children. In: Starke JR, Donald PR, editors. Handbook of child and adolescent tuberculosis. New York: Oxford University Press; 2016. p. 177–99.
6. Penn R, Steehler MK, Sokohl A, Harley EH. Nontuberculous mycobacterial cervicofacial lymphadenitis--a review and proposed classification system. Int J Pediatr Otorhinolaryngol. 2011;75:1599–603.
7. Lindeboom JA, Smets AM, Kuijper EJ, van Rijn RR, Prins JM. The sonographic characteristics of nontuberculous mycobacterial cervicofacial lymphadenitis in children. Pediatr Radiol. 2006;36:1063–7.
8. Robson CD, Hazra R, Barnes PD, Robertson RL, Jones D, Husson RN. Nontuberculous mycobacterial infection of the head and neck in immunocompetent children: CT and MR findings. Am J Neuroradiol. 1999;20:1829–35.
9. Cruz AT, Ong LT, Starke JR. Mycobacterial infections in Texas children: a 5-year case series. Pediatr Infect Dis J. 2010;29:772–4.
10. Haimi-Cohen Y, Zeharia A, Mimouni M, Amir J. Skin indurations in response to tuberculin testing in patients with nontuberculous mycobacterial lymphadenitis. Clin Infect Dis. 2001;33:1786–8.
11. Hermansen TS, Thomsen VØ, Lillebaek T, Ravn P. Non-tuberculous mycobacteria and the performance of interferon-gamma release assays in Denmark. PLoS One. 2014;9(4):e93986.
12. Saggese D, Compadretti GC. Burnelli R nontuberculous mycobacterial adenitis in children: diagnostic and therapeutic management. Am J Otol. 2003;24:79–84.
13. Bayazit YA, Bayazit N, Namiduru M. Mycobacterial cervical lymphadenitis. J Otorhinolaryngol Relat Spec. 2004;66:275–80.
14. Lindeboom JA, Kuijper EJ, van Coppenraet B, Lindeboom R, Prins JM. Surgical excision versus antibiotic treatment for nontuberculous mycobacterial cervicofacial lymphadenitis in children: a multicenter, randomized, controlled trial. Clin Infect Dis. 2007;44:1057–64.
15. Lindeboom JA. Surgical treatment for nontuberculous mycobacterial (NTM) cervicofacial lymphadenitis in children. J Oral Maxillofac Surg. 2012;70:345–8.
16. Griffith DE, Aksamit T, Brown-Elliott BA, et al. An official ATS/IDSA statement: diagnosis, treatment, and prevention of nontuberculous mycobacterial diseases. Am J Respir Crit Care Med. 2007;175:367–416.
17. Lindeboom JA, Kuijper EJ, Bruijnesteijn van Coppenraet ES, Lindeboom R, Prins JM. Surgical excision versus antibiotic treatment for nontuberculous mycobacterial cervicofacial lymphadenitis in children: a multicenter, randomized, controlled trial. Clin Infect Dis. 2007;44:1057–64.
18. van Ingen J, Totten SE, Heifets LB, Boeree MJ, Daley CL. Drug susceptibility testing and pharmacokinetics question current treatment regimens in Mycobacterium simiae complex disease. Int J Antimicrob Agents. 2011;39:173–6.
19. Wallace RJ Jr, Brown-Elliott BA, Ward SC, Crist CJ, Mann LB, Wilson RW. Activities of linezolid against rapidly growing mycobacteria. Antimicrob Agents Chemother. 2001;45:764–7.
20. Wallace RJ Jr, Bedsole G, Sumter G, et al. Activities of ciprofloxacin and ofloxacin against rapidly growing mycobacteria with demonstration of acquired resistance following single-drug therapy. Antimicrob Agents Chemother. 1990;34:65–70.
21. Nash KA, Brown-Elliott BA, Wallace RJ Jr. A novel gene, erm(41), confers inducible macrolide resistance to clinical isolates of mycobacterium abscessus but is absent from Mycobacterium chelonae. Antimicrob Agents Chemother. 2009;53:1367–76.
22. Reuss A, Drzymala S, Hauer B, von Kries R, Haas W. Treatment outcome in children with nontuberculous mycobacterial lymphadenitis: a retrospective follow-up study. Int J Mycobacteriol. 2017;6:76–82.

Influenza in Children

61

Nihal Yaman Artunç, Melda Çelik, and Michael Rudenko

61.1 Introduction

Influenza is a respiratory tract disease that can be seen in a variety of ways, ranging from an asymptomatic mild clinical course to severe infections resulting in death. There are approximately 1 billion influenza cases per year worldwide and 3–5 million of these are severe cases, while 290,000–650,000 cause influenza-related respiratory deaths. It can be life-threatening especially in the elderly, children, pregnant women, and individuals with underlying chronic diseases [1].

61.2 Etiology

The influenza virus contains a genome composed of single-stranded ribonucleic acids (RNAs) and belongs to the *Orthomyxoviridae* family. There are 3 types that cause infections in humans: Type A, Type B, and Type C. It is not known whether type D can infect humans [2]. The genetic structure, host types, epidemiology, and clinical findings of these three types are different from each other. While influenza

N. Y. Artunç (✉)
Section of Pediatrics, Dr. Sami Ulus Children's Hospital, University of Health Sciences, Ankara, Turkey
e-mail: nihalyaman@hacettepe.edu.tr

M. Çelik
Division of Social Pediatrics, Department of Pediatrics, Faculty of Medicine, Hacettepe University, Ankara, Turkey

M. Rudenko
Section of Pediatric Allergy and Immunology, The London Allergy and Immunology Centre, London, UK

A and B viruses are the main pathogens that bring about seasonal epidemics, influenza C mostly causes mild upper respiratory tract disease [3].

61.3 Pathogenesis

Influenza viruses are divided into serotypes according to the surface proteins called hemagglutinin (HA) and neuraminidase (NA). Hemagglutinin lets the virus to bind to glycoproteins and glycolipids containing sialic acid on the host cell surface so that the virus enters the host cell. After viral replication, NA separates its substrate, sialic acid, from infected cell surfaces, so enables the release of new viruses that occur inside the cell [4].

Numerous subtypes of influenza viruses have been defined according to the combinations of antigenic differences in HA and NA. 16 subtypes of HA (H1–H16) and 9 subtypes of NA (N1 – N9) have been described in influenza A viruses [5].

The type A viruses are the most virulent human pathogens among the three influenza types and cause the most severe disease. The serotypes that have been confirmed in humans, ordered by the number of known human pandemic deaths, are [6]:

- H1N1 caused "Spanish flu" in 1918 and "Swine flu" in 2009.
- H2N2 caused "Asian Flu".
- H3N2 caused "Hong Kong Flu".
- H5N1, "avian" or "bird flu".
- H7N7 has unusual zoonotic potential.
- H1N2 infects pigs and humans.
- H9N2, H7N2, H7N3, H10N7.

Since there is little variation among the antigens of influenza B and C viruses, there is no defined subtype [3]. The influenza virus constantly changes these antigenic structures and escapes from host immunity. Antigenic drift takes place due to point mutations in HA and NA proteins without causing changes in viral subtypes. This event causes annual influenza outbreaks. Antigenic shift is the significant alterations in these surface proteins that cause new viral subtypes. It only occurs in influenza A virus, and if the host immune system does not respond adequately and there is a human-to-human transmission, it can potentially result in a pandemic [7].

61.4 Epidemiology

Influenza virus is a highly contagious virus that causes illness in people of all ages. However, pregnant women, young children under 5 years old, the elderly, people with underlying chronic diseases (e.g., chronic heart, lung, kidney) and individuals with immunosuppressive conditions, and healthcare workers are especially at high risk [2].

In terms of influenza, disease transmission occurs in three ways as aerosol, droplet, and close contact. Droplets released after sneezing or coughing and aerosols can stay in the air for minutes to hours but are affected by environmental changes such as temperature and humidity. Contact transmission may also occur through hands from contaminated objects to mucosal areas [8].

Annual influenza epidemics occur in outbreaks in winters. Although it varies from country to country and between years, it is generally seen between November and May. These outbreaks often last 4–8 weeks or longer [7].

The incubation period is on average 2 days (1–4 days). The amount of virus excretion is greatest 1–3 days after inoculation, but contagiousness in children may extend up to 7–10 days. Children using immunosuppressive drugs or those with immunodeficiency can be contagious for a longer time [9].

Influenza epidemics affect 5–15% of the annual world population. However, complications and hospitalizations related to the disease are more common in children [10]. In children under 18 years of age, the influenza attack rate ranges from 10 to 40%, and the estimated influenza incidence is about 9% [11, 12]. In a study supported by World Health Organization (WHO), in 2018, 109.5 million influenza virus cases, 10.1 million influenza virus-associated acute lower respiratory tract infection (ALRI) cases, 870,000 influenza virus-related hospitalizations, 15,300 in-hospital deaths, and a total of 34,800 influenza virus-associated ALRI deaths have been estimated in children under 5 years of age globally. 7% of ALRI cases, 5% of ALRI hospitalizations, and 4% of ALRI deaths in children under 5 years of age were influenza-related [13]. According to the data collected by the CDC, the number of influenza-related pediatric deaths during the 2017–2018 influenza season was 171, 111 in 2018–2019, and 148 in 2019–2020 [14].

61.5 Clinical Features

Influenza typically begins with high fever, chills, headache, anorexia, malaise, and myalgia. These first manifestations are followed by a sore throat, coryza, and a nonproductive cough. Less common clinical manifestations can include conjunctivitis, parotitis, rash, abdominal pain, nausea, vomiting, and diarrhea. As respiratory system involvement, it can lead to croup, bronchiolitis, or pneumonia [15]. Most of the children with mild upper respiratory tract disease symptoms can recover within 3–7 days without any medical intervention. However, dry cough can be more severe in some cases and can last for 2 weeks or more [9].

Influenza-related illness can range from mild to severe and even death. When we look at the complications of influenza in children, otitis media, sinusitis, croup, worsening of the underlying chronic lung disease, pneumonia, respiratory failure, secondary bacterial infections, myositis, cardiac complications (such as myocarditis and pericarditis), toxic shock syndrome, Guillain-Barré syndrome, CNS complications (febrile seizures, aseptic meningitis, postinfectious encephalitis, and acute mental status changes, etc.), and Reye's syndrome can be encountered [16–19].

61.6 Diagnosis

Influenza is not easily diagnosed in children, especially those under 3 years old [20]. The most important point in the diagnosis of influenza is to bear in mind the suspicion that the patient may have influenza. In a child during the influenza season, if there is,

- Fever of unknown origin.
- Severe sick appearance with fever or hypothermia.
- Signs and symptoms of acute respiratory infection with fever, whether the child is hospitalized or not.
- Fever and exacerbation of the existing chronic pulmonary disease and at any time of the year, if there are,
- Immunocompromised children who present signs and symptoms of acute respiratory infection with fever influenza should be suspected [21].

Although some hematological and radiological changes such as neutrophil-to-lymphocyte ratio or interstitial infiltration, consolidation and ground-glass opacities and can be seen [22, 23], routine laboratory tests are not required for the diagnosis of influenza. However, it becomes difficult to clinically differentiate influenza, as other respiratory viruses also present with similar symptoms [2]. Molecular diagnostic tests can change treatment decisions in patients hospitalized with suspected or confirmed diagnosis of influenza [24]. However, the decision to initiate antiviral therapy should be a clinical decision regardless of whether molecular tests are performed to confirm the diagnosis in a child with symptoms and signs that suggests a diagnosis of influenza and/or is at high risk for complications (Table 61.1). The test result should not be expected for the decision to start treatment.

Laboratory diagnosis of influenza is based on the isolation of influenza virus or detection of virus fragments (virus proteins or virus RNA). Several diagnostic tests are available to confirm influenza (Table 61.2). Since serological tests based on antibody detection method cannot be performed in the acute period, it is not

Table 61.1 Children at higher risk for influenza complications recommended for antiviral treatment

• children younger than 2 years of age[a]
• people with chronic pulmonary (including asthma), cardiovascular (except hypertension alone), renal, hepatic, hematological (including sickle cell disease), and metabolic disorders (including diabetes mellitus), or neurologic and neurodevelopmental conditions (including disorders of the brain, spinal cord, peripheral nerve, and muscle, such as cerebral palsy, epilepsy [seizure disorders], stroke, intellectual disability, moderate to severe developmental delay, muscular dystrophy, or spinal cord injury)
• people with immunosuppression, including those caused by medications or by HIV infection
• adolescents who are pregnant or postpartum (within 2 weeks after delivery)
• people younger than 19 years old who are receiving long-term aspirin- or salicylate-containing medications
• American Indians/Alaska natives
• people who are extremely obese (i.e., body mass index is equal to or greater than 40)
• residents of chronic care facilities

Adopted from Centers for Disease Control and Prevention (CDC): *Influenza antiviral medications: summary for clinicians*. Available at https://www.cdc.gov/flu/professionals/antivirals/summary-clinicians.htm#summary.
Current for 2020–2021 influenza season.
[a]Although all children younger than 5 years old are considered at higher risk for complications from influenza, the highest risk is for those younger than 2 years old, with the highest hospitalization and death rates among infants younger than 6 months old.

Table 61.2 Diagnostic tests for influenza

Diagnostic test	Types detected	Acceptable specimen	Test time
Rapid influenza diagnostic tests (antigen detection)	A and B	Nasopharyngeal (NP) swab, aspirate or wash, nasal swab, aspirate or wash, throat swab	<15 min
Rapid molecular assay (influenza viral RNA or nucleic acid detection)	A and B	NP swab, nasal swab	15–30 min
Immunofluorescence, direct (DFA) or indirect (IFA) fluorescent antibody staining (antigen detection)	A and B	NP swab or wash, bronchial wash, nasal or endotracheal aspirate	1–4 h
RT-PCR(singleplex and multiplex; real-time and other RNA-based) and other molecular assays (influenza viral RNA or nucleic acid detection)	A and B	NP swab, throat swab, NP or bronchial wash, nasal or endotracheal aspirate, sputum	Varies by assay (1–8 h)
Rapid cell culture (shell vials; cell mixtures; yields live virus)	A and B	NP swab, throat swab, NP or bronchial wash, nasal or endotracheal aspirate, sputum	1–3 days
Viral tissue cell culture (conventional; yields live virus)	A and B	NP swab, throat swab, NP or bronchial wash, nasal or endotracheal aspirate, sputum	3–10 days

NP nucleoprotein, *RT-PCR* reverse transcription-polymerase chain reaction.
Adopted from Centers for Disease Control and Prevention (CDC): Influenza virus testing methods.
Available at https://www.cdc.gov/flu/professionals/diagnosis/table-testing-methods.htm.

recommended to be used in confirming the diagnosis of influenza, but can be useful in clinical research and epidemic studies [8]. It gives more accurate results by obtaining respiratory specimens (e.g., nasopharyngeal swab, nasal wash, or aspirates) within 72–96 h after symptoms appear [25].

61.7 Treatment

Influenza is an illness that usually regresses spontaneously in healthy children. Supportive care recommendations are often given for uncomplicated disease. According to the results of clinical and observational studies, early initiation of antiviral drugs reduces the symptoms of the disease and the possibility of complications [26]. The recommendation of the Centers for Disease Control and Prevention (CDC) and the American Academy of Pediatrics is that antiviral treatment should be initiated as soon as possible for all children hospitalized with a diagnosis of influenza [27]. For outpatients with suspected influenza clinically, if antiviral medications are given within 48 h after the onset of disease, the most clinically effective response is obtained [28].

Anti-influenza drugs used in the therapy and prophylaxis in children are NA inhibitors including oseltamivir, zanamivir, peramivir, and baloxavir, which is an inhibitor of influenza cap-dependent endonuclease activity [28] (Tables 61.3, 61.4).

Table 61.3 Antiviral drugs used in the prophylaxis and treatment of influenza virus infections

Antiviral drug	Activity against	Use	Recommended for	Not recommended for use in	Adverse effects
Oral oseltamivir	Influenza A and B	Treatment Prophylaxis	Any age[a] 3 months and older[a]	N/A N/A	Nausea, vomiting, headache. Postmarketing reports of serious skin reactions and sporadic, transient neuropsychiatric events[b]
Inhaled Zanamivir	Influenza A and B	Treatment Prophylaxis	7 years and older 5 years and older	People with underlying respiratory disease (e.g., asthma, COPD)[c] People with underlying respiratory disease (e.g., asthma, COPD)[c]	Risk of bronchospasm, especially in the setting of underlying airways disease; sinusitis, and dizziness. Postmarketing reports of serious skin reactions and sporadic, transient neuropsychiatric events[b]
Intravenous Peramivir	Influenza A and B[d]	Treatment Prophylaxis[e]	2 years and older[d] Not recommended	N/A N/A	Diarrhea. Postmarketing reports of serious skin reactions and sporadic, transient neuropsychiatric events[b]

Table 61.3 (continued)

Antiviral drug	Activity against	Use	Recommended for	Not recommended for use in	Adverse effects
Oral Baloxavir	Influenza A and B[f]	Treatment Prophylaxis[e]	12 years and older[f] Approved for post-exposure prophylaxis in persons 12 years and older[e]	N/A	None more common than placebo in clinical trials

N/A not applicable, *COPD* chronic obstructive pulmonary disease.

Adopted from Centers for Disease Control and Prevention (CDC): *Influenza antiviral medications: summary for clinicians.* Available at https://www.cdc.gov/flu/professionals/antivirals/summary-clinicians.htm#summary.

[a]Oral oseltamivir phosphate is approved by the FDA for treatment of acute uncomplicated influenza within 2 days of illness onset in people 14 days and older, and for chemoprophylaxis in people 1 year and older. Although not part of the FDA-approved indications, the use of oral oseltamivir for treatment of influenza in infants less than 14 days old, and for chemoprophylaxis in infants 3 months to 1 year, is recommended by the CDC and the American Academy of Pediatrics. If a child is younger than 3 months old, the use of oseltamivir for chemoprophylaxis is not recommended unless the situation is judged critical due to limited data in this age group.

[b]Self-injury or delirium; mainly reported among Japanese pediatric patients.

[c]Inhaled zanamivir is contraindicated also in patients with a history of allergy to lactose or milk protein.

[d]Intravenous peramivir is approved by the FDA for the treatment of acute uncomplicated influenza within 2 days of illness onset in people 2 years and older. Peramivir efficacy is based on clinical trials versus placebo in which the predominant influenza virus type was influenza A; in one trial, a very limited number of subjects infected with influenza B virus were enrolled.

[e]There are no data for use of peramivir for chemoprophylaxis of influenza. On November 23, 2020, FDA approved baloxavir for post-exposure prophylaxis of influenza in persons aged 12 years and older.

[f]Oral baloxavir marboxil is approved by the FDA for treatment of acute uncomplicated influenza within 2 days of illness onset in people 12 years and older who are otherwise healthy, or at high risk of developing influenza-related complications. The safety and efficacy of baloxavir for the treatment of influenza have been established in pediatric patients 12 years and older weighing at least 40 kg. Baloxavir efficacy is based on clinical trials in previously healthy outpatients 12–64 years old [29]. However, there are no available data for baloxavir treatment of influenza in pregnant women, immunocompromised people, or in people with severe influenza. There are no available data from clinical trials for baloxavir treatment of hospitalized patients with influenza.

Adamantanes (also called M2 inhibitors) that function through the M2 protein of influenza A, including amantadine and rimantadine, are not preferred in treatment and prophylaxis due to resistance in circulating influenza strains [35].

61.8 Influenza Vaccines

Immunization is the most important way of protection from flu [36]. The reason why vaccination is required every year is that the immunity provided by the vaccine declines in the following year. Influenza vaccines are re-prepared each year to

Table 61.4 Recommended dosage and duration of antiviral drugs used in the prophylaxis and treatment of influenza virus infections

Antiviral drug	Use	Children	Adults
Oral oseltamivir	Treatment (5 days)[a]	If younger than 1 year old[b]: 3 mg/kg/dose twice daily[c,d] If 1 year or older, dose varies by child's weight: 15 kg or less, the dose is 30 mg twice a day >15–23 kg, the dose is 45 mg twice a day >23–40 kg, the dose is 60 mg twice a day	75 mg twice daily
	Prophylaxis (7 days)[5]	>40 kg, the dose is 75 mg twice a day If child is 3 months or older and younger than 1 year old[b] 3 mg/kg/dose once daily[c] If 1 year or older, dose varies by child's weight: 15 kg or less, the dose is 30 mg once a day >15–23 kg, the dose is 45 mg once a day >23–40 kg, the dose is 60 mg once a day >40 kg, the dose is 75 mg once a day	75 mg once daily
Inhaled Zanamivir[f]	Treatment (5 days)	*Children 7 years or older* 10 mg (two 5-mg inhalations) twice daily	10 mg (two 5 mg inhalations) twice daily
	Prophylaxis (7 days)[e]	Children 5 years or older 10 mg (two 5-mg inhalations) once daily	10 mg (two 5 mg inhalations) once daily
Intravenous Peramivir[g]	Treatment (1 day)[a]	*Children 2–12 years of age* One 12 mg/kg dose, up to 600 mg maximum, via intravenous infusion for a minimum of 15 min	One 600 mg dose, via intravenous infusion for a minimum of 15 min
	Prophylaxis[h]	*Children 13–17 years of age* One 600 mg dose, via intravenous infusion for a minimum of 15 min Not recommended	N/A
Oral Baloxavir[i]	Treatment (1 day)[a]	*Children 12 years and older, dose varies by weight:* <80 kg, one 40 mg dose ≥80 kg, one 80 mg dose[i]	<80 kg, one 40 mg dose ≥80 kg, one 80 mg dose[i]

Table 61.4 (continued)

Antiviral drug	Use	Children	Adults
	Prophylaxi[h]	*Children 12 years and older, dose varies by weight*: <80 kg, one 40 mg dose ≥80 kg, one 80 mg dose	<80 kg, one 40 mg dose ≥80 kg, one 80 mg dose[h]

N/A not approved.

Adopted from Centers for Disease Control and Prevention (CDC): *Influenza antiviral medications: summary for clinicians.* Available at https://www.cdc.gov/flu/professionals/antivirals/summary-clinicians.htm#summary.

[a]Longer treatment duration may be needed for severely ill patients.

[b]Oral oseltamivir is approved by the FDA for treatment of acute uncomplicated influenza within 2 days of illness onset with twice-daily dosing in people 14 days and older, and for chemoprophylaxis with once-daily dosing in people 1 year and older. Although not part of the FDA-approved indications, use of oral oseltamivir for treatment of influenza in infants less than 14 days old, and for chemoprophylaxis in infants 3 months to 1 year of age, is recommended by the CDC and the American Academy of Pediatrics.

[c]This is the FDA-approved oral oseltamivir treatment dose for infants 14 days and older and less than 1 year old, and provides oseltamivir exposure in children similar to that achieved by the approved dose of 75 mg orally twice daily for adults. The American Academy of Pediatrics has recommended an oseltamivir treatment dose of 3.5 mg/kg orally twice daily for infants 9–11 months old, based on data which indicated that a higher dose of 3.5 mg/kg was needed to achieve the protocol-defined targeted exposure for this cohort as defined in the CASG 114 study [30]. It is unknown whether this higher dose will improve efficacy or prevent the development of antiviral resistance. However, there is no evidence that the 3.5 mg/kg dose is harmful or causes more adverse events to infants in this age group.

[d]Current weight-based dosing recommendations are not appropriate for premature infants. Premature infants might have slower clearance of oral oseltamivir because of immature renal function, and doses recommended for full-term infants might lead to very high drug concentrations in this age group. CDC recommends dosing as also recommended by the American Academy of Pediatrics [31]: limited data from the National Institute of Allergy and Infectious Diseases Collaborative Antiviral Study Group provide the basis for dosing preterm infants using their postmenstrual age (gestational age + chronological age): 1.0 mg/kg/dose, orally, twice daily, for those <38 weeks postmenstrual age; 1.5 mg/kg/dose, orally, twice daily, for those 38 through 40 weeks postmenstrual age; 3.0 mg/kg/dose, orally, twice daily, for those >40 weeks postmenstrual age.

[e]If child is younger than 3 months old, use of oseltamivir for chemoprophylaxis is not recommended unless the situation is judged critical due to limited data in this age group.

[f]Inhaled zanamivir is approved for the treatment of acute uncomplicated influenza within 2 days of illness onset with twice-daily dosing in people 7 years and older, and for chemoprophylaxis with once-daily dosing in people 5 years and older

[g]Intravenous peramivir is approved for the treatment of acute uncomplicated influenza within 2 days of illness onset with a single dose in people 2 years and older. Daily dosing for a minimum of 5 days was used in clinical trials of hospitalized patients with influenza [32, 33].

[h]There are no data for use of peramivir for chemoprophylaxis of influenza. One study of baloxavir post-exposure prophylaxis (PEP) of influenza in household members aged 12 years and older (73% received baloxavir within 24 h of onset of symptoms in the index household case who received antiviral treatment) reported that the risk of laboratory-confirmed influenza was significantly lower, by 86%, among those who received baloxavir PEP than among those who received placebo (1.9% [7 of 374] vs. 13.6% [51 of 375]; adjusted risk ratio, 0.14; 95% confidence interval [CI], 0.06 to 0.30; P < 0.001) [34].

[i]Oral baloxavir marboxil is approved by the FDA for treatment of acute uncomplicated influenza within 2 days of illness onset in people 12 years and older who are otherwise healthy, or at high risk of developing influenza-related complications. Baloxavir marboxil should not be administered with dairy products, calcium-fortified beverages, polyvalent cation-containing laxatives, antacids or oral supplements (e.g., calcium, iron, magnesium, selenium, or zinc); co-administration with polyvalent cation-containing products may decrease plasma concentrations of baloxavir which may reduce efficacy. There are no available published data from clinical trials for baloxavir treatment of influenza in patients who are pregnant, immunocompromised, have severe disease, or in hospitalized patients.

Table 61.5 Types of influenza vaccines licensed for children in 2020–2021 season

Vaccine type	Available formulation	Age indication	Route
Inactivated influenza vaccines	Quadrivalent	Although the indications for age vary, there are many brands to be applied from the sixth month. However, in all cases, an age-appropriate vaccine should be used	Intramuscular
Live attenuated influenza vaccine	Quadrivalent	2–49 years	Intranasal

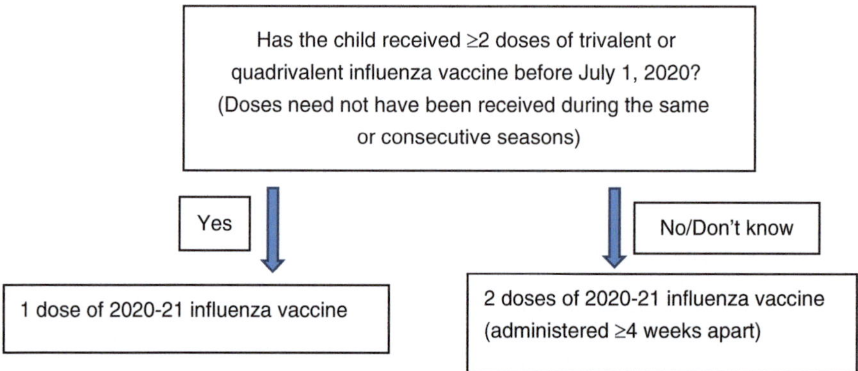

Fig. 61.1 Influenza vaccination algorithm for children aged 6 months to 8 years. https://www.cdc.gov/flu/pdf/professionals/acip/acip-2020-21-summary-of-recommendations.pdf

contain different proportions of influenza A and B subtypes that are predicted to be mostly circulating in the next influenza season.

According to the report published by the American Academy of Pediatrics for the period 2020–21, seasonal influenza vaccines applied to children are quadrivalent [37] (Table 61.5). Influenza vaccines used for children are of two types: inactivated influenza vaccine (IIV) applied intramuscularly and live attenuated vaccine (LAIV) applied intranasally. While IIV can be applied to anyone over 6 months, LAIV is only approved for people between the ages of 2 and 49 who do not have any illnesses and are not pregnant [38]. A routine annual influenza vaccine is advised by the end of October [39].

The most common adverse effects of influenza vaccines are regional reactions such as pain, tenderness, or swelling from the injection and runny nose or nasal congestion after a nasal spray [40, 41]. Rarely, fever, malaise, myalgia, and other systemic symptoms may be observed. These findings may begin 6–12 h after vaccination and continue for 24–48 h [41].

In the 2020–2021 influenza season, the first dose of the vaccine is determined according to the age of the child and the number of vaccine doses taken in previous seasons. The number of doses between 6 months and 8 years is as shown below (Fig. 61.1). People aged 9 and over only need one dose for 2020–2021, but if the child has reached the age of 9 between dose 1 and dose 2, a second dose is recommended. The flu vaccine is not given to children under 6 months of age [42].

Advisory Committee on Immunization Practices (ACIP) publishes guidelines for vaccine formulations every year, and it is important to apply to them in terms of vaccine types, formulations, and contraindications for each new season.

References

1. World Health Organization Global Influenza Strategy 2019–2030: World Health Organization; 2019. https://www.who.int/influenza/global_influenza_strategy_2019_2030/en/.
2. Organization WH. Influenza (seasonal): World Health Organization; 2018; https://www.who.int/news-room/fact-sheets/detail/influenza-(seasonal).
3. Havers FP, Campbell AJP. Influenza viruses. In: Kliegman RM, Stanton BMD, Geme JS, Schor NF, editors. Nelson textbook of pediatrics. 21st ed. Philadelphia: Elsevier; 2019.
4. Gamblin SJ, Skehel JJ. Influenza hemagglutinin and neuraminidase membrane glycoproteins. J Biol Chem. 2010;285(37):28403–9.
5. Brook I. Pediatric influenza: medscape. 2020; https://emedicine.medscape.com/article/972269-overview#a3.
6. Atkinson W, Hamborsky J, McIntyre L, Wolfe S. Epidemiology and prevention of vaccine-preventable diseases. 10th ed. Washington DC: Centers for Disease Control and Prevention; 2007.
7. Carr S. Seasonal and pandemic influenza: an overview with pediatric focus. Adv Pediatr Infect Dis. 2012;59(1):75–93.
8. Paules C, Subbarao K. Influenza. Lancet. 2017;390(10095):697–708.
9. Kumar V. Influenza in children. Indian J Pediatr. 2017;84(2):139–43.
10. Jané M, Vidal MJ, Soldevila N, Romero A, Martínez A, Torner N, et al. Epidemiological and clinical characteristics of children hospitalized due to influenza a and B in the south of Europe, 2010-2016. Sci Rep. 2019;9(1):12853.
11. Kimberlin DW, Brady MT, Jackson MA, Long SS. Influenza. In: Red Book: 2018–2021 report of the Committee on Infectious Diseases. Itasca: American Academy of Pediatrics; 2018. p. 31.
12. Tokars JI, Olsen SJ, Reed C. Seasonal incidence of symptomatic influenza in the United States. Clin Infect Dis. 2018;66(10):1511–8.
13. Wang X, Li Y, O'Brien KL, Madhi SA, Widdowson M-A, Byass P, et al. Global burden of respiratory infections associated with seasonal influenza in children under 5 years in 2018: a systematic review and modelling study. Lancet Glob Health. 2020;8(4):e497–510.
14. Influenza-associated pediatric mortality. Fluview, Weekly U.S. Influenza Surveillance Report: Centers for Disease Control and Prevention; https://gis.cdc.gov/GRASP/Fluview/PedFluDeath.html.
15. Clinical signs and symptoms of influenza: Centers for Disease Control and Prevention; 2020. https://www.cdc.gov/flu/professionals/acip/clinical.htm.
16. Heikkinen T. Influenza in children. Acta Paediatr. 2006;95(7):778–84.
17. Silvennoinen H, Peltola V, Lehtinen P, Vainionpää R, Heikkinen T. Clinical presentation of influenza in unselected children treated as outpatients. Pediatr Infect Dis J. 2009;28(5):372–5.
18. Brook I. Pediatric influenza clinical presentation: medscape; updated August 07, 2020. https://emedicine.medscape.com/article/972269-clinical#b3.
19. Newland JG, Laurich VM, Rosenquist AW, Heydon K, Licht DJ, Keren R, et al. Neurologic complications in children hospitalized with influenza: characteristics, incidence, and risk factors. J Pediatr. 2007;150(3):306–10.
20. Peltola V, Reunanen T, Ziegler T, Silvennoinen H, Heikkinen T. Accuracy of clinical diagnosis of influenza in outpatient children. Clin Infect Dis. 2005;41(8):1198–200.
21. Harper SA, Bradley JS, Englund JA, File TM, Gravenstein S, Hayden FG, et al. Seasonal influenza in adults and children--diagnosis, treatment, chemoprophylaxis, and institutional out-

break management: clinical practice guidelines of the Infectious Diseases Society of America. Clin Infect Dis. 2009;48(8):1003–32.

22. Han Q, Wen X, Wang L, Han X, Shen Y, Cao J, et al. Role of hematological parameters in the diagnosis of influenza virus infection in patients with respiratory tract infection symptoms. J Clin Lab Anal. 2020;34(5):e23191.

23. Liu CY, Wang JD, Yu JT, Wang LC, Lin MC, Lee HF, et al. Influenza B virus-associated pneumonia in pediatric patients: clinical features, laboratory data, and chest X-ray findings. Pediatr Neonatol. 2014;55(1):58–64.

24. Gaitonde DY, Moore FC, Morgan MK. Influenza: diagnosis and treatment. Am Fam Physician. 2019;100(12):751–8.

25. Kondrich J, Rosenthal M. Influenza in children. Curr Opin Pediatr. 2017;29(3):297–302.

26. Ghebrehewet S, MacPherson P, Ho A. Influenza. BMJ. 2016;355:i6258.

27. Murphy A, Lindegren ML, Schaffner W, Johnson D, Riley L, Chappell JD, et al. Improving influenza testing and treatment in hospitalized children. Hosp Pediatr. 2018;8(9):570–7.

28. Influenza antiviral medications: summary for clinicians: Centers for Disease Control and Prevention; 2020. https://www.cdc.gov/flu/professionals/antivirals/summary-clinicians. htm#summary.

29. Hayden FG, Sugaya N, Hirotsu N, Lee N, de Jong MD, Hurt AC, et al. Baloxavir Marboxil for uncomplicated influenza in adults and adolescents. N Engl J Med. 2018;379(10):913–23.

30. Kimberlin DW, Acosta EP, Prichard MN, Sánchez PJ, Ampofo K, Lang D, et al. Oseltamivir pharmacokinetics, dosing, and resistance among children aged <2 years with influenza. J Infect Dis. 2013;207(5):709–20.

31. Pediatrics AAo. Committee on Infectious Diseases. Recommendations for prevention and control of influenza in children , 2017–2018. Pediatrics. 2018;141:1.

32. de Jong MD, Ison MG, Monto AS, Metev H, Clark C, O'Neil B, et al. Evaluation of intravenous peramivir for treatment of influenza in hospitalized patients. Clin Infect Dis. 2014;59(12):e172–85.

33. Ison MG, Fraiz J, Heller B, Jauregui L, Mills G, O'Riordan W, et al. Intravenous peramivir for treatment of influenza in hospitalized patients. Antivir Ther. 2014;19(4):349–61.

34. Ikematsu H, Hayden FG, Kawaguchi K, Kinoshita M, de Jong MD, Lee N, et al. Baloxavir Marboxil for prophylaxis against influenza in household contacts. N Engl J Med. 2020;383(4):309–20.

35. Antiviral drugs for seasonal influenza: Centers for Disease Control and Prevention; updated November 30, 2020. https://www.cdc.gov/flu/professionals/antivirals/links.htm.

36. Trombetta CM, Montomoli E. Influenza immunology evaluation and correlates of protection: a focus on vaccines. Expert Rev Vaccines. 2016;15(8):967–76.

37. Committee on Infectious Diseases. Recommendations for prevention and control of influenza in children, 2020–2021. Pediatrics. 2020;146:4.

38. Types of seasonal influenza vaccine: World Health Organization Regional Office for Europe. https://www.euro.who.int/en/health-topics/communicable-diseases/influenza/vaccination/ types-of-seasonal-influenza-vaccine.

39. Grohskopf LA, Alyanak E, Broder KR, Blanton LH, Fry AM, Jernigan DB, et al. Prevention and control of seasonal influenza with vaccines: recommendations of the advisory Committee on immunization practices United States, 2020-21 influenza season. MMWR Recomm Rep. 2020;69(8):1–24.

40. Mohn KG, Smith I, Sjursen H, Cox RJ. Immune responses after live attenuated influenza vaccination. Hum Vaccin Immunother. 2018;14(3):571–8.

41. Fiore AE, Uyeki TM, Broder K, Finelli L, Euler GL, Singleton JA, et al. Prevention and control of influenza with vaccines: recommendations of the Advisory Committee on Immunization Practices (ACIP), 2010. MMWR Recomm Rep. 2010;59:1–62.

42. Prevention and Control of Seasonal Influenza with Vaccines: Recommendations of the Advisory Committee on Immunization Practices (ACIP)—United States, 2020–21. Summary of Recommendations: Centers for Disease Control and Prevention. https://www.cdc.gov/flu/pdf/professionals/acip/acip-2020-21-summary-of-recommendations.pdf.

Pertussis in Children

62

Adem Karbuz, Emin Sami Arısoy, and Sheldon L. Kaplan

62.1 Introduction

Pertussis, also known as "whooping cough," is an acute respiratory tract infection caused primarily by *Bordetella pertussis* and much less frequently by other *Bordetella* species. As a human disease, it can affect susceptible individuals in all age groups. Pertussis, a highly contagious and severe infectious disease, is endemic mainly in middle- and low-income countries and occurs most commonly in unprotected infants younger than 6 months of age and neonates. However, surveillance of pertussis is insufficient for precisely estimating the numbers of cases or deaths in many countries. Pertussis remains a significant health issue for children worldwide, although it has been among the vaccine-preventable diseases for a very long time.

62.2 Etiology

Currently, 10 species are known in the genus *Bordetella,* which belongs to the family of Alcaligenaceae. The classic species that cause pertussis are *B. pertussis, Bordetella bronchiseptica,* and *Bordetella parapertussis. B. bronchiseptica* generally causes disease in animals; it also leads to pertussis-like syndromes, mainly

A. Karbuz (✉)
Section of Pediatric Infectious Diseases, Prof. Dr. Cemil Taşçıoğlu City Hospital, İstanbul, Turkey

E. S. Arısoy
Division of Pediatric Infectious Diseases, Department of Pediatrics, Faculty of Medicine, Kocaeli University, Kocaeli, Turkey

S. L. Kaplan
Section of Infectious Diseases, Department of Pediatrics, Baylor College of Medicine, and Infectious Disease Service, Texas Children's Hospital, Houston, TX, USA

C. Cingi et al. (eds.), *Pediatric ENT Infections,*
https://doi.org/10.1007/978-3-030-80691-0_62

735

in immune-compromised individuals. *B. parapertussis* typically and much less frequently causes milder pertussis. *Bordetella holmesii* causes pertussis-like respiratory symptoms and invasive infections like bacteremia, endocarditis, and septic arthritis [1–6].

Bordetella species are small, thin, pleomorphic, strictly aerobic (except *Bordetella petrii*) gram-negative coccobacilli. They grow optimally at 35 °C to 37 °C. *B. pertussis* is a nonmotile, catalase- and oxidase-positive, nitrate reduction- and urease production-negative species; however, *B. parapertussis* is a nonmotile, catalase- and urease production-positive and oxidase- and nitrate reduction-negative species [1, 2, 4].

Although many *Bordetella* spp. have relatively simple requirements, sulfides, metal ions, peroxides, and fatty acids prevent the growth of *B. pertussis* in numerous laboratory media. *B. pertussis* is extremely sensitive and requires special media comprising starch, blood, or charcoal for isolation. *Bordetella* species are resistant to cephalexin, except *B. holmesii*. Therefore, cephalexin frequently is added to culture media for inhibition of growth of the other pathogens. Bordet-Gengou agar and Regan-Lowe agar are the selective culture mediums for isolation of *B. pertussis* [1, 2, 4, 5].

62.3 Epidemiology

In 2018, 151,074 pertussis cases were reported worldwide [7]. However, many pertussis cases are not diagnosed and, therefore, not reported. In line with a modeling study in 2014, approximately 24 million pertussis cases and 160,000 childhood deaths because of pertussis in children aged less than 5 years old were estimated to have occurred worldwide, mostly in low- and middle-income countries [8].

Before the introduction and nationwide use of a whole-cell pertussis vaccine in the United States (US) in the 1940s, pertussis was a major childhood illness. Pertussis was reported to frequently exceed 100,000 cases every year, with peaks of the disease occurring in 3- to 5-year cycles. Following the routine use of the pertussis vaccine, the number of cases declined by 99%. The 1010 patients reported in 1976 were the lowest number of cases in the USA. A gradual increase in the number of recorded cases occurred in the 1980s. In 2012, there were overall 48,277 cases, the highest number of pertussis patients in the USA since 1955. The number of reported cases decreased gradually within the following years and was reported to be 15,609 in 2018 [9].

The Pertussis Annual Epidemiological Report of the European Centre for Disease Prevention and Control (ECDC) for 2018 includes data from 30 European countries between 2014 and 2018 [10]. There were 35,627 cases of pertussis in 2018, the lowest number of annual cases over the 5 year study period reported by the 30 European countries. Germany, the Netherlands, Norway, Spain, and the United Kingdom reported 72% of the cases.

Pertussis is transmitted via respiratory droplets generated by coughing or sneezing. Pertussis is a highly contagious disease with an expected R_0 of 12 to 17, defined as secondary cases produced by a primary patient in a completely vulnerable population [11, 12]. The transmission risk is related to repeated or prolonged exposure and closeness of contact with the index case. Attack rates among susceptible individuals are very high. However, studies found attack rates higher in household contacts than in school contacts; the family members usually infect children [1, 4, 13, 14]. The environmental conditions are not suitable for *B. pertussis* to survive for a long time. Fomites do not play a role in transmission. Pertussis can affect susceptible individuals in all age groups [6, 14, 15].

Pertussis is reported commonly in summer and fall as most cases are observed in August, September, and October, and the smallest number of cases occurs in January [16]. In a study conducted between 2008 and 2018 in Germany, *B. pertussis* infection was reported mostly in the months from June to September [17]. Pertussis cases peaked every summer in European countries between 2014 and 2018 [10]. Cyclical epidemics continue to occur every 3–5 years in the vaccine era too. A study from Italy reported the highest pertussis infection incidence in 2012–2013 and 2016–2017 [18].

Pertussis continues to be a crucial public health issue worldwide, particularly in low- and middle-income countries and where immunization coverage is insufficient. Herd immunity, the minimum percentage threshold to be immunized in a community for eliminating infection, is 92–94% for pertussis [12]. In 2019, approximately 85% of infants (116 million infants) worldwide had received three doses of diphtheria-tetanus-pertussis (DTP3) vaccine, and 125 member states of the World Health Organization (WHO) provided at least 90% coverage for the DTP3 vaccine [19].

Increased pertussis rates were seen in adolescents and adults in the last decade, with the illness still seriously affecting children aged <6 months. In 2018, 62% of reported pertussis cases in 30 European countries were seen in children over the age of 14 years [10]; 54% of patients in the USA were over 11 years in 2019 [20]. Adolescents and adults with undiagnosed pertussis are an essential reservoir for infection in infants and children. The actual incidence of pertussis based on the seroprevalence results was significantly higher than the clinically reported incidence in the Czech Republic [21]. Despite widespread vaccination programs, whooping cough continues to be one of the major health issues worldwide.

In addition to an increase in whooping cough cases in general, patients also have been appearing at older ages in many countries in recent years. Multiple factors have likely contributed to the change in the epidemiology of pertussis: increased vaccine failures resulting from genetic changes in circulating *B. pertussis* strains, increased pertussis disease awareness combined with the use of better diagnostic tests, such as polymerase chain reaction (PCR) testing, not achieving complete protection with previous infection or vaccination, the change of whole-cell pertussis vaccine to acellular pertussis vaccine, waning immunity, improved surveillance and reporting of pertussis, vaccine refusal, inadequate vaccination schedules, and decreases in vaccination coverage [1, 3, 5, 22, 23].

62.4 Pathogenesis

Pertussis is mainly a toxin-mediated disease. Pathogenesis of pertussis comprises five essential steps; exposure, attachment, escape from host defenses, local impairment, and systemic findings. Adhesins and toxins responsible for the clinical manifestations are virulence factors expressed by *B. pertussis*. The infection starts with the adhesion of *B. pertussis* to the human respiratory tract's ciliated epithelial cells. Adhesins are implicated in facilitating the attachment process. Once attached, various virulence factors allow evasion of host immune factors and destruction of the epithelial cells. Some toxins produced by *B. pertussis* and anoxia due to coughing paroxysms lead to systemic manifestations of illness without the direct effect of bacteria [1, 2, 4, 5, 16].

The main virulence factors of *B. pertussis* are pertussis toxin (PT), filamentous haemagglutinin, agglutinogens, fimbriae type 2 and type 3, adenylate cyclase toxin, tracheal cytotoxin, pertactin, dermonecrotic toxin, and lipooligosaccharide. The virulence determinants and their impacts are shown in Table 62.1 [1, 2, 4, 5, 16].

Table 62.1 Virulence factors of *Bordetella pertussis*[a]

Virulence factors	
Filamentous hemagglutinin (FHA)	Required for tracheal colonization Highly immunogenic
Fimbriae (FIM)	Serves as adhesin (facilitate attachment) Required for persistent tracheal colonization
Pertactin (PRN)	Adversely affects the innate immune response Promotes adherence of *B. pertussis* to the upper respiratory epithelium
Pertussis toxin (PT)	Potent adjuvant and primary component of pertussis vaccines Evasion from the immune system Responsible for the systemic manifestations (leukocytosis with lymphocytosis, hyperinsulinemia with resultant hypoglycemia, sensitization to histamine and serotonin, pertussis-associated encephalopathy)
Adenylate cyclase (CyaA)	Acts as an anti-inflammatory and antiphagocytic factor during infection Impairs phagocytosis Local tissue damage (induces apoptosis of the cell)
Dermonecrotic toxin (DNT)	Plays a role in local tissue damage Leads to the characteristic skin lesion when injected into test animals
Tracheal cytotoxin (TCT)	Local tissue damage to ciliated epithelial cells (kills the tracheal epithelial cells) Inhibits the regeneration of the respiratory tract epithelium.
Lipooligosaccharide (LPS)	Facilitates attachment Pyrogenic, mitogenic, and toxic

[a]Adopted from Refs. [1, 2, 4, 5, 16].

62.5   Clinical Manifestations

The median incubation period is 7–10 days (range: 5–21 days). Patients may disseminate microorganisms for weeks or months. *B. pertussis* can generally cause mild illness in adults and life-threatening disease in unimmunized infants [1, 4, 15]. The classic clinical presentation of pertussis is composed of catarrhal, paroxysmal, and convalescent phases. The duration of these phases depends on the patient's age and immunization status. Infection is highly contagious in the catarrhal stage and the early period of the paroxysmal stage.

The clinical spectrum of pertussis ranges from asymptomatic or mild disease to life-threatening illness. The severity varies depending on the patient's age, previous vaccination or natural infection, the transplacental transfer of maternal antibodies, use of appropriate antimicrobial therapy, respiratory coinfection, and other situations such as the level of exposure, host immunity, the genotype of the circulating strain, and virulence factors of the bacteria [1–3].

The initial catarrhal stage usually continues for 1–2 weeks and resembles a common cold but has a more extended incubation period. This stage is characterized by slight fever, mild cough, rhinorrhea, sneezing, and conjunctival erythema. Pertussis disease may not be suspected during this stage, and then the frequency and severity of cough gradually increase [1, 2, 4, 16, 24].

The paroxysmal stage is characterized by bouts of repeated coughing with 5–10 or more violently and exhausting coughs during one paroxysm, which generally leads to a clinical consideration of pertussis diagnosis. The character of the cough is dry, intermittent, and irritative. At the end of the paroxysms, strong inspiratory breathing occurs when there is no extra air in the lungs, so a distinctive high-pitched whooping voice emerges. During paroxysms, the patients usually appear to be very tired, dizzy, and apathetic. The attacks lead to cyanosis, the prominence of protruding eyes, lacrimation, outthrust of the tongue, salivation, and the appearance of petechiae on the face. The paroxysms are associated with the accumulation of thick and viscous mucus plugs in the airways and may end with these plugs' expulsion. At the end of the coughing paroxysm, post-tussive vomiting is common. The paroxysms are particularly more frequent and severe at night. Paroxysms of coughing may develop spontaneously or precipitated by external factors such as eating, drinking, yawning, sneezing, cold air, inhaled irritants, or physical exertion. The patients are entirely normal and may not appear ill between attacks if complications do not occur. The paroxysmal stage generally continues for 4–6 weeks but may last for up to 10 weeks in some patients [1, 2, 4, 5, 16, 24].

The convalescent phase, the respiratory tract recovery stage, is characterized by a decline in severity, duration, and coughing attack frequency. It generally continues from weeks to months and is often exacerbated by subsequent respiratory infections but does not occur due to recurrent disease or reactivation of *B. pertussis* [4, 22].

The illness of whooping cough in adolescents, adults, and children partially immunized by vaccination may represent a disease ranging from a mild to intractable cough or one without symptoms. The pertussis diagnosis is usually not considered in adolescents and adults previously vaccinated who generally do not manifest classic pertussis presentation with paroxysms. However, pertussis should be considered in the presence of a cough lasting longer than 3 weeks in this age group [4].

It is also difficult to diagnose pertussis solely with clinical suspicion in children less than 1-year of age. In one study, pertussis was diagnosed with clinical suspicion only in 34.8% of the patients at admission [18]. Also, diagnosis with clinical suspicion was much lower in children under 3 months of age. Severe morbidity and mortality resulting from pertussis often occur in young infants, especially <3 months [3, 16, 18]. Infants usually present with nonspecific signs such as nonspecific coughs, apnea, and poor feeding. The initial findings are frequently apnea and cyanosis, and the characteristic cough attacks may not be seen, especially in the early period in newborn and young infants. Seizures in association with apnea, caused by hypoxia and severe pulmonary hypertension, are relatively common in this age group. Also, the length of hospitalization and intensive care unit admissions increase in these infants. Severe complications associated with respiratory, nutritional, and neurological problems can be fatal [3, 16, 18].

62.6 Complications

Complications frequently occur by severe coughing spells leading to hypoxia, pressure effects of severe paroxysms, secondary to feeding difficulties, and post-tussive vomiting, mostly during the paroxysmal stage. Pneumonia is the most frequent complication and the prevalent cause of pertussis-associated death, particularly in younger infants. Dehydration, sleeping difficulty, pulmonary hypertension, conjunctival bleeding, epistaxis, subdural hematoma, hernias, pneumothorax, pneumomediastinum, subcutaneous emphysema, rectal prolapse, urinary incontinence, syncope, apnea, neurologic complications such as seizures and encephalopathy, and otitis media are the other not infrequently encountered complications. Furthermore, *B. pertussis* infection is associated with sudden infant death syndrome [1, 2, 16, 22, 24].

62.7 Differential Diagnosis

A pertussis-like disease with a prolonged cough occurs during several respiratory tract infections caused by viruses, *Mycoplasma pneumoniae, Chlamydia trachomatis,* and *Chlamydia pneumoniae. Mycoplasma* infection is considered with the presence of symptoms such as malaise, fever, headache, rales in lung examination, and an occasional maculopapular rash. *C. trachomatis* causes *a* repetitive *staccato* cough, tachypnea, and rales in an afebrile, very young infant. Non-exudative pharyngitis and pulmonary rales are found in the *C. pneumoniae* illness. Respiratory syncytial virus (RSV) is distinguished by the presence of wheezing and seasonal presentation. Adenoviral infection can be considered in patients with fever, sore throat, and conjunctivitis [1, 5, 6].

A total of 543 patients with respiratory symptoms were analyzed by reverse transcriptase (RT)-PCR in a study [25]. Rhinovirus, *B. pertussis*, RSV, adenovirus, parainfluenza viruses, metapneumovirus, bocavirus, coronavirus, influenza virus, and enteroviruses were determined in most patients. The remaining patients (21.4% of the total) had a negative PCR result for pertussis and viral infections. This study is important as it explained that pertussis could often be confused with viral respiratory infections [25]. However, pertussis is rare in infants hospitalized with acute bronchiolitis that is frequently caused by respiratory tract viruses [26]. The cough associated with gastroesophageal reflux or related to a foreign body in the airway can also be confused with pertussis [1, 6].

62.8 Diagnosis and Laboratory Findings

Early pertussis symptoms and signs are often nonspecific, especially in young infants, making the diagnosis difficult in catarrhal stages. Microbiological, molecular, and serology methods are helpful for the diagnosis in these situations.

The diagnosis of pertussis depends on the combination of clinical features and laboratory findings. Pertussis should be considered in any individual with a persistent cough. The features such as fever, malaise, myalgia, rash, sore throat, and hoarseness are not expected in patients with pertussis. And the systemic physical examination findings are usually normal if the complications do not occur [1, 6].

The Centers for Disease Control and Prevention (CDC) has a pertussis case definition for public health surveillance (Table 62.2) [27].

The growth of *B. pertussis* obtained from nasopharyngeal specimens on the appropriate media is the "gold standard" for the diagnosis of disease. However, this remains a nonsensitive method for several reasons: fastidious growth of bacteria, the requirement of specific swabs and media, and culture [1, 2, 15]. The appropriate specimen for culture can be obtained by swabbing the nasopharynx with polyester, dacron, or calcium alginate swabs, not cotton and rayon swabs, washing, or nasopharyngeal aspiration.

Specimens are collected from the posterior nasopharynx containing the ciliated respiratory epithelial cells to which *B. pertussis* adheres. Specific media such as Regan-Lowe transport medium, Bordet-Gengou agar, and modified Stainer-Scholte broth are required for the growth of *B. pertussis*. The rate of *B. pertussis* isolation on selective media is the highest within the catarrhal and early paroxysmal stages [1, 2, 15].

Laboratory diagnosis of pertussis can be made by demonstrating a specific antibody titer rise between two blood samples obtained at least 2 weeks apart or an elevated single-serum antibody titer against *B. pertussis*. Pertussis toxin, a robust, specific *B. pertussis* protein as antigen, has an essential role in immune response, is also the most frequently used antigen for serologic diagnosis. But not all infected people, especially young infants, develop antibody responses to PT [3]. On the other

Table 62.2 The US CDC surveillance case definition for pertussis (2020) (Adopted from Ref. [27]

Clinical criteria	Laboratory criteria
In the absence of a more likely diagnosis, a cough illness lasting ≥2 weeks, with at least one of the following signs or symptoms: • Paroxysms of coughing, OR • Inspiratory whoop, OR • Post-tussive vomiting, OR • Apnea (with or without cyanosis)	Confirmatory laboratory evidence: • Isolation of *Bordetella pertussis* from a clinical specimen • Positive polymerase chain reaction (PCR) for *B. pertussis*
Epidemiologic linkage Contact with a laboratory-confirmed case of pertussis	
Case classification	

Probable:
In the absence of a more likely diagnosis, an illness meeting the clinical criteria
OR
Illness with cough of any duration, with
• At least one of the following signs or symptoms:
  – Paroxysms of coughing, OR
  – Inspiratory whoop, OR
  – Post-tussive vomiting, OR
  – Apnea (with or without cyanosis)
AND
Contact with a laboratory-confirmed case (epidemiologic linkage)
	Confirmed:
	• Acute cough illness of any duration with
	Isolation of *pertussis* from a clinical specimen
	OR
	• PCR positive for *B. pertussis*

US United States, *CDC* Centers for Disease Control and Prevention.

hand, the first blood specimen is generally taken too late in the course of illness to demonstrate a specific antibody titer rise to establish an early diagnosis. Hence, monitoring a specific antibody titer rise is not helpful for the acute diagnosis of pertussis.

B. pertussis immunoglobulin (Ig) G test is the best-standardized and the most widely used diagnostic serologic test. IgG titer usually increases 2–3 weeks after the onset of infection or primary immunization. PT IgG level >90 or 100 IU/mL in a single serum sample suggests a recent illness and often is positive in the middle of the paroxysmal phase [5, 6, 15]. Distinguishing between antibody responses secondary to infection or recent immunization might not be possible, and thus, serological methods should not be performed if the pertussis vaccine was administered within the last year. Serology is unreliable in infants due to maternal antibodies and is insensitive in children ≤10 years old [2].

Nucleic acid amplification tests, including PCR assay, are the most commonly used diagnostic laboratory method for detecting *B. pertussis* because of their much higher sensitivity and rapid results. The PCR test requires collecting an appropriate nasopharyngeal specimen obtained by dacron or rayon or nylon-flocked swabs or by nasopharyngeal wash or aspirate. For PCR tests, calcium alginate and cotton swabs can be inhibitory and should not be used [2, 15, 28].

62.9 Treatment

Management of pertussis disease consists of antimicrobial therapy and supportive care. Antibiotic treatment aims to reduce the severity, duration, and frequency of symptoms and prevent infection transmission. On the other hand, antibiotics started late in the illness have a limited effect on the disease during the paroxysmal stage. However, antimicrobial treatment will eradicate the bacteria from the nasopharynx, and so communicability will decrease. Thus, antimicrobial therapy should be initiated immediately based on clinical suspicion without awaiting laboratory confirmation.

A 5-day course of azithromycin is the recommended first-line antibiotic regimen for treatment and postexposure prophylaxis. Other macrolides (erythromycin, clarithromycin), fluoroquinolones, and trimethoprim-sulfamethoxazole (TMP-SMX) are alternative preferred antibiotics. Erythromycin is not recommended in newborns (<1 month of age) because of the risk of infantile hypertrophic pyloric stenosis (Table 62.3) [2, 4–6, 15].

Penicillins, amino-penicillins (ampicillin, amoxicillin), cephalosporins, and tetracyclines are not recommended for treatment or chemoprophylaxis of pertussis because of ineffectiveness. Resistance to macrolides is rare in *B. pertussis* strains. The low rate of antibiotic-resistant *B. pertussis* strains may be explained partly by the infrequent isolation of *B. pertussis* isolated (related to the insensitive culture methods and greater reliance on PCR for diagnosing illness), thus inadequacy of data on antibiotic susceptibility tests. Resistance to macrolides was reported sporadically from China, Japan, Iran, and France since the first erythromycin-resistant *B. pertussis* case was detected in 1995. Resistance to erythromycin is dependent on a mutation in the 23S rRNA gene of *B. pertussis* [4, 30–34].

Supportive care, which includes the balance of fluid and nutrition and management of cough, is essential. Intravenous hydration, feeding by nasogastric tube, aspiration of secretions, and oxygen supplementation during attacks may be required. Exchange transfusion may be necessitated for hyperleukocytosis in severe cases of pertussis. Criteria for considering exchange blood transfusion in infants with pertussis less than 60 days of age have been proposed [35]. Symptomatic therapies with bronchodilators, corticosteroids, pertussis-specific immunoglobulin, antihistamines, and antitussive agents are not recommended for whooping cough. In a Cochrane review, diphenhydramine and salbutamol did not change the frequency of coughing episodes per 24 h [36]. The external factors that can trigger cough may be avoided [1–4, 6, 15].

62.10 Prognosis

The prognosis of pertussis is closely related to the age and vaccination status of the patient. The morbidity and mortality rates are highest in neonates and susceptible infants. Older children, adolescents, and adults have a better prognosis with a milder disease course or a prolonged cough. Antibiotics do not affect the disease's course

Table 62.3 Recommended antimicrobial treatment and postexposure prophylaxis for pertussis (Adopted from Refs. [2, 4–6, 15, 29])

Age group	When is treatment initiated	When is chemoprophylaxis initiated	Azithromycin	Erythromycin	Clarithromycin	TMP-SMX
<1 month	Suspected or proven pertussis anytime after the onset of symptoms	Exposed to a case of pertussis within 21 days of onset of cough in the index case	10 mg/kg/day in a single dose for 5 days	Not recommended Associated with infantile hypertrophic pyloric stenosis	Not recommended	Not recommended <2 months of age risk for kernicterus
1–5 months	Suspected or proven pertussis within 42 days of onset of symptoms	Exposed to a case of pertussis within 21 days of onset of cough in the index case	10 mg/kg/day in a single dose for 5 days	40–50 mg/kg/day in 4 divided doses for 14 days	15 mg/kg/day in 2 divided doses for 7 days	For infants age ≥ 2-month: TMP 8 mg/kg/day plus SMX 40 mg/kg/day in two divided doses for 14 days
6–12 months	Suspected or proven pertussis within 42 days of onset of symptoms	Exposed to case of pertussis within 21 days of onset of cough in index case	10 mg/kg in a single dose on day 1 (max. 500 mg), then 5 mg/kg/day (max. 250 mg) on days 2–5	40–50 mg/kg/day (max. 2 g/day) in 4 divided doses for 14 days	15 mg/kg/day in 2 divided doses (max. 1 g/day) for 7 days	TMP 8 mg/kg/day plus SMX 40 mg/kg/day in two divided doses (max. TMP: 320 mg/day) for 14 days
Infants (aged ≥12 months) and children	Suspected or proven pertussis within 21 days of onset of symptoms	Exposed to case of pertussis within 21 days of onset of cough in index case	10 mg/kg in a single dose on day 1 (max. 500 mg), then 5 mg/kg/day (max. 250 mg) on days 2–5	40–50 mg/kg/day (max. 2 g/day) in 4 divided doses for 14 days	15 mg/kg/day in 2 divided doses (max. 1 g/day) for 7 days	TMP 8 mg/kg/day plus SMX 40 mg/kg/day in 2 divided doses (max. TMP: 320 mg/day) for 14 days

[a]*Max* maximum, *TMP-SMX* trimethoprim-sulfamethoxazole.

since antibiotics are generally started in the advanced stages; however, the use of antibiotics limits contagiousness [1, 2].

Life-threatening and severe complications such as apnea, secondary bacterial pneumonia, seizures, pulmonary hypertension, and encephalopathy can occur mostly in unvaccinated or incompletely immunized infants younger than 6 months. The mortality rate is highest in neonates and infants younger than 2 months. During admission to the hospital, high levels of mean heart rate, coinfection of RSV, leukocytosis, and lymphocytosis are poor prognostic criteria. The presence of acute respiratory failure, leukocytosis, and pulmonary hypertension, which define malignant pertussis, is almost always fatal [1, 37–39].

In patients with severe pertussis, neurodevelopmental problems can also be seen in long-term follow-up. In a study including pertussis cases requiring the intensive care unit, the patients' cognitive developments were evaluated by the Mullen Scales of Early Learning (considers gross motor, visual reception, and receptive and expressive language) at the end of the first year [40]. In 37% of the patients, abnormal scores were detected in at least one domain; language development was the most frequently affected area.

62.11 Prevention and Control

In addition to standard precautions in hospitalized patients, droplet precautions are recommended 5 days after effective therapy is initiated [15].

Postexposure chemoprophylaxis is frequently recommended for asymptomatic close contacts, high-risk individuals, and close contacts who may contact high-risk individuals. Also, active immunization of incompletely vaccinated exposed persons of all ages should be provided. The high-risk individuals include infants-age <1 year, pregnant women in the third trimester, individuals with various immune-deficiency disorders, or certain underlying medical conditions. Preferred chemoprophylactic antibiotics, dosages, and chemoprophylaxis duration are similar to treatment regimens (Table 62.3) [2, 4–6, 15, 29].

Immunization is the single most effective method of protection against pertussis infections. Whole-cell vaccines, the first pertussis vaccines, have been used worldwide since the 1940s. Purified acellular-component pertussis vaccines were initially introduced in 1997. The acellular pertussis vaccines contain three or more *B. pertussis* antigens: inactivated PT, filamentous hemagglutinin, fimbrial proteins, and pertactin. In the subsequent years, they were replaced with whole-cell vaccines in many countries. Whole-cell and acellular pertussis vaccines have a difference regarding the duration of immunity they induce. The whole-cell pertussis vaccines protect for 5–14 years, and acellular vaccines protect for 4–7 years. This difference is mainly based on their distinct way of producing immunity. The whole-cell pertussis vaccines induce the T helper (Th)-1 and Th-17 cellular immune responses, whereas the acellular pertussis vaccines induce a predominantly Th-2 cellular immune response [1, 4, 6, 15].

Five doses of diphtheria and tetanus toxoid and acellular pertussis (DTaP) vaccines are recommended in children age <7 years. The first four doses should be administered before the age of 2, and the fifth dose is recommended before kindergarten and after the age of 4. The first dose can be administered at 6 weeks at the earliest. There should be 4 weeks between each dose of the first three doses, and there should be at least a 6-month interval for the subsequent doses [6, 15].

DTaP vaccines are licensed to use in children under 7 years of age. Tdap vaccines include "the adolescent or adult type of acellular pertussis vaccine (ap)" composed of diminished amounts of pertussis antigens and should not be administered instead of DTaP. If the Tdap vaccine is administered mistakenly for the initial 3 doses of pertussis vaccination instead of DTaP in a child less than 7 years of age, it is not accepted as a valid vaccination. Thus, the DTaP vaccine should be administered for revaccination at an appropriate time. However, more than six doses of vaccines that contain diphtheria and tetanus vaccines should not be administered before the age of 7 years. If this does occur, adverse reactions, including mostly local reactions, can be observed [6, 15].

Immunization is generally performed at 2, 4, 6, 15–18 months, and 4–6 years of age for protection against pertussis in many countries. However, neither vaccination nor previous infection protects children lifelong against pertussis or reinfection. Thus, vaccination is recommended in children who have had the disease as well. DTaP vaccine is protective for 2 years following four doses of the vaccine, and then immunity decreases over the years. Hence, a Tdap booster dose is recommended at 11–12 years old [15, 41].

Local reactions such as redness, swelling, and pain and systemic reactions such as fever ($\geq$38.6 °C [100.1 °F]), fussiness, drowsiness, anorexia, and vomiting are not uncommon after pertussis vaccination. More severe adverse events such as seizures, hypotonic-hyporesponsive episodes, fever 40.5 °C (104.8 °F) or higher, or prolonged crying ($\geq$3 hours) are rare. Local reactions (i.e., limb swelling) increase slightly in frequency and severity after administration of the fourth and fifth doses of vaccines. These conditions are not contraindications for the next dose(s). Most local and systemic reactions are significantly less common with acellular pertussis vaccines than with whole-cell pertussis vaccines. A severe allergic reaction (e.g., anaphylaxis) or encephalopathy within 7 days after administration of a previous pertussis vaccine is a contraindication for the next dose(s) [1, 6, 15].

Severe pertussis and related deaths occur mostly in the first months of life. In this period, infants have not been vaccinated, or only the first dose vaccine has been administered. This situation makes the infants at this age the most vulnerable and unprotected population. Experts consider two strategies to protect this population [42]. In the cocoon strategy, vaccination is recommended for all caregivers or close contacts of this age group. Transmission to infants usually occurs through close contacts who are caregivers, especially mothers and fathers [43]. Prevention of transmission tried by the cocoon strategy provides indirect protection. This strategy is recommended in some countries, including the USA, Belgium, France, and Germany. However, there is limited data about the effectiveness of the cocoon strategy [42]. A study reported from Australia showed that the risk of pertussis was reduced by 51% in those younger than 4 months whose mother and father are vaccinated [44].

Computer modeling methods have been used to assess the effectiveness of the cocoon strategy. It has been reported that the cocoon strategy is not effective in regions where the incidence is low. And a large number of individuals need to be vaccinated to obtain favorable results regarding the disease of pertussis [42]. A study reported that the number of required parental immunizations to prevent hospitalization, intensive care unit admission, and death of one case from pertussis was 10,000, 100,000, and one million, respectively [45]. Therefore, the cocoon strategy was not found to be cost-effective. In addition, a minimum of 2 weeks is required for maximal antibody development in vaccinated individuals. If vaccination is administered immediately after delivery, it should be kept in mind that the newborn will still be at risk for the first 2 weeks [42].

The second strategy aims to increase the protective antibodies transmitted to the fetus by the maternal vaccination during pregnancy. Thus, the passive transfer of maternal antibodies results in sufficient protective antibody levels against severe pertussis infection in the neonatal period and first months of life. During pregnancy, the maternal pertussis vaccination program is recommended in many countries, including the USA (the preferred strategy), the United Kingdom, New Zealand, Australia, and Israel [42, 46, 47].

Eberhardt et al. showed that maternal Tdap immunization administered in the early second-trimester significantly increased neonatal antibodies [48]. In the United Kingdom, initially in 2012, maternal vaccination as a single dose of Tdap was recommended to all women for each pregnancy at 28–38 gestational weeks. Subsequently, in 2016 maternal vaccination was recommended between 20 and 32 gestational weeks, the earliest at 16 weeks. In this way, more pregnant women are vaccinated, and more premature newborns are protected [46].

A case-control study was conducted by Dabrera et al. in the United Kingdom to estimate vaccination effectiveness during pregnancy. The adjusted efficacy of vaccination in infants <8 weeks of age was 93% [49]. Maternal immunization during pregnancy is preferred over the cocoon strategy. If it is not possible, a complete cocoon strategy is performed. If this is not possible, both parents' vaccination should be administered, especially mothers' [42].

A systematic review showed that vaccination during pregnancy did not adversely affect the course of the pregnancy, the developmental features of the fetus, and neonatal outcomes. Self-limiting mild local and systemic reactions were reported, and vaccination was well tolerated during pregnancy [50].

There is no risk in vaccination of nursing mothers or pregnant women planning to breastfeed. Some studies report increased pertussis antibodies in the breast milk of women vaccinated during pregnancy, at delivery, or in the early postpartum period. Pertussis antibodies can be detected even at 8 weeks postpartum in the breast milk of women vaccinated during pregnancy and may help reduce the risk of developing illness in younger infants [46, 51–53].

62.12 Conclusion

Even though the pertussis vaccine coverage is high in infants worldwide, the current immunization programs and the acellular vaccines used in most countries are insufficient to control the illness. Therefore, the development of new-generation pertussis vaccines should be targeted, or the currently available vaccines with various immunization programs should be enhanced [4].

References

1. Cherry JD, Heininger U. Pertussis and other Bordetella infections. In: Cherry JD, Harrison GJ, Kaplan SL, Steinbach WJ, Hotez PJ, editors. Feigin and Cherry's textbook of pediatric infectious diseases. 8th ed. Philadelphia: Elsevier; 2019. p. 1159–78.
2. Waters V, Halperin SA. Bordetella pertussis. In: Bennett JE, Dolin R, Blaser MJ, editors. Mandell, Douglas and Bennett's principles and practice of infectious diseases. 9th ed. Philadelphia: Elsevier; 2020. p. 2793–802.
3. Nieves DJ, Heininger U, Cherry JD. Bordetella pertussis and other Bordetella spp. infections. In: Wilson CB, Nizet V, Maldonado YA, Remington JS, Klein JO, editors. Remington and Klein's infectious diseases of the fetus and newborn infant. 8th ed. Philadelphia: Elsevier; 2016. p. 598–616.
4. Kilgore PE, Salim AM, Zervos MJ, Schmitt H-J. Pertussis: microbiology, disease, treatment, and prevention. Clin Microbiol Rev. 2016;29:449–86.
5. Long SS, Edwards KM, Mertsola J. Bordetella pertussis (pertussis) and other species. In: Long SS, Prober CG, Fischer M, editors. Principles and practice of pediatric infectious diseases. 5th ed. Philadelphia: Elsevier; 2018. p. 890–8.
6. Souder EL, Long SS. Pertussis (Bordetella pertussis and Bordetella parapertussis). In: Kliegman RM, St Geme III JW, Blum NJ, Shah SS, Tasker RC, Wilson KM, editors. Nelson textbook of pediatrics. 21st ed. Philadelphia: Elsevier; 2020. p. 1492–6.
7. World Health Organization. Pertussis. https://www.who.int/health-topics/pertussis#tab=tab_1. Accessed 30 Dec 2020.
8. Yeung KHT, Duclos P, Nelson EAS, Hutubessy RCW. An update of the global burden of pertussis in children younger than 5 years: a modelling study. Lancet Infect Dis. 2017;17:974–80.
9. Centers for Disease Control and Prevention. Pertussis (Whooping Cough): Surveillance & Reporting. Reported national notifiable diseases surveillance system pertussis cases: 1922–2018, http://www.cdc.gov/pertussis/surv-reporting.html. Accessed 30 Dec 2020.
10. European Centre for Disease Prevention and Control. Pertussis—annual epidemiological report for 2018. Stockholm: ECDC; 2020. p. 1–8. https://www.ecdc.europa.eu/sites/default/files/documents/AER_for_2018_pertussis.pdf. Accessed 30 Dec 2020
11. Diekmann O, Heesterbeek JAP, Metz JAJ. On the definition and the computation of the basic reproduction ratio R_0 in models for infectious diseases in heterogeneous populations. J Math Biol. 1990;28:365–82.
12. Fine PE. Herd immunity: history, theory, practice. Epidemiol Rev. 1993;15:265–302.
13. Kowalzik F, Barbosa AP, Fernandes VR, et al. Prospective multinational study of pertussis infection in hospitalized infants and their household contacts. Pediatr Infect Dis J. 2007;26:238–42.
14. Shehab ZM. Pertussis. In: Taussig LM, Landau LI, editors. Pediatric respiratory medicine. 2nd ed. Philadelphia: Elsevier; 2008. p. 589–95.
15. American Academy of Pediatrics. Pertussis (whooping cough). In: Kimberlin DW, Brady MT, Jackson MA, Long SS, editors. Red Book: 2018 Report of the committee on infectious diseases. 31st ed. Itasca: American Academy of Pediatrics; 2018. p. 620–34.

16. Mattoo S, Cherry JD. Molecular pathogenesis, epidemiology, and clinical manifestations of respiratory infections due to Bordetella pertussis and other Bordetella subspecies. Clin Microbiol Rev. 2005;18:326–82.
17. Hitz DA, Tewald F, Eggers M. Seasonal Bordetella pertussis pattern in the period from 2008 to 2018 in Germany. BMC Infect Dis. 2020;20(1):474.
18. Camillo CD, Vittucci AC, Antilici L, et al. Pertussis in early life: underdiagnosed, severe, and risky disease. A seven-year experience in a pediatric tertiary-care hospital. Hum Vaccin Immunother. 2020;5:1–9.
19. World Health Organization. Factsheet immunization coverage; 2020. https://www.who.int/news-room/fact-sheets/detail/immunization-coverage. Accessed 30 Dec 2020.
20. Centers for Disease Control and Prevention. National Center for Immunization and Respiratory Diseases, Division of Bacterial Diseases. Provisional pertussis surveillance report; 2019 https://www.cdc.gov/pertussis/downloads/pertuss-surv-report-2019-508.pdf. Accessed 30 Dec 2020.
21. Chlibek R, Smetana J, Sosovickova R, et al. Seroepidemiology of whooping cough in the Czech Republic: estimates of incidence of infection in adults. Public Health. 2017;150:77–83.
22. Daniels HL, Sabella C. Bordetella pertussis (pertussis). Pediatr Rev. 2018;39:247–57.
23. Saadatian-Elahi M, Plotkin S, Mills KHG, et al. Pertussis: biology, epidemiology and prevention. Vaccine. 2016;34:5819–26.
24. Centers for Disease Control and Prevention. Pertussis. In: Hamborsky J, Kroger A, Wolfe S, editors. Epidemiology and prevention of vaccine-preventable diseases – pink book. 13th ed. Washington: Public Health Foundation; 2015. p. 261–78. https://www.cdc.gov/vaccines/pubs/pinkbook/pert.html. Accessed: Dec. 30, 2020.
25. Tozzi AE, Gesualdo F, Rizzo C, et al. A data driven clinical algorithm for differential diagnosis of pertussis and other respiratory infections in infants. PLoS One. 2020;15(7):e0236041.
26. Efendiyeva E, Kara TT, Erat T, et al. The incidence and clinical effects of Bordetella pertussis in children hospitalized with acute bronchiolitis. Turk J Pediatr. 2020;62:726–33.
27. Centers for Disease Control and Prevention National Notifiable Diseases Surveillance System (NNDSS). Surveillance Case Definitions. Pertussis. Case definition 2020. https://wwwn.cdc.gov/nndss/conditions/pertussis/case-definition/2020/ Accessed 30 Dec 2020.
28. Centers for Disease Control and Prevention. Best practices for health care professionals on the use of polymerase chain reaction (PCR) for diagnosing pertussis. https://www.cdc.gov/pertussis/clinical/diagnostic-testing/diagnosis-pcr-bestpractices.html. Accessed 30 Dec 2020.
29. Centers for Disease Control and Prevention. Recommended antimicrobial agents for the treatment and postexposure prophylaxis of pertussis. MMWR. 2005;54(RR14):1–16.
30. Wang Z, Cui Z, Li Y, et al. High prevalence of erythromycin-resistant *Bordetella pertussis* in Xi'an, China. Clin Microbiol Infect. 2014;20:O825–30.
31. Yamaguchi T, Kawasaki Y, Katsukawa C, Kawahara R, Kawatsu K. The first report of macrolide-resistant Bordetella pertussis isolation in Japan. Jpn J Infect Dis. 2020;73:361–2.
32. Fereshteh S, Masoumeh NL, Vajiheh SN, et al. The first macrolide-resistant Bordetella pertussis strains isolated from Iranian patients. Jundishapur J Microbiol. 2014;7(6):e10880.
33. Sophie G, Ghislaine D, Yves G, Jérome E, Daniel F, Nicole G. Macrolide-resistant *Bordetella pertussis* infection in newborn girl. France Emerg Infect Dis. 2012;18:966–8.
34. Lewis K, Saubolle MA, Tenover FC, Rudinsky MF, Barbour SD, Cherry JD. Pertussis caused by an erythromycin-resistant strain of Bordetella pertussis. Pediatr Infect Dis. 1995;14:388–91.
35. Cherry JD, Wendorf K, Bregman B, et al. An observational study of severe pertussis in 100 infants ≤120 days of age. Pediatr Infect Dis J. 2018;37:202–5.
36. Bettiol S, Wang K, Thompson MJ, et al. Symptomatic treatment of the cough in whooping cough. Cochrane Database Syst Rev. 2012;5:CD003257.
37. Palvo F, Fabro AT, Cervi MC, Aragon DC, Ramalho FS, Carlotti APCP. Severe pertussis infection: a clinicopathological study. Medicine (Baltimore). 2017;96(48):e8823.
38. Şık G, Demirbuğa A, Annayev A, Çıtak A. The clinical characteristics and prognosis of pertussis among unvaccinated infants in the pediatric intensive care unit. Turk Pediatri Ars. 2020;55:54–9.

39. Bouziri A, Hamdi A, Khaldi A, et al. La coqueluche maligne: une maladie sous diagnostiquée [Malignant pertussis: an underdiagnosed illness]. Med Trop (Mars). 2010;70:245–8.
40. Berger JT, Villalobos ME, Clark AE, et al. Cognitive development one year after infantile critical pertussis. Pediatr Crit Care Med. 2018;19:89–97.
41. Centers for Disease Control and Prevention. Pertussis (whooping cough): pertussis 41. Frequently asked questions, https://www.cdc.gov/pertussis/about/faqs.html. Accessed 30 Dec 2020.
42. Forsyth K, Plotkin S, Tan T, Wirsing von König CH. Strategies to decrease pertussis transmission to infants. Pediatrics. 2015;135:e1475–82.
43. Wendelboe AM, Njamkepo E, Bourillon A, et al. Transmission of Bordetella pertussis to young infants. Pediatr Infect Dis J. 2007;26:293–9.
44. Quinn HE, Snelling TL, Habig A, Chiu C, Spokes PJ, McIntyre PB. Parental Tdap boosters and infant pertussis: a case-control study. Pediatrics. 2014;134:713–20.
45. Skowronski DM, Janjua NZ, Tsafack ER, Quakkki M, Hoang L, De Serres G. The number needed to vaccinate to prevent infant pertussis hospitalization and death though parent cocoon immunization. Clin Infect Dis. 2012;54:318–27.
46. Public Health England. Vaccination against pertussis (whooping cough) for pregnant women. London: Public Health England; 2020. p. 1–19.
47. State of Israel Ministry of Health. Vaccines for women before pregnancy, during pregnancy and after childbirth. https://www.health.gov.il/English/Topics/Pregnancy/during/Pages/vaccine_pregnant.aspx. Accessed 30 Dec 2020.
48. Eberhardt CS, Blanchard-Rohner G, Lemaitre B, et al. Maternal immunization earlier in pregnancy maximizes antibody transfer and expected infant seropositivity against pertussis. Clin Infect Dis. 2016;62:829–36.
49. Dabrera G, Amirthalingam G, Andrews N, et al. A case-control study to estimate the effectiveness of maternal pertussis vaccination in protecting newborn infants in England and Wales, 2012–2013. Clin Infect Dis. 2015;60:333–7.
50. D'Heilly C, Switzer C, Macina D. Safety of maternal immunization against pertussis: a systematic review. Infect Dis Ther. 2019;8:543–68.
51. Halperin BA, Morris A, Mackinnon-Cameron D, et al. Kinetics of the antibody response to tetanus-diphtheria-acellular pertussis vaccine in women of childbearing age and postpartum women. Clin Infect Dis. 2011;53:885–92.
52. Abu Raya B, Srugo I, Kessel A, et al. The induction of breast milk pertussis specific antibodies following gestational tetanus-diphtheria-acellular pertussis vaccination. Vaccine. 2014;32:5632–7.
53. Sara DS, Kirsten M, Lesley B, Ingrid DM, Pierre VD, Elke L. Quantification of vaccine-induced antipertussis toxin secretory iga antibodies in breast milk: comparison of different vaccination strategies in women. Pediatr Infect Dis J. 2015;34:e149–52.

Diphtheria in Children

63

Kamile Arıkan, Marwan Alqunaee, and Ateş Kara

63.1 Introduction

Diphtheria is an acute infectious disease caused by *Corynebacterium diphtheriae.* The toxin released by *C. diphtheriae* causes the disease. Nontoxigenic strains also may cause less severe disease. *Corynebacterium pseudotuberculosis,* which primarily infects animals, rarely causes a diphtheria-like disease in humans.

Hippocrates mentioned diphtheria in the work, *Epidemics,* written 2500 years ago as a winter epidemic of an upper respiratory tract infection followed by peripheral nervous system complications [1]. In 1826, Pierre Bretonneau applied the first tracheostomy for a patient with diphtheria. Brettoneau used the origin of the modern term *diphtheria* from the Greek word *diphthera* [2]. The bacillus was discovered by Klebs in smears in 1883, and 1 year later, Löffler grew the organism on an artificial media, Tindale medium (tellurite medium with cystine). Roux and Yersin purified toxin at end of the eighteenth century. Antitoxin used to treat children with diphtheria at the turn of the twentieth century resulted in one of the largest decreases in mortality rates.

K. Arıkan (✉)
Section of Pediatric Infectious Diseases, İzmir Dr. Behçet Uz Children's Hospital, University of Health Sciences, İzmir, Turkey

M. Alqunaee
Division of Otolaryngology, Head and Neck Surgery, Saint Paul's Sinus Center, Vancouver General Hospital, University of British Columbia, Vancouver, BC, Canada

A. Kara
Division of Pediatric Infectious Diseases, Department of Pediatrics, Faculty of Medicine, Hacettepe University, Ankara, Turkey

© The Author(s), under exclusive license to Springer Nature Switzerland AG 2022
C. Cingi et al. (eds.), *Pediatric ENT Infections,*
https://doi.org/10.1007/978-3-030-80691-0_63

63.2 Pathogen

Corynebacteria are gram-positive, nonmotile, nonsporulating bacilli [3]. *C. diphtheriae* primarily infects humans, and *Corynebacterium ulcerans* and *C. pseudotuberculosis* may infect some animals. *C. diphtheriae* can survive on dry surfaces for several months. The organism can be recovered most readily on a sheep blood agar-based medium containing fosfomycin and Tindale medium [4, 5]. Three *C. diphtheriae* colony types can be distinguished: *mitis, gravis,* and *intermedius* on the selective medium. *Mitis* colonies are blackish, smooth, and hemolytic, and they do not ferment glycogen. *Gravis* colonies are gray, and usually are not hemolytic; they ferment glycogen. *Intermedius* colonies are small, black centrally; they do not ferment starch or glycogen and are not hemolytic. There is no difference in the clinical presentation of different types of *C. diphtheriae* [3–5].

Diphtheria exotoxin *is* encoded by the tox gene of the β-prophage and is the most important virulence factor of C. *diphtheriae*. The diphtheria exotoxin has A and B parts. After the entrance of the non-toxic B fragment into the host cell, fragment A is detached, inhibits protein synthesis, and leads to apoptosis. The β-prophage can infect nontoxigenic strains of *Corynebacterium,* C. *ulcerans,* and C. *pseudotuberculosis*, converting them into a toxigenic strain [6].

Diphtheria toxin is lethal to humans in an amount of approximately 130 μg/kg body weight [3]. Only strains that produce toxin cause myocarditis and neuritis whereas both toxigenic and nontoxigenic strains of *C. diphtheriae* can cause the disease of diphtheria [3–6].

63.3 Epidemiology

Infection by *C. diphtheriae* is acquired by contact with either a carrier or an individual with active disease. The bacteria may be transmitted via droplets during coughing. Transmission may also occur via contagious cutaneous diphtheria lesions. Cutaneous diphtheria is more common in warmer climates and conditions with poor hygiene and overcrowding [3, 4]. Asymptomatic human carriers serve as a reservoir for *C. diphtheriae.*

Throughout history, diphtheria has been one of the most feared infectious diseases globally causing devastating epidemics with high case-fatality rates, mainly affecting children. During major diphtheria epidemics in Europe and the United States (US) in the 1880s, the case-fatality rates of respiratory diphtheria reached 50% in some areas. Case-fatality rates in Europe had dropped to about 15% during the First World War, mainly as a result of widespread use of diphtheria antitoxin (DAT) treatment. Diphtheria epidemics during the Second World War caused about one million cases and 50,000 deaths. Diphtheria toxoid-based vaccines became available in the late 1940s in Europe and North America and were shown to reduce outbreaks in vaccinated populations. In the 1970s, before vaccination, an estimated one million cases of diphtheria including approximately 60,000 deaths occurred each year in low-income countries [7]. The largest from the Russian Federation and former Soviet Republics in the 1990s caused more than 157,000 cases and 5000 deaths because of the reason for decreasing immunization rates in the population [8, 9]. A female predominance of cases reported in several outbreaks among adults in the 1940s and outbreaks in the 1990s was attributed to lower susceptibility among men vaccinated during military service [10]. A mass immunization program was initiated in Russia in 1993, with a resultant 10% decrease in the number of new cases reported between 1994 and 1995. As cases also began to increase in Europe with increasing frequency, the European Laboratory Working Group on Diphtheria (ELWGD) decided to assist in routine screening for diphtheria [9].

Diphtheria remains a significant health problem in countries with poor routine vaccination coverage. In the period 2011–2015, India had the largest total number of reported cases each year, with a 5-year total of 18,350 cases, followed by Indonesia and Madagascar with 3203 and 1633 reported cases, respectively. The South-East Asia Region was the source of 55–99% of all reported cases each year during this period [10]. After the establishment of the Expanded Programme on Immunization (EPI) in the 1970s, with the diphtheria vaccine as one of the original six EPI vaccines, the incidence of diphtheria decreased dramatically worldwide. The total number of reported diphtheria cases was reduced by >90% during the period 1980–2000 [9].

Approximately 86% of children in the world receive the recommended three doses of routine diphtheria-containing vaccine during infancy and 14% of children are undervaccinated [11]. Maternal antibodies seem to protect infants up to 6 months. As a result of the increase in vaccination coverage, the majority of cases occur in adolescents and adults. After the introduction of a primary series of childhood diphtheria vaccination in a diphtheria endemic population, the shift of disease incidence from pre-school to school-age children at first, and then to adolescents and young adults were seen [11].

The incidence of diphtheria peaks during the cooler months [3]. Several epidemics in the northern hemisphere occurred in late summer and fall and corresponded to a high prevalence of *C. diphtheriae* skin infections. Diphtheria was reported to be seen in low socioeconomic conditions and poor hygiene. In a 1993–1994 outbreak in St. Petersburg, Russia, 69 percent of a total of 42 deaths occurred in individuals classified as chronic alcoholics [8].

In recent years, only sporadic cases of diphtheria have been reported in Europe, most of which were cutaneous, and only 4 of 17 cases with toxigenic *C. diphtheriae* had classical respiratory diphtheria. A total of 18 *C. diphtheriae* and 21 *C. ulcerans* cases were reported in 2017 with an overall notification rate below 0.01/100,000 population. Latvia is the sole European country still reporting indigenous *C. diphtheriae* cases since 2012 [12]. However, there has recently been an increase of the disease in many regions of the world, mainly due to wars and movement of populations combined with the breakdown of immunization programs, for example, in Bangladesh, Yemen, and Syria [13–16].

63.4 Pathogenesis and Pathology

C. diphtheriae enters through the nose or mouth and remains localized on the mucosal surfaces of the upper respiratory tract. The bacilli can infect preexisting skin lesions. After a 2- to 4-day period of incubation, lysogenic strains may elaborate toxin. Diphtheria toxin is secreted as a single peptide with 535 amino acids with a molecular weight of 58,342 D [6]. The toxin is composed of two subunits: a large B subunit that is involved in receptor binding and an enzymatically active portion of the toxin A subunit. The toxin binds a receptor on the cell membrane and then undergoes receptor-mediated endocytosis. Then it undergoes a conformational change with subsequent release of the A subunit into the cytoplasm. The A subunit transfers an adenosine diphosphate (ADP)-ribosyl group to elongation factor 2 and inhibits protein synthesis.

C. diphtheriae causes toxin-mediated tissue necrosis and local inflammatory response. The inflammatory response coupled with the necrotic tissue produces a patchy exudate. The increased production of toxin causes a centrifugal widening of the area of infection and resulting in a fibrinous exudate. As a result of the coagulation of the exudate, the adherent membrane develops. The color of the pseudomembrane which is white initially becomes dirty gray during the time. Late in the course of the infection, areas of necrosis seen as green or black spots appear on the membrane. Analysis of the pharyngeal pseudomembrane shows fibrin; inflammatory cells, especially neutrophils, red blood cells, and colonies of organisms; and epithelial cells. With severe infections, significant vascular congestion, interstitial edema, fibrin exudate, and intense neutrophilic infiltration develop [17–19]. The pseudomembrane firmly adherent to the tissue may cause bleeding as a result of detachment. The edematous tissue and the diphtheritic membrane may block the airway. The membrane sloughing may occur during the acute phase of the illness, leading to aspiration. Respiratory suffocation may occur, as a result of the involvement of the upper respiratory tract. Bronchopneumonia may develop if the exudate enters the small airways and alveoli. Occasionally, secondary bacterial infection (usually with *Streptococcus pyogenes*) develops. Infections of the esophagus and stomach, with pseudomembranous lesions indistinguishable from lesions found in the respiratory tract, have been reported [3–5].

The toxin may distribute throughout the body via the bloodstream and the lymphatics mostly as a result of the diphtheritic membrane on the pharynx and tonsils. Clinical manifestations are seen after a period of 10–14 days for myocarditis and 3–7 weeks for manifestations in the nervous system, such as peripheral neuritis. The most prominent pathologic finding of myocarditis is hyaline degeneration of the myocardium. The myocardium also appears edematous as a result of infiltration with mononuclear cells. Also, fatty accumulation in muscle fibers and the conducting system may be observed. The toxin may be observed within the myocardial cells with fluorescent antibody staining [6]. With time muscle regeneration and interstitial fibrosis can be seen secondary to *C. diphtheriae* infections.

In peripheral neuropathy, histologic studies have shown degeneration of myelin sheaths and axons. Toxic neuritis with fatty degeneration of paranodal myelin may be encountered [6]. Axonal damage may be complicated by external pressure from the swollen Schwann cell cytoplasm and myelin. *C. diphtheriae* infections, also rare, can cause hyaline degeneration of the liver. Adrenal hemorrhage and acute tubular necrosis of the kidney also rarely have been reported as disease course [3, 6].

63.5 Clinical Manifestations

Clinical severity of diphtheria changes according to the site of infection, systemic distribution of the toxin, and the immunization status. The incubation period ranges from 1 to 10 days. Diphtheria may be in clinical forms of respiratory, cutaneous, or systemic diphtheria. Transmission of *C. diphtheriae* may occur through droplets and close physical contact of cutaneous diphtheria lesions. Cutaneous diphtheria is more commonly seen in warmer climates with poor hygiene [3, 4, 17–21]. Nontoxigenic *C. diphtheriae* frequently results in an asymptomatic pharyngeal carriage or mild clinical disease.

After an incubation period of 2–5 days, the clinical symptoms of respiratory diphtheria are seen. Clinical forms of respiratory disease are nasal, pharyngeal (the most common form), and laryngeal. Clinical severity of the respiratory disease changes according to the anatomical site of infection, the extent of the mucosal lesions, and time interval before treatment. The onset is characterized by mild fever and exudative pharyngitis. The exudate is known as pseudomembrane that may be seen in the nose, pharynx, tonsils, or larynx. The firmly attached pseudomembrane is asymmetrical, grayish-white, and may bleed with the attempts of detachment. The extent of membrane formation depends on the immune status of the host. The pseudomembrane may obstruct the airways, as a result of extension into the nasal cavity and the larynx. "Bull-neck" appearance may be seen secondary to anterior cervical lymphadenomegaly and edema of surrounding tissues [18]. The heart, kidneys, and peripheral nerves may be damaged as a result of toxemia.

63.5.1 Nasal Diphtheria

Nasal diphtheria is a mild form of the disease attributable to the slow absorption of the toxin. Nasal diphtheria is characterized by mild rhinorrhea and systemic symptoms similar to upper respiratory tract infection. With time the nasal discharge becomes serosanguineous and then mucopurulent. A foul odor may be noticed, and careful inspection reveals a white membrane on the nasal mucosa. In severe cases, the infection may damage the nares and upper lip. Rarely, *C. diphtheriae* can involve the paranasal sinuses and present similarly to acute sinusitis with symptoms of nasal obstruction, facial pressure, and thick mucopurulent discharge. This has been reported in endemic countries. Although *Corynebacterium diphtheriae* is the most common causative organism, toxigenic variants of *Corynebacterium ulcerans*, which can acquire Beta-phage that codes for the diphtheria toxin, has been isolated in immunocompromised adult patients with invasive sinusitis with the potential of causing severe diphtheria like fulminant illness [19].

63.5.2 Pharyngeal and Tonsillar Diphtheria

Pharyngeal and tonsillar diphtheria begins with symptoms of anorexia, malaise, low-grade fever, and pharyngitis, membrane developing in 1 or 2 days. The white or gray adherent membrane may cover the tonsils and pharyngeal walls and extend on to the uvula and soft palate or down on to the larynx and trachea. The detachment of the membrane may cause bleeding. Cervical lymphadenitis with edema of the soft tissues of the neck may be so severe that it gives the appearance of a "bull neck." In an epidemic seen in the 1970s, "erasure" edema of the neck characterized by obliteration of the sternocleidomastoid muscle border, the mandible, and the median border of the clavicle was mentioned in patients with pharyngeal diphtheria [1, 3]. Erasure edema was noted in 29% of immunized patients and 30% of under-immunized patients. It occurred most commonly in children older than 6 years and generally was associated with infection by the *gravis* or *intermedius* strain of *C. diphtheriae*.

The course of pharyngeal diphtheria depends on the amount of the toxin and the extent of the membrane. Respiratory and circulatory collapse may be seen in severe cases. The paralysis of the palate associated with difficulty swallowing and nasal regurgitation of swallowed fluids may be experienced. In severe cases, stupor, coma, and death may occur within 7–10 days. In mild cases, the membrane sloughs off in 7–10 days.

63.5.3 Pharyngeal and Laryngeal Diphtheria

Laryngeal diphtheria results from the downward extension of the membrane from the pharynx. Noisy breathing, progressive stridor, hoarseness, and cough may be noted. Suprasternal, subcostal, and supraclavicular retractions may cause death. Although rare, a partially detached piece of the pseudomembrane may occlude the airway. In severe cases, the membrane may extend downward and invade the entire tracheobronchial tree (Table 63.1).

The cutaneous disease caused by nontoxigenic strains occurs most commonly on the extremities. Cutaneous diphtheria is more contagious than respiratory diphtheria. Thus, cutaneous diphtheria may be an important source of person-to-person transmission of diphtheritic organisms. The skin lesions start as vesicles or pustules, then progress to typical ulcers with sharply defined borders with erythema and edema. For the first 1–2 weeks, the lesions are painful. Spontaneous healing generally takes 6–12 weeks.

After distribution diphtheria toxin may affect any system, but myocarditis and involvement of the nervous system are most common. Myocarditis most commonly appears in the second week of the disease up to the sixth week of illness. Generally,

Table 63.1 Diphtheria classification according to the site of infection

Nasal Diphtheria	Clinical presentation is similar to upper respiratory tract infection and is usually characterized by a mucopurulent nasal discharge. A white membrane usually develops on the nasal septum
Pharyngeal diphtheria	The most common presentation of diphtheria. Malaise, sore throat, anorexia, and low-grade fever are the most prominent symptoms. Within 2–3 days, bluish-white membrane forms and extends through the surrounding tissue
Laryngeal diphtheria	Laryngeal diphtheria can occur as a result of the extension of the pharyngeal form. Symptoms include fever, hoarseness, and a barking cough. The membrane can lead to airway obstruction, coma, and death
Cutaneous diphtheria	Skin infections are quite common in warm climates. Skin infections may be manifested with ulcers with clearly demarcated edges and membrane
Other mucous membranes	The mucous membranes of the conjunctiva and vulvovaginal area, as well as the external auditory canal, may be affected

it develops in patients in whom the administration of antitoxin is delayed. Also rare, *C. diphtheriae* may cause meningitis, endocarditis, osteomyelitis, and hepatitis. These infections occur in patients with underlying risk factors. Although rare, several cases of septic arthritis caused by nontoxigenic *C. diphtheriae* have been reported.

Neurologic complications appear after a variable latent period. Approximately 75% of patients with severe diphtheria may develop neuropathies. The incidence of neurologic sequelae, usually bilateral and motor, has been shown to correlate with the severity of respiratory symptoms; 1 in 5 of all patients with respiratory problems develop polyneuritis. Paralysis of the soft palate generally appears after second week. Due to ocular paralysis, blurring of vision and difficulty with accommodation usually occurs after 1 month. Paralysis of the diaphragm, peripheral neuropathy, loss of deep tendon reflexes, gastritis, hepatitis, nephritis, and hemolytic-uremic syndrome are reported as rare complications of diphtheria [20, 21].

A case of pharyngeal diphtheria in a pregnant woman was reported [22]. No complications of pregnancy were noted. Severe diphtheritic toxemia in the mother was characterized by quadriparesis, from which she fully recovered. A physically normal female infant was delivered at term. In this reported case, severe diphtheritic toxemia during pregnancy was not associated with any teratogenic effect in the fetus.

63.6 Diagnosis

The presence of pseudomembranous is typical for the clinical diagnosis of diphtheria. Material cultured from the mucosal lesions and followed by prompt inoculation onto blood agar and tellurite containing media helps diagnosis. A positive culture with toxin-producing *C. diphtheriae* confirms the diagnosis. The modified Elek immunoprecipitation test may be used for the detection of the toxin. Diphtheria toxin gene (tox) can be detected directly in C. *diphtheriae* isolates using polymerase chain reaction (PCR) techniques [18].

63.7 Differential Diagnosis

Mild forms of nasal diphtheria may resemble upper respiratory tract infection. When the nasal discharge is more serosanguineous or purulent, nasal diphtheria must be distinguished from a foreign body in the nose, sinusitis, adenoiditis, or congenital syphilis. Careful examination of the nose with a nasal speculum, sinus radiographs, and appropriate serologic tests for syphilis help exclude these disorders.

Tonsillar or pharyngeal diphtheria must be differentiated from streptococcal pharyngitis. Generally, streptococcal pharyngitis is associated with more severe pain on swallowing, higher temperature, and a nonadherent membrane limited to the tonsils. Tonsillar and pharyngeal diphtheria also must be differentiated from infectious mononucleosis, nonbacterial membranous tonsillitis, primary herpetic tonsillitis, Vincent angina. Tonsillar and pharyngeal diphtheria also must be differentiated from blood dyscrasias such as agranulocytosis and leukemia, and oropharyngeal involvement by toxoplasmosis, tularemia, salmonellosis, and *Arcanobacterium haemolyticum* and cytomegalovirus infections [3, 4].

Laryngeal diphtheria must be differentiated from croup, acute epiglottitis, laryngotracheobronchitis, aspirated foreign bodies, peri-pharyngeal and retropharyngeal abscesses, and laryngeal papillomas, hemangiomas, or lymphangiomas. A careful history, followed by careful visualization in the hospital, the immune status of the patient helps diagnosis.

63.8 Prevention

Active immunization is the most appropriate way of diphtheria prevention. Diphtheria toxoid developed by formaldehyde detoxification of diphtheria toxin was produced in 1923. A more immunogenic alum-precipitated diphtheria toxoid was developed after 3 years. Diphtheria vaccines contain inactivated toxin adsorbed onto aluminum hydroxide or aluminum phosphate adjuvant. During the Second World War, diphtheria toxoid, tetanus toxoid, and pertussis antigens were combined in the diphtheria-tetanus-pertussis (DTP) vaccine [21]. Toxoid concentration is expressed as flocculation units (Lf), as the amount of toxoid that flocculates 1 unit of an international reference antitoxin. Toxoid potency is expressed as international units (IU). The higher potency of diphtheria vaccine (D) used for the immunization of children up to 6 years of age should be no less than 30 IU per dose. Diphtheria toxoid is available in combination with tetanus toxoid as pediatric DT or adult Td and combination with acellular pertussis as DTaP and Tdap [23, 24].

Combination vaccines with DTaP and inactivated poliovirus and hepatitis B, and inactivated poliovirus and *H. influenzae* type B are also present. Td and Tdap contain 2–2.5 Lf diphtheria toxoid per dose compared with 7–25 Lf in pediatric diphtheria, tetanus toxoid, and pertussis vaccine preparations (DTaP, DT). This reduction of diphtheria toxoid potency decreases reactions at the injection site but causes a sufficient antibody response in older children and adults.

For pediatric use, diphtheria toxoid is available in combination with tetanus toxoid (T) as DT, or with tetanus and pertussis antigens (DTP). Children younger than 7 years should be given the pediatric formulations of the vaccine, but children older than 7 years should receive the adult Td. Primary immunization is achieved by applying diphtheria and tetanus toxoids and pertussis vaccine, DTaP, at 2, 4, and 6 months of age, with booster doses given at 15 to 18 months and again when the child is 4–6 years of age [11].

After 7 years old, primary immunization of children may be performed with Td. Two doses are given intramuscularly at least 4 weeks apart, with a booster dose provided 1 year later. Two forms of Tdap vaccine are available: Boostrix®, approved for children 10–18 years old, and Adacel®, approved for individuals 11–64 years old [24, 25]. Booster doses with adult-type diphtheria and tetanus toxoids adsorbed (Td) are advised to be given every 10 years.

Children and adults undergoing long-term hemodialysis should use the standard immunization schedule [26]. Diphtheria toxoid-containing vaccines are administered as a 0.5 mL dose, intramuscularly. Diphtheria vaccines should be stored at 2–8 °C. Infants develop protective levels of antibody after primary three dose vaccination. After the primary series of DTP-containing vaccine, nearly 100% of children have anti-diphtheria antibody levels >0.01 IU/mL. A randomized controlled trial of a 3-dose primary series of a DTwP-Hib vaccine, starting at 6–8 weeks of age with intervals of 4 weeks between doses, showed that seroprotection ($\geq$0.1 IU/mL) was obtained in 94%–100% of the infants [25].

Diphtheria toxoid, one of the safest vaccines available, rarely cause severe reactions. However, local reactions at the site of injection are common (50%). Prophylactic administration of an antipyretic should not be given [27, 28].

Vaccination resulted in significant decreases in diphtheria incidence worldwide as a result of herd protection. Risk factors contributing to the epidemic in the 1990s in countries of the former Soviet Union were attributed to the under-vaccination and large numbers of migrants [21, 29]. It is advised that vaccine coverage of at least 80–85% must be maintained to maintain herd protection. Immunity after a 3-dose primary vaccination schedule wanes over time, because of that, booster doses are needed to maintain protection [30, 31].

Prevention of diphtheria also depends on the management of the contacts of known cases of diphtheria and carriers of the organism and on the isolation of patients to minimize the spread of disease. Close respiratory or physical contact of the index case's household may contract the disease. Eczema may increase the risk of contracting diphtheria from the index case [3]. The patient is infectious until diphtheria bacilli no longer can be cultured from the site of infection. Two or three consecutive negative cultures at least 24 h apart are required, and antibiotic therapy must be completed for 24 h before the patient is released from isolation [3, 4]. Nasal and throat cultures should be taken from all close contacts and should be kept under surveillance for 7 days. Regardless of their immunization status, all contacts should be treated with an intramuscular dose of benzathine penicillin G (600,000 U for individuals weighing <30 kg and 1.2 million U for individuals weighing >30 kg) or a 7-day course of erythromycin, 40 to 50 mg/kg/day (maximum 2 g/day) divided into four doses. The immune status of each contact should be determined; individuals for whom immune status is inadequate should receive diphtheria vaccine [32].

Because infection does not result in immunity, patients with diphtheria should be immunized. Asymptomatic carriers who previously were not immunized against diphtheria should have cultures taken, receive diphtheria toxoid and penicillin or erythromycin (as described earlier). Asymptomatic contacts that carry a toxigenic strain should be isolated and treated as the index case.

63.9 Treatment

Treatment of diphtheria is achieved with antitoxin and eradication of *C. diphtheriae* or *C. ulcerans* by the use of antibiotics. Early treatment is the first step to limit tissue damage. Disease caused by *C. ulcerans* should be treated in the same manner as *C. diphtheriae*. The decision to administer equine antitoxin should be based on the severity of clinical presentation. Antitoxin can neutralize the circulating toxin. A single dose is used to avoid the risk of developing sensitization of horse serum. Tests for sensitivity to horse serum must be performed with administration of 0.02 mL of a 1:1000 dilution of antitoxin in saline intracutaneously. Positive (histamine) and negative (isotonic saline) controls should be ready. A positive reaction consists of a wheal at least 3 mm larger than the negative control, with surrounding erythema at the site of injection, which developed in 15 to 20 minutes. The histamine control must be positive if test results are to be considered valid. Alternatively, the test may be done with a drop of serum diluted 1:100 and applied to the site of a superficial puncture on the anterior of the forearm. If no reaction has occurred, the remaining antitoxin may be given by slow intravenous infusion. Intravenous administration results in rapid excretion of antitoxin into saliva and preventing further absorption of the toxin in the oropharynx.

Pharyngeal or laryngeal disease <48 h duration should be treated with 20,000 to 40,000 U, nasopharyngeal disease with 40,000 to 60,000 U, and severe pharyngeal or laryngeal diphtheria with 80,000 to 120,000 U of antitoxin. In cutaneous disease, 20,000 to 40,000 U were recommended because toxic effects have been reported [33].

Antibiotics should be given to treat diphtheria. Penicillin and erythromycin are effective against most strains of *C. diphtheriae*. Penicillin and erythromycin also are effective in eradicating group A hemolytic streptococci, which may be present concomitantly in 30% of cases of diphtheria. Treatment is a 14-day course of penicillin or erythromycin. Penicillin may be given as aqueous penicillin G, 100,000–150,000 U/kg/day in four divided doses intravenously, or as procaine penicillin, 25,000–50,000 U/kg/day (maximum of 1.2 million U) in two divided doses intramuscularly. Patients who are sensitive to penicillin should be given erythromycin in a daily dosage of 40–50 mg/kg (maximum of 2 g/day) in four divided doses for 14 days. When the patient is able to tolerate oral medications, erythromycin or penicillin V may be given.

Follow-up cultures should be obtained at least 2 weeks after antibiotic therapy is complete; if they are positive, erythromycin should be given for an additional 10 days.

Amoxicillin, rifampin, and clindamycin provided appropriate dosages also may be effective [34, 35].

The therapy may be stopped after two to three consecutive negative cultures taken at least 24 h apart. In addition to receiving antibiotic therapy, patients with diphtheria should be immunized during convalescence because the infection may not confer immunity. The carrier state is treated effectively with a single intramuscular dose of benzathine penicillin G (600,000 U for children weighing <30 kg or 1.2 million U for individuals weighing ≥30 kg) or oral erythromycin (40–50 mg/kg/day for children and 1 g/day for adults) for 7–10 days. Carriers should have repeat pharyngeal cultures performed a minimum of 2 weeks after antibiotic therapy is complete; if the repeat cultures are positive, carriers should receive an additional course of antibiotics [3].

63.10 Prognosis

The immunization status of the host is the most important factor affecting prognosis. Also the virulence of the infecting organism and the location of infection are important prognostic factors. Morbidity and mortality rates are increased significantly in under-immunized patients. If rapid treatment is provided on the first day of the disease, the mortality rate may be reduced to less than 1%. Delay in treatment for 4 days may cause a 20-fold increase in the mortality rate. Infection with a non-toxigenic *C. diphtheriae* strain may cause disease but does not lead to myocarditis, neuritis, and other toxin-related phenomena. The toxigenic disease may vary from mild to severe. In cases of mild diphtheria, membrane sloughing and full recovery generally occur within 7 days. Disease caused by toxigenic *gravis* strains tends to be more severe with a poorer prognosis.

Although diphtheria usually affects the skin, nasopharynx, and other mucous membranes, the involvement of the larynx causes a more complicated course. Laryngeal diphtheria increases the risk of the development of airway obstruction and causes systemic absorption of the toxin. These patients require close monitoring of respiratory function. Laryngeal diphtheria is more likely to be fatal in infants.

Few laboratory parameters indicate the severity of diphtheria. The development of amegakaryocytic thrombocytopenia and leukocytosis greater than 25,000 cells/mm^3 has been associated with a poor outcome [3, 4].

At any time during the illness, complications such as laryngeal obstruction, shock, and ventricular fibrillation may occur suddenly. In patients with myocardial involvement, permanent damage to the heart, specifically fibrosis, may be seen. Also potentially severe neurologic manifestations, such as phrenic nerve paralysis, may appear late in the course of the disease.

The persistence of *C. diphtheriae* may be noted in the nasopharynx of 5–10% of patients. Immunization should be performed after the patient recovers. Before the use of antitoxin and antibiotics, the mortality rate from diphtheria was up to 50 percent. Death was most common in children younger than 4 years old and was the result of suffocation. At present, the worldwide mortality rate is 5–10%, with no clear association with age.

References

1. Lloyd GER, editor. Hippocratic writings. New York: Penguin Books; 1983. p. 118.
2. English PC. Diphtheria and theories of infectious disease: centennial appreciation of the critical role of diphtheria in the history of medicine. Pediatrics. 1985;76:1–9.
3. Stechenberg BW. Diphtheria. In: Cherry JD, Harrison GJ, Kaplan SL, Steinbach WJ, Hotez PJ, editors. Feigin & Cherry's textbook of pediatric infectious diseases. 8th ed. Philadelphia: Elsevier Saunders; 2019. p. 931–8.
4. Daskalaki I. Corynebacterium diphtheriae. In: Long SS, Prober CG, Fischer M, editors. Principles and practice of pediatric infectious diseases. 5th ed. Philadelphia: Elsevier; 2018. p. 773–8.
5. Bernard KA. Coryneform Gram-positive rods. In: Carroll KC, Pfaller MA, Landry ML, et al., editors. Manual of clinical microbiology. 12th ed. Washington: ASM Press; 2019. p. 488.
6. Tiwari TSP, Wharton M. Diphtheria toxoid. In: Plotkin SA, Orenstein WA, Offit PA, Edwards KM, editors. Plotkin's vaccines. 7th ed. Philadelphia: Elsevier; 2018. p. 261–75.
7. Walsh JA, Warren KS. Selective primary health care: an interim strategy for disease control in developing countries. N Engl J Med. 1979;301:967–74.
8. Dittmann S, Wharton M, Vitek C, et al. Successful control of epidemic diphtheria in the states of the former Union of Soviet Socialist Republics: lessons learned. J Infect Dis. 2000;181(Suppl. 1):S10–22.
9. Efstratiou A, Roure C. The European laboratory working group on diphtheria: a global microbiologic network. J Infect Dis. 2000;181(Suppl. 1):146–51.
10. Hardy IRB, Dittmann S, Sutter RW. Current situation and control strategies for resurgence of diphtheria in newly independent states of the former Soviet Union. Lancet. 1996;347:1739–44.
11. World Health Organization. Diphtheria vaccine: WHO position paper. August 2017—recommendations. Vaccine. 2018;36:199–201.
12. European Centre for Disease Prevention and Control. Diphtheria. In: Annual epidemiological report for 2017. Stockholm: ECDC; 2019.
13. Rahman R, Islam K. Massive diphtheria outbreak among Rohingya refugees: lessons learnt. J Travel Med. 2019;26(1):30407562.
14. Dureab F, Al-Sakkaf M, Ismail O, et al. Diphtheria outbreak in Yemen: the impact of conflict on a fragile health system. Confl Heal. 2019;13:19.
15. Raad II, Chaftari A-M, Wilson Dib R, Graviss EA, Hachem R. Emerging outbreaks associated with conflict and failing healthcare systems in the Middle East. Infect Control Hosp Epidemiol. 2018;39:1230–6.
16. Georgakopoulou T, Tryfinopoulou K, Doudoulakakis A, et al. A patient with respiratory toxigenic diphtheria in Greece after more than 30 years. Epidemiol Infect. 2020;148:e274.
17. Galazka A. The changing epidemiology of diphtheria in the vaccine era. J Infect Dis. 2000;181(Suppl 1):52–9.
18. Holmes R. Biology and molecular epidemiology of diphtheria toxin and the *tox* gene. J Infect Dis. 2000;181(Suppl.1):156–67.
19. Wellinghausen N, Sing A, Kern WV, Perner S, Marre R, Rentschler J. A fatal case of necrotizing sinusitis due to toxigenic Corynebacterium ulcerans. Int J Med Microbiol. 2002;292(1):59–63. https://doi.org/10.1078/1438-4221-00186.
20. Clarke KEN, Centers for Disease Control and Prevention. Review of the epidemiology of diphtheria 2000–2016; 2017. https://www.who.int/immunization/sage/meetings/2017/april/1_Final_report_Clarke_april3.pdf. Accessed 7 Dec 2020.

21. Am A, Moro PL, Hariri S, TSP T. Diphtheria. In: Pink book - epidemiology and prevention of vaccine-preventable diseases. 13th ed. Atlanta: Centers for Disease Control and Prevention; 2020. p. 107–20.
22. El Seed AM, Dafalla AA, Abboud OI. Fetal immune response following maternal diphtheria during pregnancy. Ann Trop Paediatr. 1981;1:217–9.
23. Nakayama T, Suga S, Okada K, Okabe N. Persistence of antibodies against diphtheria, tetanus, pertussis, and poliovirus types I, II, and ii following immunization with DTaP combined with inactivated wild-type polio vaccine (DTaP-wIPV). Jpn J Infect Dis. 2019;72:49–52.
24. Pichichero ME, Rennels MB, Edwards KM, et al. Combined tetanus, diphtheria, and 5-component pertussis vaccine for use in adolescents and adults. JAMA. 2005;293:3003–11.
25. Vesikari T, Van Damme P, Lindblad N, et al. An open-label, randomized, multicenter study of the safety, tolerability, and immunogenicity of quadrivalent human papillomavirus (types 6/11/16/18) vaccine given concomitantly with diphtheria, tetanus, pertussis, and poliomyelitis vaccine in healthy adolescents 11 to 17 years of age. Pediatr Infect Dis J. 2010;29:314–8.
26. Reddy S, Chitturi C, Yee J. Vaccination in chronic kidney disease. Adv Chronic Kidney Dis. 2019;26:72–8.
27. Das RR, Panigrahi I, Naik SS. The effect of prophylactic antipyretic administration on post-vaccination adverse reactions and antibody response in children: a systematic review. PLoS One. 2014;9(9):e106629.
28. Yalcin SS, Gumus A, Yurdakok K. Prophylactic use of acetaminophen in children vaccinated with diphtheria-tetanus-pertussis. World J Pediatr. 2008;4:127–9.
29. American Public Health Association. Diphtheria. In: Chin J, editor. Control of communicable diseases manual. Washington: American Public Health Association; 2000. p. 165–70.
30. Domenech de Cellès M, Rohani P, King AA. Duration of immunity and effectiveness of diphtheria-tetanus-acellular pertussis vaccines in children. JAMA Pediatr. 2019;173:588–94.
31. Pool V, Tomovici A, Johnson DR, Greenberg DP, Decker MD. Humoral immunity 10 years after booster immunization with an adolescent and adult formulation combined tetanus, diphtheria, and 5-component acellular pertussis vaccine in the USA. Vaccine. 2018;36:2282–7.
32. Klein NP, Bartlett J, Fireman B, et al. Waning protection following 5 doses of a 3-component diphtheria, tetanus, and acellular pertussis vaccine. Vaccine. 2017;35:3395–400.
33. Sharma NC, Efstratiou A, Mokrousov I, Mutreja A, Das B, Ramamurthy T. Diphtheria. Nat Rev Dis Primers. 2019;5(1):81.
34. Kharseeva GG, Scherbataya OS, Labushkina AV. The antibiotic sensitivity of Corynebacterium diphtheriae gravis tox+ in composition of mixed biofilms. Klin Lab Diagn. 2018;63:253–6.
35. Neemuchwala A, Soares D, Ravirajan V, Marchand-Austin A, Kus JV, Patel SN. In vitro antibiotic susceptibility pattern of non-diphtheriae Corynebacterium isolates in Ontario, Canada, from 2011 to 2016. Antimicrob Agents Chemother. 2018;62(4):e01776–17.

Oropharyngeal Tularemia in Children

64

Benhur Şirvan Çetin, Emin Sami Arısoy,
and Armando G. Correa

64.1 Introduction

Tularemia is a zoonotic disease found throughout most of the Northern and Southern Hemispheres [1]. In 1837, Homma Soken provided the first definition of human tularemia in Japan and described the illness as "hare meat poisoning." McCoy and Chapin isolated and characterized the organism *Bacterium tularense* from naturally infected ground squirrels in 1912. Edward Francis later isolated *Bacterium tularense* from human blood and showed the connections between the Japanese disease and McCoy and Chapin's findings in 1919 [2]. Much of the knowledge of the organism, modes of transmission, and clinical manifestations of disease originated from the work of Edward Francis. Hence, the causative agent was renamed as *Francisella tularensis* is honor.

Although there are effective treatment options, tularemia continues to be an important public health problem worldwide today. This chapter focuses on oropharyngeal tularemia, a common clinical form in children and in whom the differential diagnosis should be considered carefully.

B. Ş. Çetin (✉)
Division of Pediatric Infectious Diseases, Department of Pediatrics, Faculty of Medicine, Erciyes University, Kayseri, Turkey
e-mail: benhurcetin@erciyes.edu.tr

E. S. Arısoy
Division of Pediatric Infectious Diseases, Department of Pediatrics, Faculty of Medicine, Kocaeli University, Kocaeli, Turkey

A. G. Correa
Section of Academic General Pediatrics, Department of Pediatrics, Baylor College of Medicine, and Section of International and Destination Medicine, Texas Children's Hospital, Houston, TX, USA

64.2   Etiology and Epidemiology

Tularemia, also known as "rabbit fever," is caused by *F. tularensis*, a highly infective, virulent, non-sporulating, non-motile, aerobic, pleomorphic gram-negative coccobacillus [1]. There are four recognized subspecies of *F. tularensis*: tularensis (type A), holarctica (type B), mediasiatica, and novicida. Their pathogenicity and geographic distributions are different.

United States (US), China, Iran, Israel, Japan, and some parts of Europe (mostly Scandinavian, Balkan countries, and Turkey) are endemic areas for tularemia [1–6]. New findings have shown that *F. tularensis* subspecies and genotypes differ according to geographic regions, resulting in clinical, epidemiological, therapeutic, and prognostic variability [6]. The subspecies tularensis and holarctica are of particular clinical and epidemiological concern, and the novicida subspecies is the most common one found in Asia, Europe, and North America [7]. The clinical form and severity of tularemia depend on the route of infection, subspecies, and the virulence of the infecting organism, and the host's immune status [8].

Small and medium-sized mammals are the natural reservoirs for *F. tularensis*. However, *F. tularensis* can infect more than a hundred different animal and invertebrate species; the most important ones are vertebrates such as rabbits, hares, and some rodents, particularly voles, beavers, and muskrats [9].

Humans become infected by different mechanisms like bites by arthropods (e.g., ticks and blood-sucking flies), ingestion of contaminated food, water, or soil, contact with infected animal tissues or fluids, and inhalation of infectious aerosols. Although not able to develop spores or multiplying outside an animal host, this organism can survive in cold, moist conditions for months. The most common mode of transmission also varies for the countries. In the US, most human cases are attributed to bites of infected ticks and flies [2]. In countries like Turkey, Kosovo, and Bulgaria, the infection is mainly acquired following the ingestion of inadequately cooked meat or contaminated water [5].

The route of transmission determines the clinical form of the disease. The most frequent clinical form in North America is ulceroglandular tularemia, while in Europe and Turkey, oropharyngeal tularemia makes up the majority of the tularemia cases [8, 10, 11]. The oropharyngeal form has been most commonly reported in Turkey due to the consumption of contaminated water and food [5, 10, 12]. Contamination of the water by infected animals such as rabbits, voles, beavers, lemmings, and muskrats has led to numerous outbreaks. Farmers, veterinarians, livestock workers, hunters, cooks, and meat handlers have an increased risk for tularemia.

Children acquire tularemia by the same routes as adults. Tularemia is highly infectious, requiring as few as 10 organisms to cause disease. Microorganisms may be present in the blood for the first two weeks of disease and in skin lesions for up to one month. The incubation period usually is 3 to 5 days, with a range of 1 to 21 days [9]. Infections caused by *F. tularensis* subspecies tularensis are generally more severe than those caused by *F. tularensis* subspecies holarctica [3]. Person-to-person transmission has not been reported.

Because of its infectivity, high associated mortality, and potential for easy dissemination, tularemia is considered a potential biological weapon, most likely in an aerosolized form.

64.3 Clinical Manifestations

Clinical presentation of tularemia can be variable and is divided into categories based on the most prominent physical findings: glandular, ulceroglandular, oculoglandular, respiratory (inhalational, pneumonic), oropharyngeal, and typhoidal. However, initial symptoms are usually the same and nonspecific, including fever, arthralgia, myalgia, chills, fatigue, headache, and anorexia [9]. Other symptoms like sore throat, cough, nausea, vomiting, and chest or abdominal pain can also be seen. The most commonly identified clinical feature in children is lymphadenopathy, and it is present in 96% of children with tularemia (Figs. 64.1, 64.2, 64.3) [13].

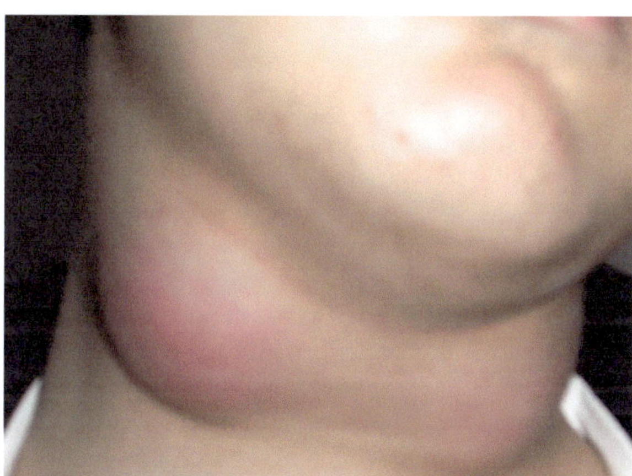

Fig. 64.1 Bilateral cervical lymphadenopathy with overlying erythema in a child with tularemia (Courtesy Solmaz Çelebi, MD)

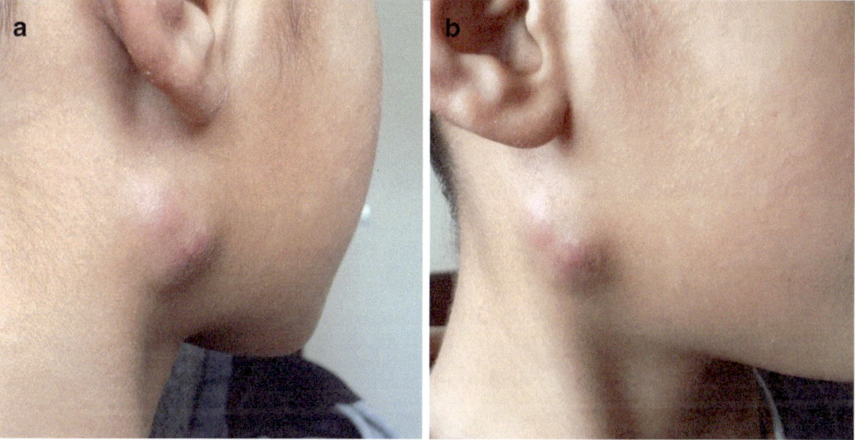

Fig. 64.2 (**a** and **b**) Chronic cervical lymphadenopathy in a child with tularemia. The same lymph node seen from different angles (Courtesy Benhur Şirvan Çetin, MD)

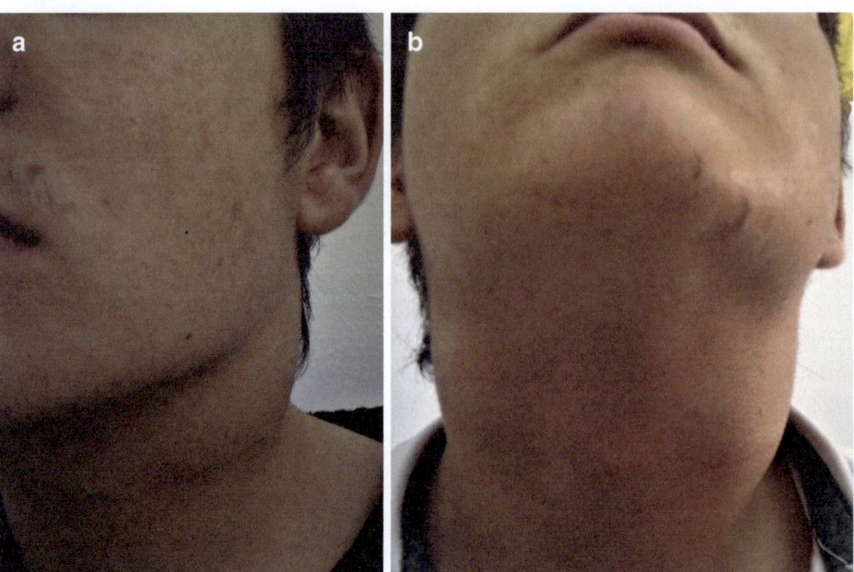

Fig. 64.3 Lymph node enlargement without any color changes on the skin in two children with tularemia. (**a**) Unilateral left cervical lymphadenomegaly. (**b**) Bilateral cervical lymph node enlargement (Courtesy Solmaz Çelebi, MD)

Fever can be continuous or biphasic, sometimes remits for a short time. Without treatment, fever may persist for 3–4 weeks, while the other findings like lymphadenopathy, weight loss, and fatigue may persist for months [1–3]. Temperature-pulse dissociation has been described in nearly half of the cases. Various types of skin rashes (maculopapular, vesicular, and pustular), erythema nodosum, and erythema multiforme may appear in all forms of tularemia and last for a few days to several weeks [2]. The features of the different clinical forms of tularemia are listed in Table 64.1.

Oropharyngeal and rarely gastrointestinal tularemia occurs by ingestion of contaminated food, including undercooked meat, contaminated water, and oral inoculation from the hands following contact with infectious content [9]. Children have been involved more often than adults, and several family members may be affected simultaneously [3]. Outbreaks can be seen due to the contaminated water source [4, 5, 8, 10, 12]. After an incubation period of 3–5 days (up to 2 weeks), oropharyngeal form comprises acute pharyngitis, sometimes with mucosal ulcers and often with swollen and painful cervical lymph nodes [14]. There can be a pseudomembrane on the tonsils, similar to diphtheria [1]. The retropharyngeal area may be affected, and there may be occasional bilateral involvement or abscess development in cervical lymph nodes or retropharyngeal regions. Abdominal pain, nausea, vomiting, diarrhea, and mesenteric lymphadenopathy can be seen if *F. tularensis* invades the lower portions of the gastrointestinal tract [11]. Fever or pharyngitis symptoms may resolve spontaneously, and cervical lymphadenopathy may become the main finding in the later course of the disease [3].

Table 64.1 Common features of the clinical forms of tularemia

Clinical form	Features
Ulceroglandular/glandular	• Generally, the most common form in children and adults • Painful lymphadenitis • With or without a papule that becomes an ulcer distal to the lymphadenitis • Tender, swollen lymph nodes, most commonly in the axillary or inguinal areas • Lymph nodes suppurate and drain in untreated cases
Oculoglandular	• Nodular conjunctivitis • Swollen, tender, and painful regional lymphadenopathy (preauricular, submaxillary, and cervical nodes) • Corneal ulceration may occur
Oropharyngeal	• Associated with ingestion of contaminated meat or water • Acute tonsillitis may be covered by an exudate or membrane-like in diphtheria • Cervical lymph nodes may suppurate • Fever is common • Oral ulcers can be seen
Pneumonic	• Caused by aerosol exposure or hematogenous dissemination to lung (most common in laboratory workers). May also be the result of a bio-terrorism attack. • Most severe and can be rapidly fatal • Rare in children
Typhoidal	• Caused by ingestion of contaminated food • Sepsis-like manifestation (toxemia, high and continuous fever, myalgia, and severe headache) • Pleuropulmonary involvement can be seen in adults

Chronic granulomatous illnesses such as tuberculosis usually exhibit painless lymphadenopathy, while lymph nodes affected in tularemia are typically painful. In tularemia, nearly 30% of patients with lymphadenopathy develop chronic lymph node suppuration, and it is often associated with a delay in starting antibiotic therapy [15]. Fistulization to the skin following suppuration can also be seen in these cases. Complications of oropharyngeal tularemia might include soft tissue abscesses, otitis media, meningitis, brain abscesses, endocarditis, peritonitis, joint infection, and other secondary locations due to the hematogenous spread of bacteria [2, 3, 8, 16]. During an outbreak of waterborne tularemia in the Republic of Georgia, symptoms such as headache, chronic fatigue, difficulty concentrating, and sleep disruption were linked to delayed diagnosis and treatment [17].

Imaging of lymph nodes in tularemia share characteristics with other infectious diseases, particularly with tuberculosis. Imaging features, such as low-density ring-enhancing lymphadenopathy showing cutaneous extension, conglomeration, and calcification involving the neck region and the retropharyngeal space, may suggest the diagnosis of oropharyngeal tularemia [18].

64.4 Differential Diagnosis

A high index of suspicion is required to diagnose tularemia since the different types of tularemia may have a nonspecific presentation and mimic a wide variety of far more common diseases. Additionally, there is not a readily available rapid and specific confirmatory test for tularemia. The differential diagnosis of tularemia depends on the clinical form of the disease. For oropharyngeal tularemia, the differential diagnosis includes streptococcal pharyngitis, adenoviral infection, infectious mononucleosis, toxoplasmosis, and diphtheria. Tularemia can be confused with an abscess of dental origin due to the location of the lymphadenopathy and the similarities of clinical signs and symptoms. Lymph nodes from patients with tularemia have shown follicular hyperplasia with conglomerates of macrophages and caseating granulomas [2, 19, 20]. Lymph nodes can fistulized if the treatment is inappropriate or delayed. With these clinicopathologic findings of affected lymph nodes and the similarity of symptoms, tularemia can be misinterpreted and diagnosed as tuberculosis. In a study, tularemia antibody positivity was confirmed in 6.75% of the patients with a diagnosis of tuberculosis lymphadenitis [21]. Hence, tularemia should be suspected in an endemic area whenever a severe sore throat or chronic cervical lymphadenopathy is unresponsive to nonspecific first-line antibiotic therapy, and routine diagnostic tests have been undiagnostic [2, 3, 5, 9]. Further history, testing, and empiric treatment for these may be indicated early in the evaluative process. Differential diagnosis of the clinical forms of tularemia is listed in Table 64.2.

Table 64.2 Differential diagnosis of the clinical forms of tularemia

Clinical form	Differential diagnosis	
Ulceroglandular/ glandular	• Bacterial adenitis • *Bartonella henselae* infection • Tuberculosis and nontuberculous mycobacterial infections • Kawasaki disease • Herpes simplex virüs (HSV) infection	• Infectious mononucleosis • Plague • *Treponema pallidum* infection • Lymphogranuloma venereum • Sporotrichosis • Anthrax
Oculoglandular	• HSV or adenovirus infections • *Coccidioides immitis* disease	• *B. henselae* infection • Other bacterial conjunctivitis
Oropharyngeal	• Streptococcal pharyngitis • Adenovirus infection	• Diphtheria
Pneumonic	• Tuberculosis • *Legionella* infection • *Mycoplasma* infection	• *Chlamydophila* infection • Fungal infections • Rickettsial diseases
Typhoidal tularemia	• *Salmonella* species infections • Brucellosis • Q fever • *Legionella* infection	• Rickettsial diseases • Fungal infections • Malaria

64.5 Laboratory Findings and Diagnosis

In tularemia, clinical findings and routine tests are generally nonspecific. Leukocytosis or high sedimentation rates may be present. If there is systemic involvement, thrombocytopenia, hyponatremia, myoglobinuria, and sterile pyuria can be seen [2]. Early suspicion is critical for the diagnosis of tularemia. Family history should be taken carefully because several family members can have the same symptoms or findings. Other points to consider in diagnosis are the endemic rate of the disease in the area, the clinical picture of the disease, and failure to respond to antibiotics that are not effective in tularemia [9, 11, 22].

The organism is rarely seen on Gram-stained smears or in biopsy specimens and does not grow in routine culture media. If special culture conditions are provided, isolation of the bacteria is possible from various clinical specimens like blood, lymph nodes, wounds, sputum, pleural fluid, and gastric aspirates. Laboratory workers are considered in the risk group for tularemia. Biosafety level 2 must be met for laboratory processing of routine clinical specimens, and biosafety level 3 requirements for processing suspected *F. tularensis* isolates [23]. In many countries, microbiological studies for tularemia are performed in selected laboratories authorized by the health authority. Samples taken for microbiological analysis of cases with suspected tularemia or isolates thought to be the *F. tularensis* agent should be carefully sent to such specialized laboratories.

Diagnosis is most commonly made on the basis of the clinical picture, and it is confirmed by serologic testing because of the difficulties in culturing *F. tularensis*. Different types of serological tests are available for antibody detection including microagglutination, tube agglutination, hemagglutination, and enzyme-linked immunosorbent assay (ELISA). Microagglutination and tube agglutination tests are standard methods. The microagglutination assay is up to 100-fold more sensitive than tube agglutination. When interpreting serologic testing, it is essential to understand that they may not provide an early diagnosis because agglutinating antibodies may not be detectable until the second week of illness [2, 3, 5, 9]. A presumptive diagnosis is supported by an acute tube agglutination titer of 1:160 or more, or an acute microagglutination titer of 1:128 or more, in the presence of compatible disease. Although these titers may also reflect past infection, it should be considered an indication for therapy in a clinically suspicious case. For definitive serologic diagnosis, a fourfold or greater rise in titer between acute and convalescent specimens is needed [2]. The agglutination tests are specific, but these antibodies may cross-react with *Brucella* spp., *Legionella* spp., *Yersinia* spp., and *Proteus OX19* [2, 3]. Antibiotic therapy does not prevent the development of agglutinating antibodies. In tularemia, immunoglobulin (Ig) M and IgG antibodies appear together and peak at 4 to 5 weeks. High titers of both IgM and IgG may persist for longer than a decade after infection. Therefore, detecting IgM antibodies are not useful for diagnosing acute infection.

Polymerase chain reaction (PCR)-based assays and direct fluorescent antibody (DFA) testing can be used for early detection of *F. tularensis* infection. Bacterial DNA can be detected from the smears and other clinical specimens like biopsy materials, urine, and blood rapidly with PCR assays, even in the early stage of the disease [24]. However, PCR assays are less sensitive than agglutination tests when applied to biologic specimens, and false-negative results may be seen [25]. These assays are not widely commercially available. However, certain laboratories authorized by public health entities may be able to provide PCR or DFA testing on certain clinical specimens.

If the diagnosis of tularemia is strongly suspected, even if the agglutination test is negative, running a PCR test on tissue samples, especially from lymph nodes itself, will increase the possibility of reaching the correct diagnosis. Before the procedure, it should be planned where and how the tissue samples will be sent for further analysis.

64.6 Treatment and Prognosis

If there is strong suspicion for tularemia or the disease is severe, antimicrobial therapy should be initiated empirically before serologic confirmation of infection. Gentamicin (5 mg/kg/day, divided twice or three times/day, intravenously or intramuscularly, with the dose adjusted to maintain the desired peak serum levels of at least 5 µg/mL) is recommended for the treatment of tularemia in children. Once-daily dosing of gentamicin is not routinely recommended for the treatment of tularemia in children because of the limited data. The duration of therapy usually is 10 days. A 5- to 7-day course may be sufficient in mild disease in which patients become afebrile within 48 h of starting antimicrobial therapy. A longer course of antimicrobial therapy is required for more severe illness.

Streptomycin (30–40 mg/kg/day, divided twice/day, intramuscularly; maximum 2 g/day) is another option for the treatment in children, but it has more adverse effects than gentamicin. Evaluation of hearing function before the treatment and monitoring during the treatment are recommended because of the possible ototoxic side effects of aminoglycosides [26]. Ciprofloxacin (30 mg/kg/day, divided twice/day, intravenously or orally, maximum 800 m/day) may be used for mild disease (10–14 days) or after relapse following aminoglycoside therapy. Tetracyclines (e.g., doxycycline) are considered a potential alternative, but they are associated with a higher relapse and treatment failure rate than other therapies. Bacteriostatic activity is the main reason for this failure, and doxycycline is not recommended for definitive therapy [26]. Doxycycline (4.4 mg/kg/day, divided twice/day, orally; maximum 200 mg/day) may be considered a combination therapy with gentamicin in tularemic meningitis. Historically, tetracyclines have been used with caution in children under 8 years of age due to the risk of permanent tooth discoloration. Photosensitivity is another side effect of doxycycline and children should avoid excess sun exposure during the therapy. Regarding the age limit for doxycycline use, recent studies suggest that doxycycline can be used safely for short durations (i.e., less than 3 weeks) in children under 8 years of age [9]. The beta-lactam antibiotics, including carbapenems, are not an option in the treatment of this infection as *F tularensis* is resistant to this class [9].

Lymph node suppuration is another problem in tularemia, and it can be seen despite antimicrobial therapy. Delays between the onset of symptoms and initiation of successful antimicrobial therapy have been correlated with a higher risk of lymph node suppuration. On the other hand, the response to antibiotics is reduced once the lymph node has suppurated. To achieve better cosmetic results, it is crucial to begin treatment promptly and, if necessary, surgical drainage of suppurative lymph nodes. Approximately 20 percent of pediatric cases of ulceroglandular or glandular tularemia have needed surgical drainage [13].

Treatment failure in tularemia is described as having at least one of the following: an increase in size or appearance of new enlarged lymph nodes, constantly elevated inflammatory markers, persistent or recurrent fever, and presence of lymph node suppuration despite being on medical treatment for at least 10 days [27]. In a multicenter study from Turkey, which reviewed the course of tularemia in 1034 adults, treatment failure was seen in 495 patients (48%) [27]. The most frequent reasons for failure were related to lymph node involvement, such as the absence of shrinkage, suppuration, and the formation of new lymphadenopathy, despite appropriate antimicrobial treatment. Although the authors did not disclose the risk factors related to the treatment failure, they stated that when medical treatment was extended in combination with surgical procedures, the infection was completely eradicated even in problematic cases. In other previous reports, initiation of therapy after 14 days, female gender, and doxycycline use were related to treatment failure [5, 28]. With proper diagnosis and treatment, the mortality risk associated with tularemia is less than 1%, except in cases of fulminant pneumonia and typhoidal disease [2].

64.7 Prevention

Prevention of exposure to the vectors or contaminated animal tissue is the critical point for preventing tularemia. In rural places, using protective clothes and repellents and avoiding contact with dead and wild animals protect from the disease. In countries where oropharyngeal forms are more common, food and beverage hygiene measures are more critical than other control measures [8]. The consumption of chlorinated water and well-cooked meat and animal products prevents contamination via the digestive system. In endemic or high-risk areas, conducting investigations into the hygienic control of water resources will help predict possible outbreaks. Postexposure antibiotic prophylaxis after a potential unknown-risk exposure such as tick bites is not recommended. For adults with suspected or proven high-risk exposure to *F. tularensis,* ciprofloxacin 500 mg or doxycycline 100 mg, given orally twice daily for 14 days is recommended. For exposed children and adults with lower-risk exposures, observation without prophylactic antibiotics is appropriate. Patients with tularemia do not need isolation because person-to-person spread does not occur [3].

Whenever tularemia is suspected or confirmed, laboratory personnel handling the patient's specimen should be notified in advance so that precautions can be taken to minimize exposure to *F. tularensis* [29].

Live attenuated vaccines based on an attenuated strain of *F. tularensis* subspecies *holarctica* was firstly used in the Soviet Union and brought to the US in 1956. The live vaccine strain (LVS) delivered by scarification was effective in reducing the severity effectively and reduces the severity of ulceroglandular disease and preventing typhoidal presentation. In the past, LVS vaccination was considered for the people who worked with *F. tularensis* and used for decades [3]. However, because of concerns about its unknown mechanisms of attenuation, stability, and production, the LVS vaccine has not been approved and is no longer available for general use in the US. Although there are some treatment options, tularemia is still a potential threat to public health and the reason why a wide range of approaches to vaccine development are being evaluated for this disease. In 2017, a phase 2 randomized clinical trial compared a new lot of tularemia live vaccine strain to the existing vaccine. This phase-2 study showed the safety, tolerability, and antibody responses exhibited by the two vaccines were similar. The results were suggesting that the new vaccine could replace the old one [30]. Despite many efforts, we currently do not have a licensed tularemia vaccine for human use. Studies are still ongoing for a safe vaccine that shows sufficient efficacy.

If a cluster of pneumonic and/or oropharyngeal cases is identified, particularly in the absence of a natural disaster or contamination, it should raise the possibility of a terroristic bioweapon attack and the appropriate authorities should be promptly notified [31].

64.8 Conclusion

Oropharyngeal tularemia in general is the most frequently seen clinical form of tularemia. Fever, sore throat, abdominal pain, mouth ulcers, inflamed tonsils, and swollen lymph nodes in the neck are the main symptoms. Additionally, chronic lymph node suppuration and fistulization to the skin following suppuration can be seen. Tularemia should be suspected when a severe sore throat or chronic cervical lymphadenopathy is unresponsive to empiric antibiotic therapy, especially in endemic regions. Early appropriate antimicrobial therapy is crucial for preventing complications and treatment failure. Gentamicin is the first-line therapy in children, and surgical drainage of suppurative lymph nodes may be needed in complicated cases. Prevention of exposure to the vectors or contaminated animal tissue, food, and beverage hygiene measures are essential in preventing tularemia.

References

1. Rubin LG. Francisella tularensis (tularemia). In: Long SS, Prober CG, Fischer M, editors. Principles and practice of pediatric infectious diseases. 5th ed. Philadelphia: Elsevier; 2018. p. 923–5.
2. Schutze G. Tularemia. In: Cherry J, Harrison GJ, Kaplan SL, Steinbach WJ, Hotez PJ, editors. Feigin and Cherry's textbook of pediatric infectious diseases. 8th ed. Philadelphia: Elsevier; 2019. p. 1193–8.

3. Auwaerter PG, Penn RL. Francisella tularensis (tularemia). In: Bennett JE, Dolin R, Blaser MJ, editors. Mandell, Douglas, and Bennett's principles and practice of infectious diseases. 9th ed. Philadelphia: Elsevier; 2020. p. 2759–73.

4. Celebi S, Hacimustafaoglu M, Gedikoglu S. Tularemia in children. Indian J Pediatr. 2008;75:1129–32.

5. Tezer H, Ozkaya-Parlakay A, Aykan H, et al. Tularemia in children, Turkey, September 2009-November 2012. Emerg Infect Dis. 2015;21:1–7.

6. Maurin M, Gyuranecz M. Tularaemia: clinical aspects in Europe. Lancet Infect Dis. 2016;16:113–24.

7. Gurcan S. Epidemiology of tularemia. Balkan Med J. 2014;33:3–10.

8. Tärnvik A, Priebe H, Grunow R. Tularaemia in Europe: an epidemiological overview. Scand J Infect Dis. 2004;36:350–5.

9. American Academy of Pediatrics. Tularemia. In: Brady M, Jackson M, Long S, editors. Red book: 2018 report of the committee on infectious diseases. 31st ed. Itasca: American Academy of Pediatrics; 2018. p. 861–4.

10. Özden K, Özden A, Albayrak A, Özkurt Z, Döneray H, Parla M. Evaluation of epidemiologic and clinical features of oropharyngeal tularemia patients in the Eastern Anatolia Region of Turkey. Mikrobiyol Bul. 2018;52:108–10.

11. Stier DM, Mercer MP. Tularemia. In: Chin RL, Frazee BW, editors. Emergency management of infectious diseases. 2nd ed. Cambridge: Cambridge University Press; 2018. p. 506–13.

12. Karakas A, Coskun O, Artuk C, et al. Oropharyngeal tularemia cases admitted to a military hospital in Ankara, Turkey. J Infect Dev Ctries. 2014;8:994–9.

13. Simonsen KA, Snowden J. Tularemia. In: Feld LG, Mahan JD, editors. Succinct pediatrics, evaluation and management for infectious diseases and dermatologic disorders. 1st ed. Elk Grove Village: American Academy of Pediatrics; 2017. p. 267–72.

14. Cağlı S, Vural A, Sönmez O, et al. Tularemia: a rare cause of neck mass, evaluation of 33 patients. Eur Arch Otorhinolaryngol. 2011;268:1699–704.

15. Maurin M, Pelloux I, Brion JP, et al. Human tularemia in France, 2006-2010. Clin Infect Dis. 2011;53:e133–41.

16. Hofinger DM, Cardona L, Mertz GJ, Davis LE. Tularemic meningitis in the United States. Arch Neurol. 2009;66:523–7.

17. Chitadze N, Kuchuloria T, Clark DV, et al. Waterborne outbreak of oropharyngeal and glandular tularemia in Georgia: investigation and follow-up. Infection. 2009;37:514–21.

18. Koçak Ö, Ayan A, Ilıca AT, et al. Clinical imaging findings of oropharyngeal tularemia: the diagnostic value of imaging findings. Muğla Sıtkı Koçman Üniversitesi Tıp Derg. 2019;6:10–5.

19. Staples JE, Kubota KA, Chalcraft LG, et al. Epidemiologic and molecular analysis of human tularemia, United States, 1964-2004. Emerg Infect Dis. 2006;12:1113–8.

20. Kirimanjeswara GS, Olmos S, Bakshi CS, Metzger DW. Humoral and cell-mediated immunity to the intracellular pathogen Francisella tularensis. Immunol Rev. 2008;225:244–55.

21. Karabay O, Kilic S, Gurcan S, et al. Cervical lymphadenitis: tuberculosis or tularaemia? Clin Microbiol Infect. 2013;19:E113–7.

22. Turhan V, Salihoglu M, Ulçay A, et al. Differential diagnosis of cervical lymphadenitis mimicking malignancy due to tularemia: our experiences. Indian J Pathol Microbiol. 2013;56:252–7.

23. Petersen J, Schriefer M, Araj G. Francisella and Brucella. In: Versalovic J, Carroll K, Funke G, et al., editors. Manual of clinical microbiology. 10th ed. Washington, DC: ASM Press; 2011. p. 751–69.

24. Sjöstedt A, Eriksson U, Berglund L, Tärnvik A. Detection of Francisella tularensis in ulcers of patients with tularemia by PCR. J Clin Microbiol. 1997;35:1045–8.

25. Johansson A, Berglund L, Eriksson U, et al. Comparative analysis of PCR versus culture for diagnosis of ulceroglandular tularemia. J Clin Microbiol. 2000;38:22–6.

26. Boisset S, Caspar Y, Sutera V, Maurin M. New therapeutic approaches for treatment of tularaemia: a review. Front Cell Infect Microbiol. 2014;4:1–8.

27. Ulu-Kilic A, Gulen G, Sezen F, et al. Tularemia in Central Anatolia. Infection. 2013;41:391–9.

28. Meric M, Willke A, Finke E-J, et al. Evaluation of clinical, laboratory, and therapeutic features of 145 tularemia cases: the role of quinolones in oropharyngeal tularemia. APMIS. 2008;116:66–73.

29. Imbimbo C, Karrer U, Wittwer M, Buettcher M. Tularemia in children and adolescents. Pediatr Infect Dis J. 2020;39:e435–8.
30. Mulligan MJ, Stapleton JT, Keitel WA, et al. Tularemia vaccine: safety, reactogenicity, "take" skin reactions, and antibody responses following vaccination with a new lot of the Francisella tularensis live vaccine strain—a phase 2 randomized clinical trial. Vaccine. 2017;35:4730–7.
31. Dennis DT, Inglesby TV, Henderson DA, et al. Tularemia as a biological weapon: medical and public health management. JAMA. 2001;285:2763.

Cervicofacial Actinomycosis in Children

65

Semra Şen, Emin Sami Arısoy, and Jeffrey R. Starke

65.1 Introduction

Actinomycosis is a slowly progressive, chronic, suppurative, granulomatous disease. The etiologic agents are *Actinomyces spp. and* cervicofacial, thoracic, and abdominal actinomycosis *are the* primary clinical forms of the disease worldwide [1]. The cervicofacial illness is the most common form (50–70%); however, actinomycosis of oral and pelvic regions, the central nervous system (CNS), and metastatic foci to other sites are also reported [2].

Nonspecific findings of cervicofacial actinomycosis are often overlooked due to empirical antibiotics for various head and neck infections. Imaging methods may not guide the initial diagnostic examination. Operative excision and histopathological diagnosis of the diseased cervicofacial or oral tissues are generally required for definitive diagnosis [3, 4]. Most of the patients with cervicofacial and oral actinomycosis recover completely with appropriate treatment. In this chapter, primarily cervicofacial actinomycosis will be highlighted.

S. Şen (✉)
Division of Pediatric Infectious Diseases, Department of Pediatrics, Faculty of Medicine, Manisa Celal Bayar University, Manisa, Turkey

E. S. Arısoy
Division of Pediatric Infectious Diseases, Department of Pediatrics, Faculty of Medicine, Kocaeli University, Kocaeli, Turkey

J. R. Starke
Section of Infectious Diseases, Department of Pediatrics, Baylor College of Medicine, and Infectious Disease Service, Texas Children's Hospital, Houston, TX, USA

                777
C. Cingi et al. (eds.), *Pediatric ENT Infections*,
https://doi.org/10.1007/978-3-030-80691-0_65

65.2 Microbiology

Actinomycosis is caused by *Actinomyces* spp., which are Gram-positive, non-acid-fast, pleomorphic, non-spore-forming rods. They require anaerobic or microaerophilic environments for growth, and demonstrate branching, often appearing as beaded filaments [5, 6]. Gram stain shows varying morphology from diphtheria bacillus-like appearance to a mycelial structure. The organisms are members of the Actinomycetales order, Actinomycetaceae family, *Actinomyces* genus [2]. *Mycobacteria* and *Nocardia* are also included in the Actinomycetales order, and histopathological and clinical differential diagnosis with the members of *Actinomyces* genus is sometimes difficult [1–3].

Genus *Actinomyces* and the very closely related genus *Nocardia* were previously considered fungi [1, 2]. The word *Actinomyces* means "ray-fungus," and the organisms resemble fungi because of their filamentous appearance. However, *Actinomyces* spp. are typical bacteria due to the structural features and antimicrobial drug susceptibility. They have much narrower filaments than the hyphae of the fungi. While the filaments of *Actinomyces* are easily fragmented, the tubular hyphae of the molds do not split and exhibit different branching patterns. Reproduction of *Actinomyces* is by binary fission, while fungi reproduce by spore and bud formation [2–4].

Actinomyces spp. are natural members of the oropharyngeal, gastrointestinal, and genitourinary system microbiota [1, 5, 7]. Dental plaques, carious teeth, periodontal pockets, gingival crevices, tonsillar crypts, and saliva are colonized by *Actinomyces* species [8, 9]. In a pediatric study performed on tonsillectomy tissue, *Actinomyces* colonization was detected at a rate of 12% [10].

Twenty-six of the 49 known *Actinomyces* species have been implicated in human infections [7]. *Actinomyces israelii* is the most frequent cause of human disease, and *Actinomyces gerencseriae*, *Actinomyces graevenitzii*, *Actinomyces meyeri*, *Actinomyces naeslundii*, *Actinomyces neuii*, *Actinomyces odontolyticus*, *Actinomyces radicidentis*, *Actinomyces radingae*, *Actinomyces turicensis*, and *Actinomyces viscosus* were reported as the other leading *Actinomyces* species causing disease in humans [1, 2, 6, 8]. Although *A. israelii* is the leading cause of actinomycosis, *A. odontolyticus* and *A. naeslundii* are the most common colonizing species in the oral cavity of children [11]. While *Actinomyces bovis* causes the disease known as "lumpy jaw" in cattle, it has been identified only in a single human case due to possible transmission via a lamb bite [12]. A study conducted in Germany found that *A. israelii* (42.0%) and *A. gerencseriae* (26.7%) were the most common species in 1997 culture-positive cases of human cervicofacial actinomycoses [13].

Actinomyces spp. are co-pathogens, and require other bacteria to multiply, explaining why they are commonly found in tissues harboring other aerobic and/or anaerobic species. Thus, *Actinomyces* species are frequently isolated from clinical specimens together with other bacteria of the polymicrobial microbiota. They synergistically inhibit the host defenses with other co-pathogens [2]. *Aggregatibacter* (*Actinobacillus*) species are frequent co-pathogens, and their isolation suggests the presence of actinomycosis [2, 5]. *Eikenella corrodens, Bacteroides, Fusobacterium,*

Capnocytophaga, and microaerophilic streptococci are other concomitant bacterial species often isolated with *Actinomyces*. However, the significance of these co-existing bacteria in the pathogenesis of actinomycosis remains unclear [1, 4, 5].

Actinomyces species grow slowly (5–20 days) at their optimal temperature of 35–37 °C (98.6 °F) and require an enriched medium. The laboratory should be alerted when there is clinical suspicion for actinomycosis [9].

65.3 Epidemiology

Actinomyces spp. are part of the normal microbiota of the human gastrointestinal tract. Actinomycosis was first reported as a fungal infection by Von Langenback in 1845 [9]. In 1878, Israel identified the human disease, then the anaerobic nature of the Actinomyces was described by Israel and Wolff in 1891 [14, 15].

Humans are the only natural host for the causative species of oral and cervicofacial actinomycosis [16]. However, actinomycosis is not considered a communicable disease. It is supposed that the endogenous nature of this bacterium already present in the normal microbiota prevents person-to-person transmission [8]. Actinomycosis in children is uncommon, representing less than 3% of reported cases [17]. Although rare in children, actinomycosis has been reported in all ages, even in newborns [18].

Actinomycosis can occur in immunocompetent and immunocompromised individuals. Breaks in the mucosal barrier, including trauma, surgery, or perforation, are frequent risk factors in children [19]. Predisposing risk factors for actinomycosis are listed in Table 65.1 [8, 20, 21].

Table 65.1 Risk factors for actinomycosis

General risk factors	Specific risk factors
Organ transplantation (pulmonary, renal)	Tooth decay and extractions
Malignancy	Secondary tooth eruption
Steroid use	Gingivitis, gingival trauma
Cancer chemotherapy	Mucositis
Biological response modifiers (anti-tumor necrosis-α inhibitors, etanercept)	Tonsillitis
	Otitis
Diabetes mellitus	Mastoiditis
Immunosuppression (including HIV)	Dental implants
Malnutrition	Bisphosphonate-associated
Low socioeconomic level Non-steroidal anti-inflammatory drug use Crohn's disease	Osteonecrosis of the jaw Head and neck surgery Trauma Irradiation

Adopted from Ref. [8, 20, and 21].

There are reports of actinomycosis in patients with human immunodeficiency virus (HIV) infection and other immunocompromising conditions, such as primary immunodeficiencies and autoimmune disorders. However, actinomycosis has been reported only rarely in pediatric hematopoietic stem cell transplantation (HSCT) and solid organ transplantation (SOT) recipients [22].

Oral and cervicofacial actinomycosis is a relatively rare disease with a global distribution regardless of race, season, age, or occupation [2, 4, 20]. However, men are affected three times more than women, and adult males with poor oral hygiene are considered the highest risk [21].

Actinomycosis has been identified in 12% of cancer patients with osteoradionecrosis, devitalization or necrosis of the jawbone caused by irradiation [23]. *Actinomyces* spp. has also been reported to play a role in bisphosphonate-associated osteonecrosis in the jaw in oncology patients [24, 25]. *Actinomyces* species isolation inform patients with bisphosphonate-associated osteonecrosis was reported to be 53–86% [24, 25].

65.4 Pathogenesis

Actinomyces spp. are generally opportunistic pathogens with low virulence and cannot penetrate healthy tissues [1, 4]. Any damage to the mucosae or tissues by penetrating or non-penetrating trauma, the presence of foreign bodies, or devitalized tissues can increase virulence [16, 20]. *Actinomyces* can directly cross tissue planes to cause soft tissue abscesses and chronic suppurative granulomatous lesions and frequently extend into the bone during the infection process [2, 21]. The fimbria can bind to collagen and cause the development of osteomyelitis. In general, the presence of biofilm is related to the chronicity of the infection, and, as a result, antibiotic therapy may be insufficient to eliminate the pathogens in long-standing infections [3, 9].

In oral and cervicofacial actinomycosis, the organisms often pass through damaged mucosa or tissues caused by dental infection, tooth extraction, endodontic treatment, and oral, maxillary, or facial trauma invade otherwise normal head and neck tissues [4, 5]. Spread into the tissue occurs independently of anatomical barriers, fascial planes or lymphatic drainage. Hematogenous spread is rare [3]. Multiple sinus tracts interconnecting abscesses can develop [20]. In rare cases, the cervicofacial disease can disseminate, or oral and cervicofacial actinomycosis can result from a disseminated infection [16, 21]. If the antimicrobial treatment is not appropriate, bloodstream-related infection, cranial invasion, and metastatic foci in other sites can occur [4].

Bacterial co-pathogens may aid the spread of *Actinomyces* spp. by inhibiting host defenses and reducing local oxygen tension [21]. Once the *Actinomyces* are established locally, they invade into surrounding tissues, leading to a chronic, indurated, suppurative infection, often with tissue fibrosis and draining sinuses. *Actinomyces* grow in clusters of tangled filaments surrounded by neutrophils within tissues. These pale yellow clusters produce sulfur granules that exude through sinus tracts and may be macroscopically visible. They are 0.1–1 mm discreet grains of hard consistency [26]. The granules are composed of an internal tangle of mycelial fragments of bacilli and a peripheral rosette of clubs. This structure is stabilized by a polysaccharide-protein complex and mineralized by the host calcium phosphate. The "sulfur-granule" term describes the yellowish color of the particles in the suppuration. However, the absence of sulfur granules does not rule out the diagnosis of actinomycosis [27], and other conditions, such as nocardiosis, have been linked to the production of sulfur granules [21].

65.5   Clinical Manifestations

Actinomycosis occurs in a spectrum, presenting as an acute, rapidly progressive process or a chronic indolent infection. However, it more often occurs as a chronic indolent disease. The clinical course of cervicofacial actinomycosis can be classified into three stages. Initially, the infection causes soft tissue enlargement in the perimandibular region. In the second phase, the enlargement hardens, becomes "woody," and spreads to adjacent tissues. Then sinus tracts develop in the third phase, and sulfur granules contained within suppuration material may drain. Patients may be complicated with bone or cranial involvement if left untreated [4].

Cervicofacial actinomycosis, also called "lumpy jaw syndrome," is the most common form of the disease in immunocompetent patients, accounting for 40%–60% of cases overall; the mandible (50%), cheeks (10%–15%), chin (10%–15%), and mandible joints (5%–10%) are most frequently affected [3, 7, 8]. The diseased tissue is most commonly at the angle of the jaw (lumpy jaw); however, it can occur anywhere on the mandible, face, or neck.

Actinomyces can invade almost any tissue around the mandibles, and involvement of the nasopharynx [28], middle ear [29, 30], paranasal sinus [31], mastoid [30], temporal bone, labyrinthine and facial nerve [32], tongue [14, 33], tonsil [10, 34], larynx [35], thyroid [36], and parotid [37] involvements also have been reported. Bone involvement develops in the late period and usually occurs in the mandible [26, 38].

Early symptoms of cervicofacial actinomycosis are variable and may include painless or painful cervicofacial enlargement, movement limitation of the neck or mandible, pain when chewing, oral lesions, trismus, fever, or weight loss [2, 3]. Dysphagia rarely occurs. The typical disease occurs as a slowly progressive, indurated, localized hardening and swelling or mass characterized by abscess formation, suppuration, draining sinuses, and tissue fibrosis [1–3]. In rare cases, especially in immunocompromised patients, the illness has a fulminant course with sudden, rapid swelling and suppurative discharge [8]. Low-grade fever may occur; other systemic signs and symptoms are uncommon in the chronic form but are sometimes seen in the acute fulminant course of the illness [16]. Pain is rarely present initially in the slow, progressive chronic clinical course, but sudden and severe pain may develop in the acute fulminant form. Typical chronic indolent lesions often develop over weeks to months; if they adhere to adjacent skin tissue, they create a blue or red-colored appearance confused with cellulitis. Over time, the sinus tracts open to the mucosa or skin surface, and yellow pus containing thick sulfur granules is exuded. Tissue fibrosis is the long-term sequelae [2, 4, 8].

The appearance of the disease often changes with time. *Actinomyces* spread independently of tissue fascia and, as a result, regional lymphadenopathy rarely occurs even in the late course. Several cold abscesses interconnected by sinuses may develop. Yellow-colored sulfur granules in the sinuses become brownish with calcium-phosphate deposition and give the appearance of sand grains in microscopic examination [8].

65.6 Diagnosis

Cervicofacial actinomycosis is a major mimicker of other chronic cervicofacial diseases [39]. Appropriate diagnosis is generally delayed due to its relative rarity and the lack of familiarity among physicians [16]. The illness is often diagnosed months after the onset of symptoms and signs. The diagnosis of actinomycosis may be suspected by histopathology without microbiological evidence [5]. Because *Actinomyces* is a member of the natural human microbiota, *Actinomyces* growth in the culture does not absolutely confirm the diagnosis, nor does the absence of growth rule out the actinomycosis [8, 21, 40–42]. Combining risk factors for actinomycosis, positive culture, and histopathology, and a consistent clinical presentation is an optimal basis for diagnosis.

In children with tooth infections, temporary clinical improvement can be obtained by short-term antimicrobial treatment. Isolation of causative agents in patients receiving antibiotics within 7–10 days is uncommon. In patients with undiagnosed actinomycosis, the course of illness becomes chronic, and fibrotic and "woody" hardening frequently resembles a malignancy. And the identification of sulfur granules becomes more difficult with the increase of fibrous tissue. The granulomatous inflammation of the diseased tissue sometimes confuses with tuberculosis or nontuberculous mycobacterial disease [43].

The laboratory findings may include mild leukocytosis, anemia, high C-reactive protein (CRP) levels, and elevated erythrocyte sedimentation rate (ESR) [2, 3, 40]. However, the white blood cell count and acute inflammation indicators, such as CRP and ESR, are often normal.

65.6.1 Gram and Acid-Fast Stains

A Gram-positive branched structure of the filaments is typical for *Actinomyces* spp. but may not be present in *A. meyeri* [5, 8]. Differentiation of *Nocardia* and *Actinomyces* cannot be made by Gram staining [2, 44]. Gram staining may be more sensitive than culture in the case of previous antibiotic use [15, 16]. *Nocardia* and mycobacteria are characteristically acid-fast, but *Actinomyces* species are not [2, 44].

65.6.2 Culture

The microbiological diagnosis necessitates the isolation of *Actinomyces* from a sterile body area. Previous antimicrobial usage can cause false-negative culture results. The best clinical samples for microbiologic investigation are pus, fine-needle aspirates, sulfur granules in the material discharged from the sinuses, and tissue biopsy samples [8].

After urgent (less than 15 minutes) transport of the samples, incubation under strict anaerobic, microaerophilic conditions is suggested for at least 2 weeks; however, the incubation period should be extended in osteomyelitis cases [4]. Brain and heart infusion blood agar enriched with carbon dioxide is preferably used [1, 2]. Growth of *Actinomyces* species begins in 5–7 days and can last up to 2–4 weeks [21]. The rate of culture confirmation is around 30 percent, probably because of inadequate sample collection, contamination, or polymicrobial growth [45]. Matrix-assisted laser desorption-ionization time-of-flight mass spectrometry (MALDI-TOF MS) is a useful technique for the rapid identification of *Actinomyces* spp. [1, 4].

65.6.3 Histopathology

Under the guidance of computed tomography or ultrasound, fine-needle aspiration and biopsy will provide diagnostic material [21]. Specimens should be taken from potential active infection areas of the lesions instead of fibrotic and/or necrotic tissues [46]. Small-sized samples generally provide nonspecific histopathological findings like inflammatory infiltration, bleeding, fibrosis, and necrosis [46, 47]. The adequate evaluation may require obtaining multiple samples from most of the patients [16]. Thus, multiple sections from at least two tissue planes should be evaluated for optimal findings. Most commonly, small abscesses with extension to form multiple sinus tracts draining yellow, gritty, purulent material (contained sulfur granules) composed of spheroidal colonies of radiating filaments club-shaped, neutrophils, granulomatous reaction, and debris are seen [2, 21, 44].

Sulfur-granules are seen in only 33% to 50% of cases and are also seen in the infections of some other agents such as *Nocardia brasiliensis, Streptomyces madurae, Peptostreptococcus,* and *Staphylococcus aureus* presenting as botryomycosis [3, 44]. Yellow color with a size of ≤1 mm can be seen directly in microscopy by staining with Gram stain or methylene blue [4, 44]. Filaments of the *Nocardia* and *Actinomyces* species are almost identical and impossible to distinguish by standard approaches such as the Grocott-Gomori-methenamine silver dye and hematoxylin-eosin-dye.

65.6.4 Monoclonal Antibody Staining, Molecular Techniques, and Serology

Usage of specific staining with fluorescent-conjugated monoclonal antibodies has shown improvement in identifying *Actinomyces* species in polymicrobial infections, even after tissue fixation with formalin [15, 21].

In addition, a wide variety of *Actinomyces* species has been reported with increasing frequency as causes of infection using newer diagnostic techniques like 16S rRNA gene sequence analysis, DNA-DNA hybridization, real-time polymerase chain reaction (PCR), MALDI-TOF MS, and whole-genome/next-generation sequencing (WGS/NGS) [5, 7, 8]. Serology does not appear to be a reliable diagnostic tool [2, 22].

65.6.5 Imaging

Ultrasonography, direct radiography, computed tomography, and magnetic resonance imaging may not be diagnostic or specific for diagnosing cervicofacial actinomycosis. Mass-like lesions, soft-tissue edema, cystic or necrotic areas, focal microabscesses, cysts, abscesses, sinus tracts, irregular demineralization and/or erosion of adjacent bones can be detected [16, 20, 44]. Computed tomography can help distinguish between inflammation and malignancy [21]. Magnetic resonance imaging can show abscesses [1]. Infection that invades across tissue planes and anatomic boundaries is highly suggestive of actinomycosis [20]. Imaging may help localize the disease, help determine the optimal location for sample taking, and be useful in evaluating treatment response [1, 3, 6].

65.7 Differential Diagnosis

Actinomycosis is characterized by nonspecific symptoms, a slow-progressing chronic indolent clinical course, and may also mimic other pathologies such as tumors, tuberculosis, nocardiosis, and fungal infections [4, 6, 8, 21]. Actinomycosis generally has a differential diagnosis in a wide range, including pyogenic abscess, pyogenic granuloma, carbuncle, suppurative lymphadenitis, lymphoproliferative disorders, oral Crohn's disease, botryomycosis, osteomyelitis, parotitis, orocutaneous fistula, etc. [1, 6, 20].

In the differential diagnosis of any mass located in the head and neck, cervicofacial and oral actinomycosis should be included, mainly when a granulomatous disease or malignancy is suspected. Within this context, patients should be assessed in terms of dental health, mouth hygiene, and chronic local infection.

The diagnosis of actinomycosis in children should be kept in mind regarding possible immunodeficiency, mainly chronic granulomatous disease (CGD) [8, 47]. In one review of ten patients with CGD, it was reported that the patients were susceptible to *Actinomyces* infection, although *Actinomyces* spp. are catalase-negative [47]. Thus, actinomycosis should be vigorously investigated and appropriately treated in patients with CGD.

65.8   Treatment

The management of cervicofacial and oral actinomycosis includes antibiotic therapy, with or without surgical debridement or excision of the lesion [1, 6]. Treatment can be planned with the consultation of a pediatric infectious diseases specialist, an ear, nose, and throat specialist, dentist, and/or maxillofacial surgeon [1, 2].

65.8.1 Medical Therapy

Treatment recommendations are based on small case series as no randomized controlled trials have been reported [2–4, 42]. The fundamental principle is to treat actinomycosis with high-dose antimicrobials for a long time because of the difficulty of penetrating antibiotics into the avascular and indurated areas of infection [47, 48]. Recent reports suggest that early and aggressive antibiotic treatment provides a high cure rate and may decrease the need for surgical intervention [40].

Actinomyces are generally susceptible to penicillin and beta-lactams but intrinsically resistant to ciprofloxacin and metronidazole [1, 2, 49]. High-dose penicillin is recommended for treatment [20]. Severe or widespread actinomycosis should be treated intravenously with penicillin G (250,000 units/kg/day, every 6 h, maximum 18–24 million units/day) or ampicillin (150 mg/kg/day, every 8 h, maximum 8 g/day) until significant improvement has occurred. Parenteral therapy for extensive infection is typically continued for 4–6 weeks. Oral penicillin V (100 mg/kg/day divided every 6 hours, peroral, maximum 4 g/day) is then used for long-term convalescent therapy and initially for mild infections without fistula tracts or severe suppuration [17, 20, 43, 49, 50]. Oral antibiotic treatment is continued for 2–6 months in mild illness and 6–12 months in severe disease [20, 43]. In cases with a rapid response to therapy or patients of non-classical actinomycosis (e.g., subcutaneous abscesses), shorter treatment regimens may be appropriate [3, 43].

Although *A. israelii* is generally sensitive to penicillin (MIC 0.03–0.05 µg/mL), resistance has been rarely reported. The drug susceptibilities should be determined for patients with severe disease and immunosuppression [2, 20, 43]. Ceftriaxone, meropenem, amoxicillin, clindamycin, erythromycin, and doxycycline are alternative antibiotics [20, 49–52]. For patients with beta-lactam allergies, clindamycin, erythromycin, and doxycycline should be recommended as alternatives. Aminoglycosides, aztreonam, co-trimoxazole, penicillin-resistant penicillins (e.g. oxacillin), cephalexin, and fluoroquinolones have poor or no efficacy in the treatment of actinomycosis [52].

Other organisms are isolated with *Actinomyces* approximately 75–95% of the time. Antimicrobial therapy does not always need to be adjusted to target other microorganisms. Treatment adjustment may be necessary when organisms isolated with *Actinomyces* are considered to be typical pathogens. In such cases, the combination of a beta-lactam and a beta-lactamase inhibitor (i.e., piperacillin-tazobactam, amoxicillin-clavulanate) offers the advantage of protection against penicillin-resistant aerobic and anaerobic pathogens [43].

65.8.2 Surgical Treatment

Surgical treatment is usually not required for mild diseases. The classical treatment for an abscess is drainage. Surgical resection may be preferred in case of extensive lesions [1]. Indications for surgery are infection in critical spaces (e.g., epidural infection, intracranial abscess); extensive necrotic tissue, fistula, and/or sinus tracts; osteomyelitis; differential diagnosis of malignant tumors; and when the patient is not responding to antibiotic therapy [3, 43]. Osteomyelitis may require multiple debridements [20]. A study in which 19 pediatric osteomyelitis cases were reported, mandibular involvement was found in 14 cases; all of them were debrided at least once, and four patients needed multiple debridements [38].

65.9   Prevention

Standard isolation measures are suitable for actinomycosis in most cases; there is no person-to-person spread. Oral hygiene and treatment of any tooth decay or disease can prevent infection [1, 2, 22]. There is no recommendation for prophylaxis associated with HSCT, SOT, cancer chemotherapy, HIV infection, or any other immuno-compromise condition [22].

References

1. Whitworth S, Pence AM, Jacobs RF. Actinomycosis. In: Cherry JD, Harrison GJ, Kaplan SL, Steinbach WJ, Hotez PJ, editors. Feigin and Cherry's textbook of pediatric infectious diseases. 8th ed. Philadelphia: Elsevier; 2019. p. 1312–6.
2. Russo TA. Agents of actinomycosis. In: Bennett JE, Dolin R, Blaser MJ, editors. Mandell, Douglas, and Bennett's principles and practice of infectious diseases. 9th ed. Philadelphia: Elsevier; 2020. p. 3071–81.
3. Valour F, Sénéchal A, Dupieux C, et al. Actinomycosis: etiology, clinical features, diagnosis, treatment, and management. Infect Drug Resist 2014;7:183–97.
4. Boyanova L, Kolarov R, Mateva L, Markovska R, Mitov I. Actinomycosis: a frequently forgotten disease. Future Microbiol. 2015;10:613–28.
5. Könönen E, Wade WG. Actinomyces and related organisms in human infections. Clin Microbiol Rev. 2015;28:419–42.
6. Feingold AR, Meislich D. Anaerobic gram-positive nonsporulating bacilli (including actinomyces). In: Long SS, Prober CG, Fischer M, editors. Principles and practice of pediatric infectious diseases. 5th ed. Philadelphia: Elsevier; 2018. p. 1019–22.
7. Gajdács M, Urbán E. The pathogenic role of Actinomyces spp. and related organisms in genitourinary infections: discoveries in the new, modern diagnostic era. Antibiotics. 2020;9(524):1–19.

8. Gajdács M, Urbán E, Terhes G. Microbiological and clinical aspects of cervicofacial actinomyces infections: an overview. Dent J (Basel). 2019;7(3):85.

9. Smego RA Jr, Foglia G. Actinomycosis. Clin Infect Dis. 1998;26:1255–63.

10. van Lierop AC, Prescott CA, Sinclair-Smith CC. An investigation of the significance of actinomycosis in tonsil disease. Int J Pediatr Otorhinolaryngol. 2007;71:1883–8.

11. Sarkonen N, Kononen E, Summanen P, Kanervo A, Takala A, Jousimies-Somer H. Oral colonization with Actinomyces species in infants by two years of age. J Dent Res. 2000;79:864–7.

12. Mansouri P, Farshi S, Khosravi A, Naraghi ZS. Primary cutaneous actinomycosis caused by Actinomyces bovis in a patient with common variable immunodeficiency. J Dermatol. 2011;38:911–5.

13. Pulverer G, Schütt-Gerowitt H, Schaal KP. Human cervicofacial actinomycoses: microbiological data for 1997 cases. Clin Infect Dis. 2003;37:490–7.

14. Jat PS, Paulose AA, Agarwal S. Lingual actinomycosis, an uncommon diagnosis of tongue lesions: a case report and review of literature. Ann Clin Case Rep. 2017;2:1381.

15. Sharma S, Hashmi MF, Valentino III DJ. Actinomycosis. StatPearls (Internet), updated Aug. 10, 2020, https://www.ncbi.nlm.nih.gov/books/NBK482151/. Accessed 21 Nov 2020.

16. Sharkawy AA, Chow AW. Cervicofacial actinomycosis. In: Calderwood SB, Bloom A (eds). Uptodate.com; 2020, https://www.uptodate.com/contents/cervicofacial-actinomycosis. Accessed 21 Nov 2020.

17. Wacharachaisurapol N, Bender JM, Wang L, Bliss D, Ponrartana S, Pannaraj PS. Abdominal actinomycosis in children: a case report and literature review. Pediatr Infect Dis J. 2017;36:e76–9.

18. Alsohime F, Assiri RA, Al-Shahrani F, Bakeet H, Elhazmi M, Somily AM. Premature labor and neonatal sepsis caused by Actinomyces neuii. J Infect Public Health. 2019;12:282–4.

19. Rolfe R, Steed LL, Salgado C, Kilby JM. Actinomyces meyeri, a common agent of actinomycosis. Am J Med Sci. 2016;352:53–62.

20. Fisher BT. Actinomyces. In: Kliegman RM, St Geme III JW, Blum NJ, Shah SS, Tasker RJ, Wilson KM, editors. Nelson textbook of pediatrics. 21st ed. Philadelphia: Elsevier; 2020. p. 1465–7.

21. Quinonez MJ. Pediatric actinomycosis. In: Steele RW (ed). Medscape; 2016. https://emedicine.medscape.com/article/960759-overview. Accessed 21 Nov. 2020.

22. Paulsen GC, Sue PK. Nocardia and Actinomyces. In: Steinbach WJ, Green MD, Michaels MG, Danziger-Isakov LA, Fisher BT, editors. Pediatric transplant and oncology infectious diseases. Philadelphia: Elsevier; 2021. p. 233–40.

23. Curi MM, Dib LL, Kowalski LP, Landman G, Mangini C. Opportunistic actinomycosis in osteoradionecrosis of the jaws in patients affected by head and neck cancer: incidence and clinical significance. Oral Oncol. 2000;36:294–9.

24. Kos M, Kuebler JF, Luczak K, Engelke W. Bisphosphonate-related osteonecrosis of the jaws: a review of 34 cases and evaluation of risk. J Craniomaxillofac Surg. 2010;38:255–9.

25. Schipmann S, Metzler P, Rössle M, et al. Osteopathology associated with bone resorption inhibitors - which role does Actinomyces play? A presentation of 51 cases with systematic review of the literature. J Oral Pathol Med. 2013;42:587–93.

26. Sharkawy AA. Cervicofacial actinomycosis and mandibular osteomyelitis. Infect Dis Clin North Am. 2007;21:543–56.

27. Lerner PI. The lumpy jaw. Cervicofacial actinomycosis. Infect Dis Clin North Am. 1988;2:203–20.

28. Daamen N, Johnson JT. Nasopharyngeal actinomycosis: a rare cause of nasal airway obstruction. Laryngoscope. 2004;114:1403–5.

29. Kullar PJ, Yates P. Actinomycosis of the middle ear. J Laryngol Otol. 2013;127:712–5.

30. Kakuta R, Hidaka H, Yano H, et al. Identification of Actinomyces meyeri actinomycosis in middle ear and mastoid by 16S rRNA analysis. J Med Microbiol. 2013;62:1245–8.

31. Woo HJ, Bae CH, Song SY, Choi YS, Kim YD. Actinomycosis of the paranasal sinus. Otolaryngol Head Neck Surg. 2008;139:460–2.

32. Mehta D, Statham M, Choo D. Actinomycosis of the temporal bone with labyrinthine and facial nerve involvement. Laryngoscope. 2007;117:1999–2001.

33. Sadeghi S, Azaïs M, Ghannoum J. Actinomycosis presenting as macroglossia: case report and review of literature. Head Neck Pathol. 2019;13:327–30.
34. Takasaki K, Kitaoka K, Kaieda S, Hayashi T, Abe K, Takahashi H. A case of actinomycosis causing unilateral tonsillar hypertrophy. Acta Otolaryngol. 2006;126:1001–4.
35. Lensing F, Abele T, Wiggins R 3rd, Quigley E. Laryngeal actinomycosis. Proc (Bayl Univ Med Cent). 2014;27:35–6.
36. Karatoprak N, Atay Z, Erol N, et al. Actinomycotic suppurative thyroiditis in a child. J Trop Pediatr. 2005;51:383–5.
37. Hensher R, Bowerman J. Actinomycosis of the parotid gland. Br J Oral Maxillofac Surg. 1995;23:128–34.
38. Robinson JL, Vaudry WL, Dobrovolsky W. Actinomycosis presenting as osteomyelitis in the pediatric population. Pediatr Infect Dis J. 2005;24:365–9.
39. Rankow RM, Abraham DM. Actinomycosis: masquerader in the head and neck. Ann Otol Rhinol Laryngol. 1978;87:230–7.
40. Wong VK, Turmezei TD, Weston VC. Actinomycosis. BMJ. 2011;343:6099.
41. Hansen JM, Fjeldsøe-Nielsen H, Sulim S, Kemp M, Christensen JJ. Actinomyces species: a Danish survey on human infections and microbiological characteristics. Open Microbiol J. 2009;3:113–20.
42. Bonnefond S, Catroux M, Melenotte C, et al. Clinical features of actinomycosis: a retrospective, multicenter study of 28 cases of miscellaneous presentations. Medicine (Baltimore). 2016;95(24):e3923.
43. Brook I. Treatment of actinomycosis. In: Calderwood SB, Bloom A (eds). Uptodate.com; 2020, https://www.uptodate.com/contents/treatment-of-actinomycosis. Accessed: Nov. 21, 2020.
44. Okulicz JF. Actinomycosis. In Bronze MS (ed). Medscape; 2019. https://emedicine.medscape.com/article/211587-overview Accessed 21 Nov 2020.
45. Volante M, Contucci AM, Fantoni M, Ricci R, Galli J. Cervicofacial actinomycosis: still a difficult differential diagnosis. Acta Otorhinolaryngol Ital. 2005;25:116–9.
46. Bartell HL, Sonabend ML, Hsu S. Actinomycosis presenting as a large facial mass. Dermatol Online J. 2006;12:20.
47. Reichenbach J, Lopatin U, Mahlaoui M, et al. Actinomyces in chronic granulomatous disease: an emerging and unanticipated pathogen. Clin Infect Dis. 2009;49:1703–10.
48. Sudhakar SS, Ross JJ. Short-term treatment of actinomycosis: two cases and a review. Clin Infect Dis. 2004;38:444–7.
49. American Academy of Pediatrics. Actinomycosis. In: Kimberlin DW, Brady MT, Jackson MA, Long SS, editors. Red book: 2018 report of the committee on infectious diseases. 31st ed. Itasca: American Academy of Pediatrics; 2018. p. 205–6.
50. American Academy of Pediatrics. Antimicrobial therapy according to clinical syndromes: miscellaneous systemic infections. In: Bradley JS JS, Nelson JD, Barnett ED, et al., editors. 2020 Nelson's pediatric antimicrobial therapy. 26th ed. Itasca: American Academy of Pediatrics; 2020. p. 123–9.
51. Smith AJ, Hall V, Thakker B, Gemmell CG. Antimicrobial susceptibility testing of Actinomyces species with 12 antimicrobial agents. J Antimicrob Chemother. 2005;56:407–9.
52. Lancella A, Abbate G, Foscolo AM, Dosdegani R. Two unusual presentations of cervicofacial actinomycosis and review of the literature. Acta Otorhinolaryngol Ital. 2008;28:89–93.

Cervicofacial Nocardiosis in Children

66

Ayşe Büyükçam, Emin Sami Arısoy,
and Armando G. Correa

66.1 Introduction

Nocardiosis is a suppurative and granulomatous infectious disease in animals and humans caused by *Nocardia* spp. [1, 2]. *Nocardia* species are found extensively in soil, organic matter, and aquatic habitats throughout the world. Considered an opportunistic infection, *Nocardia* spp. can cause both local and disseminated disease in children and adults, primarily occurring in immunosuppressed patients or after trauma [1, 3, 4].

66.2 Etiology

Nocardia spp. are filamentous and branched gram-positive bacteria included among the actinomycetes. They grow more slowly than other aerobic and facultatively anaerobic bacteria. They commonly produce a fungus-like mycelium that fragments or breaks up into bacillary or coccoid forms [1, 5]. *Nocardia* spp. are characterized by an ability to form aerial hyphae, and grow in media containing lysozyme, and by an inability to grow at 50 °C [1]. *Nocardia* spp. grow slowly on various culture

A. Büyükçam (✉)
Section of Pediatric Infectious Diseases, Gaziantep Cengiz Gökçek Maternity and Children's
Hospital, Gaziantep, Turkey

E. S. Arısoy
Division of Pediatric Infectious Diseases, Department of Pediatrics, Faculty of Medicine,
Kocaeli University, Kocaeli, Turkey

A. G. Correa
Section of Academic General Pediatrics, Department of Pediatrics, Baylor College of
Medicine, and Section of International and Destination Medicine, Texas Children's Hospital,
Houston, TX, USA

media, including simple blood agar, brain-heart infusion agar, and Lowenstein-Jensen media. Mature colonies usually are light orange and have a velvety appearance. *Nocardia* species appear to have similar morphological characteristics to *Actinomyces* species. The most distinguishing feature of the *Nocardia* is their partial acid fastness; cells stain positively with a modified acid-fast (Ziehl-Neelsen or Kinyoun) stain, differentiating them from *Actinomyces* [5, 6].

The use of molecular microbiology methods has led to the description of more than 100 *Nocardia* species, with over 30 clinically significant species identified in humans [3, 5, 7]. *Nocardia abscessus, Nocardia asteroides, Nocardia brasiliensis, Nocardia brevicatena-paucivorans* complex, *Nocardia farcinica, Nocardia nova* complex, *Nocardia otitidiscaviarum* complex, *Nocardia pseudobrasiliensis, and Nocardia transvalensis* complex have been reported as the most medically important *Nocardia* species [1, 3, 5].

Historically, many conventional microbiologic techniques were used to identify Nocardia, including microscopic and colonial morphology, biochemical tests, chemotaxonomic methods, and antimicrobial susceptibility patterns. Analyzing *Nocardia* spp. with molecular techniques has led to reclassification and renaming of many *Nocardia* isolates. Currently, 16S rRNA gene sequencing, multilocus sequence analysis, and polymerase chain reaction (PCR) restriction fragment length polymorphism (RFLP) analysis are the methods most frequently used for *Nocardia* species identification. Also, techniques such as 16S rDNA PCR or matrix-assisted laser desorption/ionization–time of flight mass spectrometry (MALDI-TOF MS) can more efficiently speciate *Nocardia* [3, 5, 8, 9]. Species identification is essential because of the variability in antibiotic susceptibility profiles and virulence among species [3, 6].

66.3 Epidemiology

Nocardia species are ubiquitously found environmental saprophytes worldwide [1, 10]. Nocardial human infections are usually acquired via inhalation of the organism or direct inoculation of the skin or soft tissues [6, 10]. *Nocardia* spp. cause suppurative infections ranging from localized cutaneous or lung involvement to disseminated disease [1, 2, 11]. The illness can become systemic by hematogenous spread [1, 2, 4]. Species distribution varies with a geographic region. Respiratory and disseminated infections occur predominately in immunocompromised hosts. Clusters of invasive nocardiosis in oncology and transplantation units have been described [1]. Person-to-person and animal-to-human transmission are not known to occur. The incubation period is unknown [10].

Except for cutaneous nocardiosis cases, almost all patients with the nocardial disease have one or more severe underlying conditions and/or are immunocompromised [1, 3, 11, 12]. Nocardiosis has been reported in patients of all ages. Cellular immune deficiency or suppression is the most critical risk factor in pediatric patients. However, nocardiosis has also been reported in patients without an identified immune defect [2, 3, 5]. The incidence of nocardiosis has been estimated to be six cases per 100,000 hospital admissions. The incidence is much higher in immunosuppressed hosts such as solid-organ transplant recipients, in whom the rate is as high as 20 per 1000 transplants [3]. In one comprehensive review of 1050 cases of nocardiosis, the body sites most commonly involved were: pulmonary (39%), systemic ($\geq$2 sites affected) (32%), central nervous system (9%), cutaneous or lymphocutaneous (8%), and single-site extrapulmonary (e.g., eyes, bone) (12%) [12].

66.4 Pathogenesis

Human infections are usually acquired by inhalation of the organism or direct cutaneous inoculation. *Nocardia* infections can be local or disseminate from the primary infection site to any organ or musculoskeletal location [3–5]. The immune response to *Nocardia* has multiple mechanisms. Neutrophils and local macrophages give the first host response and inhibit the organisms; however, they cannot kill the bacteria. This inhibition limits the spread of infection until an adequate cell-mediated immune response develops. Immune T cells are significant for clearing *Nocardia* [5]. Gamma delta T lymphocytes may have a particular role in the host defenses against *Nocardia* spp. Although it is clear that T cells, macrophages, and cell-mediated immunity are significant in host resistance to *Nocardia* spp., there is less information on the B cells' role [1, 2].

Nocardia may survive inside neutrophils and macrophages by inhibiting phagosome-lysosome fusion and production of catalase and superoxide dismutase [5]. Also, mycolic acid polymers are associated with virulence. The genomes of pathogenic *Nocardia* spp. contain the genes related to catalases, superoxide dismutase, two types of putative determinants of mammalian cell entry, secreted siderophores, and toxins. *Nocardia* has a capacity for a heavy growth of biofilms on the surface of central venous catheter segments in vitro [1].

66.5 Clinical Manifestations

Cutaneous disease is usually acquired by direct inoculation of the organism due to trauma, surgery, a vascular catheter, intralesional infection, or an animal or insect bite [5, 12–15]. It seems that cutaneous *Nocardia* inoculation is relatively common. When inoculation happens, *Nocardia* breaches the integrity of the skin and results in either cellulitis or pyoderma. In some instances, this infectious process is progressive, but most frequently appears to be self-limited. Four cutaneous disease patterns have been observed: primary cutaneous, lymphocutaneous, cutaneous involvement from a disseminated focus, and mycetoma [5, 12].

Cutaneous and subcutaneous infections manifest as cellulitis, pustules, pyoderma, or localized abscesses have the same appearance as diseases caused by other pyogenic bacteria such as *Staphylococcus aureus* and *Streptococcus pyogenes*.

Also, there may be secondary lesions along the course of the lymphatic drainage system. *N. brasiliensis* is isolated from approximately 80% of cases of primary cutaneous or subcutaneous nocardiosis.

Nocardia may spread through the lymphatics to the regional lymph nodes, resulting in lymphocutaneous nocardiosis [12, 15]. The lymphocutaneous form as a variant of cervicofacial nocardiosis is associated with localized lymphadenitis. Cutaneous nocardiosis typically involves the lower and upper extremities but also the face and neck.

Mycetoma is a chronic infection involving the skin, subcutaneous tissues, and deeper tissues, including bone, resulting from traumatic inoculation by various bacteria and fungi. Traumatic implantation of *Nocardia* into deep subcutaneous tissue may result in actinomycotic mycetoma. *N. brasiliensis* is the most frequently recognized cause of *Nocardia* induced mycetomas [5, 15].

Nocardia infections of the face and neck are rare. Localized facial abscess and lymphocutaneous form have been shown as major clinical presentations. Classic pediatric cervicofacial nocardiosis begins with an erythematous pustule, most often in the nasolabial region, which progresses to involve draining lymph nodes, typically the submandibular or cervical chain [4, 11]. Fever, swelling, superficial cellulitis, and mycetomas of the face can present with pediatric cervicofacial nocardiosis. Extension of infection from the face to the surrounding soft tissue and bone has been reported [10, 11, 16].

There are limited pediatric cervicofacial nocardiosis cases reported in the literature to date [4, 11]. A case series by Fergie et al. [17] described nocardiosis in 31 children, 19 of which were hospitalized for treatment. Lesions were most commonly found on the legs (47% of patients), followed by the trunk (32%), arms (14%), buttocks (11%), and head (5%). There was only one case with facial involvement (cellulitis, infraorbital).

Lampe et al. [16] reported three pediatric cases of cervicofacial nocardiosis. One patient was a 22-month-old Caucasian girl, hospitalized because of a pustular facial lesion and swelling in the left submandibular area. The second patient, a 5-year-old Caucasian boy, first developed an erythematous papule on his left cheek. And a 3-year-old Asian girl developed progressive swelling in the left submandibular area followed by a small draining pustule on the left naris with fever. *N. brasiliensis* and *Nocardia caviae* were pathogens identified. All three patients did not have any underlying disease and no history of unusual or recurrent infections.

A few other isolated cases have been described. In the case report of Beckmeyer [18], a 3-year-old child was presented with cervicofacial lymphocutaneous nocardiosis caused by *N. asteroides*, including left cheek papule and submandibular lymphadenopathy. In the case series of Law and Marks [19], *N. brasiliensis* was isolated from six immunologically competent children, five of whom had localized, uncomplicated, cutaneous infections (lymphocutaneous form and abscess). One child developed osteomyelitis following a compound skull fracture. All cases were cured. Kumar et al. [20] reported a 1-year-old child with lymphocutaneous form caused by *N. asteroides*, forehead and external auditory canal involvement, and submandibular lymphadenopathy.

N. brasiliensis has been reported as the main species responsible for nocardial infections of the face and neck in children [4, 17, 19–21]. A major risk factor has not been identified in most case reports of pediatric cervicofacial nocardiosis [4, 11].

66.6 Diagnosis and Laboratory Tests

Diagnosis of nocardiosis is mostly established by isolation of *Nocardia* spp. from respiratory secretions, aspirate from an abscess, and biopsy specimens [1]. For cutaneous nocardiosis, tissue biopsy specimens are preferred for culture. Histopathologic staining of such samples may reveal branching, beaded, weakly gram-positive, or modified acid-fast filamentous bacteria. Filaments may fragment to form rods and cocci. "Sulfur granules" may be seen in nocardial mycetomas [1, 3]. The identification of characteristic "sulfur granules" or "grains," which contain the infectious organisms, confirms the diagnosis of the type of mycetoma [22, 23].

Standard blood culture media support the growth of *Nocardia*, but routine aerobic cultures usually require 5–21 days for detection [1, 5]. However, *Nocardia* colonies may not be detected because of the more rapidly growing bacteria. The growth is increased by selective media, such as Thayer-Martin agar with antibiotics or paraffin agar [1]. For these reasons, the microbiology laboratory should be informed when the nocardial infection is suspected [5]. *Nocardia* spp. are differentiated from most other aerobic actinomycetes by testing resistance to lysozyme's action and their morphology on tap water agar [1].

Laboratory tests for humoral immunologic responses to diagnose nocardiosis are not sufficient because of the high degree of serologic cross-reactivity among *Mycobacteria, Streptomyces,* and *Nocardia* species [1, 24].

Many new *Nocardia* species have been identified, and traditional biochemical tests are insufficient to identify new members [1, 5]. Molecular techniques (e.g., DNA probes, PCR and PCR-RFLP molecular analyses, DNA sequencing, pyrosequencing, and ribotyping) and MALDI-TOF MS can help identify most *Nocardia* isolates and recognize new species [1, 5]. The use of 16S rDNA PCR or MALDI-TOF technologies in identifying *Nocardia* spp. has increased dramatically [2, 3].

Imaging studies: Immune-compromised patients with cutaneous nocardiosis may have central nervous system involvement without symptoms, so they should undergo brain imaging. Immunocompetent patients with primary cutaneous nocardiosis rarely have disseminated disease, so brain imaging decisions should be made on an individual basis [1–3].

In Vitro Susceptibility Testing: The Clinical and Laboratory Standards Institute (CLSI, formerly the National Committee for Clinical Laboratory Standards [NCCLS]) has approved broth microdilution methods for antimicrobial susceptibility testing of aerobic actinomycetes and has set interpretive breakpoints for commonly used antimicrobials. The optimal method for antimicrobial susceptibility testing for *Nocardia* spp. is the microdilution method. Others are the E-test (AB Biodisk©) and BACTEC radiometric methods. Disk diffusion may be performed following broth microdilution if the MIC result is questionable [1, 25]

66.7 Management

Cervicofacial nocardiosis management principles are similar to those in the body's other sites [1–5]. Drainage and surgical debridement of the abscess and the infected tissue combined with antibacterial therapy are the mainstays of treatment. The site and severity of infection, the host immune status, potential for drug interactions and toxicity, the *Nocardia* species, and their susceptibility testing are significant factors for the initial selection of a therapeutic regimen [1–3, 10, 11, 15]. Also, the initial clinical response is important for the dose and antimicrobial treatment duration [3]. Because an optimal antimicrobial regimen has not been established, susceptibility testing is the best available guide for selecting appropriate combination therapy [5]. Treatment based on in vitro susceptibility is often effective [1].

66.7.1 Antimicrobial Treatment

Trimethoprim-sulfamethoxazole (TMP-SMX, co-trimoxazole) is commonly used (8 mg/kg/day of TMP, every 12 h) for 6–12 weeks or longer as the first-line antibiotic recommended for the treatment of pediatric nocardiosis [26]. TMP-SMX is well absorbed orally and has excellent penetration into most tissue compartments of the body [1, 2]. TMP-SMX resistance rates range from 3% to 10% [3, 15]. Alternative antimicrobial agents should be considered in *Nocardia* infections clinically failing with TMP-SMX therapy or if there is hypersensitivity or toxicity due to TMP-SMX [1, 3, 4]. Amoxicillin-clavulanate, ceftriaxone, clarithromycin, amikacin, ciprofloxacin, imipenem, linezolid, and doxycycline are some of the other antibacterial agents with in vitro activity against many *Nocardia* spp. [3–5, 15, 26].

Because *Nocardia* species show the least resistance against linezolid than other antimicrobials, some experts consider it an essential choice for empiric treatment of a *Nocardia* infection until antibiotic susceptibility test results are known [3]. However, myelosuppression, lactic acidosis, retrobulbar optic neuritis, peripheral neuropathy, and serotonin syndrome may be seen in individuals receiving linezolid, particularly when administered for longer than 2 weeks. In addition to its high cost, these side effects may limit the potential use of linezolid in the prolonged treatment course required for most nocardiosis cases [1, 2, 5, 15].

It is not well known whether parenteral administration of antibiotics is superior to enteral formulations for nocardiosis treatment. However, most clinicians usually prefer the parenteral option in more severe disease [1, 3]. Although current clinical data is insufficient to confirm the need for combination therapy [3], many experts administer empiric combination drug therapies for patients with severe disease, central nervous system nocardiosis, or disseminated nocardiosis, and immunosuppressed patients as mortality rates with sulfonamide monotherapy are greater than 50% in these patients [11]. *Nocardia* species have intrinsic resistance to multiple drugs, so the essential tool for a successful combination therapy depends on antimicrobial susceptibility testing [10]. Combination therapy choice should be made according to susceptibility test results of the clinical isolate of *Nocardia* [3].

66.7.2 Treatment of Cervicofacial Nocardiosis

Typical cervicofacial nocardiosis in children has frequently resolved with antimicrobial therapy alone [4, 5, 11]. In the absence of underlying immune-suppression, TMP-SMX is generally successful in localized infections as a single agent [4, 26]. Other agents, including amoxicillin-clavulanate, fluoroquinolones, and macrolides, have been used depending on the susceptibility of isolate in the localized or isolated cutaneous disease [1, 2]. An oral or intravenous formulation choice depends on the severity of infection [11]. Generally, superficial cutaneous infection requires at least 6–12 weeks of antimicrobial treatment [1].

66.7.3 Treatment of Mycetoma

Treatment of nocardial mycetoma usually involves antibiotics alone. Surgical excision may be undertaken before diagnosis [23]. Mycetoma in an immunocompetent host can be treated with oral TMP-SMX monotherapy [1]. However, intravenous imipenem alone or in combination with amikacin may be a good choice in patients with more severe disease or nocardial mycetoma refractory to TMP-SMX treatment [1, 27].

66.7.4 Treatment of Disseminated Disease and Nocardiosis in Immunosuppressed Patients

Combination therapy is necessary for immunosuppressed patients or brain involvement or disease involving multiple sites [1, 28]. The initial combination of imipenem (or meropenem) *plus* amikacin is a suitable regimen, but it should be noted that carbapenems are not active against many strains of *N. brasiliensis* [1, 10]. Amikacin has also been used successfully in combination with TMP/SMX in immunocompromised patients.

Alternatively, three-drug regimens consisting of TMP-SMX, *plus* amikacin, *plus* a carbapenem or a third-generation cephalosporin (e.g., ceftriaxone), have been used for high-risk patients; however, there is no clear data of increased efficacy [1, 11, 26, 28]. Meropenem is an alternative to imipenem because it has good in vitro activity against most *Nocardia* species. There is not enough clinical experience in its use in cutaneous cervicofacial nocardiosis and nocardial neck infections [11].

In general, systemic nocardiosis is treated for 6–12 months [1–3]. Immune-compromised patients with cutaneous disease should be treated for a minimum of 1 year. Patients with human immunodeficiency virus (HIV) infection may need even more prolonged therapy [5, 10].

Clinical improvement is expected within 3–10 days after the initiation of appropriate therapy. An insufficient response to initial treatment is related to primary drug resistance, inadequate penetration of the drug into infection sites, patient non-compliance, or host immune status [11]. Prolonged therapy is often necessary for patients with mycetoma, although cure has occurred in some patients after 3 months of treatment. Patients should be monitored for at least 6–12 months after completing therapy to detect late relapses [1, 5, 28].

66.7.5 Surgical Management

Nocardial infection site and extent of disease are essential factors for surgical approach [1, 28]. Surgical drainage of abscesses is important because metastatic abscesses can appear even while receiving adequate therapy until surgical drainage is achieved [5]. Many patients with cervicofacial nocardiosis require incision and drainage of the lesion or abscess, depending on the location and size. In addition, lesions that progress despite antimicrobial therapy are candidates for surgical intervention [1, 11].

66.8 Prognosis and Prevention

Pediatric cervicofacial nocardiosis is rare. Isolated cervicofacial nocardiosis has nearly a 100% cure rate with appropriate antibiotic treatment [1]. Generally, the 10–20% case-fatality attributed to Nocardia infections has been associated with disseminated and visceral disease. Early diagnosis and appropriate treatment reduce the morbidity and mortality of nocardiosis, particularly in immunocompromised patients [3]. For prevention, those at increased risk should be advised to cover their skin when working with soil [10, 15].

Pediatricians should keep in mind the possibility of cervicofacial nocardiosis in children with face and neck infections, mainly if there has been a prolonged or complicated course [4, 20].

References

1. Chen SCA, Watts MR, Maddocks S, Sorrell TC. Nocardia species. In: Bennett JE, Dolin R, Blaser MJ, editors. Mandell, Douglas and Bennett's principles and practice of infectious diseases. 9th ed. Philadelphia: Elsevier; 2020. p. 3059–70.
2. Spelman D. Clinical manifestations and diagnosis of nocardiosis. In: Sexton DJ, Mitty J (eds). Uptodate; 2020. https://www.uptodate.com/contents/clinical-manifestations-and-diagnosis-of-nocardiosis. Accessed 15 Dec 2020.
3. Fisher BT. Nocardia. In: Kliegman RM, St Geme III JW, Blum NJ, Shah SS, Tasker RC, Wilson KM, editors. Nelson textbook of pediatrics. 21st ed. Philadelphia: Elsevier; 2020. p. 1467–9.
4. Bennett NJ. Pediatric nocardiosis. In: Steele RW (ed). Medscape; 2018. https://emedicine.medscape.com/article/966919-overview. Accessed 15 Dec 2020.

5. Harik N, Jacobs RF. Nocardia. In: Cherry JD, Harrison GJ, Kaplan SL, Steinbach WJ, Hotez PJ, editors. Feigin and Cherry's textbook of pediatric infectious diseases. 8th ed. Philadelphia: Elsevier; 2019. p. 1013–6.

6. Hall GS, Woods GL. Medical bacteriology. In: McPherson RA RA, Pincus MR, editors. Henry's clinical diagnosis and management by laboratory methods. 23rd ed; 2017. p. 1114–52.

7. Lebeaux D, Bergeron E, Berthet J, et al. Antibiotic susceptibility testing and species identification of Nocardia isolates: a retrospective analysis of data from a French expert laboratory, 2010-2015. Clin Microbiol Infect. 2019;25:489–95.

8. Cloud JL, Conville PS, Croft A, Harmsen D, Witebsky FG, Carroll KC. Evaluation of partial 16S ribosomal DNA sequencing for identification of Nocardia species by using the MicroSeq 500 system with an expanded database. J Clin Microbiol. 2004;42:578–84.

9. Farfour E, Leto J, Barritault M, et al. Evaluation of the Andromas matrix-assisted laser desorption-time of flight mass spectrometry system for identification of aerobically growing Gram-positive bacilli. J Clin Microbiol. 2012;50:2702–7.

10. American Academy of Pediatrics. Nocardiosis. In: Kimberlin DW, Brady MT, Jackson MA, Long SS, editors. Red book: 2018 report of the committee on infectious diseases. 31st ed. Itasca: American Academy of Pediatrics; 2018. p. 575–7.

11. Outhred AC, Watts MR, Chen SC, Sorrell TC. Nocardia infections of the face and neck. Curr Infect Dis Rep. 2011;13:132–40.

12. Beaman BL, Beaman L. Nocardia species: host-parasite relationships. Clin Microbiol Rev. 1994;7:213–64.

13. Lederman ER, Crum NF. A case series and focused review of nocardiosis: clinical and microbiologic aspects. Medicine (Baltimore). 2004;83:300–13.

14. Baek JO, Kim JS, Lee SK, Ji H, Jeong JH, Lee MJ, Seo IH. Two cases of primary cutaneous nocardiosis caused by intralesional injection. Dermatol Ther. 2019;32:e12775.

15. Srour ML, Wong V, Wyllie S. Noma, actinomycosis and nocardia. In: Farrar J, Hotez PJ, Junghanss T, Kang G, Lalloo D, White NJ, editors. Manson's tropical diseases. 23rd ed; 2014. p. 379–84.

16. Lampe RM, Baker CJ, Septimus EJ, Wallace RJ Jr. Cervicofacial nocardiosis in children. J PediatrJ Pediatr. 1981;99:593–5.

17. Fergie JE, Purcell K. Nocardiosis in South Texas children. Pediatr Infect Dis J. 2001;20:711–4.

18. Beckmeyer WJ. Nocardiosis; report of a successfully treated case of cutaneous granuloma. Pediatrics. 1959;23(1 Pt 1):33–9.

19. Law BJ, Marks MI. Pediatric nocardiosis. Pediatrics. 1982;70:560–5.

20. Kumar TS, Scott JX, Viswanathan S, Agarwal I, Raj PM, Lalitha MK. Cervicofacial nocardiosis in an immunocompetent child. Acta Paediatr. 2005;94:1342–3.

21. Bates RR, Rifkind D. Nocardia brasiliensis lymphocutaneous syndrome. Am J Dis Child. 1971;121:246–7.

22. Shanbhag NU, Karandikar S, Deshmukkh PA. Disseminated orbital actinomycetoma: a case report. Indian J Ophthalmol. 2010;58:60–3.

23. Arenas R, Ameen M. Giant grains of Nocardia actinomycetoma. Lancet Infect Dis. 2010;10(1):66.

24. Boiron P, Stynen D. Immunodiagnosis of nocardiosis. GeneGene. 1992;115:219–22.

25. Clinical and Laboratory Standards Institute. Susceptibility testing of aerobic actinomycetes. In: Woods GL, Brown-Elliott BA, Conville PS, et al., editors. Susceptibility testing of mycobacteria, nocardiae, and other aerobic actinomycetes. 2nd ed. Wayne: CLSI; 2011. p. 29–33.

26. American Academy of Pediatrics. Antimicrobial therapy according to clinical syndromes: miscellaneous systemic infections. In: John S, Bradley JS, Nelson JD, Barnett ED, et al., editors. Nelson's pediatric antimicrobial therapy. 26th ed. Itasca: American Academy of Pediatrics; 2020. p. 123–9.

27. Ameen M, Arenas R, Vasquez del Mercado E, et al. Eff icacy of imipenem therapy for Nocardia actinomycetomas refractory to sulfonamides. J Am Acad Dermatol. 2010;62:239–46.

28. Spelman D. Treatment of nocardiosis. In: Sexton DJ, Mitty J (eds). Uptodate; 2020. https://www.uptodate.com/contents/treatment-of-nocardiosis. Accessed: 15 Dec 2020.

Anthrax in the Ear, Nose, and Throat Area in Children

67

Gülsüm İclal Bayhan, Emin Sami Arısoy,
and Morven S. Edwards

67.1 Introduction

Anthrax is a zoonosis that causes disease in herbivores. Human anthrax most often occurs in agricultural areas where anthrax is common in animals. However, the global importance of *Bacillus anthracis* has increased as a potential bioterrorism agent following the "anthrax letter" events of 2001 in the United States (US) [1]. Human cases acquired through natural routes are usually associated with contact with infected animals or contaminated animal products [1]. Anthrax has three main clinical forms, depending on the type of exposure: cutaneous, gastrointestinal, and inhalation anthrax. Each can lead to a visit to a pediatrician or an ear, nose, and throat (ENT) specialist.

67.2 Etiology

Bacillus anthracis is a gram-positive, aerobic, spore-forming bacillus. *Bacillus anthracis* is one of the largest pathogenic bacteria with a length of 3–8 μm and a width of 1–1.5 μm [1]. The ends of the bacilli are usually concave and slightly

G. İ. Bayhan (✉)
Section of Pediatric Infectious Diseases, Ankara City Hospital, Ankara Yıldırım Beyazıt University, Ankara, Turkey

E. S. Arısoy
Division of Pediatric Infectious Diseases, Department of Pediatrics, Faculty of Medicine, Kocaeli University, Kocaeli, Turkey

M. S. Edwards
Section of Infectious Diseases, Department of Pediatrics, Baylor College of Medicine, and Infectious Disease Service, Texas Children's Hospital, Houston, TX, USA

© The Author(s), under exclusive license to Springer Nature Switzerland AG 2022
C. Cingi et al. (eds.), *Pediatric ENT Infections*,
https://doi.org/10.1007/978-3-030-80691-0_67

swollen, making the anthrax bacillus chain have a "bamboo rod"-like appearance [2]. The microorganism appears as nonhemolytic, rapidly growing colonies in sheep blood agar. Anthrax bacillus colonies are large and gray-white. The periphery of the colonies has a rough appearance with a curved or hair-like structure, giving them a "Medusa head" appearance. *Bacillus anthracis* differs from most other aerobic pathogenic bacteria in that it is spore-forming [1]. It has two life stages with distinct biological features as the spore and the vegetative form. *Bacillus anthracis* is mainly found in its spore form, which is metabolically inactive and shows no replication for extended periods, in nature [1, 3]. The spores are quite resistant as long as they are not exposed to ultraviolet light and stay viable for decades in soil. Germination develops once the spores enter the host and the bacillus then enters the vegetative form.

67.3   Epidemiology

Most mammals can serve as hosts for anthrax. All animals are susceptible to varying degrees but the disease is most commonly seen among herbivores (cattle, sheep, horses, deer, and goats) [4]. Anthrax has a severe course in herbivores with a mortality rate of approximately 80% in cattle and sheep [5].

Bacillus anthracis is almost global in distribution. It is highly endemic in Central America and South America and southern and eastern Europe, Asia, Africa, the Caribbean, and the Middle East [6, 7]. However, there has been a significant decrease in anthrax prevalence in many industrialized countries as the result of active control measures and widespread animal vaccination programs initiated in the first half of the twentieth century [3].

Most human infections result from environmental exposure. Less commonly, transmission can occur by inhalation through bioterrorism attacks. This intentional release of anthrax has, to date, been rare but can cause panic as the results are difficult to predict and control [8, 9].

Anthrax transmission to humans occurs through contact with infected animals or contaminated animal products (cutaneous anthrax). Rarely, it can present as oropharyngeal or gastrointestinal anthrax following the ingestion of meat that has not been well cooked. Anthrax cases acquired via the respiratory route, historically called woolsorters' disease, have been associated with the large-scale processing of hides and wool in closed factory areas where aerosolized anthrax spores can be inhaled [1, 7]. Transmission from mother to infant through skin-to-skin contact has also been reported [10].

The biological weapon potential of anthrax due to its transmission via inhalation has long been recognized [11]. In September 2001, letters containing anthrax spores sent to various addresses in the US led to five deaths and 22 cases, one-half of which were cutaneous and one-half inhalation anthrax. This outbreak demonstrated the potential of using anthrax spores as a biological weapon [12].

67.4 Pathogenesis

The two main virulence factors of *B. anthracis* are the toxin complex and the polypeptide capsule. The capsule increases the virulence of the organism by making it resistant to phagocytosis. It plays an important role in the infection stage. *Bacillus anthracis* is resistant to phagocytosis, and germination can therefore occur within the macrophage at the point of entry following phagocytosis of the spores by the macrophage, with the bacillus then converted into the vegetative form. The non-encapsulated variants of *B. anthracis* are not virulent [1, 5, 6].

The toxin complex is composed of a protective antigen, lethal factor, and edema factor polypeptides [6]. Protective antigen enables binding to cell surface receptors. Following proteolytic cleavage, the protective antigen acts as a binding region for the two other components. Edema factor is a calmodulin-dependent adenyl cyclase and has been shown to create edema when injected under the skin. The lethal factor is a protease and promotes tumor necrosis factor-alpha (TNF-α) and interleukin-1beta (IL-1β) secretion by macrophages following macrophage stimulation, resulting in potentially fatal systemic shock. The toxin complex is secreted during the multiplication of vegetative bacilli and is responsible for the development of the characteristic signs and symptoms of anthrax [5, 9, 13, 14].

The cutaneous infection starts following inoculation of spores through a skin scrape or the mucosa, gastrointestinal anthrax following ingestion of meat contaminated with the bacillus and not well cooked, and inhalation anthrax following the access of inhaled spores to the alveoli [6, 8]. The bacilli are ingested by macrophages at the point of entry, and germination into the vegetative form takes place. The bacteria start to rapidly multiply and produce anthrax toxins. The early stage of the infection progresses with the capsule inhibiting the phagocytosis of bacteria and immune cells becoming inactive with the effect of anthrax toxins. The late-stage develops with a high degree of bacterial entry into the circulation [15]. Cutaneous anthrax usually causes local edema and necrosis at the lesion region while the gastrointestinal and inhalation forms can result in sepsis and shock-like vascular collapse [6, 15]. The reason for the sepsis and meningitis is the lymphohematogenous spread of *B. anthracis* from the primary involvement area.

67.5 Clinical Presentation

67.5.1 Cutaneous Anthrax

Cutaneous anthrax makes up 95% of anthrax cases and is the most common form [1, 7]. The mortality has decreased significantly with antibiotic treatment, and death from the cutaneous form is rare [1]. The anthrax lesion develops in exposed areas of the skin and especially the head, neck, and extremities [16]. The regions involved in the order of frequency in one report in young children were head and neck (52%), trunk (28%), and extremities (20%), and in older children head and neck (70%), trunk (16%) and extremities (14%) [17]. Patients usually present with a single cutaneous lesion but two or more lesions are also sometimes encountered [9].

Spore inoculation develops through a scratch or scrapes in the skin. A primary lesion in the form of a painless, itchy papule develops 1–12 days after entry. Vesicles filled with clear or serosanguineous fluid develop around the papule within 1 or 2 days. The vesicles contain a few leukocytes and many large, gram-positive bacilli [1, 8, 18, 19]. The vesicle content is not purulent. The vesicles have a thin wall and can rupture easily, with the development of a black eschar at the ulcer base. The characteristic black color becomes more prominent as the ulcer becomes more mature (Figs. 67.1, 67.2, 67.3). There is significant edema around the eschar. Such diffuse edema is not seen with other skin infections and edema disproportionate to the lesion itself is a sign of anthrax. The anthrax lesion itself is painless as long as there is no secondary infection [1].

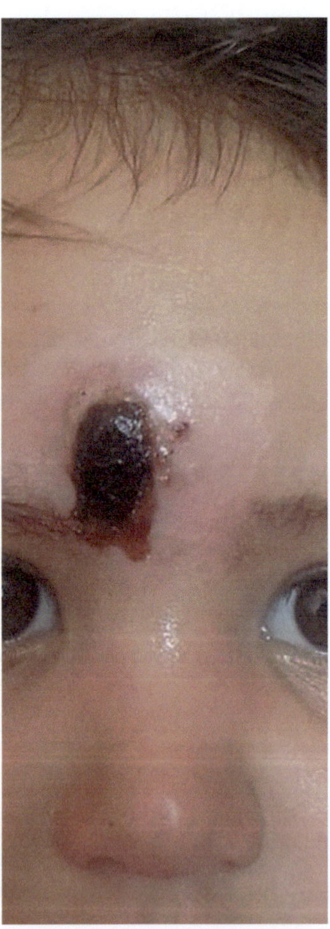

Fig. 67.1 A black eschar surrounded by an erythematous-edematous halo on the forehead (Courtesy Gülsüm İclal Bayhan, MD)

Fig. 67.2 A black necrotic lesion on the right eyelid with surrounding extensive edema (Courtesy Gülsüm İclal Bayhan, MD)

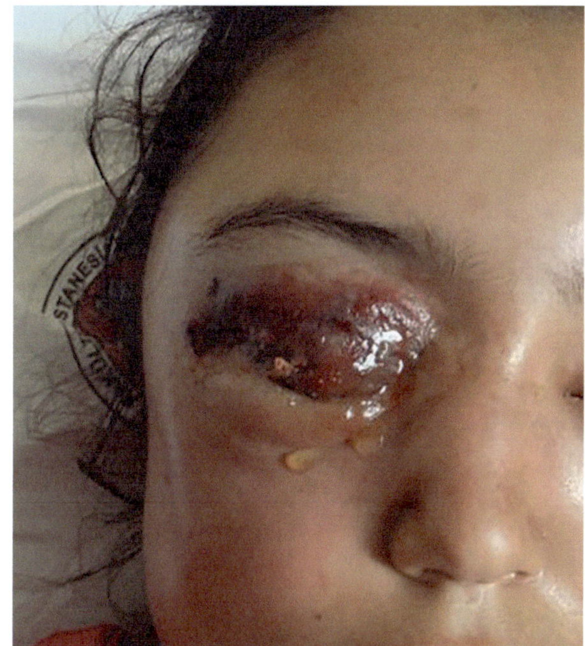

Fig. 67.3 The anthrax lesion on the nose (Courtesy Gülsüm İclal Bayhan, MD)

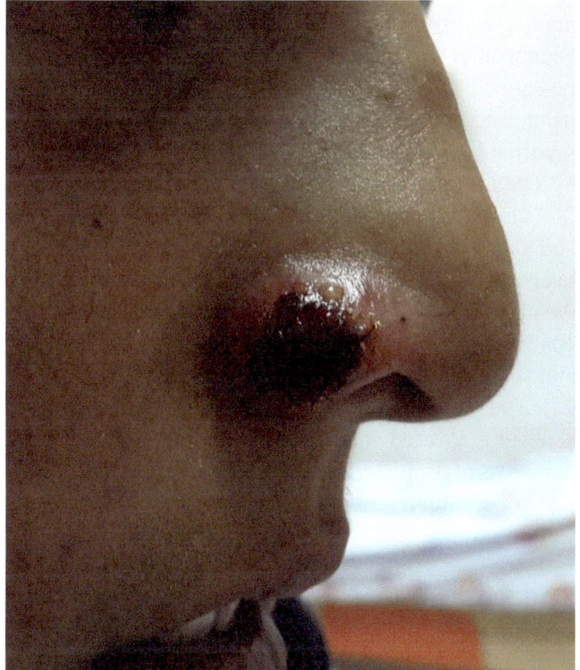

After the extremities, the head and neck are commonly involved areas. An important feature of head and neck lesions is that the edema can be massive if the lesions are on the face or neck. The edema may spread to involve the head, neck, shoulder, and chest and can lead to shortness of breath or even airway obstruction. Treatment may require corticosteroids, intubation, or tracheostomy [14].

Surgical intervention should be avoided in the acute inflammatory period of cutaneous anthrax as it can increase the risk of bacteremia. A lesion in the acute stage should be covered with sterile gauze. The edema starts to resolve within 2–3 days with appropriate antibiotic treatment but it can take weeks for the scar to dry and separate. Low-grade fever and malaise are common, whereas small children can present with a temperature of 39–40 °C [6, 8].

67.5.2 Oropharyngeal Anthrax

Gastrointestinal anthrax has two types: oropharyngeal and intestinal [20]. The oropharyngeal form is less common and has a better prognosis than the intestinal, but it can still be fatal [3, 9]. Oropharyngeal anthrax is underreported because it is difficult to diagnose without a high index of suspicion.

Oropharyngeal anthrax develops following the deposition and germination of spores in the oropharynx. The symptoms and signs start 1–7 days after ingestion of undercooked meat containing spores and include fever, sore throat, dysphagia, odynophagia, diffuse edema of the tonsils, oropharynx, and neck, and cervical lymphadenopathy [1, 7, 8, 21]. The oral lesions usually are localized on the tonsils, posterior pharyngeal wall, or the hard palate and can progress to involve the soft palate and uvula in severe cases [22]. Lesions on the tongue and lip have also been reported [23, 24].

The lesions show edema and congestion in the early stage. Lesions usually are 2–3 cm in diameter but are surrounded by a wide area of edema. Central necrosis and ulcers develop at the end of the first week. A pseudomembrane frequently forms over the ulcers in the second week. When the infection is localized on the tonsils, the affected tonsil shows intense edema and is covered by a pseudomembrane. The condition leads to severe throat pain. Painful neck swelling due to lymphadenitis and soft tissue edema is usually present and can lead to respiratory distress [5, 23, 25]. The physical findings can suggest a peritonsillar abscess but purulent material is never recovered when an attempt is made to drain the lesion [1]. The differential diagnosis of oropharyngeal anthrax also includes diphtheria, complicated tonsillitis, streptococcal pharyngitis, Vincent angina, and Ludwig angina [9].

67.5.3 Gastrointestinal Anthrax

Anthrax lesions can occur in any area of the gastrointestinal system but usually are found in the ileum and cecum [20]. The lesions are generally ulcerative, usually multiple and superficial, and surrounded by edema.

The initial symptoms of intestinal anthrax are nonspecific with nausea, vomiting, loss of appetite, mild diarrhea, and fever. A diagnosis of intestinal anthrax is unlikely at this stage as many other agents can cause similar symptoms. Fluid and electrolyte imbalance, intestinal bleeding, and, ultimately, shock can develop in later stages. The result can be intestinal obstruction and perforation. The condition can cause massive ascites. Bloody diarrhea and abdominal pain can sometimes be present with a clinical presentation resembling an acute abdomen. Shock, sepsis, or death may result in severe cases. Death is due to intestinal perforation and anthrax toxemia [1, 6, 7].

The patient's history is very important when making a diagnosis of gastrointestinal anthrax. Physicians should query the ingestion of raw or improperly cooked meat in patients who come from endemic regions [9].

67.5.4 Inhalational Anthrax

Inhalational anthrax is rare and has a high mortality rate. It classically has two phases. Following an incubation period of 1–7 days after natural exposure or potentially as long as 43 days after very low dose exposure, the first stage begins as a nonspecific influenza-like illness with mild fever, malaise, myalgia, and nonproductive cough [8, 18]. The primary lesion of the inhalation form can, rarely, appear in the nasal mucosa. There are significant associated facial edema and a thick and gelatinous nasal secretion [8].

The disease progresses to the second stage within 2 or 3 days. This stage has an abrupt onset characterized by fever, acute respiratory distress, sweating, and cyanosis. Some patients may experience stridor due to external tracheal compression from enlarged lymph nodes and subcutaneous edema of the chest and neck. The second stage is rapidly progressive, associated with hypothermia, and ends in death within 24–36 h [8]. The chest radiograph can show infiltration, pleural effusion, mediastinal lymphadenopathy, and mediastinal widening [20]. Death results from respiratory failure, sepsis, and shock [1].

The symptoms are nonspecific in the first stage and can suggest a common cold or viral infection. A history of exposure to spores is therefore very important in making the diagnosis of inhalation anthrax [9]. The possibility of anthrax increases with the detection of the typical radiological findings of mediastinal bleeding or mediastinal widening together with a rapidly progressive clinical picture in the second stage. Clinical deterioration is rapid after this stage and the success rate of treatment is low [5].

67.5.5 Injection Anthrax

Injection anthrax, as has been described in heroin users, can cause extensive edema at the injection site without a typical eschar. It can cause severe tissue damage and can result in systemic infection [26].

67.6   Laboratory Diagnosis

Gram staining is widely available and can enable a rapid presumptive diagnosis of anthrax. Gram stain of fluid aspirated from a skin lesion, from the eschar, or a punch biopsy sample can reveal the gram-positive bacilli. A few polymorphonuclear leukocytes usually are also present [1, 8].

In the case of an oropharyngeal lesion, Gram stain of a swab sample from the lesion shows the presence of many polymorphonuclear leukocytes and gram-positive bacilli [9, 14]. It is possible to grow *B. anthracis* by the culture of samples obtained from oropharyngeal lesions. The culture is frequently positive if obtained before antibiotic therapy is initiated [1, 8]. The microorganism can be isolated from blood, skin, respiratory secretion, pleural fluid, feces, or cerebrospinal fluid samples, depending on the type of anthrax involvement [18].

Although Gram stain and culture of the lesion are valuable for anthrax diagnosis, previous antibiotic treatment rapidly converts the Gram stain and culture of the lesions to negative, so cultures should be obtained before antibiotics are administered. Silver staining and immunohistochemical testing of punch biopsy samples obtained from the border of the lesion are valuable, especially if antibiotics have been administered [27]. Direct fluorescent antibody (DFA), polymerase chain reaction (PCR), and an enzyme-linked immunosorbent assay (ELISA) that measures antibody to protective antigen also can confirm the diagnosis [1].

67.7   Treatment

Despite the historical use of penicillin, isolates with a natural resistance to this antibiotic can be encountered and penicillin therapy by itself is therefore not currently recommended for empiric anthrax treatment [2]. *Bacillus anthracis* is susceptible to many antimicrobials such as macrolides, clindamycin, vancomycin, aminoglycosides, rifampin, imipenem, meropenem, ciprofloxacin, ofloxacin, levofloxacin, and tetracyclines in vitro. However, it is resistant to cephalosporins such as cefuroxime, cefotaxime, ceftazidime, and also to trimethoprim-sulfamethoxazole [6, 8].

The first-line treatment of uncomplicated and naturally acquired cutaneous anthrax is

ciprofloxacin or an equivalent fluoroquinolone, or doxycycline. If the isolate is susceptible, penicillin and clindamycin are alternative treatment options [6]. A single antibiotic is sufficient and the treatment duration for uncomplicated, naturally acquired cutaneous anthrax without systemic symptoms is 7–10 days [6, 28]. Bioterrorism-associated cutaneous disease without systemic symptoms should be initially treated with ciprofloxacin (30 mg/kg/day orally in two divided doses, maximum 1000 mg/day), or doxycycline ($\geq$8 years of age 100 mg orally 2 times/day; or <8 years of age 4.4 mg/kg/day in two divided doses with a maximum of 200 mg/day), until susceptibility results are available [6, 28]. The antimicrobial regimen should continue for 60 days to provide postexposure prophylaxis.

Multidrug intravenous treatment is recommended if systemic symptoms or diffuse edema of the head and neck are present. A triple antibiotic combination is recommended for all anthrax types with systemic signs, consisting of two bactericidal agents with central nervous system penetration (a fluoroquinolone [ciprofloxacin] *plus* a beta-lactam [meropenem] or glycopeptide [vancomycin]) *plus* a protein synthesis inhibitor (linezolid) to decrease toxin production [2, 6]. Levofloxacin or moxifloxacin are alternatives to ciprofloxacin. If the strain shown susceptible, penicillin G or ampicillin are equivalent alternative beta-lactam agents. When meningitis has been excluded, treatment consists of two antimicrobials including a bactericidal agent (ciprofloxacin [preferred] with levofloxacin, meropenem, imipenem, vancomycin as acceptable alternatives) and a protein synthesis inhibitor (clindamycin [preferred] with linezolid, doxycycline, or rifampin as acceptable alternatives). If the strain is susceptible, penicillin G or ampicillin are acceptable alternatives as the bactericidal agent [28]. Dependent on clinical recovery, treatment can be converted to an oral regimen to complete in 2 weeks or longer total duration. If meningitis is present, the treatment should continue by the intravenous route for 2–6 weeks [2]. In the case of bioterrorism-associated exposure, antimicrobial therapy should be continued to complete a 60-day course by mouth, to provide postexposure prophylaxis, after initial treatment is discontinued [6, 11].

Administration of an antitoxin product (either anthrax immunoglobulin or raxibacumab) should be considered in addition to antimicrobial treatment to treat systemic or progressive disease. Corticosteroids are suggested when systemic anthrax is accompanied by meningitis, widespread edema, and respiratory failure; when cutaneous anthrax is associated with diffuse edema of the head and neck region; and in case of adrenal failure associated with the disease [2].

Antibiotic treatment eradicates bacteria from tissue within 24–48 h in cutaneous lesions. It can take weeks for the lesions to heal as they are the result of damage induced by the toxins. Antibiotic treatment should not be prolonged until cutaneous lesions resolve and surgery should not be attempted although lesion recovery will be slow [20]. Topical treatment is not useful [11]. Systemic anthrax infection should be considered as a medical emergency while planning the treatment.

67.8 Prognosis

The most commonly reported complications of anthrax are deep tissue necrosis and tissue loss. The tissue loss may require reconstructive surgery. The associated edema can also cause airway obstruction that can result in death [1, 7].

Although rare in cutaneous anthrax, all three forms can cause meningitis and sepsis, and the outcome can be fatal [7, 20]. The mortality rate is high in systemic anthrax with rates of 50–100% for gastrointestinal anthrax, and almost 100% for inhalation anthrax reported [6]. The typical appearance of the lesion allows for early diagnosis of the cutaneous form but early diagnosis is difficult in the non-cutaneous forms and a delayed diagnosis can contribute to mortality. However, all three types of anthrax can be effectively treated following early diagnosis [6, 11, 20].

67.9 Infection Control in Hospital Settings

Abiding by standard precautions during patient care is recommended [1]. Human-to-human transmission is possible through contact of non-intact skin with cutaneous lesions, and observing contact isolation methods is therefore recommended during the care of patients with draining cutaneous lesions [8, 11, 18]. Skin lesions should be covered at the time of presentation. Vegetative bacilli are no longer present in cutaneous lesions following 24 h of antibiotic treatment [18]. Respiratory isolation is not necessary as the person-to-person transmission does not occur through the air [11].

Alcohol-based antiseptics are not recommended following contact with spores, as alcohol does not have sporicidal activity. Ensuring hand hygiene by washing with soap and water or 2% chlorhexidine gluconate is recommended [29].

67.10 Prevention

Prevention of anthrax in humans requires effective anthrax control in animals first. This can be achieved by vaccinating animal herds in endemic areas and burning or burying animals that have died from the disease [30]. One of the most common challenges to infection control is when farmers involved in animal husbandry slaughter animals at the first sign of infection and then use their meat, hide, and wool [9]. It is not possible to fully eradicate anthrax as the organism's spores can remain viable in the soil for many years. Infection risk also remains from bioterrorism attempts [30].

67.10.1 Vaccine

Anthrax vaccines for humans and animals are available. The only vaccine approved for human use and available in the US is the cell-free filtrate of a non-encapsulated, attenuated strain of *B. anthracis* (Anthrax vaccine adsorbed [AVA] BioThrax®). The Centers for Diseases Control and Prevention (CDC) Advisory Committee on Immunization Practices (ACIP) recommends the use of AVA together with antimicrobials in adults aged 18–65 years exposed to aerosolized *B. anthracis* spores [31]. There are also vaccines with investigational new drug status that are not yet licensed. The AVA is recommended for workers with the risk of repeated exposure to anthrax spores through contact with animal hide, hair, or textile products and those with potential occupational exposure, including selected military personnel and laboratory workers [2, 30].

References

1. Martin GJ, Friedlander AM. *Bacillus anthracis* (anthrax). In: Bennett JE, Dolin R, Blaser MJ, editors. Mandell, Douglas, and Bennett's principles and practice of infectious diseases. 9th ed. Philadelphia: Elsevier; 2020. p. 2550–69.
2. Bratcher DF. *Bacillus* species (anthrax). In: Long SS, Prober CG, Fischer M, editors. Principles and practice of pediatric infectious diseases. 5th ed. Philadelphia: Elsevier; 2018. p. 770–3.

3. Pilo P, Frey J. Pathogenicity, population genetics and dissemination of *Bacillus anthracis*. Infect Genet Evol. 2018;64:115–25.
4. Cooper IA, Russell P, Thwaite JE. *Bacillus*: anthrax; food poisoning. In: Barer MR, Irving W, Swann A, Perera N, editors. Medical microbiology: a guide to microbial infections. 9th ed. Philadelphia: Elsevier; 2021. p. 169–77.
5. Bradley PJ, Ferlito A, Brandwein MS, Benninger MS, Rinaldo A. Anthrax: what should the otolaryngologist know? Acta Otolaryngol. 2002;122:580–5.
6. Edwards MS. Anthrax. In: Cherry JD, Harrison GJ, Kaplan SL, Steinbach WJ, Hotez PJ, editors. Feigin and Cherry's textbook of pediatric infectious diseases. 8th ed. Philadelphia: Elsevier; 2019. p. 938–41.
7. Doganay M, Metan G. Human anthrax in Turkey from 1990 to 2007. Vector Borne Zoonotic Dis. 2009;9:131–40.
8. Swartz MN. Recognition and management of anthrax--an update. N Engl J Med. 2001;345:1621–6.
9. Doganay M, Demirarslan H. Human anthrax as a re-emerging disease. Recent Pat Antiinfect Drug Discov. 2015;10:10–29.
10. Freedman A, Afonja O, Chang MW, et al. Cutaneous anthrax associated with microangiopathic hemolytic anemia and coagulopathy in a 7-month-old child. JAMA. 2002;287:869–74.
11. Inglesby TV, O'Toole T, Henderson DA, Working Group on Civilian Biodefense, et al. Anthrax as a biological weapon, 2002: updated recommendations for management. JAMA. 2002;287:2236–52.
12. Kman NE, Nelson RN. Infectious agents of bioterrorism: a review for emergency physicians. Emerg Med Clin North Am. 2008;26:517–47.
13. Bhatnagar R, Batra S. Anthrax toxin. Crit Rev Microbiol. 2001;27:167–200.
14. Wirtschafter A, Cherukuri S, Benninger MS. Anthrax: ENT manifestations and current concepts. Otolaryngol Head Neck Surg. 2002;126:8–13.
15. Moayeri M, Leppla SH, Vrentas C, Pomerantsev AP, Liu S. Anthrax pathogenesis. Annu Rev Microbiol. 2015;69:185–208.
16. Akbayram S, Doğan M, Akgün C, et al. Clinical findings in children with cutaneous anthrax in eastern Turkey. Pediatr Dermatol. 2010;27:600–6.
17. Heyworth B, Ropp ME, Voos UG, Meinel HI, Darlow HM. Anthrax in the Gambia: an epidemiological study. BMJ. 1975;4:79–82.
18. Bradley JS, Peacock G, Krug SE, et al. American Academy of Pediatrics Committee on infectious diseases and disaster preparedness advisory council. Pediatric anthrax clinical management. Pediatrics. 2014;133:e1411–36.
19. Karahocagil MK, Akdeniz N, Akdeniz H, et al. Cutaneous anthrax in eastern Turkey: a review of 85 cases. Clin Exp Dermatol. 2008;33:406–11.
20. World Health Organization Anthrax Working Group. Anthrax in humans. In: Turnbull P, editor. Anthrax in humans and animals. 4th ed. Geneva: World Health Organization; 2008. p. 36–52.
21. Navacharoen N, Sirisanthana T, Navacharoen W, Ruckphaopunt K. Oropharyngeal anthrax. J Laryngol Otol. 1985;99:1293–5.
22. Veraldi S, Nazzaro G, Çuka E, Drago L. Anthrax of the lower lip. Oral Surg Oral Med Oral Pathol Oral Radiol. 2013;116:e490–2.
23. Sirisanthana T, Brown AE. Anthrax of the gastrointestinal tract. Emerg Infect Dis. 2002;8:649–51.
24. Doganay M, Almac A, Hanagasi R. Primary throat anthrax. A report of six cases. Scand J Infect Dis. 1986;18:415–9.
25. Sirisanthana T, Navachareon N, Tharavichitkul P, Sirisanthana V, Brown AE. Outbreak of oral-oropharyngeal anthrax: an unusual manifestation of human infection with *Bacillus anthracis*. Am J Trop Med Hyg. 1984;33:144–50.
26. Hicks CW, Sweeney DA, Cui X, Li Y, Eichacker PQ. An overview of anthrax infection including the recently identified form of disease in injection drug users. Intensive Care Med. 2012;38:1092–104.
27. Bell DM, Kozarsky PE, Stephens DS. Clinical issues in the prophylaxis, diagnosis, and treatment of anthrax. Emerg Infect Dis. 2002;8:222–5.

28. American Academy of Pediatrics. Anthrax. In: Kimberlin DW, Brady MT, Jackson MA, Long SS, editors. Red Book: 2018: report of the committee on infectious diseases. 31st ed. Itaska: American Academy of Pediatrics; 2018. p. 214–20.
29. Siegel JD, Rhinehart E, Jackson M, Chiarello L, the Healthcare Infection Control Practices Advisory Committee. 2007 Guideline for isolation precautions: preventing transmission of infectious agents in healthcare settings, June 2007, http://www.cdc.gov/ncidod/dhqp/pdf/isolation2007.pdf. Accessed 21 Nov 2020.
30. Murray PR, Rosenthal KS, Pfaller MA. Bacillus. In: Murray PR, Rosenthal KS, Pfaller MA, editors. Medical microbiology. 9th ed. Philadelphia: Elsevier; 2021. p. 210–6.
31. Bower WA, Schiffer J, Atmar RI, et al. Use of anthrax vaccine in the United States: recommendations of the advisory committee on immunization practices, 2019. MMWR. 2019;68:1–14.

COVID19 Pandemic and Children

Selçuk Yıldız, Sema Zer Toros, and Philippe Rombaux

68.1 Introduction

On December 31, 2019, "an unknown viral pneumonia" was initially noticed in Wuhan, China. Since December 2019, the epidemic that started in Wuhan, China has spread quickly over an extensive field [1]. On January 10, 2020, a recent type of coronavirus genome was isolated from a patient's tracheal secretion. Then, the World Health Organization (WHO) temporarily named the virus "2019 novel Coronavirus" [2, 3]. The disease was included in "Class B infectious diseases" by "National Health Commission of the People's Republic of China" on January 20, 2020 [4]. This new agent formally clept as "SARS-CoV-2 infection Coronavirus Disease 2019 (COVID-19)" and "Severe Acute Respiratory Syndrome Coronavirus-2 (SARS-CoV-2)" by WHO on February 11, 2020. WHO described this as a "Public Health Emergency of International Concern (PHEIC)" [5].

There have been two serious coronavirus epidemics in recent years. "Severe Acute Respiratory Syndrome (SARS-CoV)" outbreak was in 2003 and "Middle East Respiratory Syndrome (MERS-CoV)" outbreak was in 2012 [6].

The "2019 novel coronavirus" was entitled "SARS-CoV-2" because of its genomic identity to SARS-CoV (~ 80%). SARS-CoV, which had a high mortality rate, also caused acute respiratory distress syndrome [7].

The SARS-CoV-2 epidemic has extended throughout China and around globally [8–11]. WHO declared "pandemic condition" following the assessment of the

S. Yıldız (✉) · S. Z. Toros
Section of Otorhinolaryngology, Head and Neck Surgery, İstanbul Haydarpaşa Numune Training and Research Hospital, İstanbul, Turkey

P. Rombaux
Department of Otorhinolaryngology, and Institute of Neurosciences, Saint Luc University Clinics, Catholic University of Louvain, Brussels, Belgium

C. Cingi et al. (eds.), *Pediatric ENT Infections*,
https://doi.org/10.1007/978-3-030-80691-0_68

COVID-19 epidemic on March 12, 2020 [12]. COVID-19 affects a great count of people globally. Outbreak is notified to have spread in about 200 climes and regions [13, 14].

Most coronaviruses entail ailments in their own host types which may infect humans by way of interspecies transmission [15].

SARS-CoV-2 causes a variety of diseases, from mild symptoms of upper respiratory tract infection to more serious conditions like seen in the epidemics of MERS-CoV and SARS-CoV [16].

SARS-CoV-2 has an identical pathophysiology with SARS-CoV. Both viruses cause illness through potentially damaging vital organs like the liver, heart, kidneys, and lungs. In addition, SARS-CoV-2 infection with a high prevalence of pneumonia poses a significant risk for patients [17]. The general symptoms of SARS-CoV-2 infection in adults contain fever, breath shortness, cough, anosmia, dysgeusia, and respiratory distress. Critical patients can lead to pneumonia, kidney insufficiency, severe acute respiratory syndrome (SARS), and death [18].

In the onset of the COVID-19 outbreak, pediatric patients who were considered not be susceptible to this virus, were observed quite rarely. However, children affected by COVID-19 infection gradually appeared with the emergence of familial clustering. Most pediatric cases have epidemiological links with adult patients. They are mostly household contact cases. According to epidemiological studies, the mortality rate was higher in elderly patients [19–21]. In addition, epidemiological studies suggested that the incidence is lower in children [19–21]. Compared to adults with COVID-19 infection, most COVID-19 infected children experience a slighter clinical process [20]. Several patients of pneumonia have been noticed in SARS-CoV-2 infected children. Pneumonia is the primary reason of death in pediatric population [22]. Children may develop different immunological responses to viral infections and this may cause serious damage to vital organs [23]. Sidiq et al. suggest that humoral immunity created by MMR vaccine provides advantageous protection against COVID-19 to children [24].

68.2 Epidemiology

In children with COVID-19, clinical analysis is insufficient and the spread is rapid. Therefore, the outbreak features of pediatric population in the MERS-CoV, and SARS-CoV periods, should be considered to supply hints for efficient precaution. A comprehensive literature study has shown that MERS-CoV was infrequent in children. Thirty-one patients were reported between 2012 and 2016 [25]. Cause of this situation is that the transmission is largely dependent on animal exposure and direct contact at home or in healthcare facilities. As a whole, coronavirus disease which previously occurred with two major epidemics did not affect children extensively due to the short-lived outbreak of SARS-CoV and the narrow mode of spread of MERS-CoV.

As the epidemic transmission, it was approved by stages that SARS-CoV-2 could infect places like houses or health care centers. SARS-CoV-2 could even spread among cities and also among countries. Pediatric population is a very specific bunch, usually because of adjacent household relationships, and may be prone to cross-infection. Compared to adults, there are limited studies on children with SARS-CoV-2 infection [10, 26–29]. Previous studies in literature haven't found any cases in children who were formerly considered less sensitive [30]. Pursuant to the present trend, familial clusters develop as a result of person-to-person transmission [31]. According to the available epidemiological datum, 56% of SARS-CoV-2 infected children showed obvious proof of spread through family meetings [32]. The latest literature knowledge suggests that all age groups, also children, are usually sensitive against SARS-CoV-2 infection [31, 33]. Moreover, children show specific characteristics and cannot directly identify their complaints or contact histories. This leads to serious difficulties in the protection, diagnosis, and treatment of this population [34].

Since the onset of the epidemic, the rate of children among total SARS-CoV-2 infected patients was low. Considering to data reported in February 2020, as stated by "Chinese Center for Disease Control and Prevention" data, children who were aged 19 years and under accounted for 1% of the entire SARS-CoV-2 infected individuals [35]. Aged 19 years and under population exemplify 20% of the entire population. Thus, it may be stated that COVID-19 is less common in children. Given that fewer tests are performed in children due to fewer symptoms, however, it can be concluded that this alleviates the true incidence in the pediatric population.

In "Korean Center for Disease Control and Prevention" data, 6.3% of all patients diagnosed SARS-CoV-2 infection were children [36]. Italian data issued on March 2020 stated that just 1.2% of 22,512 patients with SARS-CoV-2 infection were children [37]. On April 2020, "US Center for Disease Control and Prevention" published 2572 SARS-CoV-2 infected patients among children under the age of 18 [38]. Although this age group accounts for 22% of the US population, it accounts for only 1.7% of the total cases reported in the USA.

The study which has the highest number of SARS-CoV-2 infected patients was prepared by "Chinese Novel Coronavirus Pneumonia Emergency Response Epidemiology Team" with 72,314 cases. This study found that approximately 2% of 44,672 approved COVID-19 cases were children aged between 0 and 19 years [39]. At the time of diagnosis, 0.9% of patients were under the age of 10 [39].

Median age was found to be 6.7 and 7 years in pediatric patients in the largest pediatric case series published in China (20, 40, respectively). COVID-19 can infect all children at all ages. Also infants and young children can be infected by SARS-CoV-2 [40]. The youngest one among the approved pediatric patients to date was only 30 hours old [1].

Even though the Chinese series show an identical size of patients among adult female and male population, the datum suggest that male patients suffer from more serious illness and die [41, 42]. There are studies reporting a higher incidence in males compared to females (0.31/100,000 vs. 0.27/100000, respectively) [43]. In pediatric group gender difference was prominent. In a study consisting of 2143 cases, 56.6% of patients were reported to be boys [44].

Children represent approximately 2% of the patients diagnosed in China [39], 1.2% of the patients diagnosed in Italy [37], and 5% of patients with SARS-CoV-2 infection in the United States of America [45]. In this outbreak, low figures like the SARS-CoV epidemic in 2003 draw attention [46].

COVID-19 has a mortality rate of about 2% at all ages; however, children with the critical illness have also been reported. Disease which has an acute progress is self-limiting [47, 48]. Compared to the SARS-CoV-2 outbreak, the number of confirmed pediatric cases during the SARS-CoV outbreak was not more than 0.02% of the entire patients. Besides the percentage of children with a serious illness was about 7.9% during the SARS-CoV epidemic [47, 48]. The most of them had a history of household exposure or contact with grown-up patients, while a small group of them had a travel history and a history of hospital exposure in the epidemic regions [47, 48]. Of 1621 confirmed MERS-CoV cases reported globally, the proportion of children under the age of 19 years is 2.2% [49].

There were fewer pediatric patients during the SARS-CoV epidemic. The complaints of pediatric patients were significantly milder in children compared to grown-up patients [50–53]. Similarly, official data showed that children with COVID-19 are relatively infrequent. Besides, their general signs are significantly mild [54]. Also, all schools in China were on a spring festival holiday at the time of the COVID-19 epidemic, which may have forestalled children from being exposed to contagion origins. After spreading of the virus to other countries, countries closed schools as a precaution, and this reduced the exposure of children.

68.3 Etiology and Pathogenesis

Coronaviruses are the largest single-stranded RNA viruses known [55]. Coronaviruses are classified as "Alphacoronaviruses," "Betacoronaviruses," "Gammacoronaviruses," and "Deltacoronaviruses" [56–58]. "Alphacoronaviruses" and "Betacoronaviruses" infect only mammals [59]. HCoV2-229E, HCoV2-HKU1, HCoV2-OC43, and HCoV2-NL63 are four of the coronaviruses generally spread among humans [60, 61]. Mentioned four viruses which spread among humans are deemed to be reproduced initially from cattles, dromedary camels, and bats [62–65]. Coronaviruses are talented of rapid recombination and mutation. Due to these properties, it leads to new coronaviruses. Thus, these new coronaviruses can spread from animals to humans. Due to these features, they caused the epidemic of SARS-CoV [15, 66–68], which was thought to be transmitted to humans from musk cats or bats in 2002, and to the epidemic of MERS-CoV [69, 70], which was spread to humans from dromedary camels in Saudi Arabia in 2012. SARS-CoV and MERS-CoV are Betacoronaviruses [71]. The 2019 novel coronavirus which is now causing a global pandemic is a new Betacoronavirus [72]. It is closely related to the coronavirus which was isolated from horseshoe bats in China [10, 72].

"Attachment," "Penetration," "Biosynthesis," "Maturation," and "Release" are the steps of the life cycle of the virus. In the "Attachment" step, the virus binds to host cell receptors. The step which virus enters into the host cells through membrane fusion or endocytosis is called "Penetration." Then the viral content is released into the host cell. Viral RNA goes to the host cell nucleus for replication. The step which viral RNA is replicated in the host cell nucleus is called "Biosynthesis." The viral particles produced mature and are released out of the host cell. These steps are called "Maturation" and "Release," respectively.

"Membrane (M)," "Spike (S)," "Nucleocapsid (N)," and "Envelope (E)" are the four constructional proteins of coronaviruses. [73]. The spike protein protruses on the viral surface. The spike protein states the variety of tropism between host and coronaviruses. The spike protein consists of two physiological subunits. S1 is in charge for binding, and S2 for fusion of membranes. ACE-2 has been stated as a binding point for SARS-CoV [74]. Also the spike protein of SARS-CoV-2 binds to ACE-2 according to the structural and functional analyses [75–77]. The urinary bladder, lungs, ileum, heart, and kidneys are the organs with high ACE-2 expression [78]. Expression of ACE-2 is high in epithelial cells in the upper segments of the lungs and in the nasopharynx. Because of this, the virus can enter these cells and cause destruction. [79, 80]. This situation explains why early lung damage is common in the distal airway. Endothelial cells also express ACE-2 [81, 82]. As the endothelium has an important duty in organization of thrombosis, increased clotting profiles in severe disease most likely report important endothelial damage [83]. Zhang et al. identified the virus by single-cell transcription. After that they investigated the SARS-CoV-2 infection pathway and the duty of ACE-2 in the gastrointestinal system, and the expression rate of ACE-2 in healthy human lungs and gastrointestinal tract [84]. They found that ACE-2 is expressed not just in lung alveolar epithelial cells. Besides, epithelial cells in the proximal esophagus, ileal epithelial cells and epithelial cells in the colon express ACE-2. Therefore, intestinal symptoms of COVID-19 can be explained by the spreading over by SARS-CoV-2 due to the ACE-2 expression capabilities of intestinal epithelial cells [84]. Detection of the RNA of SARS-CoV-2 in the stool of cases supports that the development of destruction also occurs in the gastrointestinal tract [85].

Similarly, official data to date show that children with COVID-19 are relatively infrequent, and their signs are significantly mild [54]. The main causes of this situation might be as follows: (1) they are primarily contaminated by grown-up family members, and the area of efficiency for children is relatively small. Like other RNA viruses, the SARS-CoV-2 virus can also cause proliferation, mutation, and survival errors without being recognized by the immune system. As a result, a reduction in virulence may occur. Therefore, infection with a new generation virus leads milder symptoms; (2) there may be variations in immune reactions of pediatric population check against to grown-ups. The innate immune response inclines to be more effective in pediatric population. The innate immune response is the early response to a broad group of pathogens. The first response to pathogens is given by the innate immune system. The cells in this system reply instantly to foreign pathogens. Children can fight COVID-19 just like other coronaviruses, including MERS-CoV and SARS-CoV, more easily compared to grown-ups and experience only mild symptoms thanks to the innate immune response is powerful [86]; (3) The function or number of ACE-2 receptors in children is not as appropriate as in grown-ups.

Latterly, a study has searched the role of the ACE-2 receptor. Authors suggest that SARS-CoV-2 uses cellular protease TMPRSS2 and ACE-2 for entry into target cells [87]. The ACE-2 receptors distribute differently in different systems and demographic groups. Therefore, children and adults can suffer different severity of illness because of different levels or functions of receptors in; (4) Other causes: children have lesser cigarette exposure, children have a lesser chronic diseases, and children have more potent self-healing capability. Another reason for the mild course in pediatric patients may be the fact that the level of expression of ACE-2 differs between pediatric population and grown-ups. Another research suggested that ACE2 was more plenty of expressed in well-diversified ciliary cells because of continuity of human lung and epithelial cells' development [80]. Also, sex can affect ACE-2 expression. The gene of ACE-2 is spotted on the X-chromosome. The levels of ACE-2 are higher in males compared to females [88]. This may partially be responsible for the variation in mortality and severity in terms of gender in all age groups [38, 41, 42].

SARS-CoV-2 is extremely infectious. In general, all individuals are sensitive. Besides, contact and respiratory droplets are the primary transmission lanes [89, 90]. Generally, the incubation period is considered to range averagely from 3 to 7 days (minimum 1 day and maximum 14 days) [33, 89, 91]. In children, the incubation period is usually about 2 days and varies between 2 and 10 days [92].

Some certain live vaccines like measles, BCG, and oral polio vaccine stimulate heterologous preservation toward pathogens. They demonstrate these effects by increasing transcriptional, epigenetic, and functional reprogramming of congenital immune cells and increasing congenital immune responses, also called "trained immunity." There are studies suggesting that initiation of immunity accustomed by all pathogen vaccines can be a significant instrument to reduce the sensitivity and severity of SARS-CoV-2 [34, 93, 94]. Covian et al., suggest that where BCG vaccination is given at birth, this is followed by a lower transmission rate and fewer SARS-CoV-2 infection-related deaths [94].

68.4 Clinical Characteristics

SARS-CoV-2 infected children may not be symptomatic. Besides, they could have symptoms like fatigue, fever, and dry cough. Children may also show superior respiratory tract symptoms, like runny nose, nasal obstruction and chemosensory dysfunction [95]. Some of the patients also have gastrointestinal system symptoms such as diarrhea, nauseation, spewing, and abdominal pain. The most common symptoms have been reported as cough, sore throat, and fever [20, 21, 44, 96]. Less common symptoms have been reported as diarrhea, fatigue, runny nose, and vomiting [20, 97]. Some children and newborns experience vomiting, diarrhea, and other gastrointestinal symptoms, or atypical symptoms that are only manifested as asthma and shortness of breath [34, 98]. Also myocarditis, heart failure, and arrhythmias are among the possible symptoms. There are studies reporting acute myocarditis manifestations following SARS-CoV-2 infection. Acute myocarditis manifestation following SARS-CoV-2 infection progresses as intense systemic inflammation and atypical Kawasaki disease [99–101].

Most children with COVID-19 have mild symptoms. Also their prognosis is well. Most children with COVID-19 got well 1–2 weeks after onset. Progression to lower respiratory infections is very rare. Patients with severe condition may advance to coagulation dysfunction, acute respiratory distress syndrome, refractory metabolic acidosis, and septic shock. However, this much severity is rare in pediatric population [89, 102]. The primary child case with critical illness was noticed in Wuhan Children's Hospital [102]. The patient, who was followed up in the intensive care unit for a total of 10 days, recovered completely [102]. It is clear from the report that pediatric population is also sensitive to SARS-CoV-2 infection, and that serious infections may occur.

Although SARS-CoV-2 infected patients are rare in infants, infants requiring hospitalization for treatment, have been reported [40]. It has been reported that the incidence of severe and critical diseases is higher in patients younger than 1 year [44, 103].

Diagnostic criteria for cases are defined as follows [104]: Diagnostic criteria for asymptomatic cases: individuals with COVID-19 who remain without any symptoms during infection, with or without abnormal thorax CT signs; Diagnostic criteria of mild patients: mild clinical signs, no thorax CT signs of pneumonia; Diagnostic criteria of common patients: fever, respiratory symptoms, and thorax CT signs of pneumonia; Diagnostic criteria of severe patients: (1) respiratory distress, tachypnea; (2) hypoxemia while resting; and (3) arterial partial oxygen pressure (PaO2) / fraction of inspired oxygen (FiO2) $\leq$ 300 mmHg; Diagnostic criteria of critical patients: (1) respiratory insufficiency and mechanical ventilation are required; (2) shock; and (3) complicated by different organ failures that require intensive care. According to these criteria, the asymptomatic, mild, or moderate disease was detected in more than 90% of one of the largest pediatric case series [44]. The remaining 5.2% had a serious illness and 0.6% had a critical illness [44].

The rate of hospitalization was 1.6% to 2.5% in US children, and there were no children in need of intensive care [45]. The approximative hospitalization percentage for children is at most 14% [38].

In late April 2020, reports from Europe identified the emergence of a new febrile pediatric entity that involved multi-organ involvement, cardiogenic shock, and hypotension, requiring pediatric ICU care in the most cases. Initially, this syndrome, which was called Kawasaki syndrome and Kawasaki-like syndrome, progressed with persistent fever, systemic hyperinflammation, and pronounced and severe gastrointestinal symptoms [105]. This new syndrome associated with COVID-19 was soon realized to be very different from Kawasaki disease or Kawasaki shock syndrome. This syndrome, which affects different demographic characteristics and shows great differences in clinical and laboratory parameters, was named Multisystem Inflammatory Syndrome (MIS-C) [106].

Symptoms may be mild, such as mild fever, sore throat, headache, conjunctival injection, abdominal pain, vomiting and rash. However, necrotizing pneumonia, myocardial dysfunction, shock, kidney damage, coronary artery aneurysms, and severe cases resulting in death may also occur [106]. Gastrointestinal system involvement is seen in 92% of patients [107]. As of July 2020, children and adolescents accounted for a small proportion (1% -5%) of a total of 12,274,654 laboratory-confirmed COVID-19 cases reported worldwide [108, 109]. CRP, BNP and troponin are often increased in the laboratory [110]. Anemia, lymphopenia, neutrophilia, thrombocytopenia can be observed [110]. Diagnostic suspicion should be raised in the presence of unexplained persistent fever with unexplained symptomatology following exposure to COVID-19 [111].

68.5 Diagnosis and Diagnostic Tests

The basic diagnostic test for the diagnosis of coronavirus infections is "real-time polymerase chain reaction (RT-PCR)" in respiratory tract secretions [60, 112–119]. PCR is the current gold standard diagnostic test for SARS-CoV-2 infection. However, negative PCR results cannot rule out SARS-CoV-2 infection for patients [120, 121]. SARS-CoV-2 is usually diagnosed using upper respiratory tract swabs or blood samples that are definitive for nucleic acid of the 2019-nCoV on RT-PCR tests. For SARS-CoV-2, SARS-CoV, and MERS-CoV higher viral burdens were picked out in examples obtained from the tracheal secretion crosschecked to the nasopharyngeal or oropharyngeal secretion [72, 122]. So, in patients with clinical signs that primarily give negative results in upper respiratory tract swabs, retesting of the nasopharyngeal or oropharyngeal samples or rather of the tracheal secretion examples must be tested. RT-PCRs in feces examples may also be definitive. However they are not used for routine diagnosis for coronaviruses [114, 123, 124]. A few cases with positive PCR in blood samples have been noticed for SARS-CoV-2 and SARS-CoV [72, 125]. Patients with MERS-CoV and SARS-CoV infection has been diagnosed with serology. But serology is not beneficial in the early stage of coronavirus infection. Antibodies toward SARS-CoV have been noticed to have cross-reactivities against common coronaviruses [126].

Laboratory findings of children with COVID-19 are similar to infections caused by different coronaviruses. Either leukocyte count is usually ordinary or derogated lymphocyte and neutrophil counts can be observed [51, 52, 97, 127–129]. It has been shown that decreased lymphocyte counts are a common laboratory finding, especially in severe cases [28, 130]. Thrombocytopenia may be observed [51, 52, 127, 129, 131]. Levels of procalcitonin and C-reactive protein are usually standard [97]. In patients with severe disease, increased liver enzymes increased lactate dehydrogenase levels, increased D-dimers, and abnormal coagulation have been noticed [28, 51, 52, 97, 127, 129]. Lactate dehydrogenase levels were increased by 30% of the cases [96]. In patients with severe disease, increased "granulocyte-colony stimulating factor," "macrophage inflammatory protein 1α," plasma concentrations of "proinflammatory cytokines," "tumor necrosis factor-α," and "monocyte chemoattractant protein 1" have been reported [130, 132–134].

Children with SARS-CoV-2 infection mostly show bilateral irregular airspace consolidations, peribronchial thickening, and ground-glass opacities in the periphery of the lungs on chest radiography [51, 52, 127, 129, 131, 135, 136].

Ground-glass opacities and airspace consolidations are the mostly seen findings on lung computed tomography (CT) [137]. CT changes of children with COVID-19 are spotted and nodular ground-glass opacities, bilateral multiple patches, and oozing shades in the central and peripheral zones of lungs or below the pleura [96, 120, 138]. None of the mentioned findings are specific. CT findings of children with COVID-19 are milder compared to CT findings of adults [138–140].

We can identify some factors that may be associated with illness severity in children with COVID-19. Most importantly, CT findings in more than 3 segments indicates the severe lung harm which poses the maximum risk for exacerbation of SARS-CoV-2 infection in children. Secondly, an overactivated immune response to COVID-19 particularly increased IL-6 is related to severe disease. At the last stage, organ damage like intravascular coagulation and hepatobiliary dysfunction may indicate multiple organ failure [132].

68.6 Treatment

In the treatment of children infected with coronaviruses, additional therapy should be used. This treatment is including adequate calorie and liquid intake, and supplemental oxygen support. The aim is to prevent organ dysfunction, acute respiratory distress syndrome, and secondary bacterial superinfections. If there is a bacterial infection suspected, broad-spectrum antibiotics can be used. Empirically cephalosporins can be utilized. Most of the studies about treatment suggested additional therapy such as supplemental oxygen therapy and empirical antibiotics for secondar bacterial infections [92]. Till the results of ongoing clinical trials are revealed, there is no certain proof to base on the treatment of patients with COVID-19.

It is recommended to use intravenous immunoglobulin, oral lopinavir/ritonavir, and nebulized interferon-alpha-2b for severe cases, and corticosteroids for complications such as acute respiratory distress syndrome, septic shock, hemophagocytic syndrome, or encephalitis [97].

Neither WHO nor "US Centers for Disease Control and Prevention" recommend any special therapy for any age groups [141, 142]. The effectiveness of antiviral agents is not certain in pediatric population, and antibiotics apply just to cases with probable or approved secondary bacterial superinfections. However, in one of the studies, 59% of children with COVID-19 were applied with lopinavir/ritonavir [96].

Despite of their variety, coronaviruses have many similar proteins between different types that help in the think up of novel species. One of these is the spike protein [143]. Function of glycoprotein S is virus-cell interaction [143]. Monoclonal antibodies against spike glycoprotein S (obtained from healing plasma) have been proved to block the binding of coronaviruses with host cells and reduce severity in patients infected with SARS-CoV [144–150]. Although not a monoclonal antibody, a protein which has solely been tested in animal trials also blocks spike glycoprotein S. This protein was obtained from red algae called Griffithsia [151].

Aminopeptidase N, O-acetylated sialic acid, ACE-2, and dipeptidyl peptidase 4 are also binding points for coronaviruses. Monoclonal antibodies to be developed toward mentioned receptors can also be the target of therapy [74, 152–154]. However, the rapid mutation ability of coronaviruses is a potential problem for using monoclonal antibodies in treatment [145].

The entry of viruses inside host cells can be decreased by blocking the proteases which are responsible [155–157]. Papain-like proteases which are inclusive in the replication phase of coronaviruses are another probable aims for therapy. Many papain-like protease inhibitors have been shown. However, any of these -like protease inhibitors were approved in vivo studies [158, 159]. Also, papain-like protease enzymes differ between coronavirus types. This situation renders papain-like protease inhibitors narrow-spectrum antiviral drugs against coronaviruses [160]. Another protein inclusive in viral replication is the coronavirus parent protein, which is inhibited by lopinavir. Also, lopinavir (plus ritonavir) is effective against coronaviruses in animals and SARS-CoV infected humans in nonrandomized studies, as mentioned earlier [161, 162].

Chloroquine widely used against autoimmune diseases and malaria also inhibits virus-cell fusion by increasing endosomal pH and is whence a probable broad-spectrum antiviral agent [163]. Besides, it is effective in the glycosylation stage of cells SARS-CoV receptors. [164]. Also, in vitro studies suggest that chloroquine blocks the entrance of SARS-CoV-2 inside cells, and postentry stages [165]. Also, chloroquine has an immune-modulating activity that can increase its antiviral effect in vivo [165].

Immucillin-A is a recently developed adenosine analog. It blocks the RNA polymerase of a large variety of RNA viruses, such as MERS-CoV and SARS-CoV. Immucillin-A may be helpful in the therapy of another coronaviruses [166]. In addition, helicase inhibitors may be beneficial in the therapy of coronaviruses [167]. RNA synthesis inhibitors are the plate-mark of SARS-CoV-2 replication and also decrease the creation of double-membrane vesicles. RNA synthesis inhibitors identified as probable antiviral agents [168, 169]. A double-stranded RNA-activated caspase oligomerizer (DRACO) aims extended viral double-stranded RNA and stimulates apoptosis of infected cells however protects healthy cells. DRACO may also be helpful in the therapy of coronaviruses [170].

In addition, the authors suggested treatment with cyclosporine A, interferons, levamisole, thymopentin, thymosin alpha-1, and intravenous gamma globulin [171].

Various vaccines against coronaviruses are being developed to prevent infection and to reduce viral spread and severity of disease. The spike protein or this protein's connection area are the main antigens for vaccine development [172]. Besides, the tendency of coronaviruses to rapid mutation and recombination poses a potential problem in terms of vaccine progress [173–175]. In addition, advanced disease that developed after viral difficulties following vaccination was observed in animal models [176–178].

Treatment approaches should be different in neonatal cases, because newborns may have a more severe clinical course [44, 102]. All probable or laboratory-approved neonatal COVID-19 patients must have therapy in the neonatal intensive care unit. High-dose pulmonary surfactant, high-frequency oscillating ventilation, and nitric oxide inhalation should be used for newborn with SARS-CoV-2 infection. Parenteral application of immunoglobulins or glucocorticoids, extracorporeal membrane oxygenation, and sustainable kidney replacement may be used for critical neonates with COVID-19 [179].

68.7   Prognosis

According to initial data, the mortality rate in patients with COVID-19 is 2.38% for China and 0.25% for another countries. The mortality rates for MERS-CoV and for SARS-CoV were 9.6% and 34%, respectively [180]. When the mortality rates were compared, it was found that the mortality rates were lower in SARS-CoV-2 patients [180]. Death cases have been noticed also in children [20, 39, 44].

The disease shows a mild course in the pediatric population as mentioned above. One study reported that 149 (87.1%) of 171 children hospitalized in January–February, were discharged in the first week of March [20]. In addition, Cao et al. contended that most of the 398 pediatric cases got healed about 7–14 days [181].

We can identify some factors that may be associated with disease severity in children with COVID-19. Most importantly, CT findings in more than 3 segments indicates the severe lung harm which poses the maximum risk for exacerbation of SARS-CoV-2 infection in pediatric population. Secondly, an overactivated immune response to SARS-CoV-2 particularly increased IL-6 is related to severity of disease. Finally, organ damage such as intravascular coagulation dysfunction and hepatobiliary, multiple organ failure are important markers that are related to severity of disease [132].

Wang et al. suggested that the closure of schools and the closure of children to their homes may have negative consequences on children's mental and physical situation. This kind of negative effects include less healthy diets which result in longer screening times, irregular sleep, obesity, and loss of cardiovascular compatibility [182].

68.8   Conclusion

Influence of SARS-CoV-2, SARS-CoV, and MERS-CoV-2 infections on pediatric population is less frequent and less severe compared to grown-ups. Regarding SARS-CoV-2, a previously published study showed that pediatric population was as likely to get this virus like grown-ups. However, they are unlikely to exhibit symptoms or improve serious clinical manifestations [183]. This may be due to less exposure of children to main sources of contamination (disproportionately nosocomial to date) or less exposure to animals. However, children being less symptomatic or having less severe symptoms may cause less testing. This may cause the number of infected children to be underestimated. In addition, the significance of children in viral transmission is still unclear. Although the rate of transmission of undiagnosed (undocumented) cases is lower, higher numbers suggest that they may be the origin in 79% of asymptomatic cases [184].

The COVID-19 epidemic is a living issue that affects people around the world. In the absence of basic therapeutic interventions, current management involves the reduction of viral transmission and supportive treatment for symptomatic patients. There is an immediate requirement to improve targeted treatments. Although the reported number of pediatric patients consists in a small portion of all patients at this point, children are undefended to outbreak. More emphasis should be placed on raising awareness, strengthening infection control measures, and managing family health. Understanding the difference between responses of pediatric population and adult population to this novel coronavirus can help guide immune-based treatments.

References

1. Jiatong S, Wenjun L. Epidemiological characteristics and prevention and control measures of corona virus disease 2019 in children. J Trop Med. 2020;20:153–6.
2. World Health Organization. Coronavirus disease (COVID-19) outbreak; 2020. https://www.who.int/emergencies/diseases/novelcoronavirus-2019. Accessed 15 Feb 2020.
3. World Health Organization Novel coronavirus – China; 2020. https://www.who.int/csr/don/12-january-2020-novelcoronaviruschina/en/. Accessed 15 Feb 2020.
4. National Health Commission of the People's Republic of China. Notice of the National Health Council of the People's Republic of China [EB/OL]; 2020. http://www.nhc.gov.cn/jkj/s7916/202001/44a3b8245e8049d2837a4f27529cd386.shtml. Accessed 20 Jan 2020.
5. WHO. Coronavirus. https://www.who.int/emergencies/diseases/novel-coronavirus-2019. Accessed 11 Feb 2020.
6. Donnelly CA, Ghani AC, Leung GM, et al. Epidemiological determinants of spread of causal agent of severe acute respiratory syndrome in Hong Kong. Lancet. 2003;361:1761–6.
7. Ksiazek TG, Erdman D, Goldsmith CS, et al. A novel coronavirus associated with severe acute respiratory syndrome. N Engl J Med. 2003;348:1953–66.
8. Chinese Center For Disease Control and Prevention. Coronavirus disease (COVID-19) situation reports. http://2019ncov.chinacdc.cn/2019-nCoV/index.html. Accessed 11 Feb 2020.
9. Chinese Center For Disease Control and Prevention. Coronavirus disease (COVID-19) situation reports. http://2019ncov.chinacdc.cn/2019-nCoV/global.html. Accessed 19 Feb 2020.
10. Zhu N, Zhang D, Wang W, et al. A novel coronavirus from patients with pneumonia in China, 2019. N Engl J Med. 2020;382:727–33.
11. Hui DS, IAzhar E, Madani TA, et al. The continuing 2019-nCoV epidemic threat of novel coronaviruses to global health: the latest 2019 novel coronavirus outbreak in Wuhan, China. Int J Infect Dis. 2020;91:264–6.
12. World Health Organization (WHO). WHO characterizes COVID-19 as a pandemic [EB/OL]. Geneva: World Health Organization; 2020.
13. Zheng M, Gao Y, Wang G, et al. Functional exhaustion of antiviral lymphocytes in COVID-19 patients. Cell Mol Immunol. 2020;17:533–5.
14. Zhang J, Litvinova M, Wang W, et al. Evolving epidemiology and transmission dynamics of coronavirus disease 2019 outside Hubei province, China: a descriptive and modelling study. Lancet Infect Dis. 2020;20:793–802.

15. Shi Z, Hu Z. A review of studies on animal reservoirs of the SARS coronavirus. Virus Res. 2008;133:74–87.
16. de Wit E, van Doremalen N, Falzarano D, et al. SARS and MERS: recent insights into emerging coronaviruses. Nat Rev Microbiol. 2016;14:523–34.
17. Hamming I, Timens W, Bulthuis ML, et al. Tissue distribution of ACE2 protein, the functional receptor for SARS coronavirus: a first step in understanding SARS pathogenesis. J Pathol. 2004;203:631–7.
18. Malave A, Elamin EM. Severe acute respiratory syndrome (SARS)- lessons for future pandemics. Virtual Mentor. 2010;12:719–25.
19. Zhou F, Yu T, Du R, et al. Clinical course and risk factors for mortality of adult inpatients with COVID-19 in Wuhan, China: a retrospective cohort study. Lancet. 2020;395:1054–62.
20. Lu X, Zhang L, Du H, et al. SARS-CoV-2 infection in children. N Engl J Med. 2020;382:1663–5.
21. Qiu H, Wu J, Hong L, et al. Clinical and epidemiological features of 36 children with coronavirus disease 2019 (COVID-19) in Zhejiang, China: an observational cohort study. Lancet Infect Dis. 2020;20:689–96.
22. Dagan R, Bhutta ZA, de Quadros CA, et al. The remaining challenge of pneumonia: the leading killer of children. Pediatr Infect Dis J. 2011;30:1–2.
23. Campbell H, Nair H. Child pneumonia at a time of epidemiological transition. Lancet Glob Health. 2012;3:e65–6.
24. Sidiq K, Sabir DK, Ali SM, et al. Does early childhood vaccination protect against COVID-19? Front Mol Biosci. 2020;7:120.
25. Al-Tawfiq JA, Kattan RF, Memish ZA. Middle East respiratory syndrome coronavirus disease is rare in children: an update from Saudi Arabia. World J Clin Pediatr. 2016;5:391–6.
26. Lu H, Stratton CW, Tang YW. Outbreak of pneumonia of unknown etiology in Wuhan China: the mystery and the miracle. J Med Virol. 2020;92:401–2.
27. Paules CI, Marston HD, Fauci AS. Coronavirus infections—more than just the common cold. JAMA. 2020;323:707. https://doi.org/10.1001/jama.2020.0757.
28. Chen N, Zhou M, Dong X, et al. Epidemiological and clinical characteristics of 99 cases of 2019 novel coronavirus pneumonia in Wuhan, China: a descriptive study. Lancet. 2020;395:507–13.
29. Wang D, Hu B, Hu C, et al. Clinical characteristics of 138 hospitalized patients with 2019 novel coronavirus–infected pneumonia in Wuhan. JAMA. 2020;323:1061–9.
30. Li Q, Guan X, Wu P, et al. Early transmission dynamics in Wuhan, China, of novel coronavirus-infected pneumonia. N Engl J Med. 2020;382:1199–207.
31. Chan JF-W, Yuan S, Kok K-H, et al. A familial cluster of pneumonia associated with the 2019 novel coronavirus indicating personto-person transmission: a study of a family cluster. Lancet. 2020;395:514–23.
32. Feng F, Xiaoping L. Facing the pandemic of 2019 novel coronavirus infections: the pediatric perspectives. Chin J Pediatr. 2020;58:81–5.
33. National Health Commission of the People's Republic of China (2020) Diagnosis and treatment of novel coronavirus pneumonia (trial version 7 revised version). [EB/OL]. http://www.nhc.gov.cn/yzygj/s7653p/202003/46c9294a7dfe4cef80dc7f5912eb1989.shtml. Accessed 3 Mar 2020.
34. Lifen Y, Zhenyuan D, Mengqi D, et al (2020) Suggestions for medical staff from department of pediatrics during the treatment of 2019-nCoV infection/pneumonia J N Med (PrePrint). 10.3969/j.issn.0253-9802.2020.02.001.
35. Wu Z, McGoogan JM. Characteristics of and important lessons from the coronavirus disease 2019 (COVID-19) outbreak in China: summary of a report of 72314 cases from the Chinese Center for Disease Control and Prevention. JAMA. 2020;323:1239. https://doi.org/10.1001/jama.2020.2648.
36. Brodin P. Why is COVID-19 so mild in children? Acta Paediatr. 2020;109:1082–3.
37. Livingston E, Bucher K. Coronavirus disease 2019 (COVID-19) in Italy. JAMA. 2020;323:1335. https://doi.org/10.1001/jama.2020.4344.

38. Yuki K, Fujiogi M, Koutsogiannaki S. COVID-19 pathophysiology: a review. Clin Immunol. 2020;215:108427.
39. Zhang Y. The epidemiological characteristics of an outbreak of 2019 novel coronavirus diseases (COVID-19)—China, 2020. Chin J Epidemiol. 2020;41:145.
40. Wei M, Yuan J, Liu YU, et al. Novel coronavirus infection in hospitalized infants under 1 year of age in China. JAMA. 2020;323:1313–4.
41. Wenham C, Smith J, Morgan R. Gender and C-W group, COVID-19: the gendered impacts of the outbreak. Lancet. 2020;395:846–8.
42. Jin J, Bai P, He W, et al. Gender differences in patients with COVID-19: focus on severity and mortality. Front Public Health. 2020;8:152.
43. Yang Y, Lu Q, Liu M, et al. Epidemiological and clinical features of the 2019 novel coronavirus outbreak in China. Med Rxiv. 2020; https://doi.org/10.1101/2020.02.10.20021675.
44. Dong Y, Mo XI, Hu Y, et al. Epidemiological characteristics of 2143 pediatric patients with 2019 coronavirus disease in China. Pediatrics. 2020;16:16.
45. Bialek S, Boundy E, Bowen V, et al. Severe outcomes among patients with coronavirus disease 2019 (COVID-19) — United States. MMWR Morb Mortal Wkly Rep. 2020;69:343–6.
46. Caselli D, Arico M. 2019-nCoV: polite with children! Pediatric Rep. 2020;12:8495.
47. Xu Z, Shi L, Wang Y, et al. Pathological findings of COVID-19 associated with acute respiratory distress syndrome. Lancet Respir Med. 2020;8:420–2.
48. Feng K, Yun YX, Wang XF, et al. First case of severe childhood novel coronavirus pneumonia in China. Chin J Pediatr. 2020;58:179–83.
49. Mei Z, Xiaowen Z, Jianshe W. 2019 novel coronavirus infection: pediatric professionals perspectives and action. Chin J Infect Dis. 2020;38:E003.
50. Ng PC, Leung CW, Chiu WK, et al. SARS in newborns and children. Biol Neonate. 2004;85:293–8.
51. Chiu WK, Cheung PCH, Ng KL, et al. Severe acute respiratory syndrome in children: experience in a regional hospital in Hong Kong. Pediatr Crit Care Med. 2003;4:279–83.
52. Hon KL, Leung CW, Cheng WT. Clinical presentations and outcome of severe acute respiratory syndrome in children. Lancet. 2003;361:1701–3.
53. Spicuzza L, Spicuzza A, La Rosa M, et al. New and emerging infectious diseases. Allergy Asthma Proc. 2007;28:28–34.
54. The Novel Coronavirus Pneumonia Emergency Response Epidemiology Team. The epidemiological characteristics of an outbreak of 2019 novel coronavirus diseases (COVID-19) in China. Chin J Epidemiol. 2020;4:145–51.
55. Cui J, Li F, Shi Z-L. Origin and evolution of pathogenic coronaviruses. Nat Rev Microbiol. 2019;17:181–92.
56. Woo PC, Lau SK, Chu CM, et al. Characterization and complete genome sequence of a novel coronavirus, coronavirus HKU1, from patients with pneumonia. J Virol. 2005;79:884–95.
57. Woo PC, Lau SK, Lam CS, et al. Discovery of seven novel mammalian and avian coronaviruses in the genus deltacoronavirus supports bat coronaviruses as the gene source of alphacoronavirus and betacoronavirus and avian coronaviruses as the gene source of gammacoronavirus and deltacoronavirus. J Virol. 2012;86:3995–4008.
58. Lau SK, Woo PC, Li KS, et al. Discovery of a novel coronavirus, China Rattus coronavirus HKU24, from Norway rats supports the murine origin of Betacoronavirus 1 and has implications for the ancestor of Betacoronavirus lineage A. J Virol. 2015;89:3076–92.
59. Rabi FA, Al Zoubi MS, Kasasbeh GA, et al. SARS-CoV-2 and coronavirus disease 2019: what we know so far. Pathogens. 2020;9:23.
60. Gaunt ER, Hardie A, Claas EC, et al. Epidemiology and clinical presentations of the four human coronaviruses 229E, HKU1, NL63, and OC43 detected over 3 years using a novel multiplex real-time PCR method. J Clin Microbiol. 2010;48:2940–7.
61. Davis BM, Foxman B, Monto AS, et al. Human coronaviruses and other respiratory infections in young adults on a university campus: prevalence, symptoms, and shedding. Influenza Other Respi Viruses. 2018;12:582–90.

62. Huynh J, Li S, Yount B, et al. Evidence supporting a zoonotic origin of human coronavirus strain NL63. J Virol. 2012;86:12816–25.
63. Pfefferle S, Oppong S, Drexler JF, et al. Distant relatives of severe acute respiratory syndrome coronavirus and close relatives of human coronavirus 229E in bats, Ghana. Emerg Infect Dis. 2009;15:1377–84.
64. Corman VM, Eckerle I, Memish ZA, et al. Link of a ubiquitous human coronavirus to dromedary camels. Proc Natl Acad Sci U S A. 2016;113:9864–9.
65. Vijgen L, Keyaerts E, Moës E, et al. Complete genomic sequence of human coronavirus OC43: molecular clock analysis suggests a relatively recent zoonotic coronavirus transmission event. J Virol. 2005;79:1595–604.
66. Drosten C, Günther S, Preiser W, et al. Identification of a novel coronavirus in patients with severe acute respiratory syndrome. N Engl J Med. 2003;348:1967–76.
67. Wang M, Yan M, Xu H, et al. SARS-CoV infection in a restaurant from palm civet. Emerg Infect Dis. 2005;11:1860–5.
68. Luk HKH, Li X, Fung J, et al. Molecular epidemiology, evolution and phylogeny of SARS coronavirus. Infect Genet Evol. 2019;71:21–30.
69. de Groot RJ, Baker SC, Baric RS, et al. Middle East respiratory syndrome coronavirus (MERS-CoV): announcement of the coronavirus study group. J Virol. 2013;87:7790–2.
70. Ommeh S, Zhang W, Zohaib A, et al. Genetic evidence of Middle East respiratory syndrome coronavirus (MERS-Cov) and widespread seroprevalence among camels in Kenya. Virol Sin. 2018;33:484–92.
71. Ceraolo C, Giorgi FM. Genomic variance of the 2019-nCoV coronavirus. J Med Virol. 2020;92:522–8.
72. Chan JF, Yuan S, Kok KH, et al. A familial cluster of pneumonia associated with the 2019 novel coronavirus indicating person-to person transmission: a study of a family cluster. Lancet. 2020;395:514–23.
73. Bosch BJ, van der Zee R, de Haan CA, et al. The coronavirus spike protein is a class I virus fusion protein: structural and functional characterization of the fusion core complex. J Virol. 2003;77:8801–11.
74. Li W, Moore MJ, Vasilieva N, et al. Angiotensin-converting enzyme 2 is a functional receptor for the SARS coronavirus. Nature. 2003;426:450–4.
75. Chen Y, Guo Y, Pan Y, Zhao ZJ. Structure analysis of the receptor binding of 2019-nCoV. Biochem Biophys Res Commun. 2020;525:135–40.
76. Walls AC, Park YJ, Tortorici MA, et al. Structure, function, and antigenicity of the SARS-CoV-2 spike glycoprotein. Cell. 2020;181:281–92.
77. Letko M, Marzi A, Munster V. Functional assessment of cell entry and receptor usage for SARS-CoV-2 and other lineage B betacoronaviruses. Nat Microbiol. 2020;5:562–9.
78. Zou X, Chen K, Zou J, et al. Single-cell RNA-seq data analysis on the receptor ACE2 expression reveals the potential risk of different human organs vulnerable to 2019-nCoV infection. Front Med. 2020;14:185–92.
79. Hamming I, Timens W, Bulthuis ML, et al. Tissue distribution of ACE2 protein, the functional receptor for SARS coronavirus. A first step in understanding SARS pathogenesis. J Pathol. 2004;203:631–7.
80. Jia HP, Look DC, Shi L, et al. ACE2 receptor expression and severe acute respiratory syndrome coronavirus infection depend on differentiation of human airway epithelia. J Virol. 2005;79:14614–21.
81. Lovren F, Pan Y, Quan A, et al. Angiotensin converting enzyme-2 confers endothelial protection and attenuates atherosclerosis. Am J Physiol Heart Circ Physiol. 2008;295:1377–84.
82. Sluimer JC, Gasc JM, Hamming I, et al. Angiotensin-converting enzyme 2 (ACE2) expression and activity in human carotid atherosclerotic lesions. J Pathol. 2008;215:273–9.
83. Wang M, Hao H, Leeper NJ, et al. Thrombotic regulation from the endothelial cell perspectives. Arterioscler Thromb Vasc Biol. 2018;38:e90–5.

84. Zhang H, Kang Z, Gong H, et al. The digestive system is a potential route of 2019-nCov infection: a bioinformatics analysis based on single-cell transcriptomes. 2020; https://doi.org/10.1101/2020.01.30.927806.

85. Holshue ML, DeBolt C, Lindquist S, et al. First case of 2019 novel coronavirus in the United States. N Engl J Med. 2020;382:929–36.

86. https://www.livescience.com/whykids-missing-coronavirus-cases.html.

87. Hoffmann M, Kleine-Weber H, Krüger N, et al. The novel coronavirus 2019 (2019-nCoV) uses the SARS coronavirus receptor ACE2 and the cellular protease TMPRSS2 for entry into target cells. bioRxiv (PrePrint). 2020; https://doi.org/10.1101/2020.01.31.929042.

88. Patel SK, Velkoska E, Burrell LM. Emerging markers in cardiovascular disease: where does angiotensin-converting enzyme 2 fit in? Clin Exp Pharmacol Physiol. 2013;40:551–9.

89. Li Q, Guan X, Wu P, et al. Early transmission dynamics in Wuhan, China, of novel coronavirusinfected pneumonia. N Engl J Med. 2020;382:1199–207.

90. Munster VJ, Koopmans M, van Doremalen N, et al. A novel coronavirus emerging in China d key questions for impact assessment. N Engl J Med. 2020;382:692e4.

91. Guan WJ, Ni ZY, Hu Y, et al. Clinical characteristics of 2019 novel coronavirus infection in China. MedRxiv. 2020; https://doi.org/10.1101/2020.02.06.20020974.

92. Cai J, Xu J, Lin D, et al. A case series of children with 2019 novel coronavirus infection: clinical and epidemiological features. Clin Infect Dis. 2020;28:28.

93. Netea MG, Giamarellos-Bourboulis EJ, Domínguez-Andrés J, et al. Trained immunity: a tool for reducing susceptibility to and the severity of SARS-CoV-2 infection. Cell. 2020;181:969–77.

94. Covián C, Retamal-Díaz A, Bueno SM, et al. Could BCG vaccination induce protective trained immunity for SARS-CoV-2? Front Immunol. 2020;11:970.

95. Chan JF, Yuan S, Kok KH, et al. A familial cluster of pneumonia associated with the 2019 novel coronavirus indicating person-to-person transmission: a study of a family cluster. Lancet. 2020;395:514e23.

96. Wang XF, Yuan J, Zheng YJ, et al. Clinical and epidemiological characteristics of 34 children with 2019 novel coronavirus infection in Shenzhen. Zhonghua Er Ke Za Zhi. 2020;58:E008.

97. Chen ZM, Fu JF, Shu Q, et al. Diagnosis and treatment recommendations for pediatric respiratory infection caused by the 2019 novel coronavirus. World J Pediatr. 2020;16:240–6.

98. Hu T, Fang L, Junling W, et al. Clinical characteristics of 2019 novel coronavirus (2019-nCoV) infection in children and family prevention and control. Med J Wuhan Univ. 2020;81:11. https://doi.org/10.14188/j.1671-8852.2020.6020.

99. Grimaud M, Starck J, Levy M, et al. Acute myocarditis and multisystem inflammatory emerging disease following SARS-CoV-2 infection in critically ill children. Ann Intensive Care. 2020;10:69.

100. Sanna G, Serrau G, Bassareo PP, et al. Children's heart and COVID-19: up-to-date evidence in the form of a systematic review. Eur J Pediatr. 2020;179:1079–87.

101. Alsaied T, Aboulhosn JA, Cotts TB, et al. Coronavirus disease 2019 (COVID-19) pandemic implications in pediatric and adult congenital heart disease. J Am Heart Assoc. 2020;9:e017224.

102. Hong H, Wang Y, Chung HT, et al. Clinical characteristics of novel coronavirus disease 2019 (COVID-19) in newborns, infants and children. Pediatr Neonatol. 2020;61:131–2.

103. Cui Y, Tian M, Huang D, et al. A 55-day-old female infant infected with COVID 19: presenting with pneumonia, liver injury, and heart damage. J Infect Dis. 2020;221:1775–81.

104. Du W, Yu J, Wang H, et al. Clinical characteristics of COVID-19 in children compared with adults in Shandong Province, China. Infection. 2020;48:445–52.

105. Rivas MN, Porritt RA, Cheng MH, et al. COVID-19 Associated Multisystem Inflammatory Syndrome in Children (MIS-C): a novel disease that mimics Toxic Shock Syndrome. The superantigen hypothesis. J Allergy Clin Immunol. 2020;16:31414–7.

106. Whittaker E, Bamford A, Kenny J, et al. Clinical characteristics of 58 children with a pediatric inflammatory multisystem syndrome temporally associated with SARS-CoV-2. JAMA. 2020;324:259–69.

107. Feldstein LR, Rose EB, Horwitz SM, et al. Multisystem inflammatory syndrome in U.S. children and adolescents. N Engl J Med. 2020;383:334–46.
108. Dong Y, Mo X, Hu Y, et al. Epidemiology of COVID-19 among children in China. Pediatrics. 2020;145:e20200702.
109. Bialek S, Gierke R, Hughes M, et al. Coronavirus disease 2019 in children—United States, February 12–April 2, 2020. Morb Mortal Wkly Rep. 2020;69:422–6.
110. Kaushik A, Gupta S, Sood M, et al. A systematic review of multisystem inflammatory syndrome in children associated with SARS-CoV-2 infection. Pediatr Infect Dis J. 2020;39:e340–6.
111. Jackson RJ, Chavarria HD, Hacking SM. A case of multisystem inflammatory syndrome in children mimicking acute appendicitis in a COVID-19 pandemic area. Cureus. 2020;12(9):e10722.
112. Vabret A, Mourez T, Gouarin S, et al. An outbreak of coronavirus OC43 respiratory infection in Normandy, France. Clin Infect Dis. 2003;36:985–9.
113. Vabret A, Mouthon F, Mourez T, et al. Direct diagnosis of human respiratory coronaviruses 229E and OC43 by the polymerase chain reaction. J Virol Methods. 2001;97:59–66.
114. Cheng PK, Wong DA, Tong LK, et al. Viral shedding patterns of coronavirus in patients with probable severe acute respiratory syndrome. Lancet. 2004;363:1699–700.
115. Chim SS, Chiu RW, Lo YM. Genomic sequencing of the severe acute respiratory syndrome-coronavirus. Methods Mol Biol. 2006;336:177–94.
116. Chim SS, Tong YK, Hung EC, et al. Genomic sequencing of a SARS coronavirus isolate that predated the metropole hotel case cluster in Hong Kong. Clin Chem. 2004;50:231–3.
117. Lee JS, Ahn JS, Yu BS, et al. Evaluation of a real-time reverse transcription-PCR (RT-PCR) assay for detection of Middle East respiratory syndrome coronavirus (MERS-CoV) in clinical samples from an outbreak in South Korea in 2015. J Clin Microbiol. 2017;55:2554–5.
118. Kim MN, Ko YJ, Seong MW, et al. Analytical and clinical validation of six commercial Middle East respiratory syndrome coronavirus RNA detection kits based on real-time reverse-transcription PCR. Ann Lab Med. 2016;36:450–6.
119. Al Johani S, Hajeer AH. MERS-CoV diagnosis: an update. J Infect Public Health. 2016;9:216–9.
120. Xia W, Shao J, Guo Y, et al. Clinical and CT features in pediatric patients with COVID-19 infection: different points from adults. Pediatr Pulmonol. 2020;55:1169–74.
121. Xie X, Zhong Z, Zhao W, et al. Chest CT for typical 2019-nCoV pneumonia: relationship to negative RT-PCR testing. Radiology. 2020;2020:200343. https://doi.org/10.1148/radiol.2020200343.
122. Memish ZA, Al-Tawfiq JA, Makhdoom HQ, et al. Respiratory tract samples, viral load, and genome fraction yield in patients with Middle East respiratory syndrome. J Infect Dis. 2014;210:1590–4.
123. Jevšnik M, Steyer A, Zrim T, et al. Detection of human coronaviruses in simultaneously collected stool samples and nasopharyngeal swabs from hospitalized children with acute gastroenteritis. Virol J. 2013;10:46.
124. Zhou J, Li C, Zhao G, et al. Human intestinal tract serves as an alternative infection route for Middle East respiratory syndrome coronavirus. Sci Adv. 2017;3:4966.
125. Hung IF, Cheng VC, Wu AK, et al. Viral loads in clinical specimens and SARS manifestations. Emerg Infect Dis. 2004;10:1550–7.
126. Che XY, Qiu LW, Liao ZY, et al. Antigenic cross-reactivity between severe acute respiratory syndrome-associated coronavirus and human coronaviruses 229E and OC43. J Infect Dis. 2005;191:2033–7.
127. Bitnun A, Allen U, Heurter H, et al. Other members of the Hospital for Sick Children SARS investigation team. Children hospitalized with severe acute respiratory syndrome-related illness in Toronto. Pediatrics. 2003;112:e261.
128. Cheng FW, Ng PC, Chiu WK, et al. A case-control study of SARS versus community acquired pneumonia. Arch Dis Child. 2005;90:747–9.
129. Leung CW, Kwan YW, Ko PW, et al. Severe acute respiratory syndrome among children. Pediatrics. 2004;113:e535–43.

130. Huang C, Wang Y, Li X, et al. Clinical features of patients infected with 2019 novel coronavirus in Wuhan, China. Lancet. 2020;395:497–506.
131. Alfaraj SH, Al-Tawfiq JA, Altuwaijri TA, et al. Middle East respiratory syndrome coronavirus in pediatrics: a report of seven cases from Saudi Arabia. Front Med. 2019;13:126–30.
132. Wang Y, Zhu F, Wang C, et al. Children hospitalized with severe COVID-19 in Wuhan. Pediatr Infect Dis J. 2020;39:e91–4.
133. Zhou Y, Fu B, Zheng X, et al. Pathogenic T cells and inflammatory monocytes incite inflammatory storm in severe COVID-19 patients. Natl Sci Rev. 2020;7:998–1002.
134. Qin C, Zhou L, Hu Z, et al. Dysregulation of immune response in patients with COVID-19 in Wuhan, China. Clin Infect Dis. 2020;2020:248.
135. Babyn PS, Chu WC, Tsou IY, et al. Severe acute respiratory syndrome (SARS): chest radiographic features in children. Pediatr Radiol. 2004;34:47–58.
136. Chung M, Bernheim A, Mei XY, et al. CT imaging features of 2019 novel coronavirus (2019-nCoV). Radiology. 2020;295:202–7.
137. Li AM, Ng PC. Severe acute respiratory syndrome (SARS) in neonates and children. Arch Dis Child Fetal Neonatal Ed. 2005;90:F461–5.
138. Feng K, Yun YX, Wang XF, et al. Analysis of CT features of 15 children with 2019 novel coronavirus infection. Zhonghua Er Ke Za Zhi. 2020;58:E007.
139. Kanne JP. Chest CT findings in 2019 novel coronavirus (2019-nCoV) infections from Wuhan, China: key points for the radiologist. Radiology. 2020;295:16–7.
140. Song F, Shi N, Shan F, et al. Emerging coronavirus 2019-nCoV pneumonia. Radiology. 2020;295:210–7.
141. World Health Organization. WHO interim guidance on clinical management of severe acute respiratory infection when novel coronavirus (nCoV) infection is suspected. 2020. https://apps.who.int/iris/handle/10665/330893. Accessed 5 Mar 2020.
142. Centers for Disease Control and Prevention CfDCaP. Interim clinical guidance for management of patients with confirmed 2019 novel coronavirus (2019-nCoV) infection; 2020. https://www.cdc.gov/coronavirus/2019-ncov/hcp/clinical-guidance-management-patients.html. Accessed 21 Feb 2010.
143. Zumla A, Chan JF, Azhar EI, et al. Coronaviruses - drug discovery and therapeutic options. Nat Rev Drug Discov. 2016;15:327–47.
144. Cheng Y, Wong R, Soo YO, et al. Use of convalescent plasma therapy in SARS patients in Hong Kong. Eur J Clin Microbiol Infect Dis. 2005;24:44–6.
145. Jiang L, Wang N, Zuo T, et al. Potent neutralization of MERS-CoV by human neutralizing monoclonal antibodies to the viral spike glycoprotein. Sci Transl Med. 2014;6:234ra59.
146. Ying T, Du L, Ju TW, et al. Exceptionally potent neutralization of Middle East respiratory syndrome coronavirus by human monoclonal antibodies. J Virol. 2014;88:7796–805.
147. Tang XC, Agnihothram SS, Jiao Y, et al. Identification of human neutralizing antibodies against MERS-CoV and their role in virus adaptive evolution. Proc Natl Acad Sci U S A. 2014;111:E2018–26.
148. Channappanavar R, Lu L, Xia S, et al. Protective effect of intranasal regimens containing peptidic Middle East respiratory syndrome coronavirus fusion inhibitor against MERS-CoV infection. J Infect Dis. 2015;212:1894–903.
149. Soo YO, Cheng Y, Wong R, et al. Retrospective comparison of convalescent plasma with continuing high-dose methylprednisolone treatment in SARS patients. Clin Microbiol Infect. 2004;10:676–8.
150. Pang H, Liu Y, Han X, et al. Protective humoral responses to severe acute respiratory syndrome-associated coronavirus: implications for the design of an effective protein-based vaccine. J Gen Virol. 2004;85:3109–13.
151. Barton C, Kouokam JC, Lasnik AB, et al. Activity of and effect of subcutaneous treatment with the broad-spectrum antiviral lectin griffithsin in two laboratory rodent models. Antimicrob Agents Chemother. 2014;58:120–7.
152. Raj VS, Mou H, Smits SL, et al. Dipeptidyl peptidase 4 is a functional receptor for the emerging human coronavirus-EMC. Nature. 2013;495:251–4.

153. Huang X, Dong W, Milewska A, et al. Human coronavirus HKU1 spike protein uses O-acetylated sialic acid as an attachment receptor determinant and employs hemagglutinin-esterase protein as a receptor-destroying enzyme. J Virol. 2015;89:7202–13.
154. Vijgen L, Keyaerts E, Zlateva K, et al. Identification of six new polymorphisms in the human coronavirus 229E receptor gene (aminopeptidase N/CD13). Int J Infect Dis. 2004;8:217–22.
155. Shirato K, Kawase M, Matsuyama S. Middle East respiratory syndrome coronavirus infection mediated by the transmembrane serine protease TMPRSS2. J Virol. 2013;87:12552–61.
156. Zhou Y, Vedantham P, Lu K, et al. Protease inhibitors targeting coronavirus and filovirus entry. Antiviral Res. 2015;116:76–84.
157. Kawase M, Shirato K, van der Hoek L, et al. Simultaneous treatment of human bronchial epithelial cells with serine and cysteine protease inhibitors prevents severe acute respiratory syndrome coronavirus entry. J Virol. 2012;86:6537–45.
158. Báez-Santos YM, St John SE, Mesecar AD. The SARS-coronavirus papainlike protease: structure, function and inhibition by designed antiviral compounds. Antiviral Res. 2015;115:21–38.
159. Ratia K, Pegan S, Takayama J, et al. A noncovalent class of papain like protease/deubiquitinase inhibitors blocks SARS virus replication. Proc Natl Acad Sci U S A. 2008;105:16119–24.
160. Lee H, Lei H, Santarsiero BD, et al. Inhibitor recognition specificity of MERS-CoV papainlike protease may differ from that of SARS-CoV. ACS Chem Biol. 2015;10:1456–65.
161. Chan KS, Lai ST, Chu CM, et al. Treatment of severe acute respiratory syndrome with lopinavir/ritonavir: a multicentre retrospective matched cohort study. Hong Kong Med J. 2003;9:399–406.
162. Chan JF, Yao Y, Yeung ML, et al. Treatment with lopinavir/ritonavir or interferon-β1b improves outcome of MERS-CoV infection in a nonhuman primate model of common marmoset. J Infect Dis. 2015;212:1904–13.
163. Savarino A, Di Trani L, Donatelli I, et al. New insights into the antiviral effects of chloroquine. Lancet Infect Dis. 2006;6:67–9.
164. Vincent MJ, Bergeron E, Benjannet S, et al. Chloroquine is a potent inhibitor of SARS coronavirus infection and spread. Virol J. 2005;2:69.
165. Wang M, Cao R, Zhang L, et al. Remdesivir and chloroquine effectively inhibit the recently emerged novel coronavirus (2019-nCoV) in vitro. Cell Res. 2020;30:269–71.
166. Warren TK, Wells J, Panchal RG, et al. Protection against filovirus diseases by a novel broadspectrum nucleoside analogue BCX4430. Nature. 2014;508:402–5.
167. Adedeji AO, Singh K, Kassim A, et al. Evaluation of SSYA10-001 as a replication inhibitor of severe acute respiratory syndrome, mouse hepatitis, and Middle East respiratory syndrome coronaviruses. Antimicrob Agents Chemother. 2014;58:4894–8.
168. Lundin A, Dijkman R, Bergström T, et al. Targeting membrane-bound viral RNA synthesis reveals potent inhibition of diverse coronaviruses including the Middle East respiratory syndrome virus. PLoS Pathog. 2014;10:e1004166.
169. Rappe JCF, de Wilde A, Di H, et al. Antiviral activity of K22 against members of the order Nidovirales. Virus Res. 2018;246:28–34.
170. Rider TH, Zook CE, Boettcher TL, et al. Broad-spectrum antiviral therapeutics. PLoS One. 2011;6:e22572.
171. Zhang L, Liu Y. Potential interventions for novel coronavirus in China: a systematic review. J Med Virol. 2020;92:479–90.
172. He Y, Li J, Du L, et al. Identification and characterization of novel neutralizing epitopes in the receptor-binding domain of SARS-CoV spike protein: revealing the critical antigenic determinants in inactivated SARS-CoV vaccine. Vaccine. 2006;24:5498–508.
173. Su S, Wong G, Shi W, et al. Epidemiology, genetic recombination, and pathogenesis of coronaviruses. Trends Microbiol. 2016;24:490–502.
174. Kim DW, Kim YJ, Park SH, et al. Variations in spike glycoprotein gene of MERS-CoV, South Korea, 2015. Emerg Infect Dis. 2016;22:100–4.
175. Sohrab SS, Azhar EI. Genetic diversity of MERS-CoV spike protein gene in Saudi Arabia. J Infect Public Health. 2020;13:709–17.

176. He Y, Zhou Y, Siddiqui P, et al. Inactivated SARS-CoV vaccine elicits high titers of spike protein-specific antibodies that block receptor binding and virus entry. Biochem Biophys Res Commun. 2004;325:445–52.
177. Hashem AM, Algaissi A, Agrawal AS, et al. A highly immunogenic, protective, and safe adenovirus-based vaccine expressing Middle East respiratory syndrome coronavirus S1-CD40L fusion protein in a transgenic human dipeptidyl peptidase 4 mouse model. J Infect Dis. 2019;220:1558–67.
178. Czub M, Weingartl H, Czub S, et al. Evaluation of modified vaccinia virus Ankara based recombinant SARS vaccine in ferrets. Vaccine. 2005;23:2273–9.
179. Wang J, Qi H, Bao L, et al. A contingency plan for the management of the 2019 novel corona-virus outbreak in neonatal intensive care units. Lancet Child Adolesc Health. 2020;4:258–9.
180. Special Expert Group for Control of the Epidemic of Novel Coronavirus Pneumonia of the Chinese Preventive Medicine Association. An update on the epidemiological characteristics of novel coronavirus pneumonia (COVID-19). Chin J Epidemiol. 2020;41:139–44.
181. Cao Q, Chen Y-C, Chen C-L, et al. SARS-CoV-2 infection in children: transmission dynamics and clinical characteristics. J Formos Med Assoc. 2020;119:670–3.
182. Wang L, Shi Y, Xiao T, et al. Chinese expert consensus on the perinatal and neonatal management for the prevention and control of the 2019 novel coronavirus infection (first edition). Ann Trans Med. 2020;8:47.
183. Bi Q, Wu Y, Mei S, et al. Epidemiology and transmission of COVID-19 in 391 cases and 1286 of their close contacts in Shenzhen, China: a retrospective cohort study. Lancet Infect Dis. 2020;3099(20):30287–5. https://doi.org/10.1016/S1473-3099(20)30287-5.
184. Li R, Pei S, Chen B, et al. Substantial undocumented infection facilitates the rapid dissemination of novel coronavirus (SARS-CoV2). Science. 2020;368:489–93.

Ophthalmological Perspective on Pediatric Ear, Nose, and Throat Infections

69

Furkan Kırık and Mehmet Hakan Özdemir

69.1 Introduction

The majority of the tissues and organs that fall into the area of expertise of ear, nose and throat (ENT) specialists are adjacent to the orbit, and therefore to the globe. As a result of this contiguity, ENT diseases can spread to the orbit and present with various orbital complications. While these complications can be mild, they can also manifest as severe morbidities that lead to permanent loss of vision. In addition, ENT diseases can also spread to the cranium as well as the orbit, and lead to severe intracranial complications that may result in mortality. Such intracranial complications may also manifest with findings in an ophthalmological examination, as many cranial nerves (CNs) are also associated with the orbital structures. This is why ENT specialists commonly encounter ophthalmological findings as a result of both the orbital and cranial complications of infectious ENT diseases. In addition, ophthalmological examination findings are useful for diagnosis, as some infectious agents can cause a common infection both in the ocular and head-neck region.

Most infectious ENT diseases can be self-limited with relevant treatment without leading to any complications. However, they can also cause various morbidities and even mortality, although this is rare. While questioning symptoms can help lead to diagnosis in adult patients, it may not always be possible to exactly and reliably ascertain the symptoms of a disease in pediatric patients. The clinical presentation and findings therefore become particularly important in pediatric patients.

As the spectrum of ocular findings in infectious ENT diseases can range from mild palpebral edema to severe complications that may result in loss of vision, it is important to recognize the ophthalmological signs and to associate them with the clinical presentation for early diagnosis.

F. Kırık (✉) · M. H. Özdemir
Department of Ophthalmology, Faculty of Medicine, Bezmialem Vakıf University, İstanbul, Turkey

© The Author(s), under exclusive license to Springer Nature Switzerland AG 2022
C. Cingi et al. (eds.), *Pediatric ENT Infections*,
https://doi.org/10.1007/978-3-030-80691-0_69

69.2 Ophthalmological Evaluation

Eye examination is recommended in infectious ENT diseases in order to assist with diagnosis, to monitor disease progression, to plan the treatment and to follow the treatment response, and thereby help to prevent possible morbidity and mortality [1]. It is beneficial for ENT specialists to know some basic steps of the ophthalmological examination and diagnostic tests, in addition to the meaning of examination findings that coexist with ENT diseases.

Ophthalmological examinations require cooperation and attention, particularly in pediatric patients [1]. Therefore, a quiet, comfortable, and safe examination environment should be provided, and objects that could cause distraction should be moved away from the visual field of children. In order to conduct a systematic eye examination and prevent confusion of the obtained findings, another examination step should not be applied before the current step is finished, each eye should be examined separately (monocular), and the monocular exam should preferably be initiated with the right eye. Diligent clinical documentation is essential to monitor disease progression.

69.2.1 Evaluation of Vision

Regardless of the patient's age, an evaluation of their vision should first be performed with both eyes open (binocular), followed by separate monocular examinations for each eye, with one eye closed. From 8 to 12 weeks to 3 years of age, children's vision is evaluated according to the child's ability to focus on an object (the object should be able to attract the child's attention) and to follow it (fixation) [2, 3]. It is not possible to make a measurable visual acuity assessment in children in this age group. If there is decreased vision in one eye, during a monocular exam the child will feel uncomfortable when the other eye is closed and try to overcome the obstacle in front of the closed eye by turning/moving their head away [4]. On the other hand, the child will not exhibit severe discomfort when the eye with low vision is closed. However, a child may also show discomfort and cry when one of the eyes is closed regardless of whether there is decreased vision or not, due to the fact that feel uncomfortable during the examination. In such cases, the exam should be stopped and reattempted after the child has been soothed. In the preverbal period, various commercial cards and symbols can be used to evaluate visual acuity in children. For children over 4 years old, and depending on the reading skills of the child, a quantifiable visual acuity can be obtained using Snellen charts and Tumbling E tests, which consist of various figures, letters and numbers [1]. In addition, it is also beneficial to use contrast sensitivity, the Amsler grid, and color vision tests in suspected cases, as these tests can highlight optic nerve and retinal disorders. However, it should be known that these tests can be difficult to administer in children.

69.2.2 External Examinations (Palpebrae, Orbit, Periorbita, Lacrimal Apparatus)

In a healthy person, the upper palpebra covers the upper border of the cornea by 1–2 mm, whereas the lower palpebral border is located at the corneoscleral junction, wherein the palpebral structure should be symmetrical in both eyes. Blepharoptosis or ptosis refers to the condition in which the upper palpebra covers the cornea more than it normally should [5]. While mild blepharoptosis that does not cover the pupil only causes cosmetic or refractive problems in children, long-term blepharoptosis that obstructs the visual axis may lead to amblyopia, thereby causing ocular morbidity in early childhood [6].

Childhood ptosis, which is mostly congenital, can also occur due to a variety of causes [6–8]. Secondary ptosis observed in infectious ENT diseases is frequently of the mechanical type, occurring due to inflammatory palpebral edema, whereas neurogenic ptosis can also be encountered occasionally as a result of an affected oculomotor nerve [9–11]. Determining the function of the levator muscle, which is primarily responsible for the elevation of the upper eyelid, and investigating the presence of other ocular findings coexisting with blepharoptosis are essential for distinguishing the etiology.

The skin on the eyelids is the thinnest skin in the body, wherein eyelid edema can also be encountered in inflammatory events involving the periocular or ocular structures [12]. Hyperemia, pain, increased skin temperature, conjunctival injection, chemosis (subconjunctival edema), and abnormal appearance of the scleral-episcleral vascular structures concomitant with palpebral edema (increased tortuosity) should be evaluated. The presence of chemosis, cellulitis, and fluctuation primarily suggest inflammatory pathologies. Identifying the localization of eyelid edema (diffuse, localized medially, or superiorly) is also important in terms of predicting the location of a possible infectious disease. Investigating the presence of increased skin temperature, hyperemia, and pain coexisting with palpebral edema is necessary in order to recognize inflammatory pathologies. In addition, for the differential diagnosis, it is important to know that hordeolum (accompanied by painful and more severe inflammation) and chalazions (less inflammation and minimal pain or no pain) may also cause palpebral edema and localized eyelid swelling [13].

Proptosis (exophthalmos) can be defined as the forward protrusion of the globe. There are two main types. While intraorbital proptosis is caused primarily by the intraorbital tissues, extraorbital proptosis occurs as a result of the effect of extraorbital structures on the orbit (spread, invasion or metastasis). Moreover, extraorbital proptosis can be divided into two subgroups: intracranial and extracranial. Proptosis encountered as a result of infectious ENT diseases in particular is of extraorbital-extracranial origin [14]. It is important to question the presence of pain and the duration of its development (distinguishing between acute and chronic). In order to roughly determine proptosis, centers of the cornea can be compared from over the patient's head by positioning oneself behind the patient while the patient is looking forward with their head straight on. The severity of proptosis can be evaluated quantitatively with special equipment (Hertel exophthalmometer, etc.). While a difference of more than 2 mm between the eyes is considered significant, it should be kept in mind that bilateral exophthalmos may also be present. In severe cases of proptosis, it may not be possible to completely close the eyelids, in which case corneal ulcers that threaten vision and corneal drying due to lagophthalmos may be encountered (exposure keratopathy).

The lacrimal gland, located anteriorly below the superotemporal orbital rim, secretes the aqueous layer of tears [15]. The produced tear first wets the ocular surface and is then guided to the lacrimal sac via the canaliculi and puncta located medial to the upper and lower eyelids. The lacrimal sac is located in the lacrimal fossa formed by the anterior and posterior lacrimal crests at the inferomedial aspect of the anterior orbital bone wall. The lacrimal sac continues as the nasolacrimal canal and opens into the inferior nasal meatus below the inferior nasal turbinate [16, 17]. Congenital nasolacrimal duct obstruction (CNLDO) has been reported in approximately 10% of newborns [18]. These patients present with epiphora due to insufficient tear drainage. In addition, purulent discharge from the puncta as a result of pressure applied on the lacrimal sac area, conjunctivitis, and hyperemia on the eyelid skin due to irritation can be seen in these patients. Tears accumulating in the lacrimal sac provide an ideal environment for bacterial colonization, particularly in nasolacrimal canal obstruction. Dacryocystitis may therefore be encountered as the result of an infected lacrimal sac [19]. In rare cases, there may be a congenital obstruction in both the proximal and distal opening of the lacrimal sac, which may lead to dacryocystocele as a result of amniotic fluid filling the lacrimal sac [20]. Lacrimal gland infections (primary or secondary) can also be rarely seen.

69.2.3 Ocular Motility and Ocular Alignment

Ocular motility disorders or alignment anomalies may suggest severe orbital, intraocular, or intracranial pathologies. When evaluating eye movement, movement of the child's head must be restricted. It is important to hold the head still for more accurate evaluation of eye movement, as children will try to follow a moving object with both their eyes and head. The eyes can be first examined for misalignment with tests such as the corneal light reflex test (Hirschberg test) and cover-uncover test [21, 22]. In addition to determining alignment, this method is also used to determine globe displacement caused by an external effect. When conducting the Hirschberg test, the patient and the examiner should sit facing each other with their eyes at the same level. Then, a light source is shined across the patient's eye. The light reflection will be visible from the slightly nasal of the central cornea if both the eyes can fix on the light source (Fig. 69.1). If ocular alignment or ocular displacement disorders are present, corneal light reflex will occur from a location other than the center of the cornea in the affected eye. For instance, in a patient with unilateral exotropia (outward turn of the eye), corneal reflection will occur from the center in the healthy eye, while the light reflex in the other eye with ocular misalignment will be from the nasal cornea (Fig. 69.2). As another example, if an abscess has formed

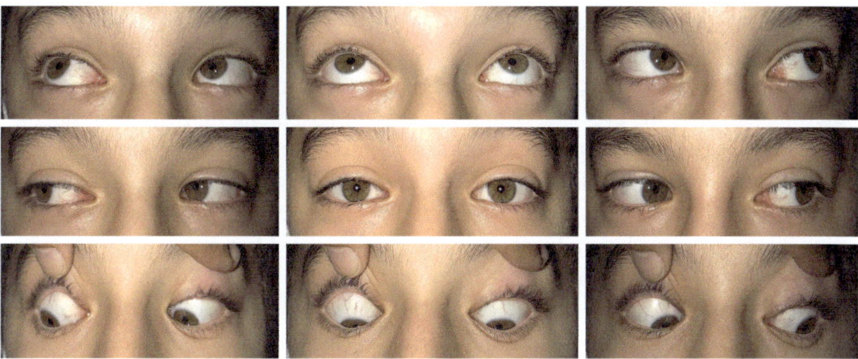

Fig. 69.1 Ocular movements and alignments in nine cardinal positions of gaze in a healthy child, and normal corneal light reflex in primary position (photo in the center of the figure)

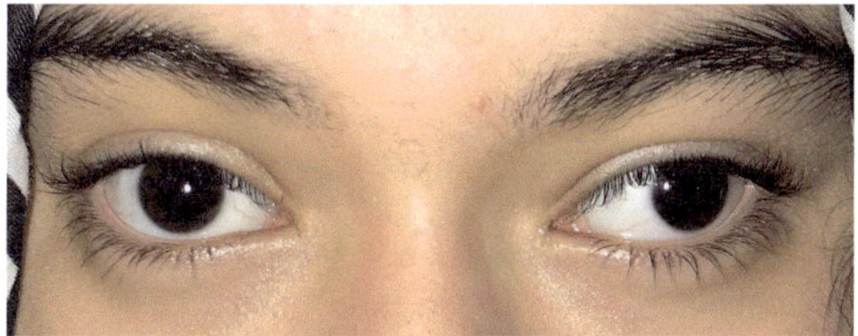

Fig. 69.2 Ocular misalignment in the left eye. Normal corneal light reflex (slightly nasal from the center of the cornea) in the right eye, and light reflection in the nasal cornea due to exotropia (outward deviation) in the left eye

in the superior aspect of the orbit, corneal light reflection will occur from the superior aspect of the center of the cornea due to the inferior displacement of the globe.

After evaluating primary position, eye movement and alignment should be evaluated in eight cardinal gaze positions [23] (Fig. 69.1). If an anomaly is detected in these movements, movement of each eye should be evaluated separately. Ocular motility disorders frequently stem from restrictive conditions or paralytic causes, and they can be distinguished with a forced duction test. The test can be applied under topical or general anesthesia. To evaluate vertical gaze positions, the conjunctivae neighboring the nasal and temporal limbus are held with opposing forceps, and to evaluate horizontal gaze positions, the conjunctivae neighboring the superior and inferior limbus are held. The eye is moved towards the direction of gaze limitation with the forceps [24]. While movement of the eye in the desired direction cannot be completely achieved in conditions that lead to the restriction of extraocular muscles, eye movement can be achieved without any discomfort in conditions associated with paralytic causes. It is important for the patient to try not to move the eye voluntarily in topical treatment. Otherwise, they may experience discomfort trying to move the eye during examination and restrictive pathology could be accidentally diagnosed. The presence of ocular misalignment and a head position coexisting with eye movement disorders should also be evaluated.

69.2.4 Cornea and Conjunctivae

The cornea is a transparent, dome-shaped avascular tissue located at the front of the outermost layer of the eye. The conjunctivae is a transparent, thin vascular mucosal tissue that covers the scleral surface of the eyeball that can be seen from the outside and the inner surface of the eyelids. The conjunctivae and cornea are always kept moist by tears and the effect of the blink reflex [25, 26]. Specialized devices used by ophthalmologists, such as a biomicroscope, are required for detailed evaluation of both structures. In an illuminated environment or with the help of a light source, increased conjunctival vascularization, characteristics of secretion (purulent or serous, mild or heavy discharge), and the presence of distinct chemosis (edema in the subconjunctival area) can be observed externally. Moreover, a disruption in the transparent structure of the cornea indicates corneal pathology.

69.2.5 Pupils

It is possible to conduct a macroscopic evaluation of the appearance and function of the pupils with the aid of a light source. Pupil diameter, shape, response to direct/ indirect light and presence of anisocoria (a difference in pupil diameter of more than 1 mm between the eyes) should be evaluated. If anisocoria is detected, it should also be specified which pupil is smaller or larger than normal [27]. The relative difference between two pupils in terms of response to light is evaluated with the swinging-flashlight test, which can reveal the presence of relative afferent pupil defect [28]. The patient should be asked whether they have used any ocular medication recently before starting a pupil examination. This is because the pupils can be dilated, visual acuity can be affected, and response to light decreased for several days in a patient who has been administered atropine (a drug that causes the pupils to dilate) by an ophthalmologist for a detailed eye exam.

69.2.6 Ophthalmoscopic Examination of the Posterior Segment

The red reflex test can also be performed with a direct ophthalmoscope, which is used to evaluate the optic disc and retinal vasculature in the posterior pole. The location of the optic disc can be determined in a direct ophthalmoscopic examination by following the retinal vasculature (indirect ophthalmoscopy is a special examination method that requires special devices and lenses). A normal optic disc is oval or circular, pink or orange in color, and located at the same level as the retinal surface (there may be a 1/3–1/2 depression in the central part of the optic disc), in addition to having clearly visible margins [29, 30]. Optic disc pallor or blurred margins require attention. It is diagnostically important to distinguish unilaterality or bilaterality for optic disc edema. It is also recommended that the retinal vasculature and the retinal areas in between are evaluated. Increased vessel tortuosity and diameter, the presence of hemorrhagic foci in the retina, or retinal pallor may indicate severe pathologies (Fig. 69.3).

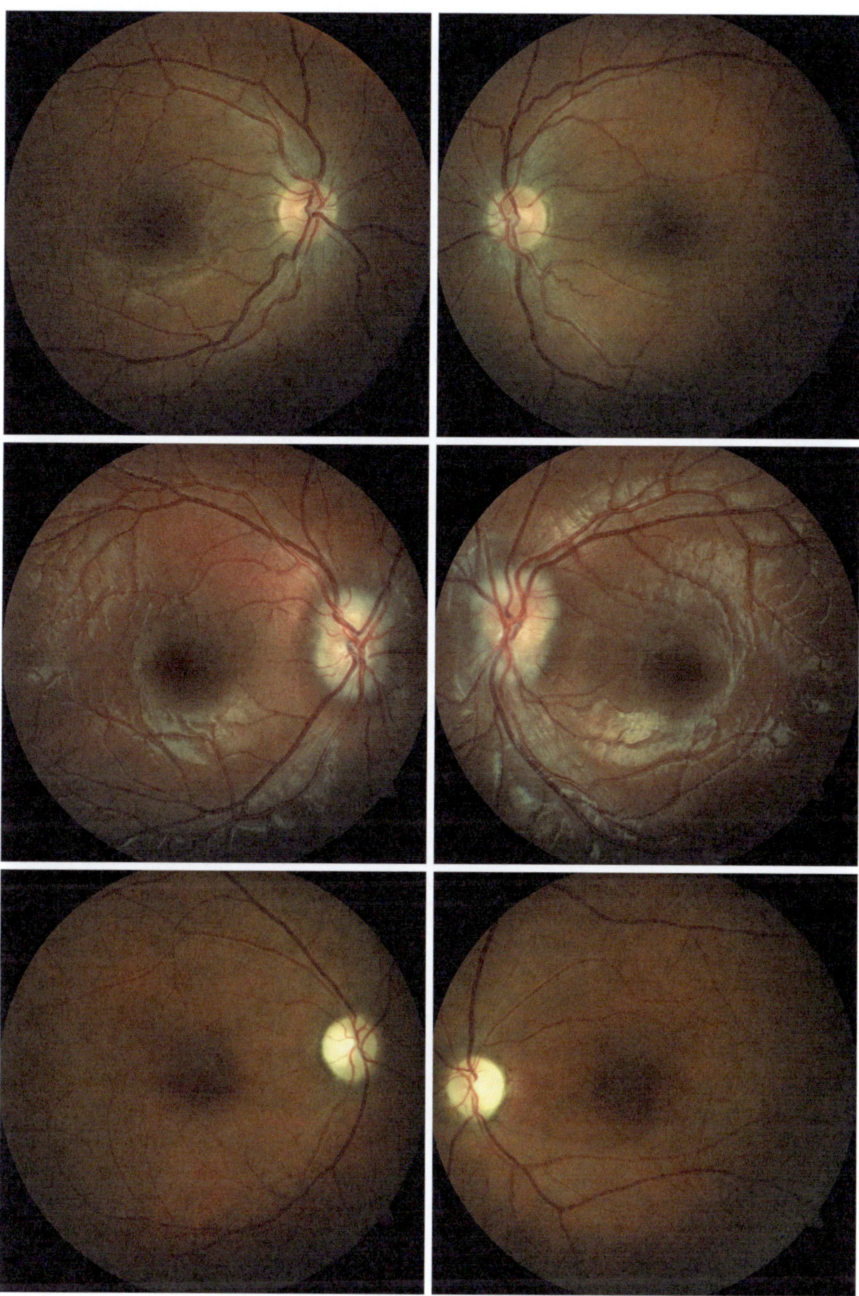

Fig. 69.3 Appearance of the macula and optic disc on color fundus photographs of three patients. Optic disc and macula in a healthy eye (top), papilledema due to increased intracranial pressure (middle), and optic disc pallor in a patient with a history of bilateral optic neuropathy (bottom)

69.2.7 Examination of the Cranial Nerves Associated with Orbital Structures [31, 32]

- *Optic nerve (second CN):* The optic nerve enables the transmission of the image on the retina to the primary visual cortex in the brain. It is also the afferent nerve for light reflex. In the ophthalmoscopic (direct or indirect) examination, it is located nasal to the macula at the same level as the retinal surface, has clear margins, and is orange/pink in color. Ophthalmoscopic examination of the optic disc can provide an idea about optic nerve involvement by also evaluating vision, color vision, and the pupil and its reactions to light. However, further examinations (diagnostic tests such as the visual field test, contrast sensitivity test, peripapillary nerve fiber analysis with optical coherence tomography, and visual evoked potential test, which require specialist knowledge to interpret the results) are necessary if a pathological finding is detected in one or more of these evaluations. Impaired light reflex, visual field defects, and impaired color vision and contrast sensitivity are expected if there is a problem with the optic nerve. In addition, optic disc elevation, blurred optic disc margin, and optic disc pallor indicate various orbital and/or neuro-ophthalmological pathologies (Fig. 69.2).
- *Oculomotor nerve (third CN):* The oculomotor nerve is the efferent of light reaction. It innervates the oblique muscle with the medial, superior, and inferior recti. Moreover, it helps keep the eyelid open by innervating the levator palpebrae superioris muscle, i.e., the main elevator muscle of the upper eyelid. Limited adduction with the upward and downward gaze movement of the globe, ptosis, and mydriasis are observed in cases where the oculomotor nerve is affected. Moreover, as the muscle that provides movement in the opposite direction is dominant in the event of paralysis of the nerve that affects the extraocular muscle (or muscles), the eye will shift towards the direction of the movement of the muscle that has a more dominant impact (Fig. 69.4). For instance, in a patient with medial rectus paralysis secondary to third CN palsy, the eye will deviate laterally if the sixth CN functions.
- *Trochlear nerve (fourth CN):* The trochlear nerve innervates the superior oblique muscle. This nerve is responsible for abduction, depression, and internal rotation in the inferolateral gaze position of the eye. Therefore, vertical, horizontal, and torsional ocular misalignment are observed when this nerve is affected.
- *Trigeminal nerve (fifth CN):* The ophthalmic (V1) and maxillary (V2) branches of the trigeminal nerve in particular, which has three branches, play a role in the sensory innervation of ocular structures. The V1 branch supplies sensory innervation to the lacrimal gland, upper eyelid skin, bulbar and upper eyelid conjunctiva, and the cornea. It is an afferent of the corneal reflex. The V2 branch affects the sensory innervation of the skin and conjunctiva of the lower eyelid. If this nerve is affected, decreased corneal reflex as well as hypoesthesia of the other dermatomes that are supplied with sensory innervation by this nerve are observed, depending on the affected branch.

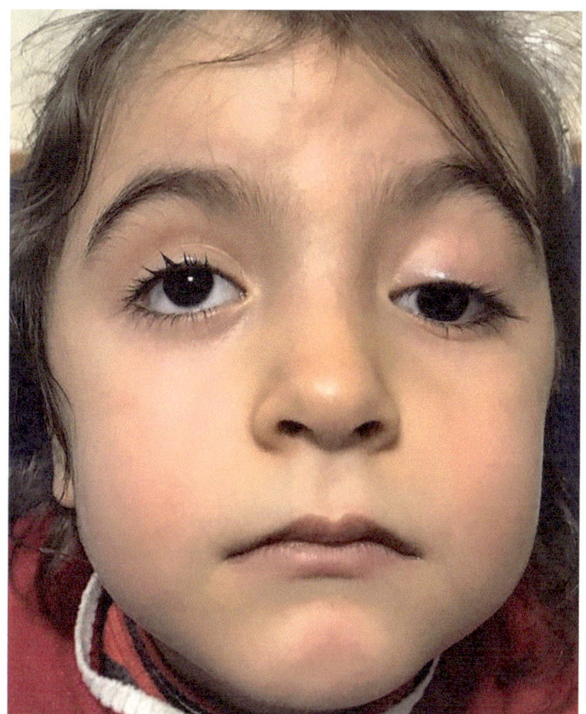

Fig. 69.4 Partial oculomotor nerve (third cranial nerve) palsy in the left eye. Blepharoptosis and upward gaze palsy are present in the affected eye, and the globe is deviated downward as the inferior rectus muscle function is preserved

- *Abducens nerve (sixth CN):* The abducens nerve provides motor innervation of the lateral rectus muscle. It is responsible for the lateral gaze position of the eye in the midline. Gaze limitation is observed in the event of abducens nerve palsy.
- *Facial nerve (seventh CN):* The facial nerve is responsible for the closure of the eyelids by providing motor innervation of the orbicularis oculi muscle. In addition, the fibers that have a role in the parasympathetic innervation of the lacrimal gland are carried by the facial nerve. Facial nerve paralysis is divided into two categories: peripheral and central. Findings detected in ophthalmological examination associated with peripheral facial nerve paralysis, which has various symptoms, lagophthalmos or consist of difficulty closing the eye, droopy eyebrows, and dry eye (Fig. 69.5).

69.3 Ophthalmological Manifestations of Infectious Sinonasal Diseases

69.3.1 Bacterial Paranasal Sinusitis

Although there are no exact figures regarding its prevalence in children, 5–10% of children who have acute upper respiratory tract infection have been shown to develop acute rhinosinusitis [33, 34]. With appropriate medical treatment, acute

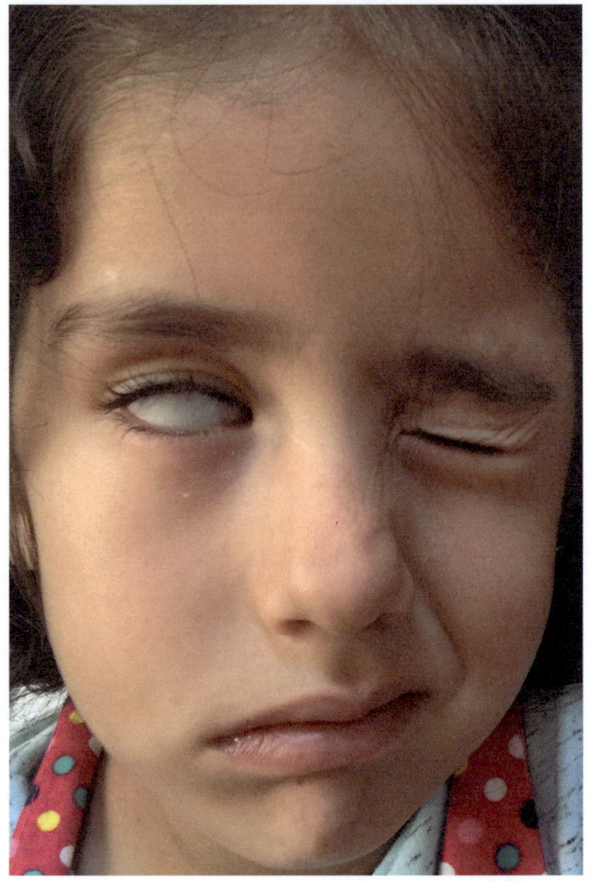

Fig. 69.5 Right peripheral facial nerve (seventh cranial nerve) palsy due to complicated otitis media. Positive Bell's phenomenon is seen in the affected eye

rhinosinusitis is a self-limiting disease. However, it may also lead to serious morbidities such as loss of vision, neurological damage, and even death by causing orbital complications in up to 15% of children and intracranial complications in nearly 3% of children, if left untreated [35, 36]. Complications of acute sinusitis can be divided into two main groups: intracranial and extracranial. Extracranial complications also include orbital and osseous complications. Patients with complicated pediatric rhinosinusitis most frequently present with orbital complications [37].

Attempts have been made to explain the complications associated with acute sinusitis through various pathophysiological mechanisms. The most important cause is the destruction of bony structures by inflammation in the sinuses, which then reaches the adjacent structures. Another cause is a septic thrombophlebitis reaching the neighboring tissues via retrograde flow through the valveless blood vessels. Congenital or acquired defects in bony structures also constitute a risk factor for such spread, although they are rare [38–40]. While the most common cause of complications is ethmoid sinusitis in children under 10 years of age, the same is frontal sinusitis in older children [14, 41]. As the lamina papyracea is a thin bony structure that separates the ethmoid sinus and the orbit, this bony structure may undergo erosion, thereby easily leading to orbital spread in advanced ethmoid sinusitis cases. While ethmoid sinusitis mainly causes orbital complications, frontal sinusitis is associated with intracranial complications [38, 42]. Complications caused by maxillary and sphenoid sinusitis are less frequently encountered in children.

An ophthalmological examination should be conducted carefully, as expecting ocular findings only in orbital involvement could lead to possible intracranial pathologies being overlooked. For instance, in a patient with severe palpebral edema due to orbital inflammation, the diagnosis of cavernous sinus thrombosis can be delayed unless the eyelids are opened to check for corneal reflex or eye movements. In this respect, ENT specialists and pediatricians should know which ophthalmological manifestations to look for and what these manifestations mean from a clinical aspect in patient follow-up. ENT specialists and pediatricians should therefore always be in contact with ophthalmologists and the changes in the clinical presentation of a patient should be evaluated by all physicians specializing in the relevant branches. In brief, pediatric patients with acute sinusitis essentially require a multidisciplinary approach.

69.3.2 Orbital Complications

Although orbital complications secondary to acute rhinosinusitis are more common in pediatric patients compared to adults, the prognosis is better in children [43]. Such complications are more prevalent among boys than girls [37, 44]. Microbiological agents vary depending on age in cases where inflammation has invaded through the orbit, which is also important for determining treatment. While sterile or single aerobic bacteria have been detected as the agent in children under 9 years of age, there are reports of anaerobic microorganisms having been isolated in older children who exhibited orbital complications. Previously, the most commonly isolated pathogen in pediatric orbital complications was the Streptococcus genus. However, with the inclusion of pneumococcal vaccination in clinical practice, pathogens of the Staphylococcus genus have become the most commonly encountered, wherein a significant increase has also been reported in methicillin-resistant S. Aureus infections [45–47]. Moreover, complications associated with fungal sinusitis can also be observed less frequently.

In 1970, Chandler et al. divided orbital complications into five classes [40]:

- Class 1: Preseptal cellulitis
- Class 2: Orbital cellulitis
- Class 3: Subperiosteal abscess
- Class 4: Orbital abscess
- Class 5: Cavernous sinus thrombosis

1. *Preseptal cellulitis*: In Chandler's classification system, a distinction is made in relation to the orbital septum. The orbital septum is a thin, fibrous fascia that originates from the periosteum in the arcus marginalis and extends to the tarsus. It separates the superficial orbital structures (skin and orbicularis oculi muscle) from deep orbital tissues and acts as a barrier between the superficial and deep orbital structures. In Chandler's class 1 complication, i.e., preseptal cellulitis, periorbital edema is limited to the skin and subcutaneous tissues. 15% of acute rhinosinusitis cases present with preseptal cellulitis [35]. While various prevalence rates have been reported, preseptal cellulitis is the most common orbital complication [48–50]. Such patients are expected to have palpebral edema, periocular erythema, and increased temperature and pain. However, findings such as proptosis, conjunctival injection, pain when moving the eye, ophthalmoplegia, and papilledema are not encountered as inflammation does not the reach intraorbital structures. Imaging is required for all patients, unless they are known without doubt to have preseptal cellulitis [38].

2. *Orbital cellulitis*: Orbital cellulitis can also be referred to as postseptal cellulitis. Inflammation and infection secondary to sinusitis have now reached the posterior structures of the orbital septum and started to affect the orbital structures. From this stage onward, ophthalmologists should also be involved in patient follow-up. Visual acuity, optic nerve functions, and intraocular pressure should be closely monitored. While nearly 50% of patients with preseptal cellulitis have fever, the same rate has been reported as 94% in patients with a postseptal infection [51]. In addition, from this stage, it is possible to observe ophthalmoplegia, proptosis, chemosis, conjunctival injection, diplopia, loss of vision, and optic nerve involvement (can be transient or permanent) at varying severities as a result of orbital inflammation [52]. In a study by Patt et al., it was reported that retinal arterial occlusion due to increased intraorbital pressure, ischemia caused by thrombophlebitis in the orbital veins, and optic neuropathy resulting from infectious inflammation in proximity to the optic nerve can lead to loss of vision [53]. Progression to blindness was reported in nearly 3% of the patients with orbital infection due to sinusitis [54]. There is controversy over the necessity of imaging in patients with orbital cellulitis. Some clinicians prefer to use imaging modalities (contrast-enhanced computed tomography) if there is no treatment response after initiating 24–48 h of intravenous (IV) antibiotic therapy in patients with a mild version of the disease who do not exhibit decreased visual acuity [38].

3. *Subperiosteal abscess*: This refers to an abscess developing between the bone wall and periosteum of the orbital bone structure [40]. A subperiosteal abscess is among the most frequently observed intraorbital complication of acute bacterial rhinosinusitis [55]. At this stage, it is possible to observe eyeball displacement that leads to diplopia (children can express this condition from the verbal period onward) and/or compensatory head posture (in order to eliminate diplopia resulting from ocular misalignment) at varying degrees depending on abscess localization, in addition to the signs of orbital cellulitis [37, 39]. A definitive diagnosis should be made with the use of imaging if there is any clinical suspicion. A cor-

relation between the orbital localization of inflammation and abscess formations to the optic nerve, severity of the compression effect caused by increased intra-orbital pressure on the optic nerve, and the involvement of optic nerve functions can be observed. For example, a small subperiosteal abscess localized in the anteromedial aspect of the orbit and a large orbital abscess in proximity to the optic nerve secondary to ethmoid sinusitis can have different effects on optic nerve functions.

4. *Orbital abscess*: This is an intraconal and/or extraconal abscess formation observed in the orbit. There may be a single or multiple abscess formation. In the previous three stages, the signs are more severe and there is marked proptosis. It is possible to observe reduced vision, impaired color vision, decreased pupil response to light (presence of a relative afferent pupil defect), and optic disc edema as a result of an affected optic nerve directly by an infection or indirectly by increased intraorbital pressure [39]. According to the data published in 2010 and thereafter, i.e., the period since pneumococcal vaccination was included in clinical practice, the rate of orbital abscess has dropped significantly [56].

5. *Cavernous sinus thrombosis*: Although class 5 is referred to as an intraorbital complication according to Chandler's classification, some authors include it in the intracranial complications category as it represents an intracranial pathology [49, 55–58]. Cavernous sinus thrombosis resulting from a septic thrombophlebitis reaching the cavernous sinus through the valveless superior ophthalmic vein leads to a high mortality (up to 30%) [59, 60]. Moreover, it may also cause various ophthalmological morbidities secondary to affected CNs neighboring the cavernous sinus. In addition to the signs of orbital inflammation/infection, it can also manifest with decreased corneal reflex, pain, hypoesthesia in dermatomes that are supplied with sensory innervation by V1 and V2, ptosis, or ophthalmoplegia secondary to third, fourth, or sixth CN involvement [38, 39].

Treatment: In preseptal cellulitis, patients who have a mild condition can be followed as outpatients with oral antibiotic therapy, depending on the clinical presentation of the patient [61]. While some authors refer to the change in visual acuity when determining treatment in cases where inflammation and infection have spread to the orbit, we are of the opinion that evaluating optic nerve functions as a whole is generally more accurate. Therefore, other examination methods that evaluate the functions and structure of the optic nerve, such as color vision, pupil light reflex, and optic disc examination, should also be considered in addition to those examining visual acuity. Follow-up of visual acuity and reactions to light should be performed every 6 h for the first 48 h (can be more frequent depending on the clinical presentation) [62]. In addition, monitoring intraocular pressure is also recommended. Treatment strategies for subperiosteal abscess vary according to the age. It has been reported that 93% of children under 9 years of age who have a subperiosteal abscess can be successfully treated with IV antibiotic therapy. In children aged from 9 to 14 with a subperiosteal abscess, surgical treatment is warranted if any of the following conditions is present: frontal sinusitis, a large ($\geq$1 cm) subperiosteal abscess with a non-medial orbital localization, suspected anaerobic infection (presence of gas in the subperiosteal abscess on the CT, etc.), reaccumulation of the subperiosteal abscess after drainage, and optic neuropathy [62, 63]. Moreover, if there is optic nerve involvement (optic neuropathy) despite IV antibiotic therapy, surgical drainage of the subperiosteal abscess is recommended in cases where fever does not go down within 36 h, the clinical picture worsens within 48 h, or if there is no clinical improvement within 72 h [62]. Although rare, it has been shown that papilledema (perioptic neuritis) secondary to inflammation can be detected without suppurative complications in acute infections of the sinuses that are in close proximity to the optic nerve and that these patients can be successfully treated with IV antibiotic therapy without requiring surgery [64]. Surgical drainage should be performed in combination with IV antibiotic therapy in children older than 14 years of age with a subperiosteal abscess. Surgical drainage is recommended in combination with IV antibiotic therapy for an orbital abscess, in the presence of optic neuropathy, or when there are signs of increased intraorbital pressure [37, 62, 63]. In septic cavernous sinus thrombus, anticoagulant therapy can be considered in addition to IV antibiotics in order to prevent the spread of thrombus and ensure recanalization [38].

69.3.3 Intracranial Complications

It has been reported that intracranial complications can be observed in up to 17% of patients with acute bacterial sinusitis and that these complications have a mortality rate of 10–20% [65]. While intracranial complications frequently stem from the frontal sinus, they can also be encountered in other sinus infections. Intracranial complications include meningitis, epidural abscess and empyema, subdural abscess and empyema (most often), intraparenchymal brain abscess, encephalitis, and septic venous sinus thrombosis [36, 38, 39, 42, 66]. The diagnostic process is important for these patients, as such complications can lead to severe neurological sequelae or death. Intracranial complications can manifest alone as well as with various orbital complications [67]. Early manifestations of intracranial complications may include only headache and fever, which can be overshadowed by orbital complications and missed [39]. However, severe headache, lethargy, signs of meningeal irritation and increased intracranial pressure, neurological deficits, seizures, and even respiratory depression may occur when these complications progress. Bilateral papilledema is detected as a result of increased intracranial pressure. Therefore, these patients require regular optic nerve examinations. In addition, various ophthalmological signs (ocular misalignment, gaze palsy, ptosis, mydriasis, decreased corneal reflex) can be observed as a result of loss of the function in the CN that has been affected by increased intracranial pressure [68]. However, it should also be kept in mind that the ocular symptoms and signs can mask the symptoms of an intracranial complication in patients who both have postseptal orbital complications (Chandler's classes 2–4) and intracranial complications. At this stage, a diligent examination by the clinician is important. The findings of a thorough ophthalmological examination should be evaluated as a whole.

69.4 Other Ophthalmological Signs/Complications Secondary to Acute Bacterial Rhinosinusitis

- Papilledema and permanent loss of vision due to optic chiasm empyema [69].
- Development of third CN palsy and epidural hematoma secondary to acute sphenoid sinusitis [70].
- Lacrimal gland abscess [71, 72].
- Optic neuropathy and vision loss secondary to sphenoid sinusitis are among the most well-known potential ophthalmological complications. The possible pathophysiological causes for the development of optic neuropathy include direct spread of the infection to the optic nerve, occlusive vasculitis, and bone wall defects around the sinus [73].

69.4.1 Other Infectious Sinonasal Diseases

- Both invasive and noninvasive fungal sinusitis can lead to various ocular complications. Invasive fungal sinusitis is an opportunistic infection that has been increasing in prevalence in recent years [74]. As the name suggests, it invades through the orbit, thereby leading to various possible orbital complications [75]. It has even been shown to manifest with dacryocystitis [76]. It has been reported that up to 34% of allergic fungal sinusitis cases (a type of noninvasive fungal sinusitis) experience ophthalmological complications. Similar to bacterial sinusitis, various ophthalmological signs and symptoms are encountered as a result of inflammation and infection reaching the orbital structures. While the most common ocular sign is proptosis, it may also lead to loss of vision if left untreated [77].
- Nasal furunculosis and nasal vestibular infections has been shown to cause preseptal cellulitis, orbital abscess, ophthalmic vein thrombosis, and septic cavernous sinus thrombosis in rare cases [78–81].

69.5 Ophthalmological Manifestations of Infectious Diseases of the Ear and Related Structures

Direct orbital complications can be observed in infections of the sinonasal structures due to the spread of inflammation and infection to orbital structures. However, direct orbital complications are generally not expected in infectious diseases of the ear and its related structures due to the distance between the anatomic locations of the ear and orbit. Instead, we usually encounter indirect ophthalmological clinical findings resulting from extracranial or intracranial complications. The most common ophthalmological manifestation is facial paralysis, which results in ocular morbidities.

69.5.1 Otitis Media and Facial Paralysis

Complications of otitis media are most frequently observed in pediatric patients between 0–3 years of age, wherein the rate of facial paralysis has been reported to be 16.7% [82–84]. One of the most common infectious causes of facial paralysis in the pediatric population is acute otitis media [82, 85]. Primarily, pediatric acute otitis media as well as acute mastoiditis with osteitis, chronic suppurative otitis media, and cholesteatoma can be complicated by peripheral facial paralysis. Facial paralysis secondary to chronic otitis media is frequently caused by the direct pressure of a cholesteatoma on the facial nerve [86].

In peripheral facial paralysis, the patient will not be able to close their eyes completely as the orbicularis oculi muscle function will be impaired in the affected half of the face (Fig. 69.5). Tears always keep the corneal surface wet (cornea and conjunctiva) with closure of the eyelids/spontaneous blink reflex. However, dryness of the corneal surface is observed as these patients cannot completely close their eyes (paralytic lagophthalmos). This condition is significant as it leads to corneal exposure keratopathy/exposure keratitis, which may progress to injury in the corneal epithelium, development of keratitis, corneal vascularization, or corneal ulceration, thereby leading to loss of vision [87]. When monitoring patients in terms of exposure keratopathy, the presence of Bell's phenomenon (palpebral oculogyric reflex) and corneal sensation should also be evaluated.

Bell's phenomenon is the upward and outward movement of the globe when closing the eyelids (except for the brief blink reflex), and is described as a reflex that protects the globe and cornea. In the absence of this reflex, which exists in nearly 75% of the normal population, coexisting with lagophthalmos, the risk of exposure keratopathy is significantly increased [88, 89] (Fig. 69.5).

Slit lamp biomicroscopy is required to diagnose exposure keratopathy. In this exam, the effect on the ocular surface is evaluated with fluorescein stain and without using any dyes. In the early phase, punctate corneal dye uptake is observed, particularly in the inferior aspect of the cornea with fluorescein stain. In advanced cases, it is also possible to observe conjunctival injection, chemosis, corneal vascularization, keratitis, corneal ulceration, and even corneal perforation [90]. While pediatric patients in the verbal period can express their ocular discomfort (burning, stinging, foreign body sensation, blurred vision, etc.), it is important to monitor ocular symptoms in younger children. In general, children present with symptoms such as sensitivity to light (photophobia), watery eyes, and a desire to put their hands over their eyes or to keep their eyes closed. Complaints and symptoms may be more apparent in the morning, particularly in patients with nocturnal lagophthalmos. Moreover, corneal sensitivity should also be evaluated in patients with exposure keratopathy. This is because complaints such as burning and stinging may not be present in patients with decreased corneal sensitivity.

These patients are recommended preservative-free artificial tears and lubricant gels in medical treatment [90]. Moreover, punctal plugs that reduce tear drainage and eyepatches that cover the eyes have also been reported to be beneficial. In mild cases, treatment with artificial tears (lubricant drops and gels) can also keep the corneal surface wet. Scleral bandage contact lenses can also be recommended after considering the difficulties of getting children to use the lenses and the risk of infection [91]. Surgical treatment options that can be considered in advanced cases include ocular interventions, such as temporary or permanent tarsorrhaphy and gold weight implantation in the eyelid [92, 93]. Amniotic membrane transplantation can be considered for ocular surface reconstruction [94]. Temporary or reversible treatment options (such as temporary tarsorrhaphy) should be considered primarily in patients with peripheral facial paralysis that will possibly resolve spontaneously. In pediatric facial paralysis, ectropion is rare, as lower eyelid tightness is generally preserved. However, ectropion can be observed in severe and long-term cases due to increased eyelid laxity.

69.5.2 Infectious Causes of Pediatric Facial Paralysis Other than Otitis Media

Herpes simplex virus infection, which is among the common causes of Bell's palsy in adults, is also included among the causes of Bell's palsy in children [95, 96]. On the other hand, reactivation of varicella zoster virus can also lead to the development of facial paralysis without causing the classical skin rash and other otological findings (different from Ramsay Hunt syndrome) [97].

Herpes zoster oticus, also knowns as Ramsay Hunt syndrome type 2, occurs as a result of the reactivation of latent varicella zoster virus in the geniculate ganglion. It can manifest with acute facial paralysis coexisting with a small vesicular rash in the external auditory canal and auricle, decreased hearing and dizziness in case of eighth CN involvement, diplopia with the involvement of the abducens nerve, and limited outward gaze [98]. An ophthalmological examination for the presence of ocular herpetic lesions is beneficial in these patients [99].

Lyme disease is an infectious tick-transmitted disease caused by the spirochete Borrelia Burgdorferi. It is the most common infectious cause of facial paralysis in endemic countries [100, 101]. The disease can affect various organs and systems, and lead to facial paralysis in addition to exhibiting ocular involvement (uveitis, keratitis, scleritis/episcleritis, retinal vein occlusion, lack of accommodation, and optic neuritis) [102, 103].

In addition, human immunodeficiency virus, Epstein-Barr virus, adenovirus, rubella, mumps, cytomegalovirus and coxsackievirus have rarely been reported to cause facial paralysis [104].

69.5.3 Other Ophthalmological Manifestations Associated with Otitis Media

Otitis media may also lead to various *intracranial complications*, such as brain abscesses, subdural empyema, cavernous sinus thrombosis, meningitis, lateral sinus thrombosis, and otitic hydrocephalus. In intracranial complications, papilledema, affected CN, including abducens nerve palsy in particular, visual field defects, and diplopia can be detected due to increased cerebrospinal fluid pressure [105, 106].

Gradenigo syndrome is one of the suppurative complications of otitis media. It occurs secondary to petrous bone inflammation. The classic triad of symptoms is as follows; otitis media, ipsilateral abducens palsy, and facial retro-orbital pain (pain in the dermatomes that receive sensory supply from the first and/or second division of the trigeminal nerve) [107]. It has been shown to rarely cause proptosis, cranial sinus thrombosis, papilledema, and Horner's syndrome [106, 108].

The presentation in which acute otitis media coexists with purulent conjunctivitis is described as *conjunctivitis-otitis syndrome*. The most commonly isolated pathogen is H. influenzae, which has been detected as the causative agent in 61–89% of cases [109, 110].

69.6 Ophthalmological Manifestations of Oral Cavity, Pharynx, Upper Airway, and Neck Infections

Pathogens that lead to an infection in these ENT areas also cause ocular infections. In other words, ocular signs constitute a part of the disease spectrum and should not be considered as complications. In addition, as these infectious diseases also cause lymphadenopathy in the head-neck region, as well as various ocular manifestations (frequently conjunctivitis), they should also be considered in the differential diagnosis of patients with a neck mass.

69.6.1 Pharyngoconjunctival Fever

Forty to sixty percent of all pharyngitis cases are of viral origin and lymphadenopathy is a common sign of adenoviral pharyngitis that results from adenovirus. There is also coexisting conjunctivitis in 25–50% of cases, which is referred to as pharyngoconjunctival fever. Preauricular lymphadenopathy is also a common sign in other viral conjunctivitis cases [111].

69.6.2 Parinaud's Oculoglandular Syndrome

This disease is characterized by a unilateral granulomatous follicular conjunctivitis along with ipsilateral regional (frequently preauricular) lymphadenopathy. Parinaud's oculoglandular syndrome, which is one of the common causes of preauricular lymphadenopathy accompanying conjunctivitis, can be seen as a result of various infectious diseases (primarily cat-scratch disease). Commonly observed etiological pathogens include: Bartonella henselae (cat-scratch disease), Francisella tularensis (tularemia), Epstein-Barr virus (infectious mononucleosis), Mycobacterium tuberculosis (tuberculosis), and Treponema pallidum (syphilis) [112, 113].

69.6.3 Other Viral Diseases that Manifest with Conjunctivitis and Lymphadenopathy

Measles causes diffuse maculopapular skin rash, oral vesicles (Koplik's spots), fever, cough, non-purulent conjunctivitis, and cervical lymphadenopathy [114].

Coxsackievirus A and B, echovirus and enterovirus lead to fever, upper airway infection, herpangina, stomatitis, cervical lymphadenopathy, and conjunctivitis [115, 116].

69.6.4 Leptospirosis

Leptospirosis transmitted from infected animals causes various symptoms, such as diffuse muscle and joint pain, fever, headache, generalized lymphadenopathy, and conjunctival suffusion [117].

69.6.5 Chlamydia Trachomatis Infection

This infectious disease can be transmitted from the mother during birth or acquired later years. In children of untreated mothers, the prevalence of inclusion conjunctivitis is 25–50% and the prevalence of pneumonia is 5–30%, along with possible nasopharyngitis and generalized lymphadenopathy [118].

References

1. Committee on Practice and Ambulatory Medicine Section on Ophthalmology, et al. Eye examination in infants, children, and young adults by pediatricians: organizational principles to guide and define the child health care system and/or improve the health of all children. Ophthalmology. 2003;110(4):860–5.
2. Simons K. Preschool vision screening: rationale, methodology and outcome. Surv Ophthalmol. 1996;41(1):3–30.
3. Wasserman RC, Croft CA, Brotherton SE. Preschool vision screening in pediatric practice: a study from the pediatric research in office settings (PROS) network. Am Acad Pediatr. 1992;89(5 Pt 1):834–8.
4. Kazlas M. Pediatric ophthalmology. In: Bluestone CD, Simons JP, Healy GB, editors. Bluestone and Stool's pediatric otolaryngology. 5th ed. Shelton: People's Medical Publishing House; 2014.
5. Jubbal KT, Kania K, Braun TL, Katowitz WR, Marx DP. Pediatric Blepharoptosis. Semin Plast Surg. 2017;31(1):58–64.
6. Berry-Brincat A, Willshaw H. Paediatric blepharoptosis: a 10-year review. Eye (Lond). 2009;23(7):1554–9.
7. Pavone P, Cho SY, Praticò AD, Falsaperla R, Ruggieri M, Jin DK. Ptosis in childhood: a clinical sign of several disorders: case series reports and literature review. Medicine (Baltimore). 2018;97(36):e12124.
8. Rasiah S, Hardy TG, Elder JE, Ng CY, McNab A. Etiology of pediatric acquired blepharoptosis. J AAPOS. 2017;21(6):485–7.

9. Utheim T, Hodges RR, Dartt DA. The eyelid. In: McManus LM, Mitchell RN, editors. Pathobiology of human disease. San Diego: Academic Press; 2014.

10. Wilbanks ND, Filutowski OR, Maldonado MD, Karcioglu ZA. Isolated left upper eyelid ptosis with pansinusitis and contralateral otitis media in a 9-year-old boy. Am J Ophthalmol Case Rep. 2018;11:6–9.

11. Park DY, Baek BJ. Superior branch palsy of the oculomotor nerve caused by frontal sinusitis. J Craniofac Surg. 2016;27(3):e248–9.

12. Ha RY, Nojima K, Adams WPJ, Brown SA. Analysis of facial skin thickness: defining the relative thickness index. Plast Reconstr Surg. 2005;115(6):1769–73.

13. Hsu HC, Lin HF. Eyelid tumors in children: a clinicopathologic study of a 10-year review in southern Taiwan. Ophthalmologica. 2004;218(4):274–7.

14. Suh JD, Shapiro NL. Orbital swellings. In: Bluestone CD, Simons JP, Healy GB, editors. Bluestone and Stool's pediatric otolaryngology. 5th ed. Shelton: People's Medical Publishing House; 2014.

15. Walcott B. The lacrimal gland and its veil of tears. News Physiol Sci. 1998;13:97–103.

16. Holly FJ, Lamberts DW, Buesseler JA. The human lacrimal apparatus: anatomy, physiology, pathology, and surgical aspects. Plast Reconstr Surg. 1984;74(3):438–45.

17. Tatlisumak E, Aslan A, Cömert A, Ozlugedik S, Acar HI, Tekdemir I. Surgical anatomy of the nasolacrimal duct on the lateral nasal wall as revealed by serial dissections. Anat Sci Int. 2010;85(1):8–12.

18. Sathiamoorthi S, Frank RD, Mohney BG. Incidence and clinical characteristics of congenital nasolacrimal duct obstruction. Br J Ophthalmol. 2019;103(4):527–9.

19. Petris C, Liu D. Probing for congenital nasolacrimal duct obstruction. Cochrane Database Syst Rev. 2017;7(7):CD011109.

20. Harris GJ, DiClementi D. Congenital dacryocystocele. Arch Ophthalmol. 1982;100(11):1763–5.

21. Krimsky E. Fixational corneal light reflexes as an aid in binocular investigation. Arch Ophthalmol. 1943;30(4):505–20.

22. Thompson JT, Guyton DL. Ophthalmic prisms. Measurement errors and how to minimize them. Ophthalmology. 1983;90(3):204–10.

23. Wright KW. Anatomy and physiology of eye movements. In: Wright KW, Spiegel PH, editors. Pediatric ophthalmology and strabismus. New York: Springer; 2003.

24. Mazow ML. The four-step test for diagnosis of paralytic and/or restrictive strabismus. Ophthalmology. 1979;86(8):1397–400.

25. Gipson IK. Goblet cells of the conjunctiva: a review of recent findings. Prog Retin Eye Res. 2016;54:49–63.

26. DelMonte DW, Kim T. Anatomy and physiology of the cornea. J Cataract Refract Surg. 2011;37(3):588–98.

27. Gross JR, McClelland CM, Lee MS. An approach to anisocoria. Curr Opin Ophthalmol. 2016;27(6):486–92.

28. Wilhelm H. Disorders of the pupil. In: Kennard C, Leigh RJ, editors. Handbook of clinical neurology, vol. 102. Amsterdam: Elsevier; 2011.

29. Pensyl CD, Benjamin WJ. Ocular motility. In: Benjamin WJ, Borish IM, editors. Borish's clinical refraction. 2nd ed. Saint Louis: Butterworth-Heinemann; 2006.

30. Gloster J. The colour of the optic disc. Doc Ophthalmol. 1969;26(1):155–63.

31. Salmon JF. Neuro-ophthalmology. In: Kanski's clinical ophthalmology: a systematic approach. 9th ed. Amsterdam: Elsevier; 2019.

32. May M, Fria TJ, Blumenthal F, Curtin H. Facial paralysis in children: differential diagnosis. Otolaryngol Head Neck Surg. 1981;89(5):841–8.

33. American Academy of Pediatrics Subcommittee on Management of Sinusitis and Committee on Quality Improvement. Clinical practice guideline: management of sinusitis. Pediatrics. 2001;108(3):798–808.

34. Isaacson G. Sinusitis in childhood. Pediatr Clin North Am. 1996;43(6):1297–318.

35. Ambati BK, Ambati J, Azar N, Stratton L, Schmidt EV. Periorbital and orbital cellulitis before and after the advent of Haemophilus influenzae type B vaccination. Ophthalmology. 2000;107(8):1450–3.
36. Lerner DN, Choi SS, Zalzal GH, Johnson DL. Intracranial complications of sinusitis in childhood. Ann Otol Rhinol Laryngol. 1995;104(4 Pt 1):288–93.
37. Oxford LE, McClay J. Complications of acute sinusitis in children. Otolaryngol Head Neck Surg. 2005;133(1):32–7.
38. Marquez L, Sitton M, Dang J, Tran BH, Larrier DR. Complications of sinusitis. In: Valdez TA, Vallejo JG, editors. Infectious diseases in pediatric otolaryngology. New York: Springer; 2016.
39. Edmondson NE, Parikh SR. Complications of rhinosinusitis. In: Bluestone CD, Simons JP, Healy GB, editors. Bluestone and Stool's Pediatric Otolaryngology. 5th ed. Shelton: People's Medical Publishing House; 2014.
40. Chandler JR, Langenbrunner DJ, Stevens ER. The pathogenesis of orbital complications in acute sinusitis. Laryngoscope. 1970;80(9):1414–28.
41. Reid JR. Complications of pediatric paranasal sinusitis. Pediatr Radiol. 2004;34(12):933–42.
42. Hakim HE, Malik AC, Aronyk K, Ledi E, Bhargava R. The prevalence of intracranial complications in pediatric frontal sinusitis. Int J Pediatr Otorhinolaryngol. 2006;70(8):1383–7.
43. Nageswaran S, Woods CR, Benjamin DK Jr, Givner LB, Shetty AK. Orbital cellulitis in children. Pediatr Infect Dis J. 2006;25(8):695–9.
44. Mekhitarian Neto L, Pignatari S, Mitsuda S, Fava AS, Stamm A. Acute sinusitis in children: a retrospective study of orbital complications. Braz J Otorhinolaryngol. 2007;73(1):75–9.
45. Seltz LB, Smith J, Durairaj VD, Enzenauer R, Todd J. Microbiology and antibiotic management of orbital cellulitis. Pediatrics. 2011;127(3):e566–72.
46. McKinley SH, Yen MT, Miller AM, Yen KG. Microbiology of pediatric orbital cellulitis. Am J Ophthalmol. 2007;144(4):497–501.
47. Pena MT, Preciado D, Orestes M, Choi S. Orbital complications of acute sinusitis: changes in the post–pneumococcal vaccine era. JAMA Otolaryngol Head Neck Surg. 2013;139(3):223–7.
48. Radovani P, Vasili D, Xhelili M, Dervishi J. Orbital complications of sinusitis. Balkan Med J. 2013;30(2):151–4.
49. Siedek V, Kremer A, Betz CS, Tschiesner U, Berghaus A, Leunig A. Management of orbital complications due to rhinosinusitis. Eur Arch Otorhinolaryngol. 2010;267(12):1881–6.
50. Trivić A, Cevik M, Folić M, et al. Management of orbital complications of acute rhinosinusitis in pediatric patients: a 15-year single-center experience. Pediatr Infect Dis J. 2019;38(10):994–8.
51. Botting AM, McIntosh D, Mahadevan M. Paediatric pre- and post-septal peri-orbital infections are different diseases. A retrospective review of 262 cases. Int J Pediatr Otorhinolaryngol. 2008;72(3):377–83.
52. Hamed-Azzam S, AlHashash I, Briscoe D, Rose GE, Verity DH. Common orbital infections ~ state of the art ~ part I. J Ophthalmic Vis Res. 2018;13(2):175–82.
53. Patt BS, Manning SC. Blindness resulting from orbital complications of sinusitis. Otolaryngol Head Neck Surg. 1991;104(6):789–95.
54. Fisher RG, Boyce TG, Moffet HL. Eye, ear, and sinus syndromes. In: Moffet's pediatric infectious diseases: a problem-oriented approach. 4th ed. Lippincott: Williams & Wilkins; 2005.
55. Zeifer B. Pediatric sinonasal imaging: normal anatomy and inflammatory disease. Neuroimaging Clin N Am. 2000;10(1):137–59.
56. Zhao EE, Koochakzadeh S, Nguyen SA, Yoo F, Pecha P, Schlosser RJ. Orbital complications of acute bacterial rhinosinusitis in the pediatric population: a systematic review and meta-analysis. Int J Pediatr Otorhinolaryngol. 2020;135:110078.
57. Herrmann BW, Forsen JW Jr. Simultaneous intracranial and orbital complications of acute rhinosinusitis in children. Int J Pediatr Otorhinolaryngol. 2004;68(5):619–25.
58. Mortimore S, Wormald PJ. The Groote Schuur hospital classification of the orbital complications of sinusitis. J Laryngol Otol. 1997;111(8):719–23.

59. Southwick FS, Richardson EP Jr, Swartz MN. Septic thrombosis of the dural venous sinuses. Medicine (Baltimore). 1986;65(2):82–106.
60. Cannon ML, Antonio BL, McCloskey JJ, Hines MH, Tobin JR, Shetty AK. Cavernous sinus thrombosis complicating sinusitis. Pediatr Crit Care Med. 2004;5(1):86–8.
61. Wald ER, Applegate KE, Bordley C, Darrow DH, Glode MP, Marcy SM, Nelson CE, Rosenfeld RM, Shaikh N, Smith MJ, Williams PV, Weinberg ST. Clinical practice guideline for the diagnosis and management of acute bacterial sinusitis in children aged 1 to 18 years. Pediatrics. 2013;132(1):e262–80.
62. Garcia GH, Harris GJ. Criteria for nonsurgical management of subperiosteal abscess of the orbit: analysis of outcomes 1988-1998. Ophthalmology. 2000;107(8):1454–6.
63. Souliere CR Jr, Antoine GA, Martin MP, Blumberg AI, Isaacson G. Selective non-surgical management of subperiosteal abscess of the orbit: computerized tomography and clinical course as indication for surgical drainage. Int J Pediatr Otorhinolaryngol. 1990;19(2):109–19.
64. Kumar RK, Ghali M, Dragojevic F, Young F. Papilloedema secondary to acute purulent sinusitis. J Paediatr Child Health. 1999;35(4):396–8.
65. Nathoo N, Nadvi SS, van Dellen JR, Gouws E. Intracranial subdural empyemas in the era of computed tomography: a review of 699 cases. Neurosurgery. 1999;44(3):529–35.
66. Giannoni CM, Stewart MG, Alford EL. Intracranial complications of sinusitis. Laryngoscope. 1997;107(7):863–7.
67. Kuczkowski J, Narozny W, Mikaszewski B, Stankiewicz C. Suppurative complications of frontal sinusitis in children. Clin Pediatr (Phila). 2005;44(8):675–82.
68. Germiller JA, Monin DL, Sparano AM, Tom LW. Intracranial complications of sinusitis in children and adolescents and their outcomes. Arch Otolaryngol Head Neck Surg. 2006;132(9):969–76.
69. Jüngert JM, Uberall M, Mayer UM, Guggenbichler JP, Heininger U. Papilledema and acute bilateral amaurosis accompanying acute sinusitis. Klin Padiatr. 2001;213(6):343–6.
70. Cho KS, Cho WH, Kim HJ, Roh HJ. Epidural hematoma accompanied by oculomotor nerve palsy due to sphenoid sinusitis. Am J Otolaryngol. 2011;32(4):355–7.
71. Parvizi N, Choudhury N, Singh A. Complicated periorbital cellulitis: case report and literature review. J Laryngol Otol. 2012;126(1):94–6.
72. Patel N, Khalil HM, Amirfeyz R, Kaddour HS. Lacrimal gland abscess complicating acute sinusitis. Int J Pediatr Otorhinolaryngol. 2003;67(8):917–9.
73. Moorman CM, Anslow P, Elston JS. Is sphenoid sinus opacity significant in patients with optic neuritis? Eye (Lond). 1999;13(Pt 1):76–82.
74. Lansford BK, Bower CM, Seibert RW. Invasive fungal sinusitis in the immunocompromised pediatric patient. Ear Nose Throat J. 1995;74(8):566–73.
75. Kalin-Hajdu E, Hirabayashi KE, Vagefi MR, Kersten RC. Invasive fungal sinusitis: treatment of the orbit. Curr Opin Ophthalmol. 2017;28(5):522–33.
76. Davies BW, Gonzalez MO, Vaughn RC, Allen GC, Durairaj VD. Dacryocystitis as the initial presentation of invasive fungal sinusitis in immunocompromised children. Ophthal Plast Reconstr Surg. 2016;32(4):e79–81.
77. Alaraj AM, Al-Faky YH, Alsuhaibani AH. Ophthalmic manifestations of allergic fungal sinusitis. Ophthal Plast Reconstr Surg. 2018;34(5):463–6.
78. Cho CY, Kim KS, Kim KB. A case of cavernous sinus thrombosis due to a mistreated facial furuncle. J Korean Pediatr Soc. 1999;42(4):584–8.
79. Mahasin Z, Saleem M, Quick CA. Multiple bilateral orbital abscesses secondary to nasal furunculosis. Int J Pediatr Otorhinolaryngol. 2001;58(2):167–71.
80. Rohana A, Rosli M, Nik Rizal N, Shatriah I, Wan HW. Bilateral ophthalmic vein thrombosis secondary to nasal furunculosis. Orbit. 2008;27(3):215–7.
81. Varshney S, Malhotra M, Gupta P, Gairola P, Kaur N. Cavernous sinus thrombosis of nasal origin in children. Indian J Otolaryngol Head Neck Surg. 2015;67(1):100–5.
82. Bluestone CD, Chi DH, Klein JO. Complications and sequelae of otitis media. In: Bluestone CD, Simons JP, Healy GB, editors. Bluestone and Stool's pediatric otolaryngology. 5th ed. Shelton: People's Medical Publishing House; 2014.

83. Mattos JL, Colman KL, Casselbrant ML, Chi DH. Intratemporal and intracranial complications of acute otitis media in a pediatric population. Int J Pediatr Otorhinolaryngol. 2014;78(12):2161–4.

84. Ellefsen B, Bonding P. Facial palsy in acute otitis media. Clin Otolaryngol Allied Sci. 1996;21(5):393–5.

85. Evans AK, Licameli G, Brietzke S, Whittemore K, Kenna M. Pediatric facial nerve paralysis: patients, management and outcomes. Int J Pediatr Otorhinolaryngol. 2005;69(11):1521–8.

86. Choi JW, Park Y-H. Facial nerve paralysis in patients with chronic ear infections: surgical outcomes and radiologic analysis. Clin Exp Otorhinolaryngol. 2015;8(3):218–23.

87. MacIntosh PW, Fay AM. Update on the ophthalmic management of facial paralysis. Surv Ophthalmol. 2019;64(1):79–89.

88. Francis IC, Loughhead JA. Bell's phenomenon. A study of 508 patients. Aust J Ophthalmol. 1984;12(1):15–21.

89. Jones DH. Bell's phenomenon should not be regarded as pathognomonic sign. BMJ. 2001;323(7318):935.

90. Mathenge W. Emergency management: exposure keratopathy. Community Eye Health. 2018;31(103):69.

91. Grey F, Carley F, Biswas S, Tromans C. Scleral contact lens management of bilateral exposure and neurotrophic keratopathy. Cont Lens Anterior Eye. 2012;35(6):288–91.

92. Abell KM, Baker RS, Cowen DE, Porter JD. Efficacy of gold weight implants in facial nerve palsy: quantitative alterations in blinking. Vision Res. 1998;38(19):3019–23.

93. Demirci H, Frueh BR. Palpebral spring in the management of lagophthalmos and exposure keratopathy secondary to facial nerve palsy. Ophthal Plast Reconstr Surg. 2009;25(4):270–5.

94. Solomon A, Meller D, Prabhasawat P, et al. Amniotic membrane grafts for nontraumatic corneal perforations, descemetoceles, and deep ulcers. Ophthalmology. 2002;109(4):694–703.

95. Kanerva M, Nissinen J, Moilanen K, Mäki M, Lahdenne P, Pitkäranta A. Microbiologic findings in acute facial palsy in children. Otol Neurotol. 2013;34(7):e82–7.

96. Khine H, Mayers M, Avner JR, Fox A, Herold B, Goldman DL. Association between herpes simplex virus-1 infection and idiopathic unilateral facial paralysis in children and adolescents. Pediatr Infect Dis J. 2008;27(5):468–9.

97. Furuta Y, Ohtani F, Aizawa H, Fukuda S, Kawabata H, Bergström T. Varicella-zoster virus reactivation is an important cause of acute peripheral facial paralysis in children. Pediatr Infect Dis J. 2005;24(2):97–101.

98. Wagner G, Klinge H, Sachse MM. Ramsay Hunt syndrome. J Dtsch Dermatol Ges. 2012;10(4):238–44.

99. Musso MF, Crews JD. Infections of the external ear. In: Valdez TA, Vallejo JG, editors. Infectious diseases in pediatric otolaryngology. New York: Springer; 2016.

100. Christen HJ, Bartlau N, Hanefeld F, Eiffert H, Thomssen R. Peripheral facial palsy in childhood--Lyme borreliosis to be suspected unless proven otherwise. Acta Paediatr Scand. 1990;79(12):1219–24.

101. Cook SP, Macartney KK, Rose CD, Hunt PG, Eppes SC, Reilly JS. Lyme disease and seventh nerve paralysis in children. Am J Otolaryngol. 1997;18(5):320–3.

102. Sood SK. Lyme disease in children. Infect Dis Clin North Am. 2015;29(2):281–94.

103. Mora P, Carta A. Ocular manifestations of Lyme borreliosis in Europe. Int J Med Sci. 2009;6(3):124–5.

104. Ciorba A, Corazzi V, Conz V, Bianchini C, Aimoni C. Facial nerve paralysis in children. World J Clin Cases. 2015;3(12):973–9.

105. Vagefi MR, Fredrick DR. Papilloedema secondary to otitic hydrocephalus. Br J Ophthalmol. 2006;90(5):646.

106. Pollock TJ, Kim P, Sargent MA, Aroichane M, Lyons CJ, Gardiner JA. Ophthalmic complications of otitis media in children. J AAPOS. 2011;15(3):272–5.

107. Valles JM, Fekete R. Gradenigo syndrome: unusual consequence of otitis media. Case Rep Neurol. 2014;6(2):197–201.

108. Costa JV, João M, Guimarães S. Bilateral papilledema and abducens nerve palsy following cerebral venous sinus thrombosis due to Gradenigo's syndrome in a pediatric patient. Am J Ophthalmol Case Rep. 2020;19:100824.
109. Bingen E, Cohen R, Jourenkova N, Gehanno P. Epidemiologic study of conjunctivitis-otitis syndrome. Pediatr Infect Dis J. 2005;24(8):731–2.
110. Sugita G, Hotomi M, Sugita R, Kono M, Togawa A, Yamauchi K, Funaki T, Yamanaka N. Genetic characteristics of Haemophilus influenzae and Streptococcus pneumoniae isolated from children with conjunctivitis-otitis media syndrome. J Infect Chemother. 2014;20(8):493–7.
111. Watters K, Patil N, Russell J. Inflammatory disease of the mouth and pharynx. In: Bluestone CD, Simons JP, Healy GB, editors. Bluestone and Stool's Pediatric Otolaryngology. 5th ed. Shelton: People's Medical Publishing House; 2014.
112. Salmon JF. Conjunctiva. In: Kanski's clinical ophthalmology: a systematic approach. 9th ed. Amsterdam: Elsevier; 2019.
113. Meisler DM, Bosworth DE, Krachmer JH. Ocular infectious mononucleosis manifested as Parinaud's oculoglandular syndrome. Am J Ophthalmol. 1981;92(5):722–6.
114. Perry RT, Halsey NA. The clinical significance of measles: a review. J Infect Dis. 2004;189(Suppl 1):S4–16.
115. McNamara PS, Van Doorn HR. Respiratory viruses and atypical bacteria. In: Farrar J, Hotez PJ, Junghanss T, Kang G, Lalloo D, White NJ, editors. Manson's tropical infectious diseases. 23rd ed. London: W.B. Saunders; 2014.
116. Goldsmith AJ, Rosenfeld RM. Cervical adenopathy. In: Bluestone CD, Simons JP, Healy GB, editors. Bluestone and Stool's Pediatric Otolaryngology. 5th ed. Shelton: People's Medical Publishing House; 2014.
117. Khurana S, Gupta P, Ram J. Bilateral conjunctival suffusion: an ocular manifestation of leptospirosis. Indian J Ophthalmol. 2020;68(9):1971.
118. American Academy of Pediatrics. Chlamydia trachomatis. In: Kimberlin DW, Brady MT, Jackson MA, Long SS, editors. Red book: 2015 report of the committee on infectious diseases. 30th ed. Elk Grove Village: American Academy of Pediatrics; 2015.

Ümit Yılmaz, Aylin Gül, and Sheng-Po Hao

70.1 Introduction

It is common for ENT specialists to come across foreign bodies in children. Foreign bodies may be seen in the ear canal, nasal interior, pharynx, oesophagus or within the lower respiratory tree (larynx, trachea or bronchi). In an older child, a history of the child putting something in a body cavity is generally forthcoming, but in younger children this may not be the case and the parent or care giver may be anxious about the situation, but unable to supply an informative history. In younger children it pays to be suspicious about the possibility of a foreign body.

70.2 Foreign Bodies in the Nose

In accident and emergency departments a variety of different foreign bodies may be encountered in children's noses. Most such occurrences are not highly risky, although there are specific objects with the potential to significantly harm a child, such as a battery or magnet, which call for urgent action to remove them. It may be easy to visualise a foreign body in the nose, while, conversely, some are so hard to find that they remain in place anywhere between weeks and potentially years. A fundamental distinction is whether the foreign body consists of organic or inorganic material. Typically, an organic matter foreign body produces a higher degree of

Ü. Yılmaz (✉)
Section of Otorhinolaryngology, Selahaddin Eyyubi State Hospital, Diyarbakır, Turkey

A. Gül
Section of Otorhinolayngology, Medical Park Gaziantep Hospital, Gaziantep, Turkey

S.-P. Hao
Department of Otorhinolaryngology, Shin Kong Wu Ho-Su Memorial Hospital, Fu Jen Catholic University, Taipei, Taiwan

© The Author(s), under exclusive license to Springer Nature Switzerland AG 2022
C. Cingi et al. (eds.), *Pediatric ENT Infections*,
https://doi.org/10.1007/978-3-030-80691-0_70

irritation to the lining of the nose and patients more rapidly become symptomatic [1–4].

The usual foreign bodies encountered are pebbles, beads, nuts, pieces of chalk or other items of small size. Two organic foreign bodies that may be encountered are house fly maggots or blowfly larvae. The housefly larvae are especially prone to injure the child.

There are two points within the nasal interior where foreign bodies are especially likely to lodge: the base of the inferior turbinate or in front of the middle turbinate. The foreign body may result in no nasal trauma, but certain objects provoke mucosal oedema and may erode the nasal lining, produce an ulcer or trigger a nosebleed. Organic foreign bodies are generally responsible for such issues as they typically draw moisture from the nasal environment and increase in size. Over time the foreign body may be gradually mineralised, becoming a rhinolith and causing even further trauma.

A battery in the nasal cavity may cause injury to the septum, which may even be perforated. Batteries provoke localised inflammation and the area may undergo liquefactive necrotic change [5]. Button batteries are found in large numbers of electric devices, such as electronic toys, remote control devices, pocket calculators, hearing aids and so forth. In excess of 300 button batteries are swallowed each year by American children [6].

It is usually children who experiment with placing items inside their nose, as part of exploratory play. Below the age of 9 months, children generally cannot form a pincer grip on objects and thus they usually do not insert small objects into their nose. The usual age at which children are prone to put things into the nose is between the ages of 2 and 5 years. Males are marginally more likely to do this than females. Two thirds of foreign bodies in the nose are in the right cavity, which is likely to be connected to more children being right- than left-handed. It is often the case that a child with an autistic spectrum disorder may keep on placing items into various body openings and sometimes there will be several foreign bodies present in several orifices concurrently. A nasal foreign body increases in probability in families where another younger child is also at home [6–8].

The foreign body may result in no nasal trauma, but particular objects have a tendency to cause mucosal oedema and may erode the nasal lining, producing an ulcer or triggering a nosebleed. Organic foreign bodies are generally responsible for such issues as they typically draw moisture from the nasal environment and increase in size. Over time the foreign body may be gradually mineralised, becoming a rhinolith and causing even further trauma [7, 8].

The usual presentation of a nasal foreign body is with pus-filled rhinorrhoea from one nostril, accompanied by an unpleasant smell. Generally, the condition does not cause pain, but occasionally a child may complain of ipsilateral cephalgia. The discharge may also contain blood, or there may be a frank nosebleed.

Whilst children other than the very young often admit to placing an object in their nose, the only clue in a very young child may be irritable behaviour. When the foreign body is organic, there may be some variety in how the case presents, with a greater likelihood that both sides of the nose are affected. Such children generally complain of a blocked nose, tend to sneeze and experience cephalgia as well as rhinorrhoea. Since organic foreign bodies have the potential to cause an infection, the child may have a leucocytosis. The child may also be pyrexial.

An adequate light source is needed to enable the foreign body can be seen when the patient is examined. The patient needs to adopt the sniffing neck position. Before beginning to examine the nose it may be helpful to supply a vasoconstrictive agent, which renders the membranous nasal lining less swollen. Anterior rhinoscopy will be required, augmented as required by flexible nasopharyngeal endoscopy. If the foreign body remains alive in the nose, it is generally readily seen and there is often significant damage to the nasal lining and the cartilaginous and osseous tissues. There may be bleeding from one side of the nose or rhinorrhoea, which can be anything from watery to pus-filled in appearance [7–10].

A rhinolith appears as a grey object lying on the basal aspect of the nasal cavity.

The physical examination should also include otoscopy, to exclude inflammation of the middle ear, apparent through changes in the tympanic membrane. Auscultation may reveal wheezing, indicative of aspiration deeper within the respiratory tract.

If the child is unable to co-operate with being fully examined, it may be necessary to carry out an examination under a general anaesthetic.

70.2.1 Diagnosis

The finding that most strongly points towards the presence of a foreign body in the nose is unilateral rhinorrhoea. In the majority of disorders, rhinorrhoea affects both sides of the nose, through the action of nasal reflexes; hence unilateral rhinorrhoea is quite specific for a foreign body. Laboratory tests are not generally needed. Radiological assessment may be of value if the foreign body is suspected to be a battery or magnet, or no clear views can be obtained by direct visualisation. However, many other foreign bodies are actually radiolucent [1].

70.2.2 Treatment

Whereas diagnosing a foreign body may present difficulties, treating the patient is typically straightforward for experienced ENT specialists. Endoscopy can usually confirm where the body is lodged and its magnitude. The preferred method of removal is by use of suction, employing a nasal speculum to permit the object to be directly visualised. In circumstances where suction removal is not feasible, removal with alligator forceps via the nostril may be possible. There is a risk, if the foreign body has a round shape, that attempts to grasp it may inadvertently propel it further into the nose. If the object is pushed right through the choana, it may pass through the nasopharynx and be retrievable via the mouth. Whilst the surgeon is removing the foreign body, the child may need to be slightly sedated, or at least held down [9–11].

## 70.3	Foreign Bodies in the Ear Canal

Both paediatricians and ENT specialists often come across children who have a foreign body lodged in the external auditory meatus. The usual symptoms created by such a situation are one-sided otorrhoea, earache, blood coming from the ear, auditory impairment, ringing in the ear, coughing, feeling lightheaded or paralysis of facial muscles. In some children, there are no associated symptoms and the foreign body may only come to light when the ear undergoes a routine examination [12–14].

The nature and occurrence of symptoms from a foreign body lodged in the external auditory meatus depend closely on what the foreign body consists of, for example, whether organic or inorganic, living or non-living, metal or other material and whether the object tends to absorb water or not [15, 16].

Whilst a foreign object can frequently be extracted without difficulty, there exists a risk that the external or middle ear may suffer iatrogenic injury as a result of attempted removal. If the external auditory meatus is particularly narrow or the child or adolescent does not co-operate fully with the procedure, a foreign body may be difficult to dislodge [17–19]. There are a number of surgical instruments suitable for removing these objects, and guidance may be with the naked eye or operative microscope. In difficult cases, the patient may need sedation or even require putting under a general anaesthetic [18–20]. A patient who moves excessively during the procedure may suffer an iatrogenic injury, e.g. a tear to the ear drum or damage to the skin lining the external auditory meatus [21, 22].

The nature of the foreign body has an impact on the risk of iatrogenic injury during removal, earrings being the object associated with highest risk, whilst cotton buds are least likely to cause an injury. A living creature within the ear canal is more likely to result in complications than a non-living object [23, 24]. However, insects have not been reported to cause high rates of complication. There are a range of variables that have an influence on the likelihood of a complication, amongst which the age of the child, the type of object, the removal technique and the experience of the surgeon may be noted. The key factors that predict the likelihood of suffering a complication appear to be how old the child is and their willingness to co-operate with removal [25].

A number of surgical instruments find employment as tools to extract foreign objects from the ear, notably alligator forceps, loops or right-angled ball hooks. As long as the tympanic membrane is uninjured, the ear may be irrigated to remove objects liable to disintegration, such as insects or tissue paper. This method is not safe to use if the object is a battery or absorbs water. Some items that absorb water are vegetables, beans and other food items. Water absorption makes them swell and get more firmly lodged in the external auditory meatus [5, 26].

It is recommended that the operating microscope be used for removal of any foreign body from the external auditory meatus. If the foreign body is not adherent to the canal or consists of cotton wool, an otoscope and bayonet forceps are suitable. If the foreign body is close to the ear drum or there is an inflammatory reaction associated with it, an ENT opinion is needed. According to the literature, early referral to ENT is advisable if complications are to be avoided. Indeed, it has been reported that only 15.7% of children operated on by ENT specialists suffer complications, whereas those operated on by non-specialists had a 68.1% risk of complications [27]. It has also been reported that non-specialists may need to attempt removal repeatedly, making children less willing to co-operate and thus removal more challenging. It is evident that promptly referring a child in this situation to an ENT clinic is the way to prevent unnecessary complications [1, 5].

It has been shown recently, on the basis of claims submitted to a health insurance provider [27], that children with ADHD (attention deficit hyperactivity disorder) are especially likely to place a foreign body within the nose or ear canal. The study authors propose that the occurrence of a foreign body in the external auditory meatus should trigger investigation of any underlying reasons, especially undiagnosed ADHD. It is also recognised that there is an association between lower socioeconomic status and having a foreign body in the ear [27].

70.4   Foreign Body Aspiration in Children

The aspiration of foreign bodies by children is a global problem which may cause significant morbidity and even death. A foreign body may lodge in any portion of the airway, such as the oropharynx, hypopharynx, larynx or even down to the level of the bronchi. Some objects that are transparent may be difficult to identify by direct visualisation. The lateral walls of the hypopharynx are an area where a sharp object may get stuck. The majority of objects aspirated consist of organic material that does not show up well on X-ray. It is calculated that every year around 2000 paediatric cases of aspiration of a foreign body result in hospitalisation in the USA. Complications may occur if the case comes late to medical attention or the diagnosis is missed due to a lack of symptoms or because the pattern of symptoms does not point towards aspiration. Such complications may include an airway being completely blocked, with a potentially fatal outcome, a longstanding wheeze, development of a cough or repeated episodes of pneumonia [28].

The assessment of a child for possible aspiration of a foreign body is often triggered by a parent or carer seeing an object ingested, or witnessing choking. It is a regrettable fact that such a history is sometimes absent or the history may not be completely reliable. In the latter situation, the clinician will rely on presenting features, chest X-ray and examination of the child before consideration of bronchoscopic examination. There are studies in the literature which examine how often particular symptoms occur, what signs are expected on examination and the likely imaging appearances [27, 28]. The complication that occurs with highest frequency in paediatric patients is blockage of the oesophagus. A swallowed foreign body might also penetrate through the gut wall, with complications arising from perforation or the movement of the foreign body within the body [28].

## 70.5	Conclusion

Children might place a variety of different objects or insects into their nose or ear. When extracting such a foreign body, the choice of method depends on how old the child is and the nature of the object. Treatment aims for minimal complications. If a child or adolescent with such a foreign body cannot co-operate with removal, clinicians will be obliged to offer sedation or perform removal with the patient under a general anaesthetic.

On a global scale, the aspiration of a foreign body causes important levels of morbidity and even death. The entire airway should be checked, as a foreign body may lodge anywhere along its length. The majority of such objects consist of organic material and display radiolucency. The best safeguard against a late diagnosis is a meticulous history and detailed examination with appropriate use of imaging.

References

1. Baranowski K, Al-Aaraj MJ, Sinha V. Nasal foreign body. Treasure Island: StatPearls Publishing; 2020.
2. Koehler P, Jung N, Kochanek M, Lohneis P, Shimabukuro-Vornhagen A, Böll B. 'Lost in nasal Space': Staphylococcus aureus sepsis associated with nasal handkerchief packing. Infection. 2019;47(2):307–11.
3. Zhang T, Zhuang H, Wang K, Xu G. Clinical features and surgical outcomes of posterior segment intraocular foreign bodies in children in East China. J Ophthalmol. 2018;2018:5861043.
4. Kalan A, Tariq M. Foreign bodies in the nasal cavities: a comprehensive review of the aetiology, diagnostic pointers, and therapeutic measures. Postgrad Med J. 2000 Aug;76(898):484–7.
5. Morris S, Osborne MS, McDermott AL. Will children ever learn? Removal of nasal and aural foreign bodies: a study of hospital episode statistics. Ann R Coll Surg Engl. 2018;3:1–3.
6. Tasche KK, Chang KE. Otolaryngologic emergencies in the primary care setting. Med Clin North Am. 2017;101(3):641–56.
7. Sinikumpu JJ, Serlo W. Confirmed and suspected foreign body injuries in children during 2008-2013: a hospital-based single center study in Oulu university hospital. Scand J Surg. 2017;106(4):350–5.
8. Regonne PE, Ndiaye M, Sy A, Diandy Y, Diop AD, Diallo BK. Nasal foreign bodies in children in a pediatric hospital in Senegal: a three-year assessment. Eur Ann Otorhinolaryngol Head Neck Dis. 2017;134(5):361–4.
9. Endican S, Garap JP, Dubey SP. Ear, nose and throat foreign bodies in Melanesian children: an analysis of 1037 cases. Int J Pediatr Otorhinolaryngol. 2006;70(9):1539–45. https://doi.org/10.1016/j.ijporl.2006.03.018.
10. Mohan S, Fuller JC, Ford SF, Lindsay RW. Diagnostic and therapeutic management of nasal airway obstruction: advances in diagnosis and treatment. JAMA Facial Plast Surg. 2018;20(5):409–18.
11. Awad AH, ElTaher M. ENT foreign bodies: an experience. Int Arch Otorhinolaryngol. 2018;22(2):146–51.
12. Kim KH, Chung JH, Byun H, Zheng T, Jeong JH, Lee SH. Clinical characteristics of external auditory canal foreign bodies in children and adolescents. Ear Nose Throat J. 2019;9:145561319893164. https://doi.org/10.1177/0145561319893164.
13. Olson MD, Saw J, Visscher SL, Balakrishnan K. Cost comparison and safety of emergency department conscious sedation for the removal of ear foreign bodies. Int J Pediatr Otorhinolaryngol. 2018;110:140–3.

14. Marin JR, Trainor JL. Foreign body removal from the external auditory canal in a pediatric emergency department. Pediatr Emerg Care. 2006;22(9):630–4.
15. Bahannan AA, Aljabry AO. Aural foreign bodies among patients presenting to IBN SINA teaching hospital, Mukalla, Hadhramout province, Yemen. Indian J Otolaryngol Head Neck Surg. 2018;70(2):194–9.
16. Gold KR, Wester JL, Gold R. Foreign body in external ear canal: an unusual cause of chronic cough. Am J Med. 2017;130(4):e143–4.
17. Wada I, Kase Y, Iinuma T. Statistical study on the case of aural foreign bodies [in Japanese]. Nihon Jibiinkoka Gakkai Kaiho. 2003;106(6):678–84.
18. Ansley JF, Cunningham MJ. Treatment of aural foreign bodies in children. Pediatrics. 1998;101(4 pt 1):638–41.
19. Craig SS, Cheek JA, Seith RW, West A. Removal of ENT for- eign bodies in children. Emerg Med Australas. 2015;27(2):145–7.
20. Morris S, Osborne MS, McDermott AL. Will children ever learn? Removal of nasal and aural foreign bodies: a study of hospital episode statistics. Ann R Coll Surg Engl. 2018;100(8):632–4.
21. Al-Juboori AN. Aural foreign bodies: descriptive study of 224 patients in Al-Fallujah general hospital. Iraq Int J Otolaryngol. 2013;2013(4):401289.
22. Olajide TG, Ologe FE, Arigbede OO. Management of foreign bodies in the ear: a retrospective review of 123 cases in Nigeria. Ear Nose Throat J. 2011;90(11):E16–9.
23. Nakao Y, Tanigawa T, Murotani K, Yamashita JI. Foreign bodies in the external auditory canal: influence of age on incidence and outcomes in a Japanese population. Geriatr Gerontol Int. 2017;17(11):2131–5.
24. Sikka K, Agrawal R, Devraja K, Lodha JV, Thakar A. Hazardous complications of animate foreign bodies in otology practice. J Laryngol Otol. 2015;129(6):540–3.
25. Olajuyin O, Olatunya OS. Aural foreign body extraction in chil- dren: a double-edged sword. Pan Afr Med J. 2015;20(1):186.
26. Ng TT. Aural foreign body removal: there is no one-size-fits-all method. Open Access Emerg Med. 2018;10:177–82.
27. Schuldt T, Grossmann W, Weiss NM, Ovari A, Mlynski R. Schra- ven SP. aural and nasal foreign bodies in children - epidemiology and correlation with hyperkinetic disorders, developmental disorders and congenital malformations. Int J Pediatr Otorhinolaryngol. 2019;118:165–9.
28. Sink JR, Kitsko DJ, Georg MW, Winger DG, Simons JP. Predictors of foreign body aspiration in children. Otolaryngol Head Neck Surg. 2016;155(3):501–7. https://doi.org/10.1177/0194599816644410.

Infections After Cochlear Implantation

Emine Demir and Ş. Armağan İncesulu

71.1 Introduction

Cochlear implants are one of the most successful surgically implanted medical devices for the patients with severe-to-profound sensorineural hearing loss worldwide. Surgical procedure for implantation is a safe procedure with low rate of early and long-term complications, but besides other problems, infections may unavoidably occur.

Post-cochlear implant infections can be treated medically or revision surgery may be required. These infections are the second most common cause of revision surgeries after device failure. Some infectious such as meningitis can be life-threatening, whereas some infections may only prevent to device use. Understanding the etiology, management, and prevention of infections is of great importance for this patient population [1, 2]. When the implanted ear has an infection in the case using unilateral cochlear implant, patient may not use cochlear implant for a while or permanently and pose significant difficulties, especially in children. The child cannot communicate or may lose the progress of speech-language in a critical period of the development [2]. In addition, middle ear infection is a risk factor for postimplant meningitis [3]. Therefore, it requires to be alert to the infections and the things to be done for both diagnosis and treatment should be applied quickly.

Post-CI infections include acute otitis media (AOM), chronic suppurative otitis media (CSOM), cholesteatoma, meningitis, and wound infection.

E. Demir (✉)
Department of Otorhinolaryngology, Faculty of Medicine, Recep Tayyip Erdoğan University, Rize, Turkey
e-mail: emine.demir@erdogan.edu.tr

Ş. A. İncesulu
Department of Otorhinolaryngology, Faculty of Medicine, Eskişehir Osmangazi University, Eskişehir, Turkey

71.2 Acute Otitis Media

Acute otitis media is an acute infection of the mucosa lining the middle ear and mastoid cavity. It is very common especially in childhood and is the second most common upper respiratory tract infection. Children with CI can have an AOM attack as in the normal population. Although CI was previously thought to increase the incidence of AOM, it has recently seen that this is not true. The incidence of AOM in children with CI is approximately 10% and is similar to children without implants [3–5]. Post-CI middle ear infections can be seen at any time, and most frequently occur within the first 2 years after surgery [4].

Acute otitis media causes symptoms of otalgia, high fever, and restlessness that develop within 48 h in patients. These complaints are similar in patients with CI, but there are some differences and points to be considered. If a patient with CI has an AOM attack, persistent fever and consciousness are important because the infection can pass to perilymph and cause meningitis, which the clinician should be alert about. In addition, pain during the implant stimulation is a rare but important symptom in patients with CI. This symptom indicates device failure requiring explantation, even if the infection is eliminated. In a patient with CI presenting with acute otitis media symptoms, the diagnosis can easily be made with hyperemia and/or bulging in the tympanum during otoscopic examination [2, 5, 6] (Fig. 71.1).

Antibiotic resistance has become an increasing problem with the over-prescribing of antibiotics. Therefore, according to the AOM Guideline of the American Academy of Pediatrics (AAP), 10-day antibiotic treatment is recommended only for patients under 2 years of age with severe disease (temperature is >39 °C, significant otalgia, or toxic appearance). "Watchful waiting" is recommended for patients other than this [5, 7]. There are uncertainty and some degree of controversy about how to best management to AOM in patients with CI [2]. However, the general opinion is that

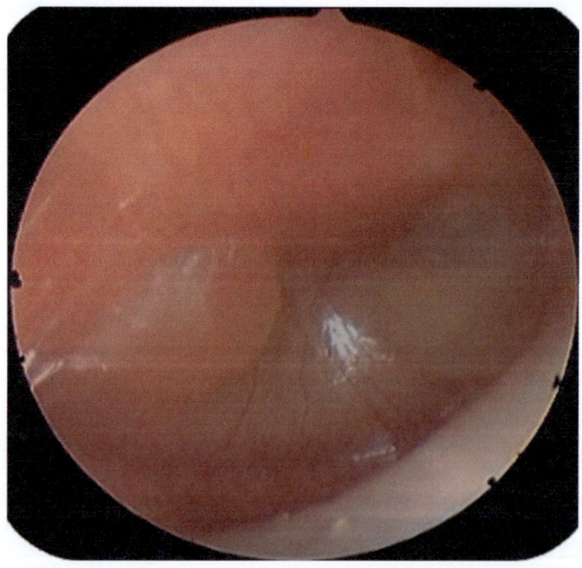

Fig. 71.1 Three-year-old girl. She was implanted bilaterally at the age of 15 months. She has acute otitis media. She was treated with oral antibiotics successfully

antibiotic treatment for AOM in children with implants should be started immediately after the diagnosis is made and the duration should be extended to 2 weeks [8]. Main reason for early and aggressive treatment of otitis media is that the infection of the middle ear cavity is considered a risk factor for postimplant meningitis. Second, this treatment is necessary to prevent the development of the retraction pocket, adhesion of the tympanic membrane, and the formation of cholesteatoma [3]. Third, otitis media in the implanted ear that is not well treated can cause device failure, leading to explantation [9].

Pathogens that cause AOM after cochlear implantation are *Streptococcus pneumoniae* (*S. pneumoniae*), *Haemophilus influenzae* (*H. influenzae*), and *Moraxella catarrhalis* (*M. catarrhalis*), which usually cause AOM in non-implanted children. Thus, most of the cases can be treated with empirical antibiotherapy without culturing. High-dose (90 mg/kg/day) amoxicillin is the first choice, but there is no consensus on oral or parenteral administration [5, 8]. There are some important factors that should be considered when directing AOM treatment in a patient with CI. Especially if AOM develops in the first 2 months after implantation since no fibrous capsule is formed around the implant and the cochleostomy, microorganisms have a high risk of both passing to the perilymph and causing meningitis and also poses a risk for implant colonization [2]. Therefore, broad-spectrum parenteral antibiotherapy is recommended for those who have AOM attack in less than 2 months postoperatively, those with inner ear anomalies, and those with systemic comorbidities [2, 10]. When an AOM attack develops in a patient with CI other than these conditions, empirical antibiotherapy can be started orally, but the patient's condition should be strictly controlled. If a communication problem with the family is suspected, parenteral antibiotherapy can be started.

When an AOM patient with CI under treatment does not improve within 72 hours, culture should be taken considering atypical microorganisms for AOM [2]. Cochlear implants like other prosthetic devices are biocompatible, but they are still foreign bodies and *Staphylococcus aureus (S. aureus)* is the most common isolated organism with the rate of 73.3% in cochlear implant cases [11]. Prostheses do not have the capacity of microcirculation and also prevent the delivery of antibiotics. Moreover, *Staphylococcus aureus (S. aureus)* can be resistant to empirical antibiotherapy and can increase the risk of device failure that requires explantation. High-dose amoxicillin-clavulanate or ceftriaxone is required until the result of culture is obtained [5, 7]. If the culture is not diagnostic in treatment-resistant cases, broad-spectrum antibiotics such as vancomycin and cefepime should be given [7]. In addition, if *S. aureus* is detected in the culture, a beta-lactam antibiotic treatment such as nafcillin is sufficient, whereas if a resistant microorganism such as *Methicillin resistant staphylococcus aureus (MRSA)* is identified, combined treatments such as rifampin and vancomycin or linezolid should be applied [2].

71.3 Mastoiditis

The incidence of acute mastoiditis after cochlear implantation is between 1 and 4.7% and more than the normal population because cortical mastoidectomy is routinely performed during CI surgery. By removing the natural anatomical barrier with cortical mastoidectomy, infection can rapidly spread to the mastoid space during AOM attacks [10].

Acute mastoiditis is characterized by persistent otalgia, fever and, retroauricular erythema, fluctuation, and auricular proptosis occurring during or immediately after an AOM attack. Diagnosis can be made by the patient's clinic and physical examination. Computed tomography (CT) is indicated when intracranial complications are suspected according to the general diagnosis and treatment protocol of acute mastoiditis. However, image artifact created by the implant makes it difficult to evaluate CT [12, 13]. Moreover, conventional CT scan delivers higher radiation doses. Cone Beam Computed Tomography with reasonable radiation exposure may be a good alternative.

Presence of acute mastoiditis in a patient with cochlear implantation requires prompt and precise medical decisions. As soon as mastoiditis is diagnosed, parenteral antibiotherapy should order immediately, regardless of the need for surgical intervention. It is recommended to continue broad-spectrum antibiotherapy, either ceftriaxone and clindamycin or vancomycin, for at least 7–10 days, and then oral antibiotics for 10–14 days [6, 12]. The necessity and timing of surgical treatment are controversial. Some authors suggest that half of the patients can be cured by antibiotherapy without the need for surgical intervention and that close follow-up may be sufficient. They argue that mastoidectomy and/or abscess drainage should be added to the treatment only if abscess formation such as subperiosteal abscess occurs [14]. However, there are those who think that early surgical intervention and application of pressure equalizing tubes (PET) together with antibiotherapy are beneficial because mastoiditis may cause the spread of bacteria from the middle ear to the inner ear in patients with CI and may increase the risk of meningitis [15, 16]. The only common opinion in cases of mastoiditis with CI is that antibiotherapy should be started immediately. It is also recognized that the key to implant protection in patients with mastoiditis is the immediate initiation of aggressive medical and, if necessary, surgical treatment. When the implant surgeon encounters such a situation, he/she must make a careful decision by considering the complications and comorbidities that may occur related to the implant [6].

71.4 Chronic Suppurative Otitis Media and Cholesteatom

While the incidence of chronic suppurative otitis media (CSOM), which is a late complication of cochlear implantation, in adults after implantation is 5.4%, it is less common in pediatric implant cases. Cholesteatoma develops in approximately 1% of the implanted cases [9, 17]. However, the follow-up periods of the studies in the literature are short. Knowing that CSOM and cholesteatoma can develop many years after implantation suggests that the actual incidence is higher.

The pathogenesis of CSOM that develops after cochlear implantation is unclear. However, the implant may create a potential focus for infection by creating a foreign body reaction and cause a predisposition to CSOM and cholesteatoma by disrupting mastoid aeration [3]. Cholesteatoma can also be seen as an iatrogenic complication after CI surgery. Damage to the posterior wall of the external auditory canal or annular ligament may result in long-term cholesteatoma formation. Therefore, it is important not to damage the posterior wall of the external auditory canal during implant surgery. It may result de novo development of CSOM and cholesteatoma independent of the implant [18, 19]. In addition, posterior wall of the external auditory canal, which becomes very thin during CI operation, may undergo bone resorption over time. Keratin accumulation in the defect may result in the development of cholesteatoma. Protection of the posterior wall of the external auditory canal and annular ligament is vital in CI surgery. If any damage develops, repair should be provided with a suitable material such as cartilage and bone pate in a way that prevents the migration of the epithelium. In addition, when placing the electrode into the mastoid cavity, ensuring that it does not contact the posterior wall of the external auditory canal can prevent bone resorption in the long term.

Otorrhea is the most common symptom of CSOM and cholesteatoma. Persistent and recurrent otorrhea, ear pain or otitis with recurrent effusion, and recurrent ventilation tube history in an implanted person should be alarming for CSOM and cholesteatoma. In addition, the surgeon should be more alert in the postimplantation follow-up of children with a history of EOM treated with a preimplantation ventilation tube [19, 20]. Patients who can be diagnosed with a visible pathology such as tympanic membrane perforation, cytokeratins, granulation tissue, or polyps by physical examination should be treated as soon as possible. In patients with persistent symptoms, if the diagnosis cannot be made by physical examination, computed tomography is helpful, although it may only define bony erosion caused by cholesteatoma in middle ear, mastoid or petrous bone and pathologic soft tissue without differentiation (Fig. 71.2). Non-echo planar diffusion-weighted magnetic resonance imaging is more recommended modality with high sensitivity and specificity to diagnose cholesteatoma especially in cases with cochlear implant surgery. Recently, most of the cochlear implants are magnetic resonance imaging compatible with recent technological development, but magnetic resonance imaging must be performed under controlled condition. Moreover, artifact generated by either cochlear implant magnet or the electrodes may impede the clear visualization of the

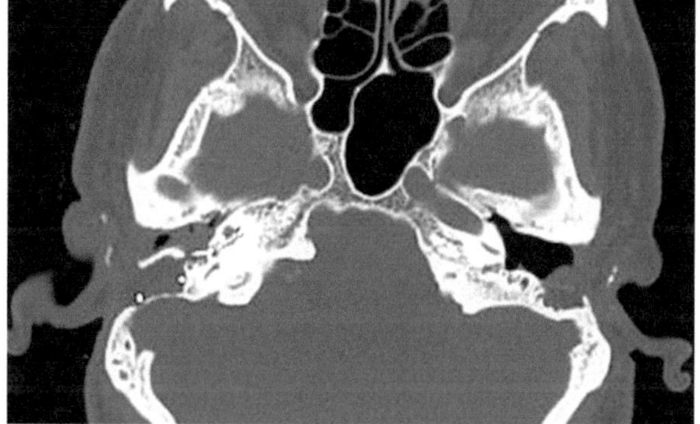

Fig. 71.2 CT scan of 39-year-old women. She had bilateral mastoid operation when she was young. Before cochlear implant surgery tympanic membrane perforation was diagnosed. It was reconstructed and cochlear implant successfully placed. 3 years later, she applied to clinic with otorrhea

cholesteatoma. If necessary, examine under general anesthesia and evaluate the middle ear in patient with intact tympanic membrane with tympanotomy [20].

Although the management of CSOM and cholesteatoma in a cochlear implanted ear has some differences, it is generally similar to the non-cochlear implanted ear. However, the presence of implants challenges the surgeon in the management of CSOM and cholesteatoma. If there is discharge, medical treatment should be started immediately after the ear is aspirated and the culture is taken [20]. Most of the time, *Pseudomonas aeruginosa (P. aeruginosa)* and *S. aureus* are the isolated microorganisms. Therefore, empirical treatment for these microorganisms should be started until the culture result is obtained. Topical ciprofloxacin 0.3% and topical dexamethasone treatment must be recommended. Systemic antibiotics are cephalexin, flucloxacillin, cloxacillin, and ciprofloxacin. Aural toilet should be performed with regular aspiration, the microorganism load should be reduced, and debris should be cleaned [21].

Surgical planning should be made with the response of the patient who is followed up with topical and systemic antibiotics. If there is no implant in a CSOM case without cholesteatoma, tympanoplasty is optional and the timing is not very important. However, if there is a cochlear implant, tympanoplasty should be applied to create a closed cavity as soon as possible by providing appropriate conditions. Cholesteatoma is more urgent condition.

Pathology should be eradicated by protecting the implant if it is possible. However, explantation of the cochlear implant and planned single or stage surgery is more appropriate management. Electrodes should be left in the cochlea to ensure reimplantation afterward during the explantation surgery. The electrode array is cut from the cochleostomy site and the portion of the implant in the mastoid cavity is removed because the removal of the electrodes causes rapid fibrosis or ossification in the cochlea and prevents reimplantation. Subtotal petrosectomy and double-blind closure of external auditory canal after the explantation of the cochlear implant in the infected ear in the first stage is recommended procedure of the authors of the chapter. If the opposite ear is suitable for implantation, the opposite ear can also be implanted in the same session [19, 20].

The key to not losing the implant due to CSOM and cholesteatoma is early diagnosis and intervention. Since these pathologies may develop years after CI, continuous medical follow-up of patients after implant and patient and parent education regarding ear discharge are important [20].

71.5   Meningitis

Bacterial meningitis after implantation is a rare but life-threatening infection. Cochlear implant surgery may increase the risk of meningitis by causing new communication between the middle ear and the subarachnoid space through the inner ear [22]. Therefore, individuals who undergo cochlear implantation are 30 times more likely to have meningitis than their age group [23]. However, many patients also have pre-existing risk factors for meningitis prior to cochlear implantation, which contributes to an increased risk. Among these are age (less than 5 years), immunodeficiency, history of preimplant meningitis, congenital inner ear anomaly, history of ventriculoperitoneal shunt, CSF leak, and history of otitis media before meningitis [24].

Meningitis develops with the spread of microorganisms directly from the middle ear (otogenic) or hematogenously to the meninges. The otogenic spread can also be classified as direct invasion of the meninges by bacteria or indirect invasion through the inner ear. In patients with cochlear implants, the spread of bacteria from the middle ear to the meninges through the inner ear is the most widely accepted view and has been the main focus of the study of infection prevention strategies in implant-associated meningitis. With the removal of the bone, soft tissue and mucosal barriers between the middle ear and inner ear with cochlear implant surgery, bacteria can access the inner ear more easily from the middle ear [24, 25]. The occurrence of meningitis is directly related to the duration and intensity of bacteremia. The bacterial threshold required for hematogenous spread to the meninges is the highest, while the threshold required for otogenous spread is the lowest. In addition, in the presence of a foreign body such as a cochlear implant electrode array in the inner ear, the threshold further decreases with the increase in the apoptotic activity of polymorphonuclear leukocytes and the decrease in the phagocytosis ability of bacteria [24, 26]. This explains why the risk of meningitis in cochlear implant patients is much higher than in the normal population. The most common microorganism identified in cerebrospinal fluid (CSF) cultures of patients with post-cochlear implant meningitis is *S. pneumoniae*. Other less common microorganisms are *H. influenzae*, *Escherichia coli*, *Streptococcus viridians*, and *staphylococcus* [24].

The typical clinical presentation of meningitis is severe, acute onset headache, fever, and nuchal rigidity. Altered mental state (Glasgow Coma Scale score <14), cranial nerve palsy, seizure, and focal neurological findings are other symptoms that may be seen. These symptoms seen in individuals with cochlear implants should be warning. In addition, since AOM history is important in individuals with CI, ear pain should be questioned and otological examination should be done carefully. If meningitis is suspected, middle ear drainage (if available) and a lumbar puncture for CSF cultures should be performed to allow diagnosis and culture-oriented treatment [12, 27].

Patients should be hospitalized and closely monitored to observe their clinical condition. Hemodynamic monitoring is important for fluid resuscitation, whereas saturation monitoring is important for providing airway support. For the treatment of increased CSF pressure, dexamethasone can be given, and the head of the bed can be elevated by 30° [27]. If meningitis is suspected after implantation, empirical antibiotics should be administered immediately until culture results are available. If meningitis develops within the first 60 days after surgery, an agent effective against gram-negative bacilli, especially intravenous vancomycin and meropenem, should be used. Meningitis that develops after this period can be treated with a standard bacterial meningitis regimen (intravenous vancomycin and ceftriaxone) [12].

The risks, causes, and management of meningitis in cochlear implant patients require careful consideration. Meningitis that occurs within the first 30 days after surgery is likely to be associated with surgery (e.g., wound infection or leaky cochleostomy site) and causes should be investigated. Between 30 days and 2 years after surgery, AOM becomes a more likely etiological factor for meningitis especially in children. Therefore, the use of intravenous antibiotics is definitely recommended in AOM attacks that develop within the first 2 months after cochlear implant surgery. After 2 months and in the absence of an electrode positioning device, empirical treatment with oral antibiotics (90 mg/kg/day amoxicillin or amoxicillin-clavulanate) can be applied in an uncomplicated otitis media environment [12].

Vaccination and use of perioperative antibiotics are important to prevent implant-related meningitis. Pneumococcal vaccination guidelines have been created to reduce the incidence of bacterial meningitis in patients with cochlear implants. However, there is no agreed practice regarding the vaccination schedule. Pneumococcal vaccine is included in the routine vaccination calendar in many countries, so it is important to know the previous vaccination status of the patients to be operated. If the patient has not been vaccinated before implantation, vaccination with pneumococcal polysaccharide vaccine (PPSV23) should be recommended. In addition, one additional dose of vaccination is recommended for patients with cochlear implants 5 years after the last PPSV23 [22]. Time of vaccination is also important. Vaccination should be completed at least 2 weeks or more before cochlear implant surgery.

71.6 Wound Site Infection (Biofilm)

Wound infections seen after cochlear implantation are one of the worst complications. The infection can be complicated by the foreign body effect of the implanted device. Post-CI infections that can be cured by conservative outpatient treatment are classified as minor complications, and those that require hospitalization and parenteral antibiotherapy as major complications. The incidence of all skin infections after CI ranges from 1.7% to 4.1% (27). Although in the form of a small localized inflammatory reaction, post-CI infections cause delay in implant use or stop the use of implants for a while. Serious infections can lead to extrusion and may require removal of the implant in most cases [28]. Therefore, even a mild infection requires serious follow-up and management.

Being a child and the presence of additional comorbidities are risk factors for wound site infection after cochlear implantation. Being a child includes a high risk for head traumas and has an immune system immaturity. Additional comorbidities may contribute to the development of local infections by adversely affecting wound site healing [28, 29]. Suture materials and application properties used in surgery may also contribute to the increase of infection risk. During wound closure, it is important to avoid long stitches close to the skin. In addition, most suture infections occur with a delayed onset due to non-absorbable polypropylene stitches. As a typical feature, a pointed polypropylene suture tip located close to the skin surface causes granuloma formation, inflammation, and infection, respectively [28]. If the patient has previously received radiotherapy to the surgical area due to head and neck tumors, the risk of wound site healing and wound site infection may increase due to decreased collagen support [30].

Prophylactic use of cefazolin 30 min before the perioperative skin incision significantly reduces the rate of wound infection within 1 month postoperatively. Clindamycin and vancomycin can be used in patients with penicillin allergy [31].

Wound site hyperemia, edema, and tenderness are symptoms of wound site infection. It is important to take a culture, if available, for the management of infection. *S. aureus* grows in the cultures of most patients. *P. aeruginosa* is one of the most common microorganisms after *S. aureus. Staphylococcus epidermidis*, which is found in the skin flora of the patient, is a less common isolated microorganism. Preoperative antiseptic cleaning and prophylactic use of perioperative antibiotics are important to minimize perioperative inoculation of pathogens from patients' own skin microflora [32, 33].

In the presence of postimplantation wound site infections, it is important to reduce the microorganism burden by draining the abscess or collection at the wound site. After the intervention, cleaning the wound with antiseptic solutions and applying pressure dressing should be done because it reduces dead spaces. Even if the culture antibiogram has been studied, intravenous empirical antibiotherapy should be started immediately until the result is obtained. Ceftazidime and tazocin or ceftriaxone and ciprofloxacin combinations can be started [34]. Treatment of an infected implant is complicated by the presence of bacterial biofilms on the surface of implanted devices. Therefore, long-term administration of intravenous antibiotics for at least 6 weeks is advocated. In addition, direct topical antibiotic application to the device may aid the treatment [35, 36].

Surgical intervention should be considered if the infection does not regress in patients who are closely followed up with medical treatment and wound site dressing. The infected area can be cleaned surgically by moving the implant body to an area of healthy skin. However, repetitive surgery sessions may be required in patients undergoing rescue surgery and iatrogenic damage may occur in the device. In addition, it should not be forgotten that the infection has the risk to be carried to the inner ear with the implant electrode and cause meningitis development. Therefore, it should be kept in mind that early explantation should be considered before the spread of infection in order to facilitate rapid wound healing. During surgery, the electrode is cut and left in the cochlea and the second operation is delayed until the infection is completely resolved [28, 37]. Although there is no consensus on the time to wait for insertion of the new device, a waiting period of at least 3 months after the infection resolves will reduce the risk of reinfection.

71.7 Biofilm

Biofilms are the most common form of microbial life in which microorganisms are found as clusters of cells in a matrix they produce. Because of this matrix, microorganisms are more likely to be resistant to the host immune system and anti-infective therapy [38]. Biofilm formation in all implanted medical devices, including the cochlear implant, causes medical treatment failure and surgical removal of the implant [29, 39].

S. aureus and *P. aeruginosa* have been shown to be responsible for the majority of biofilm-related implant infections in pathogen isolations performed microbiologically in infected cochlear implants [39, 40]. Other causative pathogens are *S. pyogenes* and *S. Epidermidis* [39]. In long-term parenteral treatment with broad-spectrum antibiotics such as vancomycin, despite repeated drainage and massive debridement, the infection cannot be cured, and the implant needs to be removed in almost all cases with biofilms. In addition, even if the infection regresses, it is possible for biofilms to cause permanent inflammation by causing an allergic reaction. In this case, biofilms may cause device malfunction and reimplantation surgery may be required [39, 40].

71.8　Conclusion

Cochlear implantation is a safe and widely accepted procedure for the cases with severe-to-profound hearing loss in all around the world. However, infections due to cochlear implant like the other medical devices and host infections can be life-threatening or result in explantation and reimplantation of cochlear implant, since implants are vital for children and adult patients in their life. Early diagnosis and meticulous management are mandatory.

References

1. Broomfield SJ, Murphy J, Wild DC, Emmett SR, O'Donoghue GM. Writing for the UK National Paediatric CI surgical audit group. Results of a prospective surgical audit of bilateral paediatric cochlear implantation in the UK. Cochlear Implants Int. 2014;15(5):246–53.
2. Vila PM, Ghogomu NT, Odom-John AR, Hullar TE, Hirose K. Infectious complications of pediatric cochlear implants are highly influenced by otitis media. Int J Pediatr Otorhinolaryngol. 2017;97:76–82.
3. Lin YS. Management of otitis media-related diseases in children with a cochlear implant. Acta Otolaryngol. 2009;129:254–60.
4. Bhatia K, Gibbin KP, Nikolopoulos TP, O'Donoghue GM. Surgical complications and their management in a series of 300 consecutive pediatric cochlear implantations. Otol Neurotol. 2004;25:730–9.
5. Shirai N, Pireciado D. Otitis media: what is new? Curr Opin Otolaryngol Head Neck Surg. 2019;27(6):495–8
6. Zawawi F, Cardona I, Akinpelu OV, Daniel SJ. Acute mastoiditis in children with cochlear implants: is explantation required? Otolaryngol Head Neck Surg. 2014;151:394–8.
7. American Academy of Pediatrics Subcommittee on Management of Acute Otitis Media. Diagnosis and management of acute otitis media. Pediatrics. 2014;113:1451–65.
8. Kempf HG, Johann K, Lenarz T. Complications in pediatric cochlear implant surgery. Eur Arch Otorhinolaryngol. 1999;256:128–32.
9. Lassig AA, Zwolan TA, Telian SA. Cochlear implant failures and revision. Otol Neurotol. 2005;26:624–34.
10. Rubin LG, Papsin B. Committee on infectious diseases and section on otolaryngology- head and neck surgery. Cochlear implants in children: surgical site infections and prevention and treatment of acute otitis media and meningitis. Pediatrics. 2010;126:381–91.

11. Cunningham CD 3rd, Slattery WH 3rd, Luxford WM. Postoperative infection in cochlear implant patients. Otolaryngol Head Neck Surg. 2004;131:109–14.
12. Raveh E, Ulanovski D, Attias J, Shkedy Y, Sokolov M. Acute mastoiditis in children with a cochlear implant. Int J Pediatr Otorhinolaryngol. 2016;81:80–3.
13. Oestreicher-Kedem Y, Ravey E, Kornreich L, Popovtzer A, Buller N, Nageris B. Complications of mastoiditis in children at the onset of a new millennium. Ann Otol Rhinol Laryngol. 2005;114:147–52.
14. Migirov L, Yakirevitch A, Henkin Y, Kaplan-Neeman R, Kronenberg J. Acute otitis media and mastoiditis following cochlear implantation. Int J Pediatr Otorhiniolaryngol. 2006;70:899–903.
15. Neely JG (1993) Complications of temporal bone infection. In: Cummings C, Fredrickson JM, Harker LA, Krause CJ, Schuller DE (Eds) Otolaryngology Head and Neck Surgery Mosby-Year Book St Louis
16. Osborn HA, Cushing SL, Gordon KA, James AL, Papsin BC. The management of acute mastoiditis in children with cochlear implants: saving the device. Cochlear Implants Int. 2013;14:252–6.
17. Kempf HG, Tempel S, Johann K, Lenarz T. Komplikationen der cochlear implant-chirurgie bei kindern und erwachsenen. Laryngorhinootologie. 1999;78:529–37.
18. Kaila R, Evans RA. Cochlear implant infection due to cholesteatoma. Cochlear Implants Int. 2005;6:141–6.
19. Bibas A, Phillips S, Bailey CM, Papsin BC. Chronic suppurative otitis media following paediatric cochlear implantation. Cochlear Implants Int. 2006;7:167–78.
20. Baruah P, Hanvey K, Irving R, Tzifa K. Impact of chronic suppurative otitis media in pediatric cochlear implant recipients-insight into the challenges from a tertiary referral center in UK. Otol Neurotol. 2017;38:672–7.
21. Morris P. Chronic suppurative otitis media. BMJ Clin Evid. 2012;0507:1–45.
22. Kahue CN, Sweeney AD, Carlson ML, Haynes DS. Vaccination recommendations and risk of meningitis following cochlear implantation. Curr Opin Otolaryngol Head Neck Surg. 2014;22:359–66.
23. Reefhuis J, Honein MA, Whitney CG, et al. Risk of bacterial meningitis in children with cochlear implants. N Engl J Med. 2003;349:435–45.
24. Wei BP, Shepherd RK, Robins-Browne RM, Clark GM, O'Leary SJ. Pneumococcal meningitis post-cochlear implantation: potential routes of infection and pathophysiology. Otolaryngol Head Neck Surg. 2010;143(5 Suppl 3):S15–23.
25. Clark GM. Cochlear implants: fundamentals and applications. New York: Springer; 2003.
26. Zimmerli W, Waldvogel FA, Vaudaux P, Nydegger UE. Pathogenesis of foreign body infection: description and characteristics of an animal model. J Infect Dis. 1982;146:487–97.
27. Putz K, Hayani K, Zar FA. Meningitis. Prim Care. 2013;40:707–26.
28. Low WK, Rangabashyam M, Wang F. Management of major post-cochlear implant wound infections. Eur Arch Otorhinolaryngol. 2014;271:2409–13.
29. Gawęcki W, Karlik M, Borucki Ł, Szyfter-Harris J, Wróbel M. Skin flap complications after cochlear implantations. Eur Arch Otorhinolaryngol. 2016;273:4175–83.
30. Waldman EH, Niparko JK. The avoidance and treatment of scalp flap complications in cochlear implant surgery. Oper Tech Otolaryngol Head Neck Surg. 2005;16:149–53.
31. Vijendren A, Borsetto D, Barker EJ, Manjaly JG, Tysome JR, Axon PR, Donnelly NP, Bance ML. A systematic review on prevention and management of wound infections from cochlear implantation. Clin Otolaryngol. 2019;44:1059–70.
32. Hopfenspirger MT, Levine SC, Rimell FL. Infectious complications in pediatric cochlear implants. Laryngoscope. 2007;117:1825–9.
33. Darouiche RO. Antimicrobial approaches for preventing infections associated with surgical implants. Clin Infect Dis. 2003;36:1284–9.
34. Kabelka Z, Groh D, Katra R, Jurovcik M. Bacterial infection complications in children with cochlear implants in the Czech Republic. Int J Pediatr Otorhinolaryngol. 2010;74:499–502.
35. Antonelli PJ, Lee JC, Burne RA. Bacterial biofilms may contribute to persistent cochlear implant infection. Otol Neurotol. 2004;25:953–7.

36. Yu KC, Hegarty JL, Gantz BJ, Lalwani AK. Conservative management of infections in cochlear implant recipients. Otolaryngol Head Neck Surg. 2001;125:66–70.
37. Zeitler DM, Budenz CL, Roland JT Jr. Revision cochlear implantation. Curr Opin Otolaryngol Head Neck Surg. 2009;17:334–8.
38. Cerca N, Martins S, Sillankorva S, Jefferson KK, Pier GB, Oliveira R, Azeredo J. Effects of growth in the presence of subinhibitory concentrations of dicloxacillin on Staphylococcus epidermidis and Staphylococcus haemolyticus biofilms. Appl Environ Microbiol. 2005;71:8677–82.
39. Höing B, Kirchhoff L, Arnolds J, Hussain T, Buer J, Lang S, Arweiler-Harbeck D, Steinmann J. Bioactive glass granules inhibit mature bacterial biofilms on the surfaces of cochlear implants. Otol Neurotol. 2018;39:985–91.
40. Kao WK, Gagnon PM, Vogel JP, Chole RA. Surface charge modification decreases Pseudomonas aeruginosa adherence in vitro and bacterial persistence in an in vivo implant model. Laryngoscope. 2017;127:1655–61.

Travel-Related Paediatric ENT Infections

72

Mehmet Arıcı, Cüneyt Yılmazer, and Oleg Khorov

72.1 Introduction

Travel-related illnesses are those which result from travel by a patient. They may be caused by the motion of travel, moving to higher elevations, an alteration in the climate or by infections that are endemic to a particular region.

The overall trend is for leisure travel, i.e. travel for recreational purposes, to keep increasing on a worldwide scale. Alongside the better-known and popular tourist destinations, more and more people are travelling to areas which are far off the beaten track and thus considered more exotic, but which also entail a number of different health risks [1–3]. A particularly challenging situation occurs when children who have grown up in a developed, urban environment visit the original homelands of their parents, which may be very different from the children's usual environment. These children then remain for lengthy periods in a developing country, where they may be exposed to considerable risks, especially if the place they visit is remote. It is common for children to develop signs of disease following such trips [2, 3].

The range of diseases associated with travel that a paediatrician or general practitioner may encounter in a child includes malaria, diarrhoeal illness, typhoid or paratyphoid fever and skin conditions, including cutaneous larva migrans. Despite the fact that there are precautions which may prevent such disorders, some

M. Arıcı (✉)
Section of Otorhinolaryngology, Adıyaman Training and Research Hospital, University of Health Sciences, Adıyaman, Turkey

C. Yılmazer
Section of Otorhinolaryngology, Adıyaman Training and Research Hospital, Adıyaman, Turkey

O. Khorov
Department of Otorhinolaryngology, Grodno State Medical University, Grodno, Belarus

© The Author(s), under exclusive license to Springer Nature Switzerland AG 2022
C. Cingi et al. (eds.), *Pediatric ENT Infections*,
https://doi.org/10.1007/978-3-030-80691-0_72

travellers, especially those who make their own travel arrangements, fail to prepare adequately, and return in a diseased state [1–3].

When evaluating a case involving a child who has been travelling, the clinician needs to bear in mind where and when the travel occurred, what kind of environment the child will have encountered and whether any precautions were taken before undertaking the journey. Thus, malaria is less likely in a child who has been fully compliant with malarial prophylaxis. A child visiting Southeast Asia may have contracted dengue if they now exhibit pyrexia. On the other hand, malaria and yellow fever are of relevance only in certain portions of the African continent. One study ascertained that children who had attended a travel clinic prior to the journey were likely to have diarrhoeal illness, abdominodynia or pyrexia when presenting on their return. The majority of illness had its onset in the initial 10 days of travelling. A large-scale study of children with travel-related diseases identified one of three regions as having the highest risk: Asia, sub-Saharan Africa or Latin America, and the most frequently occurring complaints were diarrhoeal illness, skin problems, systemic illness with pyrexia or respiratory infections. Diarrhoeal illnesses occurred in 28% of travellers and pyrexia in 23%. Sub-Saharan African travel carried the highest risk for malaria, whilst travel to Latin America was the most likely to result in skin conditions, such as cutaneous larva migrans [2–4].

It is important to remember that a child who has just come back from travel in tropical regions and is febrile may still be suffering from any of the usual infections commonly seen amongst children of that age, such as middle ear infection or pneumonia of bacterial origin. It is common not to identify a clear cause for a pyrexia of unknown origin in a child who is admitted to hospital after returning from a tropical region. Whilst they are not common amongst children with a history of overseas travel, pyogenic arthritis, pyomyositis, deep bone infections, rheumatic fever or meningitis all can and do occur [5].

Children travelling often contract an infection of the respiratory system, with influenza and parainfluenza being the most frequently occurring viral pathogens. The GeoSentinel study, which looked at disease occurrence in travellers, found that influenza was most common in travellers to the Northern hemisphere in the winter months. Travelling for longer than 30 days made influenza more likely, along with infection of the lower respiratory tract. Travellers who were visiting friends or relatives in the parents' country of origin had a sixfold increased risk of influenza [6].

Tuberculosis is not frequent as a travel-related infection. Transmission is not straightforward. The likelihood of being infected depends on the length of contact with infected individuals and the stage of the disease in that person or persons. An individual with cavitating pulmonary lesions represents the highest risk. Amongst children in the USA, a large number of tuberculosis cases are found to be refugees, foreign-born individuals, or contacts thereof. According to one study, some 80% of cases of tuberculosis in children were connected to travelling. The most significant risk factor for tuberculosis was spending time with parents or other family members in places with a high number of tuberculosis cases [5–7].

72.2 Malaria

The organisms which cause malaria are protozoal parasites of the genus *Plasmodium*, which infect red blood cells. The key species of significance to humans are *P. falciparum*, *P. vivax*, *P. ovale*, *P. malariae* and *P. knowlesi*. These organisms have an insect vector, the *Anopheles* mosquito, which is found in many parts of the globe, such as sub-Saharan Africa, Southeastern Asia and the Pacific, the Amazon region of South America, and some regions in Central America. It is also endemic to the USA. The distribution of *P. knowlesi* covers the Malay Peninsula, Borneo and the Philippines [8].

Disease control has largely failed in Africa as the malarial parasite, *P. falciparum*, has acquired resistance to the usual medications. *P. falciparum* generally possesses resistance to chloroquine, except strains found in Central America, and has acquired resistance to mefloquine in parts of Asia (in particular, the areas surrounding Thailand, Myanmar, Laos and Cambodia). Other than in Africa, malaria is usually due to *P. vivax*. The facilities to diagnose and treat malaria are usually better in Asia than in Africa, which accounts for the lower prevalence of *P. falciparum*. However, some strains of *P. vivax* are also treatment-resistant, such as those in Indonesia and Malaysia, which are no longer sensitive to chloroquine. It is unusual to isolate *P. ovale* unless there has been contact with Africa. The latest reports indicate that malarial parasites in Southeastern Asia are becoming resistant to artemisinin and its synthetic derivatives [8–10].

72.2.1 Clinical Manifestations

Generally, malaria in children presents non-specifically. Frequently noted symptoms are pyrexia, vomiting, cephalgia, feeling suddenly cold, muscular ache and loss of appetite. There may also be gut-related manifestations, such as diarrhoea, abdominodynia and bloating. A low platelet count is a common finding. Malaria is severe when the parasite becomes intracerebral, there is acute respiratory distress syndrome, a marked degree of anaemia secondary to the parasite or multiple organ systems are involved. In these cases, death is the most likely outcome in the absence of admission to hospital followed by supportive treatment and antimalarial pharmacotherapy. There is a high risk of fatality if coma, fits, metabolic acidosis, septic shock or extremely low blood sugar occurs [8]. The majority of severe cases of malaria are in patients infected with *P. falciparum*, albeit children below the age of 1 year may also become severely anaemic following infection with *P. vivax* [9–11].

72.2.2 Management

Updated guidelines were issued by the World Health Organisation in 2015 for how to manage malaria [12]. In cases due to *P. falciparum* without complications and where chloroquine resistance is present, it is recommended to treat with agents derived from artemisinin. Combinations which are currently employed across the globe are Artemether-lumefantrine, artesunate plus amodiaquine, artesunate plus mefloquine, and artesunate plus sulphadoxine-pyrimethamine. The sole combination amongst this list with FDA approval in the USA is artemether and lumefantrine, and the course duration is 3 days [13]. If malaria lacks complications, there are other licensed options with proven efficacy available in the USA, namely atovaquone-proguanil, or quinine alongside tetracycline, doxycycline or clindamycin. Some cases of *P. falciparum* malaria, where the organism does not possess resistance, can be treated with chloroquine, provided there are no complications. These cases are usually acquired in Haiti or areas of Central America lying to the west of the Panama Canal [14].

If *P. vivax* possesses sensitivity to chloroquine, the first-line management involves chloroquine plus primaquine. However, if the parasite is resistant, or thought to be, pharmacotherapy with derivatives of artemisinin is appropriate. It is advised that primaquine be administered for 2 weeks so that the hypnozoite (dormant) life stage of the parasite in the liver is prevented and thus malarial recurrence halted. A case of severe malaria secondary to *P. vivax* or *P. knowlesi* needs to be managed with pharmacotherapy based on artemisinin. Primaquine has the potential side effect of haemolysis in patients who are glucose-6-phosphate dehydrogenase deficient; thus, this metabolic abnormality should be screened for first. It is beneficial to transfuse red blood cells to paediatric cases of malaria of marked severity where there is respiratory distress or metabolic acidosis has developed. It is vital to keep checking blood glucose, as hypoglycaemia is a possibility. A seizure may result either from extremely low blood glucose or intracerebral infection [12–14].

72.3 Leishmaniasis

Leishmaniasis refers to a range of disorders, all of which result from infection by the protozoal parasitic organisms of the *Leishmania* genus. The insect vector is the sand fly (female insects only). Leishmaniasis is native to 88 countries in the world. On a global scale, it produces a high burden of disease and results in numerous deaths. Developed countries are seeing increasing numbers of cases of Leishmaniasis, linked to globalisation, population movement and the popularity of international travel. Furthermore, Leishmaniasis is being increasingly noted in patients with immunocompromise through chronic disease, cancer, post organ transplantation and as a result of AIDS. These disorders are therefore a concern for public health. Infection with *Leishmania* leads to three different types of syndromic presentation, namely cutaneous, mucocutaneous or visceral. Involvement of the mucocutaneous system may develop if the lesion extends from the cutaneous system into the mucosae. This may occur directly or spread may be haematogenous or via the lymphatic system. Mucocutaneous Leishmaniasis is generally localised to the linings of the mouth and nose, with the pharynx or larynx also sometimes affected. Painless, deforming lesions of the mouth and nose, metastasising to neighbouring areas with the appearance of mushroom and erosive ulcers on the tongue, mucous membrane of the cheeks and nose, are characteristic. Scars on the skin leave cosmetic defects and disfigure patients. Failure to diagnose and manage this syndrome may result in disfigurement, since the lesions destroy the pharyngeal, nasal and palatal tissues. Since mucocutaneous Leishmaniasis always involves the region of the body of greatest interest to ENT specialists and since children are often affected, paediatricians and otorhinolaryngologists need to have a good knowledge of how this disorder may present and be alert to the possibility, especially if a patient has travelled to the regions where Leishmaniasis is prevalent. Clinicians suspecting mucocutaneous Leishmaniasis should refer the case to an ENT specialist for appropriate evaluation and to ensure the correct management [15, 16].

Etiotropic therapy of visceral leishmaniasis includes the use of pentavalent antimony preparations. In case of insufficient effectiveness, therapy is supplemented with amphotericin B.

72.4 HIV Infection and Paediatric ENT

HIV is a retrovirus within the subgroup Lentivirus which is responsible for AIDS. HIV exists in two separate forms: HIV1 and HIV2. HIV1 is the most common form of the virus and is found all across the world, whereas HIV2 is generally endemic to West Africa and Asia. HIV2 causes a less virulent form of AIDS. There are three modes of viral transmission: through sexual intercourse, via blood transfusion or vertically (i.e. materno-foetal) [17, 18].

Sexual transmission is especially likely to occur from anal intercourse, whether between a male and female or two males, since the epithelial lining of the anus lacks the strength of the vaginal epithelium and microinjury allows for passage of the virus. Vaginal intercourse and oral sex carry a somewhat lower risk. Bloodborne transmission is one of the key routes for infection in richer countries, where intravenous drug abuse may involve the sharing of paraphernalia. Transmission may also occur due to contaminated transfusions of whole blood or blood products [17, 18].

The highest risk of materno-foetal vertical transmission occurs during birth, where there is direct contact between the baby and the mother's circulating blood. It has also been shown that HIV can cross the materno-foetal interface (i.e. the placenta) up to the end of the second trimester. Breastfeeding may also facilitate transmission, given the presence of viable virus in colostrum and breast milk of infected mothers [19, 20].

72.4.1 ENT Manifestations of HIV in Children

Whilst the various conditions associated with HIV positivity are the same in both adults and young children, there are certain conditions which are more typical in an infected child. For a young child, the most likely way for infection to have occurred is by vertical transmission from the mother. Occasionally, a child becomes infected after being sexually abused, or as a result of receiving a contaminated transfusion of whole blood or blood products. Around 40% of young children who are HIV positive show signs of the disorder in the ear, nose and throat region [16, 19, 20].

Children with HIV have a considerably higher propensity than HIV+ adults to suffer from infections by viruses or bacteria. Thus, they may suffer from repeated or chronic episodes of middle ear infection, rhinosinusitis with a persistent nasal discharge and infection of the parotid gland [16, 19, 20].

The most frequently occurring mucocutaneous manifestation of HIV in children is oral candidal infection. HIV is the underlying cause in between 60 and 75% of children who present with symptoms of oral candidiasis. Oesophageal candidiasis occurs rather less commonly, but the consequences may be more concerning, as it may lead to pain on swallowing and prevent growth of the child, particularly if the child is very young or still breastfeeding. HIV may also produce other signs in the mouth, such as herpetic cold sores or petechial haemorrhages on the palate due to a platelet deficiency [19, 20].

72.4.2 Ear Problems

Young children with HIV are not only at a higher risk of developing disorders of the middle ear, but they also have a greater risk of auditory impairment of sensorineural type [16]. One study based in the USA looked at the frequency of auditory impairment in young children who were infected with HIV or who had undergone exposure to HIV but were not HIV+ and compared the rate with children in general. The young children with HIV had a 20% risk of auditory impairment, compared with a risk of 10.5% in children with a history of exposure, but actually HIV-. Once adjusted to account for differences in educational attainment by care givers, the odds ratio for auditory impairment in a young child who is HIV+ was found to be 2.13 (CI 95%: 0.95–4.76; $p = 0.07$). Being infected with HIV at the time of birth significantly increases the chance of a child suffering from auditory impairment [16].

72.5   High Altitude Sickness Amongst Children

The most frequently occurring altitude disorder is acute mountain sickness (AMS). An individual's chances of suffering from AMS is linked to individual predisposition, the altitude travelled to and how rapidly that altitude was reached. AMS rarely affects individuals at elevations below 2000 m (6560 ft). However, around 1 in 4 adults and children experience AMS if they sleep at an altitude of between 2000 and 3000 m. A number of cities and most of the skiing locations in the west of the USA are found at such elevations [21–24]. In the majority of cases, high altitude illness (HAI) in children is preventable provided certain prophylactic measures are taken. Where it does occur, treatment can usually be initiated before the serious complications of the condition, such as pulmonary or cerebral oedema, have developed.

Some earlier studies of observational type and involving low numbers of individuals appeared to show an increased risk of AMS in children or adolescents, compared to adults, when the ascent to a high altitude (i.e. greater than 3500 m) form zero altitude happened within the space of a few hours [25, 26]. Subsequent research, with higher numbers of individuals, indicates that the true rate may be the same in adults and children, or even lower in children.

One study of observational type examined the effect of rapid ascent in several families containing a total of 157 children. All had undergone a 3450 m increase in altitude in a two-and-a-half-hour period. The highest rate of AMS was in adults, with a 45% risk, followed by a 37% risk in adolescents. The lowest risk was amongst children—just 30% [27]. AMS was clustered in families and accounted for between 25 and 50% of variability. This study was the first to show evidence of a genetic basis for the disorder [27].

A different study involved 48 children with the same pattern of rise in altitude as the previous study. After 6 h, 25% of the children had symptoms of AMS, but this fell to 21% 12 h later and was only 8% 42 h after the ascent. All the participants in the study had at most mild symptoms of AMS and no children needed to be treated by returning them to a lower altitude [28].

Finally, a third study involving the same conditions but with 118 children assessed, all between 6 and 16 years old, discovered that the risk of AMS 40 hours after ascending was 6%. Thus, it was confirmed that AMS resolves very quickly even without intervention [29].

In conclusion, then, AMS is no more likely in a child than an adult, and may actually be less likely. Moreover, ascending at a more leisurely pace makes AMS less likely to occur.

72.5.1 Clinical Manifestations

Young children suffering from AMS do not have any specific presenting features, although they may be less willing to play, look pale, act fussily, decline food and have trouble sleeping [23, 24, 30]. Adults experiencing high altitude sickness typically experience cephalgia, possibly with dyspnoea, vertigo, insomnia, loss of appetite, excessive tiredness, nausea and vomiting. These symptoms are generally the same in an older child or adolescent [24]. The symptoms of AMS typically do not begin straightaway, usually starting between 6 and 12 h after reaching the high elevation, but their onset has been reported anytime between 1 h and 1 day after reaching high altitude [31]. There is usually a peak in symptomatic severity following the initial night at altitude and, provided the patient goes no higher, symptoms resolve within 24 h. Should the patient then ascend further, AMS may recur. Occasionally, AMS has a duration of several days, even without further increases in altitude. In this situation, where the usual therapeutic measures fail, the child will need to descend to a lower altitude.

A trial of supplementary oxygen may help to prove a putative diagnosis of AMS. If the diagnosis is correct, supplying oxygen through a nasal cannula at a rate of 2–4 L/min for a period lasting between a quarter of an hour and 20 min will cause cessation of symptoms, including cephalgia. An alternative test is to arrange for the child to spend a short period of time at a lower altitude. This is particularly effective in young children. In either case, this test should precede other measures, to ensure diagnostic clarity [29–31].

Where symptoms have only begun at least 48 h after a traveller arrives at high altitude, cephalgia is not present, shortness of breath is present even without exertion and oxygen does not induce rapid symptomatic resolution, AMS is unlikely to be the correct diagnosis. Except in cases of diagnostic difficulty, there is no need for imaging studies or laboratory tests in suspected AMS. The differential diagnosis for AMS includes carbon monoxide toxicity, migrainous headache, dehydration, gross fatigue, hyponatraemia, a viral infection, a bacterial infection (affecting the lungs or the ear) or an unnoticed injury, as may occur with an abrasion of the cornea. AMS is diagnosed in young children after exhausting all other diagnostic possibilities.

AMS does not result in pyrexia; hence an increase in body temperature in a child at high altitude should not be attributed to the disorder. It should be investigated as a pyrexia of unknown origin. Frequently, AMS is only diagnosed when other possible aetiologies have been excluded. Treating physicians need to closely monitor what happens when a child receives oxygen. If doubt persists, a lengthier period of monitoring may be beneficial in making a final diagnostic evaluation [29–31].

72.5.2 Diagnosis and Treatment

To diagnose AMS, doctors rely on a characteristic clinical presentation, in which the child vomits, feels unwell, has a headache, acts fussily and potentially experiences dyspnoea. Such a clinical picture should have developed no later than 24 h after the child ascended to high altitude. No other condition, such as middle ear infection, a lung infection or a viral episode, should be present. A swift symptomatic improvement when additional oxygen is supplied helps to confirm the diagnosis [32–37]. Management of high altitude sickness does not differ between adults and children [28–30]. Children whose symptoms do not improve or deteriorate are treated by returning them to lower altitudes. Those accompanying a patient with AMS need to monitor the situation for potential deterioration, since AMS may develop into high altitude cerebral oedema at some altitudes.

72.5.3 Prevention and Prophylactic Drug Treatment

Ascending to high altitudes gradually and allowing the body to adjust is by far the optimal way to prevent AMS. Those who ascend to high altitudes to take part in vigorous exercise, such as skiing, trekking or rock climbing, need to be advised to begin such activities gradually. It is essential to maintain sufficient fluid intake. However, excessive fluid intake runs the risk of causing hyponatraemia.

There are no studies which have examined the role of acetazolamide as a preventive treatment in paediatric patients who ascend rapidly. There is a single study conducted prospectively and with an observational methodology which involved 48 individuals, either older children or adolescents, all of whom rapidly ascended to an altitude of 3450 m. Whilst 18 individuals (38%) had symptoms of AMS in the first 3 days, no pharmacotherapy was required and no individual needed to descend to recover. The results support the notion that there is no necessity for older children or adolescents to receive pharmacotherapy prophylactically, even if gradual acclimatisation is not undertaken [30, 31].

High altitude pulmonary oedema often causes a gradually worsening cough, dyspnoea on slight or even no exertion, and sputum that contains froth and is frequently rust-coloured. On examination, patients may be tachypnoeic, cyanosed, have a raised heart rate and auscultation may reveal crackles throughout the lung fields. If an X-ray is obtained, it shows widespread interstitial changes consistent with pulmonary oedema not due to cardiac abnormalities. This condition can come on slowly over a period of hours or days, but it may also begin abruptly. It may or may not follow on from previous AMS. In some patients, pulmonary oedema develops each time they are located above a particular elevation. Thus, there may be an altitude acting as a threshold for the condition in that person. A past history of this type of pulmonary oedema indicates the presence of genetic or physiological risk factors. This is why rapidly reaching the same height triggers the disorder. If such patients need to keep ascending to the same altitude, they may avoid the development of pulmonary oedema by climbing slowly [30, 31].

It is worth observing that high altitude pulmonary oedema rarely results in an increase in body temperature exceeding 38.3 °C. Thus, a rise in temperature beyond this should prompt the search for a pyrexia of unknown origin or another underlying condition. In evaluating a young child with marked pyrexia, the age and their immunisation history need to be borne in mind. It is possible for high altitude pulmonary oedema to occur concurrently with an infective episode of the respiratory system.

In a paediatric patient, it is necessary to exclude pneumonia, cardiac failure and other conditions not related to the heart which may cause oedema in the lungs.

72.5.3.1 Diagnosis

High altitude pulmonary oedema manifests as laboured breathing and hypoxia, with an onset within 24–48 h after ascending to a high altitude. The condition may sometimes be even more abrupt. The child may cough or make a rattling noise whilst breathing. Babies and younger children may well present with the features of AMS, which are not unique to one disorder, i.e. fussy behaviour, moving less, anorexia and vomiting. An older child or an adolescent might produce sputum, which contains froth and is rust-coloured. When X-rays are available, the appearances are of widespread alteration in the interstitium of a type found in pulmonary oedema when the cause is not related to the heart.

72.5.3.2 Treatment

Treating high altitude pulmonary oedema in a child unused to being at high elevations aims to achieve the same objective as with an adult, i.e. lowering rapidly the pressure within the pulmonary arteries [31].

72.6 Epistaxis and Rhinitis

Nosebleeds occur in adults and children alike, when exposed to high altitudes. Epistaxis is caused by freezing temperature air drying out the lining of the nose to a marked degree. Small calibre blood vessels are then inclined to burst. Epistaxis is not in itself a reason to avoid high altitude pursuits, unless there is another condition present rendering epistaxis more likely to be copious, notably high blood pressure or a bleeding diathesis. Unless such a condition is well-controlled, epistaxis may escalate an individual's risk. Rhinitis often develops in paediatric patients following repeated epistaxis [34, 35].

72.7 Respiratory Tract Infections and Nasal Obstruction

Another complication of being at a high altitude is an increased susceptibility to infections of the respiratory tract. High altitudes impair the ability of leucocytes to phagocytose bacteria, which renders infection more probable. Additionally, the combined effect of hypoxia and exposure to freezing, dry air is to impair mucociliary clearance. Mucociliary clearance is a major component of innate immune function and is key to clearing away particulate matter from the airways. Impaired clearance contributes to susceptibility to infection. When a child breathes in cold air, the nasal lining becomes congested, and this then means that efficient heat transfer between the air and blood is prevented, both during inspiration and expiration. Furthermore, cold air triggers an increased level of secretion by the lining of the nose. Taken together, these alterations may mean the nose is partially obstructed. Children who are already predisposed to a degree of nasal obstruction, perhaps from abnormal nasal anatomy, are even more affected than usual by these physiological compensatory actions and thus more prone to suffer a respiratory infection [34, 35].

72.8 High Altitude Periodic Breathing of Sleep

Periodic breathing of sleep at high altitude refers to a variant of Cheyne-Stokes type respiration virtually confined in occurrence to non-REM sleep. Hyperventilation may be so marked that the patient is roused from sleep. Children are probably at lower risk for this condition than adults. One study looked at respiration in a group containing 20 children between the ages of 9 and 12 years old and their male parents. The study was observational in design. Respiratory function was compared at 3450 m and 490 m altitude. The measurements included respiratory inductive plethysmography, pulse oximetry, and end-tidal carbon dioxide level. The children had significantly lower levels of periodic breathing than adults. There was no significant difference between adults and children in terms of hyperventilation and drops in O_2 overnight [33]. Half the children were diagnosed with AMS, whilst only 30% of the adults showed symptoms of the condition during the research period. These findings may be interpreted to show that the children's respiratory pattern exhibited greater stability as a result of a diminished CO_2 threshold for the occurrence of apnoea, rather than indicating they have a higher tolerance for elevated altitudes.

References

1. Fox TG, Manaloor JJ, Christenson JC. Travel-related infections in children. Pediatr Clin North Am. 2013;60(2):507–27. https://doi.org/10.1016/j.pcl.2012.12.004.
2. Bacaner N, Stauffer B, Boulware DR, et al. Travel medicine considerations for north American immigrants visiting friends and relatives. JAMA. 2004;291:2856–64.
3. Han P, Yanni E, Jentes ES, et al. Health challenges of young travelers visiting friends and relatives compared with those traveling for other purposes. Pediatr Infect Dis J. 2012;31:915–9.
4. Zimmermann P, Mühlethaler K, Furrer H, Staehelin C. Travellers returning ill from the tropics - a descriptive retrospective study. Trop Dis Travel Med Vaccines. 2016;2:6. https://doi.org/10.1186/s40794-016-0021-1.
5. Alabi BS, Abdulkarim AA, Olatoke F, et al. Acute otitis media–a common diag- nosis among febrile children in the tropics. Trop Doct. 2006;36:31–2.
6. Leder K, Sundararajan V, Weld L, et al. Respiratory tract infections in travelers: a review of the GeoSentinel surveillance network. Clin Infect Dis. 2003;36:399–406.
7. Korzeniewski K, Nitsch-Osuch A, Lass A, Guzek A. Respiratory infections in travelers returning from the tropics. Adv Exp Med Biol. 2015;849:75–82. https://doi.org/10.1007/5584_2014_89.
8. Tripathy R, Parida S, Das L, et al. Clinical manifestations and predictors of severe malaria in Indian children. Pediatrics. 2007;120:e454–60.
9. Stauffer WM, Cartwright CP, Olson DA, et al. Diagnostic performance of rapid diagnostic tests versus blood smears for malaria in US clinical practice. Clin Infect Dis. 2009;49:908–13.
10. Poschl B, Waneesorn J, Thekisoe O, et al. Comparative diagnosis of malaria infections by microscopy, nested PCR, and LAMP in northern Thailand. Am J Trop Med Hyg. 2010;83:56–60.
11. Nkrumah B, Agyekum A, Acquah SE, et al. Comparison of the novel Partec rapid malaria test to the conventional Giemsa stain and the gold standard real-time PCR. J Clin Microbiol. 2010;48:2925–8.
12. World Health Organization. Guidelines for the treatment of malaria. 3rd ed. Geneva: World Health Organization; 2015.
13. Stover KR, King ST, Robinson J. Artemether-lumefantrine: an option for malaria. Ann Pharmacother. 2012;46:567–77.
14. Kopel E, Marhoom E, Sidi Y, et al. Successful oral therapy for severe falciparum malaria: the World Health Organization criteria revisited. Am J Trop Med Hyg. 2012;86:409–11.
15. Marra F, Chiappetta MC, Vincenti V. Ear, nose and throat manifestations of mucocutaneous Leishmaniasis: a literature review. Acta Biomed. 2014;85(1):3–7.
16. Scasso F, Ferrari G, De Vincentiis GC, Arosio A, Bottero S, Carretti M, Ciardo A, Cocuzza S, Colombo A, Conti B, Cordone A, De Ciccio M, Delehaye E, Della Vecchia L, De Macina I, Dentone C, Di Mauro P, Dorati R, Fazio R, Ferrari A, Ferrea G, Giannantonio S, Genta I, Giuliani M, Lucidi D, Maiolino L, Marini G, Marsella P, Meucci D, Modena T, Montemurri B, Odone A, Palma S, Panatta ML, Piemonte M, Pisani P, Pisani S, Prioglio L, Scorpecci A, Scotto DI Santillo L, Serra A, Signorelli C, Sitzia E, Tropiano ML, Trozzi M, Tucci FM, Vezzosi L, Viaggi B. Emerging and re-emerging infectious disease in otorhinolaryngology. Acta Otorhinolaryngol Ital. 2018;38(suppl. 1):S1–S106. https://doi.org/10.14639/0392-100X-suppl.1-38-2018.
17. Leigh JE, Shetty K, Fidel PL Jr. Oral opportunistic infections in HIV-positive individuals: review and role of mucosal immunity. AIDS Patient Care STDS. 2004;18:443–56.
18. Cassone A, Cauda R. Candida and candidiasis in HIV-infected patients: where commensalism, opportunistic be- havior and frank pathogenicity lose their borders. AIDS. 2012;26:1457–72.

19. Scully C, de Almeida OP, Sposto MR. The deep mycoses in HIV infection. Oral Dis. 1997;3:S200–7.
20. Robinson PG. The significance and management of periodontal lesions in HIV infection. Oral Dis. 2002;8:91–7.
21. Kohler M, Kriemler S, Wilhelm EM, et al. Children at high altitude have less nocturnal periodic breathing than adults. Eur Respir J. 2008;32:189.
22. Yaron M, Waldman N, Niermeyer S, et al. The diagnosis of acute mountain sickness in preverbal children. Arch Pediatr Adolesc Med. 1998;152:683.
23. Yaron M, Niermeyer S, Lindgren KN, Honigman B. Evaluation of diagnostic criteria and incidence of acute mountain sickness in preverbal children. Wilderness Environ Med. 2002;13:21.
24. Theis MK, Honigman B, Yip R, et al. Acute mountain sickness in children at 2835 meters. Am J Dis Child. 1993;147:143.
25. Moraga FA, Osorio JD, Vargas ME. Acute mountain sickness in tourists with children at Lake Chungará (4400 m) in northern Chile. Wilderness Environ Med. 2002;13:31.
26. Moraga FA, Pedreros CP, Rodríguez CE. Acute mountain sickness in children and their parents after rapid ascent to 3500 m (Putre, Chile). Wilderness Environ Med. 2008;19:287.
27. Kriemler S, Bürgi F, Wick C, et al. Prevalence of acute mountain sickness at 3500 m within and between families: a prospective cohort study. High Alt Med Biol. 2014;15:28.
28. Bloch J, Duplain H, Rimoldi SF, et al. Prevalence and time course of acute mountain sickness in older children and adolescents after rapid ascent to 3450 meters. Pediatrics. 2009;123:1.
29. Allemann Y, Stuber T, de Marchi SF, et al. Pulmonary artery pressure and cardiac function in children and adolescents after rapid ascent to 3,450 m. Am J Physiol Heart Circ Physiol. 2012;302:H2646.
30. Carpenter TC, Niermeyer S, Durmowicz AG. Altitude-related illness in children. Curr Probl Pediatr. 1998;28:181.
31. Major SA, Hogan RJ, Yeates E, Imray CH. Peripheral arterial desaturation is further exacerbated by exercise in adolescents with acute mountain sickness. Wilderness Environ Med. 2012;23:15.
32. Altundag A, Salihoglu M, Cayonu M, Cingi C, Tekeli H, Hummel T. The effect of high altitude on nasal nitric oxide levels. Eur Arch Otorhinolaryngol. 2014 Sep;271(9):2583–6. https://doi.org/10.1007/s00405-014-3170-8.
33. Altundağ A, Salihoglu M, Çayönü M, Cingi C, Tekeli H, Hummel T. The effect of high altitude on olfactory functions. Eur Arch Otorhinolaryngol. 2014;271(3):615–8. https://doi.org/10.1007/s00405-013-2823-3.
34. Cingi C, Erkan AN, Rettinger G. Ear, nose, and throat effects of high altitude. Eur Arch Otorhinolaryngol. 2010;267(3):467–71. https://doi.org/10.1007/s00405-009-1016-6.
35. San T, Polat S, Cingi C, Eskiizmir G, Oghan F, Cakir B. Effects of high altitude on sleep and respiratory system and theirs adaptations. Scientific World Journal. 2013;17:241569. https://doi.org/10.1155/2013/241569.
36. Cingi C, Selcuk A, Oghan F, Firat Y, Guvey A. The physiological impact of high altitude on nasal and lower airway parameters. Eur Arch Otorhinolaryngol. 2011;268(6):841–4. https://doi.org/10.1007/s00405-010-1468-8.
37. Oghan F, Cingi C, Seren E, Ural A, Guvey A. Assessment of the impact of altitude on nasal airflow via expiratory nasal sound spectral analysis. Eur Arch Otorhinolaryngol. 2010;267(11):1713–8. https://doi.org/10.1007/s00405-010-1252-9.

Tracheotomy in Children

Muhammet Dilber, Fazilet Altın, and Peter Catalano

73.1 Introduction

Tracheotomy is a combination of Latin words meaning trachea and opening to create a new communication between the airway tract below the larynx level and environment for medical purposes [1]. Although the concepts of tracheotomy/tracheostomy are different, they are widely used interchangeably today and define the temporary or permanent opening of the trachea. It is one of the oldest surgical procedures performed that originates in ancient Greece [1]. Although the tracheotomy procedure is a lifesaving procedure in many conditions, it can cause high mortality and morbidity if the indication and technique is not taken into account due to anatomical differences in adult and pediatric patients. In this section, the indications, techniques, and complications of pediatric tracheotomy will be discussed.

73.2 History of Pediatric Tracheotomy

The first elective tracheotomy mentioned in history was done in Rome in 100 BC by Asclepiades of Bithynia [2, 3]. As the laryngeal anatomy is described in more detail over time, in 340 AD, Antyllus of Rome described a tracheotomy between the third and fourth cartilaginous rings of trachea by a transverse incision due to difficult

M. Dilber (✉)
The Dilber Ear, Nose, and Throat Diseases and Surgery Clinic, İstanbul, Turkey

F. Altın
Section of Otorhinolaryngology, Haseki Training and Research Hospital, University of Health Sciences, İstanbul, Turkey

P. Catalano
Department of Otolaryngology, School of Medicine, St. Elizabeth's Medical Center, Tufts University, Boston, MA, USA

© The Author(s), under exclusive license to Springer Nature Switzerland AG 2022
C. Cingi et al. (eds.), *Pediatric ENT Infections*,
https://doi.org/10.1007/978-3-030-80691-0_73

breathing [4]. In 1546 Antonio Musa Brasavola described the use of tracheotomy in the case of a submental-submandibular space abscess [2]. Up until this time, the procedure was named as a "laryngotomy" and "bronchotomy," but Lorenz Heister named the operation as tracheotomy in 1718 and this term became commonly accepted by the nineteenth century [3, 4].

Nicholas Habicot reported an emergency tracheotomy to relieve the obstruction on a 14-year-old boy [4], but the first successful pediatric tracheotomy was performed on a seven-year-old child by Caron to remove foreign body [1]. In 1833, Armand Trousseau reported more than 200 tracheotomies in pediatric patients with diphtheria and saved the lives of 50 children [5]. But during this period, tracheotomy still had high morbidity and mortality. In 1909, Chevalier Jackson analyzed the tracheotomy technique to define the factors leading to complications [6]. After redefinition of correct technique and postoperative care recommendations by Jackson in 1921, a significant decrease in mortality and morbidity due to tracheotomy was observed [7].

73.3 Indications, Technique, and Complications of Pediatric Tracheotomy

The indications for tracheotomy in children have changed considerably in the last 20 years. Until nasotracheal intubation developed in the late 1970s, tracheotomy was used in the treatment of epiglottitis and laryngotracheobronchitis [8, 9]. Acute upper respiratory tract obstructions due to bacterial infection were the most important indications for tracheotomy until the 1980s [10, 11]. After developments of vaccines and antibiotics, the number of upper airway obstructions from infections was dramatically reduced resulting in decrease in the indications of tracheotomy. Another reason is the usage of flexible fiberoptic endoscope allowing quicker and safer oral or nasal intubation than tracheotomy in acute patients. Campisi et al. [12] evaluated indications for the pediatric tracheotomy cases and found infections were a common cause of tracheotomy in 49% of patients between 1963 and 1970, while it decreased to 14% of patients with vaccination in the 1980s and to 3% in 2000s. Similarly, Özmen et al. [13] examined indications for tracheotomies performed between 1960 and 1980, and the study showed that acute respiratory tract obstruction due to infection was the most common indication in the 1960s, while it was replaced by prolonged mechanical ventilation in the 1980s. In a study including a large series of 1130 trachcotomics, Goldcnbcrg ct al. [14] showed that indications for tracheotomies were prophylactic in 76% of patients with prolonged mechanical ventilation, 6% of patients with upper airway obstruction, and only 0.26% of patients on an emergency basis. The most important reason of this is the increase in survival rates of patients who were in neonatal and pediatric intensive care units due to current technological advances.

Pediatric tracheotomy has become important especially in recent years due to surgical advances in patients with congenital cardiac and pulmonary pathologies, and also due to prolonged mechanical ventilation support in patients with neurological pathologies [15]. Although tracheotomy can be performed in all age groups, it was shown in studies that the majority of pediatric tracheotomies were performed under age 1 [10, 16, 17]. Due to the increase in ventilated newborns, the frequency of subglottic stenosis increased and the number of tracheotomies performed to correct it also increased [18]. Nevertheless, improvement of new techniques to correct subglottic stenosis decreased the need for tracheotomy in those patients.

The decision to perform a tracheotomy on a pediatric patient depends on many factors such as the severity of airway obstruction, the difficulty and duration of intubation, and the state of the underlying disease. Nowadays, the common indications for tracheotomy can be classified as upper airway obstruction, the need for prolonged mechanical ventilation and pulmonary care [10, 19, 20]. Most of the primary causes of upper respiratory tract obstruction in children are congenital, such as Pierre-Robin sequence, and CHARGE syndrome [21, 22]. Also complex congenital heart diseases can be a cause of tracheotomy due to its ability to lead to mechanical ventilator dependency for a long time or due to the development of diaphragm paralysis after cardiac surgery [23, 24].

Tracheotomy in patients with prolonged mechanical ventilation support is important to facilitate patient care, to clean tracheobronchial secretion and plugs, to prevent development of tracheal stenosis and facilitating the process of weaning from the mechanical ventilator by reducing the dead space [25, 26]. Indication of tracheotomy in children with mechanical ventilator support varies according to child's age, difficulty and duration of intubation, and underlying disease causing prolonged intubation. If the underlying disease is progressive or if very long ventilation is required, a tracheotomy should be performed early. In patients with the expectation of extubation, intubation trauma should be followed closely by flexible fiberoptic endoscopy, and if seen, tracheotomy should be considered without delay [27].

Although it has similarities with adult tracheotomy, pediatric tracheotomy has some differences. General anesthesia should be preferred as cooperation cannot be achieved in children. When possible, pediatric tracheotomy should be performed under operating room conditions, under general anesthesia, after the patient is intubated, with the appropriate team and surgical equipment. If intubation is not possible, a ventilation with laryngeal mask or a face mask can be used. It should not be forgotten that the trachea is small in diameter, shorter, less stabilized, and located more superiorly in pediatric patients when compared with the adult anatomy [28]. Skin and trachea incision, subcutaneous tissue removal, and maturation specific to pediatric tracheotomy and tracheal stay suture techniques vary from surgeon to surgeon. Generally, vertical or horizontal incisions are preferred as skin incision, and a vertical incision is preferred in the trachea itself [29].

Many different surgical techniques have been described to reduce complications associated with tracheotomy. Studies have shown that vertical tracheal incision is preferred because suprastomal collapse and tracheal stenosis are higher in patients with horizontal, "T" versus "H" tracheal incisions and in patients who underwent tracheal wall resection [30, 31]. A vertical incision is made in the 3-4-5 tracheal rings, the trachea is retracted with the help of sutures, the intubation tube is pulled up, and the suitable tracheotomy cannula is placed [28]. Then, the inside of the cannula is aspirated and the patient is ventilated through the cannula to check position of the cannula. If there is an asymmetric ventilation present, it should be kept in mind that the tracheotomy tube may be too long, the right main bronchus may have been selectively intubated, or the patient has developed pneumothorax [32].

Pediatric tracheotomy complication rates vary between 11 and 51% in the literature [33–35]. Among the early complications (in the postoperative first 7 days) are bleeding, infection, pneumothorax, tube obstruction, and accidental decannulation. Late complications of tracheostomy are airway stenosis, failure of breathing after decannulation, and suprastomal granulation development that result in airway obstruction [34, 35]. Less common late complications are tracheomalacia, tracheo-innominate artery fistula (TIF), tracheoesophageal fistula (TEF), pneumonia, and aspiration, and each can be associated with significant morbidity and mortality [36, 37]. Tracheostomy-related mortality is commonly due to accidental decannulation and blockage of the tracheostomy tube [16, 20, 35].

73.4 Postoperative Care of Pediatric Tracheotomy

Tracheotomy care begins in the operating room at the end of the surgical procedure. It is vital to ensure airway safety by the surgical team and anesthesia team during transport in order to minimize the problems that may occur during the transportation of the patient. Since accidental decannulation is the most common cause of mortality after tracheotomy, an intubation tube and spare cannula must be available at the head of the patient's bed and during transport [38].

After the patient is transferred to the service, chest radiography should be performed to show the correct placement of the cannula and to rule out pneumothorax [39]. The patient should be monitored and followed up by a trained nurse. Care should be taken to fix the cannula and its occlusion should be prevented by frequent aspiration and proper humidification of the respiratory air [40]. Tracheobronchial secretion increases in the first days due to tracheal irritation after tracheotomy. Therefore, tracheal aspiration should be performed hourly on the first day and every 2–3 h on the next 2 days. Tracheal aspirations should be done gently so as not to cause tracheal damage. Aspiration should be done with a soft aspiration catheter, closed while pushing into the trachea, and opened while retracting and gently rotating. In cases where secretions are thick, irrigation-aspiration can be performed with saline; otherwise occlusion of cannula can be seen. The patient should lie in a neutral position and the patient's neck should not be in extension or flexion.

The International Pediatric Otolaryngology Group has a comprehensive postoperative care recommendation for pediatric patients undergoing a tracheotomy [41]. Accordingly, during the postoperative period, important suggestions should be considered to provide airway safety, patient comfort, protection of cervical skin, and nutrition. Cannula and skin injuries due to cannula bands in children are more commonly seen compared to adults; therefore cannula bands should be neither loose nor tight [42]. If an infection develops, swabs are taken from this area for culture and the appropriate i.v. and antibiotic ointment should be applied and the wound should be meticulously cleaned.

The tracheostomy cannula should be changed due to colonizations that may develop within the tubes and plugs that cannot be easily cleaned. Although there are different opinions, the first cannula change should generally be done 1 week after the operation. During this time, the tracheotomy tract is epithelialized, allowing the procedure to be performed more efficiently and safely. The first cannula replacement must be done by or under the supervision of an otolaryngologist. The intubation set must be kept ready during the change. During the first cannula change after the previous cannula is removed, collapsing the passage or inability to see the tracheal window can be experienced especially in pediatric patients. In this case, a tracheotomy set is used, the wound lips are opened to expose the tracheal lumen with the help of retractors and clamps and a new cannula is applied. If still unsuccessful, performing endolaryngeal intubation is lifesaving.

Under observation, the patient can take a bath in water that does not exceed the abdominal level. Again, attention should be paid to the aspiration of the splashing water. Bath toys such as buckets and water guns should not be allowed. While washing the hair, the neck should be protected with a waterproof protector [43]. For children who will be monitored at home and will have tracheotomy for a long time, at least one of the parents should be educated about tracheostomy care, humidification and suctioning the cannula, and emergency conditions of tracheotomy. The home environment should be adapted to the child and his needs. A regular relationship should be established between family, children, and experienced healthcare professionals [44]. In a study conducted by Mac Cormick et al., it was observed that approximately 40% of patients followed at home with tracheotomy applied to the emergency department for various reasons in the first month after discharge [45]. In the same study, the main problems experienced by families regarding tracheotomy were mucus plugs, unwanted decannulation, insufficiency of home healthcare, and problem with equipment used (ventilator, aspirator, etc.). Therefore, parents of patients should be adequately educated and informed.

Because of the functional, psychological, and financial burdens of long-term tracheotomy care, decannulation has been the ultimate goal after tracheotomy and should be considered, especially when the underlying condition disappears or is corrected. The decannulation rate in pediatric tracheotomies is around 30% [11]. In the statement published by the American Academy of Otorhinolaryngology Head and Neck Surgery, if a patient does not need mechanical ventilation for at least 3 months, decannulation could be considered [46]. Before decannulation, bronchoscopy should check the airway patency and determine whether there is suprastomal granulation and it must be a patent glottic zone with at least one mobile vocal cord. There should be no history of aspiration that prevents decannulation. A similar decannulation protocol was described by Wirtz et al. [46]. In this protocol, patients who did not need a mechanical ventilator for 2 months were evaluated in the operating room with flexible endoscopy, patients with suitable airway patency were followed up in the hospital for 24 h after they were decannulated, and the patients without any problem were discharged.

73.5 Conclusion

Successful pediatric tracheotomy requires appropriate surgical technique and adequate postoperative care to minimize the complication rates. Today the most common indication for pediatric tracheotomy is prolonged intubation. Success of pediatric tracheotomy is directly related to the quality of the relationship that is established between family, patient, and doctor. Mortality generally parallels the course of the underlying disease.

References

1. Gooddal EW. The story of tracheotomy. Br J Child Dis. 1934;31:167–76.
2. Wetmore RF. Tracheotomy. In: Bluestone CD, Stool SE, Alpes CM, Arjmand EM, Casselbrant ML, Dohar JE, et al., editors. Pediatric otolaryngology. 4th ed. Philadelphia: Saunders; 2003. p. 1583–98.
3. Stock CR. What is past is prologue: a short history of the development of tracheostomy. Ear Nose Throat J. 1987;66:166–9.
4. Frost EAM. Tracing the tracheostomy. Ann Otol Rhinol Laryngol. 1976;85(5 Pt. 1):618–24.
5. Trosseau A. In: Cormack JR, editor. Lectures on clinical medicine, Delivered at the Hôtel-Dieu, Paris. Philadelphia: Lindsay and Blakiston; 1869. p. 598.
6. Jackson C. Tracheotomy. Laryngoscope. 1909;19:285–90.
7. Jackson C. High tracheotomy and other errors: the chief causes of chronic laryngeal stenosis. Surg Gynecol Obstet. 1921;32:392–8.
8. Gerson CR, Tucker GF Jr. Infant tracheotomy. Ann Otol Rhinol Laryngol. 1982;91(4 Pt1):413–6.
9. MacRae DL, Rae RE, Heeneman H. Pediatric tracheotomy. J Otolaryngol. 1984;13(5):309–11.
10. Carron JD, Derkay CS, Strope GL, Nosonchuk JE, Darrow DH. Pediatric tracheotomies: changing indications and outcomes. Laryngoscope. 2000;110:1099–104.
11. Funamura JL, Durbin-Johnson B, Tollefson TT, Harrison J, Senders CW. Pediatric tracheotomy: indications and decannulation outcomes. Laryngoscope. 2014;124(8):1952–8.
12. Campisi P, Forte V. Pediatric tracheostomy. Semin Pediatr Surg. 2016;25:191–5.
13. Ozmen S, Ozmen OA, Unal OF. Pediatric tracheotomies: a 37-year experience in 282 children. Int J Pediatr Otorhinolaryngol. 2009;73:959–61.
14. Goldenberg D, Ari EG, Golz A, et al. Tracheotomy complications: a retrospective study of 1130 cases. Otolaryngol Head Neck Surg. 2000;123:495–500.
15. Acar B, Acar M, Yıldız E, Karaşen RM. Çocuk Trakeostomi: Endikasyonlar, Komplikasyonlar ve 20 Olgunun İncelenmesi. J Turgut Ozal Med Cent. 2014;211:41–3.
16. Wetmore RF, Marsh RR, Thompson ME, Tom LW. Pediatric tracheostomy: a changing procedure? Ann Otol Rhinol Laryngol. 1999;108(7 Pt 1):695–9.
17. Corbett HJ, Mann KS, Mitra I, Jesudason EC, Losty PD, Clarke RW. Tracheostomy – a 10 year experience from a UK pediatric surgical center. J Pediatr Surg. 2007;42:1251–4.
18. Alladi A, Rao S, Das K, Charles AR, D'Cruz AJ. Pediatric tracheostomy: a 13-year experience. Pediatr Surg Int. 2004;20:695–8.
19. Trachsel D, Hammer J. Indications for tracheostomy in children. Paediatr Respir Rev. 2006;7(3):162–8.
20. Midwinter KI, Carrie S, Bull PD. Paediatric tracheostomy: Sheffield experience 1979-1999. J Laryngol Otol. 2002;116(7):532–5.
21. Roger G, Morisseau-Durand MP, Van Den Abbeele T, Nicollas R, Triglia JM, Narcy P, Abadie V, Manac'h Y, Garabedian EN. The CHARGE association: the role of tracheostomy. Arch Otolaryngal Head Neck Surg. 1999;125(1):33–8.

22. Sculerati N, Gottlieb MD, Zimbler MS, Chibbaro PD, McCarthy JG. Airway management in children with major craniofacial anomalies. Laryngoscope. 1998;108(12):1806–12.
23. Hoskote A, Cohen G, Goldman A, Shekerdemian L. Tracheostomy in infants and children after cardiothoracic surgery: indications, associated risk factors, and timing. J Thorac Cardiovasc Surg. 2005;130(4):1086–93.
24. LoTempio MM, Shapiro NL. Tracheotomy tube placement in children following cardiothoracic surgery: indications and outcomes. Am J Otolaryngol. 2002;23(6):337–40.
25. Mahadevan M, Barber C, Salkeld L, Douglas G, Mills N. Pediatric tracheotomy: 17 year review. Int J Pediatr Otorhinolaryngol. 2007;71(12):1829–35.
26. Davis MG. Tracheostomy in children. Paediatr Respir Rev. 2006;7:S206–9.
27. Kremer B, Botos-Kremer AI, Eckel HE, Schlöndorff G. Indications, complications, and surgical techniques for pediatric tracheostomies--un update. J Pediatr Surg. 2002;37(11):1556–62.
28. Cochrane LA, Bailey CM. Surgical aspects of tracheostomy in children. Paediatr Respir Rev. 2006;7(3):169–74.
29. Gallagher TQ, Hartnick CJ. Pediatric tracheotomy. Adv Otorhinolaryngol. 2012;73:26–30.
30. Ruggiero FP, Carr MM. Infant tracheotomy: results of a survey regarding technique. Arch Otolaryngol Head Neck Surg. 2008;134(3):263–7.
31. Antón-Pacheco JL, Villafruela M, López M, García G, Luna C, Martínez A. Surgical management of severe suprastomal cricotracheal collapse complicating pediatric tracheostomy. Int J Pediatr Otorhinolaryngol. 2008;72(2):179–83.
32. Stool SE, Beebe JK. Tracheotomy in infants and children. Curr Probl Pediatr. 1973;3:3–33.
33. Lewis CW, Carron JD, Perkins JA, Sie KC, Feudtner C. Tracheotomy in pediatric patients: a national perspective. Arch Otolaryngol Head Neck Surg. 2003;129(5):523–9.
34. Jaryszak EM, Shah RK, Amling J, Peña MT. Pediatric tracheotomy wound complications: incidence and significance. Arch Otolaryngol Head Neck Surg. 2011;137(4):363–6.
35. Carr MM, Poje CP, Kingston L, Kielma D, Heard C. Complications in pediatric tracheostomies. Laryngoscope. 2001;111(11 Pt1):1925–8.
36. Epstein SK. Late complications of tracheostomy. Respir Care. 2005;50(4):542–9.
37. D'Souza JN, Levi JR, Park D, Shah UK. Complications following pediatric tracheotomy. JAMA Otolaryngol Head Neck Surg. 2016;142(5):484–8.
38. Akcan FA. Pediatrik trakeotomi. Endikasyondan Dekanülasyona Süreç Yönetimi KBB ve BBC Dergisi. 2018;26(1):17–25.
39. Greenberg JS, Sulek M, de Jong A, Friedman EM. The role of postoperative chest radiography in pediatric tracheostomy. Int J Pediatr Otorhinolaryngol. 2001;60(1):41–7.
40. Gupta A, Cotton RT, Rutter MJ. Pediatric suprastomal granuloma: management and treatment. Otolaryngol Head Neck Surg. 2004;131(1):21–5.
41. Strychowsky JE, Albert D, Chan K, Cheng A, Daniel SJ, De Alarcon A, et al. International pediatric otolaryngology group (IPOG) consensus recommendations: routine peri-operative pediatric tracheotomy care. Int J Pediatr Otorhinolaryngol. 2016;86:250–5.
42. Bressler K, Coladipietro L, Holinger LD. Protection of the cervical skin in the pediatric patient with a recent tracheostomy. Otolaryngol Head Neck Surg. 1997;116(3):414–5.
43. Sherman JM, Davis S, Albamonte-Petrick S, Chatburn RL, Fitton C, Gren C, Johnston J, Lyrene RK, Myer C 3rd, Othersen HB, Wood R, Zach M, Zander J, Zinman R. Care of the child with a chronic tracheostomy. This offical statement of the American Thoracic Society was adopted by the ATS Board of Directors,July 1999. Am J Respir Crit Care Med. 2000;161(1):297–308.
44. Oberwaldner B, Eber E. Tracheostomy care in the home. Paediatr Respir Rev. 2006;7(3):185–90.
45. McCormick ME, Ward E, Roberson DW, Shah RK, Stachler RJ, Brenner MJ. Life after tracheostomy: patient and family perspectives on teaching, transitions, and multidisciplinary teams. Otolaryngol Head Neck Surg. 2015;153(6):914–20.
46. Mitchell RB, Hussey HM, Setzen G, Jacobs IN, Nussenbaum B, Dawson C, et al. Clinical consensus statement: tracheostomy care. Otolaryngol Head Neck Surg. 2013;148(1):6–20.

Gastroesophageal Reflux and Respiratory Diseases in Children

74

Mustafa Şahin, Sema Başak, and Yvan Vandenplas

74.1 Introduction

Gastroesophageal reflux (GER) is the backflow of gastric contents towards the esophagus, and this may be accompanied by regurgitation/vomiting. GER can be seen in children of all ages without any diseases [1]. In the pediatric age group, GER is most common in infancy, especially between 1 and 4 months. GER, which is a physiological entity in newborns and infants, gradually decreases in the first year of life [2].

GER has been associated with a variety of respiratory symptoms and disorders in the pediatric age group. When GER causes troublesome symptoms and complications, it is referred to as gastroesophageal reflux disease (GERD). The main classical symptoms of pathologic pediatric GER (GERD) are vomiting, retching, dysphagia, wheezing, choking attacks, and a delay in growth [3]. In routine clinical practice, antireflux measures/treatments to prevent delayed recovery and mucosal edema that may be caused by GER/GERD before and after airway surgeries is almost a general rule practiced by clinicians [4, 5].

GERD-related symptoms can be gastrointestinal, neurobehavioral, and respiratory origin. It has been suggested that GERD is associated with common symptoms such as heartburn and chest pain in the pediatric age group, as well as respiratory problems such as cough, stridor, wheezing, and pneumonia [4]. It is seen that the scientific evidence on the relationship between respiratory diseases and GERD has intensified in the last 30 years [3]. In a study conducted by Junqueira and Penna, the results of nasopharyngeal pH measurement in children with chronic respiratory

M. Şahin (✉) · S. Başak
Department of Otorhinolaryngology, Faculty of Medicine, Aydın Adnan Menderes University, Aydın, Turkey

Y. Vandenplas
Department of Pediatrics, University Hospital Brussels, Vrije University Brussels, KidZ Health Castle, Brussels, Belgium

C. Cingi et al. (eds.), *Pediatric ENT Infections*,
https://doi.org/10.1007/978-3-030-80691-0_74

problems had lowered (acidic) compared to the children in the control group. However, no data/theory has been provided on the pathophysiological mechanism that may be the cause of this finding [6].

It is also seen that clinicians' search for solutions to airway problems that may be associated with GERD is reflected more frequently in their daily practice. One study found that GERD diagnoses in infants increased more than threefold between 2000 and 2005 [2]. To reduce airway problems that may be associated with gastric acid content, clinicians are increasingly prescribing acid suppressant drugs such as proton pump inhibitors (PPIs), and PPIs are among the most prescribed drug classes today [4, 7].

Various theories have been proposed regarding the relationship between GER and the development of airway problems [3, 4]. First, in 1892, Osler suggested that these two entities may interact. Accordingly, GER may play a role in the development of a reactive airway disease, as well as reactive airway diseases such as asthma and the antiasthmatic drugs may cause GER to exacerbate [8]. Another proposed mechanism in the development of gastroesophageal reflux-mediated airway problems is the microaspiration of the gastric contents that are refluxed into the mouth and are then aspirated into the lower airway tract. This can cause irritation, inflammation, and spasms in the affected airway part. However it is very challenging to prove the aspiration that occurs in this way [9, 10]. Rosen et al. studied bacterial microflora of gastric, bronchoalveolar lavage, and oropharyngeal fluids in 116 children aged 1 to 18. In this study, it was reported that the bacterial composition of the gastric and lung fluid was much more alike than the oropharyngeal flora. These results support the idea that full column GER can alter the bacterial microflora of the lungs. This result also suggested that there was direct communication between the stomach and the lower respiratory tract, independent of the oropharynx. This study is important because it supports reflux as a valid mechanism for the development of lung disease in GERD patients. Considering these data, it suggests that a patient's lung bacterial profile may serve as a future biomarker of reflux-associated lung disease [11].

The laryngotracheoalveolar system develops by dissociating from the embryogenic origin common with the gastrointestinal tract. Not only do these two systems (aerodigestive systems) intersect luminal anatomy, but neurons, receptors, and reflexes are also interconnected [12]. It is highly possible that these interconnections are involved in irritative bronchospasm associated with GER. GER may play an important inflammatory cofactor role during the development of airway disorders [13]. Another proposed mechanism that derives from this knowledge postulated that activation of proximal airway receptors in children by gastroesophageal reflux-related materials such as acid and pepsin can increase airway resistance and may lead to the development of reactive airway disease [14].

Considering all these proposed mechanisms, GER/GERD can theoretically cause airway obstruction in the following four main ways and so trigger or exacerbate the development of different airway diseases:

1. Mucus oversecretion as a result of inflammation and/or reflexive stimulation.

2. Intraluminal mucosal edema caused by chemical/inflammatory mediators or stimulation of neural pathways.
3. Direct obstruction by aspirated refluxate material.
4. Bronchospasm as a result of peribronchial muscle spasm caused by local irritation and/or reflex pathways.

It should also be kept in mind that airway diseases themselves can increase GER through similar ways and interactions and cause GERD development. Therefore, treatment success can be increased by considering both airway disease and reflux when necessary [13–19].

74.2 GER Evaluation in Children with Respiratory Disorders

The most child-friendly and simplest method in evaluating GER is questionnaires. However, there is no validated and reliable questionnaire that is universally used in the evaluation of pediatric GER [20, 21]. In addition, as we learn from studies in adults, the correlation between GER/GERD questionnaires and investigations such as endoscopy and pH monitoring is quite weak [22].

Physical examination and flexible endoscopic examination, which are frequently used in otolaryngology practice, are of very limited value in detecting GER in the pediatric age group [23]. No classical physical examination findings specific to gastroesophageal reflux have been identified in the pediatric population. Posterior glottic erythema, posterior glottic edema, laryngomalacia, and subglottic stenosis have been reported as the most common flexible endoscopic examination findings in pediatric patients with GERD [20, 24, 25].

The barium swallow test can be used in the evaluation of accompanying swallowing disorder, aspiration, and anatomical structural problems, but its usefulness in detecting GERD is very limited [26]. Ultrasound is advantageous in that it is noninvasive, but it has limitations in terms of experience and subjective aspects of the performer. It is not useful in detecting GERD, except to show structural problems. Scintigraphy may be useful in detecting pulmonary aspiration, but its use in daily routine practice for this purpose is rare [27]. Upper gastrointestinal endoscopy has the advantages of direct examination of the esophageal lumen, detecting hernia and performing biopsy when necessary but is inadequate in detecting GER. Endoscopy and biopsy are the gold standard in the diagnosis of eosinophilic esophagitis, which is an important diagnostic dilemma for the pediatric age group [28]. Manometry is valuable in detecting mechanisms that may be the underlying cause of GER, not GER itself [29]. The two most valuable contemporary investigations used in the diagnosis of GERD are esophageal pH monitorization test (pHmetry), which can detect acidic liquid reflux, and impedance tests that can detect both liquid and gas acidic/nonacidic reflux. [27] The pHmetry with double-electrode probe has been the most commonly used test evaluating of otolaryngologic/respiratory manifestations of GER [30]. However, impedance is the method of choice in evaluating the response of children receiving antacid therapy and respiratory tract problems that may be associated with persistent non-acid reflux. Therefore, impedance is currently the recommended clinical test tool for use in research [31]. Although impedance is a valuable test in detecting reflux episodes and their types, its routine application and advantages in evaluating airway problems with GERD in children are controversial because of the heterogeneity of the studies, technical differences, diversity in the parameters evaluated, and the insufficiency of normative data [32]. Studies which have more common and homogeneous inclusion criteria, analyzed parameters, baseline, and prospective symptom features are needed to draw precise and clinically useful conclusions.

The results of the Bilitec test, which can detect esophageal reflux of bile content, are still insufficient [33]. Investigations analyzing samples taken from airway secretions can also be used in the diagnosis of reflux-related airway disorders. The sensitivity and specificity of detecting fat-laden macrophages or their index is quite low [34]. Instead, it has been reported that pepsin screening has higher sensitivity and specificity in bronchial secretion samples. It has been reported that acid detection in oropharyngeal secretions, which are cheaper, easier, and less invasive than these aforementioned tests, may be useful in detecting acid reflux in infants [32].

It has been suggested that a genetic variant may be effective in the development of GERD, especially in its severe or chronic forms. Hu et al. investigated inheritance pattern of patients with GERD and mapped the genetic locus for severe pediatric GERD to identify a gene for GERD. Their study reported that the severe pediatric GERD gene matches chromosome 13q14. Such studies may provide new diagnostic and treatment strategies for GERD in the future [35].

74.3 GERD and Respiratory Symptoms/Disorders

The relationship between GERD and respiratory problems and diseases has been an interesting area of research in recent decades. It has been suggested that GERD may be an important cause of the symptoms in a substantial proportion of children with persistent respiratory problems. There have been increased awareness of GERD as a cause of pediatric respiratory problems and data in the literature showing an increased incidence of GERD in children with a certain type of respiratory tract disorders [36, 37]. GERD could be a causative etiologic factor in reactive airway diseases, recurrent croup, chronic bronchitis, apnea, chronic cough, and subglottic stenosis [38]. However, there are limitations to the documentation and evidence for this relationship in the pediatric age group. One of the most important issue in reflux-related airway pathologies is the inadequacy of normative data belonging to different age, gender, and ethnic groups [7, 32]. Radiological tests, which are less invasive in the evaluation of pediatric GER, are generally performed in the postprandial period, but have limited value in the diagnosis of GERD due to the high prevalence of GER in the postprandial period [4, 27].

In their study Wenzl et al. suggested that there is a strong relationship between GER and respiratory symptoms [39]. However, it has been stated that there is a strong correlation between respiratory problems and reflux occurring in nonacidic type rather than acidic and impedancemetry test should be performed to determine this. The cutoff values for impedancemetry test have not yet been determined to distinguish normal children from GERD patients [4, 40]. Rosen et al. evaluated reflux using multi-canal intraluminal impedance in 28 children with chronic respiratory disease with a mean age of 6.5 years. In their study, they found a stronger correlation between chronic airway symptoms and non-acid reflux episodes compared to acid reflux episodes. They concluded that chronic respiratory manifestations such as coughing and wheezing are correlated with GERD in their pediatric patients group. They also reported that the closer the gastric reflux content to the proximal levels of the esophagus, the more respiratory symptoms increased [11].

Jein et al. evaluated children with persistent and/or recurrent respiratory problems between 3 months and 3 years with a median age of 14 months for GER by performing upper gastrointestinal endoscopy, biopsy, gastroesophageal scintigraphy, and 24 h esophageal pH monitoring tests. The results of this study suggest that GER may be a possible causal contributing factor in children with recurrent and persistent respiratory problems [41].

Yellon et al. reported significant relationship between presence of histologic esophagitis and chronic cough in children suspicious for GER-related symptoms [28]. In addition, during the cough associated with airway disease and GERD, the intra-abdominal pressure increases and this triggers GER and thus a vicious circle may occur. It was found that the thoracoabdominal expiratory pressure level increased in rats with partial airway obstruction [42].

GERD is considered to be a contributing factor for croup, but this relationship has not been clearly established yet. Waki et al. performed scintiscan, barium swallow, esophagoscopy, and pHmetry tests on 32 children with recurrent croup and reported that they detected GERD in 15 children (47%). In another study in which pharyngeal and esophageal pH monitoring was used simultaneously, Contencin and Narcy reported that GERD was detected in all eight children with recurrent croup [43, 44].

GERD can cause stridor, which has been called pseudolaryngomalacia by some authors because of similar symptoms [45]. Intermittent stridor occurring only during GER attacks has been demonstrated by intraesophageal pH measurements in infants [46]. Reflux associated with GER in young children may not be directly related to airway involvement but may also be associated with agitation caused by pain caused by acidic reflux [47].

Pediatric subglottic stenosis may develop as a result of many different reasons such as infection, trauma, congenital, autoimmune diseases, and sometimes a cause may not be documented [48]. GERD is one of the factors included in this etiological spectrum. However, the evidence on this subject has mostly derived from experimental animal studies. In a study conducted in canines, subglottic stenosis created experimentally significantly aggravated after gastric content application [49]. Gaynor reported ulceration and necrosis in histopathological evaluation after exposing rabbit tracheas to synthetic gastric content for periods of 1–4 h [50]. In another canine study, Koufman reported that when pepsin with acid was applied to the area of subglottic mucosal trauma, recovery was better than the group applied saline with acid [5]. In an experimental pig model study, Yellon et al. evaluated the effects of short-term contact of gastric content with healthy subglottic mucosa by reverse transcriptase polymerase chain reaction and histologically. The direct effects of this interaction on intact subglottic mucosa were ulceration, basal epithelial hyperplasia, and downregulation of epidermal growth factor receptor messenger RNA production [51]. Based on limited information, no benefit has been reported in performing diagnostic GERD tests or administering GERD therapy in subglottic stenosis surgery. However, many surgeons use GERD treatment very aggressively during the management of subglottic stenosis [4, 7, 13].

Studies of GERD as a factor that triggers or aggravates pediatric asthma have increased over the past decades. In experimental studies, it has been shown that bronchial spasm increases with increasing intraesophageal pH level by a vagal pathway [1–4]. In some epidemiological studies, the prevalence of GERD in pediatric asthma patients has been reported to be at least 50% [3, 7, 8]. GERD is more common in pediatric patients with asthma with nocturnal exacerbations and more severe asthma. It has been reported that severity of asthma symptoms decreases after pharmacotherapeutic treatment. Patients in the pediatric age group with a higher chance of responding to antireflux therapy are those with classic reflux symptoms such as heartburn and regurgitation, and those with nocturnal and non-allergic asthma [3, 8]. Particular attention should be given to nocturnal control of reflux in children with asthma who are scheduled for antireflux therapy. Children with severe asthma or symptoms that are difficult to control may require steroid use. It should not be forgotten that reflux will worsen asthma in this patient group. Conservative and medical measures should be initiated before steroid therapy in these patients [8, 10].

Further prospective clinical studies are needed to establish a definite cause-and-effect relationship between GERD and these respiratory symptoms/disorders and to determine how effective antireflux treatment methods are in controlling such respiratory problems.

74.4　GERD and Apnea

Although the exact mechanism of GERD-induced apnea is not known, some theories have been proposed. One possible mechanism is that gastric content reaching the respiratory tract (glottis, subglottis, tracheobronchial system) causes laryngospasm. The other is reflex-mediated neural mechanisms, which were mentioned earlier in this section [36, 39]. With the use of intraesophageal pH probe technology, clinicians have had the opportunity to show that there may be an association between cyanotic apnea episodes and GER (acid reflux type) in infants. In a study evaluating 1400 babies with apneic episodes, Kahn et al. reported that they detected excessive acid reflux in about half of the babies [52]. Afterward, different studies were carried out using pH probe and polysomnography to support the temporal relationship between apnea or hypoxemia and reflux. However, on the other hand, it is seen that studies showing the opposite of these findings and rejecting the mentioned significant relationship between reflux and apnea are presented to the literature [53]. These types of studies have various technical difficulties and handicaps. In addition, apnea occurs as a result of infants' response to a number of different neurosensory stimuli. Although it is thought that reflux is a possible stimulus in the formation of apnea, it is very difficult to prove the exact mechanism. Data from some experimental studies have reported that an increase in intraesophageal acidity may cause apnea in some susceptible subjects [54, 55]. In different studies focusing on reflux as the cause of infantile apnea, there are studies reporting the results of conservative approaches, medical treatment, and fundoplication as reflux treatment. Considering that infantile apnea resolves spontaneously in many cases, it is necessary to be very careful when choosing such modalities. Nevertheless, it is necessary not to avoid performing antireflux therapy to some infants with apnea episodes [56]. The history taken from the family/caregiver is very important in making this decision. The main features of apnea that may be associated with GERD and increase the chance of benefiting from antireflux therapy occur when the baby is awake, in the supine position, and about the first hour after feeding. In addition, the presence of tension in the baby's body, bending, redness and bruising, respiratory effort, and nutrient presence in the mouth and/or nose in the history of the baby should be especially questioned [53–56]. In apnea, which may be associated with GER, it is very difficult to decide which babies need further tests, which babies can be followed up at home, and which babies should be given antireflux therapy. Proper positioning, increasing the consistency of the food, and reducing the volume given during feeding should primarily be the preferred methods and are often effective and sufficient [56–58].

74.5 Treatment of GER-Related Respiratory Symptoms/Disorders

There are studies reporting that respiratory symptoms associated with GER can be significantly improved with antireflux therapy [59]. Jein et al. reported that in most of the children with persistent respiratory complaints, they found significant improvement after 3–6 months after antireflux treatment (frequent and low volume feeding with viscous foods, upright positioning, prokinetic and H2 blocker drugs) [3, 4]. However, it has been stated that this treatment may change the bacterial content of the gastrointestinal and respiratory systems' microbial environment. Therefore, antireflux medications (especially PPIs) used to reduce respiratory symptoms can worsen the problem. It has been reported that prolonged gastric acid suppression in adults may cause impaired nutrient absorption and pneumonia. It can be thought that suppression of gastric content, which also has antibacterial properties, may cause similar problems in children [2, 7, 10]. Rosen et al. in their study found that the gastric contents of children under acid suppression had higher concentrations of acid-sensitive bacteria, which may play a role in some upper airway infections and pneumonia, compared to children not under acid suppression. Gastric acid suppression drugs alter the gastric bacterial profile which can also affect the airway microbiome via high level GER. [11]

74.6 Conclusion

The complexity of interactions between the upper gastrointestinal tract and the airway still contains many unknowns to be explained. Although it is considered as a high probability that GER/GERD is associated with airway symptoms and disorders in pediatric patients in clinical practice, the scientific evidence of this relationship is not strong enough yet. Knowledge on the current literature consists largely of the results of studies with significant methodological deficiencies such as insufficient diagnostic workup for GER, biased patients selection/population, and limited statistical analysis. Studies to understand and elucidate these problems will allow children with morbidity due to respiratory diseases to be managed optimally. Understanding and preventing airway problems caused by GER/GERD means capturing one of the pieces to the advantage of winning this challenging game of chess.

References

1. McGuirt WF Jr. Gastroesophageal reflux and the upper airway. Pediatr Clin North Am. 2003;50(2):487–502. https://doi.org/10.1016/s0031-3955(03)00033-6.
2. Rosen R, Vandenplas Y, Singendonk M, Cabana M, DiLorenzo C, Gottrand F, Gupta S, Langendam M, Staiano A, Thapar N, Tipnis N, Tabbers M. Pediatric gastroesophageal reflux clinical practice guidelines: joint recommendations of the north American Society for Pediatric Gastroenterology, Hepatology, and Nutrition and the European Society for Pediatric Gastroenterology, Hepatology, and Nutrition. J Pediatr Gastroenterol Nutr. 2018;66(3):516–54. https://doi.org/10.1097/MPG.0000000000001889.
3. Vandenplas Y, Devreker T, Hauser B. Gastroesophageal reflux and chronic respiratory disease: past, present, and future. J Pediatr. 2007;83(3):196–200. https://doi.org/10.2223/JPED.1633.
4. Yellon RF, Goldberg H. Update on gastroesophageal reflux disease in pediatric airway disorders. Am J Med. 2001;111(Suppl 8A):78S–84S. https://doi.org/10.1016/s0002-9343(01)00861-0.
5. Koufman JA. The otolaryngologic manifestations of gastroesophageal reflux disease (GERD): a clinical investigation of 225 patients using ambulatory 24-hour pH monitoring and an experimental investigation of the role of acid and pepsin in the development of laryngeal injury. Laryngoscope. 1991;101(4 Pt 2 Suppl 53):1–78. https://doi.org/10.1002/lary.1991.101.s53.1.
6. Junqueira JC, Penna FJ. Nasopharyngeal pH and gastroesophageal reflux in children with chronic respiratory disease. J Pediatr. 2007;83(3):225–32. https://doi.org/10.2223/JPED.1634.
7. Gonzalez Ayerbe JI, Hauser B, Salvatore S, Vandenplas Y. Diagnosis and management of gastroesophageal reflux disease in infants and children: from guidelines to clinical practice. Pediatr Gastroenterol Hepatol Nutr. 2019;22(2):107–21. https://doi.org/10.5223/pghn.2019.22.2.107.
8. Richter JE. Gastroesophageal reflux disease and asthma: the two are directly related. Am J Med. 2000;108(Suppl 4a):153S–8S. https://doi.org/10.1016/s0002-9343(99)00356-3.
9. Diaz DM, Winter HS, Colletti RB, et al. Knowledge, attitudes and practice styles of north American pediatricians regarding gastroesophageal reflux disease. J Pediatr Gastroenterol Nutr. 2007;45:56–64.
10. Orenstein SR. Management of supraesophageal complications of gastroesophageal reflux disease in infants and children. Am J Med. 2000;108(4A):139S–43S.
11. Rosen R, Hu L, Amirault J, Khatwa U, Ward DV, Onderdonk A. 16S community profiling identifies proton pump inhibitor related differences in gastric, lung, and oropharyngeal microflora. J Pediatr. 2015;166(4):917–23. https://doi.org/10.1016/j.jpeds.2014.12.067.

12. Mansfield LE. Embryonic origins of the relation of gastroesophageal reflux disease and airway disease. Am J Med. 2001;111(Suppl 8A):3S–7S. https://doi.org/10.1016/s0002-9343(01)00846-4.
13. Herbella FA, Patti MG. Gastroesophageal reflux disease: from pathophysiology to treatment. World J Gastroenterol. 2010;16(30):3745–9. https://doi.org/10.3748/wjg.v16.i30.3745.
14. Jadcherla SR, Hogan WJ, Shaker R. Physiology and pathophysiology of glottic reflexes and pulmonary aspiration: from neonates to adults. Semin Respir Crit Care Med. 2010;31(5):554–60. https://doi.org/10.1055/s-0030-1265896.
15. Richter J. Do we know the cause of reflux disease? Eur J Gastroenterol Hepatol. 1999;11(Suppl 1):S3–9.
16. Boeckxstaens GE. Review article: the pathophysiology of gastro-oesophageal reflux disease. Aliment Pharmacol Ther. 2007;26(2):149–60. https://doi.org/10.1111/j.1365-2036.2007.03372.x.
17. Molyneux ID, Morice AH. Airway reflux, cough and respiratory disease. Ther Adv Chronic Dis. 2011;2(4):237–48. https://doi.org/10.1177/2040622311406464.
18. Özdemir P, Erdinç M, Vardar R, Veral A, Akyıldız S, Özdemir Ö, Bor S. The role of microaspiration in the pathogenesis of gastroesophageal reflux-related chronic cough. J Neurogastroenterol Motil. 2017;23(1):41–8. https://doi.org/10.5056/jnm16057.
19. Meyer KC. Gastroesophageal reflux and lung disease. Expert Rev Respir Med. 2015;9:4383–5. https://doi.org/10.1586/17476348.2015.1060858.
20. Gilger MA. Pediatric otolaryngologic manifestations of gastroesophageal reflux disease. Curr Gastroenterol Rep. 2003;5(3):247–52. https://doi.org/10.1007/s11894-003-0027-5.
21. Venkatesan NN, Pine HS, Underbrink M. Laryngopharyngeal reflux disease in children. Pediatr Clin North Am. 2013;60(4):865–78. https://doi.org/10.1016/j.pcl.2013.04.011.
22. Prachuapthunyachart S, Jarasvaraparn C, Gremse DA. Correlation of gastroesophageal reflux disease assessment symptom questionnaire to impedance-pH measurements in children. SAGE Open Med. 2017;5:2050312117745221. https://doi.org/10.1177/2050312117745221.
23. Vandenplas Y, Hauser B, Devreker T, Mahler T, Degreef E, Wauters GV. Gastro-esophageal reflux in children: symptoms, diagnosis and treatment. J Pediatr Sci. 2011;3(4):e101.
24. Lightdale JR, Gremse DA. Gastroesophageal reflux: management guidance for the pediatrician. Pediatrics. 2013;2013:e1684–96.
25. Caruso G, Passali FM. ENT manifestations of gastro-oesophageal reflux in children. Acta Otorhinolaryngol Ital. 2006;26(5):252–5.
26. Martigne L, Delaage PH, Thomas-Delecourt F, et al. Prevalence and management of gastro-esophageal reflux disease in children and adolescents: a nationwide cross-sectional observational study. Eur J Pediatr. 2012;171:1767–73.
27. van der Pol RJ, Smits MJ, Venmans L, Boluyt N, Benninga MA, Tabbers MM. Diagnostic accuracy of tests in pediatric gastroesophageal reflux disease. J Pediatr. 2013;162(5):983–7.
28. Yellon RF, Coticchia J, Dixit S. Esophageal biopsy for the diagnosis of gastroesophageal reflux-associated otolaryngologic problems in children. Am J Med. 2000;108(Suppl 4a):131S–8S. https://doi.org/10.1016/s0002-9343(99)00352-6.
29. Jain M, Agrawal V. Role of esophageal manometry and 24-h pH testing in patients with refractory reflux symptoms. Indian J Gastroenterol. 2020;39:165. https://doi.org/10.1007/s12664-020-01032-z.
30. Shin MS. Esophageal pH and combined impedance-pH monitoring in children. Pediatr Gastroenterol Hepatol Nutr. 2014;17(1):13–22. https://doi.org/10.5223/pghn.2014.17.1.13.
31. Rosen R, Lord C, Nurko S. The sensitivity of multichannel intraluminal impedance and the pH probe in the evaluation of gastroesophageal reflux in children. Clin Gastroenterol Hepatol. 2006;4:167–72.
32. Heitlinger LA. Guideline for management of pediatric gastroesophageal reflux. JAMA Otolaryngol Head Neck Surg. 2018;144(8):755–6.
33. Barrett MW, Myers JC, Watson DI, Jamieson GG. Detection of bile reflux: in vivo validation of the Bilitec fibreoptic system. Dis Esophagus. 2000;13(1):44–50. https://doi.org/10.1046/j.1442-2050.2000.00062.x.

34. Rudolph CD, Mazur LJ, Liptak JS, et al. Guidelines for evaluation and treatment of gastroesophageal reflux in infants and children: recommendations of the north American Society for Pediatric Gastroenterology and Nutrition. J Pediatr Gastroenterol Nutr. 2001;32:1–22.
35. Hu FZ, Preston RA, Post JC, White GJ, Kikuchi LW, Wang X, Leal SM, Levenstien MA, Ott J, Self TW, Allen G, Stiffler RS, McGraw C, Pulsifer-Anderson EA, Ehrlich GD. Mapping of a gene for severe pediatric gastroesophageal reflux to chromosome 13q14. JAMA. 2000;284(3):325–34. https://doi.org/10.1001/jama.284.3.325.
36. Tolia V, Vandenplas Y. Systematic review: the extra-oesophageal symptoms of gastro-oesophageal reflux disease in children. Aliment Pharmacol Ther. 2009;29:258–72.
37. Poddar U. Gastroesophageal reflux disease (GERD) in children. Paediatr Int Child Health. 2019;39(1):7–12. https://doi.org/10.1080/20469047.2018.1489649.
38. Halstead LA. Role of gastroesophageal reflux in pediatric upper airway disorders. Otolaryngol Head Neck Surg. 1999;120(2):208–14. https://doi.org/10.1016/S0194-5998(99)70408-0.
39. Wenzl TG, Schenke S, Peschgens T, Silny J, Heimann G, Skopnik H. Association of apnea and nonacid gastroesophageal reflux in infants: investigations with the intraluminal impedance technique. Pediatr Pulmonol. 2001;31(2):144–9. https://doi.org/10.1002/1099-0496(200102)3 1:2<144:aid-ppul1023>3.0.co;2-z.
40. Gaude GS. Pulmonary manifestations of gastroesophageal reflux disease. Ann Thorac Med. 2009;4(3):115–23. https://doi.org/10.4103/1817-1737.53347.
41. Jain A, Patwari AK, Bajaj P, Kashyap R, Anand VK. Association of gatroesophageal reflux disease in young children with persistent respiratory symptoms. J Trop Pediatr. 2002;48:39–42.
42. Wang W, Tovar JA, Eizaguirre I, Aldazabal P. Airway obstruction and gastroesophageal reflux: an experimental study on the pathogenesis of this association. J Pediatr Surg. 1993;28(8):995–8. https://doi.org/10.1016/0022-3468(93)90500-k.
43. Waki EY, Madgy DN, Belenky WM, Gower VC. The incidence of gastroesophageal reflux in recurrent croup. Int J Pediatr Otorhinolaryngol. 1995;32(3):223–32. https://doi.org/10.1016/0165-5876(95)01168-b.
44. Contencin P, Narcy P. Gastropharyngeal reflux in infants and children. A pharyngeal pH monitoring study. Arch Otolaryngol Head Neck Surg. 1992;118(10):1028–30. https://doi.org/10.1001/archotol.1992.01880100018006.
45. Uzun H, Alagoz D, Okur M, Dikici B, Kocabay K, Senses DA, Ozkan A, Kaya M. Do gastrointestinal and respiratory signs and symptoms correlate with the severity of gastroesophageal reflux? BMC Gastroenterol. 2012;12:22. https://doi.org/10.1186/1471-230X-12-22.
46. Nielson DW, Heldt GP, Tooley WH. Stridor and gastroesophageal reflux in infants. Pediatrics. 1990;85(6):1034–9.
47. Orenstein SR, Kocoshis SA, Orenstein DM, Proujansky R. Stridor and gastroesophageal reflux: diagnostic use of intraluminal esophageal acid perfusion (Bernstein test). Pediatr Pulmonol. 1987;3(6):420–4. https://doi.org/10.1002/ppul.1950030608.
48. Orenstein SR, Orenstein DM. Gastroesophageal reflux and respiratory disease in children. J Pediatr. 1988;112(6):847–58. https://doi.org/10.1016/s0022-3476(88)80204-x. Erratum in: J Pediatr 1988 Sep;113(3):578.
49. Richter GT, Mehta D, Albert D, Elluru RG. A novel murine model for the examination of experimental subglottic stenosis. Arch Otolaryngol Head Neck Surg. 2009;135(1):45–52. https://doi.org/10.1001/archoto.2008.516.
50. Gaynor EB. Gastroesophageal reflux as an etiologic factor in laryngeal complications of intubation. Laryngoscope. 1988;98(9):972–9. https://doi.org/10.1288/00005537-198809000-00012.
51. Yellon RF, Szeremeta W, Grandis JR, Diguisseppe P, Dickman PS. Subglottic injury, gastric juice, corticosteroids, and peptide growth factors in a porcine model. Laryngoscope. 1998;108(6):854–62. https://doi.org/10.1097/00005537-199806000-00014.
52. Kahn A, Rebuffat E, Franco P, N'Duwimana M, Blum D. Apparent life-threatening events and apnea of infancy. In: Beckerman R, Brouilette R, Hunt C, editors. Respiratory control disorders in infants and children. Baltimore: Williams & Wilkins; 1992. p. 178–89.
53. Harris P, Muñoz C, Mobarec S, Brockmann P, Mesa T, Sánchez I. Relevance of the pH probe in sleep study analysis in infants. Child Care Health Dev. 2004;30(4):337–44. https://doi.org/10.1111/j.1365-2214.2004.00432.x.

54. Seyed RA, Samur H. The results of uvulopalatopharyngoplasty in patients with moderate obstructive sleep apnea syndrome having cardiac arrhythmias. Multidisciplin Cardiovasc Ann. 2020;11(2):1–7. https://doi.org/10.5812/mca.103810.

55. Xavier SD, Eckley CA, Duprat AC, de Souza Fontes LH, Navarro-Rodriguez T, Patrocínio J, Tridente D, Lorenzi-Filho G. Temporal association between respiratory events and reflux in patients with obstructive sleep apnea and laryngopharyngeal reflux. J Clin Sleep Med. 2019;15(10):1397–402. https://doi.org/10.5664/jcsm.7960.

56. Slocum C, Hibbs AM, Martin RJ, Orenstein SR. Infant apnea and gastroesophageal reflux: a critical review and framework for further investigation. Curr Gastroenterol Rep. 2007;9(3):219–24. https://doi.org/10.1007/s11894-007-0022-3.

57. Molloy EJ, Di Fiore JM, Martin RJ. Does gastroesophageal reflux cause apnea in preterm infants? Biol Neonate. 2005;87(4):254–61. https://doi.org/10.1159/000083958.

58. Orenstein SR, McGowan JD. Efficacy of conservative therapy as taught in the primary care setting for symptoms suggesting infant gastroesophageal reflux. J Pediatr. 2008;152(3):310–4. https://doi.org/10.1016/j.jpeds.2007.09.009.

59. van der Pol RJ, Smits MJ, van Wijk MP, Omari TI, Tabbers MM, Benninga MA. Efficacy of proton-pump inhibitors in children with gastroesophageal reflux disease: a systematic review. Pediatrics. 2011;127(5):925–35. https://doi.org/10.1542/peds.2010-2719.

Obstructive Sleep Apnea in Children: ENT Perspective

Ceren Günel, Yeşim Başal, and Tania Sih

75.1 Introduction

Pediatric sleep-disordered breathing (SDD) is a wide range of diseases that evacuate part or complete obstruction of the airway and increased airway resistance during sleep. Sleep-disordered breathing can cause morbidity in children, such as growth failure, neurocognitive and behavioral abnormalities, cardiovascular dysfunction, and rarely death [1].

Childhood obstructive sleep apnea (OSA) is defined as part or complete obstruction of the upper respiratory tract during sleep and is often associated with sleep disruption, hypoxia, hypercapnia, and symptoms throughout the day. Simple snoring is a condition that has no clinical significance and does not meet OSA criteria. Upper airway air resistance is characterized by snoring in children and increased upper respiratory airway resistance (URAR), characterized by paradoxal breathing without classical apnea and hypopnea [2] (Table 75.1).

75.2 Epidemiology

While simple snoring is 8% in the pediatric population, the prevalence of OSA has been reported as 1.2–5% [3]. The frequency of OSA peaks in the age group 2–6 when adenotonsillar hypertrophy reaches its greatest extent. Boys are more common than girls and black children are more common than others. Allergic rhinitis,

C. Günel (✉) · Y. Başal
Department of Otorhinolaryngology, Faculty of Medicine, Aydın Adnan Menderes University, Aydın, Turkey

T. Sih
Department of Pediatric Otolaryngology, School of Medicine, University of São Paulo, São Paulo, Brazil

Table 75.1 Spectrum of upper airway resistance (UAWR) and obstruction

increased UAWR		Result
	Causing only snoring	Snoring
	Sufficient to cause symptoms	UAW resistance syndrome
	Sufficient to elevate PaCo2 or lower SpO2	Obstructive hypoventilation or obstructive hypopnea
	Intermittent complete UAW obstruction	Intermittent complete UAW obstruction

asthma, and cigarette exposure have also been reported to be risk factors for OSA [4]. However, there is disagreement between studies [5–7].

75.3 Etiology and Pathogenesis

When viewed structurally, the pediatric OSA is associated with dynamic narrowing of the upper airway at different levels. The structures belonging to the Waldeyer circle in childhood, including tonsils, adenoids and lingual tonsils, are sites of airway narrowing. In general, these lymphoid tissues reach the most voluminous level between the ages of 3 and 6, and their size is expected to decrease with age [1].

Obesity is another independent risk factor in the etiology of the pediatric population [7]. In these individuals, pharyngeal adipose tissue increases collapse by narrowing the pharyngeal airway from the periphery. In addition, increased thoracic adipose tissue indirectly reduces respiratory functions. This situation also explains the residual OSA after adenotonsillectomy operation. Each 1 kg/m² increase in the body mass index causes a 12% increase in OSA risk. However, we should also point out that 45% of obese children with OSA also have evidence of adenotonsillar hypertrophy [8, 9].

Craniofacial abnormalities can also change the airway opening by changing the shape of the facial bones and tongue position. Again, neuromuscular disorders such as neuromuscular diseases or laryngomalacia cause both hypotonia in the pharyngeal muscles and collapse by neuromuscular incoordination [10].

The exact role of genetics in the pathogenesis of pediatric OSAS is still controversial. Some clinical syndromes such as Down, Prader–Willi, and Beckwith–Wiedemann are strongly associated with OSAS. Studies mostly focus on gene polymorphisms, e.g., ApoE4 allele, TNFa 308G gene polymorphism, and NADPH polymorphism have been associated with OSAS. Again, other genetic syndromes that may be related have been reported as Achondroplasia, Ehlers–Danlos syndrome, Pierre Robin sequence/complex, Ellis–van Creveld syndrome, sickle cell disease, and Noonan syndrome [1–10].

Table 75.2 Pathogenesis of obstructive sleep apnea

Anatomical factors	Obesity	Muscle tone	Others
Enlarged tonsils	Fatty infiltrates	Arousal responses	Inflammation
Enlarged adenoids	Decreased lung compliance	Neural drive	Gentic factors
Pharyngeal structure	Alterations in functional mechanisms of upper air way track	UAW reflexes	
Retrognathia		Load compensation	
Hyperglossal/ retropositioned tongue			
Ethnicity			

The relationship between OSA triggers systemic inflammation and OSA is known. Analysis studies performed in tonsillar tissue revealed that leukotriene C4 synthesis and leukotriene receptors 1 and 2 increased. Many studies have shown the effect of leukotriene receptor antagonists on adenoid and tonsil hypertrophy [11]. Moreover, increased secretion of proinflammatory cytokines tumor necrosis factor (TNF)-α, interleukin (IL)-6, and IL-1α has been reported in tonsillar tissue of OSA patients. It is thought that insulin resistance and fatty liver increase the release of proinflammatory mediators, especially in obese children. This can be attributed to the ability of the airway muscles to relax against the narrowing.

It is known that only one factor that we look at the general picture does not cause sleep disturbance (Table 75.2). The presence of patients with adenoid and tonsillar hypertrophy but without OSA findings may not only be due to upper airway obstruction. This can be attributed to the ability of the airway muscles to relax against the narrowing. Adenotonsillar hypertrophy alone is not sufficient for the diagnosis of OSA. Adenotonsillar hypertrophy accompanying abnormal upper airway motor control and tone results in OSA in these children [12].

75.4 Clinical Findings

75.4.1 Nighttime Symptoms

Snoring is the most common symptom of SDS and OSA. Families also frequently present with this complaint. However, apnea periods, frequency of waking up from sleep, sleep position, restlessness, and open mouth sleep should be questioned. It would be a more correct approach to identify apnea and question families.

Nocturnal enuresis is seemed secondary to OSA and SDS must be questioned in cases lasting more than 6 months [13]. Hormone secretion and bladder pressure increase that regulates fluid regulation are shown as causes of enuresis [14]. Also, in children with sickle cell disease who present with enuresis should be evaluated by an otolaryngology for SBD [15].

75.4.2 Daytime Symptoms

Open mouth breathing is also common during the day in children with adenoid hypertrophy. Hyponasal speech may accompany rhinorrhea. In this case, it should be questioned whether there are symptoms at night. Chronic sinusitis and serous otitis media due to adenoid hypertrophy can be the reason for the application of families. Compared to their peers, growth retardation and lack of appetite can be expressed by families. Ahlqvist-Rastad found growth retardation that greatly improved following adenotonsillectomy in 10% of children with OSA and 42–56% of infants [16].

Daytime sleepiness is more common in adolescent children. Still, this rate is between 13% and 20% compared to adults. Decreased school performance, conscious and cognitive difficulties can be expected. The first study on this subject was conducted by Gozal, and education success was low grade found in children with OSA. Moreover, it was found that school success increased dramatically in the treated children [17]. Hyperactivity, attention deficit, social maladjustment, and aggressive behavior may appear as behavioral problems in untreated children [18]. It would be wrong to say behavioral problems in all children with OSA, and many OSA patients are treated for behavioral problems without diagnosis [19]. Learning and behavioral problems are largely improved with OSA treatment. However, in some behavioral patterns, partial or reversible disorder due to late treatment may continue. In this sense, it is meaningful to diagnose and treat OSA as soon as possible [20]. Systemic hypertension can be detected in 10% to 25% of children with OSA. Studies investigating the association between systemic hypertension and OSA revealed a tendency to have higher diastolic blood pressure than systolic blood pressure [21]. The degree of blood pressure increase during rapid eye movement (REM) sleep has been shown to correlate with the severity of OSA. This is probably attributed to the tendency of apnea episodes to occur during REM sleep and the fact that arterial blood pressure fluctuations occur with respiratory changes [22]. Amin et al. found that the blood pressure surge, blood pressure load, and 24-h ambulatory blood pressure control group were significantly higher in children with SDD, independent of body mass index [23].

Unlike adults, pulmonary hypertension and ventricular failure are less common problems. This may cause early diagnosis to result in improvement in circulatory disturbance or cause less accumulation of chronic, moderate intermittent hypoxia in the pulmonary system [24]. Clinical findings are summarized in Table 75.3.

75.4.3 History

The assessment of the pediatric OSA patient should include a clinical evaluation including detailed history, questionnaires, endoscopic examination, and PSG. The positive predictability of OSA diagnosis by history and clinical examination was reported as 46–65%. In addition, it is decided which patients will undergo PSG based on the clinical examination [25].

There are questionnaires defined for the pediatric population. The pediatric sleep questionnaire described by Charvin has been validated in many languages. Although

Table 75.3 Clinic findings

Nighttime	Daytime	General
Snoring	Mouth breathing	Poor growth or failure to thrive
Apneic pauses	Hyponasality	Pulmonary hypertension/cor pulmonale/ventricular dysfunction
Diaphoresis	Chronic rhinorrhea	Systemic hypertension
Gasping	Dysphagia	
Frequent arousals and awakenings	Nasal obstruction	
Restless sleep	Daytime sleepiness	
Neck extension	Poor school performance	
Unusual sleeping positions	Behavior and neurocognitive difficulties	
Enuresis		
Paradoxic chest wall motion		
Parasomnias		

questionnaire which is described by Brouilette is useful, it is not too blunted by PSG results. Epworth Sleepiness Scale pediatric form and I'm sleepy questionnaire are valid surveys [26].

75.4.4 Clinical Examination

The general appearance of the child should be assessed by measuring height, weight, and blood pressure. Craniofacial structure, retrognathia, and micrognathia should be evaluated for midface hypoplasia. The clinic characterized by open mouth, long face, and mandibular hypoplasia is defined as adenoid face. In oropharyngeal examination, tonsil size, tongue size, palate position, tooth structure, and the presence of any structural abnormalities should be examined. While the patient is sitting in the supine position, the Mallampati classification and tonsil size should be noted. The nose should be examined in terms of its structural presence, and evaluated in terms of nasal passage, septum deviation, polyp, and allergic rhinitis [12].

In addition to an experienced ENT, an experienced anesthesiologist who can simulate periods of sleep, including deep sleep, is also important. It allows observation of the level of obstruction and sleep-dependent pathologies such as palatine collapse and laryngomalacia. However, it is still controversial whether sedation mimics real sleep. It is the reality of the physiological information determined in another discussion [27].

75.5 Imaging

In some cases, lateral neck radiography may be useful in locating the upper airway stenosis. Three-dimensional computed tomography can also be used in diagnosis and treatment plans in patients with craniofacial anomalies.

75.6 Pulse Oximeter

The fact that it is a cheap and easy method has increased its use in diagnosis. During a 10–30 minute sleep period, a decrease in O2 saturation at least five times, more than 4%, is defined as cluster. The diagnosis is made when O2 saturation is below 90% at least 3 times and/or at least three desaturation clusters occur [12]. However, there are contradictory publications about its compatibility with PSG.

75.7 PSG

The main diagnostic method in the diagnosis of OSA is polysomnography. In very young infants, "nap" sleep studies during the day may also be adequate [28]. Polysomnography is recommended prior to adenotonsillectomy for selected children with premorbid conditions and for otherwise healthy children for whom the need for surgery is uncertain or for whom there is a discordance between tonsil size and reported severity of symptoms. It is based on the multi-channel recording principle during sleep in accredited sleep laboratories. A typical montage would include several electroencephalography (EEG) channels, chin and anterior tibial electromyography (EMG), bilateral electrooculography, pulse oximeter and pulse waveform, nasal pressure transducer, oronasal airflow thermistor, end-tidal capnography, chest and abdominal respiratory inductance plethysmography, body position sensor, microphone, and real-time synchronized video monitoring [27].

Apnea is defined as a decrease in air flow by more than 90% for at least two respiratory cycles. Hypopnea is defined as a 3% decrease in oxygen saturation or at least two respiratory cycles, a decrease of airflow >30. Whether or not inspiratory effort determines the type of apnea. If there is inspiratory effort during the whole period, if there is no obstructive, central type apnea is in favor. Unlike adults, even a single apnea/hypopnea period is considered pathological in children. While evaluating, the number of apnea and hypopnea (AHI) per hour and respiratory disturbance index (RDI) are used for the total number of apnea, hypopnea, and respiratory effort related arousal (RERA). OSA severity is evaluated according to AHI. AHI 1–4 is considered mild, 4–10 is moderate, and >10 severe. End-tidal CO2 pressure is not expected to rise above 50 mm Hg in a normal sleep. An increase in end-tidal CO2 pressure above 50 mm Hg in more than 8–10% of sleep is defined as obstructive hypoventilation [29].

Upper respiratory airway resistance is assessed by esophageal pressure. Awake esophageal pressure is usually between 10 and 5 cm. Increasingly, negative esophageal pressure is detected with repetitive breathing in PSG [30]. Home-type PSG is not recommended today, but it can be used to evaluate in the absence of a sleep laboratory [31].

If polysomnography is not available, alternative diagnostic tests such as night video recording, nocturnal oximetry, and daytime nap polysomnography may be ordered.

75.8 Treatment

75.8.1 Nonsurgical Treatment

Topical nasal steroids can be used in the treatment of SBD. Nasal fluticasone helps recovery from pediatric obstructive sleep apnea by reducing the frequency of mixed and obstructive apneas-hypopneas [32]. In cases with mild OSAS, it was observed that the use of intranasal budesonide for 6 weeks reduced the severity of apnea and reduced underlying adenoid hypertrophy, and this effect continued for 2 months after the treatment was completed [33].

Three months of oral use of montelukast reduced the severity of OSAS and reduced the size of adenoid tissue in children with mild OSAS [34]. It is known that the use of oral prednisone for a short time, such as 5 days, does not change AHI and does not reduce adenoid hypertrophy and open the airway [35].

Although it is known that chronic tonsil hypertrophy decreases with the use of oral amoxicillin clavulanate for a month, its effect on AHI has not been studied [36]. Oral azithromycin has an effect on temporarily improving OSAS due to adenotonsillar hypertrophy, it does not reduce the need for surgery [37]. The use of PPI in OSAS patients with GER provides improvement in sleep quality without changing AHI [38]. Nasal steroids, montelukast, and PPIs can be used in supportive therapy in mild OSA [39].

Environmental irritants, allergens, and smoking exposure should be avoided in all children with OSAS. Because exposure can increase nasal congestion. Weight loss should be supported and obesity should be treated.

Attention should be paid to sleep hygiene and the use of pillows that prevent sleeping in the supine position should be recommended. Supplemental oxygen can be given in addition to PAP therapy in patients with hypercapnia. For hypercapnia, nasal expiratory resistor device can also be used in adolescent children.

PAP therapy is the most commonly used nonsurgical treatment in cases with AHI >1. In addition, the first treatment recommended for persistent OSAS after surgery is PAP therapy. CPAP and BiPAP will be explained in different sections. CPAP and BiPAP are also recommended in OSAS not indicated for adenotonsillectomy or despite ongoing adenotonsillectomy. Supplemental oxygen therapy is not recommended as the only treatment modality. Weight loss is recommended in obese children as it reduces additional comorbidities. Rapid maxillary expansion can be used in the treatment of posttonsillectomy persistent OSA or OSA that continues despite mandibular advancement with the oral appliance [40].

Another treatment option that can be used in persistent OSAS after adenotonsillectomy or in children with OSAS with small adenotonsil tissue is rapid maxillary expansion (RME). With this orthodontic treatment, the palate and nasal passage expand, thus increasing the airway opening and reducing nasal congestion. With the combined use of RME and adenotonsillectomy, 94% of OSAS was treated [41].

75.8.2 Surgical Treatment

Since adenotonsillar hypertrophy is a common problem in childhood, tonsillectomy and/or adenoidectomy is an effective treatment method in OSAS. However, adenoidectomy alone or tonsillectomy alone is not recommended for OSAS treatment. In the presence of adenoids and tonsillar hypertrophy, adenotonsillectomy is the first option in pediatric OSAS treatment.

While evaluating the patients with pediatric OSAS preoperatively, it is sufficient to question the detailed history and family history in terms of bleeding disorder. If the patient does not have any risk factors, additional hematological and cardiac evaluation is not required.

However, pediatric expert opinion should be obtained for children with special conditions such as Down syndrome, Pierre Robin syndrome, neuromuscular disease, mucopolysaccharidosis, sickle cell anemia, cerebral palsy, and morbid obesity. Obese children under 3 years of age with abnormal upper airway tone, congenital syndrome, or craniofacial anomaly are at high risk for perioperative complications and posttonsillectomy residual OSAS [42]. Children with increased risk of postoperative respiratory complications should be followed at least one night after surgery in a unit (service or intensive care) that has experience in caring for children with airway problems.

The effect of the surgery should be controlled by evaluating the patient 8–12 weeks after the operation. Patients who continue to snore after surgery, have high preoperative AHI, and have craniofacial and neurological anomalies should be evaluated again by polysomnography. In addition, if there are adenotonsil tissue regrowth after surgery and excessive weight gain, patients should be re-evaluated in terms of OSAS.

Although cure rates vary after adenotonsillectomy, success was 59.8% when AHI <1 and 66.3% when AHI <5 [43]. According to the CHAT study comparing watchful waiting and adenotonsillectomy, symptoms regress, quality of life increases, behavioral disorders improve, and PSG results improve in children who undergo adenotonsillectomy in the early period [44]. Adenotonsillectomy improves the quality of life in mild to moderate OSAS. Children with moderate OSA see the greatest benefit in behavioral and nocturnal symptoms [45]. Obese, severe OSAS, asthma, or children over 7 years old are at risk for residual OSAS after adenotonsillectomy [46].

Tonsillectomy can be performed by using the cold knife technique as conventional, monopolar cautery, bipolar cautery, coblator, harmonic scalpel or tonsillotomy (intracapsular tonsillectomy). Tonsillotomy can be done using many different tools, including microdebrider. Pain and postoperative bleeding are less common in tonsillotomy than tonsillectomy. Tonsillotomy is a safe treatment method in children with OSA [47]. However, in tonsillotomy, unlike classical tonsillectomy, there is a risk of tonsillar regrowth due to feeding with a sugary diet and having frequent postoperative upper respiratory tract infections [48].

Lingual tonsillectomy is a surgical method that can be used in the treatment of persistent OSAS with lingual tonsil hypertrophy. It is not recommended to be performed simultaneously with adenotonsillectomy as initial therapy. Because in the upper airway, it can cause circumferential scar tissue that is very difficult to treat [49].

Postop respiratory complications can be seen more frequently in children with OSA. Respiratory complications are more common in children with morbid obesity, craniofacial anomalies, pulmonary HT, cardiac failure, growth retardation, severe apnea, or OSA under 3 years of age [39]. In the postoperative period, it is necessary to avoid narcotic analgesics. Paracetamol should be the first choice for pain relief. NSAID use is controversial. Ketorolac use has no superiority in pain control over high-dose paracetamol, and its use is not recommended because of higher hemorrhage rates compared to paracetamol [49].

Although there is no consensus about the use of postoperative antibiotics, it is frequently prescribed to prevent bleeding, pain, halitosis, fever, and postop infections. However, it has been demonstrated that antibiotics do not reduce pain, do not reduce the rates of primary and secondary hemorrhage, but only help control fever [50]. It is known that the use of peroperatively dexamethasone reduces vomiting in the postoperative period [51].

While deciding on surgery, it is necessary to pay attention to the severity of symptoms, the age of the child, the presence of underlying diseases, the presence of risk factors, the condition in PSG, and the presence of OSAS-related complications. Which surgical method to choose should be decided according to the patient's condition and the advantages and disadvantages of the technique. Surgical techniques that can be used are summarized in Table 75.4 [52].

Table 75.4 Surgery options in children with OSA

Surgery procedure	Patient	Advantage	Complications
Adenotonsillectomy	Tonsil and/or adenoid hypertrophy	Effective Mostly well tolerated	Ache, difficulty in oral intake Postop bleeding
Tonsillotomy +adenoidectomy	Tonsil and/or adenoid hypertrophy	Fast recovery	Its effectiveness in OSAS treatment is not clear Regrowth rates in OSAS are unknown
Lingual tonsillectomy	Persistent OSAS + lingual tonsil hypertrophy after AT	Effective treatment of residual OSAS	Concentric scar in the airway, no consensus of efficacy
Tracheostomy	Children with OSAS with no other treatment options	Very efficient	Tracking difficulty at home Tracheotomy complications
Bariatric surgery	Obese adolescent children with OSAS	High success rate in selected patient group	Long-term results are uncertain
Craniofacial surgery	Children with OSAS and craniofacial anomaly	High success rate in selected patient group	High morbidity Success rate depends on the center and the chosen technique

Other surgical methods can be used in OSA patients with comorbidities or in patients whose OSA does not improve after adenotonsillectomy. Sleep endoscopy or cine MRI can be used to determine the level of obstruction. Persistent OSAS may be caused by regrowth of adenoid tissue or by concha hypertrophy, lingual tonsil hypertrophy, macroglossia, laryngomalacia, and lateral pharyngeal wall collapse. It is known that the level of obstruction is multilevel in residual OSAS after adenotonsillectomy. Unlike adults, single-session multilevel surgeries are not recommended in children due to complications. The most common procedures in this patient group are lingual tonsillectomy and supraglottoplasty [53]. However, UPPP, tongue reduction, tongue root surgeries, hypoglossal nerve stimulation, expansion sphincter pharyngoplasty, mandibular distraction osteogenesis, bariatric surgery, or tracheotomy can also be performed.

Mandibular distraction osteogenesis can be used successfully in the treatment of severe OSAS in cases of micrognathia/mandibular hypoplasia as in Pierre Robin and Treacher Collins syndrome. It can be tried as the first treatment option in patients with glossoptosis due to micrognathia before tongue lip adhesion, mandibular distraction osteogenesis, and tracheotomy to reduce morbidity and mortality [54]. Although there is no study on hyoid suspension in the pediatric age group, it can be preferred in appropriate cases because it is a successful technique used in adults. In morbidly obese adolescents, bariatric surgery is a good option in the management of metabolic syndrome and advanced OSAS [55].

Hypoglossal nerve stimulation is a safe and effective treatment modality in adolescents with Down syndrome and OSA who do not benefit from conventional treatments [56]. The level of obstruction may be root of the tongue in children who are morbidly obese, with Down's syndrome, or with neuromuscular disease. Depending on the location and severity of the obstruction, lingual tonsillectomy, posterior midline glossectomy, tongue base sling, epiglottopexy, hyoid suspension, or tongue-lip adhesion may be involved in the treatment [54].

Midline posterior glossectomy and lingual tonsillectomy are beneficial in children with persistent OSAS and PAP intolerance, normal weight and overweight Down syndrome after adenotonsillectomy. The desired level of improvement could not be achieved in obese patients [57]. Tongue base suspension performed simultaneously with adenotonsillectomy in children with OSAS and cerebral palsy is a reliable method that increases success [58, 59]. Epiglottic prolapse is rarely seen in persistent OSAS. The diagnosis is made by flexible endoscopy and DISE. The aim of treatment is to prevent epiglottis to airway obstructing. The vallecula and lingual face of the epiglottis are demucolized with a cautery, coblator, or laser, and then the epiglottis is sutured to the tongue base [54].

Tracheotomy is considered as a treatment option if RDI is >60 and desaturation is more than 70% in children with persistent advanced OSAS and PAP intolerance after adenotonsillectomy. Although adenotonsillectomy is the first treatment option in pediatric OSAS, PSG should be performed in residual OSAS, and appropriate treatment modality should be applied considering the patient's morbidity and additional problems or who have persistent daytime symptoms despite PAP.

References

1. Marcus CL. Pathophysiology of childhood obstructive sleep apnea: current concepts. Respir Physiol. 2000;119:143–54.
2. From Carroll JL. Obstructive sleep-disordered breathing in children: new controversies, new directions. Clin Chest Med. 2003;24:261–82.
3. Lumeng JC, Chervin RD. Epidemiology of pediatric obstructive sleep apnea. Proc Am Thorac Soc. 2008;5:242–52.
4. Redline S, Tishler PV, Schluchter M, et al. Risk factors for sleepdisordered breathing in children: associations with obesity, race, and respiratory problems. Am J Respir Crit Care Med. 1999;159:1527–32.
5. Calhoun SL, Vgontzas AN, Mayes SD, et al. Prenatal and perinatal complications: is it the link between race and SES and childhood sleep disordered breathing? J Clin Sleep Med. 2010;6:264–9.
6. Goldstein NA, Abramowitz T, Weedon J, et al. Racial/ethnic differences in the prevalence of snoring and sleep disordered breathing in young children. J Clin Sleep Med. 2011;7:163–71.
7. Lam YY, Chan EY, Ng DK, et al. The correlation among obesity, apnea-hypopnea index, and tonsil size in children. Chest. 2006;130:1751–6.
8. Dayyat E, Kheirandish-Gozal L, Sans Capdevila O, et al. Obstructive sleep apnea in children: relative contributions of body mass index and adenotonsillar hypertrophy. Chest. 2009;136:137–44.
9. Marcus CL, Brooks LJ, Draper KA, et al. Diagnosis and Management of Childhood Obstructive Sleep Apnea Syndrome. Pediatrics. 2012;130:576–84.
10. Gulotta G, Iannella G, Vicini C. Risk factors for obstructive sleep apnea syndrome in children: state of the art. Int J Environ Res Public Health. 2019;16:3235.
11. Tan H-L, Gozal D, Kheirandish-Gozal L. Obstructive sleep apnea in children: a critical update. Nat Sci Sleep. 2013;5:109–23.
12. Saini S, Ciorba C, Bianchini C. Assessment of obstructive sleep apnoea (OSA) in children: an update. Acta Otorhinolaryngol Ital. 2019;39:289–97.
13. Jeyakumar A, Rahman SI, Armbrecht ES, et al. The association between sleep-disordered breathing and enuresis in children. Laryngoscope. 2012;122:1873–7.
14. Bediwy AS, El-Mitwali A, Zaher AA, et al. Sleep apnea in children with refractory monosymptomatic nocturnal enuresis. Nat Sci Sleep. 2014;6:37–42.
15. Lehmann GC, Bell TR, Kirkham FJ, et al. Enuresis associated with sleep disordered breathing in children with sickle cell anemia. J Urol. 2012;188:1572–S1576.
16. Ahlqvist-Rastad J, Hultcrantz E, Melander H, et al. Body growth in relation to tonsillar enlargement and tonsillectomy. Int J Pediatr Otorhinolaryngol. 1992;24:55–61.
17. Gozal D. Sleep-disordered breathing and school performance in children. Pediatrics. 1998;102:616–20.
18. Perfect MM, Archbold K, Goodwin JL, et al. Risk of behavioral and adaptive functioning difficulties in youth with previous and current sleep disordered breathing. Sleep. 2013;36:517B–25B.
19. Kheirandish-Gozal L, Gozal D. Genotype-phenotype interactions in pediatric obstructive sleep apnea. Respir Physiol Neurobiol. 2013;189:10.
20. Gozal D, Pope DW. Snoring during early childhood and academic performance at ages thirteen to fourteen years. Pediatrics. 2001;107:1394–9.
21. Marcus CL, Greene MG, Carroll JL. Blood pressure in children with obstructive sleep apnea. Am J Respir Crit Care Med. 1998;157:1098–103.
22. Kwok KL, Ng DK, Chan CH. Cardiovascular changes in children with snoring and obstructive sleep apnoea. Ann Acad Med Singapore. 2008;37:715–21.
23. Amin R, Somers VK, McConnell K, et al. Activity-adjusted 24-hour ambulatory blood pressure and cardiac remodeling in children with sleep disordered breathing. Hypertension. 2008;51:84–91.

24. Adegunsoye A, Ramachandran S. Etiopathogenetic mechanisms of pulmonary hypertension in sleep-related breathing disorders. Pulm Med. 2012;2012:273591.
25. Brietzke SE, Katz ES, Roberson DW. Can history and physical examination reliably diagnose pediatric obstructive sleep apnea/ hypopnea syndrome? A systematic review of the literature. Otolaryngol Head Neck Surg. 2004;131:827–32.
26. Amra B, Rahmati B, Soltaninejad SF. Screening questionnaires for obstructive sleep apnea: an updated systematic review. Awat Feizi Oman Med J. 2018;33:184–92.
27. Jason L. Yu, Olufunke Afolabi-Brown (2019) updates on management of pediatric obstructive sleep apnea. Pediatr Investig. 2019;3:228–35.
28. Gipson K, Lu M, Kinane TB. Sleep-disordered breathing in children. Pediatr Rev. 2019;40:3–13.
29. Berry RB, Budhiraja R, Gottlieb DJ, Gozal, et al. The AASM manual for the scoring of sleep and associated events: rules, terminology and technical specifications. Washington: American Academy of Sleep Medicine; 2016.
30. Kheirandish-Gozal L, Gozal D. The multiple challenges of obstructive sleep apnea in children: diagnosis. Curr Opin Pediatr. 2008;20:650–3.
31. Roland PS, Rosenfeld RM, Brooks LJ, et al. Clinical practice guideline: polysomnography for sleep-disordered breathing prior to tonsillectomy in children. Otolaryngol Head Neck Surg. 2011;145:1–15.
32. Brouillette RT, Manoukian JJ, Ducharme FM, et al. Efficacy of fluticasone nasal spray for pediatric obstructive sleep apnea. J Pediatr. 2001;138:838–44.
33. Kheirandish-Gozal L, Gozal D. Intranasal budesonide treatment for children with mild obstructive sleep apnea syndrome. Pediatrics. 2008;122:149–55.
34. Goldbart AD, Greenberg Dotan S, Tal A. Montelukast for children with obstructive sleep apnea: a double-blind, placebo-controlled study. Pediatrics. 2012;130:575–80.
35. Al Ghamdi SA, Manoukian JJ, Morielli A, et al. Do systemic corticosteroids effectively treat obstructive sleep apnea secondary to Adenotonsillar hypertrophy? Laryngoscope. 1997;107:1382–138.
36. Sclafani AP, Ginsburg J, Shah MK, et al. Treatment of symptomatic chronic Adenotonsillar hypertrophy with amoxicillin/Clavulanate potassium: short- and long-term results. Pediatrics. 1998;101:675–81.
37. Don DM, Goldstein NA, Crockett DM, et al. Antimicrobial therapy for children with Adenotonsillar hypertrophy and obstructive sleep apnea: a prospective randomized trial comparing azithromycin vs placebo. Otolaryngol Head Neck Surg. 2005;133:562–8.
38. Rassameehiran S, Klomjit S, Hosiriluck N, et al. Meta-analysis of the effect of proton pump inhibitors on obstructive sleep apnea symptoms and indices in patients with gastroesophageal reflux disease. Baylor Univ Med Center Proc. 2016;29:3–6.
39. Goldstein NA, Pugazhendhi V, Rao SM, et al. Clinical assessment of pediatric obstructive sleep apnea. Pediatrics. 2004;114:33–43.
40. Pirelli P, Saponara M, Guilleminault C. Rapid maxillary expansion (RME) for pediatric obstructive sleep apnea: a 12-year follow-up. Sleep Med. 2015;16:933–5.
41. Mitchell RB, Archer SM, Ishman SL, et al. Clinical practice guideline: tonsillectomy in children. Otolayngol Head and Neck Surg. 2019;160:1–42.
42. Friedman M, Wilson M, Lin HC, et al. Updated systematic review of tonsillectomy and adenoidectomy for treatment of pediatric obstructive sleep apnea/hypopnea syndrome. Otolaryngol Head Neck Surg. 2009;140:800–8.
43. Marcus CL, Moore RH, Rosen CL, et al. A randomized trial of Adenotonsillectomy for childhood sleep apnea. N Engl J Med. 2013;368:2366–76.
44. Fehrm J, Nerfeldt P, Browaldh N, et al. Effectiveness of Adenotonsillectomy vs watchful waiting in young children with mild to moderate obstructive sleep apnea: a randomized clinical trial. JAMA Otolaryngol Head Neck Surg. 2020;146:647–54.
45. Bhattacharjee R, Kheirandish Gozal L, Spruyt K, et al. Adenotonsillectomy outcomes in treatment of obstructive sleep apnea in children. Am J Respir Crit Care Med. 2010;182:676–83.

46. Lee HS, Yoon HY, Jin HJ, et al. The safety and efficacy of powered intracapsular tonsillectomy in children: a meta-analysis. Laryngoscope. 2017;128:732–44.
47. Zagólski O. Why do palatine tonsils grow back after partial tonsillectomy in children? Eur Arch Otorhinolaryngol. 2010;267:1611617.
48. Rusy LM, Houck CS, Sullivan LJ, et al. A double-blind evaluation of ketorolac Tromethamine versus acetaminophen in pediatric tonsillectomy. Anesth Analg. 1995;80:226–9.
49. Dhiwakar M, Clement WA, Supriya M, et al. Antibiotics to reduce post-tonsillectomy morbidity. Cochrane Database Syst Rev. 2008;1:1465–858. https://doi.org/10.1002/14651858. cd005607.
50. Splinter WM, Roberts DJ. Dexamethasone decreases vomiting by children after tonsillectomy. Anesth Analg. 1996;83:913–6.
51. Manickam PV, Shott SR, Bos EF, et al. Systematic review of site of obstruction identification and non-CPAP treatment options for children with persistent pediatric obstructive sleep apnea. Laryngoscope. 2015;126:491–500.
52. Guilleminault C, Monteyrol PJ, Huynh NT, et al. Adeno-tonsillectomy and rapid maxillary distraction in pre-pubertal children, a pilot study. Sleep Breath. 2010;15:173–7.
53. Cielo CM, Gungor A. Treatment options for pediatric obstructive sleep apnea. Curr Probl Pediatr Adolesc Health Care. 2016;46:27–33.
54. Michalsky M, Kramer RE, Fullmer MA, et al. Developing criteria for pediatric/adolescent bariatric surgery programs. Pediatrics. 2011;128:65–70.
55. Caloway CL, Diercks GR, Keamy D, et al. Update on hypoglossal nerve stimulation in children with down syndrome and obstructive sleep apnea. Laryngoscope. 2019;130:263. https:// doi.org/10.1002/lary.28138.
56. Ishman SL, Chang KW, Kennedy AA. Techniques for evaluation and management of tongue-base obstruction in pediatric obstructive sleep apnea. Curr Opin Otolaryngol Head Neck Surg. 2018;26:409–16.
57. Propst EJ, Amin R, Talwar N, et al. Midline posterior glossectomy and lingual tonsillectomy in obese and nonobese children with down syndrome: biomarkers for success. Laryngoscope. 2016;127:757–63.
58. Hartzell LD, Guillory RM, Munson PD, et al. Tongue base suspension in children with cerebral palsy and obstructive sleep apnea. Int J Pediatr Otorhinolaryngol. 2013;77:534–7.
59. Kheirandish L, Goldbart AD, Gozal D. Intranasal steroids and oral leukotriene modifier therapy in residual sleepdisordered breathing after tonsillectomy and adenoidectomy in children. Pediatrics. 2006;117:61–6.

Neurobehavioral Consequences of Obstructive Sleep Apnea Syndrome in Children

Gül Yücel and Nur Yücel Ekici

76.1 Introduction

Obstructive sleep disordered breathing (SDB) is a common problem in children and includes many clinical conditions with variable severity of intermittent airway obstruction such as primary snoring, upper airway resistance syndrome (UARS), obstructive hypoventilation, and obstructive sleep apnea syndrome (OSAS) (obstructive, central, and mixed). Primary snoring is described by snoring over three nights a week, without oxyhemoglobin desaturation or sleep fragmentation. UARS is characterized by snoring with frequent sleep fragmentation and increased respiratory effort with upper airway resistance, in the absence of recognizable oxyhemoglobin desaturation. OSAS is characterized by persistent episodes of upper airway obstruction with oxyhemoglobin desaturation disruption and normal sleep pattern. Obstructive hypoventilation is considered as elevated end-expiratory carbon dioxide partial pressure without noticeable obstructive events [1–5]. Definition of obstructive hypoventilation is comprised in International Classification of Sleep Disorders [4], but American Thoracic Society [5] evaluated it within the definition of OSAS.

Knowledge on the epidemiology of obstructive SDB is limited and conflicting. Prevalence of obstructive SDB in the children differs from study to study due to a variety of methodologic issues (parent-reported snoring, parent-reported apneic events, parent-reported symptoms on the questionnaire, etc.), and heterogeneity in diagnostic criteria such as most of the studies did not estimate UARS and obstructive hypoventilation. Most studies reported the prevalence of OSAS between 1 and

G. Yücel (✉)
Section of Pediatric Neurology, Konya Training and Research Hospital, University of Health Sciences, Konya, Turkey

N. Y. Ekici
Section of Otorhinolaryngology, Adana City Training and Research Hospital, University of Health Sciences, Adana, Turkey

C. Cingi et al. (eds.), *Pediatric ENT Infections*,
https://doi.org/10.1007/978-3-030-80691-0_76

4% [6]; however, the conclusion of a meta-analysis which was given by Lumeng et al. [2] indicated the rate of snoring in children is 7.45% and while OSAS occurs in 0.1–13%. According to this meta-analysis, higher prevalence of obstructive SDB symptoms was found in boys. Also, African-American ethnicity and obesity are among high risk factors for SDB in children [2].

OSAS in children is associated with cardiovascular morbidity (severe pulmonary hypertension and cor pulmonale), morbidity from the central nervous system (excessive daytime sleepiness, inattention/hyperactivity, cognitive deficits/learning problems and behavioral problems), and nocturnal enuresis, delay of growth, decreased quality of life, and also increased health care utilization. These morbidity and conditions coexisting with OSAS emphasize the importance of recognition, detection, and treatment. The diagnosis should be considered and diagnosed with overnight polysomnography (PSG) in children with representative symptoms (e.g., signs of upper airway obstruction such as snoring, fragmented sleep, oral breathing, excessive daytime sleepiness, or hyperactivity) and risk factors (obesity, tonsillar hypertrophy, mandibular hypoplasia, neuromuscular/craniofacial/neurologic or genetic disorders). In this section, the neurobehavioral consequences of OSAS in children were summarized to draw attention to the presence of symptoms and concerns about a child's learning capacity and school performance, attention, memory, hyperactivity, or emotion regulation.

76.2 Neuropathogenesis of OSAS

OSAS is described by repeated events of partial or complete obstruction during sleep and induced deterioration of the gas exchange (hypoxemia and hypercarbia), sleep fragmentation, repeated arousals, inadequate sleep efficiency, and episodic cerebral perfusion alterations. Long-time repetition of these events leads to neuronal cell losses in selective brain regions, as well as affects the brain functional response, particularly in developing brain. Regional blood flow modification during sleep, recurrent hypoxia-re-oxygenation events with apneic episodes, that causes to elevated oxidative damage and inflammation process, lipid peroxidation, and ensuing neuronal damage might be responsible for neurocognitive deficits [7–11]. Genetic and environmental factors are also effective. In experimental animal models, subjected animal to repeated intermittent hypoxia has been shown to induce neuronal damage in regional brain regions, axons inside of white matter tracts, and nerve fibers in gray matter, just as in human model [10, 12]. Also, elevated inflammatory markers, lipid peroxidation products, and oxidative damage have been demonstrated in many brain regions [10, 11].

Previous studies indicated substantially reduced gray matter volume in the caudate nucleus, insular region, hippocampal region, the frontal and temporo-parieto-occipital cortices, and cerebellar regions [13, 14]. The other studies reported that children with OSAS showed tissue damage in white matter integrity and functional activation in anterior, mid, posterior corpus callosum [9, 15]. A number of axonal tracts among such brain structures would reduce integrity, and also modify the function of these structures. The emotional expression could be affected due to injury to limbic areas (e.g., the anterior cingulate and insula, and interconnections to the amygdala and hippocampus). Damage in the limbic structure, as well as abnormal functional connectivity between hippocampus and cerebellum, may contribute to mood disorders and impaired memory process. Moreover, the possible cause of cognitive dysfunction in children with OSAS may be the structural changes in the anterior cingulate cortex, hippocampus, fornix, cerebellum, and frontal cortex [9, 16].

The prefrontal cortex is regarded as an important part of the cerebral cortex that contributes to a wide variety of executive functions such as higher cognition, planning, proper social behavior, and personality. Beebe et al. [17] proposed a model that linked to daytime cognitive and behavioral deficits in OSAS through disruption of prefrontal cortical processes. Sleep disruption, intermittent hypoxia, and hypercarbia modify the metabolism and neurochemistry of the prefrontal cortical region, and then lead to mentally manipulating information, emotional lability, poor decision-making, and deficit in attention and memory [17].

The results of the publications, mentioned above, indicate that various brain structures and their associated neuronal pathways are susceptible to OSAS complications. Disruption of the function and integrity of the related brain structures associated with neuronal damage may lead to the neurocognitive impairment in children with OSAS.

76.3   Excessive Daytime Sleepiness

Excessive daytime sleepiness (EDS), a sudden uncontrollable impulse to sleep, is an important symptom in children with OSAS. EDS is caused by a wide range of sleep-related causes and distinct conditions such as insomnia, nocturnal seizures, chronic pain, and movement disorders. Sleep-related causes of EDS are classified under four main headings, namely inefficient sleep duration (insomnia), disturbed/fragmented sleep (behavioral, SDB, movement disorder, medical problems disturbing sleep, environmental disturbances), circadian misalignment (Circadian rhythm disorder), and primary disorders that increased need for sleep (head trauma, increased intracranial pressure, hypersomnia, hypothalamic lesions).

EDS is the most frequent symptom among children and adolescents by a progressive increment with age and pubertal maturation. Female dominance occurs after mid-puberty [18]. Despite the exact prevalence of sleep-related causes of EDS in children with OSAS is unclear due to different assessment methods, studies have reported the prevalence of EDS, ranging from 10% to 20% in prepubertal children and 16% to 47% in adolescents [18, 19]. In studies conducted with Multiple Sleep Latency Test (MSLT), the prevalence of EDS was reported as 13–20% and was more prone to being obese [19–21].

EDS in children is rarely recognized by parents and physicians as sleepiness may not be verbalized by the child. They usually present to the physicians with different symptoms such as increased hyperactivity, mood disorders, behavioral problems, impairments in neurocognitive function, diminished learning capabilities, or academic difficulties. Childhood and adolescence are characterized by major developmental changes in physiological, social, and psychological fields. Some learning, behavior, mood, or sleep disorders that occur in these constantly changing periods can lead children and adolescence to seek psychiatric care. It is then very important to accurately determine which symptoms are related to sleep disorders. Otherwise, some sleepy children may be mistakenly considered lazy, hyperactive, or depressed. For these reasons, diagnosis of EDS requires a detailed systematic approach in children. A comprehensive history and physical examination are of prime importance for evaluating these children. Screening instruments such as Epworth Sleepiness Scale, Pittsburg Sleep Quality Index, Pediatric Daytime Sleepiness Scale, and Children's Report of Sleep Pattern-Sleepiness Scale can help confirm the subjective EDS in children. In the history, sleep behaviors (daily sleep duration or patterns), sleep hygiene (bedtimes, use of mobile devices, or snacking before bed), past medical history (e.g., epilepsy, asthma, neuromuscular disorders, migraine, or autism), use of medications that may affect sleep, family history of sleep disorders, snoring, or pauses in breathing during sleep should be questioned. Physical examination should include assessments of growth and development, body mass index (BMI), neurologic function, presence of the genetic condition, and ear/nose/throat examination. Objective measures include actigraphy (indicating wakefulness or sleep and estimates total sleep time), PSG, and MSLT. Lateral neck X-rays or endoscopy helps to show adenoidal hypertrophy.

PSG is the gold standard tool for evaluating OSAS and EDS [1]. PSG includes: (1) description of total sleep time, sleep latency, arousals, leg movements; (2) electroencephalography (EEG) to record sleep stages with brain wave activity, and also record seizures; (3) electromyography (EMG) to record skeletal muscle movement and electrooculography (EOG) for eye movements to determine rapid eye movement (REM) sleep; (4) monitors oxygen, CO2, and gas exchange via pulse oximetry and end-tidal CO2; and (5) monitors respiration including nasal and mouth breathing. Sleep-related breathing disorders are generally associated with hypertrophic tonsils and adenoids and sometimes incorporated with increased BMI in children, as well as chronic wheezing, nasal allergies, sinus problems, and craniofacial disorders. In accordance with the International Classification of Sleep Disorders [22], symptoms and evidence of pediatric OSAS associated with nocturnal symptoms such as snoring, oral breathing, snorting, gasping, pauses in breathing, and daytime outcomes (sleepiness, hyperactivity, inattention) should be existing. The criteria of PSG for pediatric OSAS requires either (1) ≥ 1 obstructive event (apnea or hypopnea) per hour of sleep or (2) obstructive hypoventilation, represented by $PaCO_2 > 50$ mmHg for more than 25% of sleep time [22].

The management of SDB-related EDS includes optimization of sleep hygiene and treating the cause of SDB, efficiently. Positive airway pressure (PAP) is an effective treatment choice in improving EDS for children with persistent sleepiness despite therapy [23].

76.4   Neurobehavioral Consequences of OSAS

Untreated OSAS symptoms in children are associated with a number of cognitive and behavioral effects which are generally described as "neurobehavioral." Neurobehavioral consequences of OSAS are thought to be the outcome of long-term intermittent hypoxemia with apneic events and sleep deprivation. While behavioral results are associated with inattention/hyperactivity symptoms, emotional lability, mood disorders, anxiety, and depressive symptoms, cognitive results are associated with intelligence, learning and academic difficulties, attention, executive function, memory, and language. These morbidities affect the physical health of the child, and also the quality of life for both the child and family.

Interest in neurobehavioral effects has been accelerated in recent years. Although meta-analyses on this topic frequently criticized the methodologic and conceptual issues of some researches, a number of studies have linked significant association with habitual snoring and OSAS to behavioral deficits such as emotional lability, anxiety, and depressive symptoms, especially to symptoms of attention deficit/hyperactivity disorder (ADHD) [1, 6, 17, 24–30].

ADHD is the most common behavioral disorder in children, and characterized by hyperactivity, attention deficit, and impulsivity. Children with OSAS are frequently misdiagnosed as ADHD, due to the overlap symptoms. Hyperactive and inattentive behaviors occur in almost 30% of children with habitual snoring and OSAS [20, 31]. According to parent-reports, sleep disturbances have been reported in more than 70% of children with ADHD. However, when evaluating the ADHD children by PSG, only 20% of children have reported sleep disturbance [20]. Additionally, ADHD children usually have persistent behavioral sleep problems, such as bedtime resistance, longer time to falling asleep, easily aroused sleep, and difficult to fall asleep. Several studies have demonstrated that the rate of SDB is higher in ADHD children, and also symptoms of ADHD are improved following treatment for OSAS [27–30]. A prospective and longitudinal population-based cohort study by Perfect et al. [32] indicated that children with SDB may show symptoms comparative with ADHD-like symptoms and disruptive behaviors, unless they are not treated. Wu et al. [31] reported that approximately 30% of children accompanying ADHD, and the prevalence of ADHD is increasing with age, and also the incidence of ADHD in boys with OSAS is higher than in girls. The effects of fragmented and restricted sleep have been assessed in several systematic reviews and meta-analyses. They reported that the OSAS could lead to neurobehavioral deficits associated with ADHD, and also SDB could be manifested or misdiagnosed as ADHD in some children [24–26]. Hypoxia may be an important causing factor for ADHD; therefore the assessment of sleep remains a crucial component from the perspective of clinicians in the evaluation of ADHD [25, 31].

Data on the emotional functioning of children with OSAS were based on self-reported and parent-reported symptoms, which may not be vulnerable to an objective mood [6, 33]. Degree of hypoxemia may point to the possible mechanism for increased depression in children [33, 34]. Hodges et al. [33] declared that children with OSAS have shown an increased risk for depressive symptoms, and revealed different demographic variables such as race, BMI, and maternal education. Furthermore, they declared that the arterial oxygen desaturation is strongly associated with depressive symptoms [33]. A recent study which was directed by Geckil et al. [34] noticed that the REM-related OSAS which is related to frequent apneas and hypopneas have higher rates of anxiety and depression symptoms compared to non-REM-related OSAS.

Children with OSAS may have cognitive impairments such as intelligence, learning, memory, language, attention, as well as school performance and academic difficulties [1, 35–39]. Some studies which did not evaluate the PSG findings revealed that the children with have an increased incidence of cognitive impairment and academic difficulties [37, 39]. Bourke et al. [35] reported that although the neurocognitive deficits are higher in children with OSAS compared with normal controls, they did not find the relationship between the severity of SDB and neurocognitive impairment. Furthermore, they suggested that hypoxic brain injury and sleepiness are critical factors in decreasing cognitive and academic function in these children [35]. On the contrary, Brockmann et al. [39] investigated the association of primary snoring and neurocognitive impairments and indicated that significant neurocognitive impairment may exist in children with non-hypoxic and non-apneic. The results of a large population-based cohort study conducted by Calhoun et al. [40] demonstrated that there is no significant impairment in intelligence, attention, executive functioning, and memory compared with children without OSAS although these associations were not controlled for variables known to be incorporated with learning problems such as parent education, socioeconomic status, environmentally changes, or individual genetic factors. Alchanatis et al. [41] and Olaithe et al. [42] declared that individual differences in cognitive reserve, which reflect that innate intelligence or inter-individual differences allow some individuals to deal with progressive brain damage and cognitive stressors better than other patients, may clarify the discrepancy of results in previous studies related to neurocognitive impairment in children with OSAS. According to this theory, high intelligence children with OSAS have a preventive effect against OSAS induced neurocognitive morbidity, by allowing a greater tolerance for brain injury and maintaining better cognitive and behavioral tasks [41]. Therefore, OSAS effects may differ from child to child due to the different functional plasticity of the brain.

Some cross-sectional studies revealed that the emergence of specific SDB-related neurobehavioral impairments may modify according to the child age. In a long-term SDB, children aged 3–5 years showed behavioral deficits, but no neurocognitive deficits, while children aged 7–12 years showed reduced neurocognitive skills [35, 43]. These studies demonstrated that the children with any severity of PSG defined SDB which may affect neurobehavioral condition is important to identify and treat, timely.

## 76.5	Effects of OSAS Treatment on Morbidity from Central Nervous System

There are many treatment methods for OSAS, depending on the age of the child, underlying medical problems, and the main cause of the upper airway obstruction such as adeno-tonsillar hypertrophy, craniofacial abnormalities, or neuromuscular disorders. Hypertrophy of the tonsils and adenoids is the most common cause of

OSAS in childhood. This incidence of this condition is higher in the preschool years, when the lymphoid tissue is largest relatively to upper airway size [44]. If adeno-tonsillar hypertrophy is present, adenotonsillectomy (AT) is the first-line treatment option for OSAS with the remarkably improved symptoms and PSG parameters of OSAS. Obesity in children is an independent risk factor for OSAS. Weight reduction in obese children is consolidated with improved metabolic effects and potential benefits concerning OSAS. Furthermore, obesity is a substantial risk factor for moderate to severe OSAS persistence after AT [1]. PAP which maintains the upper airway patency is a good alternative choice for treatment of children with moderate to severe OSAS as well as residual OSAS after AT. PAP therapy reduces snoring, arousals associated with obstructive events and the obstructive apnea hypopnea index (AHI), and also normalizes the oxygen saturation. Adherence to PAP therapy in childhood is a very common problem especially in children with developmental delays or behavioral problems. Further surgical treatment such as uvulo-palato-pharyngoplasty, tongue-lip adhesion, or mandibular advancement may be considered, but it has shown poor efficacy so far [45]. It should be remembered that upper airway dimensions may improve over time in children. For this reason, advanced surgeries, which have relatively lower success and higher complication rates, may be postponed to later times. Tracheostomy, which has the highest efficiency in the treatment of OSAS, is usually used only in severe OSAS, particularly in the presence of severe craniofacial anomalies, neuromuscular diseases causing severe hypotonia, or other surgical and nonsurgical interventions are contraindicated. Tracheostomy remains permanent in many of these children. But sometimes it can be used temporarily until awaiting appropriate surgical treatment.

Neurobehavioral impairments may notably improve with convenient OSAS management [1, 15, 27–30, 46–49]. Continues positive airway pressure (CPAP) is frequently used in children for whom surgical treatment is inappropriate or insufficient, such as craniofacial anomalies or neuromuscular disorders. Additionally, residual OSAS after AT, especially children with obesity, craniofacial anomalies, or neuromuscular disorders, leads to an increased number of children requiring CPAP. Complications of CPAP are including nasal congestion, epistaxis, facial erythema and ulcer, and rarely midface deformity. Nonetheless, the most important problem in children is patient adherence. Previous studies demonstrated the positive effects of PAP on neurobehavioral outcomes, sleepiness, school performance, quality of life, besides being improvements in gas exchange [1, 27, 46]. Marcus et al. [27] reported the significant amelioration in neurobehavioral function, excessive daytime sleepiness, and quality of life in children who were treated for 3 months with PAP therapy. Bee et al. [46] emphasized the importance of PAP adherence in adolescents and reported that adolescents with an average of 57% PAP adherence demonstrated improved attention and school performance while non-adherent group showed a tendency to decline in academic and school performance. Management of complications, behavioral modification, parent-directed care, and proper device usage may improve patient adherence. However, there is still insufficient evidence in the literature, regarding hours of per night of CPAP use and its effect on daytime sleepiness, further strategies to improve poor adherence in children.

AT is considered a suitable treatment choice for most cases of children with OSAS. Normalization of PSG parameters is more frequent in children with moderate to severe OSAS than in children with mild OSAS. Also, reduction in central apnea index has been shown in children with OSAS and mild central sleep apnea after AT [1, 45]. A number of studies demonstrated that the neurobehavioral morbidity tends to greatly improve 6–12 months after AT [27–29, 44–46]. Friedman et al. [48] who organized a prospective study to assess the neurocognitive function of children with OSAS before and after AT and to compare the results with healthy controls reported that neurocognitive function improved considerably 6–10 months after AT, reaching the levels of the control group; thus, they indicated that deterioration of neurocognitive function is mostly reversible. In a meta-analysis on neurophysiological functioning including attention-executive function, memory, and verbal ability after AT, Yu et al. [47] demonstrated a significant effect in children with OSAS when compared to their baseline level. But no significant effect was observed in attention-executive function and memory between children with OSAS and healthy ones. Studies concerning the PSG parameters of baseline OSAS and its following improvement after AT did not associate clearly with behavioral problems, cognitive deficits or sleepiness and they do not clarify the improvement neurobehavioral outcomes after AT [1, 28, 50, 51]. The Childhood Adenotonsillectomy Trial (CHAT) which was a randomized controlled study to evaluate a large of the cohort of school-aged children either early tonsillectomy (eAT) or seven months of watchful Waiting with Supportive Care (WWSC), reported that convalescence in the attention and executive function objective scores from baseline to follow up did not significantly differ between eAT and WWSC group after a period of 7 months as measured by psychometrician-measured neurocognitive testing, but improved the secondary outcomes of the teacher-reported behavior, caregiver-reported measures of executive function, quality of life and PSG parameters [50]. According to Cochrane systematic reviews [52], there is high-quality evidence that AT is beneficial for PSG parameters in 5–9 aged children with mild to moderate OSAS; however, the evidence in terms of quality of life and behavior is moderate quality. Additionally, high quality of evidence has shown no efficacy in regarding objective attention and measures of cognitive function compared to watchful waiting. They suggested that clinicians and parents carefully evaluate the benefits and risks of AT in these children, as PSG parameters of nearly half of children undergoing no-surgical treatment return to normal limits within 7 months [52].

Two systematic reviews concluded a significant deterioration in sleepiness, behavioral problems, attention deficit and hyperactivity symptoms, neurocognitive skills and quality of life scores of patients irrespective of preoperative OSAS severity [53, 54]. The parents completed 22 item SDB scale of Pediatric Sleep Questionnaire (PSQ) may be a useful tool since it may predict neurobehavioral morbidity from OSAS and its improvement after AT better than the AHI [1, 55]. Washtenaw Country Adenotonsillectomy Cohort [53] evaluated the effectiveness of SDB scale of PSQ by comparison with polysomnographic findings in the prediction of OSAS-related treatment responsive neurobehavioral morbidity and reported that its sensitivity and specificity for the diagnosis of OSAS are 78% and 72%, respectively. They suggested that SDB scale of PSQ provides greater clinical benefit than the more detailed PSG in terms of clinically relevant neurobehavioral health outcomes [55].

Although other surgical interventions such as maxillary or midface advancement, uvulo-palato-pharyngoplasty, and tongue-hyoid advancement are used in the treatment of severe OSAS, they have not been studied extensively in terms of neurobehavioral outcomes in the literature [1].

76.6 Conclusion

Neurobehavioral deficits which are associated with OSAS may well be multifactorial in origin with individual genetic factors, environmentally changes, socioeconomic status, parent education, age of the child, and also the severity of nocturnal events. Evidence on literature reinforces the need for increased awareness, early detection, and timely intervention by physicians and parents in pediatric OSAS to minimize the damage and optimize the neurobehavioral outcomes.

References

1. Kaditis AG, Alonso Alvarez ML, Boudewyns A, et al. Obstructive sleep disordered breathing in 2- to 18-year-old children: diagnosis and management. Eur Respir J. 2016;47(1):69–94.
2. Lumeng JC, Chervin RD. Epidemiology of pediatric obstructive sleep apnea. Proc Am Thorac Soc. 2008;5(2):242–52.
3. Balbani AP, Weber SA, Montovani JC. Update in obstructive sleep apnea syndrome in children. Braz J Otorhinolaryngol. 2005;71(1):74–80.
4. American Academy of Sleep Medicine. International classification of sleep disorders: diagnostic and coding manual. 2nd ed. Westchester, IL: American Academy of Sleep Medicine; 2005.
5. American Thoracic Society. Standards and indications for cardiopulmonary sleep studies in children. Am J Respir Crit Care Med. 1996;153(2):866–78.
6. Beebe DW. Neurobehavioral morbidity associated with disordered breathing during sleep in children: a comprehensive review. Sleep. 2006;29(9):1115–34.
7. Huang X, Tang S, Lyu X, et al. Structural and functional brain alterations in obstructive sleep apnea: a multimodal meta-analysis. Sleep Med. 2019;54:195–204.
8. Luo YG, Wang D, Liu K, et al. Brain structure network analysis in patients with obstructive sleep apnea. PLoS One. 2015;10(9):e0139055.
9. Macey PM, Kumar R, Woo MA, et al. Brain structural changes in obstructive sleep apnea. Sleep. 2008;31(7):967–77.
10. Veasey SC, Davis CW, Fenik P, et al. Long-term intermittent hypoxia in mice: protracted hypersomnolence with oxidative injury to sleep-wake brain regions. Sleep. 2004;27(2):194–201.
11. Zhu Y, Fenik P, Zhan G, et al. Selective loss of catecholaminergic wake active neurons in a murine sleep apnea model. J Neurosci. 2007;27(37):10060–71.
12. Pae EK, Chien P, Harper RM. Intermittent hypoxia damages cerebellar cortex and deep nuclei. Neurosci Lett. 2005;375(2):123–8.
13. Joo EY, Tae WS, Lee MJ, et al. Reduced brain gray matter concentration in patients with obstructive sleep apnea syndrome. Sleep. 2010;33(2):235–41.
14. Yaouhi K, Bertran F, Clochon P, et al. A combined neuropsychological and brain imaging study of obstructive sleep apnea. J Sleep Res. 2009;18(1):36–48.

15. Sweet LH, Jerskey BA, Aloia MS. Default network response to a working memory challenge after withdrawal of continuous positive airway pressure treatment for obstructive sleep apnea. Brain Imaging Behav. 2010;4(2):155–63.
16. Hastings RS, Parsey RV, Oquendo MA, et al. Volumetric analysis of the prefrontal cortex, amygdala, and hippocampus in major depression. Neuropsychopharmacology. 2004;29(5):952–9.
17. Beebe DW, Gozal D. Obstructive sleep apnea and the prefrontal cortex: towards a comprehensive model linking nocturnal upper airway obstruction to daytime cognitive and behavioral deficits. J Sleep Res. 2002;11(1):1–16.
18. Liu Y, Zhang J, Li SX, et al. Excessive daytime sleepiness among children and adolescents: prevalence, correlates, and pubertal effects. Sleep Med. 2019;53:1–8.
19. Owens JA, Babcock D, Weiss M. Evaluation and treatment of children and adolescents with excessive daytime sleepiness. Clin Pediatr (Phila). 2020;59(4–5):340–51.
20. Gozal D. Obstructive sleep apnea in children: implications for the developing central nervous system. Semin Pediatr Neurol. 2008;15(2):100–6.
21. Gozal D, Wang M, Pope DW Jr. Objective sleepiness measures in pediatric obstructive sleep apnea. Pediatrics. 2001;108(3):693–7.
22. Sateia MJ. International classification of sleep disorders-third edition: highlights and modifications. Chest. 2014;146(5):1387–94.
23. He K, Kapur VK. Sleep-disordered breathing and excessive daytime sleepiness. Sleep Med Clin. 2017;12(3):369–82.
24. Cortese S, Faraone SV, Konofal E, et al. Sleep in children with attention-deficit/hyperactivity disorder: meta-analysis of subjective and objective studies. J Am Acad Child Adolesc Psychiatry. 2009;48:894–908.
25. Sadeh A, Pergamin L, Bar-Haim Y. Sleep in children with attention-deficit hyperactivity disorder: a meta-analysis of polysomnographic studies. Sleep Med Rev. 2006;10:381–98.
26. Sedky K, Bennett DS, Carvalho KS. Attention deficit hyperactivity disorder and sleep disordered breathing in pediatric populations: a meta-analysis. Sleep Med Rev. 2014;18:349–56.
27. Marcus CL, Radcliffe J, Konstantinopoulou S, et al. Effects of positive airway pressure therapy on neurobehavioral outcomes in children with obstructive sleep apnea. Am J Respir Crit Care Med. 2012;185(9):998–1003.
28. Chervin RD, Ruzicka DL, Giordani BJ, et al. Sleep-disordered breathing, behavior, and cognition in children before and after adenotonsillectomy. Pediatrics. 2006;117(4):e769–78.
29. Dillon JE, Blunden S, Ruzicka DL, et al. DSM-IV diagnoses and obstructive sleep apnea in children before and 1 year after adenotonsillectomy. J Am Acad Child Adolesc Psychiatry. 2007;46(11):1425–36.
30. Garetz SL, Mitchell RB, Parker PD, et al. Quality of life and obstructive sleep apnea symptoms after pediatric adenotonsillectomy. Pediatrics. 2015;135(2):e477–86.
31. Wu J, Gu M, Chen S, et al. Factors related to pediatric obstructive sleep apnea-hypopnea syndrome in children with attention deficit hyperactivity disorder in different age groups. Medicine (Baltimore). 2017;96(42):e8281.
32. Perfect MM, Archbold K, Goodwin JL, et al. Risk of behavioral and adaptive functioning difficulties in youth with previous and current sleep disordered breathing. Sleep. 2013;36:517B–25B.
33. Hodges E, Marcus CL, Kim JY, et al. Depressive symptomatology in school-aged children with obstructive sleep apnea syndrome: incidence, demographic factors, and changes following a randomized controlled trial of adenotonsillectomy. Sleep. 2018;41(12):180.
34. Geckil AA, Ermis H. The relationship between anxiety, depression, daytime sleepiness in the REM-related mild OSAS and the NREM-related mild OSAS. Sleep Breath. 2020;24(1):71–5.
35. Bourke R, Anderson V, Yang JS, et al. Cognitive and academic functions are impaired in children with all severities of sleep-disordered breathing. Sleep Med. 2011;12(5):489–96.
36. Gottlieb DJ, Chase C, Vezina RM, et al. Sleep-disordered breathing symptoms are associated with poorer cognitive function in 5-year-old children. J Pediatr. 2004;145:458–64.
37. Miano S, Paolino MC, Urbano A, et al. Neurocognitive assessment and sleep analysis in children with sleep-disordered breathing. Clin Neurophysiol. 2011;122:311–9.

38. Kheirandish L, Gozal D. Neurocognitive dysfunction in children with sleep disorders. Dev Sci. 2006;9(4):388–99.
39. Brockmann PE, Urschitz MS, Schlaud M, et al. Primary snoring in school children: prevalence and neurocognitive impairments. Sleep Breath. 2012;16:23–9.
40. Calhoun SL, Mayes SD, Vgontzas AN, et al. No relationship between neurocognitive functioning and mild sleep disordered breathing in a community sample of children. J Clin Sleep Med. 2009;5:228–34.
41. Alchanatis M, Zias N, Deligiorgis N, et al. Sleep apnea-related cognitive deficits and intelligence: an implication of cognitive reserve theory. J Sleep Res. 2005;14(1):69–75.
42. Olaithe M, Pushpanathan M, Hillman D, et al. Cognitive profiles in obstructive sleep apnea: a cluster analysis in sleep clinic and community samples. J Clin Sleep Med. 2020;16(9):1493–505.
43. Jackman AR, Biggs SN, Walter LM, et al. Sleep-disordered breathing in preschool children is associated with behavioral, but not cognitive, impairments. Sleep Med. 2012;13(6):621–31.
44. Ahn YM. Treatment of obstructive sleep apnea in children. Korean J Pediatr. 2010;53(10):872–9.
45. Bitners AC, Arens R. Evaluation and management of children with obstructive sleep apnea syndrome. Lung. 2020;198(2):257–70.
46. Beebe DW, Byars KC. Adolescents with obstructive sleep apnea adhere poorly to positive airway pressure (PAP), but PAP users show improved attention and school performance. PLoS One. 2011;6:e16924.
47. Yu Y, Chen YX, Liu L, et al. Neuropsychological functioning after adenotonsillectomy in children with obstructive sleep apnea: a meta-analysis. J Huazhong Univ Sci Technolog Med Sci. 2017;37(3):453–61.
48. Friedman BC, Hendeles-Amitai A, Kozminsky E, et al. Adenotonsillectomy improves neurocognitive function in children with obstructive sleep apnea syndrome. Sleep. 2003;26(8):999–1005.
49. Owens J, Spirito A, Marcotte A, et al. Neuropsychological and behavioral correlates of obstructive sleep apnea syndrome in children: a preliminary study. Sleep Breath. 2000;4(2):67–78.
50. Marcus CL, Moore RH, Rosen CL, et al. Childhood Adenotonsillectomy trial (CHAT). A randomized trial of adenotonsillectomy for childhood sleep apnea. N Engl J Med. 2013;368(25):2366–76.
51. Thomas NH, Xanthopoulos MS, Kim JY, et al. Effects of Adenotonsillectomy on parent-reported behavior in children with obstructive sleep apnea. Sleep. 2017;40(4):zsx018.
52. Venekamp RP, Hearne BJ, Chandrasekharan D, et al. Tonsillectomy or adenotonsillectomy versus non-surgical management for obstructive sleep-disordered breathing in children. Cochrane Database Syst Rev. 2015;14(10):CD011165.
53. Garetz SL. Behavior, cognition, and quality of life after adenotonsillectomy for pediatric sleep-disordered breathing: summary of the literature. Otolaryngol Head Neck Surg. 2008;138:19–S26.
54. Kohler MJ, Lushington K, Kennedy JD. Neurocognitive performance and behavior before and after treatment for sleep-disordered breathing in children. Nat Sci Sleep. 2010;2:159–85.
55. Chervin RD, Weatherly RA, Garetz SL, et al. Pediatric sleep questionnaire: prediction of sleep apnea and outcomes. Arch Otolaryngol Head Neck Surg. 2007;133:216–22.
56. Baldassari CM, Kepchar J, Bryant L, et al. Changes in central apnea index following pediatric adenotonsillectomy. Otolaryngol Head Neck Surg. 2012;146:487–90.

Işıl Eser Şimşek, Metin Aydoğan, and Ayşe Engin Arısoy

77.1 Introduction

Acute bronchiolitis caused by a viral infection of small airways is the leading reason for hospital admission in children younger than 1 year of age [1, 2]. There is no definite age limitation of bronchiolitis. According to the different guidelines, the upper age limit varies from 6 or 12 months up to 2 years. Still, the term is broadly used for infants who experienced an episode of wheezing before the first birthday [3, 4]. Approximately one-third of infants will develop clinical bronchiolitis episodes, in particular, caused by respiratory syncytial virus (RSV) during winter months [5].

Most cases infected with RSV, responsible for up to 80% of patients with bronchiolitis younger than age 2 years, have mild upper respiratory tract illness, and can be managed conservatively at home. But approximately 30% of first infections evolve in the lower respiratory tract, such as bronchiolitis and/or pneumonia [6]. Greater disease severity has been reported in infants with risk factors such as comorbid conditions. There are no effective treatment strategies for viral bronchiolitis; the mainstay of management continues to be purely respiratory and feeding support [2, 7]. It is essential to identify risk factors associated with severe illness because

I. E. Şimşek (✉) · M. Aydoğan
Division of Pediatric Allergy and Immunology, Department of Pediatrics, Faculty of Medicine, Kocaeli University, Kocaeli, Turkey

A. E. Arısoy
Division of Neonatology, Department of Pediatrics, Faculty of Medicine, Kocaeli University, Kocaeli, Turkey

C. Cingi et al. (eds.), *Pediatric ENT Infections*,
https://doi.org/10.1007/978-3-030-80691-0_77

RSV-related hospital admissions can be reduced by using preventive treatments such as prophylactic RSV-specific monoclonal antibody.

77.2 Epidemiology

Acute bronchiolitis is recognized as a leading reason for emergency department (ED) visits and hospitalizations in infants [3, 6]. The disease's epidemiology is similar to that of RSV infection, which occurs in up to 80% of cases [3]. In the United States (US), approximately 20% of the annual birth cohort require outpatient visits with a diagnosis of bronchiolitis, and 2% of these children are hospitalized in the first year of life. Thus, acute bronchiolitis was responsible for approximately 100.000 hospitalizations at an estimated $1.73 billion cost in 2009 [1, 3, 8]. Around 5% to 9% of hospitalized children will progress to admission to the intensive care unit (ICU) because of either respiratory failure or apnea [7]. Despite the high prevalence of bronchiolitis, mortality risk is relatively low in otherwise healthy children and accounts for fewer than 125 deaths in young children annually in the USA [6].

Bronchiolitis is seen as a seasonal illness because RSV causes most cases in annual epidemics [3, 6]. These seasonal epidemics' peak and duration vary in countries but remain the same year-to-year within a country [9]. RSV occurs during winter and early spring in temperate climates, typically from late October to April in the northern hemisphere, with a peak in January or February, while winter-time epidemics in the Southern hemisphere occur from May to September [10]. Viral transmission may be facilitated in cold weather by increasing indoor crowding, especially in regions with a high population. The impairing effect on the airway mucosa and cilia of cold and dry air inhalation and the impairment of temperature-dependent antiviral responses constitute other factors affecting host defenses related to weather [3, 9].

77.3 Risk Factors

Although bronchiolitis in otherwise healthy children is mostly a self-limited disease, approximately 1–3% of all children ≤ 1 year old with bronchiolitis will be hospitalized [11]. The highest percentage of hospitalization are between 1 and 3 months of age when protective maternal antibodies wane; the chronologic age is the critical predictor of the likelihood of severe bronchiolitis. However, some patients may have risk factors associated with progression to severe disease, such as underlying disease or environmental factors (Table 77.1) [9, 12–15].

A limited number of previous reports indicate no difference in hospitalization risk between black and white children [3]. The presence of tachypnea (respiratory rate ≥ 60 per minute) on admission has been associated with severe illness risk in some studies [12, 13]. The more severe disease observed among infants born early in the RSV season may be related to lower maternal RSV antibodies (when wane protective maternal antibodies are occurring from infection during the previous season).

Table 77.1 Factors associated with severe or complicated bronchiolitis

Underlying conditions
Prematurity (especially gestational age <29 weeks)
Younger chronologic age (<2–3 months)
Male sex (due to differences in lung and airway development)
Hospitalization for episodes of the previous wheezing
Chronic pulmonary diseases (particularly bronchopulmonary dysplasia)
Hemodynamically significant congenital heart disease (especially those with pulmonary hypertension or congestive heart failure)
Immunodeficiency
Neurologic disease
Anatomic defects of the airway
Low birth weight ($\leq$2.5 kg)
Environmental and other risk factors
Daycare attendance
Having older siblings
In utero smoke exposure
Passive smoking
Not breastfeeding

77.4 Pathogenesis

Respiratory viruses like RSV are transmitted person to person by direct contact with contaminated secretions or aerosol particles' inhalation and binds nasal epithelial cells [6]. Viral replication triggers an excessive inflammatory response via direct cellular damage, with an influx of natural killer cells, lymphoid cells, and granulocytes to the site of infection. Viral replication then follows in the lower respiratory tract's epithelial cells by aspiration of nasopharyngeal secretions in one-third of infected patients [2, 9].

Bronchiolitis is characterized by airway edema, increased mucus secretion, necrosis, and sloughing in the airway's epithelial cells by the combined effect of the virus and an exaggerated immune response [1]. These pathological changes cause bronchiolar obstruction, air trapping, and atelectasis.

77.5 Etiology

RSV remains the most commonly identified etiologic agent in acute bronchiolitis, followed by rhinovirus. Other viruses involved are human metapneumovirus, adenovirus, coronavirus, influenza virus, and parainfluenza virus [6]. Approximately one-third of children hospitalized with bronchiolitis have coinfections with two viruses [1]. Studies have investigated whether disease severity is associated with infectious etiology, but the evidence is conflicting. Some studies have shown that RSV is the sole pathogen involving a more severe course. In contrast, other studies point to more significant disease severity with the presence of viral coinfections [9, 16].

77.6 Diagnosis

77.6.1 History and Physical Examination

It is important to differentiate bronchiolitis from other diseases where clinical features overlap, such as virus-induced wheezing, pneumonia, and asthma, by detailed history and physical examination [5]. Bronchiolitis is characterized by a constellation of clinical symptoms and signs in children younger than 2 years, particularly during winter months [2]. The classic initial symptoms as nasal congestion and rhinorrhea progress over 2–4 days to the lower respiratory tract illness presented with the symptoms of cough, wheezing, and increased breathing work as manifested by tachypnea, use of accessory muscles, nasal flaring, and apnea [3].

Low-grade fever can appear in about 30% of patients. Infants with bronchiolitis can present poor feeding and dehydration due to upper respiratory tract obstruction and tachypnea, which reduces the fluid and food intake and increases the need related to fever. Apnea, lethargy, and irritability with minimal respiratory symptoms may be seen as an initial presentation in infants younger than 2 months, particularly in premature and/or low birth weight (LBW, ≤2.5 kg) babies [2, 6]. In a prospective observational study that included infants presented to the ED due to bronchiolitis, subsequent apnea occurred in 5% of patients. It was associated with parental report of apnea, previous history of apnea, congenital heart disease, LBW, lower weight, and age ≤6 weeks [17]. Another multicenter prospective study reported apnea in 5% of patients hospitalized with bronchiolitis [18]. The identification of underlying conditions such as prematurity, hemodynamically significant congenital heart disease, chronic lung disease (CLD) of prematurity, particularly bronchopulmonary dysplasia (BPD), and immunodeficiency in history is important as they cause severe clinical course [1].

Physical examination findings associated with bronchiolitis can include fever, increased respiratory rate, diffuse wheezing, crackles, and prolonged expiratory phase. The clinical findings may change minute to minute due to cleaning of mucus from the airways by cough reflex or as the child's state changes with crying, agitation, and sleep. Also, upper airway obstruction contributes to difficulty breathing and may complicate physical examination due to transmitted upper airway sounds. The variable and dynamic course of bronchiolitis requires serial observations to assess clinical status, and nasal suctioning may improve the examination quality [1]. Various clinical scoring systems have been proposed to predict infants with risk for respiratory distress progress, but none has been widely accepted [1, 9].

77.6.2 Diagnostic Tests

Bronchiolitis is diagnosed clinically by history and physical examination findings [1, 5, 19].

Complete blood counts, blood cultures, and blood gas measurements should not be routinely obtained in infants with bronchiolitis unless an assessment for sepsis is required in infants younger than 1–2 months or if there are signs of severe respiratory distress. Most national guidelines advise against routine viral testing in the diagnosis or management of bronchiolitis due to inadequate evidence for any effect on management [1, 5, 19]. If breakthrough RSV infection is identified in a patient receiving RSV-specific monoclonal antibody (palivizumab) prophylaxis, the treatment should be ceased as the possibility of reinfection for that year is very rare. The RSV testing is only recommended for this condition in the American Academy of Pediatrics (AAP) practice guideline [1].

Likewise, routine chest radiography is not recommended for patients in which alternative diagnosis to bronchiolitis such as pneumonia is not suspected, based on history and physical examination, or when a child is not severely ill, or symptoms are not progressing. Increasing in inappropriate use of antibiotics after performing radiographs is observed [20].

Radiographic features of bronchiolitis are nonspecific findings, including hyperinflation, peribronchial thickening, and patchy atelectasis due to airway narrowing. Ultrasound usage for pulmonary diseases in children has expanded in recent years [9]. One observational study of infants with bronchiolitis reported the lung ultrasound findings to correlate with the need for supplementary oxygen with a specificity of 98.7% [21]. Yet, few studies are associated with ultrasound use for assessing severity in bronchiolitis, and further studies are needed.

77.7 Management: Non-Pharmacological

77.7.1 Respiratory Support

77.7.1.1 Monitoring and Supplemental Oxygen

Several studies and national practice guidelines have focused on measure oxygen saturation by pulse oximetry to guide admission and determine the need for supplemental oxygen. The previous studies showed that arbitrary thresholds for supplemental oxygen based on continuous pulse oximetry measurements, independent of other factors such as the sign of respiratory distress, may lead to increased length of stay, ICU admission, and further intervention, and decreased use of oximetry does not lead to an increase in adverse effects [1, 9, 22, 23].

In a prospective study, most otherwise stable infants with bronchiolitis have transient hypoxemia, particularly during sleep, suggesting that measuring oxygen saturation by pulse oximetry should not be used as the only factor to decision admission and predict progression of the disease [24]. The AAP guideline recommends the use of pulse oxygen saturation (SpO_2) <90% as the threshold to administer supplemental oxygen in infants with bronchiolitis (<92% in the United Kingdom [UK] National Institute for Health and Care Excellence [NICE] and Australasian Bronchiolitis—Paediatric Research in Emergency Departments International Collaborative [PREDICT] guidelines) and the continuous pulse oximetry monitoring for non-hypoxic infants not receiving supplemental oxygen may not be required [1, 5, 19].

77.7.1.2 High-Flow Nasal Cannula (HFNC) and Continuous Positive Airway Pressure (CPAP)

Humidified high flow (usually 1–2 L/kg per min) nasal cannula oxygen is a well-tolerated noninvasive new treatment approach to improve oxygenation and ventilation for bronchiolitis. This medical device is widely used in all clinical settings, including the ED, ICU, and inpatient units. Although there are data to suggest that it may decrease respiratory effort, intubation rates, and the need for escalation of care due to deterioration, its efficacy has not been conclusively proved in randomized trials [25, 26]. Conflicting data about the effectiveness of HFNC precludes specific recommendations by guidelines.

CPAP is used to reduce the work of breathing and the need for endotracheal intubation in infants and children with impending respiratory failure despite oxygen therapy. Cochrane Systemic Review 2019 suggests that CPAP improves breathing in children with bronchiolitis, uncertain for other outcomes due to limited data [27]. The NICE and PREDICT guidelines recommend considering CPAP if signs of impending respiratory failure, such as persistently increased respiratory effort and hypoxemia despite standard oxygen, are present [5, 19].

77.7.2 Nutrition and Hydration

Dehydration can occur due to increased work of breathing and nasal congestion impeding oral intake and increased insensible needs related to tachypnea and fever; thus, hydration remains a mainstay of therapy [3, 9]. Support for dehydration in infants without feeding difficulty with mild respiratory distress may be in the form of encouraging frequent small amounts of oral feeding. Nasal suctioning before feeding can be performed if oral intake is affected by nasal secretions, and breast-feeding maintenance should be supported. Most guidelines recommend either nasogastric or intravenous fluids to maintain hydration in infants with severe bronchiolitis who cannot maintain hydration orally [1, 5, 19]. Management with isotonic fluids to avoid the risk of hyponatremia related to the production of antidiuretic hormone (ADH) should be preferred if required.

77.7.3 Nasal Suction

The nasopharynx's deep suctioning to remove airway blockage is not recommended because of studies reporting an association with a longer length of stay [2]. Although superficial nasal suction may provide temporary relief in those with respiratory distress and feeding difficulties, guidelines concluded that there are insufficient data to recommend routine practice in the management of infants with bronchiolitis [1, 19].

77.7.4 Chest Physiotherapy

A recent Cochrane Collaboration review demonstrated no evidence of enough benefit of chest physiotherapy in patients with bronchiolitis [28]. No published guidelines recommend chest physiotherapy to treat previously healthy infants with bronchiolitis, as there is insufficient evidence to warrant a general recommendation.

77.8 Management: Pharmacological

77.8.1 Bronchodilators

The bronchodilators such as short-acting beta-2-agonists (salbutamol [albuterol]) and ipratropium bromide) are not recommended in infants with bronchiolitis in the clinical practice guidelines, based on data from one Cochrane Systematic Review, indicating no benefit in disease resolution outcomes, decreasing hospital admission, or shortening length of stay despite transient improvement in clinical symptom scores [29]. The current AAP guideline no longer recommends a trial of short-acting beta-2-agonists, previously included as an option, due to the side effects such as tachycardia and tremors and evidence demonstrating strength no benefit. Another Cochrane meta-analysis and a large multicenter randomized controlled trial systematically evaluated the use of nebulized epinephrine for bronchiolitis in children hospitalized and found no benefit in hospital length of stay or other outcomes [30, 31]. The current evidence does not support the use of nebulized epinephrine in outpatients, although Cochrane review suggested administering nebulized epinephrine on the day of the ED visit reduces hospitalization. The results from these studies and meta-analysis support the recommendation of guidelines against using nebulized epinephrine in patients with bronchiolitis.

77.8.2 Hypertonic Saline

A 2017 Cochrane review concluded that hypertonic saline may decrease hospital stay length in children with bronchiolitis and may also reduce the hospitalization rates in emergency settings [32]. In the recent randomized clinical trial and meta-analysis, the reduction in length of stay is attributed to older trials with the length of stay more than 3 days included in the Cochrane review [33–35]. The AAP practice guideline, highlighting the inconsistency between studies, concluded that hypertonic saline should not be used routinely in the infant with bronchiolitis in the ED to reduce hospitalization but may be considered as potentially decrease the length of stay for inpatients, mainly when administered in patients with a length of stay >3 days.

77.8.3 Corticosteroids

Similarly, systemic or inhaled corticosteroids are not recommended in treating bronchiolitis by multiple clinical practice guidelines based on data from a 2013 Cochrane review, showing no benefit in reducing admission rates and length of stay [36].

77.8.4 Antibiotics

Children with bronchiolitis have a lower risk of infections such as bacteremia and meningitis, except for acute otitis media (AOM), which can be seen in 60% of patients. Nonetheless, infants with bronchiolitis frequently continue receiving antibacterial therapy because of fever, concern for undetected bacterial infection, and nonspecific findings on chest radiograph. A randomized controlled trial showed that routine antibacterial treatment in children with bronchiolitis does not affect the duration of symptoms, length of hospital stay, or hospital readmission [37]. Based on this evidence, the guidelines do not recommend using antibiotics in patients with bronchiolitis unless there is evidence of bacterial coinfection.

77.9　Prognosis

Bronchiolitis is a self-limited illness and often resolves relatively good prognosis in approximately 2 weeks for most previously well-infants. A subset of patients experience severe disease course and may be life-threatening in those with preexisting cardiac or chronic respiratory disease.

Numerous studies have documented that severe bronchiolitis in infants is more likely associated with an increased risk of recurrent wheezing and asthma later in life, especially after rhinovirus or RSV bronchiolitis. The reported risk of developing recurrent wheezing later following severe bronchiolitis with RSV in infancy varies from 17% to 60% [9, 38]. A prospective study reported that lower respiratory tract infection with RSV increased the likelihood of subsequent wheezing; this finding was lost by 13 years old. Whether severe lower respiratory infections at an early age cause some cases of asthma through damage of normal airway or whether infants with predisposing factors to asthma such as dysregulation of the immune response or airway dysfunction might be firstly presented with severe bronchiolitis is not known [3].

77.10　Prevention

Palivizumab is a neutralizing humanized monoclonal antibody against the RSV fusion protein, preventing fusion of the plasma membrane of the respiratory epithelial cell [6].

Monthly prophylaxis may be considered at 15 mg/kg/dose (maximum of 5 doses) to protect during the RSV season in the first year of life in a high-risk population. Palivizumab is recommended for preterms born before 29 weeks and for infants born before <32 week who develop CLD of prematurity and hemodynamically significant congenital heart disease [1, 6, 9]. Use of palivizumab in the second year is recommended only for infants who continue to require treatment for CLD of prematurity within 6 months before the start of the RSV season.

Palivizumab should not be prescribed in cystic fibrosis, neuromuscular disorder, or immunodeficiency if no other indications are present due to insufficient evidence. If breakthrough RSV infection is identified in a patient receiving prophylaxis, palivizumab should be ceased as the possibility of reinfection for that year is very rare [6].

77.11 Conclusion

Bronchiolitis refers to an acute infection starting with coryza followed by signs of the lower respiratory tract illness. The conditions associated with severe bronchiolitis are prematurity, CLD of prematurity, and congenital heart disease. Routine laboratory tests and chest radiographs are not recommended because of minimal diagnostic use in most cases. The management of bronchiolitis is supportive and focuses on fluid and oxygen administration and nasal suctioning in selected cases. There is inconclusive evidence regarding deep suctioning, hypertonic saline, short-acting beta-2-agonists, epinephrine, antibiotics, and systemic corticosteroids in RSV bronchiolitis and are not recommended for the treatment.

References

1. Ralston SL, Lieberthal AS, Meissner HC, et al. Clinical practice guideline: the diagnosis, management, and prevention of bronchiolitis. Pediatrics. 2014;134:e1474–502.
2. Silver AH, Nazif JM. Bronchiolitis. Pediatr Rev. 2019;40:568–76.
3. Meissner HC. Viral bronchiolitis in children. N Engl J Med. 2016;374:62–72.
4. Jartti T, Smits HH, Bonnelykke K, et al. Bronchiolitis needs a revisit: distinguishing between virus entities and their treatments. Allergy. 2019;74:40–52.
5. National Institute for Health and Care Excellence. Bronchiolitis: diagnosis and management of bronchiolitis in children, Clinical Guideline NG9; 2015. www.nice.org.uk/guidance/ng9. Accessed 21 Nov 2020.
6. American Academy of Pediatrics. Respiratory syncytial virus. In: Kimberlin DW, Brady M, Jackson M, Long S, editors. Red book: 2018 report of the committee on infectious diseases. 31st ed. Itasca: American Academy of Pediatrics; 2018. p. 682–92.
7. Sinha IP, McBride AKS, Smith R, Fernandes RM. CPAP and high-flow nasal cannula oxygen in bronchiolitis. Chest. 2015;148:810–23.
8. Hasegawa K, Tsugawa Y, Brown DFM, Mansbach JM, Camargo CA. Trends in bronchiolitis hospitalizations in the United States, 2000–2009. Pediatrics. 2013;132:28–36.
9. Florin TA, Plint AC, Zorc JJ. Viral bronchiolitis. Lancet. 2017;389:211–24.
10. Obando-Pacheco P, Justicia-Grande AJ, Rivero-Calle I, et al. Respiratory syncytial virus seasonality: a global overview. J Infect Dis. 2018;217:1356–64.

11. Cavaye D, Roberts DP, Saravanos GL, et al. Evaluation of national guidelines for bronchiolitis: agreements and controversies. J Paediatr Child Health. 2019;55:25–31.
12. Hasegawa K, Pate BM, Mansbach JM, et al. Risk factors for requiring intensive care among children admitted to ward with bronchiolitis. Acad Pediatr. 2015;15:77–81.
13. Butler J, Gunnarsson R, Traves A, Marshall H. Severe respiratory syncytial virus infection in hospitalized children less than 3 years of age in a temperate and tropical climate. Pediatr Infect Dis J. 2019;38:6–11.
14. Behrooz L, Balekian DS, Faridi MK, Espinola JA, Townley LP, Camargo CA. Prenatal and postnatal tobacco smoke exposure and risk of severe bronchiolitis during infancy. Respir Med. 2018;140:21–6.
15. Hall CB, Weinberg GA, Blumkin AK, et al. Respiratory syncytial virus-associated hospitalizations among children less than 24 months of age. Pediatrics. 2013;132:e341–8.
16. Hasegawa K, Jartti T, Mansbach JM, et al. Respiratory syncytial virus genomic load and disease severity among children hospitalized with bronchiolitis: multicenter cohort studies in the United States and Finland. J Infect Dis. 2015;211:1550–9.
17. Walsh P, Cunningham P, Merchant S, et al. Derivation of candidate clinical decision rules to identify infants at risk for central apnea. Pediatrics. 2015;136:e1228–36.
18. Schroeder AR, Mansbach JM, Stevenson M, et al. Apnea in children hospitalized with bronchiolitis. Pediatrics. 2013;132:1194–201.
19. Paediatric Research in Emergency Departments International Collaborative (PREDICT). Australasian Bronchiolitis Guideline. Melbourne: PREDICT; 2016. https://www.predict.org.au/publications/2016-pubs/. Accessed 21 Nov 2020.
20. Ecochard-Dugelay E, Beliah M, Boisson C. Impact of chest radiography for children with lower respiratory tract infection: a propensity score approach. PLoS One. 2014;9:e96189.
21. Basile V, Di Mauro A, Scalini E, et al. Lung ultrasound: a useful tool in diagnosis and management of bronchiolitis. BMC Pediatr. 2015;15:63.
22. Schuh S, Freedman S, Coates A, et al. Effect of oximetry on hospitalization in bronchiolitis: a randomized clinical trial. JAMA. 2014;312:712–8.
23. Cunningham S, Rodriguez A, Adams T, et al. Oxygen saturation targets in infants with bronchiolitis (BIDS): a double-blind, randomised, equivalence trial. Lancet. 2015;386:1041–8.
24. Principi T, Coates AL, Parkin PC, Stephens D, DaSilva Z, Schuh S. Effect of oxygen desaturations on subsequent medical visits in infants discharged from the emergency department with bronchiolitis. JAMA Pediatr. 2016;170:602–8.
25. Sinha IP, McBride AK, Smith R, Fernandes RM. CPAP and high-flow nasal cannula oxygen in bronchiolitis. Chest. 2015;148:810–23.
26. Franklin D, Babl FE, Schlapbach LJ, et al. A randomized trial of high-flow oxygen therapy in infants with bronchiolitis. N Engl J Med. 2018;378:1121–31.
27. Jat KR, Mathew JL. Continuous positive airway pressure (CPAP) for acute bronchiolitis in children. Cochrane Database Syst Rev. 2019;1:CD010473.
28. Roqu i Figuls M, Gin Garriga M, Granados Rugeles C, Perrotta C, Vilar J. Chest physiotherapy for acute bronchiolitis in paediatric patients between 0 and 24 months old. Cochrane Database Syst Rev. 2016;2:CD004873.
29. Gadomski AM, Scribani MB. Bronchodilators for bronchiolitis. Cochrane Database Syst Rev. 2014;6:CD001266.
30. Hartling L, Fernandes RM, Bialy L, et al. Steroids and bronchodilators for acute bronchiolitis in the first two years of life: systematic review and meta-analysis. BMJ. 2011;342:d1714.
31. Skjerven HO, Hunderi JO, Brügmann-Pieper SK, et al. Racemic adrenaline and inhalation strategies in acute bronchiolitis. N Engl J Med. 2013;368:2286–93.
32. Zhang L, Mendoza-Sassi RA, Wainwright C, Klassen TP. Nebulised hypertonic saline solution for acute bronchiolitis in infants. Cochrane Database Syst Rev. 2017;12(12):CD006458.
33. Silver AH, Esteban-Cruciani N, Azzarone G. 3% hypertonic saline versus normal saline in inpatient bronchiolitis: a randomized controlled trial. Pediatrics. 2015;136:1036–43.
34. Badgett RG, Vindhyal M, Stirnaman JT, Gibson CM. Halaby R.a living systematic review of nebulized hypertonic saline for acute bronchiolitis in infants. JAMA Pediatr. 2015;169:788–9.

35. Brooks CG, Harrison WN, Ralston SL. Association between hypertonic saline and hospital length of stay in acute viral bronchiolitis: a reanalysis of 2 meta-analyses. JAMA Pediatr. 2016;170:577–84.
36. Fernandes RM, Bialy LM, Vandermeer B, et al. Glucocorticoids for acute viral bronchiolitis in infants and young children. Cochrane Database Syst Rev. 2013;6:CD004878.
37. Beigelman A, Isaacson-Schmid M, Sajol G, Baty J, Rodriguez OM, Leege E. Randomized trial to evaluate azithromycin's effects on serum and upper airway IL-8 levels and recurrent wheezing in infants with respiratory syncytial virus bronchiolitis. J Allergy Clin Immunol. 2015;135:1171–8.
38. Balekian DS, Linnemann RW, Hasegawa K, Thadhani R, Camargo CA Jr. Cohort study of severe bronchiolitis during infancy and risk of asthma by age 5 years. J Allergy Clin Immunol Pract. 2017;5:92–6.

İbrahim Güven Coşğun, Biray Harbiyeli, and Evda Vevecka

78.1 Acute Bronchitis

78.1.1 Introduction

Acute bronchitis is the term used for un acute respiratory infection that is manifested predominantly by cough with or without phlegm production that last for up to 3 weeks and without evidence of pneumonia, the common cold, acute asthma, or an acute exacerbation of chronic bronchitis. Acute bronchitis is most often caused by a viral infection. The most commonly identified viruses are rhinovirus, enterovirus, influenza A and B, parainfluenza, coronavirus, human metapneumovirus, and respiratory syncytial virus. Bacteria are detected in 1–10% of cases of acute bronchitis. Atypical bacteria, such as *Mycoplasma pneumoniae*, *Chlamydophila pneumoniae*, and *Bordetella pertussis*, are rare causes of acute bronchitis [1, 2].

İt is important in patients with acute cough and sputum production suggestive of acute bronchitis to rule out pneumonia as the cause of cough. Pneumonia should be suspected in patients with tachypnea, tachycardia, dyspnea, or lung findings suggestive of pneumonia, and radiography is warranted.

İ. G. Coşğun (✉)
Section of Pulmonology, Afyonkarahisar University of Health Sciences Hospital,
Afyonkarahisar, Turkey

B. Harbiyeli
Section of Pulmonology, Adana Seyhan State Hospital, Adana, Turkey

E. Vevecka
Division of Pediatric Pneumology, Department of Pediatrics, Faculty of Medicine,
University of Medicine, Tirana, Albania

Pertussis should be suspected in patients with cough persisting for more than 2 weeks that is accompanied by symptoms such as paroxysmal cough, whooping cough, and post-tussive emesis, or recent pertussis exposure. The cough associated with acute bronchitis typically lasts about 2–3 weeks, and this should be emphasized with patients. Acute bronchitis is usually caused by viruses, and antibiotics are not indicated in patients without chronic lung disease. Antibiotics have been shown to provide only minimal benefit, reducing the cough or illness by about half a day, and have adverse effects, including allergic reactions, nausea and vomiting, and *Clostridium difficile* infection. Evaluation and treatment of bronchitis include ruling out secondary causes for cough, such as pneumonia; educating patients about the natural course of the disease; and recommending symptomatic treatment and avoidance of unnecessary antibiotic use [1, 2].

78.1.2 Diagnosis

Cough is the predominant and defining symptom of acute bronchitis. The primary diagnostic consideration in patients with suspected acute bronchitis is ruling out more serious causes of cough, such as asthma, exacerbation of chronic obstructive pulmonary disease, heart failure, or pneumonia. The diagnoses that have the most overlap with acute bronchitis are upper respiratory tract infections and pneumonia. Whereas acute bronchitis and the common cold are self-limited illnesses that do not require antibiotic treatment, the standard therapy for pneumonia is antibiotics.

Besides cough, other signs and symptoms of acute bronchitis include sputum production, nasal congestion, headache, and fever. The first few days of an acute bronchitis infection may be indistinguishable from the common cold. Patients may have substernal or chest wall pain when coughing. Fever is not a typical finding after the first few days, and presence of a fever greater than 100 °F (37.8 °C) should prompt consideration of influenza or pneumonia. Production of sputum, even purulent, is common and does not correlate with bacterial infection [3–5].

Because the cough associated with bronchitis is so bothersome and slow to resolve, patients often seek treatment. Patients and clinicians may underestimate the time required to fully recover from acute bronchitis. The duration of acute bronchitis-related cough is typically 2–3 weeks, with a pooled estimate of 18 days in one systematic review. This corresponds to results of a prospective trial, which found that patients who had a cough for at least 5 days had a median of 18 days of coughing [4, 5].

On physical examination, patients with acute bronchitis may be mildly ill-appearing, and fever is present in about one-third of patients. Lung auscultation may reveal wheezes, as well as rhonchi that typically improve with coughing. It is important to rule out pneumonia. High fever; moderate to severe ill-appearance; hypoxia; and signs of lung consolidation, such as decreased breath sounds, bronchial breath sounds, crackles, egophony, and increased tactile fremitus, are concerning for pneumonia [6, 7].

78.1.3 Treatment of Acute Bronchitis

Supportive care and symptom management are the mainstay of treatment for acute bronchitis. The role of antibiotics is limited. Since 2005, the National Committee for Quality Assurance has recommended avoidance of antibiotic prescribing for acute bronchitis as a Healthcare Effectiveness Data and Information Set Measure. All major guidelines on bronchitis, including those from the American College of Chest Physicians, recommend against using antibiotics for acute bronchitis unless the patient has a known pertussis infection. The American Academy of Pediatrics recommends that antibiotics not be used for apparent viral respiratory illnesses, including sinusitis, pharyngitis, and bronchitis. Despite these recommendations, antibiotics are often prescribed for acute bronchitis [8–10].

78.2 Protracted Bacterial Bronchitis (PBB)

78.2.1 Introduction

Cough is the most common reason for primary care physician visit and, when chronic, a frequent indication for specialist referrals. In children a chronic cough (>4 weeks) is associated with increased morbidity and reduced quality of life. One common cause of childhood chronic cough is protracted bacterial bronchitis (PBB).

Protracted bacterial bronchitis (PBB) is characterized by chronic wet or productive cough that lasts more than 4 weeks without signs of an alternative cause and can improve with appropriate antibiotic therapy.

78.2.2 Definitions

Protracted bacterial bronchitis can be defined in various ways, depending on whether supplementary tests are included in the diagnostic evaluation. Nonetheless the practical definition is based purely on clinical criteria described in Box 78.1 [8, 11].

Box 78.1: Definition of Protracted Bacterial Bronchitis After Chang et al.

Clinical definition of protracted bacterial bronchitis
- Chronic wet cough for more than 4 weeks
- Absence of symptoms or signs of other chronic pulmonary disease
- Improved after 2 weeks of treatment with antibiotics

Microbiologically based definition of protracted bacterial bronchitis. As above, but in addition
- Lower respiratory tract infection, positive bacterial culture ($\geq 10^4$cfu/ml) in sputum or bronchoalveolar lavage fluid

Recurrent protracted bacterial bronchitis
- More than three episodes annually

Clinical Phenotype

By definition all children with a chronic wet cough were more likely to have attended childcare. Children with protracted bacterial bronchitis typically appear well. They have normal growth and development and lack signs of underlying chronic suppurative lung disease such as digital clubbing, chest wall deformity, and adventitial auscultatory chest findings. Although occasionally a rattly chest or crackles are heard. The chest radiograph is normal or near normal, showing only peri-bronchial changes.

İn children, differentiation between acute bronchitis and protracted bacterial bronchitis is based on the fact that acute bronchitis cough usually resolves within 2–3 weeks. Nevertheless, difficulties arise while recurrent episodes need to be differentiated from bronchiectasis. Although cause and effect were unproven, some repeated PBB may result in progress to bronchiectasis. A study revealed 13 children with PBB were diagnosed with bronchiectasis after 2 years follow-up in a prospective cohort study with 161 patients; Hi infection and recurrent PBB were the major risks for bronchiectasis. Therefore, the possibility of bronchiectasis should be paid attention to patients with Hi infection and repeated PBB [8, 12, 13].

78.2.3 Treatment of Protracted Bacterial Bronchitis

In PBB, the child's cough resolves only after a prolonged (2 weeks) course of appropriate antibiotics. When a typical 5–7-day course of antibiotics is prescribed, the cough either relapses or does not resolve completely. However, some children require up to 4 weeks of treatment. Many of the children whose cough was not cured by 2 weeks of antibiotics had underlying tracheo-bronchomalacia and needed a longer course of antibiotics before their cough disappeared.

The 2008 British Thoracic Society (BTS) cough guidelines suggest all children with PBB should receive 4–6 weeks of antibiotics. This recommendation, however, was based upon expert opinion as at the time no supportive high-quality studies existed. Further studies are now needed to help identify whether those with PBB requiring a longer course of antibiotics are different from those responding to shorter courses [14, 15].

While some children with PBB may need longer antibiotic treatment, the 2008 British Thoracic Society (BTS) cough guidelines still advocate the shorter 2-week course initially. This reflects the principles of good antimicrobial stewardship and should also reduce drug-related adverse events. The most widely used first-line empiric antibiotic is amoxicillin-clavulanate (as commonly associated pathogens such as H. *Influenzae* and M. *Catarrhalis* can be amoxicillin resistant) although alternative such as an oral cephalosporin, trimethoprim-sulfamethoxazole, or an oral macrolide may be used. Ideally, a lower airway specimen for microbiologic testing is obtained before treatment. Indeed, the BTS guidelines recommend that before making a diagnosis of PBB, sputum should be cultured first and other underlying conditions excluded. However, most children with chronic wet cough are young and unable to expectorate, even following sputum induction. Thus, obtaining reliable lower respiratory secretions requires bronchoscopy, which will be impractical in most clinical settings. Nevertheless, if a bronchoscopy is performed, purulent secretions and evidence of bronchitis are usually present [16–18].

The BTS guidelines also suggest physiotherapy for children with PBB. While this may be beneficial, the evidence to support this recommendation is limited. Furthermore, the time required for performing airway clearance techniques should not be underestimated [19, 20].

References

1. Kinkade S, Long NA. Acute bronchitis. Am Fam Physician. 2016;94(7):560–5.
2. Øymar K, Mikalsen IB, Crowley S. Protracted bacterial bronchitis in children. Tidsskr Nor Laegeforen. 2017;137:14–5. https://doi.org/10.4045/tidsskr.16.0843.
3. Steurer J, Held U, Spaar A, et al. A decision aid to rule out pneumo- nia and reduce unnecessary prescriptions of antibiotics in primary care patients with cough and fever. BMC Med. 2011;9:56.
4. Ebell MH, Lundgren J, Youngpairoj S. How long does a cough last? Comparing patients' expectations with data from a systematic review of the literature. Ann Fam Med. 2013;11(1):5–13.
5. Ward JI, Cherry JD, Chang SJ, APERT Study Group, et al. Efficacy of an acellular pertussis vaccine among adolescents and adults. N Engl J Med. 2005;353(15):1555–63.
6. Metlay JP, Schulz R, Li YH, et al. Influence of age on symptoms at pre- sentation in patients with community-acquired pneumonia. Arch Intern Med. 1997;157(13):1453–9.
7. Evertsen J, Baumgardner DJ, Regnery A, Banerjee I. Diagnosis and man- agement of pneumonia and bronchitis in outpatient primary care prac- tices. Prim Care Respir J. 2010;19(3):237–41.
8. Chang AB, Marchant JM. Protracted bacterial bronchitis is a precursor for bronchiectasis in children: myth or maxim? Breathe (Sheff). 2019;15:167–70. https://doi.org/10.1183/2073473 5.0178-2019.
9. American Academy of Pediatrics. Fifteen things physicians and patients should question. http://www.choosingwisely.org/wp-content/uploads/2015/02/AAP-Choosing-Wisely-List. pdf. Accessed 15 Sept 2020.
10. Barnett ML, Linder JA. Antibiotic prescribing for adults with acute bronchitis in the United States, 1996-2010. JAMA. 2014;311(19):2020–2.
11. Zhang XB, Wu X, Nong GM. Update on protracted bacterial bronchitis in children. Ital J Pediatr. 2020;46(1):38. https://doi.org/10.1186/s13052-020-0802-z.
12. Chen AC, Pena OM, Nel HJ, Yerkovich ST, Chang AB, Baines KJ, et al. Airway cells from pro- tracted bacterial bronchitis and bronchiectasis share similar gene expression profiles. Pediatr Pulmonol. 2018;53:575–82. https://doi.org/10.1002/ppul.23984.
13. Wurzel DF, Marchant JM, Yerkovich ST, Upham JW, Petsky HL, Smith-Vaughan H, et al. Protracted bacterial bronchitis in children: natural history and risk factors for bronchiectasis. Chest. 2016;150:1101–8. https://doi.org/10.1016/j.chest.2016.06.030.
14. Shields MD, Bush A, Everard ML, McKenzie SA, Primhak R. British thoracic society guide- lines recommendations for the assessment and management of cough in children. Thorax. 2008;63:1–15.
15. Goyal V, Grimwood K, Marchant JM, Masters IB, Chang AB. Does failed chronic wet cough response to antibiotics predict bronchiectasis? Arch Dis Child. 2014;99:522–5.
16. van Vugt SF, Verheij TJ, de Jong PA, GRACE Project Group, et al. Diag- nosing pneumonia in patients with acute cough: clinical judgment com-pared to chest radiography. Eur Respir J. 2013;42(4):1076–82.
17. Altiner A, Wilm S, Däubener W, et al. Sputum colour for diagnosis of a bacterial infection in patients with acute cough. Scand J Prim Health Care. 2009;27(2):70–3.

18. Chang AB, Upham JW, Masters IB, et al. Protracted bacterial bronchitis: the last decade and the road ahead. Pediatr Pulmonol. 2016;51(3):225–42. https://doi.org/10.1002/ppul.23351.
19. Marchant JM, Morris P, Gaffney J, Chang AB. Antibiotics for prolonged moist cough in children. Cochrane Database Syst Rev. 2005;19(4):CD004822.
20. Marchant JM, Masters IB, Champion A, Petsky HL, Chang AB. Randomised controlled trial of amoxycillin-clavulanate in children with chronic wet cough. Thorax. 2012;67:689–93.

Pneumonia in Children

Alev Ketenci, Laura Gochicoa-Rangel, and Özge Yılmaz

79.1 Introduction

The most frequent reason for death in children worldwide who are under the age of 5 years is pneumonia. It is estimated that 808,000 children died due to pneumonia in 2017 (WHO), representing higher than five deaths to pneumonia per 1000 live births [1]. This child mortality disproportionately affects lower- and middle-income nations, but even in developed countries pneumonia still causes considerable morbidity and healthcare costs. Epidemiological research carried out in the USA ascertained a rate of 15.7 cases of community-acquired pneumonia per 10,000 children resulting in admission to hospital. The highest risk for this event was amongst children aged below 2 years [1–3].

Pneumonia refers generally to a situation in which the pulmonary tissues, particularly the alveoli, are inflamed. The characteristic symptomatic presentation in children is with fever, cough (productive or dry), and dyspnoea. The severity of clinical presentation may range from mild to severe, a number of pathogens can cause pneumonia in the paediatric age group: bacterial, atypical bacteria (especially *Mycoplasma pneumoniae*), fungal and viral [1–4].

Pneumonia may frequently be diagnosed with careful history and physical examination, with further investigations (chest X-ray, venous bloods, microbiological culture of sputum) helping to confirm the diagnosis. Pneumonia is often categorised

A. Ketenci (✉)
Section of Pulmonology, Başakşehir Pine and Sakura City Hospital, İstanbul, Turkey

L. Gochicoa-Rangel
National Institute of Respiratory Diseases, Mexico City, Mexico

Ö. Yılmaz
Division of Pediatric Allergy and Pulmonology, Department of Pediatrics, Faculty of Medicine, Manisa Celal Bayar University, Manisa, Turkey

© The Author(s), under exclusive license to Springer Nature Switzerland AG 2022
C. Cingi et al. (eds.), *Pediatric ENT Infections*,
https://doi.org/10.1007/978-3-030-80691-0_79

as community-acquired (CAP), nosocomial or healthcare-associated. If food or drink, vomitus or saliva is aspirated into the lungs, an aspiration pneumonia may also develop [1, 2].

Although pneumonia has high prevalence and is associated with significant burden to healthcare systems, correct and timely diagnosis as well as treatment may be challenging in many cases [1–4].

The main risk factors to present pneumonia in a child are presence of anatomical congenital abnormalities, immunological deficiencies, alterations of the mucociliary system, broncho-aspirations, prolonged hospitalisation, previous viral infection, neuromuscular disease, pain from trauma or surgery of the abdomen or chest, and artificial airway. Additionally, the risk increases if the patient is malnourished, has a low socioeconomic status, passive smoking, or go to nurseries or day care.

79.2 Aetiology

Isolation of the causative agent in paediatric pneumonia is not possible in most of the cases but viral aetiology accounts for more than 50% of cases. "Etiology of Pneumonia in the Community" [EPIC] is a population-based multicentre study carried out by the Centers for Diseases Control and Prevention using an active surveillance technique to identify cases of CAP. The results of this study showed that a viral pathogenic agent was the aetiology in 66.2% of CAP cases that necessitated hospital admission. The most common viral agents identified were respiratory syncytial virus (RSV, 28.0% of cases), rhinovirus (RV, 27.3% of cases) and human metapneumovirus (hMPV, 12.8% of cases) [1, 4, 5].

Pyogenic bacteria are not the common etiological agents of paediatric CAP but may be associated with severe disease and complications with high mortality. Pyogenic bacteria were implicated in 7.3% of paediatric pneumonia cases in the EPIC study. The most frequently isolated bacteria were *Streptococcus pneumoniae* followed by *Staphylococcus aureus* and *Streptococcus pyogenes*, with frequencies of 3.6%, 1.0% and 0.7%, respectively. *M. pneumoniae*, was isolated in 8% of cases of CAP, especially more frequently in children aged 5 and older [2, 4, 5].

The multicentre, prospective, observational cohort study, CHIRP (Children's Hospital's Initiative for Research in Pneumonia), enrolled 441 participants aged ≥2 months to 18 years old, diagnosed to have CAP. Both admitted patients and outpatients were enrolled (13.8% and 86.2%, respectively). The initial analysis of the data showed that a viral pathogen was present in 55.6% of cases, with 3.6% of cases caused by pyogenic bacteria and 8.8% by atypical bacterial organisms. The division of cases into viral and bacterial pneumonia was similar to that seen in the EPIC study [4, 5].

The PERCH (Pneumonia Etiology Research for Child Health) study involved 4232 paediatric patients under 5 years of age with pneumonia of marked severity in developing countries. The findings of the PERCH study concerning pathogen and epidemiological risk factors differed somewhat from those reported on CAP paediatric cases in advanced economies [4] Table 79.1.

Table 79.1 Bacterial pneumonia aetiology according to age

Age	Bacteria
Newborn	Group B Streptococcus Escherichia coli Klebsiella pneumoniae Listeria monocytogenes Proteus
1–3 months	Chlamydia trachomatis Group B Streptococcus Staphylococcus aureus Haemophilus influenzae Streptococcus pneumoniae
3 months to 5 years old	Streptococcus pneumoniae Haemophilus influenzae Staphylococcus aureus Mycoplasma pneumonia
Older than 5 years old	Streptococcus pneumonia Mycoplasma pneumoniae Staphylococcus aureus Haemophilus influenzae Moraxella catarrhalis Legionella pneumonia

79.2.1 Viral–Bacterial Interaction

The rate at which infections due to a virus and a bacterium co-occur in CAP has been reported as 7.0% (EPIC study) and 3.9% (CHIRP study). It is probable that these figures are underestimated due to the low sensitivity of bacterial detection methods used (such as blood culture). According to the EPIC study, concurrent viral and bacterial pneumonia cases were more likely to have high white cell count, pulmonary consolidation on chest X-ray, pleural effusion, intensive care admission with mechanical ventilation support and prolonged duration of hospitalisation [4]. One interaction of particular significance is co-infection by RSV and *S. pneumoniae* in IPD (invasive pneumococcal disease), which increases the severity and alters the likely outcome [6, 7].

Research using mice with a concurrent RSV and streptococcal pneumonia has shown that pulmonary inflammation is more severe, bacteraemia more common and death more common than either pathogen alone [8, 9]. A recent case-control study [9] compared the presence of potentially pathogenic bacteria (PPB) in nasopharyngeal swab cultures of children with bronchiolitis and healthy controls younger than 2 years age. Prevalence of PPB isolation was higher in the patients with RSV bronchiolitis than in the healthy children. Moreover, detection of *S. pneumoniae* or *H. influenzae* in the bronchiolitis group was associated with more severe disease. These findings point towards the potential role played by PBB within the upper respiratory tract in mediating the course and severity of pneumonia secondary to RSV [9] (Fig. 79.1).

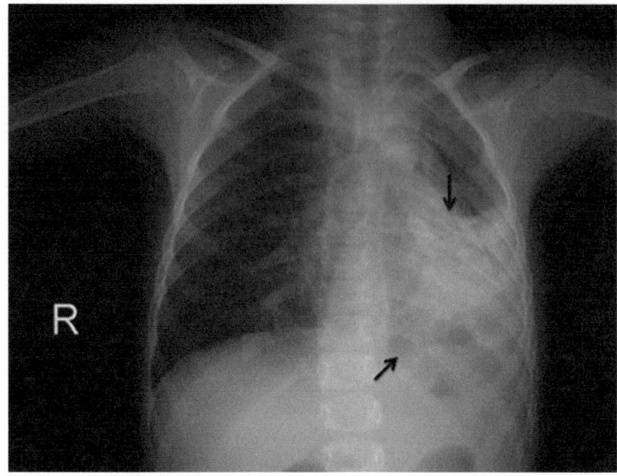

Fig. 79.1 Left lower lobe pneumonia in a 4-year-old girl with chest pain, fever and cough. Chest X-ray shows a large opacity (arrow) in the left mid and lower lung zones

79.3 Diagnosis

The clinical characteristics of pneumonia are fever, cough and dyspnoea. It is very important to identify if the patient is breathing fast (>50 breaths per minute in children from 2 to 12 months, >40 breaths per minute in those from 12 months to 5 years old and >30 breaths per minute in children older than 5 years), and if he/she has lower chest wall indrawing. Although, it is possible to diagnose pneumonia on the basis of the clinical presentation and chest X-ray, differential diagnosis especially from bronchiolitis in children may be challenging. The etiological microbiological agent cannot be isolated in majority of the subjects. Development of microbiological diagnostic methods with higher specificity and sensitivity may result in targeted pharmacotherapy, elimination of unwarranted investigations and perhaps lower morbidity and mortality [10] (Fig. 79.2).

The clinical presentation in paediatric cases of pneumonia secondary to atypical bacteria may resemble those of viral pneumonia, as may the results of laboratory testing and imaging. Indeed, pneumonia secondary to pyogenic bacteria may also present in a way that resembles viral pneumonia at the beginning, i.e. symptoms affecting the upper airways may predominate, inflammatory markers may not be very elevated and chest X-ray may reveal interstitial infiltrates [11]. Measurement of C-reactive protein levels and procalcitonin can be helpful in evaluation of treatment response when pneumonia is of high severity, but so far no clear cut-off value has been established that indicates the infection is of bacterial origin [10].

A further difficulty in identifying the causative agent in paediatric pneumonia arises from the fact that specimens for culture are challenging to procure from a child. Since pneumonia is a pulmonary condition, suitable specimens need to originate in the lung or the fluid contained within the alveoli. Thoracocentesis and bronchoalveolar lavage involve a high degree of invasiveness and are therefore not typically carried out in paediatric CAP cases. In younger children it is a challenge to procure a suitable sample for Gram staining and microbiological culture; hence

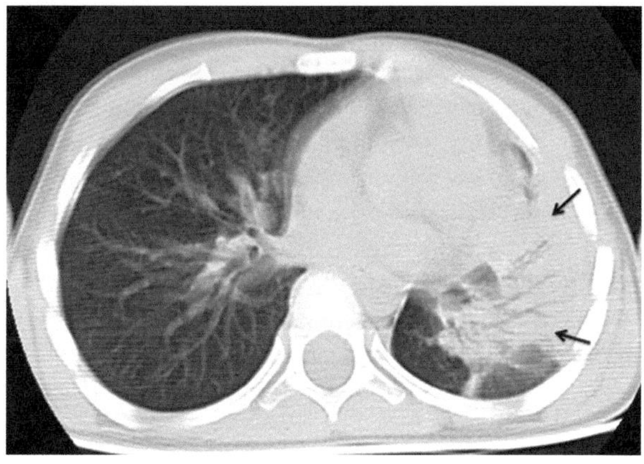

Fig. 79.2 Left lower lobe pneumonia in a 4-year-old girl with chest pain, fever and cough. Axial chest CT image with lung window settings demonstrates pulmonary consolidation with air bronchograms (arrows) in the left lower lobe (Courtesy of Esin Kurtulus Ozturk, MD)

these are not common investigations, either. Analysis of aspirate from thoracocentesis is of value in identifying causative pathogens, but in the majority of cases of CAP, there is insufficient fluid generated to permit aspiration. Thoracocentesis is therefore generally considered too invasive and the risk of complications too high. This leaves blood culture as the only feasible way of isolating pyogenic bacteria in paediatric CAP. However, it is a test of low sensitivity. Furthermore, since there seems to be an increased risk of co-infection with bacteria when a viral infection of the respiratory tract exists, isolation of a viral pathogen cannot preclude a bacterial aetiology also being present. Unfortunately, this situation frequently leads to clinicians over-employing antibiotic treatment and needlessly admitting patients to hospital [10, 11].

To diagnose *M. pneumoniae*, the method often employed is PCR (polymerase chain reaction) sequencing. Various researchers have cast doubt on the benefit to diagnosis of PCR sequencing [12], but it was considered a useful test by the researchers involved in the EPIC and CHIRP studies, applicable in various circumstances. If a viral aetiology is suspected in a child, nasopharyngeal swabs or aspirated fluid may be submitted for real-time PCR sequencing. However, it needs to be considered that PCR can also detect some of these viral pathogens in asymptomatic children and therefore the presence of viral pathogenic DNA need not prove aetiology. Viruses may persist for lengthy periods after resolution of an infection and may become active again following a different pathological event, especially rhinovirus or adenoviruses. It is unusual to detect other respiratory viruses, namely RSV, influenza or hMPV, unless symptoms of an infection are present [13].

Despite these limitations, being able to identify a viral respiratory pathogen in cases of paediatric CAP does offer assistance with management, since it is reasonable to withhold antibiotics if the clinical features, laboratory investigations and imaging results do not suggest co-occurring bacterial infection [11]. It is clear from the CHIRP study that the probability of being sent home from hospital and not started on antibiotic pharmacotherapy was higher in cases where there was proof of a viral aetiology and no evidence to support a bacterial aetiology [14].

79.4 Treatment

Pneumonia of bacterial origin without complications may be managed with oral antibiotic treatment on the outpatient basis. Provided a case of bacterial pneumonia is of no more than moderate degree, antibiotic therapy may be commenced empirically. There is no need to seek further investigations into aetiology unless there are other reasons to hospitalise the child. Possible reasons for admitting a child to hospital might be low oxygen saturation levels, moderate respiratory distress, age younger than 1 year and pleural effusion of at least moderate size. Moreover, lack of cooperation of the family and child for outpatient treatment and monitoring are relative indications for hospitalisation [15].

79.4.1 Outpatient Management

The vital element in treating cases effectively outside hospital is to find the most suitable antibiotic and the optimal dose. Treatment of choice depends on the probable etiological agent, the age of the child, contact with other cases, previous medical problems, drug allergy (if present) and the data available on local resistance patterns. Even though pneumococcal vaccination is now widespread, an agent needs to be chosen with activity against *S. pneumoniae*, as it is still the leading cause of bacterial pneumonia [16]. The treatment of choice currently is amoxicillin. Many clinicians tend to assume that per oral cephalosporin is a better choice to cover pneumococcal pneumonia, but this is an incorrect assumption. Whilst it is true that some strains of pneumococcus are penicillin-resistant, but are sensitive to ceftriaxone, cephalosporins given by mouth suffer from a brief half-life, low absorption from the gut, are predominantly protein-bound within the circulation and doses are frequently far apart. Accordingly, the concentration in plasma is inadequate to eradicate the pathogen, as can be seen by comparison of the plasma concentration and the usual minimum inhibitory concentration (MIC) for the pathogen, unless the strain has a low MIC. Oral amoxicillin, in comparison, achieves a greater plasma concentration and binds to protein to a lesser degree, which allows the MIC to be reached for a longer period. Amoxicillin is thus effective against pneumococci provided the bacterium is susceptible and the MIC achievable at an intermediate dosage level. Given the relatively unfavourable pharmacokinetic characteristics of cephalosporins versus amoxicillin, the former should only be used if the child has a penicillin allergy or the pathogen targeted is sensitive to cephalosporins but not amoxicillin, namely *M. catarrhalis* or an *H. influenzae* strain expressing a beta-lactamase [8, 17].

Another important element to consider when using beta-lactam antibiotics is the time between doses. It is not often appreciated that putting doses closer together can lengthen the "killing time" (i.e. period when plasma concentration exceeds the MIC), and thus be useful where a strain has a marginally higher than usual MIC. To give an illustration: suppose that the MIC for a certain strain of pneumococcus is 2.0 mg.mL^{-1}. If a dose of 90 mg/kg body weight is given b.d., this will eradicate the organism in 65% of cases, whereas the same dose given t.d.s. will be effective in 90% of cases [18, 19]. Hence, to achieve a higher bioavailability a high dosage (between 90-100 mg/kg daily) should be administered t.d.s. rather than b.d. This rationale applies where strains of *S. pneumoniae* possessing resistance are prevalent or perhaps in any case of lobar CAP treated outside of hospital and where there is a risk of deterioration or complications [19]. The half-life of amoxicillin within ear fluid is longer than in the serum (4 h, rather than 1.2 h), which explains why treatment for otitis media is effective with b.d. dosing, whereas t.d.s. dosing is required for pneumonia of bacterial origin, since the killing time depends on the half-life of the drug at the site of action [20].

In the majority of cases, the antibiotic chosen empirically does not need to cover *H. influenzae* or *M. catarrhalis*. Where these pathogens are present, however, there is a 30% chance that *H. influenzae* will express a beta-lactamase, and all strains of *M. catarrhalis* do so. Thus, they will be resistant to amoxicillin. Generally, these organisms are sensitive to co-amoxiclav and cephalosporin agents. CAP may also potentially result from an infection of *S. aureus* or *S. pyogenes*, but the pneumonia that results is usually of a severity necessitating hospitalisation [15].

Diffuse and lobar CAP are sometimes due to infection by *M. pneumoniae*, but just how useful antibiotics are in this situation is still the subject of debate [21, 22]. The features of the history and findings on physical examination are an unreliable guide in distinguishing *M. pneumoniae* infections from other pathogens, which may result in unwarranted attempts to cover this organism. National guidelines advocate treating all children over the age of 5, but this may be unwarranted, since the benefits of this course of action are still not fully established. There needs to be clinical judgement used in interpreting advice from guidelines, rather than a blanket approach to treatment, which ignores cases where the pattern of symptoms fits a viral infection or another bacterium is already being treated. Attempts in adult patients to cover both typical and atypical bacterial infections have led to massive overemployment of fluoroquinolones, which the FDA is at pains to prevent [23]. Azithromycin has become the second most frequently used antibiotic by paediatricians treating non-hospitalised patients, who want to provide cover for more usual bacteria, alongside *Mycoplasma*. However, this agent has low efficacy against the more usual pathogens [24]. It has recently been proposed by researchers that the use of azithromycin in younger children has a protective effect on the later development of wheeze [25], but the research findings have some limitations and even if there is a clear advantage, the prescribing physician should also consider the downsides, in particular the hazards of dual treatment, higher burden of adverse effects, potentially contributing to bacterial resistance and the disturbance of the normal healthy microbial flora that results [26, 27].

Treatment courses for CAP lacking complications should last a maximum of 7 days, with evidence that a 3-day course is adequate in CAP of no more than moderate degree [28]. The benefit from a 7-day course has been shown to be similar to when a 10-day course was used, or even a 5-day course. Research concerned with treating CAP has a tendency to suffer from positivity bias (the so-called "Pollyanna phenomenon"), but the accumulating evidence gathered from trials of brief treatment courses, taken alongside the advantages of shorter treatment durations (i.e. less development of resistant bacteria, lower adverse effect burden and greater patient concordance with treatment) ought to mean that a course of treatment between 5 and 7 days in duration becomes standard practice [29–31].

Treatment failure in cases of CAP treated outside hospital may be defined as a deterioration in clinical presentation in spite of treatment for two full days with an appropriate agent at the correct dose. Just because pyrexia is still present (generally, for 2 days more) [32], treatment failure should not be deemed to have occurred, provided other indicators (oral intake, slower respiratory rate, more participation in usual activities) point towards a clinical improvement.

79.4.2 Inpatient Management

There are two different categories of patients hospitalised for CAP. The first group consists of children who have pneumonitis of viral origin, in whom CAP may additionally have occurred. The second group consists of children in whom there is clear evidence of CAP of bacterial type, and some of whom also have a parapneumonic process. The first group of patients has been discussed earlier, and details are available in Table 79.1 about the diagnostic process, how they should be managed outside hospital and the criteria for admission. In the second group, with more straightforwardly diagnosed bacterial CAP, there are some key issues to bear in mind when treating. The first issue is the need to establish the aetiology through further investigations. The choice of antibiotic pharmacotherapy needs careful consideration, too, and any complications will need to be addressed [missing reference].

In a case of CAP where hospitalisation has occurred, the most likely aetiology is pneumococcal infection. However, in particular instances, other pathogens should be suspected. A child suffering from influenza, in whom CAP then develops, is likely to be infected with *S. aureus*. If there is rapid clinical deterioration, with or without indications of sepsis or toxic shock, the treating physician should suspect *S. aureus* or *S. pyogenes*. Ampicillin is efficacious in treating S. pyogenes, but some *S. aureus* strains are methicillin resistant (i.e. MRSA), the risk depending on the resistance characteristics in the area and how severe the disease is. It is still a matter of controversy whether treatment should provide cover for *H. influenzae* and *M. catarrhalis* in an admitted patient without immunodeficiency. Data comparing management in inpatients using ampicillin I/ amoxicillin versus the older use of broader spectrum agents indicates no major difference in benefit, even though the newer regimens do not cover 30% of *H. influenzae* strains or *M. catarrhalis* [33]. Parapneumonic processes have been observed in infection by *S. pneumoniae*, *S. pyogenes* and *S. aureus*.

All cases of bacterial CAP beyond those of mild degree result in inflammation, and research has focused on treatment to dampen down a florid inflammatory response. Macrolides and corticosteroids have been examined in this context. However, since there have been no studies up to the present involving the use of steroids in children with CAP, a cautious approach is appropriate. In children with known asthma who develop CAP and whose airways show evidence of reversible obstruction, corticosteroid treatment for between 5 and 7 days is reasonable. Although azithromycin is a macrolide and thus potentially anti-inflammatory, currently it is not recommended to employ this agent in CAP.

79.4.2.1 Prevention

To reduce the morbidity and mortality from pneumonia, it is important to implement effective prevention measures, the main ones that has shown some evidence are: (1), immunisation against those organisms that causes pneumonia (H. influenzae type b, Pneumococcal conjugate vaccines, as well as measles, and pertussis); (2) adequate nutrition, undernutrition in children 0–4 years old contributes to more than one million pneumonia deaths per year; (3) exclusive breastfeeding, those under 6 months old who are not breastfed are at five times the risk of dying from pneumonia; (4) zinc intake has proven that helps to reduce the incidence of pneumonia and the severity of disease [34–38].

References

1. https://www.who.int/health-topics/pneumonia#tab=tab_1. Accessed December 2020.
2. Yun KW, Wallihan R, Juergensen A, Mejias A, Ramilo O. Community-acquired pneumonia in children: myths and facts. Am J Perinatol. 2019;36(02):S54–7. https://doi.org/10.1055/s-0039-1691801.
3. Hooven TA, Polin RA. Pneumonia. Semin Fetal Neonatal Med. 2017;22(4):206–13. https://doi.org/10.1016/j.siny.2017.03.002.
4. O'Brien KL, Baggett HC, Brooks WA, et al. Introduction to the epidemiologic considerations, analytic methods, and foundational results from the pneumonia etiology research for child health study. Clin Infect Dis. 2017;64(Suppl 3):S179–84.
5. Marzec S, Ambroggio L, Desai A. et al. Impact of viral testing on duration of antibiotic therapy in children hospitalized with community acquired pneumonia (CAP) in a multicenter study. 2018 Pediatric academic societies annual meeting, May 5–8; 2018. Toronto, Canada.
6. Zar HJ, Andronikou S, Nicol MP. Advances in the diagnosis of pneumonia in children. BMJ. 2017;358:j2739. https://doi.org/10.1136/bmj.j2739.
7. Jain S, Williams DJ, Arnold SR, et al. CDC EPIC study team. Community-acquired pneumonia requiring hospitalization among U.S. children. N Engl J Med. 2015;372(09):835–45.
8. Bradley JS, Byington CL, Shah SS, Alverson B, Carter ER, Harrison C, Kaplan SL, Mace SE, GH MC Jr, Moore MR, St Peter SD, Stockwell JA, Swanson JT, Pediatric Infectious Diseases Society and the Infectious Diseases Society of America. The management of community-acquired pneumonia in infants and children older than 3 months of age: clinical practice guidelines by the Pediatric Infectious Diseases Society and the Infectious Diseases Society of America. Clin Infect Dis. 2011;53(7):e25–76. https://doi.org/10.1093/cid/cir531.
9. Diaz-Diaz A, Garcia-Maurino C, Jordan-Villegas A, Naples J, Ramilo O, Mejias A. Viral bacterial interactions in children: impact on clinical outcomes. Pediatr Infect Dis J. 2019;38(6S Suppl 1):S14–9. https://doi.org/10.1097/INF.0000000000002319.
10. Bradley JS, Byington CL, Shah SS, et al. Pediatric Infectious Diseases Society and the Infectious Diseases Society of America. The management of community-acquired pneumonia in infants and children older than 3 months of age: clinical practice guidelines by the Pediatric Infectious Diseases Society and the Infectious Diseases Society of America. Clin Infect Dis. 2011;53(07):e25–76.

11. Virkki R, Juven T, Rikalainen H, Svedström E, Mertsola J, Ruuskanen O. Differentiation of bacterial and viral pneumonia in children. Thorax. 2002;57(05):438–41.

12. Spuesens EB, Fraaij PL, Visser EG, et al. Carriage of Mycoplasma pneumoniae in the upper respiratory tract of symptomatic and asymptomatic children: an observational study. PLoS Med. 2013;10(05):e1001444.

13. Self WH, Williams DJ, Zhu Y, et al. Respiratory viral detection in children and adults: comparing asymptomatic controls and patients with community-acquired pneumonia. J Infect Dis. 2016;213(04):584–91.

14. Ramilo O, Mejías A. Shifting the paradigm: host gene signatures for diagnosis of infectious diseases. Cell Host Microbe. 2009;6(03):199–200.

15. Messinger AI, Kupfer O, Hurst A, Parker S. Management of pediatric community-acquired bacterial pneumonia. Pediatr Rev. 2017;38(9):394–409. https://doi.org/10.1542/pir.2016-0183.

16. Byington CL, Bradley JS. Feigin and Cherry's textbook of pediatric infectious diseases. New York: Saunders; 2014. p. 283–94.

17. Parker S, Mitchell M, Child J. Cephem antibiotics: wise use today preserves cure for tomorrow. Pediatr Rev. 2013;34(11):510–23.

18. Bradley JS, Garonzik SM, Forrest A, Bhavnani SM. Pharmacokinetics, pharmacodynamics, and Monte Carlo simulation: selecting the best antimicrobial dose to treat an infection. Pediatr Infect Dis J. 2010;29(11):1043–6.

19. Bradley JS, Nelson J. Nelson's pediatric anti-microbial therapy. Elk Grove Village: American Academy of Pediatrics; 2015.

20. Dagan R. The use of pharmacokinetic/pharmacodynamic principles to predict clinical outcome in paediatric acute otitis media. Int J Antimicrob Agents. 2007;30(Suppl 2):S127–30.

21. Meyer Sauteur PM, Unger WW, Nadal D, Berger C, Vink C, van Rossum AM. Infection with and carriage of Mycoplasma pneumoniae in children. Front Microbiol. 2016;7:329.

22. Gardiner SJ, Gavranich JB, Chang AB. Antibiotics for community-acquired lower respiratory tract infections secondary to Mycoplasma pneumoniae in children. Cochrane Database Syst Rev. 2015;1:CD004879.

23. Mandell LA, Wunderink RG, Anzueto A, et al. Infectious Diseases Society of America/American Thoracic Society consensus guidelines on the management of community-acquired pneumonia in adults. Clin Infect Dis. 2007;44(Suppl 2):S27–72.

24. Diaz MH, Benitez AJ, Cross KE, et al. Molecular detection and characterization of Mycoplasma pneumoniae among patients hospitalized with community-acquired pneumonia in the United States. Open Forum Infect Dis. 2015;2(3):ofv106.

25. Bacharier LB, Guilbert TW, Mauger DT, et al. National Heart, Lung, and Blood Institute's AsthmaNet. Early administration of azithromycin and prevention of severe lower respiratory tract illnesses in preschool children with a history of such illnesses: a randomized clinical trial. JAMA. 2015;314(19):2034–44.

26. Saari A, Virta LJ, Sankilampi U, Dunkel L, Saxen H. Antibiotic exposure in infancy and risk of being overweight in the first 24 months of life. Pediatrics. 2015;135(4):617–26.

27. Johnson CL, Versalovic J. The human microbiome and its potential importance to pediatrics. Pediatrics. 2012;129(5):950–60.

28. Haider BA, Saeed MA, Bhutta ZA. Short-course versus long-course antibiotic therapy for non-severe community-acquired pneumonia in children aged 2 months to 59 months. Cochrane Database Syst Rev. 2008;20082:CD005976.

29. Esposito S, Cohen R, Domingo JD, et al. Antibiotic therapy for pediatric community-acquired pneumonia: do we know when, what and for how long to treat? Pediatr Infect Dis J. 2012;31(6):e78–85.

30. Greenberg D, Givon-Lavi N, Sadaka Y, Ben-Shimol S, Bar-Ziv J, Dagan R. Short-course antibiotic treatment for community-acquired alveolar pneumonia in ambulatory children: a double-blind, randomized, placebo-controlled trial. Pediatr Infect Dis J. 2014;33(2):136–42.

31. Marchant CD, Carlin SA, Johnson CE, Shurin PA. Measuring the comparative efficacy of antibacterial agents for acute otitis media: the "Pollyanna phenomenon". J Pediatr. 1992;120(1):72–7.

32. Don M, Valent F, Canciani M, Korppi M. Prediction of delayed recovery from pediatric community-acquired pneumonia. Ital J Pediatr. 2010;2010:36–51.
33. Newman RE, Hedican EB, Herigon JC, Williams DD, Williams AR, Newland JG. Impact of a guideline on management of children hospitalized with community-acquired pneumonia. Pediatrics. 2012;129(3):e597–604.
34. https://apps.who.int/iris/bitstream/handle/10665/43640/9280640489_eng.pdf;jsessionid=A22 4BA19DA5A2021AA89EDF20BB3A01A?sequence=1. Accessed Dec 2020.
35. Garin N, Genné D, Carballo S, et al. β-Lactam monotherapy vs β-lactam-macrolide combination treatment in moderately severe community-acquired pneumonia: a randomized noninferiority trial. JAMA Intern Med. 2014;174(12):1894–901.
36. Wolf RB, Edwards K, Grijalva CG, et al. Time to clinical stability among children hospitalized with pneumonia. J Hosp Med. 2015;10(6):380–3.
37. Ray WA, Murray KT, Hall K, Arbogast PG, Stein CM. Azithromycin and the risk of cardiovascular death. N Engl J Med. 2012;366(20):1881–90.
38. Pneumonia: The forgotten killer of children © The United Nations Children's Fund (UNICEF)/ World Health Organization (WHO); 2006.

Diagnosis of Asthma in Children

Murat Acat and Bülent Karadağ

80.1 Introduction

The correct diagnostic approach to asthma and the exact nature of the disorder remain a matter of debate. This applies at all ages, but these issues are especially critical in childhood, the most common period for asthma to present. Over the last few decades, the concept of asthma has increasingly encompassed a more comprehensive range of presentations. It has become more heterogeneous, such that the current view of asthma is of a complicated, varied nosological concept that takes in disorders of differing aetiology yet with certain core features in common. Some researchers urge the abandonment of the term "asthma", as the concept is losing its utility. However, at present, asthma is still used as a label for conditions in which the bronchi are obstructed to varying degrees and when no other diagnosis is likely to explain the pathological features and permit a deeper aetiological understanding [1–4].

It is common for children up to the age of 1 year to have symptoms that resemble asthma, but the degree to which these symptoms persist or develop into full-blown asthma varies, to such an extent that prediction of the likely prognosis is fraught with difficulty. The difficulty in assigning a prognosis, coupled with uncertainty about the pathogenetic mechanism operating in particular cases, renders attempts to say whether a child is truly asthmatic at this age relatively futile. In older children, the diagnosis is more firmly based on symptomatic presentation than on probable

M. Acat (✉)
Department of Pulmonology, Faculty of Medicine, Karabük University, Karabük, Turkey

B. Karadağ
Division of Pediatric Pulmonology, Department of Pediatrics, Faculty of Medicine, Marmara University, İstanbul, Turkey

 965
C. Cingi et al. (eds.), *Pediatric ENT Infections*,
https://doi.org/10.1007/978-3-030-80691-0_80

aetiology, and the prognosis is less of an issue; hence diagnosing asthma in children above the age of 1 year is more straightforward. It is implicit in most guidelines published regarding asthma that asthma may be diagnosed before children reach school age, and no minimum age for diagnosing asthma is given. It has recently been noted that preschool children are being diagnosed with asthma at ever younger ages [5].

Guidelines typically suggest that asthma may be diagnosed in children of this age as long as there have been repeated episodes of symptoms consistent with asthma, such as reversible bronchoconstriction, ideally actually witnessed by the clinician, and these symptoms have responded as expected to therapy, while no competing diagnosis better accounts for the symptoms noted. Accordingly, a diagnosis of asthma in such a young child should be seen as a best guess, dependent on subjective clinical judgement, and potentially liable to being overturned later if more objective measurements allow for a more precisely informed diagnosis. Further investigations, such as radiological assessment, allergy testing, or other tests as indicated by competing differential diagnoses, are of secondary importance in diagnosis. At most, they offer indirect support for a diagnosis of asthma or a competing differential. The various indices used to predict clinical course are limited in this group since they are generally inaccurate in their predictions [6, 7]. It is considered unwarranted to subject a paediatric patient at very young ages to lung function testing, as the tests are complicated to carry out with such children, and there is a lack of experimental evidence to confirm they offer any benefit in management. However, pulmonary function testing makes a positive contribution to diagnosing suspected asthma cases in children above preschool age, since these patients can co-operate reasonably with performing forced spirometry. The occasional younger child can also carry out forced spirometry in a useful manner, even when the patient is as young as 3 years old [8–10]. On the other hand, there are other concerns about how valuable lung function tests in children of school age and even adolescents suspected of being asthmatic actually are [11, 12]. A systematic review that compared how various guidelines recommended patients with suspected asthma be evaluated diagnostically noted inconsistencies in when pulmonary function tests were suggested, both in adults and paediatric patients [12].

Clinicians are familiar with the phenomenon whereby young children appear to improve and even grow out of their asthmatic symptoms as they get older, but knowing when this will apply and indeed what the risk of recurrence is in such cases is less easy to say. The sole guideline specifically to address this phenomenon is one from Japan, where particular categories of recovery from asthma are defined as follows: "remission" implies a whole year passing without the patent being symptomatic; "clinical healing" is defined as 5 years free from asthma symptoms; and in "functional healing", the criterion for clinical healing is met, and there is a return to average values in lung function. The European Respiratory Society (ERS) is the sole guideline that proposes that asthma is an inappropriate diagnostic term to use in a child below school age who presents with an intermittent wheeze that eventually spontaneously recovers. Thus, the ERS takes a radically different stance in younger children, advocating that the diagnosis of asthma should be reserved for cases where the symptoms are attributable to chronic inflammatory processes within the airways. Since this pathogenetic mechanism is not established in the younger age range, asthma should not be diagnosed. This contrasts with the general consensus amongst other guidelines, which sees asthma as a diagnosis dependent on the clinical features [1, 13, 14].

In noting the above, it ought perhaps to be acknowledged that guidelines are not always explicit in how they view asthma, and detailed diagnostic procedures are not always offered. Indeed, guidelines have acquired a degree of notoriety from the paradox that they focus on treatment in particular groups, but the absence of clear diagnostic criteria renders it difficult for clinicians to assign patients to particular treatment groups. Thus, a straightforward answer to some of the clinicians' fundamental problems is often not answered by the guidelines, which call for a fair degree of judgement in their interpretation. In this survey of the guidelines, it must be acknowledged that the authors have drawn their own conclusions about what the guidelines are advocating, but this subjectivity has hopefully been partially offset by involving several authors in the review process. Furthermore, no survey of the guidelines available to treat asthma can include every guideline available, some of which are aimed at a specific national level only. The authors have concentrated on the critical international guidelines that are most likely to be familiar to experts in the field, and assumed that the lesser-known guidelines probably do not substantially differ in the guidance they can offer from the more widely disseminated guidelines the review has focused on [1, 13].

Over the last few decades, many researchers have questioned why there have been so few advances in treating asthma [14]. One suggestion for overcoming the apparent impasse is to conceptualize asthma as a constellation of symptoms that frequently co-occur but may not share an identical disease mechanism. According to this view, diagnosis of asthma acts as a convenient staging post towards a diagnosis reflecting aetiology, and better able to inform treatment options. An advantage of this approach is that it permits the diagnosis of even very young children, which was previously frowned upon since "asthma" is merely a convenient label for a syndrome of variable causes. The diagnosis can be made on clinical grounds and does not depend on pulmonary function test outcomes or on identifying the underlying pathophysiology. For each case, management then depends on selecting the most appropriate symptom or element to be treated. Numerous researchers have attempted a phenotypic or endotypes categorization of asthma, intending to permit a more tailored therapeutic approach [14, 15]. However, at present, the utility of the proposed subtypes has not yet been evaluated, and management principally relies on empirical trials of different agents [16–18].

80.2 Evaluation and Diagnosis

It is essential to maintain an appropriate index of suspicion for asthma in any child presenting with appropriate symptoms, but not to over-diagnose asthma. It is reported in the literature that as many as 12 to 30% of patients suffering from

Table 80.1 Comorbidities which affect asthma control [19]

• Rhinosinusitis
• Obesity
• Gastro-oesophageal reflux disorder
• Abnormal function of the vocal folds, including paralysis
• Obstructive sleep apnoea

disorders other than asthma are inappropriately labelled as uncontrolled asthma [19–22]. There are a large number of different conditions that may mimic asthma in their presentation, including abnormal function of the vocal folds, anatomical anomalies (such as tracheobronchomalacia), and disorders that lead to obstruction of the airways within the lung, notably cystic fibrosis and bronchiolitis obliterans (see Table 80.1) [20].

The critical tasks in clinical workup include assessing potential comorbid conditions, considering the possibility of non-concordance with prescribed asthma treatments, poor inhaler technique, triggers coming from the environment, and emotional or psychological elements to the presentation [21].

80.2.1 Confirming the Diagnosis of Asthma

The patient history should focus on symptoms affecting the respiratory system, especially coughing, wheezing, dyspnoea, tightness of the chest, and exacerbating or triggering factors for each symptom. Family history should be recorded concerning respiratory problems. Ask about prior therapy and how effective it was [21–23]. The patient should then be examined thoroughly and assessed using spirometry before and after administration of bronchodilator pharmacotherapy. Perform spirometry no earlier than 4 h after a short-acting bronchodilator has been administered. There also needs to be a 12-h interval between taking long-acting inhaled beta-agonists (LABA), such as salmeterol or formoterol, or oral treatment using aminophylline modified-release beta-agonists, and spirometric analysis [22]. The curves obtained from spirometry comparing airflow with volume during inspiration need to be examined so that a case of fixed or dynamic central airway obstruction is not missed. The clinician should bear in mind that a paediatric case of severe asthma may present with unremarkable pulmonary function or at most mildly obstructed airways unless currently undergoing an acute attack. The probable explanation for this paradoxical situation is that the small-calibre airways are where airflow is obstructed, not the larger airways. Hence FEV_1 may frequently fall in the reference range. There are other measures of pulmonary function, as shown by spirometry, that potentially give a better indication of how severe asthma is, in particular FEV_1/ forced vital capacity (FVC) and FEF between 25 and 75% of the standard value, or the measurement of FEV_1 after a bronchodilator has been administered [2, 23–25]. A case is considered to show a significant reversibility degree if there is a 12% or 200 mL improvement in FEV_1 following bronchodilator administration. In some recent studies, an 8% improvement in FEV_1 is suggested to be enough to signify reversibility in airway obstruction [26–28].

Where spirometry fails to show obstruction, the next stage is to try inducing bronchoconstriction by administering methacholine or arranging exercise challenge testing [20]. A chest X-ray should be obtained to exclude anatomical anomalies, if other diagnoses are suspected.

Investigations should be conducted as required to exclude any competing differential diagnoses, as revealed by atypical clinical features (Table 80.2). Some features that point away from asthma as the diagnosis are developmental abnormalities, inadequate weight gain, cough with sputum production, stridor, abrupt deterioration in pulmonary function, and where there is no allergic triggering factor [2]. In these patients, high-resolution CT, bronchoscopy accompanied by bronchoalveolar lavage (BAL), sweat chloride test, ciliary biopsy, immunology panel testing, quantification of immunoglobulins, pH testing, impedance testing, or videofluoroscopy while swallowing are all investigations that may be considered. Investigations should be performed according to the suspected diagnosis, e.g. bronchiectasis, disease affecting the pulmonary parenchyma or the airways, cystic fibrosis, primary ciliary dyskinesia, immunodeficiency, gastro-oesophageal reflux, and aspiration disorders [20, 22, 24]. Persistent bacterial bronchitis can usually be confirmed or excluded by bronchoscopic examination, coupled with BAL. Lavage specimens can be examined to assist in distinguishing between the different types of inflammation that may affect the airway in paediatric patients, namely eosinophilic, paucigranulocytic, and neutrophilic [26]. Once it has been verified that the patient has asthma, and not another condition, two different scenarios require consideration: asthma that has

Table 80.2 Differential diagnosis of severe asthma in a child [19]

Abnormal function of the vocal folds
Abnormal deglutition with repeated, unnoticed episodes of small-volume aspiration
Anatomically related, through the airway being compressed
Congenital vascular malformations
Tracheobronchomalacia
A mass within the mediastinum
Enlargement of lymph nodes
Tracheoesophageal-fistula
Cystic fibrosis
Primary ciliary dyskinesia
Persistent bacterial bronchitis
Immunodeficiency, either innate or acquired
Bronchiectasis
Bronchiolitis obliterans
Interstitial lung diseases
Connective tissue disorders
Congenital cardiac disorders
Foreign body aspiration
Hypersensitivity pneumonitis

become out of control due to co-existing disease, inadequate patient concordance, or an environmental factor; or asthma that is difficult to treat per se. The literature gives an estimated 30–50% of paediatric cases presenting as severely asthmatic who, following a comprehensive assessment, are deemed to have asthma in the difficult-to-treat category [20, 27, 28].

## 80.3	Conclusion

To conclude, it is evident that the majority of clinical guidelines concur in viewing asthma as a clinical diagnosis based on presenting features. Asthma should normally respond to therapy as expected and competing differential diagnoses must have been confidently excluded. A diagnosis of asthma then precedes an attempt to classify each case more precisely based on the phenotypic features and the genetic and environmental influences that affect the endotype. In some cases, the initial diagnosis of asthma will need to be modified to reflect aetiological evidence, such as cystic fibrosis, tracheobronchomalacia, or aortic encirclement of the trachea, amongst other potential diagnoses. Diagnosing asthma in a child of preschool age is a task undertaken by clinicians in the clear understanding that such a process differs from that employed in an older patient in various respects, principally in the fact that children of this age may be unable to co-operate with lung function testing. There is a need to consider especially carefully any competing diagnoses, that the patient may not respond particularly well to the standard therapy for asthma, and that some children are likely to grow out of the condition over time. Ideally, a consensus will eventually be reached amongst clinicians about when to use the terms "childhood wheeze", "reactive airways disease", or "asthma", perhaps eliminating the first two terms to avoid unclarity. However, the best prospect for the development of asthma management in the future will come from a more in-depth knowledge of the aetiological factors underpinning the disease, whether in children or adults [1, 18].

References

1. Moral L, Vizmanos G, Torres-Borrego J, Praena-Crespo M, Tortajada-Girbés M, Pellegrini FJ, Asensio Ó. Asthma diagnosis in infants and preschool children: a systematic review of clinical guidelines. Allergol Immunopathol (Madr). 2019;47(2):107–21. https://doi.org/10.1016/j.aller.2018.05.002.
2. Gauthier M, Ray A, Wenzel SE. Evolving concepts of asthma. Am J Respir Crit Care Med. 2015;192:660–8.
3. Holgate ST. Asthma: a simple concept but in reality a complex disease. Eur J Clin Invest. 2011;41:1339–52.
4. Warren P. Asthma as a disease concept. Lancet. 2006;368(9545):1416. https://doi.org/10.1016/S0140-6736(06)69596-2.
5. Radhakrishnan DK, Dell SD, Guttmann A, Shariff SZ, Liu K, To T. Trends in the age of diagnosis of childhood asthma. J Allergy Clin Immunol. 2014;134:1057–62.

6. Luo G, Nkoy FL, Stone BL, Schmick D, Johnson MD. A systematic review of predictive models for asthma development in children. BMC Med Inform Decis Mak. 2015;15:99.

7. Smit HA, Pinart M, Anto JM, Keil T, Bousquet J, Carlsen KH, et al. Childhood asthma prediction models: a systematic review. Lancet Respir Med. 2015;3:973–84.

8. Raywood E, Lum S, Aurora P, Pike K. The bronchodilator response in preschool children: a systematic review. Pediatr Pulmonol. 2016;51:1242–50.

9. Busi LE, Restuccia S, Torres R, Sly PD. Assessing bronchodilator response in preschool children using spirometry. Thorax. 2017;72:367–72.

10. Marín de Vicente C, de Mir Messa I, Rovira Amigo S, Torrent Vernetta A, Gartner S, Iglesias Serrano I, et al. Validación de las ecuaciones propuestas por la Iniciativa Global de Función Pulmonar (GLI) y las de Todas las Edades para espirometría forzada en preescolares sanos españoles. Arch Bronconeumol. 2018;54:24–30.

11. Murray C, Foden P, Lowe L, Durrington H, Custovic A, Simpson A. Diagnosis of asthma in symptomatic children based on measures of lung function: an analysis of data from a population- based birth cohort study. Lancet Child Adolesc Health. 2017;1:114–23.

12. Loo J, Dell S. Asthma diagnosis criteria in adult and pediatric asthma guidelines: a systematic review. Can Respir J. 2010;17:14.

13. Bisgaard H, Bonnelykke K. Long-term studies of the natural history of asthma in childhood. J Allergy Clin Immunol. 2010;126:187–97.

14. Fuchs O, Bahmer T, Rabe KF, von Mutius E. Asthma transition from childhood into adulthood. Lancet Respir Med. 2017;5:224–34.

15. Pavord ID, Beasley R, Agusti A, Anderson GP, Bel E, Brusselle G, et al. After asthma: redefining airways diseases. Lancet. 2018;391:350–400.

16. Just J, Bourgoin-Heck M, Amat F. Clinical phenotypes in asthma during childhood. Clin Exp Allergy. 2017;47:848–55.

17. Fitzpatrick AM, Jackson DJ, Mauger DT, Boehmer SJ, Phipatanakul W, Sheehan WJ, et al. Individualized therapy for persistent asthma in young children. J Allergy Clin Immunol. 2016;138:1608–18.

18. de Benedictis FM, Attanasi M. Asthma in childhood. Eur Respir Rev. 2016;25(139):41–7. https://doi.org/10.1183/16000617.0082-2015.

19. Haktanir Abul M, Phipatanakul W. Severe asthma in children: evaluation and management. Allergol Int. 2019;68(2):150–7. https://doi.org/10.1016/j.alit.2018.11.007.

20. Chung KF, Wenzel SE, Brozek JL, Bush A, Castro M, Sterk PJ, et al. International ERS/ATS guidelines on definition, evaluation and treatment of severe asthma. Eur Respir J. 2014;43:343–73. https://doi.org/10.1183/13993003.52020-2013.

21. Robinson DS, Campbell DA, Durham SR, Pfeffer J, Barnes PJ, Chung KF. Systematic assessment of difficult-to-treat asthma. Eur Respir J. 2003;22:478–83.

22. Aaron SD, Vandemheen KL, Boulet LP, McIvor RA, Fitzgerald JM, Hernandez P, et al. Overdiagnosis of asthma in obese and nonobese adults. CMAJ. 2008;179:1121–31.

23. Barsky EE, Giancola LM, Baxi SN, Gaffin JM. A practical approach to severe asthma in children. Ann Am Thorac Soc. 2018;15:399–408.

24. Guilbert TW, Bacharier LB, Fitzpatrick AM. Severe asthma in children. J Allergy Clin Immunol Pract. 2014;2:489–500.

25. Bracken M, Fleming L, Hall P, Van Stiphout N, Bossley C, Biggart E, et al. The importance of nurse-led home visits in the assessment of children with problematic asthma. Arch Dis Child. 2009;94:780–4.

26. Rajaratnam SK, Bacharier LB, Guilbert TW. Severe asthma in children. J Allergy Clin Immunol Pract. 2017;5:889–98.

27. Tse SM, Gold DR, Sordillo JE, Hoffman EB, Gillman MW, Rifas-Shiman SL, et al. Diagnostic accuracy of the bronchodilator response in children. J Allergy Clin Immunol. 2013;132:554–9.

28. Denlinger LC, Phillips BR, Ramratnam S, Ross K, Bhakta NR, Cardet JC, et al. Inflammatory and comorbid features of patients with severe asthma and frequent exacerbations. Am J Respir Crit Care Med. 2017;195:302–13.

Treatment of Asthma in Children

Fatih Alaşan, Adem Yaşar, Enrico Lombardi,
and Hasan Yüksel

81.1 Introduction

In order to keep asthma under control, it is necessary to evaluate and monitor asthma, provide asthma education to the patient and their caregivers, control environmental factors and comorbid conditions that can trigger asthma attacks, and to combine them with pharmacological treatment approaches [1]. Treatment aims to reduce/prevent asthma attacks, prevent persistent airflow restriction, and keep the side effects that may occur due to the medication within safe limits [2]. In order to achieve success in the treatment of asthma, it is important to use asthma medications and avoid the factors that trigger asthma attacks and to ensure physician-patient cooperation that will ensure success in patient follow-up in the long term [3].

In terms of compliance with the treatment, it is necessary for the patient to accept the recommendations and treatments given, to use the drugs as recommended by the doctor, and to continue using them over time [4, 5]. Asthma treatment should be personalized by considering asthma control, patient's preferences and poor compliance type [6].

In the pharmacological treatment of asthma, *controlling drugs* that control asthma with their anti-inflammatory effects, fast-acting *symptom relievers* that ensure bronchodilatation, and *additional drugs* that are not used alone and used in

F. Alaşan (✉)
Department of Pulmonology, Faculty of Medicine, Muğla Sıtkı Koçman University,
Muğla, Turkey

A. Yaşar · H. Yüksel
Division of Pediatric Allergy and Pulmonology, Department of Pediatrics, Faculty of
Medicine, Manisa Celal Bayar University, Manisa, Turkey

E. Lombardi
Pediatric Pulmonary Departmental Unit, Department of Pediatrics, Florence Meyer Pediatric
Hospital, University of Florence, Florence, Italy

C. Cingi et al. (eds.), *Pediatric ENT Infections*,
https://doi.org/10.1007/978-3-030-80691-0_81

Table 81.1 Stepwise treatment for children 5 years and younger. (Adopted from the Global Initiative for Asthma (GINA) Guideline 2020) [2]

	Preferred controller choice	Other controller options
STEP-1	As needed short-acting ß2 agonist	
STEP-2	Low-dose ICS	Daily LTRA or intermittent short courses of ICS at onset of respiratory illness
STEP-3	Double low-dose ICS	Low-dose ICS + LTRA Consider specialist referral
STEP-4	Continue controller and refer for specialist assessment	Add LTRA or increase ICS frequency, or add intermittent ICS

Table 81.2 Stepwise treatment for children 6–11 years. (Adopted from the Global Initiative for Asthma (GINA) Guideline 2020) [2]

	Preferred controller	Other controller options
STEP-1		Low-dose ICS taken whenever SABA taken[a], or daily low-dose ICS
STEP-2	Daily low-dose ICS	LTRA, or low-dose ICS taken whenever SABA taken
STEP-3	Low-dose ICS-LABA, or medium-dose ICS	Low-dose ICS + LTRA
STEP-5	Refer to phenotypic assessment + add on therapy, e.g., anti-IgE	Add on anti-IL5, or add on low-dose OCS, but consider side effects

All steps; if needed short-acting beta2-agonist, add therapy. *ICS* inhaled corticosteroid; LABA: long-acting beta2-agonist; *LTRA* leukotriene receptor antagonist; OCS: oral corticosteroids; *SABA* short-acting beta2-agonist.
[a]Off-label; separate ICS and SABA inhalers; only one study in children.

addition to controlling drugs, are used [7]. Medications for the treatment of asthma can be used thorough inhalation, orally or parenterally [1].

Inhaler therapy delivers drugs directly to the airways, providing a higher local drug concentration, which leads to a lower risk of systemic side effects. Drugs used in inhaled therapy are available in the form of a metered-dose inhaler (MDI), dry powder inhaler (DPI) and a nebulizer [1].

An important resource used in the treatment of childhood asthma is GINA. GINA recommends stepwise treatment approach for children 5 years and younger (Table 81.1) and children 6–11 years (Table 81.2) [2].

81.2 Pharmacological Treatment

81.2.1 Inhaled Corticosteroids

Airway inflammation taking an important place in asthma pathogenesis and a growing understanding of this mechanism, inhaled corticosteroids (ICS) have been recognized as a first-line controlling drug in all age groups [8]. ICSs reduce airway hyperresponsiveness, inflammation, asthma symptom load and risk of exacerbation;

besides, they prevent late phase reaction to the allergen [8, 9]. They demonstrate these effects by inhibiting the transcription of inflammatory cytokines and other proteins synthesized through nuclear receptors and inhibiting arachidonic acid metabolism, reducing the production of leukotriene and prostaglandin [2, 10].

It is a matter of concern that ICSs will affect growth negatively and may have systemic side effects [1]. However, many studies have reported that ICS treatment in children is relatively safe [11]. The negative effects of ICSs on growth potential are influenced by factors such as the dose, potency, type of device used, the child's age, gender, weight, and the individual's sensitivity to steroids [1]. However, this effect can be offset by the positive effect of ICSs on asthma control when used in the long term [12].

The most common local side effects of ICS are oropharyngeal candidiasis, hoarseness, and cough due to upper respiratory tract irritation [13, 14]. When selecting the ICS to be used in treatment, factors such as the potency of the drug to be used, the state of systemic absorption, taste, method of administration, and cost should be taken into account [1]. In a study involving patients between the ages of 6 and 66 years on the daily dose of ICS, regular, daily, low-dose ICS use in case where the asthma control was intermittent or mildly persistent has been shown to decrease asthma symptoms, airway inflammation, airway hyperresponsiveness, the risk of asthma attacks, the risk of asthma-related hospitalizations and asthma-related mortality, and to increase the quality of life and lung function [12, 15–19]. GINA recommends an increase in the dose of ICS in cases where asthma control cannot be achieved in children treated with daily ICS [2]. In the follow-up of patients using ICS, the dose should be adjusted every 3 months by following up the patient's response to treatment and the side effects of ICS [1]. Inhaled steroids should be used by finding the lowest dose which controls symptoms and has the lowest risk of attacks and side effects [1].

Daily doses of inhaled corticosteroids for 5 years and younger (Table 81.3).

Table 81.3 Daily doses of inhaled corticosteroids for 5 years and younger. (Adopted from the Global Initiative for Asthma (GINA) Guideline 2020) [1, 2]

ICS formulations	Low total daily dose (mcg)
BDP (pMDI, standard particle, HFA)	100 (ages 5 years and older)
BDP (pMDI, extrafine particle, HFA)	50 (ages 5 years and older)
Budesonide nebulized	500 (ages 5 years and older)
Fluticasone propionate (pMDI, standard particle, HFA)	50 (ages 5 years and older)
Fluticasone furoate (DPI)	Not sufficiently studied in children 5 years and younger)
Mometasone furoate (pMDI, standard particle, HFA)	100 (ages 5 years and older)
Ciclesonide (pMDI, extrafine particle, HFA)	Not sufficiently studied in children 5 years and younger

ICS inhaled corticosteroids; *BDP* beclometasone dipropionate; *DPI* dry powder inhaler; *HFA* hydrofluoroalkane propellant; *ICS* inhaled corticosteroid; *pMDI*: pressurized metered-dose inhaler (non-chlorofluorocarbon formulations); in children, pMDI should always be used with a spacer.

Table 81.4 Low, medium and high daily doses of ICS formulations for children 6–11 years and 12 years and older. (Adopted from the Global Initiative for Asthma (GINA) Guideline) [1, 2]

ICS formulations	Total daily ICS dose		
	Low (mcq)	Medium (mcq)	High (mcq)
6–11 years			
Beclometasone dipropionate (pMDI, standard particle, HFA)	100–200	>200–400	>400
Beclometasone dipropionate (pMDI, extrafine particle[a], HFA)	50–100	>100–200	>200
Budesonide (DPI)	100–200	>200–400	>400
Budesonide (nebules)	250–500	>500–1000	>1000
Ciclesonide (pMDI, extrafine particle[a], HFA)	80	>80–160	>160
Fluticasone furoate (DPI)	50		NA
Fluticasone propionate (DPI)	50–100	>100–200	>200
Fluticasone propionate (pMDI, standard particle, HFA)	50–100	>100–200	>200
Mometasone furoate (pMDI, standard particle, HFA)	100		200
12 years and older			
Beclometasone dipropionate (pMDI, standard particle, HFA)	200–500	>500–1000	>1000
Beclometasone dipropionate (pMDI, extrafine particle[a], HFA)	100–200	>200–400	>400
Budesonide (DPI)	200–400	>400–800	>800
Ciclesonide (pMDI, extrafine particle[a], HFA)	80–160	>160–320	>320
Fluticasone furoate (DPI)	100		200
Fluticasone propionate (DPI)	100–250	>250–500	>500
Fluticasone propionate (pMDI, standard particle, HFA)	100–250	>250–500	>500
Mometasone furoate (DPI)	200		400
Mometasone furoate (pMDI, standard particle, HFA)	200–400		>400

ICS inhaled corticosteroids; *DPI* dry powder inhaler; *HFA* hydrofluoroalkane propellant; *ICS* inhaled corticosteroid; *n.a.* not applicable; *pMDI*: pressurized metered-dose inhaler (non-chlorofluorocarbon formulations); ICS by pMDI should preferably be used with a spacer.
[a]See product information.

Daily doses of inhaled corticosteroids for 6–11 years and 12 years and older (Table 81.4).

81.2.2 Long-Acting Bronchodilators

Beta2-agonists provide bronchodilation by stimulating beta2-adrenergic receptors on airway smooth muscle. It also has effects such as inhibition of mediator release of mast cells and other inflammatory cells, increase of mucociliary clearance [2, 10]. If asthma control cannot be achieved with regular inhaled steroid alone and short-acting beta2-agonist used as needed, continuing the treatment with the long-acting beta2-agonist in combination with inhaled steroids is recommended [20].

Salmeterol and formoterol are two long-acting beta-agonists (LABA) that have been evaluated in children. The use of Salmeterol with a metered-dose inhaler (MDI) is approved for children aged 12 years and above, with a dry powder inhaler for children aged 4 years and above, and the use of formoterol is approved for children aged 6 years and above [1]. Although the onset of salmeterol effect (10–15 min) starts later than albuterol (5 min), the bronchodilation time of salmeterol is much longer than albuterol (12–18 h vs. 3–6 h) [11]. In a meta-analysis of several studies in patients older than 12 years, the addition of a LABA has been found to be more beneficial in reducing asthma symptoms and exacerbations and in improving lung function, compared to increasing the inhaled corticosteroid dose alone [21]. Inhaled long-acting b2-agonists have no anti-inflammatory effects and therefore the use of long-acting b2-agonists as monotherapy is contraindicated for long-term asthma control [8]. Discontinuation of ICSs after LABA initiation leads to an increase in asthma exacerbations [22]. ICS/LABA combination therapy may allow reduction of inhaled corticosteroid doses without a significant deterioration in asthma control and may be more effective without the need to increase the ICS dose, in patients 12 years of age and older [11, 22].

81.2.3 Long-Acting Muscarinic Antagonists

The effects of tiotropium, a long-acting muscarinic antagonist drug, have been studied in childhood and have recently been approved for use in children aged 6 years and older in the USA [1]. Their mechanism of action is by blockade of muscarinic receptors of the parasympathetic nervous system. Long-acting anticholinergic tiotropium can be used as an additional treatment option in steps 4 or 5 for moderate to severe persistent asthma patients who cannot be controlled with inhaled steroids and long-acting beta2-agonists [7].

81.2.4 Leukotriene Modifying Agents

In the pathogenesis of asthma, leukotrienes play a role in bronchoconstriction, increase in mucus secretion and migration of inflammatory cells to the airway [11]. Leukotriene modifying drugs 5-lipoxygenase inhibitors and leukotriene receptor antagonists used in asthma inhibit the effects of leukotrienes in the pathogenesis of asthma. In a study using montelukast as monotherapy in school-age children, it has been reported that it moderately improved lung function, allergen and exercise response, while in another study, montelukast has been reported to improve symptoms and exacerbations in children younger than 5 years compared to placebo [11, 23, 24]. However, it has been reported that ICSs are more effective on asthma symptoms, exacerbations and lung function when compared to low-dose monotherapy of inhaled corticosteroid with LTRA in children with persistent asthma [25]. In addition, those with eosinophilic/allergic signs of inflammation or those with low pulmonary function test parameters are more likely to benefit from ICS compared to LTRA [1].

Long-term safety issues related to the use of leukotriene modifiers in children have not been completely elucidated, but most of the side effects reported in clinical trials have been mild [1]. Besides, in a recent study, it has been reported that in some of young children who started using montelukast, it has caused neuropsychiatric side effects that would require drug discontinuation [26].

81.2.5 Theophylline

Theophylline is a drug methylxanthine and has bronchial dilation effect. Theophylline has been shown to be effective as monotherapy in alleviating persistent asthma in children due to its bronchodilator, antiallergic, and anti-inflammatory effects [27]. Although theophylline reduces the need for oral steroid use in children with moderate to severe persistent asthma, other data indicate that theophylline has less clinical efficacy in controlling persistent asthma compared to ICS [8, 28].

In addition, when used, serum theophylline levels should be controlled since it is a drug with a narrow therapeutic range (5–15 µg/mL).

81.2.6 Biologic Agents

Biological agents target specific molecular targets or antibody receptors that inhibit specific cell signaling pathways involved in asthma pathogenesis [1]. Omalizumab is a recombinant mouse humanized monoclonal antibody aimed at human immunoglobulin E. Omalizumab has been shown to be effective in children aged 5–18 [29–31].

Anti-IgE (omalizumab) is recommended for patients 6 years of age and older who are susceptible to perennial allergen (mite, mold, pet) with moderate to severe allergic asthma that cannot be controlled with corticosteroids (inhaled/oral) and long-acting beta2-agonists [32, 33]. Mechanism of action: The monoclonal antibody omalizumab, which binds to free IgE, is effective by blocking the interaction of the allergen with its receptor on mast cells and basophils [1]. Used as an adjunctive therapy to only ICS or ICS/LABA combination, omalizumab improves symptoms and its most important benefit in asthma is the prevention of asthma exacerbations [29, 34].

Mepolizumab, which target the IL-5 pathway in those with eosinophilic asthma, and benralizumab have been approved for adolescents, 12 years and older in the United States [1]. Anti-IL5 agents have been shown to reduce the risk of asthma exacerbation in adolescents [1]. Mepolizumab is a monoclonal antibody that binds to IL5 released from TH2 lymphocytes which cause eosinophils to mature, migrate to the bronchial mucosa, activate and prolong life, while benralizumab is a monoclonal antibody that binds to the IL5 receptor (IL5R) [35]. These antibodies can decrease eosinophil levels in both blood and airways [35].

Anti-interleukin 4 receptor α (Dupilumab) is indicated in patients with moderate to severe eosinophilic or oral steroid-dependent persistent asthma that cannot be controlled with steroids (inhaled/oral) and long-acting beta2-agonists, and it is approved for patients ≥12 years of age in Unites States and Europe [7]. Considering its side effect, although omalizumab treatment seems quite safe, since the risk of anaphylaxis has been reported (1/1000), injections should be made in centers where appropriate conditions are provided. Patients should be observed for at least 2 h in the first three applications, and at least 30 minutes in the subsequent ones [36–40]. Pharyngitis, headache, hypersensitivity reaction (such as urticaria, rash, etc.) and local reaction at the injection site are frequently (1/100) reported side effects with benralizumab [37]. Since the risk of anaphylaxis has been reported with anti-IL5s, injections should be made in centers where appropriate conditions are provided, and patients should wait at least 30 minutes after administration. Dupilumab has been observed to be well tolerated. Injection site reactions are very frequently (1/10) reported side effects, and conjunctivitis, oral herpes, eosinophilia, and headache are frequently (1/100) reported side effects with dupilumab [7].

81.3 Allergen Immunotherapy

Subcutaneous allergen-specific immunotherapy (SCIT) has been shown to reduce asthma by potentially modifying existing allergic sensitivity [41]. A meta-analysis study involving 75 pediatrics and adults have supported the efficacy of immunotherapy in asthma with a reduction in asthma burden and medication use, and improvement in bronchial hyperreactivity [42]. GINA and EPR-3 have recommended allergen immunotherapy in patients with stable asthma who are sensitive to a particular allergen if there is a clear relationship between symptoms and allergen exposure [2, 8].

81.4 Environmental Control

Previous studies have also shown the relationship between the risk of developing childhood asthma and aeroallergen sensitivity [43]. In addition, passive exposure to cigarette smoke negatively affects the incidence of asthma, airway hyperresponsiveness, asthma symptoms and exacerbations, and lung function over time [11]. Other than active and passive cigarette smoke, nitric oxide, nitrogen oxides, carbon monoxide, carbon dioxide, formaldehyde and endotoxins, which lead to indoor pollution, are other indoor air pollutants that are effective in respiratory system health [44]. Avoiding intense activity in the outdoor environment in undesirable environmental conditions such as very cold weather, low humidity or intense air pollution and not being in the environment where the air is contaminated during viral infections can be helpful [45]. Viral infections can trigger wheezing episodes in infants and children and can be a major trigger for post-disease asthma exacerbations [1]. In summary, controlling both outdoor and indoor factors is important in the general treatment of children with asthma.

81.5 Psychosocial Factors

Several observational studies have found a correlation between stress and depression and poorly controlled asthma [1]. Stress is associated with increased prevalence of asthma and asthma exacerbations [46, 47]. Emotional state may affect objective measurements of airway function, interpretation of clinical symptoms, and proper response to them [11]. It has been reported that children with asthma experience more anxiety disorders, lower self-esteem, more functional disorders, past school problems and psychiatric illnesses, and intrafamilial stress [11]. The GINA and EPR-3 recommend that patients with poorly controlled asthma should assess the potential role of the child or caregiver's stress or depression in asthma management and provide additional training on these issues [2, 8].

81.6 Physical Activity and Diet

Physical activity and a healthy diet, which are indispensable elements of a healthy life, have an important place among non-pharmacological treatment recommendations for patients with asthma. The patient should be told how and at what level physical activity should be done, and what treatment should be used in the presence of symptoms triggered by exercise. The patients should be informed in the form of recommendations about what should and should not be in a healthy diet. Weight loss in obese patients is important in terms of both lung functions and ICS response [48, 49].

81.7 Treatment of Acute Asthma Exacerbation in Children

Asthma exacerbations are the situations where asthma symptoms worsen, symptoms such as cough, wheezing, shortness of breath and chest tightness are observed, and a decrease in lung function tests or peak expiratory volume is detected, if this can be done [1]. In well-controlled asthma, the frequency of exacerbations is also reduced, however, viral infections in particular can trigger exacerbations. Acute asthma exacerbations can be treated at home, during a medical examination or, if more severe, in a hospital.

81.7.1 Treatment at Home

The management of asthma exacerbations at home prevents delays in treatment, intensification of exacerbations, and increases the child and family's sense of control over asthma. The basics of early treatment include following a written asthma action plan, recognizing early findings of an exacerbation, appropriately intensifying treatment, eliminating accelerating environmental factors or events, and training the child and their family for rapid communication with the provider to discuss. The first treatment at home is usually an assessment of the response after administration of an inhaled short-acting beta2-agonist [26]. The inhaled short-acting beta2-agonist can be given with metered-dose inhalers, dry powder inhalers or nebulizers. It should be noted that in children younger than 5 years of age, nebulizer therapy or metered-dose inhaler should be given with a connector for effective delivery of the medication [2, 8].

If the acute attack is severe and the patient does not respond to bronchodilator therapy, the family and/or patient should contact their healthcare provider [1]. Home treatment may involve administering OCSs for a short period of time, which can shorten the duration of an exacerbation and may prevent hospitalization [50]. Oral corticosteroids have been shown to be more effective than high-dose ICS in older children and adults [51]. Patients with a history of severe exacerbations should have beta-agonists and appropriate equipment (connector, nebulizer) to treat exacerbations at home [2, 8]. Increased use of SABA during an exacerbation should continue until asthma symptoms and PEFs return to the patient's baseline [1].

81.7.2 Management in Office or Emergency Service

If symptoms worsen at home despite early intervention, or if PEF does not improve, the family is instructed to contact the doctor's clinic or the hospital emergency service [1]. In the initial evaluation, a short medical history, physical examination, pulmonary function test, and oxygen saturation should be checked, if it can be done. Blood gas analysis is not required except for a severe asthma exacerbation with inadequate response to bronchodilator therapy [1]. Routine chest radiographs are not required unless possible complications (pneumothorax, pneumomediastinum, pneumonia, atelectasis, or aspiration) are suspected at the medical history or initial physical examination [11]. In a mild to moderate exacerbation (FEV1 or PEF value above 50% of the expected value, or above 50% of the best value), as an initial treatment, oxygen therapy that will keep oxygen saturation above 90% is administered with a SABA using a nebulizer or MDI with a connector, up to three doses during the first hour of patient admission, and if it does not respond to treatment, OCS may be considered to be added to the treatment [1]. In severe exacerbations (FEV1 or PEF value below 50% of the expected value or below 50% of the best value), treatment should include the rapid administration of oxygen along with high doses of inhaled SABA and continuous administration of ipratropium every 20 minutes or for the first hour, and oral corticosteroids [1]. Severe exacerbations are potentially life-threatening and therefore need hospitalization as they require close observation and repeated evaluation [1]. The bronchodilation effect with the subsequent or concomitant administration of ipratropium bromide by inhalation to SABA is controversial [1]. Some authors have reported improvement in symptoms, especially when used within the first 24 h of the exacerbation, while others have found no additional beneficial effects [27]. Although not all studies evaluating the use of intravenous theophylline in the treatment of acute exacerbations, most of them did not show any additional benefit over aggressive intervention with beta-agonists; therefore, its use in hospitalized children with asthma is also controversial [8].

81.7.3 Management in Hospital

In case of insufficient response in respiratory symptoms or lung function (FEV 1 or PEF of 40% to 69%) despite aggressive therapy, the patient should be hospitalized for close follow-up and continuous oxygen therapy with inhaled SABA and systemic corticosteroids 1. Those who respond poorly to treatment (FEV 1 or PEF below 40%, pCO2 above 42 mm Hg, severe respiratory distress, somnolence, or confusion) should be admitted to the hospital intensive care unit for oxygen, inhaled SABA, intravenous corticosteroids, and possible intubation and mechanical ventilation [1]. Particular attention should be paid to children with risk factors for fatal asthma. It may be difficult to assess the severity of an asthma exacerbation in young children and infants as the lung function tests cannot be performed or cannot provide a detailed history. Therefore, symptoms and physical examination findings should be evaluated carefully [2, 8]. A lower threshold should be used for frequent pulse oximetry and arterial blood gas monitoring because infants are more prone to hypoxia and respiratory failure than adults due to their unique ventilation/perfusion and anatomical characteristics. Hospitalization should be considered in a baby whose oxygen saturation is below 92% at room air [52]. Also, both respiratory acidosis and metabolic acidosis may occur in children during exacerbations specific to children, as metabolic acidosis is not common in adults [11].

Although intravenous use of magnesium sulfate may be beneficial in children in whom bronchodilator and corticosteroid therapy failed, double-blind, placebo-controlled studies both supported and refuted its efficacy [11]. Heliox-induced albuterol nebulization may be considered in patients with life-threatening exacerbations; however, one meta-analysis has found no significant improvement in lung function or symptoms compared to those who received treatment with oxygen or air [53]. Finally, the use of intravenous beta-agonists in the treatment of acute asthma is controversial [11].

In addition to the acute management of exacerbation, the most essential approach should be to prevent relapse of acute asthma exacerbations [1]. Asthma training is appropriate in the clinical, emergency room, and hospital settings. Trained clinical staff should review the various asthma medications' names and purposes, teach the appropriate inhaler technique and use of objective monitoring devices, schedule follow-up visits, and establish a mutually satisfactory action plan that includes both care and intervention strategies [2, 8]. Before the discharge of the patient from the emergency service or hospital, placement of a child for controller therapy, possibly with an ICS, and a follow-up appointment with an asthma care provider should be considered [2, 8]. Children who need ICU care are at an exceptionally high risk of future asthma morbidity and should be followed-up near with an asthma specialist.

References

1. Jackson DJ, Lemanske RF, Bacharier LB. Management of asthma in infants and children. Middleton's Allergy. 50:831–47.
2. Global Initiative for Asthma (GINA) 2020. https://ginasthma.org/wpcontent/uploads/2020/06/GINA-2020-report_20_06_04-1-wms.pdf.

3. Boulet LP, Vervloet D, Magar Y, Foster JM. Adherence: the goal to control asthma. Clin Chest Med. 2012;33(3):405–17.

4. Bender B, Boulet LP, Chaustre I, et al. Asthma. In: SabateÅL E, editor. Adherence to long-term therapies: evidence for action. Geneva: World Health Organization; 2003. p. 47–58.

5. Boulet LP, Vervloet D, Magar Y, et al. Adherence: the goal to control asthma. Clin Chest Med. 2012;33:405–17.

6. van Boven JF, Trappenburg JC, van der Molen T, et al. Towards tailored and targeted adherence assessment to optimise asthma management. NPJ Prim Care Respir Med. 2015;25:15046.

7. Asthma Diagnosis and Treatment Guide 2020 Update. Available from: https://www.aid.org.tr/wpcontent/uploads/2020/12/astim-rehberi-2020.pdf (Accessed online on October 27, 2021).

8. National Asthma Education and Prevention Program: Expert Panel Report 3 (EPR-3). Guidelines for the diagnosis and management of asthma-summary report 2007. J Allergy Clin Immunol. 2007;120:S94–138.

9. GINA. Scientific committee: global initiative for asthma. In: Global Strategy for Asthma Management and Prevention. Bethesda, U.S. Dept. of Health and Human Services, Public Health Service. www.ginasthma.org.

10. Turkish Thoracic Society, National Asthma Diagnosis and Treatment Guide. Thoracic Journal 2016;4–31.

11. Jackson DJ, Lemanske RF, Guilbert TW. Management of Asthma in infants and children. In: Adkinson NF, Bochner BS, Burks AW, editors. Middleton's allergy: principles and practice. Philadelphia, PA: Elsevier; 2014. p. 876–91.

12. The Childhood Asthma Management Program Research Group. Long-term effects of budesonide or nedocromil in children with asthma. N Engl J Med. 2000;343:1054–63.

13. Buhl R. Local oropharyngeal side effects of inhaled corticosteroids in patients with asthma. Allergy. 2006;61(5):518–26.

14. Roland NJ, Bhalla RK, Earis J. The local side effects of inhaled corticosteroids: current understanding and review of the literature. Chest. 2004;126(1):213–9.

15. Juniper EF, Kline PA, Vanzieleghem MA, Ramsdale EH, O'Byrne PM, Hargreave FE. Effect of long-term treatment with an inhaled corticosteroid (budesonide) on airway hyperresponsiveness and clinical asthma in nonsteroid-dependent asthmatics. The American review of respiratory disease. Am J Respir Crit Care Med. 1990;142(4):832–6.

16. Jeffery PK, Godfrey RW, Adelroth E, Nelson F, Rogers A, Johansson SA. Effects of treatment on airway inflammation and thickening of basement membrane reticular collagen in asthma. A quantitative light and electron microscopic study. The American review of respiratory disease. Am J Respir Crit Care Med. 1992;145:890–9.

17. Pauwels RA, Lofdahl CG, Postma DS, et al. Effect of inhaled formoterol and budesonide on exacerbations of asthma. Formoterol and corticosteroids establishing therapy (FACET) international study group. N Engl J Med. 1997;337(20):1405–11.

18. Suissa S, Ernst P, Benayoun S, Baltzan M, Cai B. Low-dose inhaled corticosteroids and the prevention of death from asthma. N Engl J Med. 2000;343(5):332–6.

19. Busse WW, Pedersen S, Pauwels RA, Tan WC, Chen YZ, Lamm CJ, O'Byrne PM, START Investigators Group. The inhaled steroid treatment as regular therapy in early asthma (START) study 5-year follow-up: effectiveness of early intervention with budesonide in mild persistent asthma. J Allergy Clin Immunol. 2008;121(5):1167–74.

20. Ducharme FM, Ni Chroinin M, Greenstone I, Lasserson TJ. Addition of long-acting beta2-agonists to inhaled corticosteroids versus same dose inhaled corticosteroids for chronic asthma in adults and children. Cochrane Databes Syst Rev. 2010;5:CD005535.

21. Simons FE. A comparison of beclomethasone, salmeterol, and placebo in children with asthma. N Engl J Med. 1997;337:1659–65.

22. Lemanske RF, Sorkness CA, Mauger EA, et al. Inhaled corticosteroid reduction and elimination in patients with persistent asthma receiving salmeterol: a randomized controlled trial. JAMA. 2001;285:2594–603.

23. Bisgaard H, Zielen S, Garcia-Garcia ML, et al. Montelukast reduces asthma exacerbations in 2 to 5 year old children with intermittent asthma. Am J Respir Crit Care Med. 2005;171:315–22.

24. Knorr B, Franchi LM, Bisgaard H, et al. Montelukast, a leukotriene receptor antagonist, for the treatment of persistent asthma in children aged 2 to 5 years. Pediatrics. 2001;108:E48.

25. Sorkness CA, Lemanske RF, Mauger DT, et al. Long-term comparison of 3 controller regimens for mild-moderate persistent childhood asthma: the pediatric asthma controller trial. J Allergy Clin Immunol. 2007;119:64–72.

26. Benard B, Bastien V, Vinet B, et al. Neuropsychiatric adverse drug reactions in children initiated on montelukast in real-life practice. Eur Respir J. 2017;50

27. Moss MH, Gern JE, Lemanske RF. Asthma in infancy and childhood. In: Adkinson NF, Yunginger JW, Busse WW, editors. Middleton's allergy: principles and practice. Philadelphia, PA: Mosby; 2003. p. 1225–55.

28. Nassif EG, Weinberger M, Thompson R, et al. The value of maintenance theophylline in steroid-dependent asthma. N Engl J Med. 1981;304:71–5.

29. Busse WW, Morgan WJ, Gergen PJ, et al. Randomized trial of omalizumab (anti-IgE) for asthma in inner-city children. N Engl J Med. 2011;364:1005–15.

30. Lanier B, Bridges T, Kulus M, et al. Omalizumab for the treatment of exacerbations in children with inadequately controlled allergic (IgE-mediated) asthma. J Allergy Clin Immunol. 2009;124:1210–6.

31. Each SJ, Gill MA, Togias A, et al. Preseasonal treatment with either omalizumab or an inhaled corticosteroid boost to prevent fall asthma exacerbations. J Allergy Clin Immunol. 2015;136:1476–85.

32. Humbert M, Beasley R, Ayres J, et al. Benefits of omalizumab as add-on therapy in patients with severe persistent asthma who are inadequately controlled despite best available therapy (GINA 2002 step 4 treatment): innovate. Allergy. 2005;60:309–16.

33. Normansell R, Walker S, Milan SJ, Walters EH, Nair P. Omalizumab for asthma in adults and children. Cochrane Database Syst Rev. 2014;1:CD003559.

34. Teach SJ, Gill MA, Togias A, et al. Preseasonal treatment with either omalizumab or an inhaled corticosteroid boost to prevent fall asthma exacerbations. J Allergy Clin Immunol. 2015;136:1476–85.

35. Farne HA, Wilson A, Powell C, Bax L, Milan SJ. Anti-IL5 therapies for asthma. Cochrane Database Syst Rev. 2017;9:1–123.

36. Miller CW, Krishnaswamy N, Johnston C, Krishnaswamy G. Severe asthma and the omalizumab option. Clin Mol Allergy. 2008;6:4.

37. Nucala European Union Summary of Product Characteristics (labeling information). (2015). http://www.ema.europa.eu/docs/en_GB/document_library/EPAR__Product_Information/human/003860/WC500198037.pdf

38. Fasenra European Union Summary of Product Characteristics (labeling information). (2018). https://www.ema.europa.eu/en/documents/product-information/fasenra-epar-product-information_en.pdf

39. Cinqaero European Union Summary of Product Characteristics (labeling information). (2016). https://www.ema.europa.eu/en/documents/product-information/cinqaero-epar-product-information_en.pdf

40. Chupp GL, Bradford ES, Albers FC, et al. Efficacy of mepolizumab add on therapy on health-related quality of life and markers of asthma control in severe eosinophilic asthma (MUSCA): a randomised, double-blind, placebo controlled, parallel group, multicentre, phase 3b trial. Lancet Respir Med. 2017;5:390–400.

41. American Academy of Allergy, Asthma and Immunology. Joint task force on practice parameters: allergen immunotherapy: a practice parameter. Ann Allergy Asthma Immunol. 2003;90:1–40.

42. Abramson MJ, Puy RM, Weiner JM. Allergen Immunotherapy for Asthma. New York: Wiley; 2003.

43. Halonen M, Stern DA, Wright AL, et al. Alternaria as a major allergen for asthma in children raised in a desert environment. Am J Respir Crit Care Med. 1997;155:1356–61.

44. Hussain S, Parker S, Edwards K, et al. Effects of indoor particulate matter exposure on daily asthma control. Ann Allergy Asthma Immunol. 2019;S1081-1206(19):30538–1.

45. Gautier C, Charpin D. Environmental triggers and avoidance in the management of asthma. J Asthma Allergy. 2017;10:47–56.
46. Wright RJ, Cohen S, Carey V, et al. Parental stress as a predictor of wheezing in infancy: a prospective birth-cohort study. Am J Respir Crit Care Med. 2002;165:358–65.
47. Sandberg S, Paton JY, Ahola S, et al. The role of acute and chronic stress in asthma attacks in children. Lancet. 2000;356:982–7.
48. Carpaij OA, van den Berge M. The asthma-obesity relationship: underlying mechanisms and treatment implications. Curr Opin Pulm Med. 2018;24:42–9.
49. Ozbey, Balaban S, Szener Z, et al. The effects of diet-induced weight loss on asthma control and quality of life in obese adults with asthma: a randomized controlled trial. J Asthma. 2019;57:1–9.
50. Rachelefsky G. Treating exacerbations of asthma in children: the role of systemic corticosteroids. Pediatrics. 2003;112:382–97.
51. Schuh S, Dick PT, Stephens D, et al. High-dose inhaled fluticasone does not replace oral prednisolone in children with mild to moderate acute asthma. Pediatrics. 2006;118:644–50.
52. Sole D, Komatsu MK, Carvalho KV, et al. Pulse oximetry in the evaluation of the severity of acute asthma and/or wheezing in children. J Asthma. 1999;36:327–33.
53. Ho AM, Lee A, Karmakar MK, et al. Heliox vs air-oxygen mixtures for the treatment of patients with acute asthma: a systematic overview. Chest. 2003;123:882–90.

Infections of Cervicothoracic Cystic Hygroma and Other Congenital Malformations in Children

Erdinç Çekiç, Hüsamettin Yaşar, and Oren Friedman

82.1 Introduction

Lymphatic malformations are rare congenital malformations in children. They are formed by dilated lymphatic channels in different sizes and lined by endothelial cells with lymphatic phenotype. Lymphatic malformations are classified according to the diameter of cystic lesions, categorized as macrocystic (>1 cm), microcystic (<1 cm), and mixed [1].

Cystic hygroma is first described by Wernher in 1843 and defined as macrocystic lymphatic malformation in neck region [2]. Cystic hygromas are benign structures and most frequently observed in head and neck region; other frequent locations are axilla, chest, and perineum [3].

82.2 Embryologic Mechanism

From the historical perspective different embryologic mechanisms are suggested and discussed for development of lymphovascular system. Both centrifugal and centripetal theories are competing each other more than 100 years [4–6].

Lymphatic sacs are the primary lymphatic structures in human embryo and firstly observed at the eighth week of gestation. There are total of six lymphatic sacs. Two of them are located lateral to jugular vein, two of them lateral to iliac vein, one is retroperitoneal, and the last one is cisterna chyli. These sacs are connected with

E. Çekiç (✉) · H. Yaşar
Section of Otorhinolaryngology, İstanbul Haseki Training and Research Hospital, İstanbul, Turkey

O. Friedman
Department of Otorhinolaryngology, Head and Neck Surgery, Perelman School of Medicine, University of Pennsylvania, Philadelphia, PA, USA

venous system and invaded with connective tissue and finally end up with lymph nodes. Sequestration of the lymphatic tissue from venous systems result in lymphatic malformations [7].

82.3 Clinical Features and Diagnosis

The clinical features of cystic hygroma depend on the location and extension of the lesion but as a general they are soft and easily compressible painless swellings. Stridor and dysphagia may be observed when the lesion extends to the mediastinum or aerodigestive tract and infiltrate the tongue, oropharynx, or hypopharynx.

Nowadays, many lymphatic malformations may be observed with routine prenatal ultrasonographic examinations in the second or third trimester [8]. After the birth, cystic hygromas are easily diagnosed with history and physical examination [9, 10]. Additional US (ultrasonography), CT (computerized tomography), or MRI (magnetic resonance imaging) may be required for defining the extent of the lesion, planning the treatment, and complications.

In the presence of complications such as bleeding and infection, lesion grows rapidly. Bleeding may occur due to trauma or spontaneously, and results in blue discoloration, pain, and tenderness. Intralesional bleeding may occur in up to 35% of lymphatic malformations [11]. Cystic hygromas are very sensitive to infection due to malformed lymphatic system and proteinaceous fluid content [11]. Infection may complicate the situation and progress into sepsis [12].

82.4 Treatment Modalities

Because of the benign nature of cystic hygroma, all patients do not require treatment. Asymptomatic patients with limited extension of lesion may be observed easily.

Symptomatic patients with recurrent infection attacks, extended lesions affecting the vision or aerodigestive tract resulting in life-threating conditions require urgent treatment. Patients with minor deformities and psychosocial complaints are also assessed for treatment. Treatment modalities are divided into two, as sclerotherapy and surgery. Ideal treatment is total excision of the lesion, but it is not possible in significant amount of the cases because of very extended size and distorted anatomical structures. Also, recurrence and postoperative deformity risk (iatrogenic injury to facial nerve, hypoglossal nerve and brachial plexus, etc.) make patients and physicians to search alternative treatments. Intralesional sclerosing agent injection is an easy and effective alternative treatment especially in macrocystic or mixed lesions. There are different sclerosing agents (doxycycline, ethanol, sodium tetradecyl sulfate (STS), bleomycin, and OK-432) used in the treatment of cystic hygromas [13]. Each agent has different advantage and disadvantages. Doxycycline is an antibiotic and theoretically has an anti-infective effect advantage in addition to good sclerosing effect; ethanol is cheap and effective sclerosing agent but have risk for local and systemic toxicity [14]. Bleomycin has advantages for microcystic lesions [15].

OK-432 is also effective sclerosant for unresponsive lesions but is not easily available [16]. Physician should choose the appropriate agent according to patients' necessities and personal experiences.

82.4.1 Infections of Cervicothoracic Cystic Hygroma

There is very limited information about the infection of the congenital cervical anomalies, and usually they were documented as case reports or series. There is no rate for infection of congenital cervical anomalies, but in a study conducted on 44 cases of congenital cervical anomalies, they found that the preoperative infection rate was 16.0% (n:7) [17].

Cystic hygromas are very susceptible to infection due to the malformed lymphatic system and proteinaceous fluid content [11]. Low blood flow and the malformed lymphatic channels could not be capable of removing the infective materials from the environment. Statis of fluid and intralesional bleeding make a suitable medium for microorganisms. The cyst can become infected by the blocking of the cyst orifice with these microorganisms [18]. The most common pathogens are *S. aureus* and *S. pyogenes*. Also, alpha-hemolytic streptococci, *Peptostreptococcus* spp., and anaerobic gram-negative bacilli are causative pathogens of cystic infections [19, 20]. Besides, cystic hygromas can be infected after trauma. Traumas are mainly incidental, but also after iatrogenic traumas such as the sclerotherapy procedure may have occurred.

These lesions may develop infection in the follow-up after diagnosis or may present with infection as a first presentation [21]. If cystic hygroma is infected, it might be mistaken for cervical lymphadenitis [22]. In infection setting, the lesion grows rapidly, and swelling clinically takes longer than cervical adenitis [23, 24]. These lesions can be easily distinguished from cervical lymphadenitis due to their specific anatomical location. The lesions are commonly erythematous and warm. Hoarseness, dysphagia, and odynophagia are associated with these symptoms and fever, chills, and other constitutional symptoms are uncommon [25]. Enlarged regional lymph nodes also may occur. Fluctuation may suggest abscess formation. Less commonly, congenital lesions can present as deep neck infections, and recurrences are common. Recurrent infection in the same location should lead to an evaluation of congenital anomaly [24]. However, these congenital neck masses are usually benign lesions; these infections may be associated with a high risk for infections and progress bacteremia in and sepsis in newborns [12].

The diagnosis of infected neck cysts is based on clinical presentation. Ultrasound scans can differentiate cystic from solid structures, detect abscess. If the cyst was infected, the cyst wall thickens and enhances, and inflammation gets into adjacent fat planes. Fine needle aspiration or intraoperative cultures and histopathology are the criteria for identifying infectious pathogens [19, 20]. Blood culture and aspirate cultures should be processed for aerobes, anaerobes, fungi, and mycobacteria.

Antibiotics should be targeted toward oral flora, and antibiotic regimens should be adjusted based on culture and sensitivity results. Oral antibiotics such as first-generation cephalosporins, or amoxicillin/clavulanate, in addition to clindamycin may be adequate for mild cases if the patient is not febrile. However, broadspectrum antibiotics should be given for unresponsive to oral antibiotics or severe cases such as an abscess. Incision and drainage are indicated for abscesses and if medical therapy is unsuccessful or in clinical deterioration of patient [20]. After the total resolution of the infection, complete surgical excision of the cystic hygroma must be planned. Also, physician must be alert for the risk of airway obstruction and sepsis. The family must be informed in the possible requirement of a tracheotomy. Also, surgical exploration and excision of lesion should be kept in mind to control the source of infection. To control the possible source of infection, patients with cervicothoracic cystic hygromas must be advised for good oral hygiene and avoidance of trauma. Also, prophylactic antimicrobial therapy is recommended to give after the sclerotherapy intervention.

82.5 Thyroglossal Duct Cyst

Thyroglossal duct cysts (TGDC) are the generally painless, mobile, midline masses, originating from the remnants of the embryological thyroglossal duct. TGDC are the most common congenital neck masses in children beyond the benign lymphadenopathies [26] (Fig. 82.1).

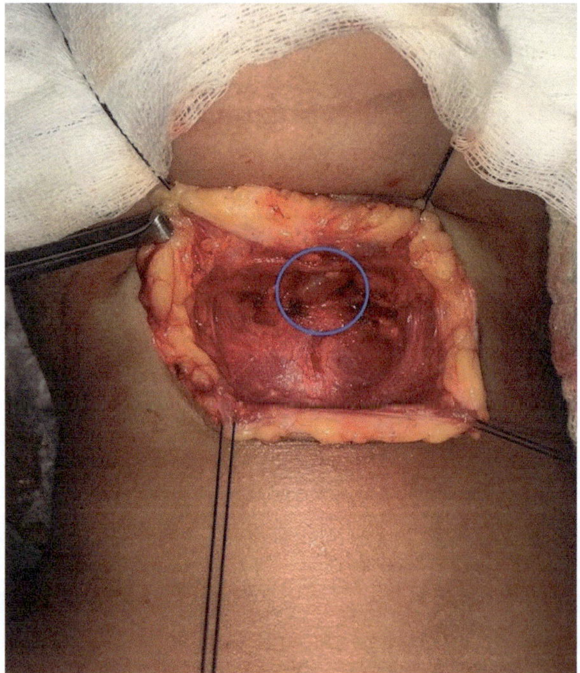

Fig. 82.1 Intraoperative view of thyroglossal duct cyst (Courtesy of Özgür Pınarbaşlı MD)

82.5.1 Embryologic Mechanism

After the formation of thyroid primordium in the base of tongue, developing thyroid gland descends in the neck, passing ventral to the developing hyoid bone and laryngeal cartilages. Finally, it ends up with its normal position in the neck. Narrow tubal connection between the tongue and thyroid gland is called thyroglossal duct. By seventh week of gestation thyroglossal duct has degenerated and disappeared. Remnants of the thyroglossal duct may persist and form the cyst [27].

82.5.2 Clinical Features and Diagnosis

Cysts may be seen anywhere along the course of thyroglossal duct. Most common clinical features of TGDC are painless, mobile, midline mass around the hyoid bone. Moving of the cyst during swallowing or tongue extraction is the typical sign of the lesion. In the presence of infection reddish discoloration and tenderness can be observed on the cyst. Patient may be febrile and painful with lesion. A perforation of the skin may occur and thyroglossal duct sinus may be appeared. It usually opens in the anterior and midline plane of the neck around the hyoid bone.

Clinical history, physical examination, ultrasonography, and thyroid function tests (TSH, fT4, fT3) are enough to diagnose the TGDC. Beside the ultrasonography, scintigraphy is also helpful to rule out ectopic or accessory thyroid tissues. Surgical removal of ectopic thyroid is controversial, because the ectopic thyroid tissue may be the only functional thyroid gland and its removal would result in permanent thyroid hormone dependent.

82.5.3 Treatment Modalities

Sistrunk procedure is the ideal treatment of the TGDC. It is defined by Sistrunk in 1920 with complete removal of cystic structures and its attachments to hyoid bone and foramen caecum [28]. Removal of attachments to hyoid bone and foramen caecum is necessary to prevent the recurrences (Figs. 82.2 and 82.3).

82.5.4 Infections of Thyroglossal Ductus Cyst

In patients with TGDC, secretions of the thyroglossal duct epithelial cells accumulate and leads to dilation of the duct and gradual development of cystic structure. Inadequate drainage of the cyst leads to bacterial overgrowth and abscess formation. Due to connection of mouth oral flora migrates to cyst cavity [18]. As it mentioned above, causative pathogens are same with cystic hygroma. The most common pathogens are *S. aureus* and *S. pyogenes*. Also, alpha-hemolytic streptococci, *Peptostreptococcus* spp., and anaerobic gram-negative bacilli (*Prevotella,*

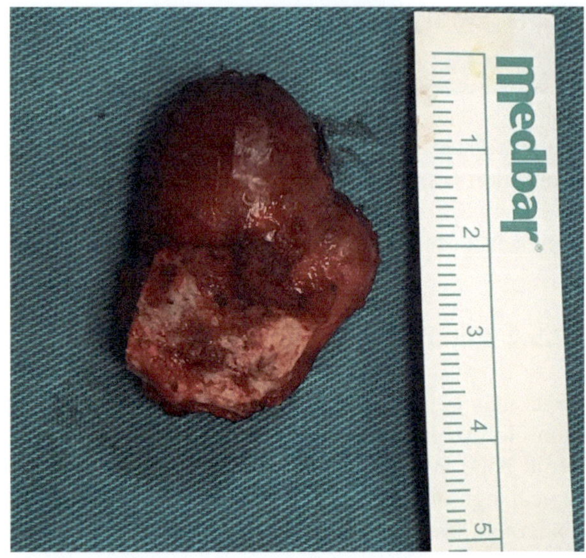

Fig. 82.2 Thyroglossal duct cyst and body of hyoid bone specimen (Courtesy of Özgür Pınarbaşlı MD)

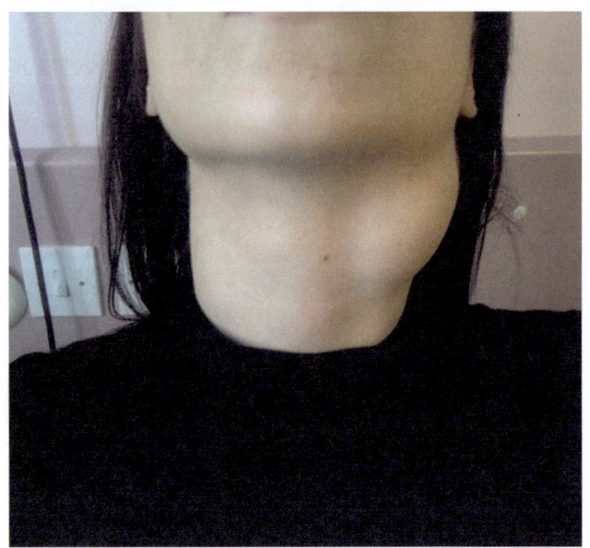

Fig. 82.3 Second branchial cleft cyst on the left side of the neck (Courtesy of Özgür Pınarbaşlı MD)

Porphyromonas, and *Bacteroides* spp.) are causative pathogens of cystic infections [19, 20, 29, 30].

In the presence of infection of TGDC red swelling and tenderness can be observed on the cyst. Also, TGDC can be painful, erythematous, and warm. The cyst often develops abscess and fluctuation may be seen. Hoarseness, dysphagia, or odynophagia and uncommonly fever, chills, and other constitutional symptoms are seen [25]. In addition, the mass moves upward with swallowing and enlarged regional lymph node also may occur. Infected thyroglossal duct cysts may suggest infected submental nodes. When perforation of the skin occurs, thyroglossal duct sinus may appear. It usually opens in the anterior and midline plane of the neck around the hyoid bone and purulent discharge may develop. In rare cases, respiratory obstruction may develop, especially if the TDC developed at the base of the tongue. This presentation can be fatal.

The diagnosis of infected neck cysts is based on clinical presentation. Most infected TGDC present with a midline neck mass that moves with swallowing, whereas others, such as branchial cleft cyst or laryngocele, are lateral. Needle aspiration is helpful for both decompression and identification of microorganism.

Antibiotics should be targeted toward oral flora and possible microorganism, and then antibiotic regimens should be adjusted based on culture and sensitivity results. Oral antibiotics such as first-generation cephalosporins, or amoxicillin/clavulanate, in addition to clindamycin may be adequate for mild cases if the patient is not febrile. In the presence of methicillin-resistant staphylococci, vancomycin may be required for the treatment. However, broad-spectrum antibiotics should be given for unresponsive to oral antibiotics or severe cases such as an abscess. Recurrent infection of the TGDC is common. Incision and drainage of the infected cyst is controversial; it is thought that it causes seeding of ductal cells and increases the recurrence risk [29]. Many authors avoid incision and drainage, unless presence of abscess. On the contrary, there are different opinions in literature that drainage does not lead to increase in the recurrence risk [30]. To prevent recurrences, surgical intervention ("Sistrunk procedure" for TGDC) is required ultimately [29]. Such surgery is delayed until an acutely inflamed cyst has resolved. Before the surgical excision of TGDC, infection should be resolved totally for the ease of the operation and prevention of the recurrence.

82.6　Branchial Cleft Cysts/Sinuses/Fistulae

Branchial anomalies originate from the remnants of pharyngeal apparatus while transforming into normal adult structures. They can be presented as cysts, sinuses, and fistulae.

82.6.1　Embryologic Mechanism

The pharyngeal apparatus consists of arches, pouches, grooves, and membranes. These structures transform into normal adult derivatives during embryologic development. Interruptions of this development result in the branchial anomalies. There are six branchial arches, five grooves, and five pouches. Last two branchial arches (fifth and sixth) are rudimentary and disappeared. Branchial arches are lined by endoderm internally, ectoderm externally, and mesoderm in between. Second branchial arch grows rapidly and covers the third and fourth arches and forms a space called the cervical sinus. If the cervical sinus does not disappear, it ends up with branchial cyst. If the cyst connects with the skin, then it is called branchial sinus. If the cyst has both internal and external connection, then it is called branchial fistulae [27].

82.6.2 Clinical Features, Diagnosis, and Treatment

Clinical features are changed according to affected pharyngeal apparatus but generally accepted as slowly growing, painless swelling in the neck (Fig. 82.3). Clinical history and physical examination are essential. Detailed examination of tonsillar fossa and pyriform sinuses are necessary. USG, CT, and MRI may be necessary for understanding the course and extension of the lesion. Fine needle aspiration (FNA) may be necessary for differential diagnosis of lesion from other congenital malformations or malignancies. There are 4 well-defined branchial cleft anomalies (Figs. 82.4, 82.5).

82.6.3 First Branchial Cleft Anomalies

First branchial arch tract extends from the skin around the submandibular fossa, superolateral to hyoid bone, ascending to the parotid gland and finally end up in the cartilage/bone junction of the external auditory canal [31]. There are two types of first branchial cleft anomalies.

Type 1 lesion is generally located around the preauricular region and parallel to the external auditory canal and lateral to the facial nerve.
Type 2 lesion is generally around the angle of mandible and close relation with parotid gland and facial nerve [32].

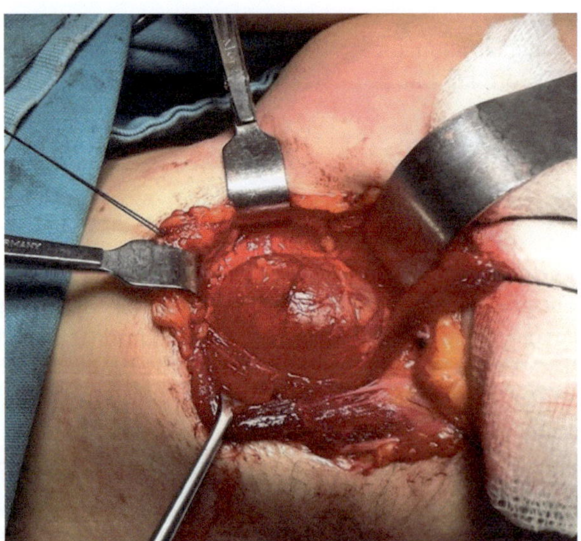

Fig. 82.4 Intraoperative view of second branchial cleft cyst (Courtesy of Özgür Pınarbaşlı MD)

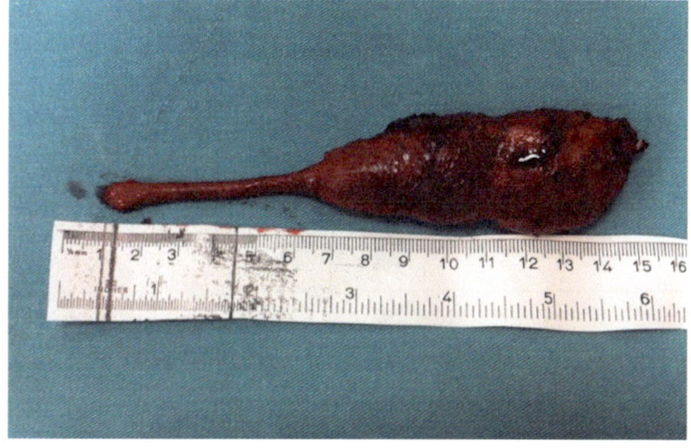

Fig. 82.5 Specimen: cyst and its tract (Courtesy of Özgür Pınarbaşlı MD)

Treatment is the same for both types, total excision of cyst, sinus, and fistula with all tract. But in type 2 lesions superficial parotidectomy and facial nerve dissection may be needed.

82.6.4 Second Branchial Cleft Anomalies

Second branchial anomalies are the most common branchial anomalies and located generally at the anterior border of sternocleidomastoid muscle. Second branchial arch tract extends from the skin of supraclavicular fossa, between the internal and external carotid arteries, and finally opens into the tonsillar fossa [32]. There are four different types of second branchial cleft anomalies.

Type I lesions are superficial and lie near the anterior border of sternocleidomastoid (SCM) muscle and no connection with carotid sheath.

Type II lesions are the most common type and lie deep to the SCM muscle, adjacent and lateral to carotid sheath.

Type III lesions lie medial to the internal and external carotid arteries, lateral to the pharyngeal wall.

Type IV lesions lie deep to carotid sheath and adjacent to the pharynx and tonsillar fossa [33, 34].

Ideal treatment is total excision of the lesion with its tract. Following a transverse cervical incision, careful dissection of fistula tract and total excision of the lesion is important to prevent the recurrence. A finger may be helpful to identify the opening in the pharynx.

82.6.5 Third and Fourth Branchial Cleft Anomalies

Third and fourth branchial anomalies are rare anomalies. It is hard to diagnose because of long course of the tract and necessity of detailed endoscopic examination of pyriform sinuses. These anomalies present with cutaneous fistula in the lower part of the neck similar to the second branchial anomalies, however internally open into the pyriform sinus below the hyoid bone. Both third and fourth branchial anomalies may appear at any age. In newborns, they may also present with tracheal compression and airway problems because of the rapid enlargement of the lesion. Other possible presentations are thyroid nodules, recurrent infections, or abscess of thyroid gland [34].

82.6.6 Infections of Branchial Anomalies

A branchial cleft anomaly generally lines with respiratory epithelium and subepithelial lymphoid aggregations [35]. These structures respond to the non-specific upper respiratory tract infection with mucus secretion. The statis of highly viscous mucus material and low lymphatic flow make the cysts sensitive to infection and progression to abscess. Infected branchial cleft cysts may be mistaken for cervical lymphadenitis. An infected branchial cyst may develop abscess form or rupture spontaneously to form a draining sinus tract [20]. Rarely manifest first presentation as an infected with swelling or draining sinus tract. Acute infections should be treated with empirical antibiotics targeting the oral flora and analgesic. Also, first branchial cleft sinus or fistula may cause aural drainage, and rarely associated with tender mass. Furthermore, in second or third branchial cleft anomalies appear with a mass in the neck and draining tract in the anterior border of the sternocleidomastoid muscle. Physicians should be familiar with the source of infection (e.g., tonsillopharyngitis, dental infection, suppurative thyroiditis) and bacteriologic profile of infected branchial anomalies. Most frequently identified microorganisms are same as TGDC or cystic hygroma *S. aureus* and *S. pyogenes*, less commonly alpha-hemolytic streptococci, *Peptostreptococcus* spp., and anaerobic gram-negative bacilli (*Prevotella, Porphyromonas,* and *Bacteroides* spp.) [19, 20, 36]. The diagnosis of infected neck cysts is based on clinical presentation. Ultrasound scans can differentiate cystic from solid structures, detect abscesses. Also, CT and MRI scans detect suppuration and identify anatomic structure before surgical intervention. Fistulography can delineate the course of the fistula and identify the level of brachial cleft involvement. Needle aspiration is helpful for culture-guided antimicrobial therapy and decompression. Incision and drainage which may complicate the future surgical plans is reserved for progression and complications. Antibiotic therapy should be targeted toward oral flora, and the possible pathogens. Oral antibiotics such as first-generation cephalosporins, or amoxicillin/clavulanate, plus clindamycin may be adequate for mild cases. Antibiotic therapy should be adjusted based on culture and sensitivity results. However, broad-spectrum antibiotics should be given for unresponsive to oral antibiotics such as methicillin-resistant staphylococci or severe cases such as an abscess. Complete resection is recommended to perform, after the total resolution of infection.

82.7   Cervical Teratoma/Dermoid Cysts

Both teratomas and dermoid cysts are benign germ cell neoplasms. Teratomas include all three germ layers but dermoid cysts are lined with stratified squamous epithelium and include skin appendages (e.g., hair, keratin, sebaceous glands) [26].

82.7.1 Clinical Features and Diagnosis

Teratomas are rare tumors and occur in 1/40000 of births. Most frequent location is sacrococcygeal region but cervicofacial lesions are also present [37]. Cervical teratomas become obvious in second trimester and most of them may be diagnosed easily with prenatal ultrasonography due to rapid growth of the tumor and polyhydramnios due to esophageal obstruction. Cesarean section is recommended for delivery [38]. Although the lesion is in benign nature, respiratory distress and dysphagia may occur due to expansile growth of the tumor. Fetal or postnatal MRI, CT may be necessary to understand the relation with vital structures (e.g., trachea, esophagus, great vessels) and differentiate the diagnosis from encephalocele or other congenital malformations [38].

Cervical dermoid cysts appear as painless, superficial masses in anterior neck region and usually move with the covering skin. They gradually increase in size because of the secretions of sebaceous glands. Clinical history, physical examination, and ultrasonography are sufficient for diagnosis. Fine needle aspiration is necessary to rule out malignancy or other congenital malformations (e.g., thyroglossal ductus cysts) [29].

82.7.2 Treatment Modalities

Cervical teratomas have increased respiratory risk, because of the mediastinum extension, tracheal compression, or pulmonary hypoplasia. Estimated mortality rate is 80% if they are left untreated [26]. After airway stabilization with either intubation or tracheotomy, complete surgical excision is the ideal treatment for cervical teratomas. Because of the benign nature of the tumor, all important structures should be preserved in the surgery [26].

Cervical dermoid cysts are easily managed with complete excision. All attachments and cyst wall should be removed to prevent the recurrence [26].

82.7.3 Infections of Cervical Teratoma and Dermoid Cysts

Both untreated cervical teratomas and dermoid cysts are susceptible to infection. In the presence of infection of dermoid cyst, lesion grows rapidly and reddish discoloration, pain, and tenderness are seen midline of the neck. Especially infected cervical teratoma can lead to life-threating respiratory distress, abscess formation, and sepsis [12]. Patients should be managed by empiric antibiotics as mentioned above and analgesics. Incision and drainage should be performed if unresponsive to the antimicrobial therapy. In order to prevent the recurrence, all attachments and cyst wall must be removed.

If suspicious of an infected cervical teratoma, patient should be hospitalized for the risk of respiratory distress, and broad-spectrum antibiotics should start promptly. Cooperation with pediatric infection disease department is essential. Needle aspiration is helpful for culture-guided antimicrobial therapy and decompression. Incision and drainage can be performed if the radiological and clinical progressions occur. After the total resolution of infection, all attachments and cyst wall should be removed.

82.8 Thymic Anomalies/Cyst

Thymus is a retrosternal lymphoid tissue that develops from the third and fourth pharyngeal pouches. The thymus is generally located in anterior mediastinum and involved in the maturation of immunocompetent T cells and implying the differentiation of sub-types of T cells [39].

82.8.1 Clinical Features and Diagnosis

Embryologic remnants of thymus may retain all along the course of primordial thymus [40]. Cervical thymic cyst is the most frequently observed thymic anomalies and originates from the remnants of thymo-pharyngeal duct or cystic degeneration of solid thymic tissue [41]. Thymic cysts present as painless swelling but may cause dysphagia, stridor, or dysphonia because of the mediastinal attachments and extensions. Because of the rarity of thymic anomalies, it is not possible to diagnose them before the surgery and histopathological examination. USG, CT, and MRI are necessary to understand the relation of the lesion with airway and vital structures. Other congenital malformations (e.g., branchial cysts, vascular malformations, cystic hygroma) must be ruled out to diagnose the thymic anomalies.

82.8.2 Treatment Modalities

Surgery is the ideal treatment for both diagnostic and therapeutic purpose. Surgeon should be aware of the mediastinal normal thymus before the ectopic thymic tissue excision. Cervical thymic cysts do not contain active lymphatic tissue, so it is not a problem to excise them.

82.8.3 Infections

Although thymic anomalies are rare congenital anomalies in children, theoretically they have potential to be infected. Due to its anatomical mediastinal location or extension, they carry the risk of mediastinitis. Therefore, infected thymic anomalies are life-threating and important infections and should be managed and treated promptly. These patients should be hospitalized and given broad-spectrum empiric antibiotic. Department of pediatric infection disease, pediatric surgery, thoracic surgery, and otolaryngology should be in coordination and intact. Cooperative management must be given for these cases.

References

1. Wassef M, Blei F, Adams D, et al. Vascular anomalies classification: recommendations from the international society for the study of vascular anomalies. Pediatrics. 2015;136:e203–14.
2. Wernher A. Die Angeborenen Kysten-Hygrome und die Ihnen verwandten. In: Geschwadste in Anatomischer, Diagnosticher and Therapeutischer Beziehung. Giessen: G. FHeyer, Vater; 1843. p. 76–91.
3. Schoinohoriti OK, Theologie-Lygidakis N, Tzerbos F, Iatrou I. Lymphatic malformations in children and adolescents. J Craniofac Surg. 2012;23:1744–7.
4. Witte MH, Bernas MJ, Martin CP, et al. (2001) wilting J. Lymphangiogenesis and lymphangiodysplasia: from molecular to clinical lymphology. The biology of lymphangiogenesis. Microsc Res Tech. 2001;55:122–45.
5. Witte MH, Dellinger MT, Mcdonald DM, Nathanson SD, Baccardo FM, Campisi CC, et al. Lymphangiogenesis and hemangiogenesis: potential targets for therapy. J Surg Oncol. 2011;103(6):489–500. https://doi.org/10.1002/jso.21714.
6. Fr S. On the origin of the lymphatic system from the veins, and the development of the lymph hearts and thoracic duct in the pig. Am J Anat. 1901;1:367–89.
7. Moore KL, TVN P. The cardiovascular system. In: The developing human, clinically oriented embryology. 8th ed. Philadelphia: Saunders; 2008.
8. Surico D, Amadori R, D'Ajello P, et al. Antenatal diagnosis of fetal lymphangioma by ultrasonography. Eur J Obstet Gynecol Reprod Biol. 2013;168:236.
9. Mulliken JB, Glowacki J. Hemangiomas and vascular malformations in infants and children: a classification based on endothelial characteristics. Plast Reconstr Surg. 1982;69:412e22.
10. Finn MC, Glowacki J, Mulliken JB. Congenital vascular lesions: clinical application of a new classification. J Pediatr Surg. 1983;18:894.
11. Padwa BL, Hayward PG, Ferraro NF, et al. Cervico-facial lymphatic malformation: clinical course, surgical intervention, and pathogenesis of skeletal hypertrophy. Plast Reconstr Surg. 1995;95:951.
12. Wiswell TE, Miller JA. Infections of congenital cervical neck masses associated with bacteremia. J Pediatr Surg. 1986;21:173.
13. Greene AK, Perlyn CA, Alomari AI. Management of lymphatic malformations. Clin Plast Surg. 2011;38:75–82.
14. Nehra D, Jacobson L, Barnes P, et al. Doxycycline sclerotherapy as primary treatment of head and neck lymphatic malformations in children. J Pediatr Surg. 2008;43:451.
15. Bai Y, Jia J, Huang XX, et al. Sclerotherapy of micro- cystic lymphatic malformations in oral and facial regions. J Oral Maxillofac Surg. 2009;67:251.
16. Smith MC, Zimmerman B, Burke DK, et al. Efficacy and safety of OK-432 immunotherapy of lymphatic malformations. Laryngoscope. 2009;119:107.

17. Charabi B, Bretlau P, Bille M, Holmelund M. Cystic hygroma of the head and neck a long-term follow-up of 44 cases. Acta Otolaryngol Suppl. 2000;543:248–50. https://doi.org/10.1080/000164800454530.

18. Al-Dajani N, Wootton SH. Cervical lymphadenitis, suppurative parotitis, thyroiditis, and infected cysts. Infect Dis Clin North Am. 2007;21(2):523.

19. Brook I. Microbiology of infected epidermal cysts. Arch Dermatol. 1989;125(12):1658–61.

20. Brook I. Microbiology and managemen t of infected neck cysts. J Oral Maxillofac Surg. 2005;63(3):392–5.

21. Myers EN, Cunningham MJ. Inflammatory presentations of congenital head and neck masses. Pediatr Infect Dis J. 1988;7(11):162–8. https://doi.org/10.1097/00006454-198811001-00009.

22. Chow AW. Infections of the oral cavity, neck, and head. In: Bennett JE, Dolin R, Blaser MJ, editors. Mandell, Douglas, and Bennett's principles and practice of infectious diseases. 9th ed. Philadelphia: Elsevier Saunders; 2020. p. 859–74.

23. Healy CM, Baker CJ. Cervical lymphadenitis. In: Cherry JD, Harrison GJ, Kaplan SL, et al., editors. Feigin and Cherry's textbook of pediatric infectious diseases. 7th ed. Philadelphia: Elsevier Saunders; 2014. p. 175.

24. Nusbaum AO, Som PM, Rothschild MA, et al. Recurrence of a deep neck infection: a clinical indication of an underlying congenital lesion. Arch Otolaryngol Head Neck Surg. 1999;125:1379.

25. Mohan P, Chokshi R, Moser R, et al. Thyroglossal duct cysts: a consideration in adults. Am Surg. 2005;71(6):508–11.

26. Enepekides DJ. Management of congenital anomalies of the neck. Facial Plast Surg Clin North Am. 2001;9:131–45.

27. Moore KL, Persaud TVN. The pharyngeal apparatus. In: The developing human, clinically oriented embryology. 8th ed. Philadelphia: Saunders; 2008.

28. Sistrunk WE. The surgical treatment of cysts of the thyroglossal tract. Ann Surg. 1920; 71:121–4.

29. Foley DS, Fallat ME. Thyroglossal duct and other congenital midline cervical anomalies. Semin Pediatr Surg. 2006;15:70–5.

30. Simon LM, Magit AE. Impact of incision and drainage of infected thyroglossal duct cyst on recurrence after Sistrunk procedure. Arch Otolaryngol Head Neck Surg. 2012;138(1):20–4. https://doi.org/10.1001/archoto.2011.225.

31. Adams A, Mankad K, Offiah C, Childs L. Branchial cleft anomalies: a pictorial review of embryological development and spectrum of imaging findings. Insights Imaging. 2016;7(1):69–76. https://doi.org/10.1007/s13244-015-0454-5.

32. Waldhausen JHT. Branchial cleft and arch anomalies in children. Semin Pediatr Surg. 2006;15:64–9.

33. Bailey H. Branchial cysts and other essays on surgical subjects in the fascio-cervical region. London: H. K Lewis & Company; 1929.

34. Acierno SP, Waldhausen JH. Congenital cervical cysts, sinuses and fistulae. Otolaryngol Clin North Am. 2007;40(1):161–76. https://doi.org/10.1016/j.otc.2006.10.009.

35. Zaifullah S, Yunus MRM, See GB. Diagnosis and treatment of branchial cleft anomalies in UKMMC: a 10-year retrospective study. Eur Arch Otorhinolaryngol. 2013;270:1501–6.

36. Hirshoren N, Fried N, Weinberger JM, Eliashar R, Korem M. The microbiology characteristics of infected branchial cleft anomalies. OTO Open. 2019;3(3):2473974. https://doi.org/10.1177/2473974X19861065.

37. Ksia A, Mosbahia S, Zrig A. Teratome cervical chez l'enfant [cervical Teratoma in a child]. Arch Pediatr. 2013;20:1133–8.

38. Paradis J, Koltai PJ. Pediatric teratoma and dermoid cysts. Otolaryngol Clin North Am. 2015;48(1):121–36. https://doi.org/10.1016/j.otc.2014.09.009.

39. Herrera Hernández AA, Aranda Valderrama P, Díaz Pérez JA. Anomalías congénitas de origen tímico en el cuello [Congenital anomalies of thymic origin in the neck]. Acta Otorrinolaringol Esp. 2008;59(5):244–9. Spanish

40. Khariwala SS, Nicollas R, Triglia JM, Garabedian EN, Marianowski R, Van Den Abbeele T, April M, Ward R, Koltai PJ. Cervical presentations of thymic anomalies in children. Int J Pediatr Otorhinolaryngol. 2004;68(7):909–14. https://doi.org/10.1016/j.ijporl.2004.02.012.
41. Zarbo RJ, McClatchey KD, Areen RG, Baker SB. Thymopharyngeal duct cyst: a form of cervical thymus. Ann Otol Rhinol Laryngol. 1983;92:284–9.

Part VI

Treatment Strategies

Principles of Appropriate Antimicrobial Therapy and Antibacterial Agents for Pediatric Ear, Nose, and Throat Infections

İlker Devrim, Nuri Bayram, and Emin Sami Arısoy

83.1　Introduction

Anti-infective drugs include a broad spectrum of pharmaceutical agents divided into subclasses such as antibacterial, antifungal, antiviral, and antiparasitic drugs [1]. This chapter mainly targets antibacterial agents and principles of the appropriate use of antimicrobial therapy in ear, nose, and throat infections. The identical principles might be applied to all or any kinds of infections in both youngsters and adults.

83.2　Pharmacokinetics and Pharmacodynamics of Antimicrobial Drugs

The clinical experience and decision about antibiotics in clinical settings depend on the pharmacodynamics and pharmacokinetics of the drugs and microbiological parameters [2]. The antibacterial agents are divided into groups depending on the mechanisms of antimicrobial activity, chemical structure, and performance. While evaluating the dosage and its frequency, the terms "concentration-dependent killing" and "time-dependent killing" are essential for antimicrobial drugs [3].

In a standard model, the height concentration of a drug (after a bolus or short rapid infusion) is mainly due to the drugs' dose and initial distribution volume [4]. The

İ. Devrim (✉) · N. Bayram
Section of Pediatric Infectious Diseases, İzmir Dr. Behçet Uz Children's Hospital, University of Health Sciences, İzmir, Turkey

E. S. Arısoy
Division of Pediatric Infectious Diseases, Department of Pediatrics, Faculty of Medicine, Kocaeli University, Kocaeli, Turkey

speed of decrease in drug concentration after the initial phase is strongly correlated with the proportion of redistribution, metabolism, or renal clearance. Pharmacokinetic and pharmacodynamics parameters are mostly evaluated by peak concentration (represents the highest concentration of a drug in the serum, cerebrospinal fluid, or target organ), minimum inhibitory concentration (MIC), and therefore the area under the concentration-time (AUC) curve at steady state over 24 h, additionally to protein binding and post-antibiotic effect. The parameters are used for optimal dosing strategies of the specific peak/MIC, time/MIC, and AUC/MIC [5].

The antimicrobials are often evaluated into two different groups, including concentration-dependent killing and time-dependent (concentration-independent) killing [6]. Aminoglycosides and fluoroquinolones show a major significant increase in bacterial killing rate with increasing concentration of antibiotics, which could be a good sample of concentration-dependent killing [4]. Higher doses lead to increased effectiveness, and dosing the aminoglycosides once a day achieves the peak concentration/MIC. On the other side, beta-lactams, glycopeptides, linezolid, clindamycin, and macrolides show time-dependent killing, and time/MIC is the preferred index for evaluation for those drugs. For these antimicrobial drugs, the clinical efficacy depends on the time in which blood concentrations of the drug remain above MIC values [4]. The effectiveness of azithromycin, tetracyclines, glycopeptides, and quinupristin-dalfopristin shows the best correlation with AUC/MIC.

One of the critical aspects of antimicrobial drug prescribing is the therapeutic index (TI), which may well be defined as a ratio that compares the blood concentration at which a drug becomes toxic and the concentration at which the drug is effective [7]. As an example, despite the aminoglycosides have a concentration-dependent killing pattern, the daily doses could not be increased even in life-threatening infections due to the narrow TI they had. It should be kept in mind that the serum antibactericidal concentrations of drugs with narrow TI should be closely monitored to decrease adverse effects. These drugs could also be more toxic than antibiotics with wider TI.

83.3   Classification of Antibacterial Agents

83.3.1 Form of Action

The classic classification of the antibacterial drugs in line with the mode of action is bactericidal or bacteriostatic agents. Bacteriostatic antibiotics inhibit the replication of bacteria without killing them. Sulfonamides, tetracyclines, and macrolides are the samples of bacteriostatic agents that mainly inhibits protein synthesis. Bactericidal drugs kill bacteria by engaging in cell walls, cell membrane, or bacterial DNA [4]. However, it should be kept in mind bactericidal or bacteriostatic features of antimicrobial drugs could change consistent with the kinds of species. Since bacteriostatic drugs only inhibit replication and do not kill bacteria, they gain time for the immune system to clear microorganisms. Thus, an intact immune system is critical for the total advantage of its actions. While treating the ear, nose, and throat infections in a patient with immunodeficiency or prolonged neutropenia (whether as a result of intensive chemotherapy or a malignancy), the employment of bactericidal drugs should be considered [8].

83.3.2 Source of Antibacterial Agents

Antibacterial drugs are often naturally achieved from fungi, while semi-synthetic agents are chemically modified antimicrobial drugs using a natural product or synthetic. Benzylpenicillin and cephalosporins are well-known samples of natural antibacterial drugs. Ampicillin and amikacin are the samples of semi-synthetic antimicrobials, and moxifloxacin could be a good sample of synthetic antibiotics. While natural antibiotics have higher toxicities, semi-synthetic and artificial antibiotics have less toxicity and better PD and PK features [9].

83.3.3 Spectrum of Activity

The activity spectrum of antibacterial drugs against the microorganisms could be classified as narrow or broad. The narrow-spectrum antibacterial drugs act on fewer species of microorganisms, such as only on gram-positive or gram-negative bacteria, or some specific bacteria but not the others [4]. However, the coverage of the broad spectrum antibacterial is wider, including both gram-positive and negative bacteria. Isoniazid and vancomycin are good samples of narrow-spectrum antibacterial drugs, while cephalosporins and carbapenems are good samples of broad-spectrum antibacterial drugs.

In clinical practice, the use of narrow-spectrum antibacterial drugs is strongly encouraged whenever possible such as if the microorganism is identified or the likely etiologic agents for a particular infection are known [10]. This recommendation's main reason is that the narrower spectrum of antibiotics does not kill many microorganisms forming the patient's microbiota, leading to less superinfection, development of antibacterial resistance, and the emergence of superbugs compared to broad-spectrum antibiotics [11].

83.3.4 Chemical Structure

Classification related to the chemical structure of the antibacterial agents is one of the well-known categories. Since the antibacterials' structure determines the effectiveness and toxicity, these features of the identical class of antibacterial drugs may need to share similar properties. The antibacterial drugs could also be classified based on their chemical structures as aminoglycosides, beta-lactams, macrolides, nitroimidazoles, quinolones, streptogramins, sulfonamides, and tetracyclines.

83.3.4.1 Beta-Lactams

This class of antibiotics had a beta-lactam ring (four-membered lactam ring). These classes of antibiotics differ from each other according to the variation of side chains or supplementary cycles. Penicillin derivatives, cephalosporins, monobactams, and carbapenems belong to this antibiotic class [12]. Here are some essential samples of beta-lactam antibiotics [13]:

1. *Penicillins*: Penicillin G, penicillin V, amoxicillin, ampicillin, oxacillin, nafcillin, piperacillin, ticarcillin.
2. *Cephalosporins*: Cephalexin, cefaclor, cefprozil, cefuroxime axetil, cefadroxil, cefdinir, cefixime, cefpodoxime, ceftibuten; cefazolin, cefuroxime, cephamycins (cefoxitin and cefotetan), cefotaxime, ceftriaxone, ceftazidime, cefoperazone, cefepime, and ceftaroline.
3. *Carbapenems*: Doripenem, ertapenem, imipenem/cilastatin, meropenem.
4. *Monobactams*: Aztreonam.
5. *Beta-lactams (BLs)-beta-lactamase inhibitors (BLIs)*: Ampicillin-sulbactam, amoxicillin-clavulanic acid, piperacillin-tazobactam, ticarcillin-clavulanic acid, ceftazidime-avibactam, ceftolozane-tazobactam, and meropenem-vaborbactam.

83.3.4.2 Aminoglycosides

These drugs' identical structure is two amino sugars connected with a glycosidic bond to an aminocyclitol [14]. Commonly prescribed aminoglycosides in clinical settings are amikacin, gentamicin, neomycin, netilmicin, kanamycin, tobramycin, and streptomycin.

83.3.4.3 Macrolides

Macrolides have a macrocyclic lactone ring, usually 14-, 15-, or 16-member to which one or more deoxy sugars may be attached. Clarithromycin, azithromycin, and erythromycin are the best-known macrolides in clinical practice [15]. These drugs have similar structural properties with erythromycin, and clarithromycin has a 14-member lactone ring, and azithromycin has a 15-member ring [13]. Consequently, these agents are not used primarily to treat serious infections like sepsis due to the macrolides' bacteriostatic effects. These drugs have affinities for binding ribosomal targets and prolonged post-antibiotic effects. The macrolides attain high concentrations within phagocytic cells. Thus, they may be prescribed against susceptible intracellular microorganisms [13].

83.3.4.4 Lincosamides

Clindamycin is the most known lincosamide that binds to the ribosome and inhibits protein synthesis by affecting tRNA movement through the peptidyl transferase center. Although its bacteriostatic efficacy, clindamycin may be used in many different sites of infections such as dental abscesses, deep neck space infections, and aspiration pneumonia [13]. Clindamycin also may be used for the treatment of soft-tissue infections caused by community-acquired *Staphylococcus aureus*.

83.3.4.5 Quinolones and Fluoroquinolones

These drugs are quinine-derived structural units, and by the addition of fluorine at position 6 to the essential quinolone, the molecule is called fluoroquinolone. While nalidixic acid is the first member of this family, many fluoroquinolones have been synthesized. New fluoroquinolones, as a more safe form, have a broader spectrum of antimicrobial activity. Fluoroquinolones include nalidixic acid, levofloxacin, ciprofloxacin, trovafloxacin, and moxifloxacin [16].

As a result of the animal models exposed to the drug, in which damage to joint cartilage was observed, fluoroquinolones' routine was not recommended in children for a long time [16–20]. Additionally, epiphyseal plate cartilage injury, especially within the weight-bearing joints, was focused on [21]. A policy statement published by the American Academy of Pediatrics (AAP) in 2006 and updated in 2011 stated the fluoroquinolones' indications were convenient for treating infections caused by multidrug-resistant microorganisms within the absence of alternative safe and effective agents [16, 17].

83.3.4.6 Nitroimidazoles

Nitroimidazoles contain a basic imidazole ring [22]. Nitroimidazoles are bactericidal, enter into the cells by passive diffusion, and form toxic metabolites; they disrupt microbial cells' DNA and inhibit nucleic acid synthesis [22].

83.3.4.7 Oxazolidinones

Linezolid is the only antimicrobial that belongs to the oxazolidinone class that may be used in children. It binds to the region the ribosomal peptidyl transferase center and inhibits the protein synthesis. The activity of linezolid is primarily to the gram-positive bacteria [13].

83.3.4.8 Streptogramins

This class includes two structurally different molecules: group A streptogramins with polyunsaturated macrolactones and group B streptogramins consisting of cyclic hexadepsipeptides. Quinupristin and dalfopristin are the members of this antimicrobial class [23, 24]. The combination of quinupristin/dalfopristin is mainly used against gram-positive cocci, including resistant microorganisms such as *Enterococcus faecium* but not *Enterococcus faecalis*.

83.3.4.9 Sulfonamides

This synthetic organic drug class has a sulfonamide functional group. The sulfonamides do not seem to be preferred in high-income countries, while they are still among the treatment choice in middle- and low-income countries because of the low cost compared to efficacy [13].

83.3.4.10 Tetracyclines

Tetracyclines contain four rings of hydrocarbons, including polyketides having an octa-hydro tetracene-2-carboxamide skeleton. Although the precursors were derived from *Streptomyces* bacteria, the recent members of these drugs are semi-synthetic.

The most ordinarily used ones in clinical practice are tetracycline and doxycycline [13].

83.3.4.11 Glycylcyclines

Glycylcyclines are semi-synthetic analogs of tetracycline and inhibit protein synthesis. Tigecycline is the most widely used glycylcycline. Glycylcyclines were modified from tetracyclines to overcome the efflux-mediated resistance mechanism, the main resistance pattern against tetracyclines.

83.3.4.12 Polymyxins

Polymyxins, produced by gram-positive bacteria belonging to the genus *Bacillus,* such as *Paenibacillus polymyxa*, are a group of cyclic non-ribosomal polypeptides. After binding to lipopolysaccharide structure in gram-negative bacteria's outer membrane, they disrupt the bacteria's membranes as a detergent-like reaction. Polymyxin B and colistin (polymyxin E) are the members of this antimicrobial class and are used to treat multidrug-resistant gram-negative bacterial infections [13].

83.3.5 Mode of Action

The antibiotics kill or inhibit the growth by affecting bacterial functions, including different mechanisms, mainly synthesis of the cell wall, protein, nucleic acid, and cell membrane functions [6].

83.3.5.1 Cell Wall Inhibitors

The bacteria incorporate cell walls different from other organisms, including humans, and a peptidoglycan structure with a polysaccharide backbone consisting of N-acetylmuramic acid and N-acetylglucosamine residues. Cell wall inhibitors prevent bacterial growth by stopping cell wall synthesis via the mechanism of inhibiting peptidoglycan synthesis. Penicillins, cephalosporins, monobactams, and carbapenems are included in this group [6].

According to the structural differences in their cell wall, gram-positive and gram-negative bacteria vary within the beta-lactam drugs' susceptibility. Gram-negative bacteria had an outer membrane that may block the antibiotics from reaching further to the cell wall and thus usually have less susceptibility to this antibiotic class. Amount of peptidoglycan, receptors, and lipids availability, nature of cross-linking, and autolytic enzymes affect the activity [25]. Resistance to cell wall inhibitors is a vitally important issue for clinicians and emerged mainly in the last years [26].

83.3.5.2 Protein Synthesis Inhibitors

Protein synthesis inhibitors target bacterial ribosomes. Bacterial cytoplasmic ribosomes are composed of the 30S and 50S subunits, while mammalian cytoplasmic ribosomes have 40S and 60S. This difference between subunits prevents drug-related adverse effects, especially in lower concentrations of the antibiotics. At the same time, higher doses of some protein synthesis inhibitors like chloramphenicol and tetracyclines may cause toxic effects by interaction with human mitochondrial ribosomes [27].

Protein synthesis inhibitors disrupt protein synthesis stages such as initiation and elongation (aminoacyl tRNA entry, proof-reading, peptidyl transfer, ribosomal translocation, and termination) [27]. Macrolides/ketolides/azalides, aminoglycosides, lincosamides (e.g., clindamycin), oxazolidinones (e.g., linezolid), tetracyclines, glycylcyclines, chloramphenicol, and quinupristin/dalfopristin are within this group [14].

83.3.5.3 Nucleic Acid Synthesis Inhibitors

The primary functional mechanism of nucleic acid synthesis inhibitors relies on the differences between enzymes that perform DNA and RNA synthesis in prokaryotic and eukaryotic cells; thus, less toxicity occurs [22]. These antibiotics are either DNA or RNA inhibitors.

RNA inhibitors interfere with the bacterial transcription process during which messenger RNA transcripts genetic material is produced for later transformation into protein. Quinolones are the DNA inhibitors, and by binding to DNA-gyrase, they inhibit the DNA replication that leads to cell damage [13]. Other antibacterial drugs like nitrofurantoin and metronidazole affect the DNA strands of anaerobic bacteria by creating metabolites.

83.4 The Principles of Antimicrobial Therapy

The general principles of antimicrobial therapy can be applied for the treatment of all infections. Before starting antimicrobial treatment, the first target should be identifying the etiologic agent. For patients with life-threatening infections such as meningitis, priorities may change, and prompt initiation of antimicrobial treatment could be even more important than identifying the etiologic agent.

Considering the characteristics of antimicrobials such as safety, efficacy, antimicrobial spectrum, compliance with therapy, dosing schedule, and cost-effectiveness are essential strategies for choosing an antimicrobial. In this part, antimicrobial therapy's general principles will be reviewed for infections by giving samples from clinical practice in ENT infections.

83.4.1 Identification of the Etiologic Agent and Determination of Antimicrobial Susceptibility

Identification of the etiologic agent(s) of the infection is crucial for the appropriate antimicrobial treatment. Sometimes a basic, older, and conventional technique such as Gram stain may be enough for the diagnosis, and in some cases more complicated molecular diagnostic techniques are required. When the microorganism is identified, its susceptibilities are known (preferably with susceptibility tests) or presumed (with the current epidemiologic data), a bactericidal, narrow-spectrum, well-tolerated, cost-effective antibacterial drug should be chosen. For example, in a child with tonsillopharyngitis, identification of group A streptococcus (*Streptococcus pyogenes*) supported by throat culture and rapid antigen detection test (RADT), benzathine penicillin G, penicillin V, or amoxicillin are appropriate drugs, and no other wide-spectrum antibiotics are required [28]. Like the Infectious Diseases Society of America (IDSA) guideline, guidelines recommend penicillin as the first-line treatment because of its proven efficacy and safety, narrow spectrum, and low cost [28–31]. An important fact for this recommendation is that penicillin-resistant *S. pyogenes* has never been documented. Clinicians sometimes prefer amoxicillin due to suspension's superior taste since the efficacy appears to be equal [28].

For patients with acute otitis media (AOM), the selection of the antimicrobial drugs is generally influenced by the previous epidemiological data, including the pathogens and their antimicrobial susceptibility results. In the patients with a toxic clinical picture, immunodeficiency, prior treatment failure, or recurrent AOM, the etiologic diagnosis is essential [32]. The same empirical approach was also appropriate for acute bacterial sinusitis. In uncomplicated cases whose clinical picture was improved with empirical antibiotics, microbiologic studies are not required and reserved for the patients with toxic-appearing, orbital or intracranial complications, immunosuppression, recurrent acute bacterial sinusitis, and treatment failures. Maxillary sinus aspiration is rarely performed at present unless the course of the infection is unusually prolonged or severe [33].

In acute and severely ill patients with unknown origin, immediate antimicrobial treatment should be started after specimens for laboratory analysis, such as materials for culture, are obtained [4]. When the microorganism and its susceptibility are not known while decision-making, the antimicrobial drug's choice is influenced by the site of infection and patient's history, including age, vaccination status, previous infections, immune status, and presence of siblings, attendance at school or day care centers, etc. For instance, in the case of AOM, the antimicrobial coverage should include *Streptococcus pneumoniae, Haemophilus influenzae,* and *Moraxella catarrhalis* which are the most commonly seen etiologic agents, and the selection of dosage as high or low, and amoxicillin versus amoxicillin-clavulanate depends on the associated risk factors of the child [32].

83.4.2 Route of Administration

The administration route of drugs generally depends on the location and severity of the infection [4]. Selection between oral versus intravenous therapy is set by the active metabolite levels required at the infection site, the severity of the disease, and absorption from the drugs by the gastrointestinal tract [6].

In case of severe life-threatening infections, parenteral administration should be selected, and treatment should be determined according to the current guidelines. However, in mild infections, oral route and outpatient follow-up should be the clinician's priority due to the economic and other issues that come with the hospitalization. Even for hospitalized patients, whenever possible, shifting towards oral therapy from intravenous therapy should be considered. For example, when considering a child with complicated orbital cellulitis, antimicrobial therapy should be given intravenously since adequate serum levels of the antimicrobial drug(s) cannot be obtained by oral administration. Intolerance to oral antibiotics is another indication for switching to the intravenous route.

One of the critical parameters in planning antimicrobial treatment is the duration of therapy. The most significant factor determining the course of the antimicrobial treatment is the clinical assessment of the patient. It should be kept in mind that the longer the antimicrobial treatment than recommended, the more likely the resistance and adverse effects occur.

83.4.3 Adverse Effects

Most adverse reactions to antibiotics, including rash, diarrhea, nausea, and vomiting, are generally minor and transient. According to how the drug is metabolized (hepatic or renal), the antimicrobial drugs show adverse effects. For example, carbapenems are associated with a transient increase in the level of hepatic transaminases, which generally recover after cessation of treatment. Aminoglycosides may cause nephrotoxicity and ototoxicity due to intracellular accumulation of the drug [34].

Among the other antibiotics, most allergic reactions are associated with beta-lactams [4] and reported in about 8% of individuals in the United States (US) [35]. A detailed drug allergy history should be taken for all patients [4]. Patients and caregivers could confuse drug allergy with rashes or the primary disease such as the rash of roseola infantum. In penicillin-allergic patients, the incidence of cross-reactivity to other beta-lactams (including cephalosporins and carbapenems) is around 10%. Carbapenems and monobactams are safely used in individuals with confirmed penicillin allergy other than type I (anaphylactic) reaction [35].

83.4.4 Resistance

Antibiotic resistance is a significant problem worldwide. Soon after introducing sulfonamides and penicillin in 1935 and 1941, resistance emerged very rapidly in a very few years. The resistance has been attributed to the misuse of antibiotics, which becomes more critical due to the absence of new antibiotic development [36–38]. The rise in the rates of resistant bacteria is decreasing the effectiveness of the antibiotics. The US Centers for Disease Control and Prevention (CDC) declared in 2013 that humankind is now in the "post-antibiotic era." In 2014, the World Health Organization (WHO) warned that the antibiotic resistance crisis is becoming dire [39]. Among the antibiotic-resistant bacteria, mainly methicillin-resistant *S. aureus*, vancomycin-resistant enterococci, extended-spectrum beta-lactamase-producing *Enterobacteriaceae*, carbapenem-resistant *Enterobacteriaceae*, multidrug-resistant *Acinetobacter* spp., and drug-resistant *Neisseria gonorrhoeae* have already spread worldwide [40]. In line with CDC data, a minimum of two million people become infected, and a minimum of 23,000 people die annually on the spot results of infections caused by antibiotic-resistant bacteria [41].

The overuse of antibiotics is one of the critical reasons behind the causes of the evolution of resistance [42]. An immediate relation between antibiotic usage and the spreading of emerging resistant bacteria strains is present. As a result of eliminating the drug-sensitive microorganisms due to antibiotics, rates of the growth in resistant bacteria increase due to natural selection. The resistance occurs due to genetic alterations or modified expression of proteins in drug-resistant organisms [43]. Briefly, primary mechanisms include modification of target sites (e.g., alteration of major protein-binding proteins leading to decreased binding of antibiotics in *S. pneumoniae* resistant to beta-lactams), decreased modification (e.g., presence of efflux pumps, and limitation of penetration of certain agents like beta-lactam antibiotics in gram-negative bacteria), and enzymatic inactivation (e.g., beta-lactamases degrading penicillins and cephalosporins, acetyltransferases inactivating aminoglycosides and esterase hydrolyzing macrolides) [6].

Antibiotics are among the principal drugs prescribed for children in community and hospital settings [44–46]. Antimicrobial drugs were prescribed for one in every five children in pediatric ambulatory [47]. Nevertheless, a considerable rate of those prescriptions is redundant or inappropriate. Moreover, broader spectrum antibiotics instead of narrow-spectrum are substantially used for children that narrower spectrum agents are recommended [47, 48]. Additionally, antibiotic prescriptions with incorrect total daily dosage and duration were common [48–50]. One of the most effective strategies for combating emerging resistance is implementing antimicrobial stewardship programs [51]. These programs should be implemented in ambulatory settings, and pediatric ENT infections, quite common, should be the foremost important target for antimicrobial stewardship programs.

83.5 Antibacterial Agents and for Pediatric Ear, Nose, and Throat Infections

83.5.1 Acute Tonsillopharyngitis

In consequence of the self-limited nature of the tonsillopharyngitis caused by group A streptococcus (GAS), initiation of antibacterial therapy is reasonable for patients that GAS is confirmed by culture or RADT [28]. However, if the clinical findings are strongly compatible with GAS pharyngitis, antimicrobial therapy may be prescribed while awaiting microbiologic confirmation. Although many antibiotics such as penicillin, amoxicillin, clindamycin, cephalosporins, or macrolides are effective in treatment, penicillin is recommended for the first-line treatment of GAS pharyngitis [28, 29]. As with many guidelines, a full 10-day course of oral penicillin—or one dose of intramuscular benzathine penicillin—is preferred in patients. Antimicrobial recommendations for GAS pharyngitis are shown in Table 83.1 [28, 29].

Table 83.1 Antimicrobial therapy for group A streptococcal tonsillopharyngitis (Adopted from Refs. [28 and 29])

Drugs	Dosage	Duration
Penicillin V, oral	Children: 250 mg two or three times daily Adolescents and adults: 250 mg four times daily or 500 mg twice daily	10 days
Amoxicillin, oral	50 mg/kg, once daily (max. 1.000 mg) or 25 mg/kg, twice daily (max. 500 mg)	10 days
Penicillin G benzathine, intramuscular	< 27 kg: 600,000 U ≥ 27 kg: 1,200,000 U	Single dose
Patients with penicillin allergy		
Cephalexin oral[a]	20 mg/kg per dose, twice daily (max. 500 mg per dose)	10 days
Cefadroxil, oral[a]	30 mg/kg, once daily (max. 1000 mg)	10 days
Clindamycin, oral	7 mg/kg per dose three times daily (max. 300 mg per dose)	10 days
Azithromycin, oral[b]	12 mg per kg once daily (max. 500 mg)	5 days
Clarithromycin, oral[b]	7.5 mg per kg per dose twice daily (max. 250 mg per dose)	10 days

[a]These agents should not be used to treat *S. pyogenes* tonsillopharyngitis in patients with type 1 hypersensitivity to beta-lactam antibiotics.
[b]Resistance of group A streptococcus to these agents is well known.

83.5.2 Acute Bacterial Sinusitis

For uncomplicated sinusitis in pediatric cases, a broader-spectrum regimen with amoxicillin was the primary choice of treatment. However, due to increasing penicillin-resistant pneumococci, higher doses of amoxicillin (90 mg/kg daily) are recommended for outpatients [33]. On the other hand, amoxicillin at a standard or high dose may not be appropriate in children with a lack of regressions in clinical findings with amoxicillin therapy in 72 h, recent treatment in the last 1 month, attendance at childcare, and uncomplicated sinusitis [52]. Furthermore, amoxicillin has no efficacy on beta-lactamase-producing *H. influenzae* and *M. catarrhalis* [53]. Therefore, amoxicillin-clavulanate instead of amoxicillin alone is the appropriate choice for the first-line treatment of acute bacterial sinusitis in these children for a duration of 10–14 days [53].

According to the IDSA guideline, higher doses of amoxicillin-clavulanate (80–90 mg/kg/day of amoxicillin with 6.4 mg/kg/day of clavulanate [14:1 formulation] twice in a day) is recommended in children who live in regions with an endemic rate of 10% or more of invasive penicillin-resistant *S. pneumoniae*, those with severe infection, children attending to day care, those who have used antibiotics within the last month, and those who are immunocompromised [53, 54]. Due to high resistance to macrolides, these antimicrobials are not recommended for empirical therapy of acute bacterial sinusitis [52, 53]. Macrolides may be considered for children with type 1 hypersensitivity reaction to beta-lactam agents. For patients with non-type I penicillin allergy, oral third-generation agents (cefixime or cefpodoxime) plus clindamycin may be prescribed. Children with acute bacterial sinusitis who require hospitalization due to severe symptoms or inability to take oral antibiotics may be treated with intravenous third-generation cephalosporins [53]. Recommendations for the treatment of acute bacterial sinusitis in children are shown in Table 83.2 [52, 53].

83.5.3 Acute Otitis Media

High dose of amoxicillin or amoxicillin-clavulanate (80–90 mg/kg/day of amoxicillin in 2 divided doses) remains the first-line therapy for children with AOM because these antibiotics achieve sufficient middle ear concentrations for treatment. Especially for patients having increased risk of beta-lactam resistance, amoxicillin-clavulanate is preferred as first-line therapy [32]. Cephalosporins other than intramuscular ceftriaxone achieves less middle ear concentration to be effective [55]. Intramuscularly administered ceftriaxone is effective for children who cannot tolerate oral antibiotics.

In children with type I penicillin allergy, either oral macrolides or oral trimethoprim-sulfamethoxazole therapies are recommended, despite acknowledging the resistance of these antimicrobials among *S. pneumoniae* isolates, and the macrolides have no activity against most of the *H. influenzae* isolates [56]. Children who have other types of allergic reactions can be treated with cefuroxime, cefdinir,

Table 83.2 Antimicrobial therapy for acute bacterial sinusitis in children (Adopted from Refs. [52 and 53])

Indication	First-line therapy	Second-line therapy
Initial therapy	Amoxicillin-clavulanate (45 mg/kg/day, orally, twice daily)	Amoxicillin-clavulanate (90 mg/kg/day, orally, twice daily)
Type 1 hypersensitivity to beta-lactams		Levofloxacin (10–20 mg/kg/day, orally, every 12–24 h)
Non-type 1 hypersensitivity to beta-lactams		Clindamycin (30–40 mg/kg/day, orally, three times a day) PLUS cefixime (8 mg/kg/day, orally, twice daily)
The risk for antibiotic resistance or failed initial therapy		Amoxicillin-clavulanate (90 mg/kg/day, orally, twice daily) Clindamycin (30–40 mg/kg/day, orally, three times a day) PLUS cefixime (8 mg/kg/day, orally, twice daily) Levofloxacin (10–20 mg/kg/day, orally, every 12–24 h)
Severe infection requiring hospitalization		Ampicillin/sulbactam (200–400 mg/kg/day, intravenous, every 6 h) Ceftriaxone (50 mg/kg/day, intravenous, every 12 h) Cefotaxime (100–200 mg/kg/day, intravenous, every 6 h) Levofloxacin (10–20 mg/kg/day, intravenous, every 12–24 h)

Table 83.3 Recommendations for antibacterial treatment of acute otitis media in children (Adopted from Refs. [32 and 57])

Initial antibacterial treatment		Antibacterial treatment after 48–72 h of failure of initial antibiotic treatment	
First-line treatment	Alternative treatment (for penicillin allergy)	First-line treatment	Alternative treatment
Amoxicillin (90 mg/kg per day in two divided doses) or Amoxicillin-clavulanate (90 mg/kg/day of amoxicillin) in 2 divided doses)	Cefdinir (14 mg/kg per day in 1 or 2 doses), Cefuroxime (30 mg/kg per day in two divided doses), Cefpodoxime (10 mg/kg per day in 2 divided doses), Ceftriaxone (50 mg/kg IM or IV per day for 1 or 3 days)	Amoxicillin-clavulanate (90 mg/kg/day of amoxicillin in 2 divided doses) or Ceftriaxone (50 mg/day IM or IV for 3 days)	Ceftriaxone (50 mg/day IM or IV for 3 days) or Clindamycin (30–40 mg/kg/day in 3 divided doses) with or without a third-generation cephalosporin

IM indicates intramuscular, *IV* intravenous.

cefpodoxime, or intramuscular ceftriaxone. Antibacterial drug recommendations for the treatment of AOM in children are shown in Table 83.3 [32, 57].

83.6 Conclusion

The appropriate use of antibiotics for ENT infections is essential for effective treatment and avoidance of serious adverse effects of medication and antibiotic resistance. The choice of antibiotics in clinical settings depends on their pharmacodynamics and pharmacokinetic properties and microbiological parameters.

Penicillin (oral penicillin V or intramuscular benzathine penicillin G) is recommended as the antibiotic of choice for GAS pharyngitis. As *S. pneumoniae, H. influenzae,* and *M. catarrhalis* are the main microorganisms causing AOM and acute bacterial sinusitis in children, amoxicillin or amoxicillin-clavulanate is recommended for the first-line treatment.

References

1. Leekha S, Terrell CL, Edson RS. General principles of antimicrobial therapy. Mayo Clin Proc. 2011;86:156–67.
2. Levison ME, Levison JH. Pharmacokinetics and pharmacodynamics of antibacterial agents. Infect Dis Clin North Am. 2009;23:791–815.
3. Downes KJ, Hahn A, Wiles J. Dose optimisation of antibiotics in children: application of pharmacokinetics/pharmacodynamics in paediatrics. Int J Antimicrob Agents. 2014;43:223–30.
4. Neely MN, Reed MD. Pharmacokinetic-pharmacodynamic basis of optimal antibiotic therapy. In: Long SS, Prober CG, Fischer M, editors. Principles and practice of pediatric infectious diseases. 5th ed. Philadelphia: Elsevier; 2018. p. 1478–98.
5. Eyler RF, Shvets K. Clinical pharmacology of antibiotics. CJASN. 2019;14:1080–90.

6. Owens RC Jr, Shorr AF. Rational dosing of antimicrobial agents: pharmacokinetic and pharmacodynamic strategies. Am J Health Syst Pharm. 2009;66(Suppl 4):S23–30.
7. Muller PY, Milton MN. The determination and interpretation of the therapeutic index in drug development. Nat Rev Drug Discov. 2012;11:751–61.
8. Nemeth J, Oesch G, Kuster SP. Bacteriostatic versus bactericidal antibiotics for patients with serious bacterial infections: systematic review and meta-analysis. J Antimicrob Chemother. 2015;70:382–95.
9. Bérdy J. Thoughts and facts about antibiotics: where we are now and where we are heading. J Antibiot (Tokyo). 2012;65:385–95.
10. Donà D, Zingarella S, Gastaldi A, et al. Effects of clinical pathway implementation on antibiotic prescriptions for pediatric community-acquired pneumonia. PLoS One. 2018;13(2):e0193581.
11. Abadi ATB, Rizvanov AA, Haertlé T, Blatt NL. World Health Organization report: current crisis of antibiotic resistance. BioNanoScience. 2019;9:778–88.
12. MacDougall C. Penicillins, cephalosporins, and other b-lactam antibiotics. In: Brunton LL, Hilal-Dandan R, Knollmann BC, editors. Goodman & Gilman's: the pharmacological basis of therapeutics. 13th ed. New York: McGraw-Hill; 2017. p. 1023–38.
13. Sauberan JB, Bradley JS. Antimicrobial agents. In: Long SS, Prober CG, Fischer M, editors. Principles and practice of pediatric infectious diseases. 5th ed. Philadelphia: Elsevier; 2018. p. 1499–531.
14. Magnet S, Blanchard JS. Molecular insights into aminoglycoside action and resistance. Chem Rev. 2005;105:477–98.
15. Zuckerman JM, Qamar F, Bono BR. Review of macrolides (azithromycin, clarithromycin), ketolids (telithromycin) and glycylcyclines (tigecycline). Med Clin North Am. 2011; 95:761–91.
16. Jackson MA, Schutze GE. Committee on infectious diseases. The use of systemic and Topical Fluoroquinolones. Pediatrics. 2016;118:1287–92.
17. Food and Drug Administration. FDA resources page. http://www.fda.gov/ohrms/dockets/ac/97/transcpt/3349t1.pdf. Accessed 27 Sep 2020.
18. Tatsumi H, Senda H, Yatera S, et al. Toxicological studies on pipemidic acid. V. Effect on diarthrodial joints of experimental animals. J Toxicol Sci. 1978;3:357–67.
19. Gough A, Barsoum NJ, Mitchell L, et al. Juvenile canine drug-induced arthropathy: clinicopathological studies on articular lesions caused by oxolinic and pipemidic acids. Toxicol Appl Pharmacol. 1979;51:177–87.
20. Patterson DR. Quinolone toxicity: methods of assessment. Am J Med. 1991;91:35S–7S.
21. Sendzik J, Lode H, Stahlmann R. Quinolone-induced arthropathy: an update focusing on new mechanistic and clinical data. Int J Antimicrob Agents. 2009;33:194–200.
22. Brook I. Management of anaerobic infection. Expert Rev Anti Infect Ther. 2004;2:153–8.
23. Mast Y, Wohlleben W. Streptogramins - two are better than one. Int J Med Microbiol. 2014;304:44–50.
24. Hershberger E, Donabedian S, Konstantinou K, et al. Quinupristin-dalfopristin resistance in gram-positive bacteria: mechanism of resistance and epidemiology. Clin Infect Dis. 2004;38:92–8.
25. Bugg TD, Braddick D, Dowson CG, et al. Bacterial cell wall assembly: still an attractive antibacterial target. Trends Biotechnol. 2011;29:167–73.
26. Fair RJ, Tor Y. Antibiotics and bacterial resistance in the 21st century. Perspect Med Chem. 2014;6:25–64.
27. Kohanski MA, Dwyer DJ, Collins JJ. How antibiotics kill bacteria: from targets to networks. Nat Rev Microbiol. 2010;8:423–35.
28. Nizet V, Arnold JC. Streptococcus pyogenes (group A streptococcus). In: Long SS, Prober CG, Fischer M, editors. Principles and practice of pediatric infectious diseases. 5th ed. Philadelphia: Elsevier; 2018. p. 715–23.
29. Shulman ST, Bisno AL, Clegg HW, et al. Clinical practice guideline for the diagnosis and management of group A streptococcal pharyngitis: 2012 update by the Infectious Diseases Society of America. Clin Infect Dis. 2012;55:1279–82.

30. Gerber MA, Baltimore RS, Eaton CB, et al. Prevention of rheumatic fever and diagnosis and treatment of acute streptococcal pharyngitis: a scientific statement from the American Heart Association Rheumatic Fever, Endocarditis, and Kawasaki Disease Committee of the Council on Cardiovascular Disease in the Young, the Interdisciplinary Council on Functional Genomics and Translational Biology, and the Interdisciplinary Council on Quality of Care and Outcomes Research: Endorsed by the American Academy of Pediatrics External. Circulation. 2009;119:1541–51.
31. Gewitz MH, Baltimore RS, Tani LY, et al. Revision of the Jones criteria for the diagnosis of acute rheumatic fever in the era of Doppler echocardiography: a scientific statement from the American Heart Association External. Circulation. 2015;131:1806.
32. Lieberthal AS, Carroll AE, Chonmaitree T, et al. The diagnosis and management of acute otitis media. Pediatrics. 2013;131:e964–99.
33. Wald ER, Applegate CB, Bordley C, et al. Clinical practice guideline for the diagnosis and management of acute bacterial sinusitis in children aged 1 to 18 years. Pediatrics. 2013;132:e262–80.
34. MacDougall C, Chambers HF. Aminoglycosides. In: Brunton LL, Hilal-Dandan R, Knollmann BC, editors. Goodman & Gilman's: the pharmacological basis of therapeutics. 13th ed. New York: McGraw-Hill; 2017. p. 1039–48.
35. Macy E. Penicillin and beta-lactam allergy: epidemiology and diagnosis. Curr Allergy Asthma Rep. 2014;14(11):476.
36. Gould IM, Bal AM. New antibiotic agents in the pipeline and how they can overcome microbial resistance. Virulence. 2013;4(2):185–91.
37. Wright GD. Something new: revisiting natural products in antibiotic drug discovery. Can J Microbiol. 2014;60:147–54.
38. Sengupta S, Chattopadhyay MK, Grossart HP. The multifaceted roles of antibiotics and antibiotic resistance in nature. Front Microbiol. 2013;4:47.
39. Michael CA, Dominey-Howes D, Labbate M. The antibiotic resistance crisis: causes, consequences, and management. Front Public Health. 2014;2:145.
40. Golkar Z, Bagazra O, Pace DG. Bacteriophage therapy: a potential solution for the antibiotic resistance crisis. J Infect Dev Ctries. 2014;8:129–36.
41. Centers for Disease Control and Prevention. Drug resistance. https://www.cdc.gov/drugresistance/index. Accessed 20 Sep 2020.
42. Read AF, Woods RJ. Antibiotic resistance management. Evol Med Public Health. 2014;2014(1):147.
43. Ventola CL. The antibiotic resistance crisis: part 1: causes and threats. Pharm Therapeut. 2015;40:277–83.
44. Gerber JS, Newland JG, Coffin SE, et al. Variability in antibiotic use at children's hospitals. Pediatrics. 2016;126:1067–73.
45. Ashiru-Oredope D, Hopkins S, English Surveillance Programme for Antimicrobial Utilization and Resistance Oversight Group. Antimicrobial stewardship: English surveillance programme for antimicrobial utilization and resistance (ESPAUR). J Antimicrob Chemother. 2013;68:2421–3.
46. Spyridis N, Syridou G, Goossens H, et al. Variation in paediatric hospital antibiotic guidelines in Europe. Arch Dis Child. 2016;101:72–6.
47. Hersh AL, Shapiro DJ, Pavia AT, et al. Antibiotic prescribing in ambulatory pediatrics in the United States. Pediatrics. 2011;128:1053–61.
48. McCaig LF, Besser RE, Hughes JM. Antimicrobial drug prescription in ambulatory care settings, United States, 1992–2000. Emerg Infect Dis. 2003;9:432–7.
49. Levy ER, Swami S, Dubois SG, et al. Rates and appropriateness of antimicrobial prescribing at an academic children's hospital, 2007–2010. Infect Control Hosp Epidemiol. 2012;33:346–53.
50. Nash DR, Harman J, Wald ER, et al. Antibiotic prescribing by primary care physicians for children with upper respiratory tract infections. Arch Pediatr Adolesc Med. 2002;156:1114–9.

51. Principi N, Esposito S. Antimicrobial stewardship in paediatrics. BMC Infect Dis. 2016;16(1):424.
52. Wald ER, DeMuri GP. Sinusitis. In: Long SS, Prober CG, Fischer M, editors. Principles and practice of pediatric infectious diseases. 5th ed. Philadelphia: Elsevier; 2018. p. 230–4.
53. Chow AW, Benninger MS, Brook I, et al. IDSA clinical practice guideline for acute bacterial rhinosinusitis in children and adults. Clin Infect Dis. 2012;54:e72–e112.
54. American Academy of Pediatrics. Principles of appropriate use of antimicrobial therapy for upper respiratory tract infections. In: Kimberlin DW, Brady MT, Jackson MA, Long SS, editors. Red Book: 2018 report of the committee on infectious diseases. 31st ed. Itasca: American Academy of Pediatrics; 2018. p. 910–3.
55. Jacobs MR. Increasing antibiotic resistance among otitis media pathogens and their susceptibility to oral agents based on pharmacodynamic parameters. Pediatr Infect Dis J. 2000;19:S47–55.
56. Suzuki HG, Dewez JE, Nijman RG, et al. Clinical practice guidelines for acute otitis media in children: a systematic review and appraisal of European national guidelines. BMJ Open. 2020;10:e035343.
57. Pelton SL. Otitis media. In: Long SS, Prober CG, Fischer M, editors. Principles and practice of pediatric infectious diseases. 5th ed. Philadelphia: Elsevier; 2018. p. 216–23.

Antiviral Agents for Pediatric Ear, Nose, and Throat Infections

84

Nurşen Belet, Emin Sami Arısoy, and Stephan Lang

84.1 Introduction

Viral infections of the upper airway tract are quite common in infants and children. Many types of viruses, mainly respiratory viruses, cause ear, nose, and throat (ENT) infections. Clinically significant respiratory viruses are respiratory syncytial virüs (RSV), rhinovirus, parainfluenza virus, coronavirus, influenza virus, adenovirus, human metapneumovirus, and bocavirus. At the end of 2019, a novel coronavirus, designated severe acute respiratory syndrome coronavirus 2 (SARS-CoV-2), the agent of coronavirus disease 2019 (COVID-19), is identified, and it also causes symptoms and signs of acute upper respiratory tract infection (URTI). Respiratory viruses affect all age groups; however, viral infection incidence is exceptionally high in infants and young children, and they have 6–8 infection episodes per year [1, 2].

The common cold is usually limited to the upper respiratory tract and self-limiting disease. The main symptoms are nasal congestion and discharge, sneezing, sore throat, and cough. Although the disease has a benign course, it has a significant economic burden due to doctor visits, treatments, absence from school, and daycare units. The common cold is the most common cause of inappropriate antibiotic use [3–5].

N. Belet (✉)
Division of Pediatric Infectious Diseases, Department of Pediatrics, Faculty of Medicine, Dokuz Eylül University, İzmir, Turkey
e-mail: nursen.belet@deu.edu.tr

E. S. Arısoy
Division of Pediatric Infectious Diseases, Department of Pediatrics, Faculty of Medicine, Kocaeli University, Kocaeli, Turkey

S. Lang
Department of Otorhinolaryngology, Head and Neck Surgery, University Hospital Essen, Essen, Germany

"

The variety of viruses that can cause a common cold is manifold, although rhinoviruses are the most common etiology in all age groups. Other possible responsible causes include RSV, parainfluenza viruses, enteroviruses, coronavirus, adenovirus, influenza, and human metapneumovirus. During an uncomplicated viral infection, symptoms peak at the 2-third day of disease and gradually disappear in 7–10 days. However, sometimes viral infections may be complicated secondary bacterial infections, hospitalization, and even mortality, especially in immunodeficient patients. Respiratory viruses frequently initiate the cascade of events causing bacterial infections such as acute otitis media and sinusitis [4].

Acute otitis media (AOM) is the most common bacterial complication of viral respiratory infection in children, occurs in nearly 20% of the viral URTIs of children. Otitis media is diagnosed frequently on the third or fourth day from the onset of upper respiratory tract symptoms. Detection of respiratory viruses in middle ear effusion has shown that viruses play an important role in the occurrence of AOM. Even though all viruses can be responsible for developing otitis media in children, the influenza virus and RSV are more pathogenic than the others [1, 3, 4]. The disruption of physiologic eustachian tube function followed by decreased middle ear pressure and fluid accumulation is the underlying cause of otitis media in viral upper respiratory disease [3, 6, 7].

Acute sinusitis is another common bacterial complication of URTI due to viruses. Viruses are responsible for 80–90% of acute rhinosinusitis. Rhinovirus, RSV, parainfluenza virus, enteroviruses, influenza virus, adenovirus, and coronavirus play an essential role in exacerbating acute rhinosinusitis. Sinusitis is present in 6–9% of children with the common cold [3, 8].

Despite the mild and self-limited course of most respiratory viral infections, specific antiviral therapy is introduced to prevent severe complications. Effective and specific treatment should shorten the disease's duration, relieve symptoms, and prevent bacterial complications. So far, various antiviral drugs with different action mechanisms against rhinoviruses were tested; however, none were found to be effective and reliable to get a license [3, 4, 9]. Unfortunately, specific antiviral therapy for respiratory viruses is commercially present for only influenza viruses currently [1, 3]. No specific antiviral treatment exists for other respiratory viruses in ENT infections, and treatment is mainly supportive [10–15]. Various antiviral agents are used in treating COVID-19 in children, but no controlled studies show their effectiveness. Therefore, antiviral agents against influenza will constitute this chapter's main subject, and antiviral treatment in COVID-19 will be briefly mentioned.

84.2　Antiviral Treatment in Influenza

Influenza is a common disease affecting many children each year. It mainly causes fever, cough, sore throat, headache, myalgia, and weakness. Symptoms can last for 1–2 weeks. Influenza is considered to be highly contagious and transmitted by droplets. Despite the disease's self-limited characteristics in most cases, it may result in lower respiratory tract infection, AOM, rhinosinusitis, febrile seizures, dehydration, and encephalopathy. Acute otitis media following influenza is seen in 20–50% of children less than 6 years of age. Most of the children who developed complications due to influenza have to be hospitalized [5].

The risk of complications due to influenza in children is higher in young children aged <2 years, children with chronic lung disease (including asthma), cardiovascular, renal, hepatic, hematologic (including sickle cell disease), or metabolic disorders (including diabetes mellitus) or neurologic and neurodevelopmental conditions (including disorders of the brain, spinal cord, peripheral nerve, and muscle such as cerebral palsy, epilepsy [seizure disorders], stroke, intellectual disability, moderate to severe developmental delay, muscular dystrophy, or spinal cord injury), children with immunosuppression, including that caused by medications or by human immunodeficiency virus (HIV) infection, children under long-term aspirin therapy, American Indian and Alaskan Native people, and residents of nursing homes and other chronic-care facilities [16].

American Academy of Pediatrics (AAP) and the United States (US) Centers for Disease Control and Prevention (CDC) Advisory Committee on Immunization Practices (ACIP) updates recommendations about influenza vaccines, antiviral drugs for influenza treatment, and prophylaxis annually. Although antiviral treatment is important for the control of influenza, it cannot substitute the effect of influenza vaccines [3, 5]. The AAP recommends urgent onset of antiviral therapy for children (1) hospitalized with presumed influenza infection, (2) hospitalized for severe, complicated, or progressive illness suggestive of influenza, or (3) at high risk of complication development regardless of the severity of the infection. Immediate antiviral treatment should be considered for any healthy child if influenza infection is possible, or influenza infection is possible, and the child lives at home with a sibling or household contact younger than 6 months or has a medical condition that predisposes to complications. If therapy can be started within 48 hours of disease, it has the most positive effects on the clinical result [3, 5, 16].

Currently, three classes of antiviral agents are available for influenza prevention and treatment: adamantane class antivirals (amantadine and rimantadine), neuraminidase inhibitors (NAIs; oseltamivir, zanamivir, peramivir, and laninamivir), and selective inhibitors of influenza cap-dependent endonuclease (baloxavir) [16]. Although adamantane class antivirals have obtained the license for the treatment of influenza A viruses, they are not recommended currently because of their missing intrinsic activity against influenza B viruses and high resistance levels of circulating influenza A viruses [5, 17–19]. Neuraminidase inhibitors act by preventing virus release from infected cells, thereby preventing the transmission to other cells. Among the four NAIs that existed, despite oseltamivir, zanamivir, and peramivir are licensed in several countries, laninamivir is licensed only in Japan but remains investigational in the USA and many other countries. Neuraminidase inhibitors are recommended for the prophylaxis and treatment of influenza [16]. Baloxavir has a different action mechanism than NAIs and blocks influenza proliferation by inhibiting mRNA synthesis initiation [20].

84.2.1 Oseltamivir

Oseltamivir was accepted as the primary drug for the treatment of influenza infection by the World Health Organization (WHO), yet, recently, its application was downgraded by WHO as "complementary" due to its limited duration the disease and potential side effects. Oral capsule and oral suspension forms of oseltamivir are present. Oral oseltamivir is absorbed by the gastrointestinal tract and converted to its active metabolite, oseltamivir carboxylate. Oseltamivir carboxylate can be detected in plasma within 30 minutes, and peak concentration is reached within 3–4 h following oral intake. Oseltamivir carboxylate is eliminated by both glomerular filtration and tubular secretion in kidneys, and dose adjustment is required in case of renal insufficiency. It is bound to protein in a low ratio, and peak concentrations in bronchoalveolar lavage (BAL), middle ear fluid, and sinuses are close to blood levels [17, 21].

Pharmacokinetics of oseltamivir varies with age, thus recommended doses for children and adults differ. The recommended doses according to age group and weight by the AAP for the 2020–2021influenza season (1) for treatment are as; in preterm infants <38-week of postmenstrual age (gestational age + chronologic age) a 5 days course of 1.0 mg/kg/dose twice daily, 38 through 40 weeks of postmenstrual age 1.5 mg/kg/dose, twice daily and >40-week of postmenstrual age 3.0 mg/kg/dose twice daily, in term infants 0–8 months old a 5 days course of 3 mg/kg/dose twice daily, 9–11-month-old 3.5 mg/kg/dose twice daily, and in those ≥1-year-old a 5 days course of 30 mg twice daily for a weight of <15 kg, 45 mg twice daily for a weight of 15–23 kg, 60 mg twice daily for a weight of 24–40 kg, and 75 mg twice daily for a weight >40 kg; (2) for chemoprophylaxis are as; in infants 3–11 months old a 7 days course of 3 mg/kg/dose once daily (oseltamivir is not recommended <3 months of age unless the situation is judged critical) and in those ≥1-year-old a 7 days course 30 mg once daily for a weight of <15 kg, 45 mg once daily for a weight of 15–23 kg, 60 mg once daily for a weight of 24–40 kg, and 75 mg once daily for a weight >40 kg. Oseltamivir can be applied in an enteral way, via either orogastric or nasogastric tube, in critically ill patients [16, 19].

Early-onset oseltamivir treatment was shown to shorten the duration of fever and the other symptoms and decrease the risk of complications [5, 22, 23]. Oseltamivir treatment has reduced the occurrence of AOM infection in children with influenza infection, and this effect was more prominent, especially in children <5 years of age [24]. Oseltamivir treatment has been shown to decrease the incidence of AOM, asthma exacerbation, and bronchiolitis significantly in children with chronic medical and neurological problems who are at risk for influenza [25]. Also, oseltamivir treatment was found to reduce both the number of complications and the antibiotic prescription incidence in children 1–12 years of age [26]. It was shown that oral oseltamivir and inhaled zanamivir were given for chemoprophylaxis were effective in people who had contact with a family member with confirmed influenza infection in randomized placebo-controlled studies [22].

The main adverse effects of oseltamivir are related to the gastrointestinal tract. Nausea and vomiting, the most common gastrointestinal adverse effects, occur in

10–15% of treated patients. Oseltamivir may cause central nervous system (CNS) side effects, especially in children and adolescents in Japan. However, no relation was detected between oseltamivir and neurological side effects in controlled clinical studies and ongoing surveillance [17, 21, 26].

Resistance to NAIs may develop due to a mutation of genes of neuraminidase or hemagglutinin, or both. H275Y mutation is the most commonly studied mutation and one of the most common determinants of resistance among N1 subtypes of influenza. During the 2019–2020 influenza season, minimal resistance to oseltamivir, zanamivir, or peramivir was identified in influenza viruses tested by the CDC [27]. Resistance is associated with lower doses than offered and described, especially in immune-suppressive patients [21, 28, 29].

84.2.2 Zanamivir

Zanamivir was approved to treat influenza infection in children ≥ 7 years of age and for post-exposure prophylaxis in children ≥ 5 years of age. Zanamivir, inhaled as a dry powder, is administered for treatment as a 5 days inhalation course of 10 mg twice a day and prophylaxis as a 7 days inhalation course of 10 mg daily. Zanamivir is usually well tolerated; however, it may cause cough, reversible decrease in pulmonary functions, and fatal bronchospasm, especially in patients with underlying pulmonary disease. Since it may result in ventilatory insufficiency and death of intubated patients, commercially available formulation should not be used for intubated patients' nebulization [16]. Intravenous zanamivir has been evaluated in clinical trials, and this form is available in the United Kingdom (UK) and Europe but is not approved in the USA [16, 29–31].

84.2.3 Laninamivir

Laninamivir is an inhaled, single-use, long-acting NAI. Laninamivir octanoate (prodrug of laninamivir) obtained license only in Japan and is also approved for use in children; however, it is not approved in other countries. Laninamivir showed efficient in vitro activity against circulating influenza A and B viruses, including H1N1 viruses, which have H275Y mutation [17].

84.2.4 Peramivir

Intravenous peramivir was approved by the Federal Drug Administration (FDA) in 2017 to treat acute uncomplicated influenza infection in non-hospitalized children ≥ 2 years of age who have been ill for no more than 2 days. It is given as a single intravenous dose, and the efficacy of peramivir in patients with severe influenza infection requiring hospitalization has not been established [16, 29].

84.2.5 Baloxavir Marboxil

Baloxavir marboxil is an inhibitor of cap-dependent endonuclease (CEN) of the influenza virus RNA polymerase, an essential enzyme in the initiation of viral mRNA synthesis. CEN produces the capped RNA primers that initiate viral mRNA synthesis. The FDA approved Baloxavir marboxil in 2018 to treat uncomplicated influenza infection in outpatient children and adolescents $\geq$12 years of age who have been ill for no more than 2 days [16]. It is given as a single oral dose for the treatment of uncomplicated influenza. Baloxavir marboxil appears to be well tolerated, and adverse events are uncommon. The primary reported side effects are diarrhea, vomiting, and hypersensitivity reactions such as anaphylaxis, urticaria, angioedema, and erythema multiforme. Although information about resistance to baloxavir marboxil is limited, it has been associated with escape mutants, especially in children [32].

84.3 Antiviral Treatment in COVID-19

COVID-19 is usually mild (upper respiratory tract involved only) or moderate course (no new or increased supplemental oxygen requirement with lower respiratory tract involved) in children. Therefore, supportive treatment is recommended in many cases. Antiviral treatment decision is made according to diseases severity, clinical course, existing evidence of efficacy, and underlying conditions that may increase disease progression risk. Many authors recommend that the treatment decision should be on a case-by-case basis and be applied in the context of clinical trials. Antiviral therapy is mainly recommended for hospitalized children with severe or critical COVID-19. Antiviral treatment can also be initiated in children with mild or moderate illnesses with an underlying disease [33].

Remdesivir is a nucleoside analog pro-drug that inhibits RNA-dependent RNA polymerase and has been approved by the FDA to treat COVID-19 requiring hospitalization in adults and children $\geq$12 years of age who weigh $\geq$40 kg. The recommendations of the multicenter panel regarding remdesivir are as follows [34]:

- Remdesivir is suggested for children with severe COVID-19.
- Remdesivir should be considered for children with critical COVID-19 unless there is a contraindication.
- Outpatients and hospitalized patients with asymptomatic, mild, or moderate COVID-19 should be managed with supportive care only, and remdesivir should be used only within the context of a clinical trial in these populations.

Nausea, vomiting, and transaminase elevations are the reported side effects of remdesivir.

However, WHO and some experts suggest not using remdesivir in hospitalized patients [35–37]

Other drugs with antiviral activity used to treat COVID-19 are hydroxychloroquine, chloroquine, and lopinavir-ritonavir. The efficacy of hydroxychloroquine and chloroquine in COVID-19 is uncertain [38]. They are not licensed for this indication and are not recommended for the treatment of COVID-19 in children, except in hospitalized patients only in the context of a clinical trial [33].

Randomized studies showing the efficacy or safety of lopinavir-ritonavir are not available in children. The multicenter panel does not recommend hydroxychloroquine and chloroquine and lopinavir-ritonavir for use in children outside of the clinical study context [34].

Oseltamivir is not effective against SARS-CoV-2.

84.4 Conclusion

In summary, oseltamivir (oral), zanamivir (inhaled), peramivir (intravenous), and baloxavir marboxil (oral) are approved by the FDA for the treatment of uncomplicated influenza infections in pediatric patients. So far, antiviral therapy's efficacy for URTIs is limited and treating physicians needs to ponder potential side effects and treatment necessity. Especially in immunocompromised patients, antiviral treatment has to be taken into consideration to prevent possible severe complications. Also, influenza and COVID-19 may not be distinguished clinically during the COVID-19 pandemic period. While waiting for the test results, antiviral therapy should be initiated in patients to indicate antiviral treatment for influenza infection.

References

1. Heikkinen T. Respiratory viruses and children. J Infect. 2016;72:29–33.
2. Liguoro I, Pilotto C, Bonanni M, et al. SARS-COV-2 infection in children and newborns: a systematic review. Eur J Pediatr. 2020;179:1029–46.
3. Heikkinen T, Järvinen A. The common cold. Lancet. 2006;361:51–9.
4. Patick AK. Rhinovirus chemotherapy. Antiviral Res. 2006;71:391–6.
5. Ruf BR, Szucs T. Reducing the burden of influenza-associated complications with antiviral therapy. Infection. 2009;37:186–96.
6. Glezen WP. Prevention of acute otitis media by prophylaxis and treatment of influenza virus infections. Vaccine. 2001;19:56–8.
7. Hayden FG. Influenza virus and rhinovirus-related otitis media: potential for antiviral intervention. Vaccine. 2001;19:66–70.
8. Tan KS, Yan Y, Ong HH, Chow VTK, Shi L, Wang D-Y. Impact of respiratory virus infections in exacerbation of acute and chronic rhinosinusitis. Curr Allergy Asthma Rep. 2017;17:24.
9. Mossad SB. Treatment of the common cold. BMJ. 1998;317:33–6.
10. Rotbart HA. Antiviral therapy for enteroviruses and rhinoviruses. Antivir Chem Chemother. 2000;11:26171.
11. Gwaltney JM. Viral respiratory infection therapy: historical perspectives and current trials. Am J Med. 2002;112:33–41.
12. Mejias A, Ramilo O. New options in the treatment of respiratory syncytial virus disease. J Infect. 2015;71:80–7.

13. Esposito S, Mastrolia MV. Metapneumovirus infections and respiratory complications. Semin Respir Crit Care Med. 2016;37:512–21.
14. Mammas IN, Theodoridou M, Kramvis A, et al. Paediatric virology: a rapidly increasing educational challenge. Exp Ther Med. 2017;13:364–77.
15. Shook BC, Lin K. Recent advances in developing antiviral therapies for respiratory syncytial virus. Top Curr Chem. 2017;375:40.
16. American Academy of Pediatrics Committee on Infectious Diseases. Recommendations for prevention and control of influenza in children, 2020–2021. Pediatrics. 2020;146(4):e2020024588.
17. Ison MG. Clinical use of approved influenza antivirals: therapy and prophylaxis. Influenza Other Respi Viruses. 2013;1:7–13.
18. Rotrosen ET, Neuzil KM. Influenza: a global perspective. Pediatr Clin North Am. 2017;64:911–36.
19. Uyeki TM. Influenza. Ann Intern Med. 2017;5:ITC33–48.
20. Heo YA. Baloxavir: first global approval. Drugs. 2018;78:693.
21. Esposito S, Principi N. Oseltamivir for influenza infection in children: risks and benefits. Expert Rev Respir Med. 2015;10:79–87.
22. Wang K, Shun-Shin M, Gill P, Perera R, Harnden A. Neuraminidase inhibitors for preventing and treating influenza in children (published trials only). Cochrane Database Syst Rev. 2012;4:CD002744.
23. Jefferson T, Jones M, Doshi P, Spencer EA, Onakpoya I, Henedgan CJ. Oseltamivir for influenza in adults and children: systematic review of clinical study reports and summary of regulatory comments. BMJ. 2014;9:348.
24. Winther B, Block SL, Reisinger K, Outkowski R. Impact of oseltamivir treatment on the incidence and course of acute otitis media in children with influenza. Int J Pediatr Otorhinolaryngol. 2010;74:684–8.
25. Piedra PA, Schulman KL, Blumentals WA. Effects of oseltamivir on influenza-related complications in children with chronic medical conditions. Pediatrics. 2009;124:170–8.
26. Whitley RJ, Hayden FG, Reisinger KS, et al. Oral oseltamivir treatment of influenza in children. Pediatr Infect Dis J. 2001;20:12733.
27. Centers for Disease Control and Prevention. Influenza antiviral drug resistance. https://www.cdc.gov/flu/treatment/antiviralresistance.htm. Accessed 20 Dec 2020.
28. Couturier BA, Bender JM, Schwarz MA, Pavia AT, Hanson KE, She RC. Oseltamivir-resistant influenza A 2009 H1N1 virus in immunocompromised patients. Influenza Other Respi Viruses. 2010;4:199–204.
29. McCullers JA. Influenza viruses. In: Cherry JD, Harrison GJ, Kaplan SL, Steinbach WJ, Hotez PJ, editors. Feigin and Cherry's textbook of pediatric infectious diseases. 8th ed. Philadelphia: Elseiver; 2019. p. 1729–44.
30. Marty FM, Man CY, van der Horst C, et al. Safety and pharmacokinetics of intravenous zanamivir treatment in hospitalized adults with influenza: an open-label, multicenter, single-arm, phase II study. J Infect Dis. 2014;209:542–50.
31. European Medicines Agency. Zanamivir (Dectova®). https://www.ema.europa.eu/en/medicines/human/EPAR/dectova. Accessed 20 Dec 2020.
32. Baker J, Block SL, Matharu B, et al. Baloxavir marboxil single-dose treatment in influenza-infected children: a randomized, double-blind, active-controlled phase 3 safety and efficacy trial (miniSTONE-2). Pediatr Infect Dis J. 2020;39:700–5.
33. Deville JG, Song E, Ouellette CP. Coronavirus disease 2019 (COVID-19): management in children. In: Edwards MS, Torchia MM (eds). Uptodate.com, https://www.uptodate.com/contents/coronavirus-disease-2019-covid-19-management-in-children. Accessed 20 Dec 2020.
34. Chiotos K, Hayes M, Kimberlin DW, et al. Multicenter interim guidance on use of antivirals for children with coronavirus disease 2019/severe acute respiratory syndrome coronavirus. J Pediatric Infect Dis Soc. 2020;22:piaa045.
35. World Health Organization. Therapeutics and COVID-19: living guideline. https://www.who.int/publications/i/item/therapeutics-and-covid-19-living-guideline. Accessed 20 Dec 2020.

36. Siemieniuk R, Rochwerg B, Agoritsas T, et al. A living WHO guideline on drugs for covid-19. BMJ. 2020;370:m3379.
37. Lamontagne F. Update to living WHO guideline on drugs for covid-19. BMJ. 2020;371:m4475.
38. RECOVERY Collaborative Group, Horby P, Mafham M, et al. Effect of hydroxychloroquine in hospitalized patients with Covid-19. N Engl J Med. 2020;383(21):2030–40.

Antifungal Agents for Pediatric Ear, Nose, and Throat Infections

Tuğçe Tural Kara, Ergin Çiftçi, and Emin Sami Arısoy

85.1 Introduction

Ear, nose, and throat (ENT) infections are common in childhood. Although many bacterial and viral agents can cause ENT infections, fungal agents are also frequently reported. Fungi are commonly responsible for superficial infections in healthy children and invasive infections in children with severe underlying disease.

Superficial fungal infections frequently seen in children are localized in keratin-containing areas, such as hair, skin, and nails. Tinea capitis, tinea pedis, mucocutaneous candidiasis, onychomycosis, and pityriasis versicolor are the most common superficial fungal infections. And *Trichophyton, Microsporum,* and *Epidermophyton* species are the most frequent causative microorganisms. The clinical course can vary according to the patient's immunological condition, localization of the infection, and the fungus' genus [1, 2]. The patient is treated with topical or systemic antifungal drugs, depending on the clinical symptoms, immunologic status, infection site, and pathogen [3].

T. T. Kara (✉)
Division of Pediatric Infectious Diseases, Department of Pediatrics, Faculty of Medicine, Akdeniz University, Antalya, Turkey

E. Çiftçi
Division of Pediatric Infectious Diseases, Department of Pediatrics, Faculty of Medicine, Ankara University, Ankara, Turkey

E. S. Arısoy
Division of Pediatric Infectious Diseases, Department of Pediatrics, Faculty of Medicine, Kocaeli University, Kocaeli, Turkey

Invasive fungal infections are the leading cause of death in immunosuppressed children. Patients at high risk for these infections include those born prematurely, with burn injuries, undergoing organ transplantation, human immunodeficiency virus (HIV) infection, receiving chemotherapy, corticosteroids, or antibiotics, with diabetes mellitus; neutropenia, and those undergoing surgery [4–6]. Early diagnosis, tissue debridement, and long-term systemic antifungal treatment are necessary for a successful recovery. Although *Candida* and *Aspergillus* species are the most frequently observed causative agents in invasive fungal infections, rare pathogens such as *Cryptococcus*, *Histoplasma*, and Zygomycetes (formerly Phycomycetes) have also been reported. Furthermore, microorganisms resistant to fluconazole (e.g., *Candida glabrata* and *Candida krusei*) resulting from routine treatment with fluconazole prophylaxis are also seen as causative agents [7].

Antifungal drugs are used as prophylaxis, empiric, and preemptive treatment of infections. Data related to the pharmacokinetics, side effects, and effectiveness of these drugs in children are limited, and adult studies' data causes difficulties in treating pediatric patients. For example, few topical antifungal drugs used for superficial fungal infections are recommended for children under the age of 13. Despite this, many antifungal agents provide effective treatment with few side effects, and most of these agents act on the ergosterol, an essential component of the fungal cell membrane.

Commonly used antifungal drugs are classified as polyenes, azoles, allylamines, pyrimidines, and echinocandins (Table 85.1).

85.2 Polyenes

Polyene antimycotics, a class of antimicrobial polyene compounds, and a subgroup of macrolides are produced from some *Streptomyces* species. Polyenes bind to ergosterol in the fungal cell membrane, thus weakens it, causing leakage of potassium and sodium ions, which may contribute to cell death. Amphotericin B and nystatin are the leading examples of polyenes.

85.2.1 Amphotericin B

Amphotericin B deoxycholate, a systemic antifungal agent presented initially in 1958, is among the leading antifungal drugs. It has also been prescribed as a drug of combination therapy with new generation antifungals [8]. However, drug companies were directed to search for new drugs because of the increasing side effects observed, such as nephrotoxicity, electrolyte abnormalities, and infusion-related adverse effects.

Amphotericin B binds to the fungal cytoplasmic membrane's ergosterol component that causes the formation of transmembrane pores. Increasing the cell membrane permeability and leakage of intracellular contents can lead to fungal cell death [9]. Amphotericin B has more affinity for the fungal ergosterol than the sterol in the

Table 85.1 Antifungal drugs used frequently to treat pediatric patients

Drug class	Antifungal drug	Age	Route	Pediatric dosing
Polyene	Amphotericin B deoxycholate		IV	1–1.5 mg/kg/day
	Liposomal amphotericin B		IV	1–5 mg/kg/day
	Amphotericin B lipid complex		IV	3–5 mg/kg/day
Pyrimidine analog	Flucytosine		Oral	150 mg/kg/day
Azole	Fluconazole		Oral/IV	6–12 mg/kg/day
	Voriconazole	2 to <12 years	IV	9 mg/kg/dose twice daily first day, then 8 mg/kg/dose twice daily
			Oral	9 mg/kg/dose twice daily
		≥12 years	IV	<50 kg: 9 mg/kg/dose twice daily first day, then 4–8 mg/kg/dose twice daily
				≥50 kg: 6 mg/kg/dose twice daily first day, then 3–4 mg/kg/dose twice daily
			Oral	<50 kg: 9 mg/kg/dose twice daily
				≥50 kg: 200 mg/dose twice daily
	Itraconazole		Oral	2.5–5 mg/kg/dose twice daily
	Posaconazole	≥13 years	Oral	200 mg/dose 3 times daily
				800 mg/day 2–4 times daily
Echinocandin	Caspofungin		IV	70 mg/m² first day, then 50 mg/m²/day
	Micafungin		IV	2–3 mg/kg/day
	Anidulafungin		IV	3 mg/kg/day first day, then 1.5 mg/kg/day

IV indicates intravenous.

human cell membranes. However, this difference disappears in organs where blood drug concentration is high. Side effects such as hypokalemia, hypomagnesemia, renal tubular acidosis, polyuria, and metabolic acidosis commonly occur in kidneys due to distal tubal destruction [10]. Nephrotoxicity is the most frequent dose-limiting adverse effect. Fortunately, it is less serious in children than in adults.

Also, amphotericin B has infusion-related side effects, such as fever, nausea, chills, and vomiting, due to the release of proinflammatory cytokines. Lipid formulations (liposomal amphotericin B, amphotericin B lipid complex, and amphotericin B colloidal dispersion) reduce all these adverse effects [11]. All amphotericin B products are used parenterally because of low oral bioavailability.

Amphotericin B deoxycholate is a broad-spectrum antifungal used to treat *Candida* spp. (excluding *Candida lusitaniae*), *Aspergillus* spp. (excluding *Aspergillus terreus* and *Aspergillus nidulans*), Zygomycetes, *Cryptococcus*, *Histoplasma capsulatum*, and *Blastomyces dermatitidis* [12, 13]. Also, it is commonly used for treating life-threatening invasive fungal infections.

The fungicidal effect of the drug depends on its level of concentration. Increased drug concentration at the infection site leads to an increased fungicidal effect until it reaches 4–10 times the minimum inhibitory concentration (MIC) required for the microorganism. However, no clinical studies have shown that a drug dose >1 mg/kg/day is required for successful treatment [3]. Amphotericin B has a sustained antifungal effect under the MIC levels; therefore, one dose per day is sufficient [14]. The recommended daily dose for neonates is 1–1.5 mg/kg/day and 0.25–0.5 mg/kg/day for infants, children, and adolescents, however, in severe infections 1.5 mg/kg/day can be given [11]. Although the primary route of excretion is unknown, a small portion is excreted through the kidneys and biliary tract. The dosage of the drug is not affected by liver and kidney failure [3].

There are increasing data on amphotericin B and lipid formulation in children with ENT infections [8]. Chakravarti et al. [15] reported three pediatric patients with mucormycosis in the nose who were successfully treated with amphotericin B. Liposomal formulations had been reported as the drug of choice for rhino-orbital-cerebral mucormycosis [9]. Liposomal amphotericin B is the primary empiric drug for acute invasive fungal rhinosinusitis [16]. The recommended doses for liposomal amphotericin B and amphotericin B lipid complex are 1–5 mg/kg/day and 3–5 mg/kg/day, respectively [17].

Treatment should be based on the causative microorganism detected by culture or histopathologically. For example, if *Aspergillus* spp. is the causative pathogen microorganism, voriconazole should be administered [18]. Some authors use topical amphotericin B in the infected area, but there are no definitive data on the optimal dose [19]. Furthermore, the topical form is expensive, and serious side effects have been reported [20].

85.2.2 Nystatin

Nystatin is a polyene antifungal drug prescribed for early, uncomplicated otomycosis and superficial *Candida* infections. It binds to the ergosterol in the fungus' cell membrane, thus augmenting cells' permeability, leading to cell death [3]. Topical and oral formulations are available. Nystatin is used for oral candidiasis. The recommended dose for neonates is 100,000 to 400,000 units/dose, 4 times per day, for infants 200,000 to 400,000 units/dose, 4 times per day or 100,000 units on both sides of the mouth 4 times per day, and for children and adolescents 400,000–600,000 units orally 4 times per day [21]. Although oral forms are well tolerated, adverse effects such as nausea, vomiting, stomach pain, and diarrhea may occur. The topical formulation can be used for cutaneous and mucocutaneous fungal infections.

85.3   Pyrimidine Analogues

The pyrimidine analogs interfere with the nucleic acid synthesis and require specialized membrane transporters for entry into cells. Intracellular enzymes convert these drugs to active metabolites. The antiproliferative effect of pyrimidine analogs is achieved by incorporating DNA, resulting in DNA synthesis inhibition. They can also interfere with nucleic acid synthesis enzymes, such as DNA polymerases and ribonucleotide reductase.

85.3.1 Flucytosine

Flucytosine has activity against fungal species by interfering with pyrimidine uptake, deaminated to 5-fluorouracil, and converted to an inhibitor of thymidylate synthetase, which interferes with DNA synthesis. Flucytosine also inhibits RNA and fungal protein synthesis. In the 1970s, flucytosine was used as an antifungal agent. However, rapid resistance development and severe side effects, such as gastrointestinal intolerance and bone marrow suppression, can lead to treatment failure. Therefore, clinicians use it in combination with other medicines. It can effectively treat *Candida* spp. and *Cryptococcus*. In sites where the penetration of amphotericin B is low, flucytosine increases its antifungal activity. Flucytosine is available only as an oral formulation, and the recommended dose is 150 mg/kg/day divided into four doses [17, 22]. It is essential to monitor serum drug levels closely, particularly in cases of renal failure.

85.4   Antifungal Triazoles

There are two groups of azole antifungal drugs: imidazoles and triazoles. Imidazoles are generally used for superficial fungal infections of the mouth, skin, and vagina in topical formulations. They are active against several filamentous fungi, including many *Candida* spp., but they are less active against *Candida krusei*. Clotrimazole, miconazole, and econazole are used for vaginal candidiasis and dermatophyte infections such as ringworm, of which the causative agents generally are *Trichophyton*, *Microsporon*, or *Epidermophyton* spp. Miconazole is also used topically for oral infections and can be given orally for intestinal infections as it is poorly absorbed from the gut [3, 9].

Triazole antifungals are often used for the treatment of systemic fungal infections. Triazoles inhibit the cytochrome p450-dependent enzyme lanosterol 14-alpha-demethylase, which converts lanosterol to ergosterol, leading to fungal cell destruction and death [17]. Triazoles are broad-spectrum antifungal drugs without severe side effects, such as nephrotoxicity. When used alone, fluconazole is effective against yeast; voriconazole, itraconazole, posaconazole, and isavuconazole have antifungal activity against molds [23].

85.4.1 Fluconazole

Fluconazole is the most frequently used antifungal drug for children. The US Federal Drug Administration (FDA) has approved using fluconazole in all age groups for candidiasis, cryptococcal meningitis, and antifungal prophylaxis in allogeneic bone marrow recipients. *Candida* is a frequent pathogen in ENT infections in children, causing infections that appear as white plaques in the mouth and throat, especially in the first few weeks of life. Fluconazole is an effective drug for oropharyngeal candidiasis. Most of the *Candida* spp. (especially *C. albicans*) are susceptible to fluconazole; however, it has no antifungal effect on mold fungi.

Oral and parenteral formulations of fluconazole are available with the same daily dose [24]. Food and gastric acidity do not affect its absorption rate when orally administered. Protein binding activity is low, and it passes to the tissues quite easily. The drug concentration in the cerebrospinal fluid and vitreous fluid can reach 80% in blood. Its concentration in urine is 10–20 times higher than in blood. Thus, fluconazole is an effective agent for treating urinary tract infections [3]. A single daily dose of 6–12 mg/kg/day is recommended (maximum dose 600 mg/day) [17]. The treatment duration and drug dose are adjusted depending on how severe the disease is. Some adverse effects, such as gastrointestinal disturbances, skin reactions, hepatitis, and abnormal hepatic function tests, can be seen. In a meta-analysis by Egunsola et al. [25], fluconazole was compared to placebo and other groups of antifungal drugs. And fluconazole was not found to be risky in terms of hepatoxicity.

85.4.2 Voriconazole

Voriconazole, a second-generation triazole with broad-spectrum antifungal activity, has fungicidal properties in treating *Candida* spp. and *Aspergillus* spp. [26]. It is the most commonly used antifungal agent for invasive aspergillosis [11]. Oral tablets, oral suspension, and parenteral formulations are available. However, only oral suspension formulation is given to patients <12 years old due to short gastric transit time. Serum drug levels are monitored for the following reasons: (1) interactions with other drugs metabolized by the cytochrome p450 2C19 enzyme in the liver are frequent and (2) drug elimination has nonlinear pharmacokinetics in children [27, 28]. It should be used at higher doses in children than adults to obtain similar serum concentrations. In a study conducted by Allegra et al. [29], 237 children received voriconazole for prophylaxis, and treatment results of invasive fungal infections were analyzed. It was determined that age, gender, and serum creatinine levels affect the drug's serum concentration. Furthermore, drug monitoring was required in children receiving voriconazole.

The FDA has approved voriconazole for treating fungal infections in children ≥2 years old. In children ≥2 to <12 years old, the recommended dose for the parenteral formulation is 9 mg/kg/dose on day 1 and 8 mg/kg/dose on the following days, twice daily, and 9 mg/kg/dose every 12 h for oral suspension. For children >12 years old, the dosage varies according to the patient's weight [30].

The duration of invasive fungal infection treatment (minimum 6–12 weeks) is based on the patient's underlying disease, the severity and localization of the disease, and clinical status [31]. The most significant side effects are reversible visual impairments (such as brightness and blurred vision), elevated liver enzymes, and skin reactions (photosensitization).

85.4.3 Itraconazole

Itraconazole, a first-generation triazole, is used orally to formulate capsule, tablet, or solution. It is considered an effective antifungal for fluconazole refractory oropharyngeal candidiasis, amphotericin B refractory or not tolerated invasive and non-invasive aspergillosis, blastomycosis, and histoplasmosis in children. Furthermore, itraconazole can prevent fungal infections in neutropenic children [22, 24].

Parenteral formulation of itraconazole is not currently available. Absorption of capsule and tablet form is limited, but it can increase with higher gastric acid levels and food intake. Conversely, oral solution absorption is quite good and is not slowed down by gastric acid and food intake [9]. Furthermore, 2.5–5 mg/kg/dose twice daily is recommended for the treatment and the same amount once daily for relapse prevention. However, it is not recommended for the eye and central nervous system infections due to low tissue penetration. Itraconazole is metabolized in the liver, and it is necessary to reduce the dose in patients with liver failure.

85.4.4 Posaconazole

Posaconazole, a second-generation triazole, is obtained by hydroxylation of itraconazole. It has a broader spectrum than voriconazole; therefore, it is also effective against Zygomycetes [10, 11]. Posaconazole prophylaxis is used to prevent invasive *Aspergillus* and *Candida* infections in children with graft-versus-host disease who underwent hematopoietic stem cell transplant (HSCT) and hematologic malignancies with prolonged neutropenia. Furthermore, posaconazole is recommended to treat fluconazole-resistant or itraconazole-resistant oropharyngeal candidiasis and invasive aspergillosis not responding to first-line antifungal therapy.

Oral suspension, delayed-release tablets, and intravenous injection formulations are available. The FDA approved oral suspension and delayed-release tablet forms in children ≥13 years old and parenteral forms in patients aged ≥18 years old [32]. For patients with prophylaxis, the preferred daily dose is 200 mg 3 times orally. The duration of prophylaxis depends on the course of immunosuppression and neutropenia. A dose of 800 mg/day 2–4 times daily is recommended for the treatment [33]. Consuming the oral suspension form with foods high in fat is recommended as it increases the absorption rate. Side effects such as arrhythmia, QT prolongation, hepatotoxicity, nausea, vomiting, diarrhea, headache, fever, hypokalemia, thrombocytopenia, rash, and abdominal pain can occur [34]. Posaconazole is commonly excreted in the feces, and it is not necessary to reduce the dose in case of renal insufficiency [35].

In the study conducted by Zhang et al. [36], pediatric patients with acute lymphoblastic leukemia who received posaconazole prophylaxis (n 70) and fluconazole prophylaxis (n 25) were analyzed. The study showed that posaconazole prophylaxis reduces invasive fungal infections and increases infection-free survival.

85.5 Echinocandins

Echinocandins, a group of cyclic lipopeptides, inhibit the synthesis of beta-glucan in the fungal cell wall via non-competitive inhibition of the enzyme 1,3-beta-glucan synthase. This enzyme's inhibition weakens the fungal cell wall, resulting in osmotic lysis and, eventually, cell death. Echinocandins class has been termed the "penicillin of antifungals" as the action mechanism resembles penicillin in bacteria. Beta-glucans are carbohydrate polymers cross-linked with other cell wall components, the fungal equivalent to bacterial peptidoglycan [14]. Caspofungin, micafungin, and anidulafungin are semisynthetic echinocandin derivatives.

Although echinocandins are fungicidal against *Candida* spp. (including fluconazole-resistant *C. glabrata* and *C. krusei*), they are fungistatic against the *Aspergillus* species. Therefore, echinocandins are recommended to be used with triazoles for treating invasive aspergillosis [22, 32]. Echinocandins are safe to use in pediatric patients due to their relatively low renal or hepatic toxicity [17].

85.5.1 Caspofungin

As an antimycotic echinocandin cyclic lipopeptide, caspofungin is semisynthetically derived from a fermentation product of the fungus *Glarea lozoyensis* [3, 9]. Caspofungin has been effective in treating fungal infections caused by *Candida* and *Aspergillus* species [14]. It is used for the treatment of esophageal and invasive candidiasis. Caspofungin is also used for the empiric antifungal therapy of febrile neutropenic patients and rescue therapy for invasive aspergillosis [37]. The FDA approved it for use in children >3 months old [32]. It is available in parenteral form only. The preferred daily dosage is 70 mg/m^2 loading on day 1, followed by 50 mg/m^2/day on subsequent days (maximum 70 mg/day). Adverse effects are uncommon compared to other groups of antifungal drugs.

85.5.2 Micafungin

Micafungin, a cyclic hexapeptide echinocandin, which dissolves in water, is derived from a natural product of the fungus *Coleophama empedri*. Like other echinocandins, micafungin noncompetitively inhibits the fungal 1,3-beta-D-glucan synthase, the essential enzyme for cell wall synthesis. The FDA approved it for the following treatments in children >4 months old: (1) esophageal candidiasis, candidemia, acute disseminated candidiasis, *Candida* peritonitis, and abscess and (2) prophylaxis of *Candida* infections in HSCT patients [38]. Micafungin has no antifungal activity for the treatment of cryptococcosis, fusariosis, and zygomycosis. A dose of 2–3 mg/kg/day once per day is recommended for the treatment. The dosage can be increased if the required response is not achieved [31]. For treating candidiasis in infants, high doses (10–15 mg/kg/day) may be needed due to pharmacokinetic differences. The recommended dose for prophylaxis is 1–3 mg/kg/day [39]. Due to the absence of cell walls in mammals, the toxic effect of micafungin acting on the fungal cell wall is expected to be minimal. However, nausea, vomiting, diarrhea, fever, infusion-related reactions, phlebitis, elevated liver enzymes, elevated alkaline phosphatase, hypoglycemia, and electrolyte disturbances have been reported [34]. In the study conducted by Leverger et al. [40], 110 pediatric patients who received micafungin for the treatment or prophylaxis of invasive fungal infections were analyzed. Adverse effects occurred in 28% of the patients, while only 1 reported serious adverse effects.

85.5.3 Anidulafungin

Anidulafungin, a semisynthetic echinocandin, like other cyclic lipopeptides, inhibits glucan synthase, an enzyme essential in synthesizing 1–3-beta-D-glucan, a major fungal cell wall component. Glucan synthase not present in mammalian cells is an attractive target for antifungal activity.

Anidulafungin is used to treat candidemia, esophageal candidiasis, and other types of Candida infections like intra-abdominal abscess and peritonitis; however, it is not approved for fungal infections in pediatric patients [37]. Anidulafungin is preferred, especially in patients with hepatic insufficiency, because it is the only echinocandin not metabolized in the liver [41].

85.6 Conclusion

Fungi are among etiologic agents of ENT infections in children. There are many antifungal drugs used for prophylaxis, empiric, and preemptive treatment of fungal infections. Although fungal infections can cause serious problems, especially in immunosuppressive children, antifungals used with appropriate indications, doses, and duration provide good clinical results.

References

1. Hawkins DM, Smidt AC. Superficial fungal infections in children. Pediatr Clin North Am. 2014;61:443–55.

2. Kovitwanichkanont T, Chong AH. Superficial fungal infections. Aust J Gen Pract. 2019;48:706–11.

3. Wattier RL, Steinbach WJ. Antifungal agents. In: Long SS, Prober CG, Fischer M, editors. Principles and practice of pediatric infectious diseases. 5th ed. Philadelphia: Elsevier; 2018. p. 1532–41.

4. Pana ZD, Roilides E, Warris A, Groll AH, Zaoutis T. Epidemiology of invasive fungal disease in children. J Pediatric Infect Dis Soc. 2017;6:3–11.

5. Ibáñez-Martínez E, Ruiz-Gaitán A, Pemán-García J. Update on the diagnosis of invasive fungal infection. Rev Esp Quimioter. 2017;30:16–21.

6. von Lilienfeld-Toal M, Wagener J, Einsele H, Cornely OA, Kurzai O. Invasive fungal infection. Dtsch Arztebl Int. 2019;116:271–8.

7. Bhattacharya S, Sae-Tia S, Fries BC. Candidiasis and mechanisms of antifungal resistance. Antibiotics (Basel). 2020;9:312–31.

8. Faustino C, Pinheiro L. Lipid systems for the delivery of amphotericin b in antifungal therapy. Pharmaceutics. 2020;12:29–76.

9. Nett JE, Andes DR. Antifungal agents: spectrum of activity, pharmacology, and clinical indications. Infect Dis Clin North Am. 2016;30:51–83.

10. Lewis RE. Current concepts in antifungal pharmacology. Mayo Clin Proc. 2011;86:805–17.

11. Cohen-Wolkowiez M, Moran C, Benjamin DK Jr, Smith PB. Pediatric antifungal agents. Curr Opin Infect Dis. 2009;22:553–8.

12. Groll AH, Rijnders BJA, Walsh TJ, Adler-Moore J, Lewis RE, Brüggemann RJM. Clinical pharmacokinetics, pharmacodynamics, safety and efficacy of liposomal amphotericin B. Clin Infect Dis. 2019;68:260–74.

13. Houšť J, Spížek J, Havlíček V. Antifungal drugs. Metabolism. 2020;10:106–22.

14. Groll AH, Piscitelli SC, Walsh TJ. Antifungal pharmacodynamics: concentration-effect relationships in vitro and in vivo. Pharmacotherapy. 2001;21:133–48.

15. Chakravarti A, Bhargava R, Bhattacharya S. Cutaneous mucormycosis of nose and facial region in children: a case series. Int J Pediatr Otorhinolaryngol. 2013;77:869–72.

16. Deutsch PG, Whittaker J, Prasad S. Invasive and non-invasive fungal rhinosinusitis-a review and update of the evidence. Medicina (Kaunas). 2019;55:319–33.

17. Watt K, Benjamin DK Jr, Cohen-Wolkowiez M. Pharmacokinetics of antifungal agents in children. Early Hum Dev. 2011;87:61–5.

18. Herbrecht R, Denning DW, Patterson TF, Invasive Fungal Infections Group of the European Organisation for Research and Treatment of Cancer and the Global Aspergillus Study Group, et al. Voriconazole versus amphotericin B for primary therapy of invasive aspergillosis. N Engl J Med. 2002;347:408–15.

19. Liu YC, Zhou ML, Cheng KJ, Zhou SH, Wen X, Chang CD. Successful treatment of invasive fungal rhinosinusitis caused by *Cunninghamella*: a case report and review of the literature. World J Clin Cases. 2019;7:228–35.

20. Head K, Sharp S, Chong LY, Hopkins C, Philpott C. Topical and systemic antifungal therapy for chronic rhinosinusitis. Cochrane Database Syst Rev. 2018;9:CD012453.

21. Hoppe JE. Treatment of oropharyngeal candidiasis and candidal diaper dermatitis in neonates and infants: review and reappraisal. Pediatr Infect Dis J. 1997;16:885–94.

22. Lestner JM, Smith PB, Cohen-Wolkowiez M, Benjamin DK Jr, Hope WW. Antifungal agents and therapy for infants and children with invasive fungal infections: a pharmacological perspective. Br J Clin Pharmacol. 2013;75:1381–95.

23. Bellmann R, Smuszkiewicz P. Pharmacokinetics of antifungal drugs: practical implications for optimized treatment of patients. Infection. 2017;45:737–79.

24. Allen U. Antifungal agents for the treatment of systemic fungal infections in children. Paediatr Child Health. 2010;15:603–15.

25. Egunsola O, Adefurin A, Fakis A, et al. Safety of fluconazole in paediatrics: a systematic review. Eur J Clin Pharmacol. 2013;69:1211–21.

26. Shi C, Xiao Y, Mao Y, Wu J, Lin N. Voriconazole: a review of population pharmacokinetic analyses. Clin Pharmacokinet. 2019;58:687–703.

27. Gastine S, Lehrnbecher T, Müller C, et al. Pharmacokinetic modeling of voriconazole to develop an alternative dosing regimen in children. Antimicrob Agents Chemother. 2017;62:e01194–17.
28. Espinoza N, Galdames J, Navea D, Farfán MJ, Salas C. Frequency of the CYP2C19*17 polymorphism in a Chilean population and its effect on voriconazole plasma concentration in immunocompromised children. Sci Rep. 2019;9:8863–9.
29. Allegra S, Fatiguso G, De Francia S, et al. Therapeutic drug monitoring of voriconazole for treatment and prophylaxis of invasive fungal infection in children. Br J Clin Pharmacol. 2018;84:197–203.
30. Boast A, Curtis N, Cranswick N, Gwee A. Voriconazole dosing and therapeutic drug monitoring in children: experience from a paediatric tertiary care centre. J Antimicrob Chemother. 2016;71:2031–6.
31. Patterson TF, Thompson GR 3rd, Denning DW, et al. Practice guidelines for the diagnosis and management of aspergillosis:2016 update by the Infectious Diseases Society of America. Clin Infect Dis. 2016;63:1–60.
32. Ramos-Martín V, O'Connor O, Hope W. Clinical pharmacology of antifungal agents in pediatrics: children are not small adults. Curr Opin Pharmacol. 2015;24:128–34.
33. Lehrnbecher T. The clinical management of invasive mold infection in children with cancer or undergoing hematopoietic stem cell transplantation. Expert Rev Anti Infect Ther. 2019;17:489–99.
34. Ramos JT, Romero CA, Belda S, et al. Fungal infection study Group of Spanish Society of Paediatric infectious disease (SEIP); Traslational research network in pediatric infectious diseases (RITIP). Clinical practice update of antifungal prophylaxis in immunocompromised children. Rev Esp Quimioter. 2019;32:410–25.
35. Vicenzi EB, Cesaro S. Posaconazole in immunocompromised pediatric patients. Expert Rev Anti Infect Ther. 2018;16:543–53.
36. Zhang T, Bai J, Huang M, et al. Posaconazole and fluconazole prophylaxis during induction therapy for pediatric acute lymphoblastic leukemia. J Microbiol Immunol Infect. 2020;1684(20):30165–1.
37. Maximova N, Schillani G, Simeone R, Maestro A, Zanon D. Comparison of efficacy and safety of caspofungin versus micafungin in pediatric allogeneic stem cell transplant recipients: a retrospective analysis. Adv Ther. 2017;34:1184–99.
38. Wasmann RE, Muilwijk EW, Burger DM, Verweij PE, Knibbe CA, Brüggemann RJ. Clinical pharmacokinetics and pharmacodynamics of micafungin. Clin Pharmacokinet. 2018;57:267–86.
39. Kusuki S, Hashii Y, Yoshida H, et al. Antifungal prophylaxis with micafungin in patients treated for childhood cancer. Pediatr Blood Cancer. 2009;53:605–9.
40. Leverger G, Timsit JF, Milpied N, Gachot B. Use of micafungin for the prevention and treatment of invasive fungal infections in everyday pediatric care in France: results of the MYRIADE study. Pediatr Infect Dis J. 2019;38:716–21.
41. Patil A, Majumdar S. Echinocandins in antifungal pharmacotherapy. J Pharm Pharmacol. 2017;69:1635–60.

Symptomatic Agents for Pediatric Ear, Nose, and Throat Infections

86

Nevin Hatipoğlu, Emin Sami Arısoy,
and Armando G. Correa

86.1 Introduction

Ear, nose, and throat (ENT) infections pose a high burden in the pediatric age group. The most common of these, also referred to as upper respiratory tract infections (URTI), are nasopharyngitis (i.e., the common cold), tonsillopharyngitis, rhinosinusitis, otitis media, and laryngotracheitis. In general, these infections are initially caused by viral agents, making antibiotics unnecessary for treatment. On the other hand, any of these conditions may cause considerable discomfort to the patient, justifying the quest to relieve symptoms and management with supportive care. Also, there is a high socioeconomic burden associated with URTI, which contributes to inappropriate use and over-prescription of medications [1].

There are many agents on the market used for the symptomatic treatment of ENT infections. Some of these agents can also be encountered in over-the-counter (OTC) medications and are approved in adults [2, 3]. Certain medications have been discouraged in young children due to a lack of proven efficacy and concerns about reliability and safety.

N. Hatipoğlu (✉)
Section of Pediatric Infectious Diseases, Bakırköy Dr. Sadi Konuk Training and Research Hospital, University of Health Sciences, İstanbul, Turkey
e-mail: nevin.hatipoglu@saglik.gov.tr

E. S. Arısoy
Division of Pediatric Infectious Diseases, Department of Pediatrics, Faculty of Medicine, Kocaeli University, Kocaeli, Turkey

A. G. Correa
Section of Academic General Pediatrics, Department of Pediatrics, Baylor College of Medicine, and Section of International and Destination Medicine, Texas Children's Hospital, Houston, TX, USA

There are not many indications for symptomatic medications in the treatment of childhood ENT infections [4]. The most common goals for their use include fever reduction, pain relief, facilitation of the flow of nasal secretions, and diminishing sore throat. Although symptomatic agents help relieve complaints and provide the patient some comfort, they do not shorten the overall duration of the disease.

86.2   Antipyretics and Pain Relievers

Pain is a prominent source of discomfort for many ENT infections. Acute otitis media (AOM) is one of the most common ENT infections for which children seek medical care. Patients with AOM frequently suffer from ear pain [5], and antibiotics do not relieve this symptom directly; only after a few days of their use may be started to see some benefit. Symptomatic treatment to reduce ear pain is recommended in some AOM guidelines [6]. Both acetaminophen and ibuprofen are appropriate for pain control in this condition; they relieve pain at a similar rate with no difference in the frequency of adverse reactions [7].

Patients with tonsillopharyngitis usually have bothersome throat pain and a resulting decrease in oral intake. Systemic analgesics help in the control of sore throat. Both acetaminophen and ibuprofen are recommended [8], though ibuprofen is more effective than acetaminophen in reducing throat pain in some trials [9].

Acetaminophen (paracetamol) is one of the most widely used medicines and is the prototype of analgesics and antipyretics. Similar to non-steroidal anti-inflammatory drugs (NSAIDs), acetaminophen inhibits cyclooxygenase (COX) activity. The antipyretic activity of acetaminophen is due to the COX-2 blockade. This, in turn, reduces the concentration of prostaglandin E_2, which results in a reduction in the hypothalamic set point for fever. Overall, acetaminophen has a slightly less analgesic effect than the NSAIDs. It shows little anti-platelet activity and has no significant toxicity to the upper gastrointestinal tract [10, 11]. The usual dose is 10–15 mg/kg of body weight orally every 4–6 h as needed (maximum single dose is 1 g, maximum daily dose is 75 mg/kg up to 4 g/day; maximum of 5 doses per day). It is tolerated well. At doses of 120–150 mg/kg of body weight, acetaminophen may be associated with liver toxicity [12].

Ibuprofen is a member of NSAIDs and is a potent inhibitor of prostaglandin synthesis, and its therapeutic and toxic effects are linked to this characteristic. Gastrointestinal side effects are more pronounced with ibuprofen compared to acetaminophen. Caution is recommended when ibuprofen is used in dehydrated patients because of the increased potential for side effects, including nephrotoxicity [9]. The recommended dose is 10 mg/kg orally every 6 h as needed (maximum single dose 600 mg; maximum daily dose 40 mg/kg up to 2.4 g/day).

Aspirin is not recommended for reducing fever or relieving pain in children because of the potential for the development of Reye's syndrome [13].

Topical analgesics, such as benzocaine, procaine, or lidocaine preparations, are other groups of pain relievers used for children with AOM over 2 years old.

Lidocaine and *benzocaine* are local anesthetics and show their action by stabilizing the neuronal membrane. They cause surface anesthesia by preventing the transmission of impulses along nerve fibers and at nerve endings. Benzocaine and lidocaine are shown more effective than placebo in reducing ear pain due to AOM in school-aged children [14, 15]. Topical anesthetics are especially useful in the first 2–3 days of therapy, but their effect after application may be of short duration, lasting for up to 30 min only. Benzocaine can cause methemoglobinemia if used in children under 2 years of age [16]. These preparations should not be instilled if the tympanic membrane is perforated [17]. Although they appear effective when used locally, the evidence in the published literature is insufficient to endorse the routine use of ear drops to relieve ear pain in AOM [18]. Of note, the Food and Drug Administration (FDA) of the United States (US) has prohibited the distribution of these topical analgesic products because no clinical trials have been conducted to prove their safety or efficacy.

In a recent meta-analysis, experts suggest that a single, low dose of **oral glucocorticoids** may be beneficial for immune-competent patients ≥ 5 years with a sore throat that is not caused by infectious mononucleosis or related to recent surgery or intubation [19]. The immediate access to rapid pain relief should be weighed against the risk of larger cumulative doses due to recurrent acute sore throat episodes [20]. Data on the risks and benefits of corticosteroids compared to NSAIDs or acetaminophen are lacking [21]. Since there are safer alternatives for managing pain, such as acetaminophen or ibuprofen (as discussed above), the routine use of corticosteroids for acute sore throat due to ENT infections in children should not be encouraged. A recent Cochrane analysis concluded that systemic corticosteroids provide a moderate effect on both resolution and improvement of sore throat in adults and children [22].

Lozenges and hard candies help to soothe the inflamed pharynx but carry a choking risk in young children (<4 years) and should be avoided [23]. There is literature support that medical lozenges may help relieve throat pain in adults [24]. However, a recent review did not show good quality evidence on the effectiveness of these medications [25]. They have the potential for allergic reactions. Benzocaine-containing lozenges may cause methemoglobinemia. Oral rinses containing topical medication for sore throat are not better than gargling with warm salt water; the latter is cheaper, easy to prepare, and lacks the risk of an allergic reaction [26]. Gargling is inappropriate for children <6 years of age. Probiotics, sorbitol, or xylitol-based chewing gum have been evaluated for symptomatic relief of acute pharyngitis but found to be ineffective [27].

86.3 Decongestants, Antihistamines, and Antitussives

Infectious inflammation of the nasal and paranasal sinus mucosa is defined as rhinosinusitis. The acute form of the disease lasts up to 4 weeks, yet it is named "acute." Irrespective of whether there is a specific therapy (i.e., antibiotics for bacterial rhinosinusitis), patients commonly desire to get rid of long-standing symptoms such as cough, nasal congestion, or nasal discharge. Acute rhinosinusitis is usually caused by respiratory viruses, and the therapy centers around symptomatic treatment. In certain situations, bacterial rhinosinusitis is also self-limited in children, and therapy can also be supportive [28].

Cough and congestion are significant symptoms of ENT infections in children [29], and in some cases, these complaints may create considerable discomfort such as feeding problems, vomiting, and sleep disturbance. Parents are eager to seek rapid solutions to improve the quality of life for these distracting symptoms.

Phenylephrine and *pseudoepinephrine* are common ingredients of systemic OTC cough and cold preparations that provide a decongestant effect. These preparations are oral or topical sympathomimetic drugs that activate alpha-1 adrenergic receptors, produce vasoconstriction, reduce nasal blood flow, and decrease nasal congestion. The effect is to lessened tissue edema and improved ostial drainage [30]. However, decreased blood flow to inflamed sinus mucosa during acute rhinosinusitis leads to increased viscosity of secretions and occluding airflow, further increasing the patient's irritability. The delivery of antibiotics to infected sinus tissue depends on proper blood flow, which may be affected due to vascular constriction induced by decongestants. Their use in young children (especially in <4 years) is not warranted because of potentially life-threatening side effects, such as convulsions, cardiac arrhythmias, and death [31].

Oxymetazoline, one of the topical decongestants, is an alpha-adrenergic receptor stimulant. It exerts its topical effect on the arterioles of the nasal mucosa to produce vasoconstriction. The drug may provide symptomatic relief of nasal mucosal congestion in patients with rhinosinusitis. Unfortunately, topical decongestants may induce rebound congestion and worsen the symptoms with the repeated intranasal application; a short course (not more than 3 days) is usually sufficient. Nasal decongestants seem to positively affect nasal congestion in adults with the common cold [32]. However, clinical evidence for their use in the symptomatic treatment of pediatric ENT infections is lacking.

Antihistamines are the other major components found in OTC cough and cold formulations. *Chlorpheniramine, brompheniramine*, and *diphenhydramine* are the most common agents included in these preparations. These first-generation antihistamines may address some of the symptoms of ENT infection, such as the itchy and runny nose, cough, and sneezing. These agents can cause sedation and mild lethargy at lower doses through their effect on the H1 histamine receptors. At higher doses, anticholinergic effects may predominate. On such effect is the drying of respiratory secretions, which in turn may lead to the inhibition of ciliary motion, decreased clearance of infected material, and impaired drainage of sinus content.

Moreover, antihistamines may prolong the duration of middle ear effusion [33]. Antihistamines have a therapeutic role in children with allergic rhinitis, and they may provide some benefits in children with ENT infections. Their wanted and unwanted net effect should be considered when deciding on their use.

Though both decongestants and antihistamines seem to ameliorate some of the annoying rhinosinusitis symptoms, they have failed to prove a significant improvement in the outcome compared to antibiotic treatment alone [34].

Dextromethorphan is a cough suppressant (antitussive) and is structurally related to codeine. It displays its effect by decreasing cough receptors' sensitivity and interrupting cough impulse transmission by depressing the medullary cough center. The product is available for systemic usage in numerous formulations and can also be obtained as an OTC product. Dextromethorphan overdose is associated with sympathomimetic symptoms (tachycardia, dilated pupils, excessive perspiration), nervousness, and hallucinations. Toxicity may cause respiratory depression, especially in young children, and coma. The lack of reliable data showing benefit in children under 4 years of age and the risks of side effects from overdosing led to the warning to avoid their use in this age group.

Codeine is also a component of some cough formulations that causes cough suppression by direct central action in the medulla and may produce generalized CNS depression. It binds to opioid receptors in the CNS, eliciting morphine-like activity. The misuse of the drug may cause serious, life-threatening, or fatal respiratory depression and death. Its use is contraindicated in children under 12 years [35].

In summary, current evidence does not support the routine use of decongestants, antihistamines, or antitussives as supportive treatment of pediatric ENT infections [28, 36]. The rate of severe adverse events associated with OTC cough and cold medicines in children is low, with no fatal cases reported when used with the therapeutic range, but rather due to unsupervised ingestions [37] or accidental overdosing.

86.4 Naso-Occlusion Relievers

Patients with allergic rhinitis are more prone to the development of bacterial rhinosinusitis due to various contributing factors, such as mucosal congestion and impaired mucociliary clearance [38]. This fact brings to mind the concept of topical corticosteroid use for bacterial rhinosinusitis, as it is one of the cornerstones in treating allergic rhinitis. *Intranasal corticosteroids* inhibit inflammation in the mucosal lining of the nasal cavity and improve sinus drainage.

Mometasone can be prescribed for children ≥2 years with allergic and seasonal rhinitis. In children ≥12 years of age with rhinosinusitis, it has been found to provide significant symptom improvement when compared to amoxicillin and placebo [39].

Budesonide was documented to be a useful ancillary treatment to antibiotics for sinusitis and effective in reducing the cough and nasal discharge of acute sinusitis earlier in the course for children 2 years and older [40]. A meta-analysis on intranasal corticosteroid use as an adjunctive therapy yields a small benefit in treating bacterial sinusitis without significant adverse events [41]. These combined data indicate that intranasal corticosteroids' routine use is not appropriate in children with bacterial rhinosinusitis without allergic comorbidity.

İntranasal *saline solutions* can be used to irrigate nasal passages to thin the viscid sinus secretions and provide patency to the ostia. Topical saline solutions are employed for mechanical wash-up containing 0.9% or hypertonic saline in the form of sprays, drops, or irrigation fluids. Nasal saline offers an adjunctive therapy that is inexpensive and with minimal side effects such as nasal discomfort and mild bleeding [42]. This treatment improves patient's comfort and is beneficial in reducing the use of nasal decongestants [43]. However, this therapy awaits additional high-quality studies to clarify its beneficial effects [44].

Humidified air has been used for moisturizing dry nasal passages. Care must be taken to avoid accidental inhalation injury due to hot air. A systemic review did not show any benefits or harms from heated, humidified air in the common cold [45].

Neither steam nor cold mist therapy should be encouraged to manage cough symptoms in patients with URTI. Steam inhalation has even been applied for the relief of coronavirus disease 2019 (COVID-19), and unfortunately this remedy has resulted in severe burn injuries in children [46].

Sore throat is a disturbing complaint to most children with pharyngitis. Topical soothing interventions are frequently applied in pediatric practice. Though the effectiveness is not studied systemically in large trials, they may give some relief.

Warm drinks help promote mucus secretion and can be used as traditional remedies with a soothing effect. Home-made remedies such as lemon and honey drinks have not been subjected to randomized controlled trials to document their effectiveness. However, they are inexpensive and do not contain potentially harmful ingredients, as may be the case with commercial preparations. According to a recent Cochrane analysis, honey seems to relieve cough symptoms better than diphenhydramine, salbutamol, or placebo [47]. Honey can be used instead of unnecessary antibiotic treatment, and thus aids in preventing antibiotic resistance [48]. Children less than 12 months should not take honey because of the risk of infantile botulism.

86.5   Other Therapies

Although found superior to placebo in some trials, the use of **mucolytics** (e.g., guaifenesin) [49], *herbal* extracts (e.g., *Pelargonium sidoides*) [50], or dietary supplements (e.g., *zinc*) as alternative therapies for ENT infections in children are not supported due to lack of reliable evidence [51–53]. A systematic review using homeopathic remedies to treat the common cold in children found no evidence to support these treatments, and safety information is insufficient [54]. Probiotics have been found to modify the severity of respiratory tract infections in some trials but no significant difference in a meta-analysis [55].

In conclusion, most of the cases of pediatric ENT infections are self-resolving [1]. Symptomatic management, not always with "symptomatic agents," but with the understanding of the disease's natural course, is the mainstay of treatment.

References

1. Jaume F, Valls-Mateus M, Mullol J. Common cold, and acute rhinosinusitis: up-to-date management in 2020. Curr Allergy Asthma Rep. 2020;20(7):28.

2. De Sutter AI, van Driel ML, Kumar AA, Lesslar O, Skrt A. Oral antihistamine-decongestant-analgesic combinations for the common cold. Cochrane Database Syst Rev. 2012;2:CD004976.

3. Taverner D, Latte J. Nasal decongestants for the common cold. Cochrane Database Syst Rev. 2007;1:CD001953.

4. van Driel ML, Scheire S, Deckx L, Gevaert P, De Sutter A. What treatments are effective for common cold in adults and children? BMJ. 2018;363:k3786.

5. Thompson M, Vodicka TA, Blair PS, Buckley DI, Heneghan C, Hay AD. TARGET programme team duration of symptoms of respiratory tract infections in children: systematic review. BMJ. 2013;347:f7027.

6. Lieberthal AS, Carroll AE, Chonmaitree T, et al. The diagnosis and management of acute otitis media. Pediatrics. 2013;13:e964–99.

7. Sjoukes A, Venekamp RP, van de Pol AC, et al. Paracetamol (acetaminophen) or non-steroidal anti-inflammatory drugs, alone or combined, for pain relief in acute otitis media in children. Cochrane Database Syst Rev. 2016;12(12):CD011534.

8. National Institute for Health and Care Excellence. Sore throat (acute): antimicrobial prescribing; 2018. https://www.nice.org.uk/guidance/ng84. Accessed 31 Dec 2020.

9. Pierce CA, Voss B. Efficacy and safety of ibuprofen and acetaminophen in children and adults: a meta-analysis and qualitative review. Ann Pharmacother. 2010;44:489–506.

10. Graham GG, Davies MJ, Day RO, Mohamudally A, Scott KF. The modern pharmacology of paracetamol: therapeutic actions, mechanism of action, metabolism, toxicity and recent pharmacological findings. Inflammopharmacology. 2013;21:201–32.

11. Kanabar DJ. A clinical and safety review of paracetamol and ibuprofen in children. Inflammopharmacology. 2017;25:1–9.

12. Alander SW, Dowd MD, Bratton SL, Kearns GL. Pediatric acetaminophen overdose: risk factors associated with hepatocellular injury. Arch Pediatr Adolesc Med. 2000;154:346–50.

13. Chapman J, Arnold JK. Reye syndrome. Treasure Island: StatPearls Publishing; 2020.

14. Hoberman A, Paradise JL, Reynolds EA, Urkin J. Efficacy of Auralgan for treating ear pain in children with acute otitis media. Arch Pediatr Adolesc Med. 1997;151:675–8.

15. Bolt P, Barnett P, Babl FE, Sharwood LN. Topical lignocaine for pain relief in acute otitis media: results of a double-blind placebo-controlled randomised trial. Arch Dis Child. 2008;93:40–4.

16. Dahshan A, Donovan GK. Severe methemoglobinemia complicating topical benzocaine use during endoscopy in a toddler: a case report and review of the literature. Pediatrics. 2006;117(4):e806–9.

17. Mujica-Mota MA, Bezdjian A, Salehi P, Schermbrucker J, Daniel SJ. Assessment of ototoxicity of intratympanic administration of Auralgan in a chinchilla animal model. Laryngoscope. 2015;125(6):1444–8.

18. Foxlee R, Johansson A, Wejfalk J, Dawkins J, Dooley L, Del Mar C. Topical analgesia for acute otitis media. Cochrane Database Syst Rev. 2006;3:CD005657.

19. Aertgeerts B, Agoritsas T, Siemieniuk RAC, et al. Corticosteroids for sore throat: a clinical practice guideline. BMJ. 2017;358:j4090.

20. Sadeghirad B, Siemieniuk RAC, Brignardello-Petersen R, et al. Corticosteroids for treatment of sore throat: systematic review and meta-analysis of randomised trials. BMJ. 2017;358:j3887.

21. Chessman AW. Guideline: experts recommend a single dose of oral steroids for pain relief in acute sore throat. Ann Intern Med. 2018;168(2):JC2.

22. de Cassan S, Thompson MJ, Perera R, et al. Corticosteroids as standalone or add-on treatment for sore throat. Cochrane Database Syst Rev. 2020;5(5):CD008268.

23. World Health Organization. Cough and cold remedies for the treatment of acute respiratory infections in young children; 2001. http://apps.who.int/iris/bitstream/10665/66856/1/WHO_FCH_CAH_01.02.pdf?ua=1&ua=1. Accessed 31 Dec 2020.

24. Cingi C, Songu M, Ural A, et al. Effect of chlorhexidine gluconate and benzydamine hydrochloride mouth spray on clinical signs and quality of life of patients with streptococcal tonsillopharyngitis: multicentre, prospective, randomised, double-blinded, placebo-controlled study. J Laryngol Otol. 2011;125:620–5.

25. Scottish Intercollegiate Guidelines Network. Management of sore throat and indications for tonsillectomy. Guideline No. 117; 2010. https://www.sign.ac.uk/our-guidelines/management-of-sore-throat-and-indications-for-tonsillectomy/. Accessed 31 Dec 2020.
26. Hopper SM, McCarthy M, Tancharoen C, Lee KJ, Davidson A, Babl FE. Topical lidocaine to improve oral intake in children with painful infectious mouth ulcers: a blinded, randomized, placebo-controlled trial. Ann Emerg Med. 2014;63:292–9.
27. Little P, Stuart B, Wingrove Z, et al. Probiotic capsules and xylitol chewing gum to manage symptoms of pharyngitis: a randomized controlled factorial trial. CMAJ. 2017;189(50):E1543–50.
28. Chow AW, Benninger MS, Brook I, et al. Infectious Diseases Society of America. IDSA clinical practice guideline for acute bacterial rhinosinusitis in children and adults. Clin Infect Dis. 2012;54(8):e72–112.
29. Wald ER, Applegate KE, Bordley C, et al. American Academy of Pediatrics. Clinical practice guideline for the diagnosis and management of acute bacterial sinusitis in children aged 1 to 18 years. Pediatrics. 2013;132(1):e262–80.
30. Leung AK, Kellner JD. Acute sinusitis in children: diagnosis and management. J Pediatr Health Care. 2004;18:72–6.
31. Food and Drug Administration (FDA). OTC cough and cold products: not for infants and children under 2 years of age. January 17, 2008, https://www.fda.gov/consumers/consumer-updates/otc-cough-and-cold-products-not-infants-and-children-under-2-years-age. Accessed 31 Dec 2020.
32. Deckx L, De Sutter AI, Guo L, Mir NA, van Driel ML. Nasal decongestants in monotherapy for the common cold. Cochrane Database Syst Rev. 2016;10(10):CD009612.
33. Chonmaitree T, Saeed K, Uchida T, et al. A randomized, placebo-controlled trial of the effect of antihistamine or corticosteroid treatment in acute otitis media. J Pediatr. 2003;143:377–85.
34. McCormick DP, John SD, Swischuk LE, Uchida T. A double-blind, placebo-controlled trial of decongestant-antihistamine for the treatment of sinusitis in children. Clin Pediatr (Phila). 1996;35:457–60.
35. Food and Drug Administration (FDA). FDA Drug Safety Communication: FDA restricts the use of prescription codeine pain and cough medicines and tramadol pain medicines in children; recommends against use in breastfeeding women; 2017, https://www.fda.gov/Drugs/DrugSafety/ucm549679.htm. Accessed 31 Dec 2020.
36. Shaikh N, Wald ER. Decongestants, antihistamines and nasal irrigation for acute sinusitis in children. Cochrane Database Syst Rev. 2014;2014(10):CD007909.
37. Green JL, Wang GS, Reynolds KM, et al. Safety profile of cough and cold medication use in pediatrics. Pediatrics. 2017;139(6):e20163070.
38. Furukawa CT. The role of allergy in sinusitis in children. J Allergy Clin Immunol. 1992;90(3 Pt 2):515–7.
39. Meltzer EO, Bachert C, Staudinger H. Treating acute rhinosinusitis: comparing efficacy and safety of mometasone furoate nasal spray, amoxicillin, and placebo. J Allergy Clin Immunol. 2005;116:1289–95.
40. Barlan IB, Erkan E, Bakir M, Berrak S, Başaran MM. Intranasal budesonide spray as an adjunct to oral antibiotic therapy for acute sinusitis in children. Ann Allergy Asthma Immunol. 1997;78:598–601.
41. Zalmanovici Trestioreanu A, Yaphe J. Intranasal steroids for acute sinusitis. Cochrane Database Syst Rev. 2013;2013(12):CD005149.
42. Wang YH, Yang CP, Ku MS, Sun HL, Lue KH. Efficacy of nasal irrigation in the treatment of acute sinusitis in children. Int J Pediatr Otorhinolaryngol. 2009;73:1696–701.
43. King D, Mitchell B, Williams CP, Spurling GK. Saline nasal irrigation for acute upper respiratory tract infections. Cochrane Database Syst Rev. 2015;4:CD006821.
44. Gallant JN, Basem JI, Turner JH, Shannon CN, Virgin FW. Nasal saline irrigation in pediatric rhinosinusitis: a systematic review. Int J Pediatr Otorhinolaryngol. 2018;108:155–62.
45. Singh M, Singh M, Jaiswal N, Chauhan A. Heated, humidified air for the common cold. Cochrane Database Syst Rev. 2017;8(8):CD001728.

46. Brewster CT, Choong J, Thomas C, Wilson D, Moiemen N. Steam inhalation and paediatric burns during the COVID-19 pandemic. Lancet. 2020;395(10238):1690.
47. Oduwole O, Udoh EE, Oyo-Ita A, Meremikwu MM. Honey for acute cough in children. Cochrane Database Syst Rev. 2018;4(4):CD007094.
48. Abuelgasim H, Albury C, Lee J. Effectiveness of honey for symptomatic relief in upper respiratory tract infections: a systematic review and meta-analysis. BMJ Evid Based Med. 2020;2020:111336.
49. Albrecht HH, Dicpinigaitis PV, Guenin EP. Role of guaifenesin in the management of chronic bronchitis and upper respiratory tract infections. Multidiscip Respir Med. 2017;12:31.
50. Bereznoy VV, Riley DS, Wassmer G, Heger M. Efficacy of extract of pelargonium sidoides in children with acute non-group a beta-hemolytic streptococcus tonsillopharyngitis: a randomized, double-blind, placebo-controlled trial. Altern Ther Health Med. 2003;9:68–79.
51. Timmer A, Günther J, Motschall E, Rücker G, Antes G, Kern WV. Pelargonium sidoides extract for treating acute respiratory tract infections. Cochrane Database Syst Rev. 2013;10:CD006323.
52. Huang Y, Wu T, Zeng L, Li S. Chinese medicinal herbs for sore throat. Cochrane Database Syst Rev. 2012;3:CD004877.
53. Singh M, Das RR. Zinc for the common cold. Cochrane Database Syst Rev. 2011;2:CD001364.
54. Hawke K, van Driel ML, Buffington BJ, McGuire TM, King D. Homeopathic medicinal products for preventing and treating acute respiratory tract infections in children. Cochrane Database Syst Rev. 2018;9(9):CD005974.
55. Robinson JL. Probiotics for modification of the incidence or severity of respiratory tract infections. Pediatr Infect Dis J. 2017;36:1093–5.

Immunomodulating Agents for Pediatric Ear, Nose, and Throat Infections

87

Can Celiloğlu, Ümit Çelik, and Fatma Levent

87.1 Introduction

Upper respiratory infections are prevalent in the childhood period. Upper respiratory tract infections (URTIs) include nasopharyngitis (common cold), pharyngitis, rhinosinusitis, laryngitis, and laryngotracheitis [1]. Viruses are responsible for the vast majority of URTIs [2]. A myriad of virus species and subspecies may cause URTIs [3]. Influenza virus, adenovirus, respiratory syncytial virus (RSV), and rhinovirus are the leading causative agents [2]. The course of the URTIs is mostly benign.

Newborns with congenital cyanotic heart disease and/or chronic lung disease (CLD) of premature and preterm ones whose gestational age under 32 weeks are recommended to have passive immunization against RSV with palivizumab, RSV specific monoclonal antibody, according to the guidelines, and susceptible children and adults are recommended to have an annual influenza vaccination. However, due to the diversity of the causative agents and lack of vaccines and other preventive approaches for each of these viruses, 4–6 URTIs annually are considered normal for a healthy child.

Among the wide variety of underlying factors for URTIs, the leadings are air pollution, cigarette smoke exposure, overcrowding, daycare attendance, early

C. Celiloğlu (✉)
Department of Pediatrics, Faculty of Medicine, Çukurova University, Adana, Turkey

Ü. Çelik
Section of Pediatric Infectious Diseases, Adana City Training and Research Hospital, University of Health Sciences, Adana, Turkey

F. Levent
Division of Pediatric Infectious Diseases, Department of Pediatrics, School of Medicine, Texas Tech University, Lubbock, TX, USA

C. Cingi et al. (eds.), *Pediatric ENT Infections*,
https://doi.org/10.1007/978-3-030-80691-0_87

weaning and lack of breastfeeding, deficiency in immune maturation, and malnutrition [4]. However, the potential of health professionals to influence all of these factors is limited. Besides the annual influenza vaccination, URTIs' management in children should focus on parents' reassurance, appropriate, mostly symptomatic treatment, and follow-up.

The unnecessary use of antibiotics for acute URTIs is a significant concern due to its contribution to antibiotic resistance, increased healthcare costs, and adverse reactions such as allergic problems and diarrhea [5]. Also, improper use of antibiotics may harm human microbiota. As demonstrated in a study from China, the percentage of antibiotic prescriptions for children less than 2 years of age diagnosed with URTIs was as high as 82% [6].

In addition to symptomatic treatment for URTIs, immunomodulatory therapies that support immune system functions may be considered. Some of these immunomodulatory agents were found useful in the literature [7]. These agents might also prevent secondary bacterial infections and decrease the need for antibiotics [8].

Immunomodulating agents are used for the immune system's proper functioning while eliminating the pathological processes caused by any microbiological etiology. The mechanisms of action of possible immunomodulatory agents may include immunosuppression, immune tolerance against particular antigens, immune potentiation, and immunological replacement.

Within this chapter, immunomodulatory agents, including e*chinacea*, bacterial derivatives, pelargonium extracts, pidotimod, beta-glucan, and propolis, are highlighted. Prednisolone therapy against periodic fever, aphthous stomatitis, pharyngitis, cervical adenitis syndrome, or the pneumococcal conjugate vaccine's role in preventing acute otitis media episodes are out of the scope of this context. Recent data on vitamin D suggest that it supports the immune system against infections. The role of vitamin D against URTIs is not discussed in this chapter.

87.2 Echinacea

Echinacea species are also referred to as coneflowers and belong to the daisy family [9]. *Echinacea* derivatives are known to be used by native Americans for pain, sore throat, and cough [10]. Echinacea may contain bioactive components such as phenolic compounds, polysaccharides, alkylamides, and glycoproteins [11].

Echinacea species have been accepted as immunostimulants after studies on *E. purpurea, E. pallida,* and *E. angustifolia* subtypes [12]. It is known that *echinacea* plant derivatives are widely consumed today in Europe and North America for common cold symptoms. *Echinacea* has also been reported to exert antiviral activity against influenza and coronavirus [13, 14].

In a study examining the mechanism of action of *Echinacea purpurea*, it was found to prevent *Haemophilus influenzae* and *Staphylococcus aureus* from adhering to the bronchial epithelium by suppressing the expression of epithelial intercellular adhesion molecule-1 (ICAM-1), fibronectin, and platelet-activating factor receptor (PAFr) [15].

Echinacea has been evaluated for both the prevention and treatment strategies of the common cold. A recent review based on several trials comparing *Echinacea*'s effectiveness against placebo found no benefits for treating the common cold [16]. However, another meta-analysis reported that *Echinacea* halved the risk of recurrent respiratory tract infections (RTIs) in susceptible individuals and lowered complications such as pneumonia, otitis media, otitis externa, tonsillitis, and pharyngitis [17]. A systematic review of randomized controlled trials (RCTs) found only limited evidence for *Echinacea*'s efficacy in children with RTIs; due to the low number of RCTs investigating preventive effects of *Echinacea*, the routine use of *Echinacea* for the prevention of RTIs was not recommended [18].

A randomized, double-blind, placebo-controlled study of healthy children revealed that treatment with *Echinacea* or placebo revealed no difference in symptom severity and URTI duration between study groups [19]. *Echinacea* has also been evaluated for prevention against URTIs and is reported not to have an overall protective effect [20].

A study in children who have a history of recurrent otitis media treatment with *Echinacea* did not decrease infection risk [21]. Although generally well tolerated, in another study, rashes were more frequent in children treated with oral *Echinacea* than placebo [19].

Echinacea may have some immunostimulating effects, but the current evidence does not support its efficacy in treating the common colds and preventing community-acquired RTIs [12, 16].

87.3 Bacterial Derived Immunomodulators

Bacterial immunomodulators are composed of bacterial lysate or bacterial cell components. Bacterial lysates have been used in Europe for a long time to prevent RTIs in children [22].

87.3.1 OM-85 BV

The most commonly used lysate derivative is OM-85 BV (Broncho-Vaxom®, Broncho-Munal®, Ommunal®, Paxoral®, and Vaxoral®), comprised of eight different bacterial agents (*Streptococcus pyogenes*, *Staphylococcus aureus*, *Streptococcus pneumoniae*, *viridans group streptococci*, *Haemophilus influenzae*, *Moraxella catarrhalis*, *Klebsiella pneumoniae*, and *Klebsiella ozaenae*) which has been shown to exert immune-stimulatory effects and improve immunological functions [23].

Bronchoalveolar lavage examinations of adults treated with OM-85 revealed an increase in helper ratio to suppressor T cells, stimulation of impaired alveolar macrophage activity, and increased interferon-gamma [24, 25]. Bacterial lysate derivatives are administered orally, intranasally, or sublingually [22]. In a study on immunostimulant use in preschool children, minor and transient adverse effects related to OM-85 were reported [23].

In a study in asthmatic children, the frequency of RTIs was significantly reduced within the OM-85 applied group, and no severe adverse reactions were encountered [26]. Another study in children with chronic rhinosinusitis concluded that bacterial lysate provided long-term prophylactic efficacy, and bacterial lysate can effectively alleviate symptoms [27]. Razi et al. reported that OM-85 might be used as a supplement to reduce the number and duration of acute RTI-induced wheezing attacks in preschool children [23]. In a meta-analysis by Yin et al., OM-85 was found to have clinical benefit in decreasing wheezing duration [28].

A meta-analysis based on eight randomized controlled trials concluded that treatment with OM-85 significantly lowered cases, and the effect is more significant in patients at increased risk of recurrent RTIs [29]. A randomized, placebo-controlled, double-blind study showed significantly lower RTIs in children receiving OM-85 for 3 months than those who received a placebo [30].

Based on the available literature, the commencement of OM-85 for preventing URTI in children may be beneficial, especially for cases with a history of recurrent respiratory infections.

87.4 Pidotimod

Pidotimod is a synthetic orally active dipeptide molecule that has activity on both innate and adaptive immune systems [31]. It stimulates immune system cells and leads to an increase in secretory immunoglobulin (Ig) A concentration. It can act on toll-like receptors (TLR) in the airway epithelium and adhesion molecules [32]. Pidotimod significantly reduced the recurrence of RTIs compared to controls over 6 months in 63 children aged 2–10 years of age [33]. The clinical efficacy of pidotimod was evaluated in a multicenter randomized trial showing reduced fever duration, the need for antibiotic treatment and recovery time, and relapse rate in children [34].

Available evidence indicates pidotimod's efficacy in children with recurrent respiratory infections; however, sufficient data for routine use in children is lacking.

87.5 Pelargonium Extracts

Historically, the traditional medical use of Pelargonium sidoides in Southern Africa was associated with diarrhea and dysentery; however, the plant gained popularity through developed countries as it was used for tuberculosis-related symptoms [35]. Today, an aqueous-ethanolic formula prepared from the roots of P. sidoides (EPs®7630) is applied widely for the treatment of URTIs of children and adults. In 2005, the Federal Institute for Drugs and Medical Devices in Germany approved it as herbal medicine to treat acute bronchitis. Numerous in vitro studies show evidence of activation of the nonspecific immune system [36].

Adhesion of bacteria to the host cell surface is essential in colonization and infection. Bacterial adhesion inhibition is useful in protecting host cells from invading pathogens. Recent studies have shown an anti-adhesive capability of EPs®7630 that prevents *S. pyogenes* (group A streptococcus) [37]. The anti-adhesive activity was reported on the inhibition of *Helicobacter pylori* [38, 39]. The exact mechanism and mode of action are yet to be elucidated.

Provided that a standardized medication is available, *P. sidoides* is thus reported to be considered an adjunctive therapy option for RTIs in children [18]. In a Cochrane analysis based on randomized controlled trials (RCTs), pelargonium extract was useful in acute rhinosinusitis and the common cold, but the evidence is low quality [40]. In another RCT review, *P. sidoides* was shown to reduce or resolve the symptoms more rapidly [41]. In a meta-analysis of six RCTs, children aged 6–10 years with acute bronchitis and acute tonsillopharyngitis, *P. sidoides* preparation (EPs®7630) improved the symptoms and accelerated recovery with decreased use of antipyretics [42]. Efficacy of EPs®7630 was significantly higher than placebo in reducing symptoms and time until recovery in children less than 6 years of age and was well tolerated [43]. In a recent study, patients with acute respiratory infections who received phytopharmaceuticals, including *P. sidoides* root extract, had a significantly reduced need for antibiotic prescriptions [44].

There is no sufficient evidence to support *P. sidoides* extract's routine use to treat common colds in children. For pediatric URTIs, *P. sidoides* extracts should be considered as an adjunct to therapy in selected cases.

87.6 Beta-Glucan

Beta (β) -glucans are groups of dietary fibers or polysaccharides naturally found in the cell wall of bacteria, fungi, algae, and higher crops [45]. Beta-glucans are composed of D-glucose monomers linked by 1,3; 1,4; or 1,6 beta-glycosidic bonds. Beta-glucans' biological and physicochemical properties may vary extensively, depending on the branching and extraction source [46]. The immunostimulatory effect of beta-glucans is suggested in animal models and human studies [46]. These immunostimulatory effects range from increased mucosal immunity and stimulation of specific chemokines to increased monocyte, natural killer (NK) cell, B cell activities [45].

Administration of beta-glucan has proven to be a potential therapeutic and preventive agent for managing and preventing recurrent RTIs in children (especially beta-glucans from *Pleurotus ostreatus*) [47]. In a prospective study, syrup containing insoluble beta-glucan isolated from *P. ostreatus* was well tolerated and reduced the number of recurrent infections and missed school days in children aged 3–7 years. No serious adverse effects were observed [48].

The protective effects of beta-glucans are considered activators of cellular immunity and effective in different experimental models of infection [49]. The molecule of beta-glucan is also considered to have antiviral activities. In a case-control study, in patients with recurrent herpes simplex virüs (HSV)-1 infection, the duration and severity of symptoms were lower in the active group versus the placebo [50]. In a double-blind, randomized, placebo-controlled study in healthy subjects, a decrease in the severity of upper respiratory infection symptoms without significant alteration of the incidence and global severity of common colds were reported [51]. Sufficient evidence for the use of beta-glucans against URTIs in children is lacking.

87.7 Propolis

Propolis is a generic name that refers to the bees' resinous substance from different types of plants. More than 300 other compounds have been revealed in propolis [52]. Propolis exerts various biological functions, which may be attributed to its antioxidant and anti-inflammatory effects [52]. Flavonoids are the main components responsible for the functional properties of propolis [53]. However, the exact molecular mechanisms are yet unknown.

Propolis may inhibit the synthesis of prostaglandins and activate the thymus as anti-inflammatory effects. Propolis also may promote phagocytic activity and stimulate cellular immunity [53]. Due to the insufficient number of RCTs, the evidence for treatment with propolis to prevent URTIs in children is lacking [54]. In a case-control study, the combination of N-acetylcysteine and propolis use has shown a reduction in symptom severity of respiratory infections in children with adenoid hypertrophy [55]. Children who presented to the emergency department with upper respiratory infections aged 5–12 years showed rapid improvement using a mixture of bee products, including propolis [56]. Randomized controlled trials favoring the routine use of propolis for treatment or prevention of pediatric URTIs are lacking.

87.8 Conclusion

Most URTIs in children are viral in origin. Most viral infections resolve spontaneously with supportive care. Prevention methods like vaccinations, hand hygiene, and pollution avoidance are helpful but might not be enough. New strategies include immunomodulators to boost the immune system and natural response to infections, especially in children with recurrent respiratory infections, to avoid complications and decrease antibiotic use. These immunomodulators are mostly used as an adjunct to current therapies. Further studies are needed to evaluate the evidence of clinical efficacy and safety of these immunomodulators in pediatric URTIs.

References

1. Grief SN. Upper respiratory infections. Prim Care. 2013;40:757–70.
2. Weintraub B. Upper respiratory tract infections. Pediatr Rev. 2015;36:554–6.
3. Papadopoulos NG, Megremis S, Kitsioulis NA, Vangelatou O, West P, Xepapadaki P. Promising approaches for the treatment and prevention of viral respiratory illnesses. J Allergy Clin Immunol. 2017;140:921–32.

4. Del-Rio-Navarro BE, Espinosa Rosales F, Flenady V, Sienra-Monge JJ. Immunostimulants for preventing respiratory tract infection in children. Cochrane Database Syst Rev. 2006;18(4):CD004974.

5. Esposito S, Soto-Martinez ME, Feleszko W, Jones MH, Shen KL, Schaad UB. Nonspecific immunomodulators for recurrent respiratory tract infections, wheezing, and asthma in children: a systematic review of mechanistic and clinical evidence. Curr Opin Allergy Clin Immunol. 2018;18:198–209.

6. Wong GWK. Reducing antibiotic prescriptions for childhood upper respiratory tract infections. Lancet Glob Health. 2017;5:e1170–1.

7. Feleszko W, Marengo R, Vieira AS, Ratajczak K, Mayorga Butrón JL. Immunity-targeted approaches to the management of chronic and recurrent upper respiratory tract disorders in children. Clin Otolaryngol. 2019;44:502–10.

8. Marrengo R, Ortega Martell JA, Esposito R. Paediatric recurrent ear, nose, throat infections and complications: can we do more? Infect Dis Ther. 2020;9:275–90.

9. Hobbs C. Echinacea: a literature review; botany, history, chemistry, pharmacology, toxicology, and clinical uses. Herbal Gram. 1994;30:33.

10. Bauer R. Echinacea: biological effects and active principles, vol. 691. New York: ACS Publications; 1998. p. 140–57.

11. Parsons JL, Cameron SI, Harris CS, Smith ML. Echinacea biotechnology: advances, commercialization and future considerations. Pharm Biol. 2018;56:485–94.

12. Saper RB. Clinical use of echinacea. In: Elmore JG, Seres D, Kunins I (eds). Massachusetts: UpToDate. (last updated: July 22, 2019). https://www.uptodate.com/contents/clinical-use-of-echinacea?source=see_link. Accessed 21 Nov 2020.

13. Pleschka S, Stein M, Schoop R, Hudson JB. Antiviral properties and mode of action of standardized Echinacea purpurea extract against highly pathogenic avian influenza virus (H5N1, H7N7) and swine-origin H1N1 (S-OIV). Virol J. 2009;6:197.

14. Signer J, Jonsdottir HR, Albrich WC, et al. In vitro virucidal activity of Echinaforce®, an Echinacea purpurea preparation, against coronaviruses, including common cold coronavirus 229E and SARS-CoV-2. Virol J. 2020;17(1):136.

15. Vimalanathan S, Schoop R, Suter A, Hudson J. Prevention of influenza virus-induced bacterial superinfection by standardized Echinacea purpurea, via regulation of surface receptor expression in human bronchial epithelial cells. Virus Res. 2017;233:51–9.

16. Karsch-Völk M, Barrett B, Kiefer D, Bauer R, Ardjomand-Woelkart K, Linde K. Echinacea for preventing and treating the common cold. Cochrane Database Syst Rev. 2014;20(2):CD00053.

17. Schapowal A, Klein P, Johnston SL. Echinacea reduces the risk of recurrent respiratory tract infections and complications: a meta-analysis of randomized controlled trials. Adv Ther. 2015;32:187–200.

18. Anheyer D, Cramer H, Lauche R, Saha FJ, Dobos G. Herbal medicine in children with respiratory tract infection: systematic review and meta-analysis. Acad Pediatr. 2017;10:S1876–2859.

19. Taylor JA, Weber W, Standish L, et al. Efficacy and safety of echinacea in treating upper respiratory tract infections in children: a randomized controlled trial. JAMA. 2003;290(21):2824–30.

20. Grimm W, Müller HH. A randomized controlled trial of the effect of fluid extract of Echinacea purpurea on the incidence and severity of colds and respiratory infections. Am J Med. 1999;106:138–43.

21. Wahl RA, Aldous MB, Worden KA, Grant KL. Echinacea purpurea and osteopathic manipulative treatment in children with recurrent otitis media: a randomized controlled trial. BMC Complement Altern Med. 2008;8:56.

22. Kearney SC, Dziekiewicz M, Feleszko W. Immunoregulatory and immunostimulatory responses of bacterial lysates in respiratory infections and asthma. Ann Allergy Asthma Immunol. 2015;114:364–9.

23. Razi CH, Harmancı K, Abacı A, et al. The immunostimulant OM-85 BV prevents wheezing attacks in preschool children. J Allergy Clin Immunol. 2010;126:763–9.

24. Emmerich B, Emslander HP, Pachmann K, Hallek M, Milatovic D, Busch R. Local immunity in patients with chronic bronchitis and the effects of a bacterial extract, Broncho-Vaxom, on T

lymphocytes, macrophages, gamma-interferon and secretory immunoglobulin a in bronchoalveolar lavage fluid and other variables. Respiration. 1990;57:90–9.

25. Emmerich B, Pachmann K, Milatovic D, Emslander HP. Influence of OM-85-BV on different humoral and cellular immune defense mechanisms of the respiratory tract. Respiration. 1992;59(Suppl 3):19–23.

26. Liao JY, Zhang T. Influence of OM-85 BV on hBD-1 and immunoglobulin in children with asthma and recurrent respiratory tract infection. Zhongguo Dang Dai Er Ke Za Zhi. 2014;16:508–12.

27. Chen J, Zhou Y, Nie J, et al. Bacterial lysate for the prevention of chronic rhinosinusitis recurrence in children. J Laryngol Otol. 2017;131:523–8.

28. Yin J, Xu B, Zeng X, Shen K. Broncho-Vaxom in pediatric recurrent respiratory tract infections: a systematic review and meta-analysis. Int Immunopharmacol. 2018;54:198–209.

29. Schaad UB. OM-85 BV, an immunostimulant in pediatric recurrent respiratory tract infections: a systematic review. World J Pediatr. 2010;6:5–12.

30. Esposito S, Bianchini S, Bosis S, et al. A randomized placebo-controlled, double-blinded, single-Centre, phase IV trial to assess the efficacy and safety of OM-65 in children suffering from recurrent respiratory tract infections. J Transl Med. 2019;17:284.

31. Riboldi P, Gerosa M, Meroni PL. Pidotimod: a reappraisal. Int J Immunopathol Pharmacol. 2009;22:255–62.

32. Ferrario BE, Garuti S, Braido F, Canonica GW. Pidotimod: the state of art. Clin Mol Allergy. 2015;13(1):8.

33. Das D, Narayanan V, Rathod R, Barkate HV, Sobti V. Efficacy of pidotimod in reducing recurrent respiratory tract infections in Indian children. Index Copernicus Int. 2017;6(2):101–10.

34. Puggioni F, Alves-Correia M, Mohamed MF, et al. Immunostimulants in respiratory diseases: focus on pidotimod. Multidiscip Respir Med. 2019;14:31.

35. Kolodziej H. Antimicrobial, antiviral, and immunomodulatory activity studies of pelargonium sidoides (EPs® 7630) in the context of health promotion. Pharmaceuticals (Basel). 2011;4:1295–314.

36. Kolodziej H. Aqueous ethanolic extract of the roots of pelargonium sidoides: new scientific evidence for an old anti-infective phytopharmaceutical. Planta Med. 2008;74:661–6.

37. Conrad A, Jung I, Tioua D, et al. Extract of pelargonium sidoides (EPs® 7630) inhibits the interactions of group a streptococci and host epithelia in-vitro. Phytomedicine. 2007;14:52–9.

38. Beil W, Kilian P. EPs 7630, an extract from pelargonium sidoides roots inhibits adherence of helicobacter pylori to gastric epithelial cells. Phytomedicine. 2007;14(Suppl 6):5–8.

39. Wittschier N, Faller G, Hensel A. An extract of pelargonium sidoides (EPs 7630) inhibits in situ adhesion of helicobacter pylori to human stomach. Phytomedicine. 2007;14:285–8.

40. Timmer A, Günther J, Motschall E, Rücker G, Antes G, Kern WV. Pelargonium sidoides extract for treating acute respiratory tract infections. Cochrane Database Syst Rev. 2013;22(10):CD006323.

41. Ceraddu D, Pettenazzo A. Pelargonium sidoides extract eps 7630: a review of its clinical efficacy and safety for treating acute respiratory tract infections in children. Intern J Gen Med. 2018;11:91–8.

42. Seifert G, Brandes-Schramm J, Zimmermann A, Lehmacher W, Kamin W. Faster recovery and reduced paracetamol use- a meta-analysis of EPs 7630 in children with acute respiratory tract infections. BMC Pediatr. 2019;19:119.

43. Kamin W, Funk P, Seifert G, Zimmerman A, Lehmacher W. EPs 7630 is effective and safe in children under 6 years with acute respiratory tract infections: clinical studies revisited. Curr Med Res Opin. 2018;34:475–85.

44. Martin D, Konrad M, Adarkwah CC, Kostev K. Reduced antibiotic use after initial treatment of acute respiratory infections with phytopharmaceuticals- a retrospective cohort study. Postgrad Med. 2020;132:412–8.

45. Bashir KMI, Choi JS. Clinical and physiological perspectives of β-glucans: the past, present, and future. Int J Mol Sci. 2017;18(9):1906.

46. Volman JJ, Ramakers JD, Plat J. Dietary modulation of immune function by beta-glucans. Physiol Behav. 2008;94:276–84.
47. Jesenak M, Urbancikova I, Banovcin P. Respiratory tract infections and the role of biologically active polysaccharides in their management and prevention. Nutrients. 2017;9(7):779.
48. Pasnik J, Slemp A, Cywinska-Bernas A, Zeman K, Jesenak M. Preventive effect of pleuran (β-glucan isolated from Pleurotus ostreatus) in children with recurrent respiratory tract infections-open-label prospective study. Curr Ped Res. 2017;21:99–104.
49. Vetvicka V, Vannucci L, Sima P, Richter J. Beta glucan: supplement or drug? From laboratory to clinical trials. Molecules. 2019;24:1251.
50. Urbancikova I, Hudackova D, Majtan J, Rennerova Z, Banovcin P, Jesenak M. Efficacy of pleuran (β-glucan from Pleurotus ostreatus) in the management of herpes simplex virus type-1 infection. Evid Based Complement Alternat Med. 2020;2020:1–8.
51. Dharsono T, Rudnicka K, Wilhelm M, Schoen C. Effects of yeast (1,3)-(1,6)-beta-glucan on severity of upper respiratory tract infections: a double-blind, randomized, placebo-controlled study in healthy subjects. J Am Coll Nutr. 2019;38:40–50.
52. Zaccaria V, Curti V, Di Lorenzo A, et al. Effect of green and brown propolis extracts on the expression levels of microRNAs, mRNAs, and proteins, related to oxidative stress and inflammation. Nutrients. 2017;9(10):1090.
53. Casaroto AR, Lara VS. Phytomedicines for Candida-associated denture stomatitis. Fitoterapia. 2010;81:323–8.
54. Yuksel S, Akyol S. The consumption of propolis and royal jelly in preventing upper respiratory tract infections and as dietary supplementation in children. J Intercult Ethnopharmacol. 2016;5:308–11.
55. Folic M, Nesic V, Arsovic N. Efficiency of propolis and N-acetylcysteine on reduction in symptom severity of respiratory infection in children with adenoid hypertrophy. J Pharm Pharmacol. 2020;8:91–8.
56. Secilmis Y, Silici S. Bee product efficacy in children with upper respiratory tract infections. Turk J Pediatr. 2020;62:634–40.

Nutritional Management of Pediatric ENT Infections

88

Z. Begüm Kalyoncu, Marina Maintinguer Norde, and Hülya Gökmen Özel

88.1 Introduction

Nutrition is the science that investigates how nutrients and food compounds nourish one's body and interact with health and disease [1]. Although the relationship between diet and disease occurrence, prevention and treatment have been studied extensively [2], the interaction between nutritional status and ENT infections has been heavily understudied, especially among pediatric populations [3]. Nutritional care should be as specialized as medicine; thus, nutritional management of ENT infections needs to be tailored towards the personalized medical needs of the patients. Healthy and balanced nutrition not only maintains proper growth and development in children, but also decreases the risk of morbidity and mortality [4]. As both health care practitioners and parents become more aware of the impact of nutrition in acute and chronic diseases, it is essential to understand nutrition's role in managing health and disease risk reduction [5]. Also, since parents feed their children daily, empowering them with the knowledge of a healthy diet would enhance their involvement and confidence in caring for the patients. Therefore, the aim of this chapter is to provide an overview of the nutritional assessment and treatment to reduce the burden of pediatric ENT infections.

Z. B. Kalyoncu (✉)
Department of Nutrition and Dietetics, Faculty of Health Sciences, Atılım University, Ankara, Turkey

M. M. Norde
Department of Nutrition, Faculty of Public Health, University of São Paulo, São Paulo, Brazil

H. G. Özel
Department of Nutrition and Dietetics, Faculty of Health Sciences, Hacettepe University, Ankara, Turkey

© The Author(s), under exclusive license to Springer Nature Switzerland AG 2022
C. Cingi et al. (eds.), *Pediatric ENT Infections*,
https://doi.org/10.1007/978-3-030-80691-0_88

88.2 The Link Between ENT Infections and Nutrition

Nutrition and lifestyle are modifiable risk factors affecting morbidity in pediatric patients undergoing ENT infections [5, 6]. On the flip side, ENT infections have also been shown to affect the nutritional status by compromising taste sensitivity, increasing energy, macronutrient and micronutrient needs to supply the acute and chronic inflammatory response, and decreasing appetite due to infections [7–9].

To begin with babies, their risk of ear infection was found to be highly correlated with excessive use of baby bottle due to the feeding position as a bedtime practice. As the contents of the baby bottle do not fully drain from the shorter and more vertical ear tubes of the infants, the liquid buildup was found to increase the risk of ear infections [8].

Bottle and pacifier use was especially associated with acute otitis media and its recurrence (Fig. 88.1). In line with that, the American Academy of Pediatrics recommends avoiding supine bottle feeding and pacifier use for reducing the acute otitis media incidence in the first year of life [10].

Moreover, cross-sectional, case-control and prospective cohort studies conducted in school age children, reviewed by Jung and colleagues, show an association between overweight and obesity and unilateral high and low frequency hearing loss along with the onset of otitis media with effusion in one or both ears [11–13]. The proposed role of obesity in hearing impairment could be due to decreased plasma adiponectin levels according to animal studies [14, 15]. Additionally, the two hypotheses that could help explaining the link between obesity and otitis media occurrence are: first, obesity is known for its underlined low-grade and systemic inflammatory state, which has been shown to impair host immune defense against infections [16]; and second, by causing gastroesophageal reflux, a well-known factor related to otolaryngologic manifestations [17].

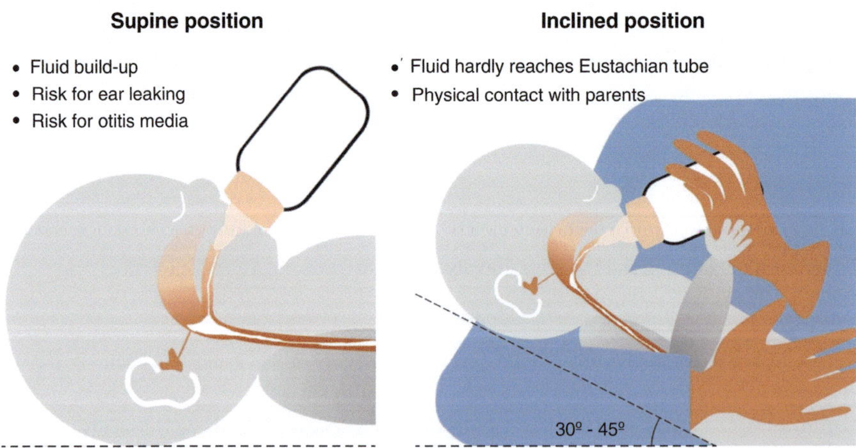

Fig. 88.1 The risk of ear infection in babies was found to be higher in supine position (Adopted from reference [10]

This relationship is particularly concerning with the alarming rise of global obesity among children and adults. According to the World Health Organization (WHO), 38 million children under the age of 5 had overweight or obesity in 2019 while 340 million people aged 5–19 years had overweight or obesity in 2016 [18]. Despite its preventable nature, pediatric overweight and obesity is independently linked with higher risk of adult obesity and hearing loss [11]. Although the hearing loss exacerbation relationship with increased body weight was mostly shown from cross-sectional studies after adjusting for possible confounding factors, the reverse causation is highly improbable [11]. Nevertheless, for otitis media, one still needs to take into account the possible damage of the chorda tympani nerve, which is responsible for taste sensitivity. Since that damage potentially raises the threshold for sweet taste satiety, a higher need for sugar intake might be needed to activate the satiety signals [9]. Therefore, health care professionals should be cognizant of the increased risk of hearing impairment among patients with pediatric overweight or obesity. Given the alarmingly increasing rate of obesity, referral of such patients to pediatric dietitians is essential for enabling efforts towards reducing obesity [19].

In addition to obesity, malnutrition has also been documented as a risk factor for current infections and hearing loss. Lack of various nutritional factors including single nutrients and the overall poor nutritional status were shown to be associated with poorer hearing status and increased susceptibility to infection [3]. Deficiency of vitamins A, B-group, C, D, and E and some minerals (zinc, magnesium, selenium, iodine, iron) and macronutrients could affect hearing negatively in pediatric populations. Higher fat, cholesterol, and carbohydrate intake coupled with low protein intake could result in poorer hearing status as opposed to higher intake of polyunsaturated fatty acids leading to better hearing status [3]. Although the pathophysiological mechanism relating hearing with the single nutritional factors still needs to be established, poor nutritional status has been documented to increase susceptibility to infection, thereby worsening the healing process.

Furthermore, Traditional Mediterranean Diet was found to decrease the recurrence of inflammatory complications of common colds and antibiotic usage significantly in children aged 1–5 years in a prospective before-after comparison study in Spain [20]. In the same study both compliance and satisfaction of the families were found to be high and the frequency of acute otitis media and rhinosinusitis was significantly lower after following a Mediterranean Diet for a year especially in the 2- to 4-year age group. Despite this study lacked a placebo group comparison, previously documented anti-inflammatory properties of Mediterranean diet could still be beneficial [21]. Supporting data from adult prospective studies, randomized controlled trials, and meta-analyses also support the anti-inflammatory properties of Mediterranean diets [22–24]. DASH diet, which is similar to the Mediterranean diet with its emphasis on foods rich in potassium, magnesium, calcium, fiber, plant-based protein could be potentially impactful in managing ENT infections in pediatric populations [25]. Adherence to DASH diet has been repeatedly shown to be effective in ameliorating the serum inflammatory biomarkers in adult populations [26]. Furthermore, based on a longitudinal cohort study of more than one million person-years follow-up in Nurses' Health Study II, higher DASH diet adherence was significantly associated with lower risk of hearing loss [27].

To sum up, proper nutrition is indispensable to prevent or manage pediatric ENT infections as it helps to control weight and supplies necessary macro and micronutrients for the immune defense. Proper nutrition helps to manage disease complications. A child that can eat orally needs to consume a well-balanced diet and following the recommendations of food-based dietary guidelines of each country. If the nutritional guidelines are followed by the family as a whole, the dietary compliance of the children could increase and the health benefits could be extended to the utter household [28]. Plus, following a healthy diet as a family would prevent the children to feel singled out [29]. However, if the children are not able to meet their energy and nutrient requirement via oral route through regular food intake, enteral or parenteral nutrition needs to be employed [30]. In order to reduce the burden of ENT infections, nutritional interventions among pediatric populations could have the potential to prevent and repair the damage before irreversible consequences occur [3].

88.3 Specific Nutritional Considerations Related with ENT Infections

88.3.1 Breastfeeding

WHO and UNICEF advocate early initiation of breastfeeding within the first hour of birth. Additionally, if possible, breastfeeding should be offered exclusively during the first 6 months of life on demand without using bottles or pacifiers. Feedings should take place every 2–3 h, amounting up to 12 feedings per day [4]. After the age of 6 months, complementary foods should be introduced alongside of breastfeeding for up to 2 years and beyond [31]. Due to having a dynamic nutrient composition, a single tabulation of human milk contents is difficult. Therefore, infant/follow on formulas can never fully mimic breastmilk in providing nutrition and immunity to the baby [32]. Unfortunately only 40% of infants under 6 months are exclusively breastfed globally [33] and the breastfeeding rates have not been distributed equally among differing sub-populations [34].

Unless the mother has untreated tuberculosis, brucellosis or infected with the human immunodeficiency virus (HIV), Ebola virus and T cell lymphotropic virus, or is undergoing treatment with drugs that can directly pass to the milk or her milk ducts were injured, all women can breastfeed. Other than the contraindications to breastfeeding such as babies having galactosemia or phenylketonuria, human milk is the optimal nourishment source for the health, growth, and development of babies [35].

Adequate breastfeeding could prevent 823.000 annual deaths in children aging 5 years or less globally, a third of all respiratory infections could be avoided, and up to 30% of all otitis media cases could be reduced among children aging 2 years or less, according to most recent meta-analysis [36]. Beyond ENT infections, longer periods of breastfeeding were associated with 26% reduction in overweight and obesity prevalence and increased intelligence quotient for children and adolescents [36].

In addition to numerous health and social benefits, exclusive breastfeeding for minimum 6 months was found to be protective against acute otitis media [37]. Another study reported exclusive breastfeeding for 6 months provided prevention against otitis media for the first 3 years of life, which is a critical period for language development [38]. Therefore, breastfeeding's protective effect against ENT infections could potentially protect the children even after the period of infancy. In another prospective longitudinal study, the relationship between breastfeeding initiation, duration, and exclusivity with maternal reports of infection including ear, throat, sinus, and upper respiratory tract was examined. Breastfeeding duration (more than 9 months), exclusivity, and timing were significantly associated with lower prevalence of ear, throat, and sinus infections [39].

All health professionals should, then, support breastfeeding, especially in the setting of high risks for general infections, including ENT infections, and obesity-related chronic non-communicable diseases.

88.3.2 Cow's Milk

Among the most common ENT infections for the first year of life is otitis media for infants, affecting 90% of the children with high treatment costs with or without surgical interventions. Therefore, studies have been conducted to understand the risk factors. In a longitudinal study that was conducted in Western Australia, early introduction of milk products (before 4 months of age) in addition to breastfeeding was found to increase the risk of acute otitis media close to 1.5 times after adjusting for possible confounders [40]. Similarly, in a case-control study that was conducted in New Zealand among children aged 3 and 4 years, the odds ratio for developing chronic otitis media with effusion was found to be 1.76 (95% CI: 1.05–2.97) for early exposure (first exposure before 13 months) to cow's milk (excluding formula or foods containing cow's milk) compared to healthy controls [41]. In contrast, fermented cow's milk in the form of probiotic was shown to be protective against common infectious diseases among children via increased levels of immunity biomarkers [42, 43].

88.4 Food Allergies

Food allergies are on the rise and affect approximately 2.5% of the general population worldwide [44]. Interestingly, they affect young children, aging less than 3 years, twice more frequently than adults and food allergy incidence peaks around 1 year of age, then declines progressively as the child grows [45]. The most common foods that are associated with food allergies also differ across age groups. Cow's milk, egg, wheat, and soybean are the main food allergens in children while fish, tree nuts, peanuts, and crustacean shellfish are the main food allergens for adults [46]. Food allergies could affect several organs including ear and they can trigger chronic otitis media in children [47]. Despite conflicting findings regarding the underlying inflammatory mechanism between otitis media with effusion and food allergy; they have been found to coexist in different studies. Furthermore, otitis media with effusion has been shown to improve with allergy treatment that combines medication and elimination diets as well as relapsing after ingesting the food allergens [45, 47]. Limited amount of research that has been done on the link between food allergies and otitis media, mostly reported heightened relationship with cow's milk, egg white, soybean, wheat, and plum allergies. However, more research is needed on larger patient groups in a longitudinal manner. Nevertheless, it would be recommendable for clinicians to inquire about the possibility of food allergies while managing pediatric patients with middle ear infections [45].

88.5 Integration of Nutrition While Caring for ENT-Infected Children

88.5.1 Nutritional Assessment

Nutritional assessment should be an integral part of the evaluation of children with acute and chronic ENT infections as conditions that limit or suspend oral intake, and hospitalization could create nutritional disturbances. Furthermore, as shown in previous sections of these chapter, overweight and obesity should be monitored as risk factors for ENT infection and severity as well. Nutritional status could be assessed using diet history, dietary intake, and by tracking the longitudinal growth in height, weight, and body mass index (BMI) [32].

For dietary assessment of infants, most suitable methods would be parents report of 24-h dietary recall, 3-day food record or health professional direct observation. Also, feeding practices and presence of supplementation need to be inquired. For dietary assessment of toddlers, 24-h dietary recall, food frequency questionnaires, and 3-day food record could be used to get the required information from parents. School-aged children and adolescents could provide information themselves to health care practitioners regarding 24-h dietary recall or food frequency questionnaires [48]. Dietary assessment requires special professional training; therefore nutritional assessment should ideally be performed by a certified dietitian [49]. Optimally, nutritional management necessitates not only evaluating patient's current nutritional status, but also knowledge on the preexisting nutritional state for understanding the metabolic requirements of the illnesses [50].

During infancy, childhood, and adolescence growth charts are used by health care practitioners. After measuring values such as weight, length, or height, they are plotted on growth charts or growth standards such as weight-for-age, height-for-age, and BMI-for-age. These charts are used to compare an individual child's development status with the general population. Health care practitioners could either use global standards that were published by WHO (Tables 88.1 and 88.2) or they can use their country-specific standards such as the cut-off values that were defined by the Centers for Disease Control in the United States, for instance [4, 8]. In order to assess pediatric underweight, overweight, and obesity, body mass index-for-age

Table 88.1 BMI-for-age percentile values for girls (kg/m²) (WHO Child Growth Standards [51, 52])

Age (years)	Age (month)	3rd p.	5th p.	15th p.	50th p.	85th p.	95th p.	97th p.
2	24	13.5	13.7	14.4	15.7	17.2	18.1	18.5
2.5	30	13.3	13.6	14.3	15.5	17	17.9	18.3
3	36	13.2	13.5	14.1	15.4	16.9	17.8	18.2
3.5	42	13.1	13.3	14	15.3	16.8	17.8	18.2
4	48	12.9	13.2	13.9	15.3	16.8	17.9	18.3
4.5	54	12.9	13.1	13.9	15.3	16.9	18	18.4
5	60	12.8	13.1	13.8	15.3	17	18.1	18.6
5.5	66	12.8	13.1	13.8	15.2	17.0	18.2	18.7
6	72	12.8	13.1	13.8	15.3	17.1	18.4	18.9
7	84	12.9	13.1	13.9	15.4	17.4	18.8	19.4
8	96	13.0	13.3	14.1	15.7	17.8	19.4	20.2
9	108	13.3	13.6	14.4	16.1	18.4	20.2	21.1
10	120	13.6	13.9	14.8	16.6	19.1	21.1	22.1
11	132	14.0	14.4	15.3	17.2	20.0	22.2	23.2
12	144	14.6	14.9	15.9	18.0	20.9	23.3	24.4
13	156	15.1	15.5	16.5	18.8	21.9	24.4	25.6
14	168	15.6	16.0	17.2	19.6	22.9	25.5	26.7
15	180	16.1	16.5	17.7	20.2	23.7	26.3	27.6
16	192	16.4	16.8	18.1	20.7	24.2	27.0	28.2
17	204	16.6	17.0	18.3	21.0	24.7	27.4	28.6
18	216	16.7	17.1	18.5	21.3	24.9	27.7	28.9

ap.: Percentile

Table 88.2 BMI-for-age percentile values for boys (kg/m²) (WHO Child Growth Standards [51, 52]

Age (years)	Age (month)	3rd p.	5th p.	15th p.	50th p.	85th p.	95th p.	97th p.
2	24	13.5	13.9	14.2	14.8	16	16.9	17.4
2.5	30	13.3	13.7	13.9	14.6	15.8	16.7	17.2
3	36	13	13.5	13.7	14.4	15.6	16.5	17
3.5	42	12.9	13.3	13.6	14.2	15.4	16.3	16.8
4	48	12.7	13.2	13.4	14.1	15.3	16.2	16.7
4.5	54	12.6	13.1	13.3	14	15.3	16.2	16.7
5	60	12.6	13	13.3	13.9	15.2	16.1	16.7
5.5	66	13.1	13.4	14.0	15.3	16.7	17.7	18.1
6	72	13.2	13.4	14.0	15.3	16.8	17.9	18.3
7	84	13.3	13.5	14.2	15.5	17.1	18.3	18.8
8	96	13.4	13.7	14.4	15.7	17.5	18.8	19.4
9	108	13.6	13.9	14.6	16.0	18.0	19.5	20.1
10	120	13.9	14.1	14.9	16.4	18.6	20.2	21.0
11	132	14.2	14.5	15.3	16.9	19.3	21.1	22.0
12	144	14.6	14.9	15.7	17.5	20.1	22.1	23.1
13	156	15.1	15.4	16.3	18.2	20.9	23.1	24.2
14	168	15.6	16.0	16.9	19.0	21.9	24.2	25.3
15	180	16.2	16.5	17.6	19.8	22.8	25.2	26.4
16	192	16.7	17.1	18.2	20.5	23.7	26.1	27.3
17	204	17.1	17.5	18.7	21.1	24.4	26.9	28.0
18	216	17.5	17.9	19.2	21.7	25.0	27.5	28.6

ap.: Percentile

Table 88.3 The cut-off points for child overweight and obesity diagnosis according to the WHO

BMI-for-age weight status	Until 5-years of age	5–19 years of age
Underweight	BMI <2 standard deviations below the WHO growth standard median	BMI >1 standard deviations above the WHO growth standard median
Overweight	BMI >2 standard deviations above the WHO growth standard median	BMI >1 standard deviations above the WHO growth standard median
Obesity	BMI >3 standard deviations above the WHO growth standard median	BMI >2 standard deviations above the WHO growth standard median

percentile could be recommended as a practical tool for children ≥2 years old [8]. For children from 2 to 19 years of age, BMI-for-age is a better index. After measuring the height and weight of the children following the standard protocols [53], BMI is calculated as weight (kg)/[height (m)]^2 [54]. The cutoff points for child overweight and obesity diagnosis according to the WHO are displayed in Table 88.3 [51, 55].

88.5.2 The Energy and Nutrient Needs of Children

Children's energy and nutrient needs should be calculated by their age, growth rate, and their body composition. Infancy is the period when growth is at the highest rate and, after the second month of postnatal life, the growth rates start to decline. Therefore, since young infants' energy needs are very high, they can be vulnerable to undernutrition [56].

The energy and nutrient needs of infants are determined by the composition of breastmilk, known to be the gold standard for meeting optimal nutrition during the first 6 months of life. Following infancy, childhood and adolescence growth happens at a slower rate and dietary reference intakes become specific for age and sex of the children [4].

Dietary recommendations have been established either by federal governments and/or professional organizations in the form of food-based dietary guidelines [8]. In general, food-based dietary guidelines advocate increasing the variety of food within diet; consuming adequate amounts of vegetables and fruits; meeting the dietary reference intakes of macronutrients (carbohydrate, fat, and protein); having breakfast every day; maintaining a diet rich in fiber and calcium; limiting sugar-sweetened beverages and energy-dense foods (see Figs. 88.2, 88.3, 88.4, 88.5 for various dietary recommendations for children) along with recommending daily moderate to vigorous physical activity for a minimum of 60 min.

Therefore, the basis of the nutritional requirements come from these guidelines. Pediatric patients undergoing ENT infections should foremost follow the dietary guidelines; otherwise, depending on their complications, their energy, nutrient, and food preparation should be adjusted to ensure optimal nutrition and hydration.

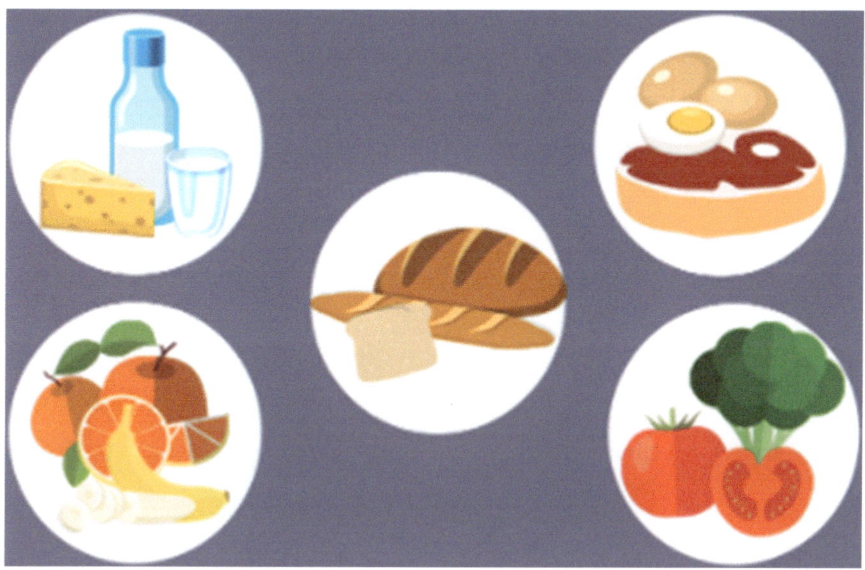

Fig. 88.2 Australian Dietary guidelines for children, 2019 [57]

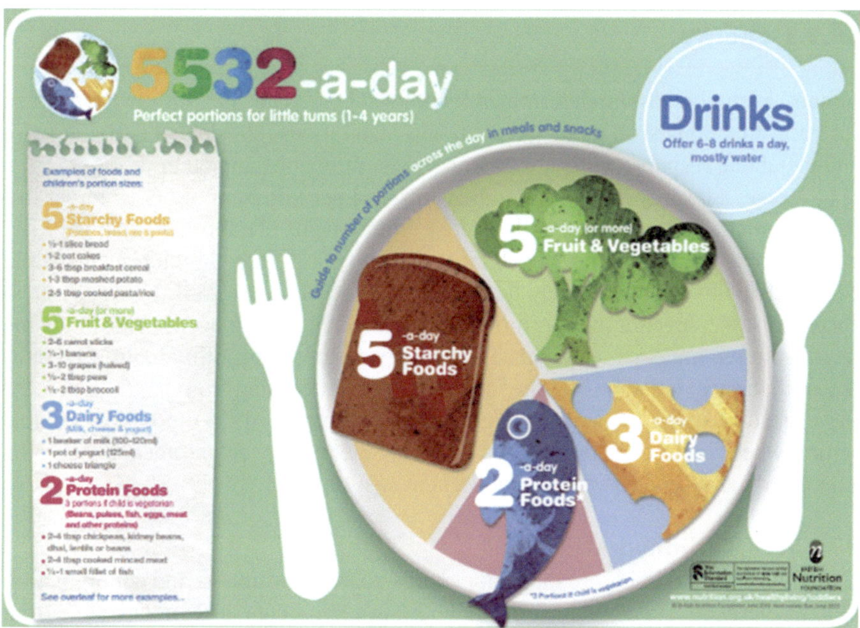

Fig. 88.3 British Nutrition Foundation's Healthy Eating for Toddlers Guideline, 2019 [58]

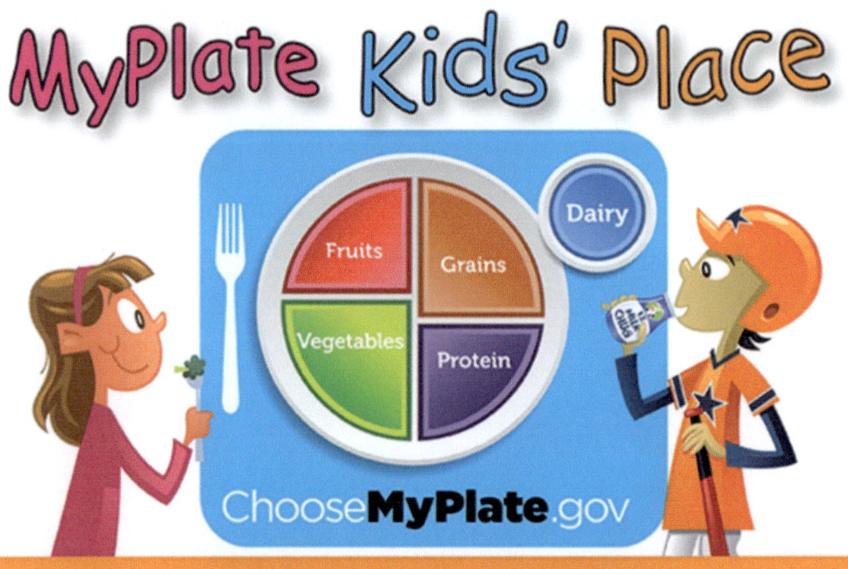

Fig. 88.4 Dietary Guidelines for Americans 2015–2020, visual for the children audiences [59]

88.5.3 Energy

Infants' energy needs are determined by basal metabolism (i.e., the energy needed for basal functions such as metabolism and respiration), physical activity, growth, and metabolic response to food and stress (e.g., infections and other diseases) [56]. On average, a healthy newborn requires 100 kcal per kilogram of body weight [4]. After 6 months, approximate daily energy requirements are about 90 kcal per kilogram of body weight till 5 years. After the first 4 years, energy requirements could be calculated by 40 kcal/kg/day until the end of adolescence [56]. However, presence of disease, fever or malnutrition could change the energy needs [4]. Among the most preferred methods to calculate the energy requirements of malnourished children is to base calculations on the ideal body weight coming from the 50th percentile instead of using the actual weight of the children [56]. In the typical clinical setting where indirect calorimetry is not available, energy requirements should be calculated via estimated energy requirement eqs. [50].

88.5.3.1 Carbohydrates

Carbohydrates and lipids are the major energy sources for infants and children. 40% of total energy intake in infants' diet and 60% in adolescents' diet should come from carbohydrate. Adequate carbohydrate intake allows protein to be used for growth and development rather than energy source [4].

For infants, the main carbohydrate is lactose from either breastmilk or infant formulas that could be digested and tolerated well [32]. In addition, milk represents an excellent source of high-quality protein, calcium, and riboflavin. In most

Kid's Healthy Eating Plate

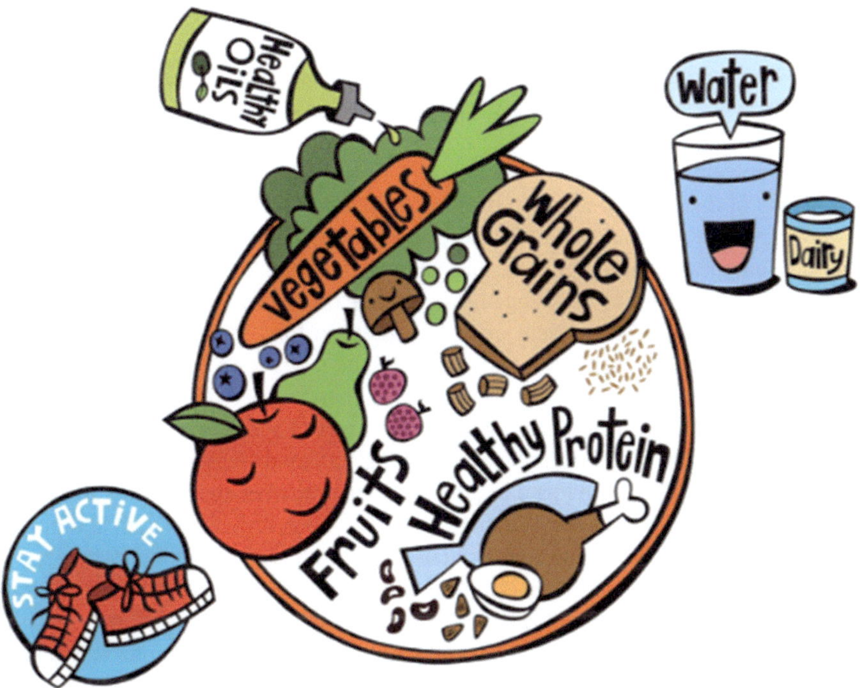

Fig. 88.5 Harvard T.H. Chan's Kid's Healthy Eating Plate [60] (Copyright © 2015 Harvard T.H. Chan School of Public Health. For more information about The Kid's Healthy Eating Plate, please see The Nutrition Source, Department of Nutrition, Harvard T.H. Chan School of Public Health, hsph.harvard.edu/nutritionsource/kids-healthy-eating-plate)

populations, even those with low lactase activity, milk can be ingested in small amounts, especially after meals with dilution by co-ingestion. Fermented dairy products can be valuable items in the diet of most people irrespective of intestinal lactase status. Often the transition from childhood to adulthood is associated with changes in dietary pattern. In developing countries, children frequently consume very high carbohydrate intakes from a single or a small number of sources, while adults have greater variety [61].

Beyond quantity, carbohydrate quality has an important role in health. WHO recommends to limit added sugar consumption to a maximum of 10% of the daily energy in order to prevent dental caries, obesity, and insulin resistance [62]. Additionally, Dietary Reference Intake (DRI) recommendation is 14 g of fiber per 1000 kcal consumed after 2 years of age. Dietary fiber is a type of carbohydrate that can be subdivided into water-soluble and water-insoluble fiber with differing functions in the body. While soluble fibers bind bile acids, reduce cholesterol absorption, and slow gastric emptying, insoluble fibers increase stool bulk and decrease gut transit time [4]. Fiber intake recommendations for children might differ in different countries or depending on the organization that the health care practitioner follows. For example, the American Academy of Pediatrics recommend age of the child in years +5 g of fiber whereas Food and Drug Agency of United States recommends 12 g of fiber per 1000 kcal consumed [63].

Previous studies have shown that both quantity and quality of carbohydrates should be assessed with respect to weight control. Jenkins et al. used the term "glycemic index" for the first time to define carbohydrate quality [64]. Glycemic index (GI) is a percentage value that ranges from 1 to 100 for each food and is defined as the ability of that food to increase blood glucose compared to a standard food such as pure glucose or white bread 2 h after consumption. Since foods with high GI cause a sharp rise in blood glucose, the fall occurs dramatically as well. Therefore, low-GI foods trigger slower changes in blood glucose levels [4]. However, since GI does not account for the amount of carbohydrate in food servings, glycemic load (GL) provides a more inclusive estimate of a food's effect on blood glucose level. The consumption of high GI and/or GL foods causes faster increase in the blood glucose and this consequently will increase the insulin secretion while lowering the glucagon level [65]. Epidemiological studies have demonstrated that higher insulin levels of the individuals are in a direct relationship with obesity [66]. Lower GI and/or GL foods, notably the ones with high in dietary fiber, resistant starch, and lipids, cause less dramatic swings in blood glucose and insulin levels (Table 88.4) [4].

Either way, the main message is that carbohydrate quantity and quality is of great importance during childhood and adolescence and health professionals should emphasize both to maintain health, development, and adequate immune response.

88.5.3.2 Lipids

Triglycerides are the main energy source for newborns and fats provide 50 to 55% of the kcals in breastmilk [56]. Human milk is rich in essential fatty acids; arachidonic acid (omage-6 fatty acid) along with eicosapentaenoic acid and docosahexaenoic acid (omega-3 fatty acids). Omega-6 and omega-3 are deemed "essential fatty acids" because they cannot be produced by the body; therefore they need to be obtained in the diet for neurological, psychomotor development, and visual acuity [4, 8]. As the child grows, fatty fish and vegetable oils provides the dietary source of omega-3 and omega-6 fatty acids [1]. Although energy requirement from fat is about 40–50% during the first year of the baby, this requirement drops to 30% for

Table 88.4 Glycemic index and glycemic load categories' classification

Classification categories	Glycemic index	Glycemic load
Low	55 or less	10 or less
Medium	56–69	11–19
High	70 or more	20 and above

children who are above 2 years of age [56]. As for carbohydrate, quantity and quality of dietary lipids are important. Energy coming from saturated fats should not exceed 10% of the total calories [1].

88.5.3.3 Protein

Similar to what is stated for energy needs, protein requirement is the highest in infancy, being close to two times the requirement of adults per kg of body weight due to high protein turnover rates [4]. Optimal growth depends on sufficient and high-quality protein intake in infants and children. The need for protein per kilogram of body weight gradually decrease as the child grows older. The Joint FAO/WHO/UNO Expert Committee recommends 2.5 g/kg/day protein for the first month, then 2.25 g/kg/day for the following 2 months, and 2 g/kg/day for the fourth month, 1.7 g/kg/day between fourth and sixth month, and 1.5 g/kg/day for the second 6 months of life [56]. Then the daily protein needs fall less than 1.1 g/kg/day after 5 years of age [4].

However, severe physical stress resulting from infections, fevers, and surgery increases the protein losses; thus, the requirements could be augmented by one-third [4]. Moreover, the protein quality is affected by the amino acid composition of the diet [1]. While breastmilk and egg, as well as the majority of animal sources, have high quality protein, wheat and rice are limited in lysine and legumes are low in methionine. Therefore, protein complementation is recommended by mixing different sources of plant proteins for achieving high quality protein whenever needed [4]. On an additional note, supplements of conditionally essential amino acids such as glutamine and arginine could function as immunonutrients in infectious complications and are associated with improvements in wound healing among patients with high risk of malnutrition [67, 68].

88.5.3.4 Vitamins and Minerals

Compared to macronutrients, the daily requirement of micronutrients is in much smaller amounts with mere milligrams or micrograms. Micronutrients do not provide the body with energy themselves, dissimilar to carbohydrates, lipids, and proteins. However, they are indispensable for extracting energy from macronutrients, maintaining the integrity of the immune system, as well as taking part in many other bodily functions [1]. Individual micronutrients frequently interact with one another and their functions could be interrelated. Therefore, deficiency of only one micronutrient could create important health problems [4].

Other than vitamins D, K, and B12 and minerals iron and fluoride, human milk provides all the needed micronutrients for the babies. However, the aforementioned micronutrients of concern during infancy are absorbed more efficiently from breastfeeding compared to formula feeding [4]. After infancy, if the child eats a healthy and balanced diet as recommended in the guidelines, most of the vitamins and minerals could easily be obtained [28]. Among younger children, two micronutrients of global concern are iron and vitamin D. To prevent iron and vitamin D deficiencies, the recommendations for vitamin D intake for infants are ranging from 5 to 30 micrograms depending on the latitudes of the countries [69] and WHO recommends daily iron supplementation in pre-school aged (24–59 months) children who are living in settings where the anima prevalence is equal or more than 40% [70]. However, unless the child has a diagnosed deficiency, malnutrition, or a condition that requires dietary restriction (such as food allergies, celiac, and phenylketonuria), they do not need to receive supplements [4]. Nevertheless, in addition to sub-optimal dietary practices found in many cultures, adolescence should be highlighted as the period that requires the most amount of macro and micronutrients. In addition to iron and vitamin D, calcium and vitamin A could be of major concern during this period [71].

Additionally, low antioxidant status among children with otitis media could exacerbate or prolong their infectious condition [72]. Specifically, acute otitis media is associated with low zinc, iron, vitamin D and vitamin A levels, leading to the hypothesis that supplementing children with known deficiencies would be especially beneficial in this case [73].

88.6 Mediterranean Diet

Mediterranean diet is a plant dominant eating pattern that is characterized by high intake of seasonal vegetables (especially green leafy vegetables) and fruits, primarily whole-grain bread and cereals, legumes, nuts, and olive oil [74]. The consumption of fermented dairy products such as yogurt and cheese are encouraged while eggs are also present in the diet a few times per week. In this eating pattern, moderate fish consumption is recommended, yet meat and sweet intake is limited to few times a month. Additionally, Mediterranean diet model advocates an active lifestyle along with strong social interaction. Evidence has been accumulating on the effect of Mediterranean diet on lowering inflammation [24]. As part of PREDIMED randomized trial, participants with high risk of cardiovascular disease had lower inflammatory biomarkers following Mediterranean diet for 12 months compared to the comparison group that consumed a low-fat diet [75]. Despite the beneficial effects of Mediterranean diet mostly shown on adult populations, reduced postprandial inflammatory response and increased adiponectin concentrations even in the absence of weight loss makes this eating pattern suitable for pediatric populations undergoing ENT infections [76]. Plus, high intake of plant foods and olive oil contribute to increased micronutrient and antioxidant intake, which could further enhance the beneficial health effects [77].

88.7 DASH Diet

Dietary Approaches to Stop Hypertension (DASH) diet provides a dietary pattern that includes high amount of vegetables, fruits, low or no fat dairy products, wholegrains, fish and seafood, beans, and nuts to maintain blood pressure control [26]. DASH eating plan is limited in foods that have high sodium and saturated fat including full-fat dairy products, fatty meats, palm and coconut oils as well as foods and beverages that contain high amount of sugar [25]. (Table 88.5).

Table 88.5 Sample Daily Menu for DASH and Mediterranean Diets (Disclaimer: The sample menus were provided as examples for DASH and Mediterranean diets and they were not arranged according to energy needs of a particular patient, therefore a registered dietitian should arrange menus tailored for the individual energy and nutrient needs of the children, taking culture and taste into consideration as well for personalized interventions)

Breakfast	
Alternative 1	Oatmeal + fruit + plant-based milk
Alternative 2	Hard-boiled egg + vegetables (tomato, cucumber) + whole wheat bread + skim milk
Mid-morning snack	
Alternative 1	Nuts (hazelnuts, walnuts, almonds) + whole wheat cracker
Alternative 2	Fruit + low-fat yogurt
Lunch	
Alternative 1	Beans or legumes + rice or bulgur + mini salad with olive oil
Alternative 2	Tuna sandwich (whole-wheat bread) + fruit
Mid-afternoon snack	
Alternative 1	Whole wheat bread or cracker + crunchy peanut butter + fruit
Alternative 2	Low-fat cheese + fruit
Dinner	
Alternative 1	Vegetable soup + grilled chicken or turkey + whole wheat pasta + lettuce / tomato
Alternative 2	Baked fish + boiled or grilled vegetables + hummus + whole-wheat bread
Evening snack	
Alternative 1	Fruit + skim milk or low-fat yogurt
Alternative 2	Nuts + fruit

88.8 Postoperative Tonsillectomy Diet

Dietary intervention could enhance children's quality of life after tonsillectomy surgery aiming to minimize the complications of pain and bleeding in the following days. The two most common dietary advice approaches regarding post-tonsillectomy are either following a diet of liquids and/or soft foods or continuing with the regular diet of children right away after the operation without imposing any dietary restrictions [78]. The disadvantages of consuming liquids solely are higher incidence rate of emesis, and feeling of restriction; however, avoiding solid foods might decrease the risk of postoperative pain, infections, and bleeding. An accepted trend has been to recommend liquids initially after the operation with a gradual progression towards a regular diet over the following days or weeks [79]. However, evidence has not been accumulated enough to clearly advocate liquid diet over the regular diet in terms of pain score and rate of hemorrhage [80]. Besides, the cold temperature of the liquids and foods did not affect the post-tonsillectomy pain among children compared to liquids and foods served at room temperature [81]. Additionally, in one study parents were found to be more satisfied with a regular diet due to their inability to obey the restrictive dietary instructions [82]. Therefore, in the light of the contemporary views, traditionalist approach of recommending a soft food diet of ice cream and jelly is not accepted as superior to regular diet [83]. Citrus fruits and milk products that could coat the mouth and throat, thereby causing the need to clear the throat, could be potential irritants after the surgery and may initiate bleeding. Hence, their consumption could be limited for the first few postoperative days in order to decrease the risk of morbidity [80].

88.9 Enteral Nutrition

Enteral nutrition support is indicated when patients have a functioning gastrointestinal system, yet energy and nutrient requirements could not be met orally [30]. Nasogastric, nasojejunal, and gastrojejunal feeding routes, gastrostomy, and jejunostomy are the most commonly used enteral nutrition routes and stomach is the preferred delivery site until patients' nutritional requirements could be met orally and age-appropriate growth is achieved [32]. Oral nutritional supplements can also be used, when energy and nutrients intake does not meet the requirements through oral diet alone. Stomach route can be replaced by post-pyloric positioning of the tube-end when the pediatric patient presents gastroparesis or gastroesophageal reflux to avoid aspiration and consequent infections in respiratory and ENT tracts [84]. If the tube feeding is anticipated to continue for more than 6 weeks, the preferred method should be the placement of endoscopic stoma/feeding tube [30]. Although both enteral and parenteral routes could be used for pediatric patients, enteral nutrition is safer with less metabolic and infectious complications (i.e., better manageability). Additionally, enteral nutrition is more physiological due to relying on gastrointestinal system and more economical compared to parenteral feedings [32]. Therefore, enteral feeding should be attempted before parenteral feeding even when the gut absorption is not fully functional [56]. Enteral nutrition should be initiated after child has hemodynamic stability within 72 hours of injury or admission [30]. For patients with severe underfeeding, such as in intensive care units, a combination of enteral and parenteral nutrition could be indicated.

88.10 Parenteral Nutrition

Only when adequate nutrition cannot be maintained orally or enterally, peripheral parenteral or total parenteral nutrition could be indicated in order to prevent malnutrition and supply for growth and development [56]. Even then, parenteral nutrition should be supplemented with enteral nutrition if the patient's gastrointestinal system can tolerate [50]. The initiation time of parenteral nutrition depends on the patient's age and size. While a single day of starvation could be detrimental for a small preterm infant, school-age children and adolescents could tolerate longer periods of insufficient nutrition [30]. Established algorithms should be followed to evaluate patients' nutritional status periodically with an aim to enhance the quality of parenteral nutrition care [56].

Peripheral parenteral nutrition is suitable for short-term feeding via a peripheral vein. However, achieving total energy and protein needs via a peripheral vein is highly improbable due to the osmolality of the required solutions. Conversely, total parenteral nutrition could be sustained for a longer time than peripheral parenteral nutrition. Yet, due to high risks of metabolic, septic, and mechanical complications, enteral nutrition should be attempted even to provide a small portion of the nutrients for preserving the integrity of the gastrointestinal mucosa and its function [56]. Since pediatric patients' energy and nutrient requirements are higher due to anabolism and growth needs compared to adults, malnutrition prevalence was found to be higher among critically ill children with an increased risk for protein-energy malnutrition. Malnutrition could increase patients' morbidity, mortality, and causes longer duration of hospitalization. Since sustaining an optimum status of micronutrients is very important in ENT related cases, nutrition support teams should provide patients with enteral micronutrient preparations. Nutritional therapies should be personalized after careful monitoring.

88.11 Conclusions

- Nutrition is a preventable risk factor for augmented morbidity in pediatric ENT infections.
- ENT infections could also impact the nutrition status of pediatric populations.
- Pediatric patients having nutritional risk factors should be referred to pediatric dietitians, who are specifically working with children and adolescents.
- Exclusive breastfeeding for the first 6 months of life, limiting the use of a bottle as part of a bedtime ritual, following the recommendations of food-based dietary guidelines, avoiding over and undernutrition are key dietary recommendations to prevent and treat ENT infections in the pediatric population.

References

1. Blake JS. Nutrition & you. New York: Benjamin Cummings; 2008.
2. Willett W. Nutritional epidemiology. Oxford: Oxford University Press; 2012.
3. Jung SY, Kim SH, Yeo SG. Association of nutritional factors with hearing loss. J Nutr. 2019;11(2):307.
4. Insel PM. Discovering nutrition. Burlington: Jones & Bartlett Publishers; 2013.
5. Bendich A. Nutrition in pediatric pulmonary disease. New York: Humana Press; 2014. p. 152.
6. Yılmaz T, Koçan EG, Besler HT. The role of oxidants and antioxidants in chronic tonsillitis and adenoid hypertrophy in children. Int J Pediatr Otorhinolaryngol. 2004;68(8):1053–8.
7. Yilmaz T, Koçcan EG, Besler HT, Yilmaz G, Gürsel BJ. The role of oxidants and antioxidants in otitis media with effusion in children. Otolaryngol Head Neck Surg. 2004;131(6):797–803.
8. Brown JE. Nutrition through the life cycle: Cengage learning; 2016.
9. Fogel A, Blissett J. Associations between Otitis media, taste sensitivity and adiposity: two studies across childhood. J Physiol Behavior. 2019;208:112570.
10. Lieberthal AS, Carroll AE, Chonmaitree T, Ganiats TG, Hoberman A, Jackson MA, et al. The diagnosis and management of acute otitis media. Pediatrics. 2013;131(3):e964–e99.
11. Kohlberg GD, Demmer RT, Lalwani AK. Adolescent obesity is an independent risk factor for sensorineural hearing loss: results from the National Health and Nutrition Examination Survey 2005 to 2010. J Neurotology. 2018;39(9):1102–8.
12. Scinicariello F, Carroll Y, Eichwald J, Decker J, Breysse PN. Association of obesity with hearing impairment in adolescents. Sci Rep. 2019;9(1):1–7.
13. Jung SY, Park DC, Kim SH, Yeo SG. Role of obesity in otorhinolaryngologic diseases. Curr Allergy Asthma Rep. 2019;19(7):34.

14. Hwang JH, Hsu CJ, Liu TC, Yang WS. Association of plasma adiponectin levels with hearing thresholds in adults. Clin Endocrinol (Oxf). 2011;75(5):614–20.

15. Tanigawa T, Shibata R, Ouchi N, Kondo K, Ishii M, Katahira N, et al. Adiponectin deficiency exacerbates age-related hearing impairment. Cell Death Dis. 2014;5(4):e1189.

16. Petrakis D, Marginǎ D, Tsarouhas K, Tekos F, Stan M, Nikitovic D, et al. Obesity-a risk factor for increased COVID-19 prevalence, severity and lethality. Mol Med Rep. 2020;22(1):9–19.

17. Yim M, Chiou EH, Ongkasuwan J. Otolaryngologic manifestations of gastroesophageal reflux. Am J Gastroenterol. 2016;2(3):236–45.

18. Organization WH. Obesity and overweight; 2020. https://www.who.int/news-room/fact-sheets/detail/obesity-and-overweight.

19. Morais A, Kelly J, Bost JE, Vaidya SS. Characteristics of correctly identified pediatric obesity and overweight status and management in an academic general pediatric clinic. Clin Pediatr. 2018;57(10):1168–75.

20. Calatayud F, Calatayud B, Gallego J, Gonzalez-Martin C, Alguacil L. Effects of Mediterranean diet in patients with recurring colds and frequent complications. Allergol Immunopathol (Madr). 2017;45(5):417–24.

21. Rodríguez JC. What are the real effects of the Mediterranean diet on recurrent colds and their complications? Allergol Immunopathol (Madr). 2017;45(5):415–6.

22. Chrysohoou C, Panagiotakos DB, Pitsavos C, Das UN, Stefanadis C. Adherence to the Mediterranean diet attenuates inflammation and coagulation process in healthy adults: the ATTICA study. J Am Coll Cardiol. 2004;44(1):152–8.

23. Urpi-Sarda M, Casas R, Chiva-Blanch G, Romero-Mamani ES, Valderas-Martínez P, Arranz S, et al. Virgin olive oil and nuts as key foods of the Mediterranean diet effects on inflammatory biomarkers related to atherosclerosis. Pharmacol Res. 2012;65(6):577–83.

24. Schwingshackl L, Hoffmann GJN. Mediterranean dietary pattern, inflammation and endothelial function: a systematic review and meta-analysis of intervention trials. Nutr Metab Cardiovasc Dis. 2014;24(9):929–39.

25. Steinberg D, Bennett GG, Svetkey L. The DASH diet, 20 years later. JAMA. 2017;317(15):1529–30.

26. Soltani S, Chitsazi MJ, Salehi-Abargouei A. The effect of dietary approaches to stop hypertension (DASH) on serum inflammatory markers: a systematic review and meta-analysis of randomized trials. Clin Nutr. 2018;37(2):542–50.

27. Curhan SG, Wang M, Eavey RD, Stampfer MJ, Curhan GC. Adherence to healthful dietary patterns is associated with lower risk of hearing loss in women. J Nutr. 2018;148(6):944–51.

28. Pekcan A, Şanlıer N, Baş M. Turkey dietary guidelines. Ankara: Republic of Turkey Ministry of Health Public Health Agency of Turkey; 2016. p. 1046.

29. Ferry RJ Jr. Management of pediatric obesity and diabetes. New York: Springer; 2011.

30. Koletzko B, Bhatia J, Bhutta ZA, Cooper P, Makrides M, Uauy R, et al. Pediatric nutrition in practice. New York: Karger; 2015.

31. Organization WH. Breastfeeding; 2020. https://www.who.int/health-topics/breastfeeding#tab=tab_1.

32. Kleinman RE, Greer FR. Pediatric nutrition. Elk Grove: American Academy of Pediatrics; 2013.

33. Unicef. The state of the world's children 2019: children, food and nutrition: growing well in a changing world. New York: Unicef; 2019

34. Organization WH. 10 facts on breastfeeding; 2017. https://www.who.int/features/factfiles/breastfeeding/en/.

35. Lawrence RM. Circumstances when breastfeeding is contraindicated. Pediatr Clin North Am. 2013;60(1):295–318.

36. Victora CG, Bahl R, Barros AJ, França GV, Horton S, Krasevec J, et al. Breastfeeding in the 21st century: epidemiology, mechanisms, and lifelong effect. Lancet. 2016;387(10017):475–90.

37. Sabirov A, Casey JR, Murphy TF, Pichichero ME. Breast-feeding is associated with a reduced frequency of acute otitis media and high serum antibody levels against NTHi and outer membrane protein vaccine antigen candidate P6. Pediatr Res. 2009;66(5):565–70.

38. Brennan-Jones CG, Eikelboom RH, Jacques A, Swanepoel D, Atlas MD, Whitehouse AJ, et al. Protective benefit of predominant breastfeeding against otitis media may be limited to early childhood: results from a prospective birth cohort study. Clin Otolaryngol. 2017;42(1):29–37.
39. Li R, Dee D, Li CM, Hoffman HJ, Grummer-Strawn LM. Breastfeeding and risk of infections at 6 years. Pediatrics. 2014;134(Suppl 1):S13–20.
40. Brennan-Jones CG, Whitehouse AJ, Park J, Hegarty M, Jacques A, Eikelboom RH, et al. Prevalence and risk factors for parent-reported recurrent otitis media during early childhood in the Western Australian Pregnancy Cohort (Raine) study. J Paediatr Child Health. 2015;51(4):403–9.
41. Walker RE, Bartley J, Flint D, Thompson JM, Mitchell EA. Determinants of chronic otitis media with effusion in preschool children: a case–control study. BMC Pediatr. 2017;17(1):4.
42. Canani RB, De Filippis F, Nocerino R, Laiola M, Paparo L, Calignano A, et al. Specific signatures of the gut microbiota and increased levels of butyrate in children treated with fermented cow's milk containing heat-killed Lactobacillus paracasei CBA L74. Appl Environ Microbiol. 2017;83:19.
43. Corsello G, Carta M, Marinello R, Picca M, De Marco G, Micillo M, et al. Preventive effect of cow's milk fermented with Lactobacillus paracasei CBA L74 on common infectious diseases in children: A multicenter randomized controlled trial. Appl Environ Microbiol. 2017;9(7):669.
44. Burks A, Tang M, Sicherer S, Muraro A, Eigenmann P, Ebisawa M, et al. ICON: food allergy. J Allergy Clin Immunol. 2012;129:906–20.
45. Mendes G, Brosseron L, Lopes I, Magalhães A. Association between food allergy and otitis media with effusion in light of current knowledge. Nascer e Crescer. 2019;28(3):126–31.
46. NIAID-Sponsored Expert Panel. Guidelines for the diagnosis and management of food allergy in the United States: report of the NIAID-sponsored expert panel. J Allergy Clin Immunol. 2010;126(6):S1–S58.
47. Nsouli T, Nsouli S, Linde R, O'mara F, Scanlon R, Bellanti J. Role of food allergy in serous otitis media. Ann Allergy. 1994;73(3):215–9.
48. Suskind D, Lenssen P. Pediatric Nutrition handbook: an algorithmic approach. New York: Wiley; 2013.
49. (BAPEN) BAfPaEN. Nutritional Assessment 2016. https://www.bapen.org.uk/nutrition-support/assessment-and-planning/nutritional-assessment?showall=1.
50. Reifen R. Pediatric nutrition. New York: Karger; 1998.
51. Organization WH. WHO child growth standards: length/height-for-age, weight-for-age, weight-for-length, weight-for-height and body mass index-for-age: methods and development. Geneva: WHO; 2006.
52. int/growthref/en/ WHOJhww. Global database on child growth and malnutrition: growth reference data for 5–19 years; 2007.
53. Organization WH. WHO child growth standards: training course on child growth assessment. Geneva: WHO; 2008.
54. Krebs NF, Himes JH, Jacobson D, Nicklas TA, Guilday P, Styne D. Assessment of child and adolescent overweight and obesity. Pediatrics. 2007;120(Supplement 4):S193–228.
55. Md O, Onyango AW, Borghi E, Siyam A, Nishida C, Siekmann J. Development of a WHO growth reference for school-aged children and adolescents. Bull World Health Organ. 2007;85:660–7.
56. Matthew A, Haemer LEP, Krebs NF. Normal childhood nutrition & its disorders. In: Hay MJL WW, Deterding RR, Abzug MJ, editors. Current diagnosis & treatment pediatrics. 24th ed. New York: Mc Graw Hill; 2018. p. 280–308.
57. Australia H. Healthy eating for children; 2019. https://www.healthdirect.gov.au/healthy-eating-for-children.
58. Foundation BN. Updated! New 5532 guide to portion size for preschoolers; 2019. https://www.nutrition.org.uk/healthyliving/toddlers/new5532.html.
59. Agriculture UDo. My Plate Kids' Place; 2020. https://www.choosemyplate.gov/browse-by-audience/view-all-audiences/children/kids.

60. Source HTHCSoPH-TN. Kid's Healthy Eating Plate; 2015. https://www.hsph.harvard.edu/nutritionsource/kids-healthy-eating-plate/.
61. World Health Organization. Carbohydrates in human nutrition report of a joint FAO/WHO expert consultation. Geneva: World Health Organization; 1998.
62. Organization WH. Guideline: sugars intake for adults and children 2015. https://www.who.int/publications/i/item/9789241549028.
63. Kranz S, Brauchla M, Slavin JL, Miller KB. What do we know about dietary fiber intake in children and health? The effects of fiber intake on constipation, obesity, and diabetes in children. Adv Nutr. 2012;3(1):47–53.
64. Jenkins D, Wolever T, Taylor RH, Barker H, Fielden H, Baldwin JM, et al. Glycemic index of foods: a physiological basis for carbohydrate exchange. Am J Clin Nutr. 1981;34(3):362–6.
65. Liese AD, Schulz M, Fang F, Wolever TM, D'Agostino RB, Sparks KC, et al. Dietary glycemic index and glycemic load, carbohydrate and fiber intake, and measures of insulin sensitivity, secretion, and adiposity in the insulin resistance atherosclerosis study. Diabetes Care. 2005;28(12):2832–8.
66. Thota P, Perez-Lopez F, Benítes-Zapata VA, Pasupuleti V, Hernandez AV. Obesity-related insulin resistance in adolescents: a systematic review and meta-analysis of observational studies. Gynecol Endocrinol. 2017;33(3):179–84.
67. Chow O, Barbul A. Immunonutrition: role in wound healing and tissue regeneration. Adv Wound Care. 2014;3(1):46–53.
68. Morris CR, Hamilton-Reeves J, Martindale RG, Sarav M, Ochoa Gautier JB. Acquired amino acid deficiencies: a focus on arginine and glutamine. Nutr Clin Pract. 2017;32:30S–47S.
69. Weiler HA, Vitamin D. Supplementation for infants—biological, behavioural and contextual rationale. Geneva: World Health Organization; 2017. https://www.who.int/elena/titles/bbc/vitamind_infants/en/
70. Organization WH. Daily iron supplementation in children 24–59 months of age 2019 [updated February 11, 2019]. https://www.who.int/elena/titles/iron-children-24to59/en/.
71. Salam RA, Hooda M, Das JK, Arshad A, Lassi ZS, Middleton P, et al. Interventions to improve adolescent nutrition: a systematic review and meta-analysis. J Adolesc Health. 2016;59(4):S29–39.
72. Cemek M, Dede S, Bayiroğlu F, Caksen H, Cemek F, Yuca K. Oxidant and antioxidant levels in children with acute otitis media and tonsillitis: a comparative study. Int J Pediatr Otorhinolaryngol. 2005;69(6):823–7.
73. Elemraid MA, Mackenzie IJ, Fraser WD, Brabin BJ. Nutritional factors in the pathogenesis of ear disease in children: a systematic review. Ann Trop Paediatr. 2009;29(2):85–99.
74. Serra-Majem L, Ribas L, Ngo J, Ortega RM, García A, Pérez-Rodrigo C, et al. Food, youth and the Mediterranean diet in Spain. Development of KIDMED, Mediterranean Diet Quality Index in children and adolescents. Public Health Nutr. 2004;7(7):931–5.
75. Casas R, Sacanella E, Urpi-Sarda M, Chiva-Blanch G, Ros E, Martínez-González M-A, et al. The effects of the mediterranean diet on biomarkers of vascular wall inflammation and plaque vulnerability in subjects with high risk for cardiovascular disease. A randomized trial. PLoS One. 2014;9(6):e100084.
76. Richard C, Couture P, Desroches S, Lamarche B. Effect of the Mediterranean diet with and without weight loss on markers of inflammation in men with metabolic syndrome. Obesity (Silver Spring). 2013;21(1):51–7.
77. Bonaccio M, Pounis G, Cerletti C, Donati MB, Iacoviello L, de Gaetano G. Mediterranean diet, dietary polyphenols and low grade inflammation: results from the MOLI-SANI study. Br J Clin Pharmacol. 2017;83(1):107–13.
78. Faramarzi M, Safari S, Roosta S. Comparing cold/liquid diet vs regular diet on posttonsillectomy pain and bleeding. Otolaryngol Head Neck Surg. 2018;159(4):755–60.
79. Hall MD, Brodsky L. The effect of post-operative diet on recovery in the first twelve hours after tonsillectomy and adenoidectomy. Int J Pediatr Otorhinolaryngol. 1995;31(2–3):215–20.
80. Millington A, Gaunt A, Phillips JJ. Post-tonsillectomy dietary advice: systematic review. Int J Pediatr Otorhinolaryngol. 2016;130(10):889.

81. Meybodian M, Dadgarnia M, Baradaranfar M, Vaziribozorg S, Mansourimanesh M, Mandegari M, et al. Effect of cold diet and diet at room temperature on post-tonsillectomy pain in children. Iran J Otorhinolaryngol. 2019;31(103):81.
82. Zagólski O. Do diet and activity restrictions influence recovery after adenoidectomy and partial tonsillectomy? Int J Pediatr Otorhinolaryngol. 2010;74(4):407–11.
83. Bannister M, Thompson CJ. Post-tonsillectomy dietary advice and haemorrhage risk: systematic review. IJoPO. 2017;103:29–31.
84. Krasaelap A, Kovacic K, Goday PS. Nutrition management in pediatric gastrointestinal motility disorders. Nutr Clin Pract. 2020;35(2):265–72.

Probiotic Use in Pediatric Ear, Nose, and Throat Infections Practice

89

Ener Çağrı Dinleyici and Yvan Vandenplas

89.1 Introduction

Probiotics are live bacterial or yeast-derived products, that when administered in adequate amounts, confer a health benefit on the host and are created using production techniques that are consistent with quality standards [1, 2]. The use of probiotics in infectious diseases started years prior to microbiota studies, and their efficacy in the treatment of acute diarrhea and antibiotic-associated diarrhea has been demonstrated in many meta-analyses and is a recommendation in many international guidelines [3–8] diseases have been largely discussed. The effects of probiotics on microbiota restoration are evaluated through the next-generation sequencing technologies and bioinformatics assessments.

89.2 Respiratory Tract Infections

The main purpose of using probiotics, in addition to the treatment infections, is to prevent relapse of disease, to reduce the use of antibiotics, and consequently to reduce the cost of disease and decrease antibiotic resistance. Probiotics are included as supportive treatments for the prevention of infectious disease in addition to

E. Ç. Dinleyici (✉)
Department of Pediatrics, Faculty of Medicine, Eskişehir Osmangazi University, Eskişehir, Turkey

Y. Vandenplas
Department of Pediatrics, University Hospital Brussels, Vrije University Brussels, KidZ Health Castle, Brussels, Belgium

current treatment and prevention strategies [9]. Ozen et al. [9] evaluated 14 randomized controlled trials up to June 2014 in a systematic review on the efficacy of probiotics in the prevention of upper respiratory tract infections in children. In this review, probiotics (especially *Lactobacillus* and *Bifidobacterium* strains) were shown to be moderately effective in the prevention of upper respiratory tract infection and in the reduction of symptom scores. Probiotics have been shown to provide significant clinical and economic benefits in upper respiratory tract infections, with a reduction of 5–10%. Ozen et al. [9] underlined that the most important difficulty to perform a meta-analysis for upper respiratory tract infections are the marked differences between the definition of infections and primary/secondary end-points. In 2015, a Cochrane meta-analysis included 12 randomized controlled trials in eight pediatric populations [10] and found that probiotics reduced the number of upper respiratory tract infection episodes by 47% versus placebo and shortened the duration of the episode of acute upper respiratory tract infection by an average of 1.9 days. It was also shown that probiotics reduced on the use of antibiotics loss of school days associated with upper respiratory tract infection. However, the quality of evidence was low or very low [10].

The meta-analysis of Wang et al. [11] concluded that probiotic use reduced the risk for upper respiratory tract infections and the number of school days lost, but without an effect on the duration of respiratory tract infections.

However, there are also studies showing that probiotics are not effective in the management of upper respiratory tract infections. The daily administration of 1×10^9 CFU of *Bifidobacterium lactis* and *Lactobacillus rhamnosus* during 6 months to 290 girls aged 8–14 months did not show a difference compared to placebo regarding the incidence of upper or lower respiratory tract infections, the frequency of diarrhea episodes, the number of doctor visits, the frequency of fever and vomiting, the duration of antibiotic use, and the frequency of parental illness [12]. According to another meta-analysis published in 2017 which included 21 studies, with 6603 patients aged 0–18 years, there was no effect of probiotics, mainly *Lactobacillus rhamnosus GG,* on the incidence of upper respiratory tract infections (amaral). It has been shown that all probiotics used in this meta-analysis are well tolerated [9–13].

89.3   Acute Otitis Media

Acute otitis media is one of the most common bacterial infections in childhood and is a major indication of antibiotic use. Seventy percent of children contract otitis at least once before the age of 2 years, and 20–30% have recurrent otitis media [14]. In a meta-analysis involving four randomized controlled trials in 2013, the use of LGG was shown to reduce the frequency of acute otitis media and antibiotic use versus placebo and LGG was considered to be safe [15]. However, Hatakka et al. showed that probiotics in patients with frequent otitis media between 10 months and 6 years had no effect on the frequency of acute otitis media and antibiotic use. There was no effect of the probiotic on nasopharyngeal carriage [16]. However, this study showed for the first time the effects of probiotic therapy on microbial balance: Probiotics did not affect the carriage of Streptococcus pneumoniae or Haemophilus influenzae, but increased the prevalence of Moraxella catarrhalis. The same study showed that recurrent upper respiratory tract infections in the group using probiotics had decreased by 12% and that the frequency of recurrent upper respiratory tract infection decreased by 45%.

It is thought that the colonization of the nasopharynx with alpha-hemolytic streptococcus may prevent the development of middle ear infections in predisposed children [17]. *Streptococcus salivarius* 24SMB (*S. salivarius 24SMB*) strain administered as a nasal spray reduces the risk of developing otitis media among otitis-prone children. Lower risk of otitis media was observed in children who are colonized in their nasopharynx with *S. salivarius* 24SMB [18]. *Streptococcus salivarius* K12 reduced the frequency of pharyngitis and otitis media, especially in day-care centers [19]. However, there is also a study showing no change in the frequency of infection with *S. salivarius* K12 [20].

There is no strong guidance of the level of dosage, form, length of use, and appropriate age group for treatment. For this reason, it will be useful to conduct a strain-specific analysis in the evaluation of the studies. A wide range of randomized controlled trials are needed to recommend the routine use of probiotics in the treatment or prevention of respiratory tract infections.

Ear, nose, and throat diseases are one of the most frequent targets of antibiotics in routine practice. It is thought that majority of the routinely used antibiotics are broad spectrum, and that they can cause significant changes in the composition of intestinal microbiota. Antibiotics, especially those with anaerobic activity, are thought to be more likely than antibiotics with aerobic activity to have negative effects on microbiota [21, 22]. Antibiotic-associated diarrhea is called diarrhea when it does not stem from other factors that occur during or after antibiotic treatment. Antibiotic-associated diarrhea is usually mild to moderate but can rarely lead to serious clinical symptoms associated with *Clostridium difficile* infection [23]. Antibiotic-associated diarrhea can comprise 35% of all cases of diarrhea. Amoxicillin-clavulanic acid and ampicillin sulbactam are frequently caused of AAD, in the level of 10–25%, while fluoroquinolones, macrolides, tetracyclines, and cephalosporins are also related with antibiotic-associated diarrhea [24, 25]. *Clostridium difficile*-associated pseudomembranous colitis is the most severe form of antibiotic-associated diarrhea. It is most commonly associated with the use of clindamycin and may occur due to changes in microbiota composition during the use of any antibiotic. The main mechanisms of antibiotic-associated diarrhea include osmotic diarrhea due to the metabolism of intestinal nutrients and the accumulation of metabolites due to the impairment of the composition of intestinal microbiota. Normally, carbohydrates reach the colon without being absorbed in the small intestines. At this point, they are transformed into short-chain fatty acids, such as butyrate, by the microbial elements of the colon. The second mechanism is the increased frequency of antibiotic-resistant bacteria (especially *Clostridium difficile*), which is the result of the loss of colonized bacteria in microbiota. In recent years, it has been shown that antibiotics have serious effects on metabolism and can lead to changes in bile acid (which is a key determinant of the Clostridium difficile life cycle), carbohydrates, and amino acid metabolism. There are also studies showing that antibiotics increase sialic acid production and enhance the development of Clostridium difficile. Another mechanism is the effect of antibiotics such as erythromycin on motility [21, 24, 26].

The main method of preventing antibiotic-associated diarrhea is the use of rational antibiotics. Antibiotic treatment is the basic approach to use at appropriate indications and at the appropriate doses. The most effective treatment available for the prevention of antibiotic-associated diarrhea is the administration of a probiotic therapy at the same time as the antibiotic therapy [6, 27–30]. The application of probiotics to selected strains simultaneously with antibiotic therapy and during treatment is evidence-based and can be found in international guidelines [5, 6]. The mechanism of action of probiotics in the prevention of antibiotic-associated diarrhea involves removing antibiotics from the negative side of microbiota [31]. The European Society of Pediatric Gastroenterology, Hepatology and Nutrition guidelines have shown that children have achieved a level of evidence of "A" with current randomized controlled trials of *Lactobacillus rhamnosus GG* and *Saccharomyces boulardii CNCM I-745* in the prevention of antibiotic-associated diarrhea [6]. In 63 randomized controlled trials of the protective effect of probiotics on the development of antibiotic-associated diarrhea, a meta-analysis of 11,811 patients showed that probiotics reduced the frequency of antibiotic-associated diarrhea by 42%. Similarly, the use of probiotics has been shown to reduce the incidence of *Clostridium difficile* infection by 66% [29]. Antibiotic-associated diarrhea usually terminates after the discontinuation of antibiotic therapy without the need for additional treatment. Antibiotics such as vancomycin or metronidazole, probiotics or fecal transplantation can be performed in the case of the development of Clostridium difficile infection [24].

References

1. Hill C, Guarner F, Reid G, Gibson GR, Merenstein DJ, Pot B, Morelli L, Canani RB, Flint HJ, Salminen S, Calder PC, Sanders ME. Expert consensus document. The International Scientific Association for Probiotics and Prebiotics consensus statement on the scope and appropriate use of the term probiotic. Nat Rev Gastroenterol Hepatol. 2014;11(8):506–14.
2. Kolaček S, Hojsak I, BerniCanani R, Guarino A, Indrio F, Orel R, Pot B, Shamir R, Szajewska H, Vandenplas Y, van Goudoever J, Weizman Z, ESPGHAN Working Group for Probiotics and Prebiotics. Commercial probiotic products: a call for improved quality control. A position paper by the ESPGHAN working Group for Probiotics and Prebiotics. J Pediatr Gastroenterol Nutr. 2017;84(1):117–24.
3. Ozen M, Dinleyici EC. The history of probiotics: the untold story. Benef Microb. 2015;6(2):159–84.
4. Hojsak I, Fabiano V, Pop TL, Goulet O, Zuccotti GV, Çokuğraş FC, Pettoello-Mantovani M, Kolaček S. Guidance on the use of probiotics in clinical practice in children with selected clinical conditions and in specific vulnerable groups. Acta Paediatr. 2018;107(6):927–37.
5. Floch MH, Walker WA, Sanders ME, Nieuwdorp M, Kim AS, Brenner DA, Qamar AA, Miloh TA, Guarino A, Guslandi M, Dieleman LA, Ringel Y, Quigley EM, Brandt

LJ. Recommendations for probiotic use--2015 update: proceedings and consensus opinion. J Clin Gastroenterol. 2015;49(Suppl 1):S69–73.

6. Szajewska H, Canani RB, Guarino A, Hojsak I, Indrio F, Kolacek S, Orel R, Shamir R, Vandenplas Y, van Goudoever JB, Weizman Z, ESPGHAN Working Group for Probiotics Prebiotics. Probiotics for the prevention of antibiotic-associated diarrhea in children. J Pediatr Gastroenterol Nutr. 2016;62(3):495–506.

7. Dinleyici EC, Eren M, Ozen M, Yargic ZA, Vandenplas Y. Effectiveness and safety of Saccharomyces boulardii for acute infectious diarrhea. Expert Opin Biol Ther. 2012;12(4):395–410.

8. Szajewska H, Guarino A, Hojsak I, Indrio F, Kolacek S, Shamir R, Vandenplas Y, Weizman Z, European Society for Pediatric Gastroenterology, Hepatology, and Nutrition. Use of probiotics for management of acute gastroenteritis: a position paper by the ESPGHAN Working Group for Probiotics and Prebiotics. J Pediatr Gastroenterol Nutr. 2014;58(4):531–9.

9. Ozen M, Kocabas Sandal G, Dinleyici EC. Probiotics for the prevention of pediatric upper respiratory tract infections: a systematic review. Expert Opin Biol Ther. 2015;15(1):9–20.

10. Hao Q, Dong BR, Wu T. Probiotics for preventing acute upper respiratory tract infections. Cochrane Database Syst Rev. 2015;2015:CD006895.

11. Wang Y, Li X, Ge T, Xiao Y, Liao Y, Cui Y, Zhang Y, Ho W, Yu G, Zhang T. Probiotics for prevention and treatment of respiratory tract infections in children: a systematic review and meta-analysis of randomized controlled trials. Medicine (Baltimore). 2016;95(31):e4509.

12. Laursen RP, Larnkjær A, Ritz C, Hauger H, Michaelsen KF, Mølgaard C. Probiotics and child care absence due to infections: a randomized controlled trial. Pediatrics. 2017;140(2):e20170735.

13. Amaral MA, Guedes GHBF, Epifanio M, Wagner MB, Jones MH, Mattiello R. Network meta-analysis of probiotics to prevent respiratory infections in children and adolescents. Pediatr Pulmonol. 2017;52(6):833–43.

14. Dinleyici EC, Yuksel F, Yargic ZA, Unalacak M, Unluoglu I. Results of a national study on the awareness of and attitudes toward acute otitis media (AOM) among clinicians and the estimated direct healthcare costs in Turkey (TR-AOM study). Int J Pediatr Otorhinolaryngol. 2013;77(5):756–61.

15. Liu S, Hu P, Du X, Zhou T, Pei X. Lactobacillus rhamnosus GG supplementation for preventing respiratory infections in children: a meta-analysis of randomized, placebo-controlled trials. Indian Pediatr. 2013;50(4):377–81.

16. Hatakka K, Blomgren K, Pohjavuori S, Kaijalainen T, Poussa T, Leinonen M, Korpela R, Pitkäranta A. Treatment of acute otitis media with probiotics in otitis-prone children-a double-blind, placebo-controlled randomised study. Clin Nutr. 2007;26:314–21.

17. Santagati M, Scillato M, Muscaridola N, Metoldo V, La Mantia I, Stefani S. Colonization, safety, and tolerability study of the Streptococcus salivarius 24SMBc nasal spray for its application in upper respiratory tract infections. Eur J Clin Microbiol Infect Dis. 2015;34(10):2075–80.

18. Marchisio P, Santagati M, Scillato M, Baggi E, Fattizzo M, Rosazza C, Stefani S, Esposito S, Principi N. Streptococcus salivarius 24SMB administered by nasal spray for the prevention of acute otitis media in otitis-prone children. Eur J Clin Microbiol Infect Dis. 2015;34(12):2377–83.

19. Di Pierro F, Risso P, Poggi E, Timitilli A, Bolloli S, Bruno M, Caneva E, Campus R, Giannattasio A. Use of streptococcus salivarius K12 to reduce the incidence pharyngo-tonsillitis and acute otitis media in children: a retrospective analysis in not-recurrent pediatric subjects. Minerva Pediatr. 2018;70(3):240–5.

20. Doyle H, Pierse N, Tiatia R, Williamson D, Baker M, Crane J. Effect of the oral probiotic Streptococcus salivarius (K12) on group a Streptococcus pharyngitis: a pragmatic trial in schools. Pediatr Infect Dis J. 2018;37(7):619–23.

21. Becattini S, Taur Y, Pamer EG. Antibiotic-induced changes in the intestinal microbiota and disease. Trends Mol Med. 2016;22(6):458–78.

22. Blaser MJ. Antibiotic use and its consequences for the normal microbiome. Science. 2016;352(6285):544–5.

23. Dinleyici M, Vandenplas Y. Clostridium difficile colitis prevention and treatment. Adv Exp Med Biol. 2019;1125:139–46.
24. McFarland LV, Ozen M, Dinleyici EC, Goh S. Comparison of pediatric and adult antibiotic-associated diarrhea and Clostridium difficile infections. World J Gastroenterol. 2016;22(11):3078–104.
25. Silverman MA, Konnikova L, Gerber JS. Impact of antibiotics on necrotizing enterocolitis and antibiotic-associated diarrhea. Gastroenterol Clin North Am. 2017;46(1):61–76.
26. Fujisaka S, Ussar S, Clish C, Devkota S, Dreyfuss JM, Sakaguchi M, Soto M, Konishi M, Softic S, Altindis E, Li N, Gerber G, Bry L, Kahn CR. Antibiotic effects on gut microbiota and metabolism are host dependent. J Clin Invest. 2016;126(12):4430–43.
27. Johnston BC, Ma SSY, Goldenberg JZ, et al. Probiotics for the prevention of Clostridium difficile-associated diarrhea: a systematic review and meta-analysis. Ann Intern Med. 2012;157(12):878–88.
28. Goldenberg JZ, Lytvyn L, Steurich J, et al. Probiotics for the prevention of pediatric antibiotic-associated diarrhea. Cochrane Database Syst Rev. 2015;5:CD004827.
29. Hempel S, Newberry SJ, Maher AR, et al. Probiotics for the prevention and treatment of antibiotic-associated diarrhea: a systematic review and meta-analysis. JAMA. 2012;307(18):1959–69.
30. Parkes GC, Sanderson JD, Whelan K. The mechanisms and efficacy of probiotics in the prevention of Clostridium difficile-associated diarrhoea. Lancet Infect Dis. 2009;9(4):237–44.
31. Kabbani TA, Pallav K, Dowd SE, Villafuerte-Galvez J, Vanga RR, Castillo NE, Hansen J, Dennis M, Leffler DA, Kelly CP. Prospective randomized controlled study on the effects of Saccharomyces boulardii CNCM I-745 and amoxicillin-clavulanate or the combination on the gut microbiota of healthy volunteers. Gut Microbes. 2017;8:17–32.

Supportive Agents for Pediatric Otolaryngological Infections

Ali Bayram, Yunus Kantekin, and Pietro Ferrara

90.1 Introduction

Upper respiratory tract infections (URTIs), otitis media, and tonsillopharyngitis are the most common pediatric otolaryngological infections during childhood. URTIs refer to any infectious diseases involving the nose, sinuses, pharynx, or larynx and they are usually caused by viral agents. Although these infections are mostly caused by viruses, diseases that last more than 7–10 days generally refer to secondary bacterial infections. Whether caused by viral or bacterial agents, pediatric otolaryngological infections constitute one of the most common reasons for doctor visits and cause considerable socioeconomic burden for the community.

Supportive agents have been used for infections since ancient times and the popularity of their use is growing among the general population. Either natural or commercially available supportive agents attract attention for overcoming several diseases including pediatric otolaryngological infections. Although there are a large number of supportive agents utilized for infectious diseases worldwide, we aimed to focus on common agents that have been used for pediatric otolaryngological infections.

90.2 Zinc and Vitamins

Zinc is an essential trace element with multiple functions related to immunity, growth and development of the human body. In addition, zinc was shown to have antiviral functions including inhibition of viral replication [1]. Kurugöz et al. [2]

A. Bayram (✉) · Y. Kantekin
Section of Otorhinolaryngology, Kayseri City Training and Research Hospital, Kayseri, Turkey

P. Ferrara
Department of Pediatrics, Faculty of Medicine and Surgery, University of Rome, Campus Bio-Medico, Rome, Italy

C. Cingi et al. (eds.), *Pediatric ENT Infections*,
https://doi.org/10.1007/978-3-030-80691-0_90

investigated the prophylactic and therapeutic effectiveness of zinc with 200 children with a common cold and found that zinc had favorable effects for the prevention and treatment of the common cold over placebo with a high safety profile.

Vitamin C (ascorbic acid) is an essential nutrient found in fresh vegetables and fruits that is the most effective water-soluble antioxidant in human plasma. Vitamin C protects host cells from oxidative stress driven by infection. Also, due to its abundance in phagocytes and lymphocytes, it is postulated that vitamin C has a significant role in immune system cells [3]. Vitamin C was reported to lower plasma histamine levels and increase neutrophil chemotaxis in healthy children.

Vitamin C has been suggested to be an effective agent for preventing URTIs and improving the symptoms due to effects on the immune system over a long period. However, accumulated data regarding the benefits of vitamin C in URTIs revealed conflicting results in the recent literature. A Cochrane review [4] showed that routine vitamin C supplementation did not reduce the common cold incidence in the general population; nevertheless, the efficacy of vitamin C for the common cold was greater in the pediatric population. According to the review, routine administration of ≥ 0.2 g/day vitamin C decreased the duration of the common cold in adults and children by 8% and 14%, respectively. Ferrara et al. [5] demonstrated that vitamin C decreased the number of infective episodes in children with recurrent respiratory tract infections (RRTIs). In their study, the reduction was significant in children who were administered 100% orange juice with a content of 70 mg of vitamin C every day compared to the control group. In a more recent meta-analysis of 3135 children with URTIs derived from eight randomized controlled trials (RCTs), Vorilhon et al. [3] reported that vitamin C had no preventive effect on pediatric URTIs but it reduced the duration of the disease. However, the authors recommended further studies with greater statistical power among children of this age. Despite the ongoing debates about the efficacy of vitamin C on URTIs, the benefit of routine supplementation of vitamin C should not be overlooked due to its safety and low cost.

Vitamin D has well-known effects in calcium and bone metabolism in the body. In addition, recent studies demonstrated that vitamin D plays a role in immune system function in the course of respiratory tract infections (RTIs). Two meta-analyses revealed that vitamin D had a protective effect in the general population with RTIs [6, 7]. In the literature, there is a consensus among most of the studies that RTIs are prevalent in children with vitamin D deficiency. However, studies investigating vitamin D supplementation revealed conflicting results in terms of benefits and optimal doses. In a meta-analysis of children, no relationship was found between the routine use of vitamin D and the prevention of acute respiratory infections [8]. In the study of Omand et al. [9], there was no association between vitamin D supplementation and health-service utilization in young children with URTIs. Although there are several studies in the literature investigating the relationship between vitamin D and RTIs, further RCTs specifically focusing on the clinical efficacy of vitamin D supplementation in pediatric URTIs may elucidate the potential benefits of vitamin D in pediatric URTIs.

90.3 Probiotics

Probiotics are live and nonpathogenic bacteria including Lactobacillus and Bifidobacterium species, Enterococcus, Propionibacterium, Streptococcus, Bacillus, Escherichia coli, Saccharomyces boulardii, and Saccharomyces cerevisiae. Probiotic products have been suggested to have broad favorable effects on human health such as bacterial growth inhibition, immunomodulation, and antiviral properties both in adults and children. They can be administered in various formulations including tablets, capsules, spray, or as a food ingredient.

In a meta-analysis, probiotics have been shown to reduce the frequency of respiratory tract infections and disease duration in children [10]. In a Cochrane review [11], probiotics were found to be better than placebo in reducing the incidence and the mean duration of URTIs episodes, cold-related school absence and antibiotic prescription, although the quality of the evidence was low or very low. Probiotics were also evaluated for preventing otitis media in children and it was shown that probiotics may be effective in preventing acute otitis media in children not prone to acute otitis media [12]. However, the underlying mechanisms of the beneficial effect of probiotics in respiratory tract infections have not yet been fully clarified. A number of studies have investigated the influence of probiotics on the immune system. According to the studies, probiotics can increase the number and activity of neutrophils, leukocytes, and natural killer cells and also help maintain higher salivary immunoglobulin A levels. Probiotics have been demonstrated to be able to affect inflammatory cytokine expression, such as increasing interleukin-10 (IL-10) and decreasing IL-1b, IL-8, and tumor necrosis factor-α (TNF-α) levels [13]. The favorable effects of probiotics on host immune systems and gut microbiota may support the resistance against pathogens [14].

There are also a number of studies in the literature investigating the favorable effects of probiotics in other pediatric otolaryngological infections. Marini et al. [15] demonstrated that oral probiotic Streptococcus salivarius K12 was effective in preventing pharyngo-tonsillar infections in children, with a decrease in school absence, antibiotic usage, and number of patients having a tonsillectomy. The treatment of recurrent Group A beta-hemolytic Streptococcus pharyngotonsillitis with an oral spray form of Streptococcus salivarius 24SMB and Streptococcus oralis 89a in children was found to reduce antibiotic use with no benefit on disease recurrence [16]. In a systematic review, the effectiveness of Streptococcus salivarius K12 on sore throat up to pharyngotonsillitis was evaluated in a systematic review [17]. The study demonstrated that concurrent prescription of probiotics with antibiotics was probably ineffective in the acute disease; however, further randomized controlled trials are required to elucidate the efficacy of Streptococcus salivarius K12 as an alternative therapy to antibiotics or prophylactic capacity in recurrent cases.

There are conflicting results in studies regarding the potential efficacy of probiotics on chronic rhinosinusitis (CRS). In a mouse sinusitis model, Staphylococcus epidermidis was shown to have probiotic properties against Staphylococcus aureus [18]. However, Mukerji et al. [19] reported no advantages of oral administration of the Lactobacillus rhamnosus R0011 strain over placebo in improving sino-nasal quality-of-life scores in patients with CRS. Although existing animal studies reported potential benefits of probiotics in CRS, human studies have yet to provide satisfactory results regarding their benefits.

90.4 Honey and Beehive Products

Honey and beehive products have been used in complementary and alternative medicine since ancient times. The most popular honeybee products that have been studied in otolaryngological diseases are honey, propolis, and royal jelly.

Honey is produced from flower nectar in the aerodigestive tract of bees. The beneficial effects of honey in wound healing are well established, including reduction of inflammation, accelerating epithelization, and pain relief [20]. Honey was shown to be effective in childhood cough and persistent post-infectious cough in children. Also, in children with oral mucositis, honey was demonstrated to accelerate complete recovery time and healing. Honey also has strong antioxidant and antibacterial effects that provide antimicrobial activity against methicillin-resistant Staphylococcus aureus and biofilm formation [21, 22].

Propolis is a mixture produced from plant resins by processes of the bee's salivary system. Propolis contains aromatic acids, polyphenols, volatile oils, and waxes and is used for protecting hives against fungi and bacteria and moisturizing and stabilizing the temperature within the hives [23]. The active ingredient of propolis, caffeic acid phenethyl ester (CAPE), is thought to have multiple beneficial effects including anti-inflammatory, immune-modulatory, antibacterial, antiviral, anticancer, and antioxidant effects. A study investigating the effect of natural propolis in the treatment of acute and chronic rhinopharyngitis in children demonstrated that the extract provided less disease episodes with no relief of rhinorrhea [24]. Although a combined therapy including propolis and zinc was applied, propolis-zinc suspension was shown to reduce acute otitis media episodes with a decrease of nasopharyngeal colonization in children with recurrent acute otitis media. However, because of the possible beneficial effect of zinc, the potential benefit cannot be attributed to the propolis alone.

Royal jelly is an acidic product of worker bees that contains a number of vitamins, minerals, and other nutritious elements to feed the queen honeybee. The active content of royal jelly, 10-hydroxy-2-decenoic acid, is known to have protective and therapeutic effects against infections [25]. Although royal jelly has bacteriostatic and antimicrobial effects due to its active ingredients such as organic acids and royalisin, there is not enough evidence regarding the routine application of royal jelly in children with respiratory infections in the literature.

90.5 Herbal Medicine

The utilization of herbal medicine provides great potential as an alternative treatment for pediatric infections with a growing interest in the medical literature. Although some of the herbal products have been shown to be beneficial, their clinical efficacy should be interpreted cautiously due to the scarcity of high-quality evidence derived from related studies.

Echinacea is one of the most used herbal products for the prevention and treatment of URTIs worldwide. A recent systematic review and meta-analysis demonstrated that commercially available Echinacea remedies likely to be effective may shorten the duration or prevent URTIs, although the majority of trials were carried out in the adult populations [26]. However, although studies are still rare, there are some reports in the literature investigating its clinical efficacy in pediatric patients. Weber et al. reported that Echinacea purpurea may have provided a beneficial effect in reducing the occurrence of subsequent URTIs in 524 children ages 2–11 [27].

Pelargonium sidoides is a traditional medicinal plant native to South Africa and its ethanolic extract known as EPs 7630 was shown to have antiviral, antibacterial, and immunomodulatory effects. The direct antiviral effect of EPs 7630 comprises a number of viral agents including respiratory syncytial viruses, rhinovirus, influenza, parainfluenza, coxsackie, and coronaviruses, whereas in vitro studies revealed that it has an inhibitory effect against several bacteria such as multi-resistant Staphylococcus aureus, Proteus mirabilis, Pseudomonas aeruginosa, Klebsiella pneumoniae, and Escherichia coli. EPs 7630 was shown to be effective in acute RTIs in adults and children [28]. In the review of Careddu and Pettenazzo [29] evaluating the studies conducted on pediatric patients, EPs 7630 was also found to be a safe and beneficial treatment modality in children and adolescents with acute RTIs. Seifert et al. [30] demonstrated that EPs 7630 relieved the fever in children with acute tonsillopharyngitis aged 6–10 years while providing less use of paracetamol.

Myrtle Essential Oil (Myrtol, ELOM-080) is a phytotherapeutic extract containing 4 rectified essential oils composed of myrtle oil, sweet orange oil, eucalyptus oil, and lemon oil. Myrtol was shown to have multiple effects on the respiratory system including bronchospasmolytic, mucolytic, antimicrobial, anti-inflammatory, and antioxidative effects [31]. In pediatric patients with acute rhinosinusitis, Myrtol was reported to be a clinically effective and safe therapeutic option [32].

In addition, many herbal therapies including traditional Chinese medicine agents, North American ginseng, pomegranate, licorice root, maoto, and guava tea were demonstrated to be effective in the treatment of URTIs but their clinical benefits in the pediatric population deserve further consideration with more RCTs.

90.6   Immunomodulators

Pidotimod (PDT, 3-L-pyroglutamyl-L-thiaziolidine-4-carboxylic acid) is a synthetic dipeptide molecule that is capable of innate and adaptive immunity alterations. PDT was investigated in a number studies regarding its effectiveness in pediatric recurrent respiratory tract infections and it demonstrated a remarkable efficacy with a high safety profile [33]. PDT treatment significantly enhances serum IgG, IgM, IgA, and T-lymphocyte subtypes (CD3+, CD4+) levels and also increases TNF-α and/or IL-12 secretion and expression of toll-like receptor 2 compared to control patients. Buongiorno and Pierossi demonstrated the benefits of PDT and bacterial lysate combination therapy in children with PFAPA (periodic fever, aphthous stomatitis, pharyngitis, and cervical adenitis) such as reducing antibiotic and antipyretic prescription and decreasing the number of school absences and tonsillectomies [34]. However, in a RCT study, PDT was not found to be significantly superior to placebo for the prevention of acute RTIs in healthy children who entered kindergarten [35].

Biologically active polysaccharides are natural immunomodulators among which β-glucans represent the most important member, comprising D-glucose monomers linked by β-glycosidic bonds. Besides the immunomodulatory properties, β-glucans also have anti-infectious and anti-inflammatory activities that have preventive and therapeutic effects in children with RRTIs with an adequate safety profile (particularly β-glucans from Pleurotus ostreatus) [36].

OM-85 (Broncho-Vaxom®; Vifor Pharma; Meyrin 2/Geneva, Switzerland) is a lysate of 21 common bacterial respiratory pathogens that can prevent RRTIs in children. In a systematic review including eight RCTs, OM-85 extract significantly reduced upper airway viral infections in children compared to placebo [37]. A recent meta-analysis involving 53 RCTs with 4851 pediatric patients demonstrated that Broncho-Vaxom had significant efficacy in the routine treatment of RRTIs; nevertheless, the authors reported that the results should be interpreted cautiously due to the low evidence levels [38]. The efficacy of OM-85 was also studied in preventing recurrent acute episodes of tonsillitis and chronic rhinosinusitis in children. Broncho-Vaxom decreased the number of acute tonsillitis episodes in the short term with a lower number of tonsillectomy requirements in long-term follow-up [39]. Similarly, Broncho-Vaxom treatment was shown to have curative and preventive effects in children with acute episodes of chronic rhinosinusitis [40]. The therapeutic effect of OM-85 BV in chronic rhinosinusitis was also demonstrated in an experimental study revealing that it is a low-cost alternative treatment option for CRS with few side effects [41].

References

1. Read SA, Obeid S, Ahlenstiel C, Ahlenstiel G. The role of zinc in antiviral immunity. Adv Nutr. 2019;10:696–710.
2. Kurugöl Z, Akilli M, Bayram N, Koturoglu G. The prophylactic and therapeutic effectiveness of zinc sulphate on common cold in children. Acta Paediatr. 2006;95:1175–81.

3. Vorilhon P, Arpajou B, Vaillant Roussel H, Merlin É, Pereira B, Cabaillot A. Efficacy of vitamin C for the prevention and treatment of upper respiratory tract infection. A meta-analysis in children. Eur J Clin Pharmacol. 2019;75:303–11.

4. Hemilä H, Chalker E. Vitamin C for preventing and treating the common cold. Cochrane Database Syst Rev. 2013;31(1):CD000980.

5. Ferrara P, Ianniello F, Bianchi V, Quintarelli F, Cammerata M, Quattrocchi E, Terranova GM, Miggiano GA, Casale M. Beneficial therapeutic effects of vitamin C on recurrent respiratory tract infections in children: preliminary data. Minerva Pediatr. 2016;68(6):487–97.

6. Bergman P, Lindh AU, Björkhem-Bergman L, Lindh JD. Vitamin D and respiratory tract infections: a systematic review and meta-analysis of randomized controlled trials. PLoS One. 2013;8(6):e65835.

7. Charan J, Goyal JP, Saxena D, Yadav P. Vitamin D for prevention of respiratory tract infections: a systematic review and meta-analysis. J Pharmacol Pharmacother. 2012;3:300–3.

8. Xiao L, Xing C, Yang Z, Xu S, Wang M, Du H, Liu K, Huang Z. Vitamin D supplementation for the prevention of childhood acute respiratory infections: a systematic review of randomised controlled trials. Br J Nutr. 2015;114:1026–34.

9. Omand JA, To T, O'Connor DL, Parkin PC, Birken CS, Thorpe KE, Maguire JL. 25-Hydroxyvitamin D supplementation and health-service utilization for upper respiratory tract infection in young children. Public Health Nutr. 2017;20:1816–24.

10. Wang Y, Li X, Ge T, Xiao Y, Liao Y, Cui Y, Zhang Y, Ho W, Yu G, Zhang T. Probiotics for prevention and treatment of respiratory tract infections in children: a systematic review and meta-analysis of randomized controlled trials. Medicine (Baltimore). 2016;95:e4509.

11. Hao Q, Dong BR, Wu T. Probiotics for preventing acute upper respiratory tract infections. Cochrane Database Syst Rev. 2015;3(2):CD006895.

12. Scott AM, Clark J, Julien B, Islam F, Roos K, Grimwood K, Little P, Del Mar CB. Probiotics for preventing acute otitis media in children. Cochrane Database Syst Rev. 2019;6:CD012941.

13. Oliva S, Di Nardo G, Ferrari F, Mallardo S, Rossi P, Patrizi G, Cucchiara S, Stronati L. Randomised clinical trial: the effectiveness of Lactobacillus reuteri ATCC 55730 rectal enema in children with active distal ulcerative colitis. Aliment Pharmacol Ther. 2012;35:327–34.

14. Hickey L, Jacobs SE, Garland SM, Pro Prems Study Group. Probiotics in neonatology. J Paediatr Child Health. 2012;9:777–83.

15. Marini G, Sitzia E, Panatta ML, De Vincentiis GC. Pilot study to explore the prophylactic efficacy of oral probiotic streptococcus salivarius K12 in preventing recurrent pharyngo-tonsillar episodes in pediatric patients. Int J Gen Med. 2019;12:213–7.

16. Andaloro C, Santagati M, Stefani S, La Mantia I. Bacteriotherapy with streptococcus salivarius 24SMB and Streptococcus oralis 89a oral spray for children with recurrent streptococcal pharyngotonsillitis: a randomized placebo-controlled clinical study. Eur Arch Otorhinolaryngol. 2019;276:879–87.

17. Wilcox CR, Stuart B, Leaver H, Lown M, Willcox M, Moore M, Little P. Effectiveness of the probiotic streptococcus salivarius K12 for the treatment and/or prevention of sore throat: a systematic review. Clin Microbiol Infect. 2019;25:673–80.

18. Cleland EJ, Drilling A, Bassiouni A, James C, Vreugde S, Wormald PJ. Probiotic manipulation of the chronic rhinosinusitis microbiome. Int Forum Allergy Rhinol. 2014;4:309–14.

19. Mukerji SS, Pynnonen MA, Kim HM, Singer A, Tabor M, Terrell JE. Probiotics as adjunctive treatment for chronic rhinosinusitis: a randomized controlled trial. Otolaryngol Head Neck Surg. 2009;140:202–8.

20. Henatsch D, Wesseling F, Kross KW, Stokroos RJ. Honey and beehive products in otorhinolaryngology: a narrative review. Clin Otolaryngol. 2016;41:519–31.

21. Maeda Y, Loughrey A, Earle JA, Millar BC, Rao JR, Kearns A, McConville O, Goldsmith CE, Rooney PJ, Dooley JS, Lowery CJ, Snelling WJ, McMahon A, McDowell D, Moore JE. Antibacterial activity of honey against community-associated methicillin-resistant Staphylococcus aureus (CA-MRSA). Complement Ther Clin Pract. 2008;14:77–82.

22. Alandejani T, Marsan J, Ferris W, Slinger R, Chan F. Effectiveness of honey on Staphylococcus aureus and Pseudomonas aeruginosa biofilms. Otolaryngol Head Neck Surg. 2009;141:114–8.

23. Yuksel S, Akyol S. The consumption of propolis and royal jelly in preventing upper respiratory tract infections and as dietary supplementation in children. J Intercult Ethnopharmacol. 2016;5:308–11.
24. Crişan I, Zaharia CN, Popovici F, Jucu V, Belu O, Dascălu C, Mutiu A, Petrescu A. Natural propolis extract NIVCRISOL in the treatment of acute and chronic rhinopharyngitis in children. Rom J Virol. 1995;46:115–33.
25. Takikawa M, Kumagai A, Hirata H, Soga M, Yamashita Y, Ueda M, et al. 10-Hydroxy-2-decenoic acid, a unique medium-chain fatty acid, activates 5'-AMP-activated protein kinase in L6 myotubes and mice. Mol Nutr Food Res. 2013;57:1794–802.
26. David S, Cunningham R. Echinacea for the prevention and treatment of upper respiratory tract infections: a systematic review and meta-analysis. Complement Ther Med. 2019;44:18–26.
27. Weber W, Taylor JA, Stoep AV, Weiss NS, Standish LJ, Calabrese C. Echinacea purpurea for prevention of upper respiratory tract infections in children. J Altern Complement Med. 2005;11:1021–6.
28. Timmer A, Günther J, Motschall E, Rücker G, Antes G, Kern WV. Pelargonium sidoides extract for treating acute respiratory tract infections. Cochrane Database Syst Rev. 2013;10:CD006323.
29. Careddu D, Pettenazzo A. Pelargonium sidoides extract EPs 7630: a review of its clinical efficacy and safety for treating acute respiratory tract infections in children. Int J Gen Med. 2018;11:91–8.
30. Seifert G, Brandes-Schramm J, Zimmermann A, Lehmacher W, Kamin W. Faster recovery and reduced paracetamol use - a meta-analysis of EPs 7630 in children with acute respiratory tract infections. BMC Pediatr. 2019;19:119.
31. Fürst R, Luong B, Thomsen J, Wittig T. ELOM-080 as add-on treatment for respiratory tract diseases - a review of clinical studies conducted in China. Planta Med. 2019;85:745–54.
32. Karpova EP, Tulupov DA, Emel'yanova MP. Use of Myrtol standardized in the treatment of children with acute rhinosinusitis. Vestn Otorinolaringol. 2016;81:47–50.
33. Niu H, Wang R, Jia YT, Cai Y. Pidotimod, an immunostimulant in pediatric recurrent respiratory tract infections: a meta-analysis of randomized controlled trials. Int Immunopharmacol. 2019;67:35–45.
34. Buongiorno A, Pierossi N. Effectiveness of pidotimod in combination with bacterial lysates in the treatment of the pfapa (periodic fever, aphthous stomatitis, pharyngitis, and cervical adenitis) syndrome. Minerva Pediatr. 2015;67:219–26.
35. Mameli C, Pasinato A, Picca M, Bedogni G, Pisanelli S, Zuccotti GV, AX-Working Group. Pidotimod for the prevention of acute respiratory infections in healthy children entering into daycare: a double blind randomized placebo-controlled study. Pharmacol Res. 2015;97:79–83.
36. Jesenak M, Urbancikova I, Banovcin P. Respiratory tract infections and the role of biologically active polysaccharides in their management and prevention. Nutrients. 2017;9(7):E779.
37. Schaad UB. OM-85 BV, an immunostimulant in pediatric recurrent respiratory tract infections: a systematic review. World J Pediatr. 2010;6:5–12.
38. Yin J, Xu B, Zeng X, Shen K. Broncho-Vaxom in pediatric recurrent respiratory tract infections: a systematic review and meta-analysis. Int Immunopharmacol. 2018;54:198–209.
39. Bitar MA, Saade R. The role of OM-85 BV (Broncho-Vaxom) in preventing recurrent acute tonsillitis in children. Int J Pediatr Otorhinolaryngol. 2013;77:670–3.
40. Zagar S, Löfler-Badzek D. Broncho-Vaxom in children with rhinosinusitis: a double-blind clinical trial. ORL J Otorhinolaryngol Relat Spec. 1988;50:397–404.
41. Tao Y, Yuan T, Li X, Yang S, Zhang F, Shi L. Bacterial extract OM-85 BV protects mice against experimental chronic rhinosinusitis. Int J Clin Exp Pathol. 2015;8:6800–6.

Murat Kar, Fazilet Altın, and Dmytro Illich Zabolotny

91.1 Introduction

Pediatric trauma refers to injuries that cause damage in infants, children, and young adolescents, which are an issue that threatens children's lives and should be carefully evaluated. Often children must be hospitalized and require immediate attention. Due to the severe anatomical and physiological differences between adults and children, trauma intervention must also be different. Due to the small body surface areas, vital organs in children are located very close to each other, so they become more sensitive to trauma than adults. Trauma is the most common cause of death in children in the United States, and it has been reported that 59.5% of child deaths under 18 years old are from trauma in 2004 [1]. The pediatric trauma approach should include the prevention of injury, the fastest transfer of the patient to the pediatric trauma center, the emergency intervention by the educated and related branches, the children's rehabilitation, and long-term follow-up. This section will discuss pediatric trauma management in terms of ear, nose, and throat.

M. Kar (✉)
Alanya Education and Research Hospital, Alanya Alaaddin Keykubat University, Alanya, Antalya, Turkey

F. Altın
Section of Otorhinolaryngology, Haseki Training and Research Hospital, University of Health Sciences, İstanbul, Turkey

D. I. Zabolotny
Institute of Otorhinolaryngology, National Academy of Medical Sciences of Ukraine, Kyiv, Ukraine

91.2   Management of Pediatric Ear Trauma

Pediatric ear trauma can occur as a result of blunt or penetrating injuries. Moreover, it occurs due to barotrauma due to air travel, diving, or blast injury [2–4]. Ear trauma includes external auditory canal middle ear and otic capsule injury. The middle ear and otic capsule injury occur in one-third of pediatric head trauma and one-half of pediatric temporal bone fractures [5, 6]. Hemotympanum, traumatic tympanic membrane perforations, hearing loss, otorrhea, traumatic perilymphatic fistula, and facial paralysis constitute pediatric ear trauma [5–9].

Cotton tip applicator related ear trauma is expected in the pediatric age group. Although it is commonly used for removing cerumen, it remains the most common penetrating injury to the tympanic membrane and external auditory canal [10]. It can cause laceration, soft tissue injury, foreign body, and bleeding, which is the common reason for applying to the emergency department [11, 12]. A foreign body in the external ear must be removed. If not removed may result in rarely brain abscess and fatal meningitis [13, 14]. Generally, most of these patients are treated at the emergency department, and there is no problem in their follow-up since they are not severe. However, some cotton tip applicator related trauma cause severe injuries such as tympanic membrane perforation, ossicular dislocation, hearing loss, perilymphatic fistula, and facial nerve paralysis [11, 15]. Sagiv et al. [16] reported that the traumatic tympanic membrane perforations in pediatric patients tend to heal spontaneously than in adults. Clinical suspicion of ossicular dislocation, perilymphatic fistula that presents with symptoms of dizziness, vertigo, sudden or fluctuating sensorineural hearing loss, and facial nerve paralysis alerts physician for immediate otolaryngology consultation for surgical evaluation within hours to prevent permanent hearing loss [17].

Although the temporal bone is a solid bone that protects the middle and inner ear structures, hearing loss, facial nerve paralysis, otorrhea, hemotympanum, and balance disturbance can often be accompanied by temporal bone fractures [18]. Temporal bone trauma can occur due to birth trauma, motor vehicle accidents, falls, biking, skateboarding, tobogganing or skiing accidents, injury by assaults, and an animal bite. The most common cause of pediatric temporal bone trauma is motor vehicle accidents. Therefore, the second cause of falls is usually associated with skull fractures such as parietal, sphenoid, frontal, occipital, ethmoid, orbital roof/wall, and others [19–21]. Waissbluth et al. [19] reported that hemotympanum, decreased or loss of consciousness, and headache were the most prevalent clinical presentation due to high impact trauma. Classically, temporal bone fractures were classified as longitudinal, transverse, and mixed concerning the fracture plane to the petrous bone axis [22]. Little et al. [23] established a newer classification based on the otic capsule involving or sparing. Both temporal bone fracture classification cannot predict hearing loss and facial paralysis for deciding surgical intervention or observation. Computed tomography (CT) is the primary diagnostic tool to evaluate initial temporal bone fracture and the associated complications and the other bone fractures [24]. The prognosis in these patients depends on the middle ear's involvement, petrous bone, otic capsule, and facial nerve canal.

CT shows fluid in the middle ear but cannot distinguish cerebrospinal fluid (CSF) and hemorrhage. In these cases, magnetic resonance imaging (MRI) may better demonstrate a fluid, and bright signaling in T1-weighted images may reveal hemorrhage in the labyrinth or middle ear; therefore, MRI is best to evaluate the membranous labyrinth [24]. The essential sequelae from temporal bone fractures include hearing loss and facial nerve injury since they are essential in the pediatric age group's emotional and social development. Fortunately, sensorineural hearing loss is less common in the pediatric group than in adults due to the more flexible and low mineralization of temporal bones that may protect the otic capsule [25]. Hearing loss, which usually occurs in the pediatric group, is a conductive type and occurs due to hemotympanum and resolves spontaneously [18]. Most pediatric temporal bone fractures are longitudinal and otic capsule sparing, resulting in less common sensorineural hearing loss, facial nerve paralysis, and cerebrospinal fluid leakage [26]. Patel et al. [27] reported that cerebrospinal fluid otorrhea resulting from pediatric temporal bone trauma usually resolves within 2 weeks without surgical intervention, and exploration is rarely required. Sensorineural, hearing loss of the pediatric population has a good prognosis. The majority of them are self-resolving, empirical steroid treatment may be beneficial, and deficient patients would be referred to cochlear implantation [28]. In pediatric temporal bone fractures, the incidence of facial nerve paralysis is very uncommon, nearly 3%, and management is similar to adults' management [27].

91.3 Management of Pediatric Nasal Trauma

The nasal bone is the prominent part of the face; therefore, it is prone to facial traumas and one of the most frequently damaged structures. The nasal bone is the third most common fractured bone of the human body and also is the second common type of facial fracture in both pediatric maxillofacial traumas [29–31]. The nasal bone of pediatric patients is less fractured than adults, as their cartilages are more elastic, contain more soft tissue, formless protrusions on the face, low impact injury due to low body weight and high cranium to face ratio in younger children [32]. Most of the nasal fractures occur at the ages of 15–17. The incidence gets lower at the age of 5 years and lower [33]. Close care of very young children by their families increased older children's involvement in outdoor and sports activities. Increased risk of motor vehicle accidents and interpersonal violence among older pediatric patients could affect the factors affecting the age distribution of nasal fracture [32, 33] (Figs. 91.1–91.3).

Pediatric patients with nasal injuries usually with high-impact mechanisms (e.g., motor vehicle) are often complicated by other more life-threatening injuries causing airway compromise, hemorrhage, and/or cervical spine trauma. Therefore, patients should be stabilized first, and fatal complications must be ruled out. How much time has passed since the trauma is important, different from adult patients in pediatric patients need reduction sooner, typically 3–7 days after trauma for minimizing secondary nasal deformities [34–36]. If the septoplasty is needed in pediatric patients

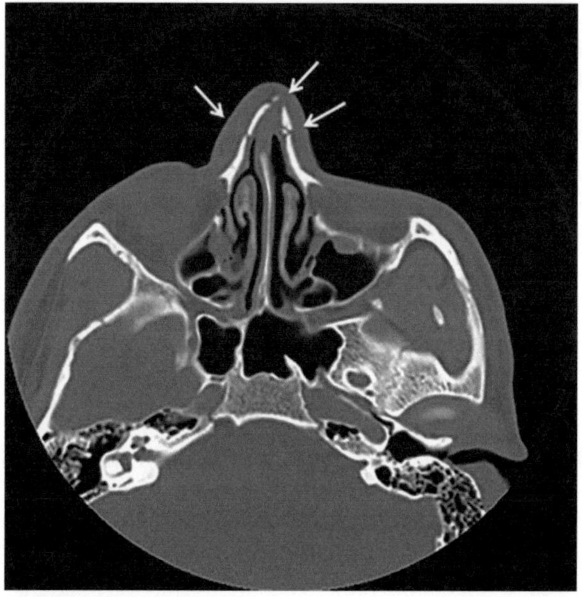

Fig. 91.1 Nasal fracture (direct graphy)

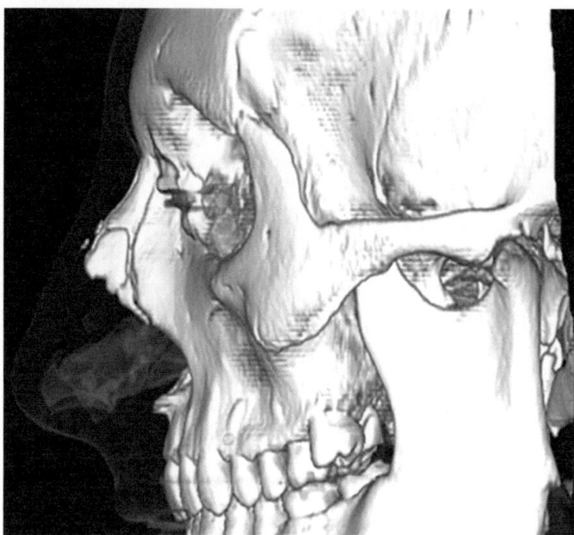

Fig. 91.2 Nasal fracture (CT, axial view)

with a nasal fracture, it must be conservative to protect the growth center of the maxilla's nasal spine; therefore, this is very important for future facial growth and development [34]. Patients should be evaluated externally and internally for soft tissue injury, ecchymosis, nasal obstruction, and epistaxis due to mucosal

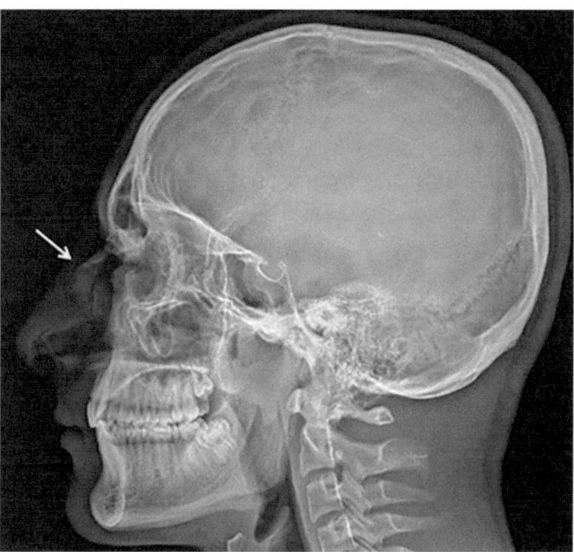

Fig. 91.3 Nasal fracture (MR view)

lacerations. If a compressible, obstructing, reddish mass is found by internal examination, the physician should be aware of a septal hematoma. Since left untreated
septal hematoma can result in avascular cartilage necrosis, subsequent loss of structural support leading saddle nose deformity, and possible septal abscess, it must be
treated by surgical drainage followed by nasal packing emergently [32]. The septal
abscess can cause possible retrograde thrombophlebitis through the valveless mid-
facial venous system. In these patients, purulent material is drained. So, the drain
should be placed, and suitable broad-spectrum intravenous antibiotic therapy is initiated according to culture [32, 34, 36]. In the case of nasal fracture, CT can be used
for diagnosis, incredibly inpatient with suspicion for associated facial fractures
[24]. Recent studies have advocated that high-resolution ultrasound proves potentially more accurate findings than CT without the associated radiation [37]. After
the displaced nasal fracture is detected, closed reduction usually or open reduction
is performed if the fracture is nonreducible [34]. Even though appropriate reduction, malunion of nasal bones can result in a cosmetic deformity that may require
secondary septorhinoplasty in the future.

91.4 Management of Pediatric Throat Trauma

There are some anatomical differences between children and adult patients. Due to
the larynx is located higher in children and a short neck, the mandibula plays a role
in protecting the larynx. The possibility of injury is lower than that of adults because
physiologically larynx is more flexible and soft in children [38]. Blunt pediatric
external laryngeal trauma usually occurs due to motor vehicle accidents and sports

injuries; less commonly, penetrating pediatric external laryngeal trauma occurs due to dog bites, falls onto objects, and penetrating stab wounds [39–41].

Laryngeal trauma can be seen in different forms, such as the fracture of the thyroid cartilage, complicated fractures involving both the thyroid and cricoid cartilages, mucosal lacerations, endolaryngeal hematoma, laceration in thyroepiglottic ligament, unilateral or bilateral recurrent laryngeal nerve injury, cricoarytenoid joint injury, and laryngotracheal dissociation [39]. Since patients may have mild symptoms despite severe trauma, laryngeal trauma should be suspected in all pediatric patients with neck trauma. The common symptoms of laryngeal injury include respiratory distress, dysphagia, hemoptysis, stridor, and subcutaneous emphysema [41]. Since most of these conditions are highly mortal, the emergency approach's most critical condition is to protect the airway in patients. CT is the gold standard and is useful when bony or soft tissue damage is considered, especially when a laryngeal fracture is suspected and CT detects the site of injury in 94% of blunt trauma [24, 42]. In pediatric patients, ultrasound is useful in evaluating laryngeal structures, cervical cartilages, and soft tissue of the neck [43].

In pediatric laryngeal trauma management, Schaefer has grouped patients according to the clinical findings for optimal treatment [44]. In group I and group II, surgical intervention is not needed; however in group III and IV, endoscopic or open laryngeal exploration must be needed. Although improvements in endoscopic techniques and technology give facility to the physician to treat complex laryngeal injuries, some patients may require an open approach for further intervention. This is important because endoscopic management reduces postoperative morbidity and recovery time [45, 46]. Early intervention in laryngeal traumas improves the voice and airway quality in later periods. However, unfortunately, in blunt laryngeal trauma, open exposure is needed in contrast to more severe injuries [41].

91.5 Conclusion

Many pediatric traumas can be prevented by sufficient parent education. There are many anatomical and physiological differences between pediatric and adult anatomy that affect a difference in managing trauma in both groups. Taking the patient to a pediatric trauma center with a fully equipped and specialist physician as soon as possible after trauma will facilitate the recovery of the child without any sequelae.

References

1. American Academy of Pediatrics Section on Orthopaedics; American Academy of Pediatrics Committee on Pediatric Emergency Medicine; American Academy of Pediatrics Section on Critical Care; American Academy of Pediatrics Section on Surgery; American Academy of Pediatrics Section on Transport Medicine; American Academy of Pediatrics Committee on Pediatric Emergency Medicine; Pediatric Orthopaedical Society of North America, Krug SE, Tuggle DW. Management of pediatric trauma. Pediatrics. 2008;121(4):849–54. https://doi.org/10.1542/peds.2008-0094.

2. Mirza S, Richardson H. Otic barotrauma from air travel. J Laryngol Otol. 2005;119:366.

3. Klingmann C, Praetorius M, Baumann I, Plinkert PK. Barotrauma and decompression illness of the inner ear: 46 cases during treatment and follow-up. Otol Neurotol. 2007;28:447.

4. Mick P, Moxham P, Ludemann J. Penetrating and blast ear trauma: 7-year review of two pediatric practices. J Otolaryngol Head Neck Surg. 2008;37:774–6.

5. Ort S, Beus K, Isaacson J. Pediatric temporal bone fractures in a rural population. Otolaryngol Head Neck Surg. 2004;131:433.

6. Brodie HA, Thompson TC. Management of complications from 820 temporal bone fractures. Am J Otol. 1997;18:188.

7. Lee D, Honrado C, Har-El G, Goldsmith A. Pediatric temporal bone fractures. Laryngoscope. 1998;108:816.

8. Zimmerman WD, Ganzel TM, Windmill IM, et al. Peripheral hearing loss following head trauma in children. Laryngoscope. 1993;103:87.

9. Kim SH, Kazahaya K, Handler SD. Traumatic perilymphatic fistulas in children: etiology, diagnosis and management. Int J Pediatr Otorhinolaryngol. 2001;60:147.

10. Ameen ZS, Chounthirath T, Smith GA, Jatana KR. Pediatric cotton-tip applicator-related ear injury treated in United States emergency departments, 1990-2010. J Pediatr. 2017;186:124–30. https://doi.org/10.1016/j.jpeds.2017.03.049.

11. Smith M, Darrat I, Seidman M. Otologic complications of cotton swab use: one institution's experience. Laryngoscope. 2012;122:409–11.

12. Marin JR, Trainor JL. Foreign body removal from the external auditory canal in a pediatric emergency department. Pediatr Emerg Care. 2006;22:630–4.

13. Chiang T, Merz M. Cerebellar abscess resulting from multiple foreign body induced otitis in a pediatric patient. Cincinnati (OH): Society for Ear, Nose, and Throat Advances in Children; 2010.

14. Goldman SA, Ankerstjerne JK, Welker KB, Chen DA. Fatal meningitis and brain abscess resulting from foreign body-induced otomastoiditis. Otolaryngol Head Neck Surg. 1998;118:6–8.

15. Neuenschwander MC, Deutsch ES, Cornetta A, Willcox TO. Penetrating middle ear trauma: a report of 2 cases. Ear Nose Throat J. 2005;84:32–5.

16. Sagiv D, Migirov L, Glikson E, Mansour J, Yousovich R, Wolf M, Shapira Y. Traumatic perforation of the tympanic membrane: a review of 80 cases. J Emerg Med. 2018;54(2):186–90. https://doi.org/10.1016/j.jemermed.2017.09.018.

17. Kravitz H, Nyhus AI, Dale DO, Laker HI, Gomberg RM, Korach A. The cotton-tipped swab. Clin Pediatr. 1974;13(11):965–70.

18. Bhindi A, Carpineta L, Al Qassabi B, Waissbluth S, Ywakim R, Manoukian JJ, Nguyen LHP. Hearing loss in pediatric temporal bone fractures: evaluating two radiographic classification systems as prognosticators. Int J Pediatr Otorhinolaryngol. 2018;109:158–63.

19. Waissbluth S, Ywakim R, Al Qassabi B, Torabi B, Carpineta L, Manoukian J, Nguyen LHP. Pediatric temporal bone fractures: a case series. Int J Pediatr Otorhinolaryngol. 2016;84:106–9. https://doi.org/10.1016/j.ijporl.2016.02.034.

20. Kang HM, Kim MG, Boo SH, Kim KH, Yeo EK, Lee SK, et al. Comparison of the clinical relevance of traditional and new classification systems of temporal bone fractures. Eur Arch Otorhinolaryngol. 2012;269:1893–9.

21. Dunklebarger J, Branstetter B 4th, Lincoln A, Sippey M, Cohen M, Gaines B, et al. Pediatric temporal bone fractures: current trends and comparison of classification schemes. Laryngoscope. 2014;124:781–4.

22. Wexler S, Poletto E, Chennupati SK. Pediatric temporal bone fractures. Pediatr Emerg Care. 2017;33(11):745–7. https://doi.org/10.1097/pec.0000000000000594.

23. Little SC, Kesser BW. Radiographic classification of temporal bone fractures: clinical predictability using a new system. Arch Otolaryngol Head Neck Surg. 2006;132:1300–4.

24. Chess MA, Chaturvedi A, Stanescu AL, Blickman JG. Emergency pediatric ear, nose, and throat imaging. Sem Ultrasound, CT MRI. 2012;33(5):449–62. https://doi.org/10.1053/j.sult.2012.06.010.

25. Kang HM, et al. Comparison of temporal bone fractures in children and adults. Acta Otolaryngol. 2013;133(5):469–74.
26. Dunklebarger J, Branstetter B, Lincoln A, et al. Pediatric temporal bone fractures: current trends and comparison of classification schemes. Laryngoscope. 2014;124:781–4.
27. Patel A, Groppo E. Management of Temporal Bone Trauma. Craniomaxillofac Trauma Reconstr. 2010;3:105–13.
28. Leung J, Levi E. Paediatric petrous temporal bone fractures: a 5-year experience at an Australian paediatric trauma centre. Australian J Otolaryngol. 2020;3:6.
29. Lee WT, Koltai PJ. Nasal deformity in neonates and young children. Pediatr Clin North Am. 2003;50:459–67.
30. Munante-Cardenas JL, Olate S, Asprino L, et al. Pattern and treatment of facial trauma in pediatric and adolescent patients. J Craniofac Surg. 2011;22:1251–5.
31. Imahara SD, Hopper RA, Wang J, et al. Patterns and outcomes of pediatric facial fractures in the United States: a survey of the National Trauma Data Bank. J Am Coll Surg. 2008;207:710–6.
32. Wright RJ, Murakami CS, Ambro BT. Pediatric nasal injuries and management. Facial Plast Surg. 2011;27:483–90.
33. Vyas RM, Dickinson BP, Wasson KL, Roostaeian J, Bradley JP. Pediatric facial fractures: current national incidence, distribution, and health care resource use. J Craniofac Surg. 2008;19:339–49.
34. Desrosiers AE 3rd, Thaller SR. Pediatric nasal fractures: evaluation and management. J Craniofac Surg. 2011;22:1327–9.
35. Ridder GJ, Boedeker CC, Fradis M, et al. Technique and timing for closed reduction of isolated nasal fractures: a retrospective study. Ear Nose Throat J. 2002;81:49–54.
36. Rohrich RJ. Adams Jr WP nasal fracture management: minimizing secondary nasal deformities. Plast Reconstr Surg. 2000;106:266–73.
37. Navaratnam R, Davis T. The role of ultrasound in the diagnosis of pediatric nasal fractures. J Craniofac Surg. 2019 Oct;30(7):2099–101.
38. Vayisoglu Y, Gorur K, Ozcan C, et al. Pediatric acute external laryngeal trauma: a case report. Turk J Emerg Med. 2007;7:36–9.
39. Yumusakhuylu AC, Topuz MF, Durgun C, Binnetoglu A, Baglam T, Sari M. Pediatric acute external laryngeal trauma. J Craniofac Surg. 2014;25(1):e70–2.
40. Butler AP, Wood BP, O'Rourke AK, et al. Acute external laryngeal trauma: experience with 112 patients. Ann Otol Rhinol Laryngol. 2005;114:361–8.
41. Sidell D, Mendelsohn AH, Shapiro NL, St. John M. Management and outcomes of laryngeal injuries in the pediatric population. Ann Otol Rhinol Laryngol. 2011;120(12):787–95.
42. Scaglione M, Romano S, Pinto A, Sparano A, Scialpi M, Rotondo A. Acute tracheobronchial injuries: impact of imaging on diagnosis and management implications. Eur J Radiol. 2006;59:336–43.
43. Jakubowska A, Zawadzka-Gaos L, Brzewski M. Usefulness of ultrasound examination in larynx traumas in children. Pol J Radiol. 2011;76:7–12.
44. Schaefer SD, Close LG. Acute management of laryngeal trauma. Ann Otol Laryngol Rhinol. 1989;98:98–104.
45. Shires CB, Preston T, Thompson J. Pediatric laryngeal trauma: a case series at a tertiary children's hospital. Int J Pediatr Otorhinolaryngol 2011;75:401–8
46. Quesnel AM, Hartnick CJ. A contemporary review of voice and airway after laryngeal trauma in children. Laryngoscope. 2009;119:2226–30.

Management of Pediatric Trauma: General View

Mustafa Salış, Mehmet Surhan Arda, and Baran Tokar

92.1 Introduction

In the pediatric age group, patients presenting with general body trauma may have ear, nose, and throat trauma concomitantly. The treatment of injuries caused by trauma to the face, head, and neck should be planned in the otorhinolaryngology department. It should not be forgotten that these patients may also have traumatic injuries in the abdomen and thoracic region; thus, a general evaluation is warranted.

Trauma is among the most frequent causes of mortality and morbidity among children globally [1]. When all age groups of children are considered, trauma is more common in boys than girls with a rate of 2: 1 and 3: 1 [2]. The etiology of traumas varies according to age groups. Falling, drowning, burns, abuse, traffic accidents in school-age children, bicycle injury, and intentional and gunshot injuries are common in infants and young children [3]. Head and neck trauma is rarely isolated to head and neck; 50–70% of those patients have multiple traumatic injuries.

High head-to-body ratio, uncompleted ossification and soft nature of bones, smaller thoracic cavity, smaller pelvis, and thinner subcutaneous tissue are the anatomical differences of infants and children so that a similar kinetic trauma might have a different effect on children comparing to adults. Mediastinum is much more flexible in children that may cause pneumothorax to turn tension pneumothorax easily. In children, even though the trauma may seem to be isolated in head and neck, other body parts should also be examined due to the possibility of thoracic, abdominal, and genitourinary traumas.

M. Salış (✉)
Department of General Surgery, Faculty of Medicine, Eskişehir Osmangazi University, Eskişehir, Turkey

M. S. Arda · B. Tokar
Department of Pediatric Surgery, Faculty of Medicine, Eskişehir Osmangazi University, Eskişehir, Turkey

C. Cingi et al. (eds.), *Pediatric ENT Infections*,
https://doi.org/10.1007/978-3-030-80691-0_92

The primary assessment in pediatric trauma patients consists of evaluating the airway, breathing, circulation, state of consciousness, and the child's relationship with the external environment [4]. The secondary evaluation phase includes a detailed review of all body parts for injury and detailed history. At this stage, appropriate radiographic and laboratory examinations are requested [5]. Finally, the third (descriptive) assessment is performed 24 hours later [4].

Laboratory tests including complete blood count, serum biochemistry, blood type, blood gas test, complete urinalysis, prothrombin time, and active partial thromboplastin time should be checked routinely [6, 7]. Laboratory investigation may not detect a severe injury in children. Results of those studies should never replace clinical evaluation in the decision-making process [8].

The radiological investigation is also one of the key elements in the evaluation of trauma in children. To determine the treatment plan, a radiological evaluation of a child with trauma should be completed in less than 24 h. In patients with multisystem trauma, cervical, chest, abdominal, pelvic, and selected extremity X-rays should be obtained. Ultrasonography is the most commonly used radiological examination used in trauma patients all over the world. Ultrasonography is preferred because it does not contain radiation and is portable and cheap [1].

Focused Assessment with Sonography for Trauma (FAST) is recommended in hemodynamically unstable pediatric trauma patients to identify pericardial effusion or intra-abdominal hemorrhage and proceed to further treatment in these patients [9, 10]. Hemodynamically unstable children with positive FAST findings may require surgical intervention [10].

The most critical step in a trauma patient's management plan is to decide whether emergency surgery or non-surgical follow-up will be required for the treatment. For the decision-making process, it is vital to determine whether any significant organ injury exists and what the degree of the injury is. For this purpose, computed tomography (CT) is a highly accurate method and is used as a reference diagnostic method in trauma worldwide [11, 12].

92.2　Thoracic Trauma

Thoracic trauma is the second most frequent cause of child mortality after head injury. While isolated thoracic trauma occurs between the rate of 4.5 and 8%, the risk of thoracic injury increases 20-fold during multi-trauma [13].

Male predominance is 2:1 or 3:1. In general, it could be classified as blunt and penetrating trauma. Soft tissue injury, rib fracture, pulmonary contusion, and trachea-bronchial tree rupture are usually identified in thoracic trauma in children. Although rare, cardiac, pericardial, great vessel, and esophageal damages should be taken into account. Traumatic diaphragmatic rupture may also occur [14].

Infants have a smaller lumen of the airway that makes them prone to obstruction with either foreign body or aspirates. Anterior-superior location of the glottis, the length of the trachea, and the distance to the carina change according to age. The size of a child is another important issue during intubation. Intubation difficulty in infants may cause iatrogenic trauma or endobronchial intubation. Iatrogenic trauma in children may cause air leaks from the respiratory system and subcutaneous emphysema on supraclavicular and neck regions.

Besides anatomical differences, increased oxygen consumption and low functional capacity are the physiologic disadvantages of children. Intra-abdominal injury and abdominal distension may affect the function of the diaphragm and that will result in difficulty of ventilation.

Thoracic trauma may not show significant findings in the first evaluation of the patient. Pneumonia or mediastinal infection may occur in such patients with delayed diagnosis. If a child having recurrent pneumonia, emphysema, and atelectasis following a thoracic or multisystem trauma, a foreign body aspiration should be suspected. A bronchoscopy might be considered in such patients.

92.2.1 Thoracic Traumatic Lesions and Treatment

Children may have isolated thoracic trauma or thorax might be involved in multisystem trauma. In all these cases, 10% of patients need surgical emergency [15]. Pulmonary contusion, hemothorax, pneumothorax, mediastinal injury, diaphragmatic rupture, and traumatic supraclavicular emphysema and asphyxia could be observed as in the adult.

Due to the flexibility of the chest wall and mediastinum, in the case of rib fracture, a pulmonary contusion is frequently seen (Fig. 92.1) [16]. According to the severity of the trauma, the patient may need intensive-care follow-up. During invasive ventilation, the pressures should be set to as low as possible so as not to cause pneumothorax. Pulmonary contusion usually heals well with conservative treatment.

Minimal pneumothorax that is not visible on chest X-ray but found on computerized tomography usually do not necessitate tube thoracostomy [17]. However, due to anatomical structural differences of the children as mentioned above, the

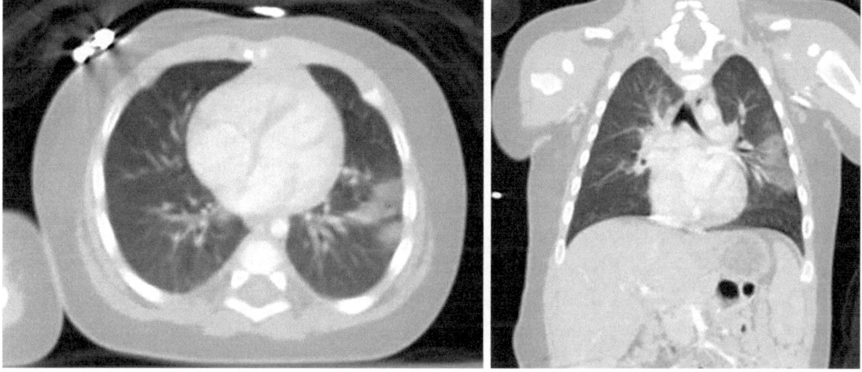

Fig. 92.1 Pulmonary contusion on the left side

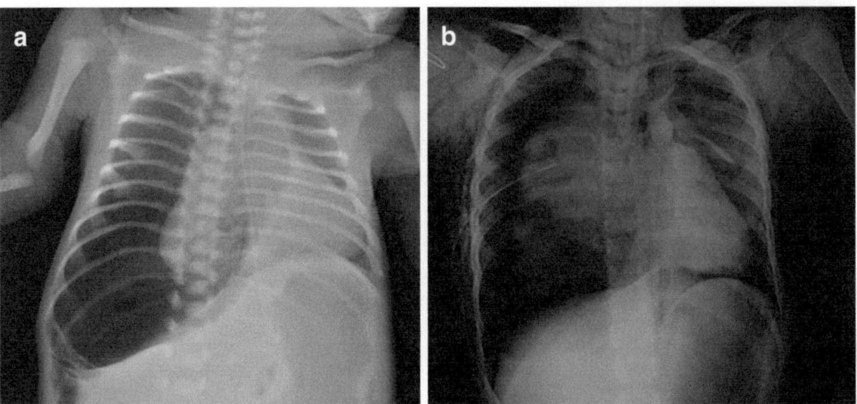

Fig. 92.2 Tension pneumothorax in an infant (**a**), and in an older child (**b**) on the left side

pneumothorax might progress to tension pneumothorax (Fig. 92.2); therefore such patients need close follow-up. If the chest X-ray shows progress in pneumothorax associated with dyspnea or respiratory difficulty, a tube thoracostomy should be performed.

Bleeding into the thoracic cavity might cause hemothorax following a traumatic thoracic injury. Drainage with tube thoracostomy is the treatment modality in children as well. If bleeding is not controlled and responding to conservative treatment, thoracotomy and surgical intervention to control bleeding might be needed.

During thoracic trauma, rib fracture is rarely seen in children due to the flexibility of the thoracic wall. If it happens, pain management should be considered.

Mediastinal injury may lead to serious consequences [18, 19]. Mediastinal pneumothorax or hemothorax may occur following a thoracic trauma in children. The tracheobronchial injuries might be the underlying reason for mediastinal pneumothorax and tube thoracostomy is the treatment modality. The mediastinal hemothorax might occur due to both penetrating and blunt trauma to the thoracic aorta. Mortality is high in such cases. In some patients, early diagnosis in the emergency room might be possible and an emergency thoracotomy should be performed.

Traumatic rupture of the diaphragm may occur in children [14, 20]. It is more common on the left side. Chest X-ray shows abdominal visceral organs in hemithorax. High-energy blunt trauma or penetrating traumas might be the underlying reason. Repair of diaphragmatic rupture could be performed by thoracotomy or laparotomy. According to the hemodynamic stability of the patient, it could also be repaired by thoracoscopy or laparoscopy.

Traumatic subcutaneous emphysema and asphyxia may also be observed in children. The injury to the tracheobronchial tree may cause mediastinal emphysema, and through the thoracic inlet, emphysema may reach the subcutaneous tissue of the supraclavicular area, neck, and head. It may also occur following difficult intubation and iatrogenic trauma to the trachea or bronchus. Children are more prone to iatrogenic trauma during intubation due to anatomical differences. Traumatic subcutaneous emphysema might be associated with pneumothorax. The patient having respiratory distress needs intensive-care follow-up with intubation. Tube thoracostomy is inserted if the pneumothorax is present.

Asphyxia is a clinical finding that is specific to children. Petechial bleeding on skin, sclera, and possibly in brain together with edema of neck and head are the clinical findings. A rapid increase of intrathoracic pressure transmits to the venous system through the vena cava superior that results in extravasation from capillary veins. The patients recover with conservative treatment but a close follow-up is needed.

92.3 Abdominal Traumas

It has been reported that abdominal traumas constitute 13% of all injuries in children, and the mortality rate is 5% [21]. In children, 85% of all abdominal traumas are blunt, and 15% are penetrating traumas [22]. The risk of a serious injury to children's internal organs is high because of the thinner chest and abdominal walls they have comparing to adults [23]. Thus, penetrating trauma can cause more severe morbidity and mortality in children, although less common than in adults [23, 24]. Of the blunt abdominal traumas, 75–80% occur in traffic accidents. Other causes are falls from height, sports injuries, bicycle accidents, and child abuse.

Some abdominal visceral injuries are more common in children than in adults. Bicycle handlebar injuries and waist-type seat belt injuries are typical injuries. Visceral contents are firmly squeezed between the anterior abdominal wall and the spine from behind. Blunt pancreatic injuries also occur with a similar mechanism. The symptoms of these injuries are generally vague; thus, diagnoses of these injuries are usually late [4, 25, 26].

Children are often frightened due to traumatic events, which makes abdominal examination difficult [27]. Repeated evaluation of abdominal inspection, auscultation, and palpation is essential in a pediatric trauma patient, as examination findings may alter over time. The clinician should evaluate the abdomen for distention, ecchymosis, presence/quality of bowel sounds, abdominal tenderness, rebound, defense, or palpable masses [28]. Following a traffic accident, the seat belt sign as a linear contusion across the abdomen might be associated with an intra-abdominal injury. Abdominal distension may be due to bleeding or intraperitoneal air, as well as gastric dilatation. Therefore, the stomach should be drained first with a nasogastric tube [8]. Gastric dilatation and distended bladder may cause abdominal tenderness [4]. The frequent abdominal examinations do not entirely exclude the possibility of intra-abdominal injury [29].

Laboratory investigation, especially complete blood count and urinalysis, should be evaluated together with clinical and radiological findings. In the radiological evaluation of abdominal trauma, an abdominal X-ray is asked. Abdominal radiography may show free air or a foreign body in the abdominal cavity. Emergency abdominal exploration might be required with positive FAST findings in hemodynamically unstable children with intra-abdominal hemorrhage. Developed from adult trauma patient outcomes, FAST is not accepted for routine use in stable children. It is an insensitive tool for detecting significant intra-abdominal injuries [30].

In hemodynamically stable children with blunt abdominal trauma, intravenous contrast-enhanced abdominal CT is the preferred imaging method for detecting intra-abdominal injury. It is very sensitive and specific in diagnosing liver, spleen, and retroperitoneal injuries [28].

Abdominal CT can be performed in pediatric trauma patients if symptoms and signs indicating intra-abdominal injury, in traumas with high kinetic energy, with *ultrasonographic* findings showing solid organ injury or free fluid in the abdomen, in the presence of macroscopic hematuria, and in patients who cannot be communicated verbally [31]. CT is highly sensitive in diagnosing solid organ injuries but is not as susceptible to injuries of the intestinal tract [8].

92.3.1 Solid Organ Injuries in Blunt Abdominal Trauma

92.3.1.1 Liver Injuries

In blunt abdominal trauma, liver injuries are the most common. Mostly the right lobe posterior segment is injured. Left lobe injuries are usually associated with duodenal-pancreatic injuries. Severe bleeding rates are higher than the spleen, as the liver receives blood from two systems [32]. Of liver injuries, 80% occur due to traffic accidents; other reasons are falling from a height, bicycle accidents, attacks, and child abuse. The most common cause of blunt liver laceration is the upper abdomen and right lower thoracic trauma. The injury occurs more in the right lobe [33].

Biliary tract injuries due to blunt abdominal trauma are infrequent, and most commonly gallbladder, liver, rib, lung, spleen, duodenum, small intestines, and pancreas injuries are associated with biliary tract injuries [34–37].

Double-contrast intravenous CT is the imaging modality that defines liver injuries at the highest rate [29]. According to the American Association's criteria for the Surgery of Trauma (AAST), liver injuries are classified as follows [38]:

- **Grade 1:** Parenchymal rupture less than 1 cm deep, subcapsular hematoma less than 1 cm thick.
- **Grade 2:** 1–3 cm deep parenchymal tear, 1–3 cm thick parenchymal or subcapsular hematoma.
- **Grade 3:** Parenchymal tear deeper than 3 cm, parenchymal or subcapsular hematoma thicker than 3 cm.
- **Grade 4:** Parenchymal or subcapsular hematoma greater than 10 cm in diameter, lobar destruction or devascularization.
- **Grade 5:** Total devascularization or destruction of the liver.
- **Grade 6:** Complete avulsion (rupture) of the liver.

Spleen and liver injuries include laceration and hematoma, which could be treated nonoperatively in up to 90% of the cases. Surgical intervention might be required in injuries extending to the hilus [39]. Although most patients with mild liver injury are followed up nonoperatively, it should be noted that blood transfusion and laparotomy are indicated when the patient is not hemodynamically stable [39, 40].

Urgent exploration is required in patients with high-grade injuries who do not respond to aggressive therapy. In patients with massive liver injury and bleeding, injury control surgery with abdominal packing is recommended. In high-grade (grade 3–5) injuries, the patient should be followed up by ultrasonography and computed tomography after discharge [41].

For biliary reconstruction, Roux-en-Y choledocoenterostomy in complete rupture biliary tract injuries [34], and laparotomy with T-tube placement in incomplete biliary tract injuries [35, 42–44] could be performed. In the treatment of isolated bile duct injuries, Endoscopic Retrograde Cholangiopancreatography (ERCP), Oddi sphincterotomy, and nasobiliary stent, an abdominal drain can be placed under ultrasonography to drain the bile with expectation of the recovery of the bile leak [36].

92.3.1.2 Spleen Injuries

Although the spleen in adults is partially protected by the ribs, in children, the spleen is larger and protruding from the lower ribs, injuring more frequently in blunt abdominal trauma than in adults [45]. The splenic injury occurs most frequently due to traffic accidents, falls from a height, and bicycle accidents [41].

Findings such as discoloration in the left upper quadrant of the abdomen or left lower thoracic region, left rib fractures and left side tenderness, abdominal tenderness, defense, distension, tachycardia, pallor, hypotension, and shock are physical examination findings of possible splenic injury. During palpation of the left upper quadrant, the feeling of pain in the left shoulder is called the "Kehr sign" [29, 46].

In blunt abdominal traumas, other organ injuries are also common. Abdominal CT should be considered following the clinical evaluation. CT shows splenic injury with approximately 100% accuracy (Fig. 92.3) [45, 47]. According to the "American Association of the Surgery for Trauma" (AAST) criteria, spleen injuries are classified as follows, as in liver injuries [48]:

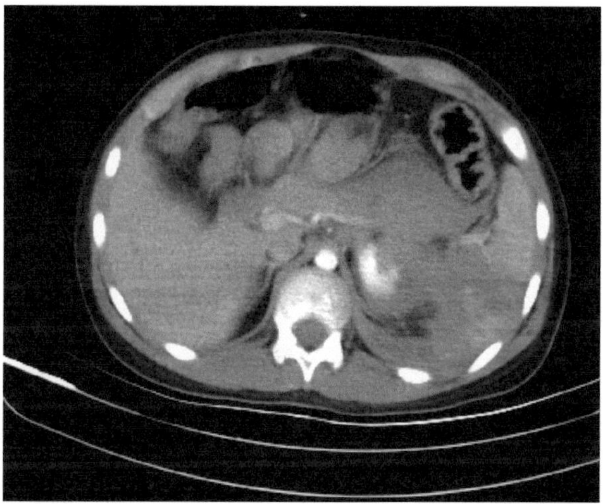

Fig. 92.3 Abdominal CT showing splenic laceration

- *Grade 1*: Subcapsular hematoma localized to less than 10% of the splenic surface area, or capsular tear less than 1 cm deep.
- *Grade 2*: Subcapsular localized to 10–50% of the splenic surface area, or intraparenchymal hematoma of less than 5 cm depth or parenchymal tear with a depth of 1–3 cm, without trabecular vessels.
- *Grade 3*: Extending or ruptured subcapsular hematoma less than 50% of the splenic surface area or an intraparenchymal hematoma greater than 5 cm deep or parenchymal tear containing trabecular vessels more massive than 3 cm in depth.
- *Grade 4*: Tear involving segmental or hilar vessels and causing devascularization of more than 25% of the spleen.
- *Grade 5*: Damage to the hilus vascular structures or ruptured spleen from the hilus.

Although organ-preserving conservative observation is generally preferred in spleen injuries, splenectomy is performed in cases of hemodynamic instability or irreparable organ damage [46]. If conservative follow-up is decided, the patient should be immobilized, and monitoring the vital signs, physical examination, and complete blood count checks with regular intervals should be performed. The clinician should be ready for an emergency surgical exploration and blood transfusion [48].

The most common nonoperative treatment complications are subcapsular hematoma, splenic abscess, splenic cyst, and splenosis. Children who underwent splenectomy should be vaccinated against Streptococcus pneumoniae, Haemophilus influenzae type B, and Neisseria meningitides [29, 49].

92.3.1.3 Pancreatic Injuries

Although the pancreatic injury is seen in less than 10% of patients with blunt abdominal trauma, abdominal trauma is the most common cause of acute pancreatitis in children (Fig. 92.4) [50].

Isolated pancreatic injuries are more common in children than in adults due to blunt abdominal trauma. Due to abdominal trauma, damage occurs by crushing the pancreas due to pressure between the lumbar vertebra and the anterior abdominal

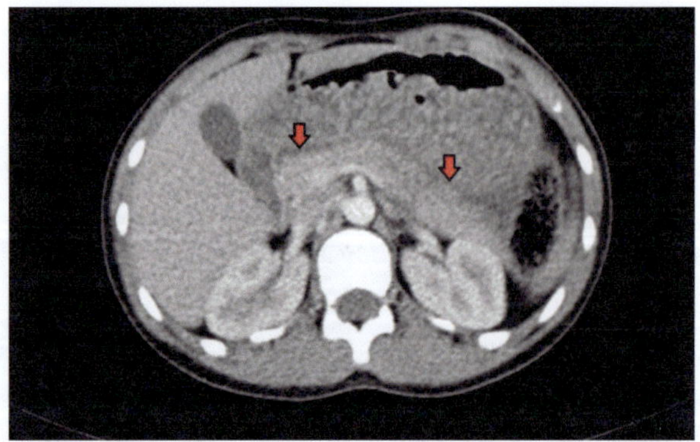

Fig. 92.4 Abdominal CT showing acute pancreatitis findings in patient with abdominal trauma

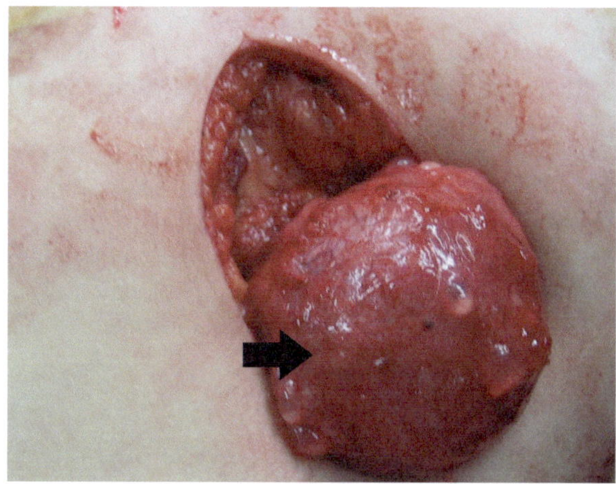

Fig. 92.5 Pancreatic pseudocyst following a blunt abdominal trauma in a child

wall. Amylase and lipase levels measurements and computed tomography imaging are the best choices, even if they are not excellent abdominal trauma indicators [51].

It is difficult to detect pancreatic injury by ultrasonography. Computed tomography shows all severe pancreatic injuries but not all mild injuries [52].

In conservative treatment, cessation of oral feeding and octreotide therapy is recommended. Also, stent placement with ERCP can be performed in patients with ductal injuries [53]. Complications such as pancreatic pseudocyst (Fig. 92.5), pancreatic acid, recurrent pancreatitis, and the intra-abdominal abscess can be seen after conservative treatment or surgery of pancreatic injuries [54].

92.3.1.4   Renal Injury

Kidneys are relatively larger comparing to adults. Size of the kidney in a child's abdominal cavity and renal fixation to retroperitoneal space with vascular pedicle, ureter, and ureteropelvic junction should be considered in the evaluation of pediatric renal injuries. Even though Gerota's fascia, perirenal fat are the protective surrounding tissue, they are thinner in infants. Distal ribs are the other important anatomical cover for the kidney, but the ribs are not ossified well and not big enough to be productive, especially at younger ages. The mobility of kidneys in children is another weak point that may cause kidneys to be effected easily by trauma. In children, isolated kidney injury is usually rare, and blunt kidney traumas are mostly associated with multisystem and other intra-abdominal organ traumas [55]. Any sign of trauma on the flank area should indicate an investigation for a renal injury.

Hematuria, rib fracture, abrasion, ecchymosis, and disruption of skin around the flank region are the clinical signs of renal injury. Abdominal tenderness, tumefaction, or palpable mass might be caused by kidney trauma.

Urine analysis, ultrasound with color doppler, and contrast-enhanced CT are the laboratory and radiological modalities that could be preferred as diagnostic studies in suspicion of renal injuries. Magnetic resonance imaging (MRI) is an alternative. However, although it is sensitive for soft tissues, it has a disadvantage in detecting the extravasation of urine MRI. Furthermore, it requires a longer time to perform due to sedation needed in children, so that it is less preferred in pediatric traumas.

In a hemodynamically stable patient, current guidelines advocate the conservative management of pediatric renal trauma [56, 57]. Expectant management was associated with acceptable rates of intervention and excellent renal salvage rates [58]. The patient immobilized and monitored for the vital signs should have a follow-up with regular physical examination, complete blood count, and urinalysis checks. The patient who does not respond to conservative treatment may need blood transfusion and emergency surgical exploration. The vascular trauma and urine extravasations are the extraordinary outcomes of kidney injury that might need intervention.

92.3.2 Hollow Abdominal Organ Injuries in Blunt and Penetrant Traumas

92.3.2.1 Gastrointestinal System Injuries

Hollow organs such as the stomach, duodenum, small intestines, and colon can be injured in blunt abdominal trauma. Serosal rupture, submucosal-subserosal hematoma, and perforation could be observed. Hollow organs are damaged due to the sudden bursting of the organ filled with gas and intestinal contents, the organ's avulsion, and the organ's crushing against the vertebral column [59].

Gastrointestinal injuries are seen in less than 10% of patients with blunt abdominal trauma [22]. Traffic accidents, bicycle accidents, and falls are the most common causes [60]. Intestinal perforations are more common on the intestine's antimesenteric side, especially where the intestines are fixed to the posterior abdominal wall, such as the ileocecal region or the Treitz ligament [22]. However, small perforations may present with delayed findings. The symptoms of peritonitis during follow-up should suggest intestinal injury [48]. The free air rate under the diaphragm has been reported as 48% in the upright abdominal X-ray in gastrointestinal injuries [41].

The mortality rate in the perforations due to blunt trauma varies depending on the accompanying additional organ injuries, the severity of the trauma, the timing of diagnosis, and surgery [59, 61].

In traumatic gastrointestinal injuries, computed tomography's sensitivity is 92%, and specificity is 94% [62]. In abdominal CT, specific bowel injury findings are intraperitoneal free fluid without solid organ injuries, lack of continuity on the intestinal wall, intraperitoneal or retroperitoneal free air, and increase in intestinal wall thickness [45].

Diagnostic laparoscopy is recommended in state of peritoneal lavage in the pediatric age group [63]. The surgical approach depends on the localization of the perforation and the patient's admission time. Either primary suture, resection anastomosis, or stoma opening is preferred [54].

Penetrating trauma may also affect gastrointestinal hollow organs by a physical trauma of foreign objects, such as a knife, gun bullet, or any sharp objects inserted through the abdominal wall. The severity of penetrant traumas is directly proportional to the kinetic energy of the object entering the body. Tissue can be damaged by low pressure and mechanical force in a small area of stab wounds. Therefore, the surrounding tissue is affected less due to the low pressure. However, in firearm injuries, the pressure is high, causing more damage to the surrounding tissues [64]. Penetrating traumas are more common in older children, especially in adolescence or post-adolescence [50]. Boys in socioeconomically low regions are particularly at risk [54].

92.3.2.2 Urinary Bladder

The incidence of urinary bladder trauma is 6.5 cases per 1.000.000 population [65, 66]. The incidence of bladder injury following blunt trauma is 0.87%, while it is 0.59% in penetrating trauma. The bladder injury is extremely rare but it should be suspected in multisystem trauma, especially if the child has a pelvic trauma associated with hematuria and/or acute abdominal findings. The lower ratio of bladder injury is attributed to the location of the urinary bladder and protection by pelvic bones [67]. On the other side, this protective bony shield might be a risk for the bladder and urethra in case of pelvic bone fractures during high energy traumas.

If a penetrating urinary bladder trauma has been identified, possibilities of injuries in the gastrointestinal tract and main vascular structures should also be considered.

The urinary bladder traumas are classified according to extravasation of urine confined only in retroperitoneum or passed transperitoneally causing peritonitis [65, 67]. This classification is highly important to decide whether to stay on the conservative side and only drain the bladder by urethral catheterization or operate. Patients having extraperitoneal injuries could have a conservative follow-up, while urinary bladder traumas causing perforation, transperitoneal urine leakage, and peritonitis need surgical repair. If the child has a pelvic fracture with a high energy trauma and/ or hematuria, one should also suspect from urethral injury [55]. Retrograde urethrogram is indicated in such patients to determine whether there is any injury to the urethra and also to define the severity of the injury. If the physician attempts to insert a urethral catheter in such patients without considering the possibility of urethral injury, an incomplete rupture of the urethra may turn into a complete rupture. Cystoscopy might be needed in urethral injuries for realignment or the decision to go on for surgical correction.

References

1. Benya EC, et al. Abdominal sonography in examination of children with blunt abdominal trauma. Am J Roentgenol. 2000;174(6):1613–6.
2. Wessen D, Stylianos S, Pearl R. Thoracic injuries, abdominal trauma. In: Pediatric Surgery, vol. 6. Philadelpia: Mosby Inc; 2006. p. 275.
3. Control, C.F.D. and Prevention. Vital signs: Unintentional injury deaths among persons aged 0–19 years-United States, 2000–2009. MMWR. 2012;61:270.
4. Galvagno SM, Nahmias JT, Young DA. Advanced trauma life support® update 2019: management and applications for adults and special populations. Anesthesiol Clin. 2019;37(1):13–32.

5. Tintanalli J, Kelen G, Stapczynski J. Emergency medicine: a comprehensive study guide. New York: McGraw-Hill; 2000.
6. Capraro AJ, Mooney D, Waltzman ML. The use of routine laboratory studies as screening tools in pediatric abdominal trauma. Pediatr Emerg Care. 2006;22(7):480–4.
7. Lindberg D, et al. Utility of hepatic transaminases to recognize abuse in children. Pediatrics. 2009;124(2):509–16.
8. Schonfeld D, Lee LK. Blunt abdominal trauma in children. Curr Opin Pediatr. 2012;24(3):314–8.
9. Stafford PW, Blinman TA, Nance ML. Practical points in evaluation and resuscitation of the injured child. Surg Clin North Am. 2002;82(2):273–301.
10. Levy JA, Bachur RG. Bedside ultrasound in the pediatric emergency department. Curr Opin Pediatr. 2008;20(3):352–242.
11. Farahmand N, et al. Hypotensive patients with blunt abdominal trauma: performance of screening US. Radiology. 2005;235(2):436–43.
12. Sivit C, Kaufman R. Commentary: sonography in the evaluation of children following blunt trauma: is it to be or not be? Pediatr Radiol. 1995;25(5):326–8.
13. Holmes JF, Sokolove PE, Brant WE, et al. A clinical decision rule for identifying children with thoracic injuries after blunt torso trauma. Ann Emerg Med. 2002;39(5):492–9.
14. Pearson EG, Fitzgerald CA, Santore MT. Pediatric thoracic trauma: current trends. Semin Pediatr Surg. 2017;26:36–42.
15. Herrera P, Langer JC. Thoracic trauma in children. In: Mikrogianakis A, Valani R, Cheng A, editors. The hospital for sick children manual of pediatric trauma. Philadelphia: Lippincott Williams & Wilkins; 2008. p. 131.
16. Goedeke J, Boehm R, Dietz HG. Multiply trauma in children: pulmonary contusion does not necessarily lead to a worsening of the treatment success. Eur J Pediatr Surg. 2014;24:508–13.
17. Ham PB, Poorak M, King RG, et al. Occult injury in the context of selective use of computed tomography (CT) in pediatric thoracic trauma. Am Surg. 2015;81:340–1.
18. Martinez L, Rivas S, Hernández F, et al. Aggressive conservative treatment of esophageal perforations in children. J Pediatr Surg. 2003;38:685–9.
19. Alemayehu H, Clifton M, Santore M, et al. Minimally invasive surgery for pediatric trauma—a multicenter review. J Laparoendosc Adv Surg Tech A. 2015;25:243–7.
20. Ramos CT, Koplewitz BZ, Babyn PS, Manson PS, Ein SH. What have we learned about traumatic diaphragmatic hernias in children. J Pediatr Surg. 2000;35:601–4.
21. Nance M, Stewart R, Rotondo M. American College of Surgeons. Chicago: American College of Surgeons; 2014.
22. Drexel S, Azarow K, Jafri MA. Abdominal trauma evaluation for the pediatric surgeon. Surgical Clinics. 2017;97(1):59–74.
23. Sandler G, et al. Body wall thickness in adults and children—relevance to penetrating trauma. Injury. 2010;41(5):506–9.
24. Bhagvan S, Ng A, Civil I. Penetrating thoraco-abdominal injuries: the Auckland City Hospital experience. ANZ J Surg. 2011;81(9):595–600.
25. Avarello JT, Cantor RM. Pediatric major trauma: an approach to evaluation and management. Emerg Med Clin North Am. 2007;25(3):803–36.
26. Santschi M, et al. Seat-belt injuries in children involved in motor vehicle crashes. Can J Surg. 2005;48(5).373.
27. Emir H. Pediatrik akut karın. Türkiye Klinikleri Cerrahi Tıp Bilimleri Dergisi. 2005;1(4):121–8.
28. Radvinsky DS, et al. Evolution and development of the advanced trauma life support (ATLS) protocol: a historical perspective. Orthopedics. 2012;35(4):305–11.
29. Keller MS. Blunt injury to solid abdominal organs. In: Seminars in pediatric surgery. Amsterdam: Elsevier; 2004.
30. Menaker J, et al. Use of the focused assessment with sonography for trauma (FAST) examination and its impact on abdominal computed tomography use in hemodynamically stable children with blunt torso trauma. J Trauma Acute Care Surg. 2014;77(3):427–32.
31. Peters E, et al. Blunt bowel and mesenteric injuries in children: Do nonspecific computed tomography findings reliably identify these injuries? Pediatr Crit Care Med. 2006;7(6):551–6.

32. Holmes JH IV, et al. The failure of nonoperative management in pediatric solid organ injury: a multi-institutional experience. J Trauma Acute Care Surg. 2005;59(6):1309–13.
33. Holmes JF, et al. Identification of children with intra-abdominal injuries after blunt trauma. Ann Emerg Med. 2002;39(5):500–9.
34. Bourque MD, et al. Isolated complete transection of the common bile duct due to blunt trauma in a child, and review of the literature. J Pediatr Surg. 1989;24(10):1068–70.
35. Rodriguez-Montes JA, Rojo E, Martín LGS. Complications following repair of extrahepatic bile duct injuries after blunt abdominal trauma. World J Surg. 2001;25(10):1313–6.
36. Sharpe RP, Nance ML, Stafford PW. Nonoperative management of blunt extrahepatic biliary duct transection in the pediatric patient: case report and review of the literature. J Pediatr Surg. 2002;37(11):1612–6.
37. Søndenaa K, Horn A, Nedrebø T. Diagnosis of blunt trauma to the gallbladder and bile ducts. Eur J Surg. 2000;166(11):903–7.
38. Van As A, Millar AJ. Management of paediatric liver trauma. Pediatr Surg Int. 2017;33(4):445–53.
39. Partrick DA, et al. Nonoperative management of solid organ injuries in children results in decreased blood utilization. J Pediatr Surg. 1999;34(11):1695–9.
40. Bond SJ, et al. Nonoperative management of blunt hepatic and splenic injury in children. Ann Surg. 1996;223(3):286.
41. Arslan S, et al. Management and treatment of splenic trauma in children. Ann Ital Di Chir. 2015;86(1):30–4.
42. Michelassi F, Ranson JH. Bile duct disruption by blunt trauma. J Trauma Acute Care Surg. 1985;25(5):454–7.
43. Ramia J, et al. Isolated extrahepatic bile duct rupture in blunt abdominal trauma. Am J Emerg Med. 2005;23(2):231–2.
44. Overhaus M, et al. Operative management of liver rupture with combined central bile duct injury in pediatric patients. J Trauma Acute Care Surg. 2005;58(6):1278–81.
45. Miele V, et al. Diagnostic imaging of blunt abdominal trauma in pediatric patients. Radiol Med. 2016;121(5):409–30.
46. Wilson R, Moorehead R. Management of splenic trauma. Injury. 1992;23(1):5–9.
47. Miele V, et al. Contrast-enhanced ultrasound (CEUS) in blunt abdominal trauma. Br J Radiol. 2016;89(1061):20150823.
48. Wegner S, Colletti JE, Van Wie D. Pediatric blunt abdominal trauma. Pediatr Clin. 2006;53(2):243–56.
49. Saraç M, Kazez A. Çocuklarda Batın Travmaları. Türkiye Klinikleri Çocuk Cerrahisi-Özel Konular. 2018;8(1):28–35.
50. Holland AJ, et al. Penetrating injuries in children: is there a message? J Paediatr Child Health. 2002;38(5):487–91.
51. Potoka DA, Saladino RA. Blunt abdominal trauma in the pediatric patient. Clin Pediatr Emerg Med. 2005;6(1):23–31.
52. Eppich WJ, Zonfrillo MR. Emergency department evaluation and management of blunt abdominal trauma in children. Curr Opin Pediatr. 2007;19(3):265–9.
53. de Blaauw I, et al. Pancreatic injury in children: good outcome of nonoperative treatment. J Pediatr Surg. 2008;43(9):1640–3.
54. Melling L, et al. Penetrating assaults in children: often non-fatal near-miss events with opportunities for prevention in the UK. Injury. 2012;43(12):2088–93.
55. Casale AJ. Urinary tract trauma. In: Gearhart J, Rink R, Mouriquand P, editors. Pediatric urology. Philadelphia: Saunders/Elsevier; 2010. p. 720–36.
56. Broghammer JA, Langenburg SE, Smith SJ, Santucci RA. Pediatric blunt renal trauma: its conservative management and pat- terns of associated injuries. Urology. 2006;67:823–7.
57. Nerli RB, Metgud T, Patil S, et al. Severe renal injuries in children following blunt abdominal trauma: selective management and outcome. Pediatr Surg Int. 2011;27:1213–6.
58. Redmond EJ, Kiddoo DA, Metcalfe PD. Contemporary management of pediatric high grade renal trauma: 10 year experience at a level 1 trauma centre. J Pediatr Urol. 2020;16(5):656.

59. Letton R, Worrell V. APSA Committee on trauma blunt intestinal injury study group delay in diagnosis and treatment of blunt intestinal injury does not adversely affect prognosis in the pediatric trauma patient. J Pediatr Surg. 2010;45(1):161–5.
60. Newman KD, et al. The lap belt complex: intestinal and lumbar spine injury in children. J Trauma. 1990;30(9):1133–8. discussion 1138
61. Chirdan L, Uba A, Chirdan O. Gastrointestinal injuries following blunt abdominal trauma in children. Niger J Clin Pract. 2008;11(3):250–3.
62. Mukhopadhyay M. Intestinal injury from blunt abdominal trauma: a study of 47 cases. Oman Med J. 2009;24(4):256.
63. Gaines BA, Rutkoski JD. The role of laparoscopy in pediatric trauma. In: Seminars in pediatric surgery. Amsterdam: Elsevier; 2010.
64. Moore K. The knife and gun club just adjourned: managing penetrating injuries in the emergency department. J Emerg Nurs. 2012;38(1):102–3.
65. Matlock K, Tyroch A, Kronfol Z, McLean S, Pirela-Cruz M. Blunt traumatic bladder rupture: a 10-year perspective. Am Surg. 2013;79:589–93.
66. Howes N, Walker T, Allorto N, Oosthuizen G, Clarke D. Laparotomy for blunt abdominal trauma in a civilian trauma service. S Afr J Surg. 2012;50:30–2.
67. Santucci RA, Mcaninch JW. bladder injuries: evaluation and management. Braz J Urol. 2000;26:408–14.